Esophageal Cancer

Principles and Practice

Esophageal Cancer

Principles and Practice

EDITED BY

Blair A. Jobe, MD, FACS
Sampson Family Endowed Associate Professor of Surgery
Division of Thoracic and Foregut Surgery
The Heart, Lung, and Esophageal Surgery Institute
University of Pittsburgh
Pittsburgh, Pennsylvania

Charles R. Thomas, Jr., MD
Professor and Chair
Department of Radiation Medicine
Professor, Division of Hematology/Oncology
Department of Medicine
Oregon Health and Science University
Portland, Oregon

John G. Hunter, MD, FACS
Mackenzie Professor and Chair
Department of Surgery
Oregon Health and Science University
Portland, Oregon

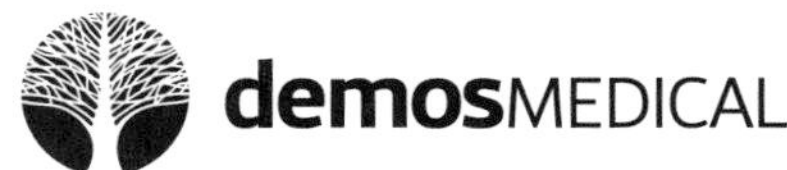

New York

Acquisitions Editor: Richard Winters
Cover Design: Steve Pisano
Copyediting, Indexing, and Composition: Apex CoVantage, LLC
Printer: Bang Printing

Visit our website at www.demosmedpub.com

Library of Congress Cataloging-in-Publication Data

Esophageal cancer : principles and practice / edited by Blair A. Jobe, Charles R. Thomas Jr., John G. Hunter.
p. ; cm.
Includes bibliographical references and index.
ISBN-13: 978-1-933864-17-4 (hardcover : alk. paper)
ISBN-10: 1-933864-17-6 (hardcover : alk. paper)
1. Esophagus—Cancer. I. Jobe, Blair A. II. Thomas, Charles R., 1957– III. Hunter, John G.
[DNLM: 1. Esophageal Neoplasms—diagnosis. 2. Esophageal Neoplasms—therapy. WI 250 E7621 2009]
RC280.E8E765 2009
616.99'432—dc22 2008048016

Special discounts on bulk quantities of Demos Medical Publishing books are available to corporations, professional associations, pharmaceutical companies, health care organizations, and other qualifying groups. For details, please contact:

Special Sales Department
Demos Medical Publishing
386 Park Avenue South, Suite 301
New York, NY 10016
Phone: 800-532-8663 or 212-683-0072
Fax: 212-683-0118
Email: orderdept@demosmedpub.com

Made in the United States of America
09 10 11 12 5 4 3 2 1

To Elizabeth, Nicolas, Patrick, Olivia, and Ian Jobe for their humor, spirit of adventure, and unwavering support of my life's passion. To my parents, Beverly and Frank Jobe, who have given me the gift of opportunity and set the example for a life lived with integrity, empathy, and a fearless pursuit of one's dreams and aspirations.

—BAJ

To my supportive wife, Muriel Elleen, our wonderful two children, Julian Franklin and Aurielle Marie, our parents, and our siblings for their love and support of my career path.

In memory of my mother, Ruth Marie Wilson Thomas, who fought gallantly in the war against cancer and whose prayers have blessed me over the past five decades.

—CRT

To the medical students, residents, fellows, and colleagues who have taught me so much and put up with much more. My success is a direct result of your many contributions to our research and the many hours spent together in the operating room. Thank you.

—JGH

Contents

Foreword

Esophageal cancer encompasses various types; the two predominant types are squamous cell cancer and adenocarcinoma. Their biologic and clinical features are compelling not only in the United States but worldwide as well. Other types of benign and malignant esophageal tumors, although less common, are of interest to both scientists and clinicians. Well-written and well-illustrated, this book is important and timely. The esteemed editors Drs. Jobe, Thomas, and Hunter have recruited over 100 experienced, expert contributing authors from diverse fields and disciplines to dissect successfully different aspects of esophageal cancer into overarching sections discussing biology, imaging/staging, principles of therapy (including specific therapies), tumor types, therapy, and palliation. Each section has specific chapters that will have broad appeal to the oncologist, surgeon, gastroenterologist, radiologist, pathologist, trainee, and allied heath personnel. A current and forward-viewing text of this type is imperative to advance the diagnosis and therapy of esophageal cancer, especially in the context of an interrelated interdisciplinary approach.

Anil K. Rustgi, MD
T. Grier Miller Professor of Medicine & Genetics
Chief of Gastroenterology
Co-Director, Tumor Biology Program
Abramson Cancer Center
University of Pennsylvania School of Medicine
Philadelphia, Pennsylvania

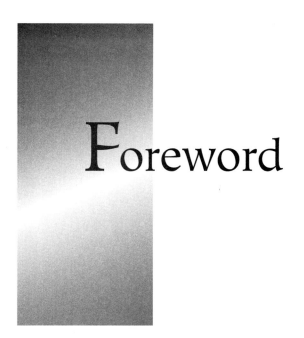

Foreword

This text is a precursor of other books that embody the concept of covering a single complex condition comprehensively.

One of the outstanding features of this volume is the attention paid to topics that are usually skimmed over by other texts but that are clinically important and difficult to manage, such as the management of recurrences, pain control, and palliative care—topics that are specific and relevant to the treatment of esophageal cancer.

Moreover, this book has not neglected the practical aspects of esophageal cancer treatment, and a significant focus has been placed on surgical techniques, which are treated in a stand-alone style for each procedure.

This volume has greatly impressed me in the following areas:

- The totality in coverage of each topic with equal emphasis on the technical as well as multidisciplinary aspects of treatment.
- The in-depth treatment of non-surgical topics in management at different phases of the disease.
- The wide-ranging attention to the disease's biologic aspects and basic science, which contribute greatly to palliative care.
- This text is technologically at the forefront and that is essential in the management of imaging, staging, minimally invasive methods, and biologic predictors.
- The information is current and up to date.
- The contributors are mostly young and rising academics who have projected fresh ideas and energy into this text.

Even in today's age of electronic search capabilities, a visit to this volume will be highly rewarding in time and effort as the relevant information is easily found. This book will be a very useful guide and reference volume for clinical and non-clinical staff and students who wish to explore or enter into this field, or who wish to access the contemporary thinking by world leaders in esophageal cancer.

John Wong, MD
Professor of Surgery
Department of Surgery
The University of Hong Kong
Hong Kong, China

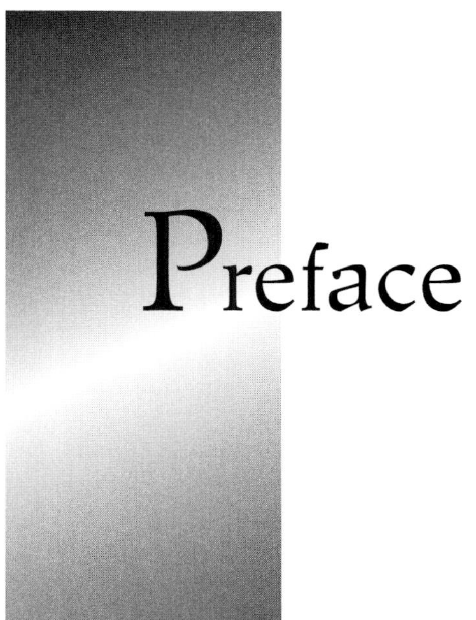

Preface

It is with great excitement that the editors and associate editors present the first edition of *Esophageal Cancer: Principles and Practice*. This text was specifically designed to address the complexities in the understanding and management of esophageal cancer with an emphasis on a multidisciplinary approach. The contributors include the major thought leaders in the world, including specialists in surgery, medical oncology, radiation oncology, gastroenterology, pathology, radiology, palliative medicine, nutrition and nurse specialists, as well as experts in basic, translational, and health services research of esophageal cancer. This work will fill a distinct void by providing a definitive synthesis of all pertinent information in this arena and has been constructed in such a way so as to remain accessible, practical, and useful to all practitioners who participate in the care of the patient with esophageal neoplasia. The genesis of this work was spawned from our own multidisciplinary esophageal cancer care team that was created to enhance communication between disciplines and provide high-quality and evidence-based treatment.

While this book focuses primarily on the two most common cancers that plague the esophagus, this text will be an opportunity to provide the first in-depth coverage of *all* types of esophageal neoplasms, regardless of incidence. Because the incidence of esophageal cancer has increased by several hundred percent over the past four decades, and because the overall mortality of this disease is near 90%, the need for a detailed and rigorous amalgam of cutting-edge information is dire. We have constructed this book to cover seven fundamental areas.

Section one is centered on the biology of esophageal cancer with a particular emphasis on the pathogenesis, molecular biology, and epidemiology of Barrett's esophagus and esophageal adenocarcinoma. In addition, we cover unique areas related to esophageal carcinogenesis, such as the link between esophageal cancer and morbid obesity and the relationship between *H. pylori* and Barrett's esophagus. It was the hope of the editors that this book will also serve as a valuable and definitive resource for esophageal cancer researchers. In this vein, there are chapters that outline the molecular biology of Barrett's esophagus and pre-clinical models for investigation.

Section two provides a detailed overview of cutting-edge esophageal imaging and staging. We have categorized the esophageal imaging components of this section into a description of the current (and future) technologies that are available to endoscopically examine the esophageal mucosa. In addition, we have separated esophageal imaging into anatomic and functional approaches in order to highlight the emphasis that is currently being placed on in-vivo measures of tumor biology. Techniques for staging have been covered from the perspective of clinical, endoscopic, and surgical approaches and highlight the utility of endoscopic mucosal resection in the staging of the esophageal nodule with the goal of providing tailored therapy. Finally, as our insights grow surrounding the natural history and the patterns of tumor progression, we have addressed the need for the modification of the current American Joint Committee on Cancer Tumor, Node, Metastasis (TNM) staging system.

Section three relates to the principles and rationale surrounding the myriad of therapeutic approaches for esophageal cancer. In order to provide a solid foundation for this section on therapy, the editors have been careful to emphasize the fundamental concepts surrounding multimodal therapy, as well as outline the principles of chemotherapy, radiation therapy, and surgical therapy. In addition, we look to the future and discuss the rationale and current standing of the rapidly evolving area of molecularly targeted therapies for esophageal cancer.

Section four consists of a series of several "mini-chapters" dedicated to describing the clinical background, gross findings, histology, and presentation of all benign and malignant neoplasms of the esophagus.

These initial four sections of *Principles and Practice* set the stage for the most comprehensive amalgam of definitive therapies for Barrett's esophagus and invasive malignancy ever assembled. Chapters 61 through 75 provide pragmatic "how-to" details of the surgical techniques used to address the various anatomical locations and stages of esophageal malignancy. Equally as important, there are several chapters which pertain to the pre and postoperative management of the esophageal cancer patient, as well as discussions surrounding the prevention and management of complications related to surgery and multimodal therapy.

Section six is entirely one of a kind in that it is dedicated solely to the techniques used to provide effective palliation for the patient with advanced locoregional or distant disease. The relief of dysphagia is perhaps one of the most critical aspects of providing effective palliation for the esophageal cancer patient. This section covers all of the techniques currently being used in the restoration of luminal patency. Three chapters in this section are dedicated to optimizing the palliation of the "entire patient" and providing maximal support and communication to the family of patients with esophageal cancer.

Section seven provides a glimpse of the future with an overview of the use of molecular markers for predicting tumor behavior and outcome. These markers may become targets for "designer chemotherapy" of esophageal cancer. Individualized cancer care will be possible once we are able to identify target genes and proteins specific to each patient's esophageal cancer.

The editors and associate editors are extremely proud of this first edition of *Esophageal Cancer: Principles and Practice,* and we wish to thank all of the contributors who have given of their time, insight, and experience to create a truly unique text that will serve as a valuable resource as we care for our patients with esophageal cancer.

Blair A. Jobe, MD, FACS
Charles R. Thomas, Jr., MD
John G. Hunter, MD, FACS

Acknowledgments

The authors wish to express their gratitude to Nichelle Tran for her dedication and tremendous assistance in assembling this work and maintaining open lines of communication between editors, associate editors, and contributors; to Richard Johnson, Richard Winters, and Demos Medical Publishing for their expert support and guidance during the development, execution, and production of this unique book; and to Olivia Jobe for her assistance with cover design.

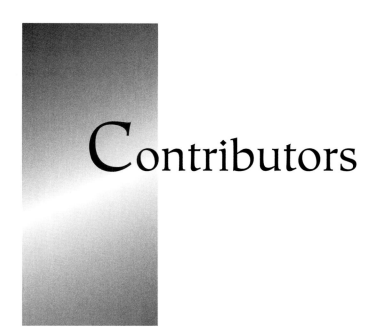

Contributors

Sajida Ahad, MD
Assistant Professor of Surgery
Department of Surgery
Southern Illinois University
Springfield, Illinois

Nasser K. Altorki, MD
Professor of Cardiothoracic Surgery
Department of Cardiothoracic Surgery
Weill Medical College of Cornell University
New York, New York

Natalia Bailey, MS, RD
Portland VA Medical Center
Portland, Oregon

Billy R. Ballard, DDS, MD
Professor and Chair
Department of Pathology
Meharry Medical College
Nashville, Tennessee

Todd Huntley Baron, MD
Professor of Medicine
Department of Gastroenterology and Hepatology
Mayo Clinic
Rochester, Minnesota

Jacques J.G.H.M. Bergman, MD, PhD
Associate Professor
Department of Gastroenterology and Hepatology
Academic Medical Center
Amsterdam, Netherlands

Rachelle E. Bernacki, MD, MS
Director of Quality Initiatives
Department of Psychosocial Oncology
Dana-Farber Cancer Institute
Brigham and Women's Hospital
Boston, Massachusetts

Yasser M. Bhat, MD
Assistant Clinical Professor of Medicine
Department of Digestive Disease
David Geffen School of Medicine at UCLA
Los Angeles, California

Sumitha Bhatia, MD
Resident in Radiation Oncology
Mayo School of Graduate Medical Education
Department of Radiation Oncology
Mayo Clinic
Rochester, Minnesota

A. William Blackstock, MD
Professor and Chair
Department of Radiation Oncology
Wake Forest University School of Medicine
Winston Salem, North Carolina

Daniel J. Boffa, MD
Assistant Professor
Department of Thoracic Surgery
Yale University School of Medicine
New Haven, Connecticut

Penelope A. Bradbury, MB, BCh, FRACP, MD
CIHR IND Fellow
Department of National Cancer Institute of Canada Clinical Trials Group
Cancer Research Institute
Queens University
Kingston, Ontario, Canada

Malcolm V. Brock, MD
Associate Professor
Department of Surgery, Oncology, and Environmental Health Sciences
Johns Hopkins Bloomberg School of Public Health
Johns Hopkins School of Medicine
Baltimore, Maryland

Linda Morris Brown, MPH, DrPH
Senior Research Epidemiologist
Department of Statistics and Epidemiology Unit
Health Sciences Department
RTI International
Rockville, Maryland

Ayesha Bryant, MSPH, MD
Assistant Professor
Department of Cardiothoracic Surgery
University of Alabama at Birmingham
Birmingham, Alabama

Daniel V. T. Catenacci, MD
The University of Chicago Medical Center
Chicago, Illinois

Robert J. Cerfolio, MD
Professor
Department of Cardiothoracic Surgery
University of Alabama at Birmingham
Birmingham, Alabama

David W. Cescon, BSc, MD
Medical Oncology Fellow
Department of Medical Oncology and Hematology
Princess Margaret Hospital
University of Toronto
Toronto, Ontario, Canada

Amitabh Chak, MD
Professor of Medicine and Oncology
Department of Gastroenterology
University Hospital—Case Medical Center
Cleveland, Ohio

Eugene Y. Chang, MD
Department of Surgery
Oregon Health and Science University
Portland, Oregon

Gregorio Chejfec, MD
Department of Pathology
University of Illinois College of Medicine
Chicago, Illinois

Xiaoxin (Luke) Chen, MD, PhD
Associate Professor
Department of Cancer Research Program
Julius L. Chambers Biomedical/Biotechnology Research Institute
North Carolina Central University
Durham, North Carolina

Mehee Choi, MD
Department of Radiation Medicine
Oregon Health and Science University
Portland, Oregon

Ezra Cohen, MD
The University of Chicago Medical Center
Chicago, Illinois

Norman A. Cohen, MD
Assistant Professor
Department of Anesthesiology and Peri-Operative Medicine
Oregon Health and Science University
Portland, Oregon

Xavier Benoit D'Journo, MD
Department of Thoracic Surgery
Université de Montréal
Montréal, Quebec, Canada

Ananya Das, MD
Associate Professor of Medicine
Department of Gastroenterology
Mayo Clinic Scottsdale
Scottsdale, Arizona

Matthew James Deeter, MD
Esophageal Research Fellow
Virginia Mason Medical Center
Seattle, Washington

Marvin Omar Delgado-Guay, MD
Palliative Care and Rehabilitation Medicine
The University of Texas MD Anderson Cancer Center
Houston, Texas

Steven R. DeMeester
Department of Surgery
University of Southern California
Los Angeles, California

Tom Ryan DeMeester, MD
Chairman Emeritus
Department of Surgery
University of Southern California
Los Angeles, California

Frank C. Detterbeck, MD
Department of Thoracic Surgery
Yale University School of Medicine
New Haven, Connecticut

Susan S. Devesa, PhD
Epidemiologist (contractor)
Department of Biostatistics Branch
Department of Cancer Epidemiology and Genetics
National Cancer Institute
National Institutes of Health
Bethesda, Maryland

Phillip M. Devlin, MD
Chief
Department of Brachytherapy
Brigham and Women's Hospital
Assistant Professor of Radiation Oncology
Harvard Medical School
Boston, Massachusetts

Attila Dubecz, MD
Department of Surgery
University of Rochester School of Medicine and Dentistry
Rochester, New York

Christy M. Dunst, MD
Director of Research
Department of Gastrointestinal and Minimally Invasive Surgery
The Oregon Clinic
Portland, Oregon

André Duranceau, MD
Department of Thoracic Surgery
Université de Montréal
Montréal, Quebec, Canada

Kai Engstad, MD
Department of Cardiothoracic Surgery
Oregon Health and Sciences University
Portland, Oregon

Pascal Ferraro, MD
Department of Surgery, Department of Thoracic Surgery
Université de Montréal
Montréal, Quebec, Canada

Jonathan Ford Finks, MD
Assistant Professor
Department of Surgery
University of Michigan
Ann Arbor, Michigan

Piero Marco Fisichella, MD
Assistant Professor of Surgery
Department of Surgery
Stritch School of Medicine
Loyola University Medical Center
Maywood, Illinois

Alexandru Gaman, MD
Research Fellow
Gastrointestinal Unit
Massachusetts General Hospital
Harvard Medical School
Boston, Massachusetts

Kenneth M. Gatter, MD, JD
Associate Professor
Department of Pathology
Oregon Health Sciences University
Portland, Oregon

Michael K. Gibson, MD
The University of Pittsburgh Cancer Institute
Pittsburgh, Pennsylvania

Sebastien Gilbert, MD
Assistant Professor of Surgery
Surgical Director, Lung Volume Reduction Surgery
VA Medical Center
Department of Heart, Lung and Esophageal Surgery Institute
University of Pittsburgh Medical Center
Pittsburgh, Pennsylvania

Gregory G. Ginsberg, MD
Professor of Medicine
Director of Endoscopic Services
Department of Gastroenterology
University of Pennsylvania Health Systems
Philadelphia, Pennsylvania

Karyn A. Goodman, MD
Department of Radiation Oncology
Memorial Sloan-Kettering Cancer Center
New York, New York

Joep J. Gondrie, MD
Research Fellow
Department of Gastroenterology and Hepatology
Academic Medical Center
Amsterdam, Netherlands

Lyall A. Gorenstein, MD
Assistant Clinical Professor of Surgery
Columbia University
New York Presbyterian Hospital
New York, New York

Jeffery A. Hagen, MD
Associate Professor of Clinical Surgery
Keck School of Medicine
University of Southern California
Los Angeles, California

Mindy Hartgers, RN, CNP
Department of Medical Oncology
Mayo Clinic
Rochester, Minnesota

Jonathan A. Hata, MD
Fellow, Minimally Invasive Surgery
Department of Surgery
Duke University
Durham, North Carolina

Robert H. Hawes, MD
Medical University of South Carolina
Charleston, South Carolina

Paul R. Helft, MD
Assistant Professor
Melvin and Bren Simon Cancer Center
Indiana University
Indianapolis, Indiana

Brenda J. Hoffman, MD
Medical University of South Carolina
Charleston, South Carolina

Wayne L. Hofstetter, MD
Associate Professor of Surgery
Department of Thoracic and Cardiovascular Surgery
MD Anderson Cancer Center
Houston, Texas

Arnulf H. Hölscher, MD
Professor of Surgery and Chairman
Department of General Visceral and Cancer Surgery
University of Cologne Medical Center
Cologne, Nordrhein-Westfalen, Germany

John Holland, MD
Department of Radiation Medicine/Radiation Oncology
Oregon Health and Science University
Portland, Oregon

Theodore Sunki Hong, MD
Director, Gastrointestinal Service
Department of Radiation Oncology
Massachusetts General Hospital and Harvard Medical School
Boston, Massachusetts

Jessica Patricia Hopkins, HonBSc, MD, MHSc
Resident
Department of Community Medicine Residency Program
McMaster University
Hamilton, Ontario, Canada

David H. Ilson, MD, PhD
Attending Physician
Department of Medicine
Memorial Sloan-Kettering Cancer Center
New York, New York

Matthew J. Iott, CNP
Oncology Nurse Practitioner
Department of Radiation Oncology
Mayo Clinic
Rochester, Minnesota

Syma Iqbal, MD
University of Southern California Norris Comprehensive Cancer Center and Hospital
Los Angeles, California

Glyn Jamieson, MD
Professor of Surgery
Royal Adelaide Hospital
North Terrace, Adelaide, Australia

Aminah Jatoi, MD
Consultant and Professor of Oncology
Department of Medical Oncology
College of Medicine
Mayo Clinic
Rochester, Minnesota

Milind Javle, MD
Associate Professor
Department of Gastrointestinal Medical Oncology
MD Anderson Cancer Center
Houston, Texas

Melenda Jeter, MD
Department of Radiation Oncology
MD Anderson Cancer Center
Houston, Texas

Blair A. Jobe, MD, FACS
Sampson Family Endowed
Associate Professor of Surgery
Division of Thoracic and Foregut Surgery
The Heart, Lung, and Esophageal Surgery Institute
University of Pittsburgh
Pittsburgh, Pennsylvania

Lisa A. Kachnic, MD
Chairperson and Associate Professor
Department of Radiation Oncology
Boston Medical Center
Boston, Massachusetts

Kimberly Marie Kaplan, MD
Oregon Health and Science University
Portland, Oregon

Andrew Y. Kee
Radiation Oncology
Mayo Clinic
Rochester, Minnesota

Kemp H. Kernstine, MD, PhD
Director
Department of Thoracic Surgery
Lung Cancer and Thoracic Oncology Program
City of Hope and Beckman
Research Institute
Duarte, California

Atif J. Khan, MD, MS
Assistant Professor
Department of Radiation Oncology
Robert Wood Johnson Medical School
University of Medicine and Dentistry of New Jersey
New Brunswick, New Jersey

Arman Kilic, BS
Medical Student
Department of Heart, Lung, and Esophageal
Surgery Institute
University of Pittsburgh School of Medicine
Pittsburgh, Pennsylvania

Jeffrey R. Kirsch, MD
Professor and Chair
Department of Anesthesiology and Peri-Operative
Medicine
Oregon Health and Science University
Portland, Oregon

Michael L. Kochman, MD
Wilmot Family Professor of Medicine
Department of Gastroenterology
University of Pennsylvania
Philadelphia, Pennsylvania

Mark J. Krasna, MD
Medical Director
St. Joseph Cancer Institute
Towson, Maryland

Geoffrey Y. Ku, MD
Memorial Sloan-Kettering Cancer Center
New York, New York

Braden Kuo, MD, MSc
Director of GI Motility Laboratory
Assistant Physician
Gastrointestinal Unit
Massachusetts General Hospital
Harvard Medical School
Boston, Massachusetts

Jesper Lagergren, MD, PhD
Professor
Upper-GI surgeon
Department of Surgery
Department of Molecular Medicine and Surgery
Karolinska Institute
Karolinska University Hospital, Solna
Unit of Esophageal and Gastric Research (ESOGAR)
Stockholm, Sweden

Rodney J. Landreneau, MD
University Of Pittsburgh Medical Center-Passavant
Pittsburgh, Pennsylvania

Simon Law, MBBChir, MA (Cantab), FRCSEd, FCSHK, FHKAM, FACS
Professor
Department of Surgery
The University of Hong Kong
Hong Kong, China

Paul C. Lee, MD
Associate Professor of Cardiothoracic Surgery
Department of Cardiothoracic Surgery
Weill Medical College
Cornell University
New York, New York

Jeffrey H. Lee, MD
Associate Professor
Department of Gastroenterology, Hepatology and
Nutrition
University of Texas MD Anderson Cancer Center
Houston, Texas

Andrew Y. Lee, MD
Senior Associate Consultant
Department of Radiation Oncology
Mayo Clinic
Rochester, Minnesota

Lawrence Leichman, MD
Desert Regional Medical Center
Palm Springs, California

Heinz-Josef Lenz, MD, FACP
Professor of Medicine and Preventive Medicine
Chair GI-Oncology
Co-Director, Colorectal Cancer Sharon A. Carpenter Laboratory
Department of Medical Oncology
University of Southern California
Norris Comprehensive Cancer Center, Keck School of Medicine
Los Angeles, California

Geoffrey Liu, MD, MSc
Alan B. Brown Chair in Molecular Genomics
Department of Medicine and Medical Biophysics
University of Toronto Princess Margaret Hospital/ Ontario Cancer Institute
Toronto, Ontario, Canada

Donald Edward Low, MD, FACS, FRCS(C)
Director, Thoracic Surgery and Thoracic Oncology
Department of General Thoracic Surgery
Virginia Mason Medical Center
Seattle, Washington

James D. Luketich, MD
Henry T. Bahnson Professor of Cardiothoracic Surgery
Director, Heart, Lung and Esophageal Surgery Institute
Chief, Department of Thoracic and Foregut Surgery
University of Pittsburgh Medical Center
Pittsburgh, Pennsylvania

Georg Lurje, MD
Research Associate
Department of Medicine
Norris Comprehensive Cancer Center
University of Southern California
Los Angeles, California

John S. Macdonald, MD, FACP, AB, MD
Lynn Wood Neag Distinguished Professor of Gastrointestinal Oncology
Department of Medicine
Aptium Oncology, Inc.
Los Angeles, California

Victor Maevsky, MD
Cardiothoracic Surgeon
Wheeling Heart Institute
Wheeling, West Virginia

Jocelyne Martin, MD
Department of Surgery
Department of Thoracic Surgery
Université de Montréal
Montréal, Quebec, Canada

Robert G. Martindale, MD, PhD
Professor of Surgery
Medical Director for Hospital Nutrition Services
Department of Surgery
Oregon Health and Science University
Portland, Oregon

Patrick I. McConnell, MD
Oregon Health and Science University
Portland, Oregon

Avedis Meneshian, MD
Fellow, Thoracic Surgery
Department of Surgery
The Johns Hopkins University School of Medicine
Baltimore, Maryland

Robert C. Miller, MD
Assistant Professor of Oncology
College of Medicine
Department of Radiation Oncology
Mayo Clinic
Rochester, Minnesota

Jessica Mitchell, RN, CNP
Department of Medical Oncology
Mayo Clinic
Rochester, Minnesota

Arta Monir Monjazeb, MD, PhD
Resident Physician
Department of Radiation Oncology
Wake Forest University School of Medicine
Winston Salem, North Carolina

Martin I. Montenovo, MD
Senior Fellow
Department of Surgery
University of Washington
Seattle, Washington

Brant K. Oelschlager, MD
Associate Professor
Department of General Surgery
University of Washington School of Medicine
Seattle, Washington

Daniel S. Oh, MD
Chief Resident
Department of Surgery
University of Southern California
Los Angeles, California

Robert W. O'Rourke, MD
Associate Professor and Director, Bariatric Surgery
Department of Surgery
Oregon Health and Science University
Portland, Oregon

Steven Z. Pantilat, MD
Director of Palliative Care Service
University of California San Francisco School of Medicine
San Francisco, California

Ashish Patel, MD
Chief Resident
Department of Radiation Oncology
University of Maryland Medical System
Baltimore, Maryland

Marco G. Patti, MD
Professor of Surgery
Department of Surgery
University of Chicago Pritzker School of Medicine
Chicago, Illinois

Subroto Paul, MD
Assistant Professor of Cardiothoracic Surgery
Department of Cardiothoracic Surgery
Weill Cornell Medical College
New York, New York

Carlos A. Pellegrini, MD
Professor and Chair of Surgery
Department of Surgery
University of Washington
Seattle, Washington

Arjun Pennathur, MD
Assistant Professor of Surgery
Department of Heart, Lung, and Esophageal Surgery
University of Pittsburgh Medical Center
Pittsburgh, Pennsylvania

Kyle A. Perry, MD
Minimally Invasive Surgery Fellow
Department of Surgery
Oregon Health and Science University
Portland, Oregon

F. P. Peters, MD
Associate Professor
Department of Gastroenterology and Hepatology
Academic Medical Center
Amsterdam, Netherlands

Jeffrey H. Peters, MD
Chairman and Seymour I. Schwartz Professor
Department of Surgery
University of Rochester
Rochester, New York

Allan Pickens, MD
Thoracic Surgery
University of Michigan
Ann Arbor, Michigan

Michael J. Pollack, MD
Advanced Endoscopy Fellow
Department of Gastroenterology
University Hospital—Case Medical Center
Cleveland, Ohio

Marek Polomsky, MD
Department of Surgery
University of Rochester School of Medicine and Dentistry
Rochester, New York

R. E. Pouw, MD
Associate Professor
Department of Gastroenterology and Hepatology
Academic Medical Center
Amsterdam, Netherlands

Aurora Pryor, MD, FACS
Assistant Professor of Surgery
Department of Surgery
Duke University Medical Center
Durham, North Carolina

David C. Rice, MD
Associate Professor
Department of Thoracic and Cardiovascular Surgery
University of Texas
MD Anderson Cancer Center
Houston, Texas

Nabil P. Rizk, MD
Assistant Attending Surgeon
Memorial Sloan-Kettering Cancer Center
Assistant Professor of Surgery
Department of Surgery
Cornell University Medical College
New York, New York

Sarah A. Rodriguez, MD
Endoscopic Therapy for Superficial Esophageal Cancer
Department of Gastroenterology
Oregon Health and Science University
Portland, Oregon

Ioannis Rouvelas, MD, PhD
Upper-GI Surgeon
Department of Surgery
Karolinska University Hospital, Solna
Unit of Esophageal and Gastric Research (ESOGAR)
Department of Molecular Medicine and Surgery
Karolinska Institutet
Stockholm, Sweden

Valerie W. Rusch, MD
Chief, Thoracic Surgery
Department of Surgery
Memorial Sloan-Kettering Cancer Center
William G. Cahan, Chair
Professor of Surgery
Cornell University Medical College
New York, New York

Richard Sampliner, MD
Southern Arizona VA Health Care
Tucson, Arizona

Parag Sanghvi, MD, MSPH
Department of Radiation Medicine
Oregon Health and Science University
Portland, Oregon

Inderpal S. Sarkaria, MD
Resident, Thoracic Surgery
Department of Surgery
Memorial Sloan-Kettering Cancer Center
New York, New York

Paul Henry Schipper, MD
Oregon Health and Science University
Portland, Oregon

David A. Schomas, MD
Resident in Radiation Oncology
Department of Radiation Oncology
Mayo Clinic
Rochester, Minnesota

Matthew J. Schuchert, MD
Assistant Professor of Surgery
Department of Heart, Lung, and Esophageal Surgery Institute
University of Pittsburgh Medical Center
Pittsburgh, Pennsylvania

Dustin V. Shackleton, MD
Oregon Health and Science University
Portland, Oregon

Scott R. Sommers, MD
Fellow
Department of Hematology/Oncology
University Hospitals
Case Medical Center
Cleveland, Ohio

Joshua R. Sonett, MD
New York-Presbyterian Hospital
New York, New York

Stephen Sontag, MD
Associate Professor
Department of Medicine
Loyola University Medical School
Maywood, Illinois

Harmik Soukiasian, MD
Minimally Invasive Thoracic Surgery Fellow
Department of Surgery
Cedars Sinai Medical Center
Los Angeles, California

Donn Spight, MD
Assistant Professor
Department of General Surgery
Oregon Health and Sciences University
Portland, Oregon

Hubert J. Stein, MD, PhD
Professor
Department of Surgery
Paracelsus Private Medical University
Salzburg, Austria

Mohan Suntharalingam, MD
Department of Radiation Oncology
University Maryland Medical Center
Baltimore, Maryland

Laura H. Tang, MD, PhD
Assistant Attending Pathologist
Department of Pathology
Memorial Sloan-Kettering Cancer Center
New York, New York

Roger P. Tatum, MD
Assistant Professor of Surgery
Department of Surgery
University of Washington
Seattle, Washington

Charles R. Thomas, Jr., MD
Professor and Chair
Department of Radiation Medicine
Professor, Division of Hematology/Oncology
Department of Medicine
Oregon Health and Science University
Portland, Oregon

George Triadafilopoulos, MD, DSc
Clinical Professor of Medicine
Department of Gastroenterology and Hepatology
Stanford University School of Medicine
Stanford, California

Wilson B. Tsai, MD
Clinical Instructor
Department of Heart, Lung, and Esophageal Surgery Institute
University of Pittsburgh Medical Center
Pittsburgh, Pennsylvania

Darren Tse, BMBS, MRCS
Physician
Departments of Otolaryngology and Medical Biophysics
The Ottawa Hospital
Ottawa, Canada
Princess Margaret Hospital
Toronto, Ontario, Canada

Shigeru Tsunoda, MD, PhD
Department of Surgery
Nagahama City Hospital
Nagahama, Japan

Paula Ugalde, MD
Assistant Professor
Federal University of Bahia
Salvador-Bahia, Brasil

Michael Ujiki, MD
Assistant Professor of Surgery
Department of Surgery
Northshore University Health System
Evanston, Illinois

Thomas K. Varghese Jr., MD
Assistant Professor
Department of Cardiothoracic Surgery
University of Washington
Seattle, Washington

Victoria M. Villaflor, MD
Assistant Professor
Department of Medicine
Section of Hematology/Oncology
University of Chicago
Chicago, Illinois

Timothy D. Wagner, MD, MBA
Captain, Medical Corps
Radiation Oncology Service
Department of Radiology
Brooke Army Medical Center
Fort Sam Houston, Texas

Jon P. Walker, MD
Assistant Professor, Clinical
The Ohio State University Medical Center
Columbus, Ohio

Malissa Warren, BA, RD, CNSD
Clinical Dietitian
Department of Nutrition and Food Services
Portland VA Medical Center
Portland, Oregon

Thomas J. Watson, MD
Associate Professor of Surgery
Chief of Thoracic Surgery
University of Rochester School of Medicine and Dentistry
Rochester, New York

Eric S. Weiss, MD
Post Doctoral Research Fellow and Resident in General Surgery
Department of Cardiac Surgery
The Johns Hopkins University School of Medicine
Baltimore, Maryland

Lawrence M. Weiss, MD
City of Hope National Medical Center
Duarte, California

Elizabeth Louise Wiley, BA, MD
Professor and Director of Surgical Pathology
Department of Pathology
University of Illinois College of Medicine
Chicago, Illinois

Douglas E. Wood, MD
Professor and Chief
Section of General Thoracic Surgery
Seattle, Washington

Cameron D. Wright, MD
Associate Professor of Surgery
Department of Thoracic Surgery
Harvard Medical School
Boston, Massachusetts

Abraham J. Wu, MD
Department of Radiation Oncology
Memorial Sloan-Kettering Cancer Center
New York, New York

Chung S. Yang, PhD
Professor and Chair
Department of Chemical Biology
Rutgers University
Piscataway, New Jersey

Gary Y. Yang, MD
Associate Professor
Department of Radiation Medicine
Roswell Park Cancer Institute
Buffalo, New York

Sai Yendamuri, MD
Associate Professor
Department of Thoracic Surgery
Roswell Park Cancer Institute
Buffalo, New York

Sriram Yennurajalingam, MD
Physician
MD Anderson Cancer Center
Houston, Texas

Harry Yoon, MD, MHS
Assistant Professor of Oncology
Mayo Clinic
Rochester, Minnesota

Lei Yu, MD
Department of Thoracic Surgery
Beijing Tongren Hospital
Beijing City, China

Esophageal Cancer

Principles and Practice

I

BIOLOGY

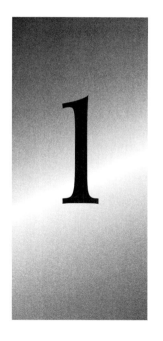

1 Esophageal Embryology and Congenital Disorders

Alexandru Gaman
Braden Kuo

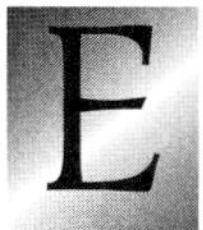

Embryologic development of the esophagus forms the foundation of the esophageal anatomy at the gross and microscopic levels. Abnormalities in the esophageal development can lead to certain important clinical conditions.

EARLY STAGES: FROM CONCEPTION TO THE PRIMORDIAL GUT

In order to have a clear understanding of the esophageal system formation, the early stages of the esophageal development are presented in the context of the entire embryonic development process.

Embryonic period is defined from conception to 8 weeks. During this period the formation of the primordial organs takes place, a process called organogenesis. Afterwards, during the fetal period (9 weeks–delivery), the organs differentiate and mature.

In the very early stages, during the embryonic period, the embryo is composed of cellular layers that later will organize progressively to form specialized structures such as organs. During the first two weeks, the embryo is formed from two cellular layers (bilaminar stage): hypo- and epiblast. The hypoblast faces the yolk sac (exocelomic cavity) and the epiblast faces the amniotic cavity. During the bilaminar stage, the embryo is totally embedded in the uterine layers, beginning with day 10 from the time of conception. In this stage, the cranial end of the hypoblast will start to thicken and form a structure called the bucopharyngeal membrane, which is a landmark in the evolution of the digestive system; it represents the cranial end of the primordial digestive system (1).

In the third week, a groove, the primary streak, appears on the surface of the epiblast and further invaginates toward the hypoblast by a process of cellular migration. The formation of the primitive streak is determined by the inductive activity of a cell population located in the posterior marginal zone of the blastiodisc (2). Inductor protein molecules such as activin (2), Vg1gene product (3), Wnt8c (4) and chordin (5) have a paracrine effect on the epiblast cell located in the vicinity of the posterior marginal zone. These factors determine the proliferation of the epiblast cells and their differentiation into the primary streak. Some other gene expression factors, such as BMP4 and Cerebrus, inhibit or lateralize the formation of the primary streak (5,6). This is the period when the embryo becomes a trilaminate structure: the epiblast will transform into ecto- and mesoderm and the hypoblast into endoderm. The mesodermal layer of the embryo has an important role in the formation of the digestive tract because it represents the origin of connective tissue, angioblasts, smooth muscles, interstitial cells of Cajal (ICC), and serosal layers in the gut (1,7).

The rapid volumetric growth of the embryo will determine craniocaudal and lateral folding at the beginning of the fourth week. The dorsal part of the yolk sac will transform into a cavity (intraembryonic cavity) lined by the endododermal columnar epithelium and form the primordium of the digestive tract. The primordial digestive tract is limited by 2 blind ends: the ectodermal-endodermal bucopharyngeal membrane at the cranial end and the ectodermal-endodermal cloacal membrane at the caudal end. Later, around the 12th week, the bulk part of the yolk sac that was not incorporated in the embryo will regress and then, at 20 weeks, will disappear completely. Failure of the yolk sac to regress totally determines the persistence of an ileal diverticulum called Meckel's diverticulum that has clinical importance especially during the infancy.

Gut development takes place in 4 major patterned axes: anterior-posterior, dorsoventral, left-right, and radial. Each axis development is based on the epithelial-mesenchymal interactions mediated by specific molecular pathways (8). Thus, growth factors such as Wnt, expressed by the mesoderm (9), and also Six2/Sox2, Bmp4, Hox are specifically involved in anterior-posterior axis development (8). As an example, Sox2 gene abnormalities have been associated with unilateral and bilateral anopthalmia but also esophageal atresia, myopathies, and genital tract abnormalities (10). These factors affect both the esophageal environment and the neural crest cells by making the environment more permissive for neural crest cells and by preparing the neural crest cells to migrate within the esophagus. The dorsoventral patterning of the gut is influenced by an asymmetrical expression of the sonic hedgehog (Shh) gene. This gene is less expressed on the ventral side of the endoderm in regions of active budding morphogenesis (8). The "master control molecules" driving the left-right asymmetry are Shh and activin: the Shh expression is restricted in the left side, while the activin is expressed more on the right side. The radial axis development is influenced by Shh and Bmp4 genes. Similar to the dorsoventral axis, the Shh gene is asymmetrically expressed along the radial axis (8).

The type of the structure that will form from the primordial gut is dictated by a strong interrelation between endoderm and splanchnic mesoderm. The mesoderm is the one that drives the formation of a specific type of lineage: as, for example, lungs in the thorax or colon in the hindgut region (11). The mechanisms involved here are probably similar to those involved in the axis development; namely, through Hox and Shh gene products. Interestingly, the expression of the Hox gene in the gut mesoderm is intimately related to the Shh expression from the endoderm. Roberts et al. (12) demonstrated that proteins expressed by the Shh genes act on the mesoderm to induce Hox expression, influencing gut development in the anterior-posterior axis.

ESOPHAGUS, FROM THE FOREGUT TO THE ADULT ORGAN

Gross Structural Development

For descriptive purposes, the primordial gut is divided in 3 regions, each of which has different roles, vascularization, and innervation: the foregut, the midgut, and hindgut (Figure 1.1).

The esophagus is derived directly from the foregut, which is the cranial division of the primordial gut. Besides the esophagus, the foregut represents the origins of pharynx, upper and lower respiratory system, stomach, and duodenum proximal to the opening of the biliary duct, as well as annex glands: liver, biliary tree, and pancreas.

The beginning of the esophageal differentiation is marked by appearance of a small diverticulum on the dorsal surface of the foregut, close to the bucopharyngeal membrane, at around 22–23 days after conception, when the embryo is around 3 mm in length (Figure 1.2). The appearance of this bud marks also the beginning of the tracheal differentiation. The esophagus is derived by the development of the foregut segment between the

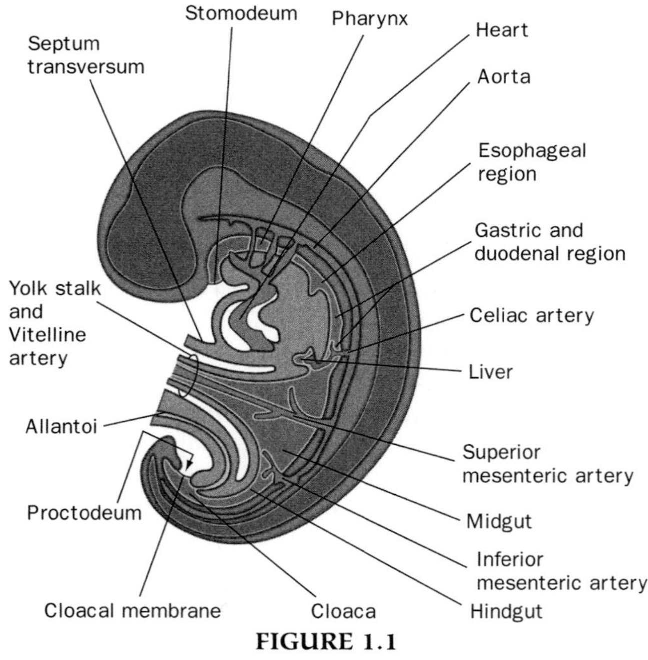

FIGURE 1.1

The primordial gut is divided in 3 regions having different roles, vascularization, and innervation.

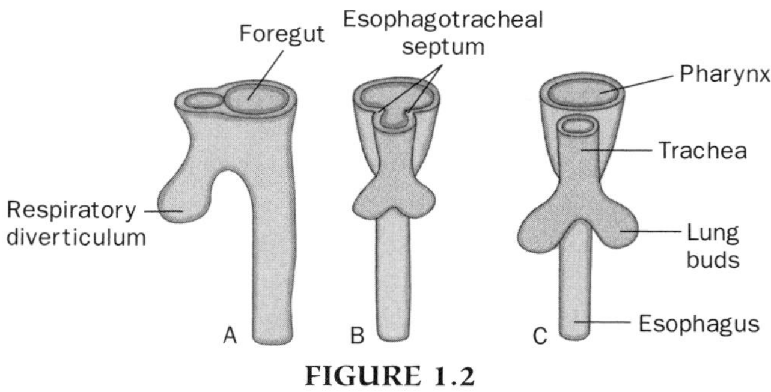

FIGURE 1.2

Successive stage in development of the respiratory diverticulum and esophagus through partitioning of the foregut. (A) At the end of the third week (lateral view). (B, C) During the fourth week (ventral view).

tracheal diverticulum and the stomach dilation. The diverticulum grows caudally and parallel with the foregut, forming a groove that is connected in the early stages to the lumen of the foregut. As previously mentioned, specific distinct differentiation into trachea or esophagus, even if these structures derive both from the endoderm, is dictated by Hox gene products and the mesoderm situated around the foregut. Sox2 is one of the genes playing a central role in generating morphologically and physiologically distinct types of epithelial cells (13). In some circumstances, the foregut may transform totally into trachea, thereby creating a condition characterized by a complete absence of the esophagus. In less severe forms, only some segments of the esophagus fail to develop generating esophageal atresia.

Shortly after the development of the primordial upper respiratory system, the cells from the lateral wall start to proliferate and to drive formation of a septum that separates the trachea from the esophagus. This separation proceeds from caudally toward cranially, and it is not completed until 34–36 days, when the embryo is about 17.5 mm (14). One of the genes proposed to play an important role in the normal process of separation is the Shh gene. Shh -/- mutants fail to develop the tracheoesophageal septum, and the esophagus and trachea fail to differentiate (15). In humans, heterozygote genotype Shh +/- is associated with major developmental defects such as cyclopia, midfacial clefting, mild hypotelorism, and holoprosencephalia (16). Failure of the septum to completely close the communication between the esophagus and the trachea will generate a condition called tracheoesophageal (TE) fistula, seen in congenital syndromes such as VACTERL (vertebral abnormalities, anal atresia, cardiac defects, TE fistula, renal abnormalities, limb abnormalities) and with the Trisomy 18 (Patau syndrome). TE fistula can be seen in Down syndrome as well, where it can be associated with an atretic esophagus. The subjects with Down syndrome have an incidence of 0.9% and a risk 30 times more than expected to develop congenital esophageal atresia (17).

When esophageal atresia is also associated with TE fistula, the amniotic fluid can circulate and reach the stomach through the trachea and polyhydramnios usually does not result. These patients present with fetal growth retardation and 40% of infants weigh less than 2,500 g at birth (18). In pure esophageal atresia without TE fistula, polyhydramnios occurs because the fetus cannot swallow and circulate the amniotic liquid during the fetal life and this accumulation of amniotic liquid results in increased fetal mortality (19).

Another condition generated by abnormalities of the septum, laryngotracheoesophageal cleft (LTEC), is a posterior midline defect described in 4 variants. Many syndromes are associated with LTECs, such as CHARGE syndrome (coloboma of the eye, heart defects, atresia of the coanae, retardation of growth and development, genital abnormalities, and urinary abnormalities), Opitz syndrome (associated with midline body defects such as cleft lip and palate, heart defects, and hypospadias), and Pallister-Hall syndrome (associated with hypothalamic abnormalities, supernumerary fingers, bifid epiglottis, and imperforate anus). It is hypothesized that the MID1 gene is involved in patterning of the left to right body axis and the development of the gut endoderm. Most males with MID1 mutated gene present with LTEC (20).

Parallel with the separation process, the primordial trachea and esophagus continue to elongate caudally because of the descent of the heart and lungs in the thorax. The elongation process carries the stomach below the developing diaphragm. Abnormalities in the elongation process can create a condition characterized by a short esophagus, where a part of the stomach may be displaced through the hiatal hernia in the diaphragm. Congenital hiatal hernia is detailed later on this chapter.

Esophageal Epithelium Development

The esophageal epithelium is derived from the pluripotent endodermal layer. Up to the eighth week, the esophageal epithelium develops to a pseudostratified columnar epithelium (21), and this development proliferates extensively until it almost but not totally occludes the lumen, for a short period of time. At around the 10th week, the recanalization process restores the esophageal lumen. Abnormalities of the recanalization process generate esophageal atresia, stenosis, and duplication (14).

At the same period, around the eighth week, ciliated cells appear in the middle third of the esophagus, as documented with scanning and transmission electron microscopy (SEM and TEM) techniques (22). The ciliated cells will migrate caudally and cranially, replacing the pseudostratified epithelium and forming a superficial layer that develops until the fourth month of the prenatal period (14). Around the 14th week, the ciliated epithelium is again replaced with a stratified squamous epithelium that initially appears in the middle third of the esophagus (21,22). This process is similar to the one previously described, where the squamous stratified epithelium extends rostrally and caudally. Immunohistochemistry showed that the replacement of the ciliated with a squamous epithelium is done through transdifferentiation, a subclass of metaplasia that irreversibly converts an already differentiated tissue with a new one, resulting in loss of one phenotype and gaining a new one (23). The electron microscopic studies showed that the glycogen granules in non-ciliated cells decrease as the differentiation of the epithelium progresses (22).

Sometimes the transdifferentiation process can be incomplete at birth and especially in premature children, patches of ciliated epithelium may be seen (24). There are reported cases of subjects with esophageal cysts covered with ciliated respiratory type of epithelium (25). Residual islands of ciliated epithelium at the proximal and distal ends of the esophagus may give rise to the superficial esophageal glands (14,26).

Esophageal Muscular Layers Development

The embryologic development of the muscular layer of the esophagus is driven by regulatory factors inducing transformation of the mesenchyme. The adult esophagus is composed of three subdivisions: the upper third with striated muscle, middle third with a mixture of smooth and striated muscle, and the lower third containing only smooth muscle.

The muscular tissue in general is derived from the embryonic mesenchyme, the middle layer of the trilaminar embryo. The muscles of the upper third of the esophagus and of the upper esophageal sphincter are derived from the mesenchyme in the caudal pharyngeal arches (4, 5, and 6), and this explains also the innervation of this area: the recurrent laryngeal nerve and the vagus nerve (27).

The process of the striated muscle differentiation in the upper third of the esophagus is still not very well understood. In the early stages of development in rats, the muscularis externa is mainly composed of differentiated smooth muscle. Some studies (28,29) suggest that the appearance of the striatal muscle is produced by transdifferentiation process, progressing in a rostrocaudal fashion. The first detected striatal fibers are found in the most rostral parts of the upper esophagus in the rat embryo in day 15 (E15). In the murine esophagus, the transdifferentiation takes place late prenatally and even after birth in the early stages of the postnatal development (30). Muscle regulatory factors (MRF) are hypothesized to be involved in the switch from one phenotype to another (28), demonstrated by the conversion of the smooth muscle cells to a skeletal phenotype with the ectopic expression of the MyoD (31).

The smooth muscle found in the lower third of the esophagus and the lower esophageal sphincter is derived from the somitic mesenchyme surrounding the foregut. The smooth muscle differentiation begins after the neural crest cells colonizes the gut. Of all the muscular layers, the circular one appears the earliest, at the beginning of the sixth week. The longitudinal smooth layer appears around the ninth week and is differentiated by week 12. The maturation of the longitudinal and circular muscular layers seem to occur as well in a rostrocaudal direction (32).

The middle third of the esophagus consists of bundles of striated and smooth muscles. How this mixed pattern of muscles develops is not fully understood.

Nerve Development

The esophagus is innervated by the autonomous nervous system (ANS) by its two divisions: sympathetic and parasympathetic. These two divisions control the esophageal activity by two nervous plexuses located in the esophageal walls: the myenteric plexus, located between the muscularis propria, and the muscularis mucosa and the submucosal plexus, located between the inner circular and outer longitudinal layers of smooth muscle. These two plexuses form the intrinsic neural system of the gut. The origin of the neural enteric system is the neural crest of the ectoderm.

The two intrinsic plexuses from the muscular wall of the esophagus are mainly derived from the cells located in the vagal neural crests, a neuroectodermal region described around somites 1–7 (33). The neural crest cells (NCC) enter the foregut at around the fourth week in human embryos (34), and they populate the primordium of the digestive tube in a rostro-caudal direction. The colonization of the digestive tube is complete by week 7 (35) in the human embryo. In order to form a mature enteric nervous system (ENS), the progenitors from the neural crest cells need to colonize the entire length of the digestive tube in a uniform fashion. The migration of the neural precursors is believed to be triggered by chemoattractant effect of glial-cell line derived neurotrophic factor (GDNF) (36,37). Mutations at the level of specific genes coding for factors such as Edn-3 (endothelin 3), NTRN (neurturin), or receptors such as EDNRB (endothelin receptor type B) have been shown to impair the neural precursor migration and to have clinical consequences such as Hirschsprung's disease (38). After colonization, the relatively small pool of neural progenitors from the foregut will proliferate to generate the millions of enteric neurons and glia present in the mature human esophagus.

The differentiation of the neural progenitors into mature neurons and glial cells begins to appear at around week 7 in the human embryo, as indicated by immunoreactivity for specific markers PGP9.5 and S100 (39) (Figure 1.3). After the differentiation, during the seventh week, the neurons start to coalesce and to form small ganglion plexuses in the myenteric space. The submucosal plexus has been shown to form from the myenteric plexus through a centripetal, inward migration process, in the inner side of the nascent smooth muscle circular layer (32). The myenteric plexus acquires cholinesterase activity at week 9.5 and is fully differentiated by 13th week. Formation of the submucosal plexus follows the myenteric one with 2–3 weeks (40) and is controlled by netrins, members of the family of laminin-related proteins. This is demonstrated with the migration of the neural crest-derived cells toward the mucosal cells that express netrin receptors, a process enhanced by netrin-1 molecules (41). The role of the intrinsic plexuses is mainly to control the esophageal peristalsis.

Esophageal peristalsis occurs as early as the first trimester of fetal life (42). High-frequency transducer ultrasonography has shown three different esophageal motility patterns in the second trimester (Figure 1.4): (a) simultaneous opening of the esophageal lumen from the oropharynx to the lower esophageal sphincter, (b) segmental, propulsive peristaltic contractions, (c) reflux-like peristalsis (43). At birth, the esophageal peristalsis is not fully matured yet, resulting in frequent regurgitation of food in infants.

The extrinsic parasympathetic innervation of the esophagus is supplied by the vagus nerve for the entire length of the esophagus. In the upper part, the recurrent laryngeal nerve supplies the somatic motor activity. This innervation can be explained by the origins in the pharyngeal arches of the upper part of the esophagus.

The vagus nerve is derived also from the neural vagal crests. The development of the vagal innervation at the esophageal levels can be traced using immunohistochemical techniques. Fibers arriving from nodose ganglia and medulla have been identified to populate the esophageal murine wall in day 12. The vagal branches populate the esophagus before the process of muscular transdifferentiation takes place (44). Similarly, in the human embryo, branches of the vagus nerve are found around the circular muscular layers at the beginning of the sixth week, before the process of muscular transdifferentiation takes place (14).

Formation of the neuromuscular connections between the vagus nerve and the esophageal muscular layers is a process that follows a specific spatiotemporal sequence (45). Diffusely spread acetylcholine (Ach) receptors arise around day 15 and eventually form clusters before the vagal branches reach the esophageal wall. The first nerve fibers to contact the Ach receptors are the vagal fibers, followed shortly by the enteric nerve terminals. This innervation process is completed in day 4 and day 10 postnatal in the mouse. As in the majority of the developmental processes, the neuromuscular junction formation takes place as well in a craniocaudal sequence.

The interstitial cells of Cajal (ICC) mediate the interaction between the nerve fibers and the muscles. These cells are spread in the muscular layers of the GI tract, from the esophagus down to the internal anal sphincter, and act as pacemakers to control the myogenic activity, mediating or amplifying the effects of motor neurons on the smooth muscle apparatus (46).

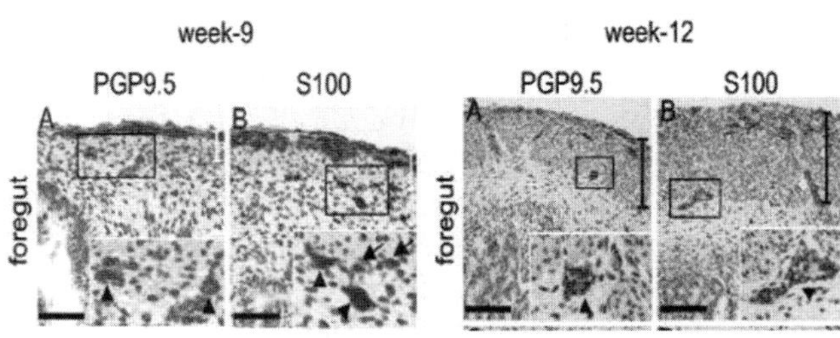

FIGURE 1.3

Immunohistochemical analysis of the spatiotemporal development of the enteric and submucosal plexuses of the human fetal foregut in weeks 9 (left) and 12 (right). The regions marked with a square are magnified in the nether side of the images. The arrowheads indicate neurons forming the submucosal plexus and the simple arrows represent single neurons and glia from the foregut wall. The scale bars indicate a depth of 100 μm.

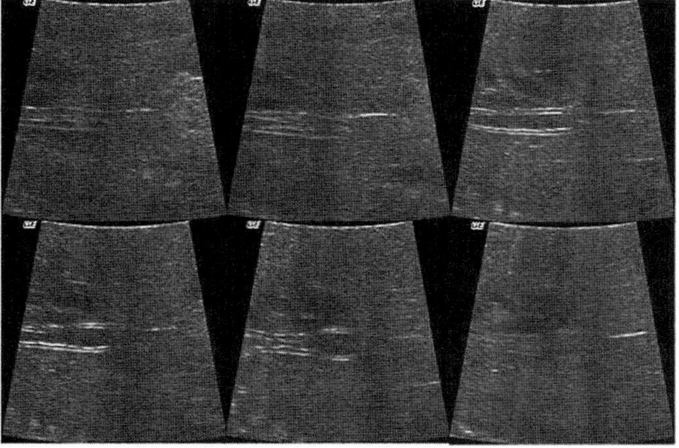

FIGURE 1.4

Series of ultrasound images demonstrating the peristalsis in the esophageal fetus with the passage of a fluid bolus. (Reproduced with the permission from John Wiley and Sons)

Developmentally, ICC are non-neuronal in origin and their differentiation starts around week 7, when they emerge from the mesenchymal layer. The maturation of ICC takes place between weeks 7 and 20, when they form plexuses in the esophageal wall (39). Development of ICC seems to be independent from the neural crest lineage. Several studies, using c-kit gene products to identify ICC, demonstrate that the differentiation of these cells is normal in aneural chick gut (47).

Development of the Esophageal Vascularization

The esophagus is supplied by thyroidal, bronchic, intercostals, and direct aortic esophageal branches. In the very early stages, the blood vessels form from the mesoderm of the yolk sac at the beginning of the third week (7). Partially, the vasculature of the esophagus is derived from the 5 and 6 aortic arches. The vascular structures deriving from the aortic arch enter the submucosa during the seventh week.

Lumen

The lumen of the esophagus changes during its development in parallel with the structural modification of the epithelial and muscular structures. In the very early stages, the esophageal lumen is round, but during the fifth week, it becomes flattened dorsoventrally. Between the 7th and 10th weeks, the lumen is partially obstructed in human embryos and because of the craniocaudal appearance of the four longitudinal folds, the esophagus assumes a Greek cross shape. The lumen becomes free again during the 10th week.

DEVELOPMENTAL ABNORMALITIES AND CLINICAL IMPLICATIONS

Tracheoesophageal fistula and esophageal atresia are the most frequent congenital esophageal abnormalities. These two conditions will be discussed together because they usually appear associated.

Tracheoesophageal fistula results from defects in the separation of the respiratory tract from the foregut by two mechanisms: arrest of the cranial growth of the septum that separates the esophagus and trachea or failure of fusion of the lateral ridges of the septum. In the later situation, only a simple TE fistula will usually be evident without esophageal atresia.

Esophageal atresia may result from failure of the primitive gut to recanalize during week 10. Five types of congenital esophageal atresia (Figure 1.5) with or without tracheoesophageal fistula have been documented (48):

- Type A—esophageal atresia with distal tracheoesophageal fistula (88.7%)
- Type B—esophageal atresia alone (6.7%)
- Type C—tracheoesophageal fistula without esophageal atresia (3.5%)
- Type D—esophageal atresia with proximal tracheoesophageal fistula (0.5%)
- Type E—esophageal atresia with proximal and distal tracheoesophageal fistula (0.5%).

Esophageal atresia with tracheoesophageal fistula occurs in 1 in 3,000 to 1 in 5,000 births. In 93% cases of esophageal atresia, there are associated malformations such as VACTERL syndrome, a condition presenting with multiple associated structural abnormalities: vertebral, anorectal, cardiac, tracheal, esophageal, renal, and limb. In type A, the upper esophagus ends in a blind pouch, and the trachea communicates with the distal esophagus, usually at the level of the carina. Air enters the GI tract via the tracheoesophageal fistula, and the newborn presents clinically with a gas-filled abdomen and frequent aspiration pneumonias due to gastric reflux into the respiratory tract through the fistula.

Congenital esophageal stenosis presents as a narrowing of the lumen at any level of the esophagus, but it usually occurs in the distal third and is associated with other anomalies, the most common being the esophageal atresia and TE fistula (49). It is a rare anomaly, occurring in 1 in every 25,000 live births.

Esophageal stenosis may be produced by: (a) incomplete recanalization of the lumen during week 10 (7); (b) an incomplete separation of the lung bud from

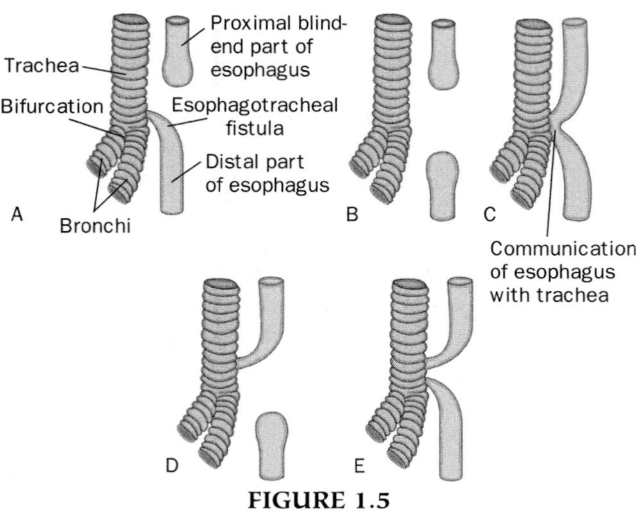

FIGURE 1.5

Variations of esophageal atresia and/or tracheoesophageal fistula.

the primitive foregut; (c) fibromuscular hypertrophy associated with impaired function of the myenteric plexus; (d) persistence of mucous remnants.

The persistence of mucous remnants related to esophageal stenosis presents as:

1. Rings (Schatzki's ring) in the distal part of the esophagus. Esophageal rings may result as a consequence of an incomplete vacuolization during week 10 and can be associated also with immunologic (50) or inflammatory conditions such as scleroderma (51). These circular structures are composed of muscosa, submucosa, and sometimes of muscular tissue.
2. Webs in the proximal and mid-esophagus, presenting as eccentric transverse membranes possible resulting from an incomplete vacuolization during the 10th week. The webs can be associated with iron-deficiency anemia (Plummer-Vinson syndrome) or gastroesophageal reflux disease (GERD) (52).

In some cases, the stenotic esophageal walls contain tracheobronchial remnants such as respiratory epithelium or hyaline cartilage, which indicate associated abnormalities of lineage.

Esophageal duplication is a rare condition occurring in 1 in 8,000 live births. They present as cystic or tubular, resulting as an abnormality of the epithelial, submucosal, or muscular layers. The structures resulting in duplication of only the epithelium of the foregut will generate the true cystic structures (Figure 1.6), which do not communicate with the luminal space. These structures can be lined with different types of epithelium, such as squamous, cuboidal, or pseudostratified and gastric mucosa, and can present with intracystic hemorrhages. This subtype of duplication is usually present in the posterior mediastinum and may complicate sometimes with rupture (53).

Another type of duplication is a consequence of development abnormalities of the submucosa or of the muscular layers. These are tubular structures, paralleling and communicating with the true esophageal lumen at both ends. They are less common than the cystic ones and they can sometimes become complicated with esophageal tumors (54) or with a foreign body producing local inflammation (55). Duplications of the esophagus can be associated with vertebral anomalies and intraspinal cysts and often are associated with intra-abdominal intestinal duplications (55). These structures may be generated by an abnormal fusion of the longitudinal mucosal folds (14).

Short esophagus results from the failure of the esophagus to lengthen in the caudal direction. True congenital short esophagus is a very rare condition and should be differentiated from the acquired hiatal hernia. Even if, clinically, these conditions are almost indistinguishable, they can be differentiated anatomically

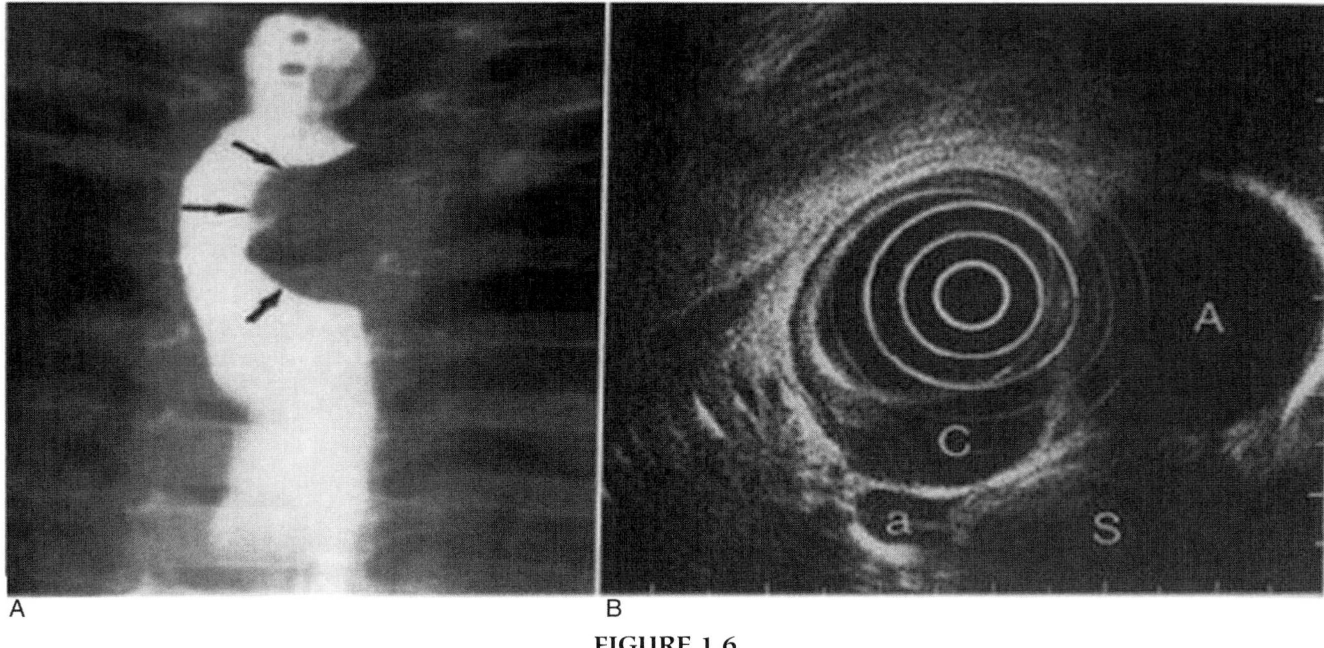

FIGURE 1.6

Esophageal duplication cyst. A. Barium esophagogram shows extrinsic compression of the wall of the esophagus (arrows). B. Endoscopic ultrasonographic image shows the distortion of the esophageal wall created by the hypoechoic cyst (C) and the cyst relationship to the other hypoechoic areas created by the aorta (A), azygos vein (a) and spine (S).

through their embryology development. In the acquired hiatal hernia, stomach vessels and protruding peritoneal sac may be seen in the thoracic cavity as a consequence of ascension of the stomach through a dilated diaphragmatic hiatus. The peritoneal sac is not protruded in the thoracic cavity with the true short esophagus.

Diverticuli are outpouchings of the esophagus located in the proximal, thoracic, or lower regions (56). Congenital true diverticuli with embryologic origins are exceedingly rarely documented (24). The biggest majority of esophageal diverticuli are not congenital but acquired because of the pulsion (i.e., Zencker's diverticulum).

References

1. Sadler TW. *Langman's Human Embryology.* 8th ed. New York: Lippincott Williams & Wilkins; 2000.
2. Khaner O, Eyal-Giladi H. The embryo-forming potency of the posterior marginal zone in stages X through XII of the chick. *Dev Biol.* 1986;115(2):275–281.
3. Seleiro EA, Connolly DJ, Cooke J. Early developmental expression and experimental axis determination by the chicken Vg1 gene. *Curr Biol.* 1996;6(11):1476–1486.
4. Hume CR, Dodd J. Cwnt-8C: a novel Wnt gene with a potential role in primitive streak formation and hindbrain organization. *Development.* 1993;119(4):1147–1160.
5. Streit A, Lee KJ, Woo I, et al. Chordin regulates primitive streak development and the stability of induced neural cells, but is not sufficient for neural induction in the chick embryo. *Development.* 1998;125(3):507–519.
6. Bertocchini F, Stern CD. The hypoblast of the chick embryo positions the primitive streak by antagonizing nodal signaling. *Dev Cell.* 2002;3(5):735–744.
7. Moore KL, Persaud TVN. *The Developing Human, Clinically Oriented Embryology.* 6th ed. Philadelphia: W.B. Saunders; 1998.
8. Roberts DJ. Molecular mechanisms of development of the gastrointestinal tract. *Dev Dyn.* 2000;219(2):109–120.
9. Lickert H, Kispert A, Kutsch S, et al. Expression patterns of Wnt genes in mouse gut development. *Mech Dev.* 2001;105(1–2):181–184.
10. Williamson KA, Hever AM, Rainger J, et al. Mutations in SOX2 cause anophthalmia-esophageal-genital (AEG) syndrome. *Hum Mol Genet.* 2006;15(9):1413–1422.
11. Grapin-Botton A, Melton DA. Endoderm development: from patterning to organogenesis. *Trends Genet.* 2000;16(3):124–130.
12. Roberts DJ, Johnson RL, Burke AC, et al. Sonic hedgehog is an endodermal signal inducing Bmp-4 and Hox genes during induction and regionalization of the chick hindgut. *Development.* 1995;121(10):3163–3174.
13. Ishii Y, Rex M, Scotting PJ, et al. Region-specific expression of chicken Sox2 in the developing gut and lung epithelium: regulation by epithelial-mesenchymal interactions. *Dev Dyn.* 1998;213(4):464–475.
14. Skandalakis JE, Gray SW. *Embryology for Surgeons.* 2nd ed. Philadelphia: W.B. Saunders; 1994.
15. Litingtung Y, Lei L, Westphal H, et al. Sonic hedgehog is essential to foregut development. *Nat Genet.* 1998;20(1):58–61.
16. Roessler E, Belloni E, Gaudenz K, et al. Mutations in the human Sonic Hedgehog gene cause holoprosencephaly. *Nat Genet.* 1996;14(3):357–360.
17. Bianca S, Bianca M, Ettore G. Oesophageal atresia and Down syndrome. *Downs Syndr Res Pract.* 2002;8(1):29–30.
18. Pearson G, Cooper J, Deslauriers J. *Esophageal Surgery.* 2nd ed. Philadelphia: Churchill Livingstone, Elsevier Science; 2002.
19. Pameijer CR, Hubbard AM, Coleman B, et al. Combined pure esophageal atresia, duodenal atresia, biliary atresia, and pancreatic ductal atresia: prenatal diagnostic features and review of the literature. *J Pediatr Surg.* 2000;35(5):745–747.
20. De Falco F, Cainarca S, Andolfi G, et al. X-linked Opitz syndrome: novel mutations in the MID1 gene and redefinition of the clinical spectrum. *Am J Med Genet A.* 2003;120(2):222–228.
21. Yu WY, Slack JM, Tosh D. Conversion of columnar to stratified squamous epithelium in the developing mouse oesophagus. *Dev Biol.* 2005;284(1):157–170.
22. Sakai N, Suenaga T, Tanaka K. Electron microscopic study on the esophageal mucosa in human fetuses. *Auris Nasus Larynx.* 1989;16(3):177–183.
23. Eguchi G, Kodama R. Transdifferentiation. *Curr Opin Cell Biol.* 1993;5(6):1023–1028.
24. Grant JC, Arneil GC. Congenital diverticulum of the esophagus: a report of two cases. *Surgery.* 1959:46:966–972.
25. Ribet M, Gosselin B, Watine O, et al. Congenital cysts of the esophageal wall with a respiratory type mucosa [in French]. *Ann Chir.* 1989:43(8):692–698.
26. Larsen W. Development of the Gastrointestinal Tract. In: Sherman LS, Potter SS, Scott WJ, eds. *Human Embryology* 3rd ed. Philadelphia, PA: Churchill Livingstone. 2001:235–264.
27. Bannister LH, Berry MM, Collins P. *Gray's Anatomy.* 38th ed. London: Churchill Livingstone; 1995.
28. Patapoutian A, Wold BJ, Wagner RA. Evidence for developmentally programmed transdifferentiation in mouse esophageal muscle. *Science.* 1995;270(5243):1818–1821.
29. Sang Q, Young HM. Development of nicotinic receptor clusters and innervation accompanying the change in muscle phenotype in the mouse esophagus. *J Comp Neurol.* 1997;386(1):119–136.
30. Ribet M, Gosselin B, Watine O, et al. Ultrastructural analysis of the transdifferentiation of smooth muscle to skeletal muscle in the murine esophagus. *Cell Tissue Res.* 2000;301(2):283–298.
31. Choi J, et al. MyoD converts primary dermal fibroblasts, chondroblasts, smooth muscle, and retinal pigmented epithelial cells into striated mononucleated myoblasts and multinucleated myotubes. *Proc Natl Acad Sci U S A.* 1990;87(20): 7988–7992.
32. Wallace AS, Burns AJ. Development of the enteric nervous system, smooth muscle and interstitial cells of Cajal in the human gastrointestinal tract. *Cell Tissue Res.* 2005;319(3):367–382.
33. Le Douarin NM, Teillet MA. The migration of neural crest cells to the wall of the digestive tract in avian embryo. *J Embryol Exp Morphol.* 1973;30(1):31–48.
34. Newgreen D, Young HM. Enteric nervous system: development and developmental disturbances—part 2. *Pediatr Dev Pathol.* 2002;5(4):329–349.
35. Fu M, Chi Hang Lui V, Har Sham M, et al. HOXB5 expression is spatially and temporarily regulated in human embryonic gut during neural crest cell colonization and differentiation of enteric neuroblasts. *Dev Dyn.* 2003;228(1):1–10.
36. Natarajan D, Marcos-Gutierrez C, Pachnis V, et al. Requirement of signalling by receptor tyrosine kinase RET for the directed migration of enteric nervous system progenitor cells during mammalian embryogenesis. *Development.* 2002;129(22):5151–5160.
37. Young HM, Hearn CJ, Farlie PG, et al. GDNF is a chemoattractant for enteric neural cells. *Dev Biol.* 2001;229(2):503–516.
38. Chakravarti A, Lyonnet S. Hirschsprung Disease. In Scriver CR, Beaudet AR, Sly W, Valle D (eds), The Metabolic and Molecular Bases of Inherited Disease, 8th ed. New York: McGraw Hill; 2001:6231–6255.
39. Fu M, Tam PK, Sham MH, et al. Embryonic development of the ganglion plexuses and the concentric layer structure of human gut: a topographical study. *Anat Embryol (Berl).* 2004;208(1):33–41.
40. Burns AJ, Thapar N. Advances in ontogeny of the enteric nervous system. *Neurogastroenterol Motil.* 2006;18(10):876–887.
41. Jiang Y, Liu MT, Gershon MD. Netrins and DCC in the guidance of migrating neural crest-derived cells in the developing bowel and pancreas. *Dev Biol.* 2003;258(2):364–384.
42. Bowie JD, Clair MR. Fetal swallowing and regurgitation: observation of normal and abnormal activity. *Radiology.* 1982;144(4):877–878.
43. Malinger G, Levine A, Rotmensch S. The fetal esophagus: anatomical and physiological ultrasonographic characterization using a high-resolution linear transducer. *Ultrasound Obstet Gynecol.* 2004;24(5):500–505.
44. Sang Q, Young HM. The origin and development of the vagal and spinal innervation of the external muscle of the mouse esophagus. *Brain Res.* 1998;809(2):253–268.
45. Breuer C, Neuhuber WL, Worl J. Development of neuromuscular junctions in the mouse esophagus: morphology suggests a role for enteric coinnervation during maturation of vagal myoneural contacts. *J Comp Neurol.* 2004;475(1):47–69.
46. Feldman M, Friedman LS, Brandt LJ. *Sleisenger and Fordtran's Gastrointestinal and Liver Disease: Pathophysiology/ Diagnosis/ Management.* 8th ed. Philadelphia: Saunders; 2006.
47. Lecoin L, Gabella G, Le Douarin N. Origin of the c-kit-positive interstitial cells in the avian bowel. *Development.* 1996;122(3):725–733.
48. Deurloo JA, Ekkelkamp S, Schoorl M, et al. Esophageal atresia: historical evolution of management and results in 371 patients. *Ann Thorac Surg.* 2002;73(1):267–272.
49. Amae S, Nio M, Kamiyama T, et al. Clinical characteristics and management of congenital esophageal stenosis: a report on 14 cases. *J Pediatr Surg.* 2003;38(4):565–570.
50. Siafakas CG, Ryan CK, Brown MR, et al. Multiple esophageal rings: an association with eosinophilic esophagitis: case report and review of the literature. *Am J Gastroenterol.* 2000;95(6):1572–1575.
51. Lovy MR, Levine JS, Steigerwald JC. Lower esophageal rings as a cause of dysphagia in progressive systemic sclerosis—coincidence or consequence? *Dig Dis Sci.* 1983;28(9):780–783.
52. Marshall JB, Kretschmar JM, Diaz-Arias AA. Gastroesophageal reflux as a pathogenic factor in the development of symptomatic lower esophageal rings. *Arch Intern Med.* 1990;150(8):1669–1672.
53. Neo EL, Watson DI, Bessell JR. Acute ruptured esophageal duplication cyst. *Dis Esophagus.* 2004;17(1):109–111.
54. Boivin Y, Cholette JP, Lefebvre R. Accessory esophagus complicated by an adenocarcinoma. *Can Med Assoc J.* 1964;90:1414–1417.
55. Stringer MD, Spitz L, Abel R, et al. Management of alimentary tract duplication in children. *Br J Surg.* 1995;82(1):74–78.
56. Jackson C, Shallow TA. Diverticula of the oesophagus, pulsion, traction, malignant and congenital. *Ann Surg.* 1926;83(1):1–19.

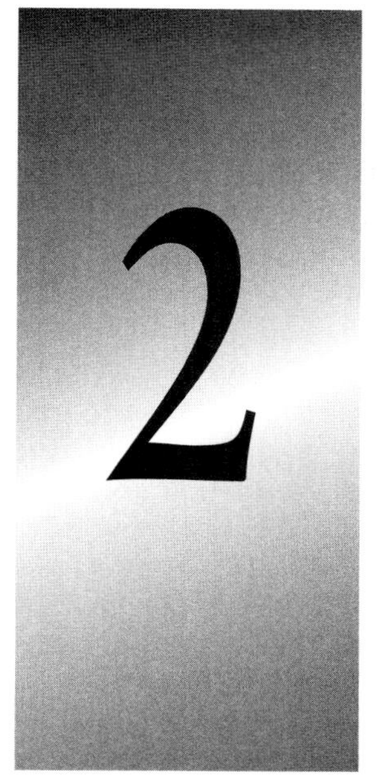

2 Esophageal Anatomy

Braden Kuo
Alexandru Gaman

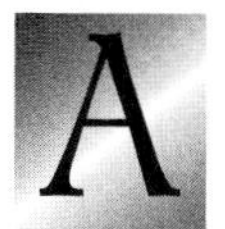

As providers who care for patients with esophageal tumors, it is critical that we have a thorough understanding of the surgical anatomy, anatomic relationships, and histology of the esophagus. This understanding must include all disciplines (surgeons, radiation oncologists, oncologists, interventional radiologists, dieticians), as the esophagus possesses unique anatomic qualities, which have profound implications for the diagnosis, treatment, and palliation of patients with esophageal malignancy. This chapter details esophageal anatomy and places its principal components into clinical context.

ANATOMIC LANDMARKS

The esophagus is a flattened muscular tube of 18 to 26 cm in length, from the upper sphincter to the lower sphincter, connecting the pharynx to the stomach. The esophagus starts at approximately 18 cm from the incisors at the pharyngoesophageal junction (C5–6 vertebral interspace at the inferior border of the cricoid cartilage) and descends anteriorly to the vertebral column spanning the superior and then the posterior mediastinum (1). After traversing the diaphragm at the diaphragmatic hiatus (T10 vertebral level), the esophagus extends through the gastroesophageal junction to end at the orifice of the cardia of the stomach (T11 vertebral level). Topographically, there are three distinct regions: cervical, thoracic, and abdominal.

The cervical esophagus extends from the pharyngoesophageal junction (C5–C6) to the suprasternal notch (T1) and is about 4 to 5 cm long. At this level, the esophagus is bordered anteriorly by the trachea, posteriorly by the vertebral column, and laterally by the carotid sheaths and the thyroid gland. The cervical esophagus is particularly vulnerable because of the lack of protective sheath between this structure and the membranous trachea that lies in very close proximity. During the surgery, special care is taken not to injure the trachea when developing the plane of dissection between the two structures (2). Periesophageal inflammation and tumoral invasion may predispose the membranous trachea to surgical injuries.

The thoracic esophagus extends from the suprasternal notch (T1) to the diaphragmatic hiatus (T10), passing posterior to the trachea, the tracheal bifurcation (T4), and the left main stem bronchus. The esophagus lies posterior and to the right of the aortic arch at the T4 vertebral level. From the level of T8 until the diaphragmatic hiatus, the esophagus lies anteriorly and medial to the aorta (3). The lower part of the thoracic esophagus runs anteriorly to the left atrium, which is the most posterior among all 4 chambers of the heart. This anatomic location may have important clinical outcomes. In mitral stenosis, the dilation of the left atrium can be seen on the barium series as an impression on the esophagus. In advanced stages of mitral stenosis, the esophagus may become obstructed, resulting in dysphagia. In this region also, the esophagus runs between the aorta and the left main bronchus, forming the broncho-aortic constriction known also as thoracic constriction. This constricted region is a common area for pill-induced strictures.

The anatomic relation of this esophageal region with the nearby structures is of relevant clinical interest. The esophageal location within defined fascial compartments allows infections from the anterior esophageal wall to spread easily via the peritracheal space down to the pericardium. Noninstrumental or spontaneous perforation of the esophagus (Boerhaave's syndrome) or leakage from the esophageal anastomosis can lead to necrotizing mediastinitis with rapid and disastrous dissemination of the sepsis and high mortality (2).

The abdominal esophagus is very short and extends from the diaphragmatic hiatus (T10) to the orifice of the cardia of the stomach (T11). The base of the esophagus transitions into the cardia sphincter of the stomach, forming a truncated cone of around 1 cm in length. The abdominal esophagus lies in the esophageal groove on the posterior surface of the left lobe of the liver. The anatomic relation of the esophagus with the diaphragmatic hiatus is also clinically important. With advancing age, the phrenoesophageal membrane, which has an anchoring role at the distal part of the esophagus, loses its elasticity because the elastic fibers in its structure are replaced by inelastic collagenous fibrous elements (4). The loss of elasticity in conjunction with a wide diaphragmatic hiatus results in herniation of the gastroesophageal junction (GEJ) and of the cardia into the thorax.

In the resting state, the esophagus is collapsed in the upper and middle parts and rounded in the lower portion (2). When the alimentary bolus passes through, the esophagus can distend to approximately 2 cm in the anteroposterior axis and 3 cm in the left-right axis.

In the course of the esophagus, three minor curvations are present. The first one, in the upper part, is from the median position toward the medial left. At the level of the T7, the esophagus shifts slightly to the right of the spine. The third angulation and the most important one is at the GEJ, where the esophagus shifts briskly to the left.

MUSCULAR LAYERS OF THE ESOPHAGUS

The muscular coat consists of an external layer of longitudinal fibers and an internal layer of circular fibers (Figure 2.1). The longitudinal fibers are arranged proximally in 3 fasciculi. The ventral fasciculus is attached to the vertical ridge on the posterior surface of the lamina of the cricoid cartilage by the tendocricoesophageus. The two lateral fasciculi are continuous with the muscular fibers of the pharynx. The longitudinal fibers descend in the esophagus and combine to form a uniform layer that covers the outer surface of the esophagus.

The circular muscle layer provides the sequential peristaltic contraction that propels food toward the stomach. The circular fibers are continuous with the inferior constrictor muscle of the hypopharynx; they run transverse at the cranial and caudal regions of the esophagus, but oblique in the body of the esophagus. The internal muscular layer is thicker than the external muscular layer. Below the diaphragm, the internal circular muscle layer thickens and the fibers become semicircular and interconnected, constituting the intrinsic component of the lower esophageal sphincter (LES).

Accessory bands of muscle connect the esophagus and the left pleura to the root of the left bronchus and the posterior of the pericardium. The muscular fibers in the cranial part of the esophagus are red and consist chiefly of striated muscle; the intermediate part is mixed; and the lower part, with rare exceptions, contains only smooth muscle.

The backflow of food and acidic gastric content is prevented at the level of two high-pressure regions: the upper and the lower esophageal sphincter. These functional zones are located at the upper and lower ends of the esophagus, but there is not a clear anatomic demarcation of the limits of the sphincters.

The upper esophageal sphincter (UES) is a high-pressure zone situated between the pharynx and the cervical esophagus (Figure 2.2). The UES is a musculocartilaginous structure composed of the posterior surface of the thyroid and cricoid cartilage, the hyoid bone, and three muscles: cricopharyngeus, thyropharyngeus, and cranial cervical esophagus. Each muscle plays a different role in UES function (5). These three muscles spread upward, posteriorly, where they insert into the esophageal submucosa after crossing the muscle bundles of the opposite side. The thyropharyngeus muscle is obliquely oriented, whereas the cricopharyngeus muscle is transversely oriented. Between these two muscles, there is a zone of sparse musculature—the Killian's triangle, of high clinical significance. Because of the low resistance, this region is prone to develop a false diverticulum named Zenker's diverticulum (6) formed only from the mucosa and submucosa.

The cricopharyngeus (CP) muscle is a striated muscle attached to the cricoid cartilage. It forms a C-shaped muscular band that produces maximum tension in the anteroposterior direction and less tension in the lateral direction (7). Structurally and mechanically, the CP is different from the surrounding pharyngeal and esophageal

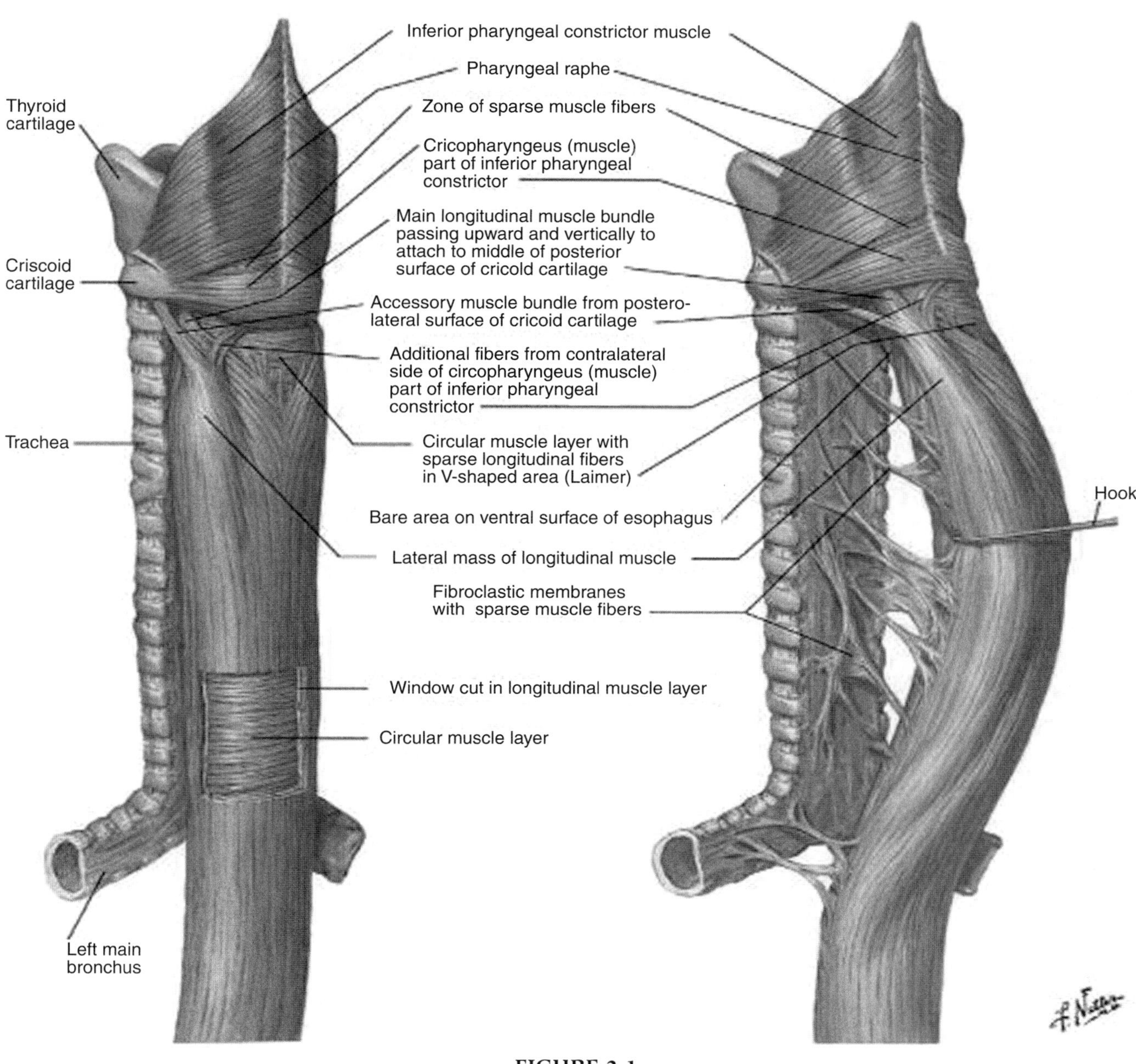

FIGURE 2.1

Muscular layers of the esophagus.

muscles. It is composed of a mixture of fast- and slow-twitch fibers, with the slow fibers being predominant and having a diameter of 25 to 35 μm (8). The CP is suspended between the cricoid (2) processes, surrounds the narrowest part of pharynx, and extends caudally where it blends with the circular muscle of the cervical esophagus. The CP can be seen as an indenting band with palpable boundaries during surgery.

Function of the UES is controlled by a variety of reflexes that involve afferent inputs to the motor neurons innervating the sphincter. These reflexes elicit either contraction or relaxation of the tonic activity of the UES. Inability of the sphincter to open or discoordination of timing between the opening of the UES with the pharyngeal push of ingested contents leads to difficulty in swallowing known as oropharyngeal dysphagia (5).

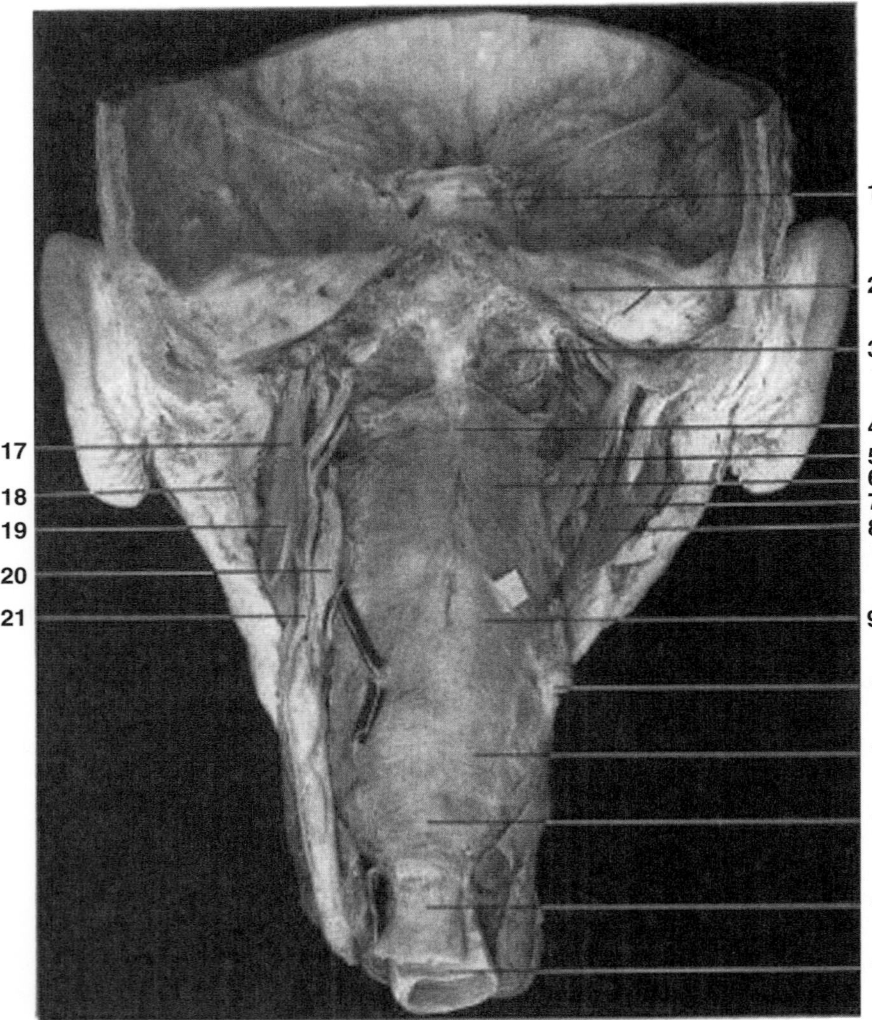

Muscles of the pharynx (posterior aspect).

1 Sella turcica
2 Internal acoustic meatus and petrous part of temporal bone
3 Pharyngobasilar fascia
4 Fibrous raphe of pharynx
5 Stylopharyngeal muscle
6 Superior constrictor muscle of pharynx
7 Posterior belly of digastric muscle
8 Stylohyoid muscle
9 Middle constrictor muscle of pharynx
10 Inferior constrictor muscle of pharynx
11 Muscle-free area (Killian's triangle)
12 Esophagus
13 Trachea
14 Thyroid and parathyroid glands
15 Medial pterygoid muscle
16 Greater horn of hyoid bone
17 Internal jugular vein
18 Parotid gland
19 Accessory nerve
20 Superior cervical ganglion of sympathetic trunk
21 Vagus nerve
22 Laimer's triangle (area prone to developing diverticula)
23 Orbicularis oculi muscle
24 Nasal muscle
25 Levator labii superioris and levator labii alaeque nasi muscles
26 Levator anguli oris muscle
27 Orbicularis oris muscle
28 Buccinator muscle
29 Depressor labii inferioris muscle
30 Hyoglossus muscle
31 Thyrohyoid muscle
32 Thyroid cartilage
33 Cricothyroid muscle
34 Pterygomandibular raphe
35 Tensor veli palatini muscle
36 Levator veli palatini muscle
37 Depressor anguli oris muscle
38 Mentalis muscle
39 Styloglossus muscle

FIGURE 2.2

Anatomic structures of the pharyngoesophageal junction.

The cervical esophagus contains predominantly striated muscle fibers and occasionally smooth fibers (5). Approximately 4 cm of the proximal end is composed exclusively of striated fibers. Between 4 and 12 cm, a mixture of smooth and striated muscle exits, and beginning with the lower border of the cricopharyngeus, only smooth muscle can be seen (1). The muscle fibers are arranged in two layers: the external layer, containing longitudinal arranged fibers, and the internal layer, containing circular or transversely arranged fibers.

The external longitudinal layer of the cervical esophagus originates from the dorsal plane of the cricoid cartilage and because of their lateral and caudal course, they delimit a weak space, called the Laimer's triangle, which is prone to developing a rare type of diverticulum (9). The external longitudinal layer courses down the length of the entire esophagus. At its distal end, the longitudinal fibers become more oblique and end along the anterior and posterior gastric wall (10). The internal circular layer of muscle originates at the level of cricoid cartilage and, while descending, forms incomplete circles (10).

The lower esophageal sphincter is a high-pressure zone located where the esophagus merges with the stomach

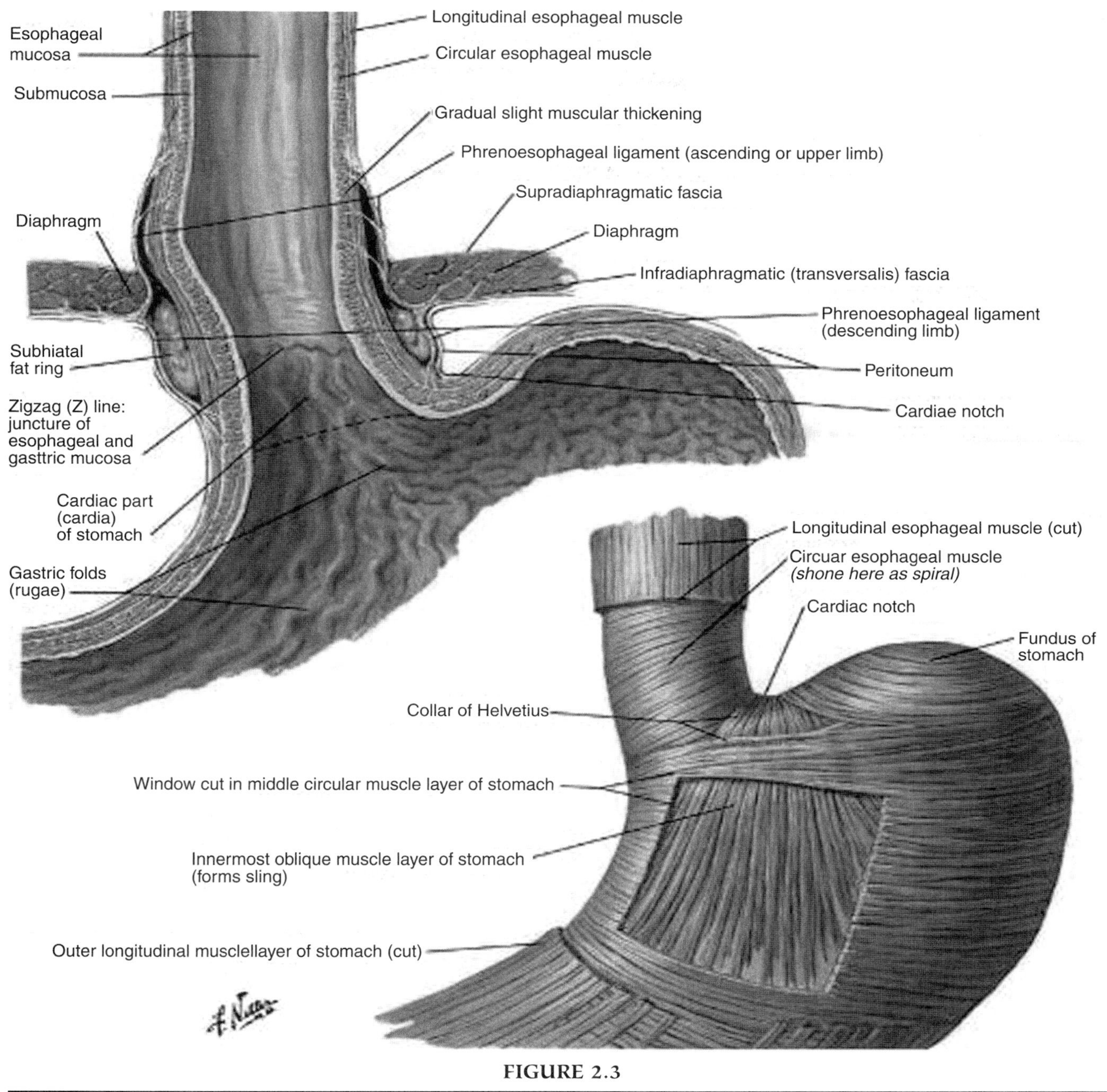

FIGURE 2.3

Anatomic structures of the gastroesophageal junction.

(Figure 2.3). The LES is a functional unit composed of an intrinsic and an extrinsic component. The intrinsic structure of LES consists of esophageal muscle fibers and is under neurohormonal influence. The extrinsic component consists of the diaphragm muscle, which functions as an adjunctive external sphincter that raises the pressure in the terminal esophagus related to the movements of respiration. Malfunction in any of these two components can cause of gastroesophageal reflux and its subsequent symptoms and mucosal changes (11).

The intrinsic component of the LES is composed of circular layers of the esophagus, clasp-like semicircular smooth muscle fibers on the right side, and sling-like oblique gastric muscle fibers on the left side (12). The circular muscles of the LES are thicker than the adjacent esophagus. The clasp-like semicircular fibers have significant myogenic tone but are not very responsive to cholinergic stimulation, whereas the sling-like oblique gastric fibers have little resting tone but contract vigorously to cholinergic stimulation (12).

The extrinsic component of the LES is composed of the crural diaphragm, which forms the esophageal hiatus, and represents a channel through which the esophagus enters into the abdomen. The crural diaphragm encircles the proximal 2 to 4 cm of the LES and determines inspiratory spike-like increases in LES pressure, as measured by esophageal manometry (13).

HISTOLOGIC ASPECTS

Macroscopically during endoscopy, the esophageal lumen appears as a smooth, pale pink tube with visible submucosal blood vessels. The transition from esophageal to gastric mucosa is known as the Z-line and consists of an irregular circumferential line between two areas of different colored mucosa. The distal gastric mucosa is darker than the more proximal pale pink esophageal mucosa.

Microscopically, the esophageal wall is composed of 4 layers: internal mucosa, submucosa, muscularis propria, and adventitia. Unlike the remainder of the gastrointenstinal (GI) tract, the esophagus has no serosa. This allows esophageal tumors to spread more easily and makes them harder to treat surgically (14). The missing serosal layer also makes luminal disruptions more challenging to repair.

Mucosa

The mucosa is thick and reddish cranially and more pale caudally. It is arranged in longitudinal folds that disappear upon distention. It consists of three sublayers.

The first sublayer is the mucous membrane: a nonkeratinized squamous epithelium. It covers the entire inner surface of the esophagus, and at the LES level, it may coexist with the columnar, gastric type epithelium. The mucous membrane is composed of stratum basale, stratum intermedium, and stratum superficialis.

Stratum basale (10%–15% of the epithelium) contains cuboidal basophilic cells, low in glycogen, attached to the basement membrane by hemidesmosomes. These cells can divide and replenish the superficial layers. In 25% of the normal population, the stratum basale contains argyrophilic-positive endocrine cells and in 4% of the normal subjects, it contains melanocytes (15). The melanocytes from this region account for the occurrence of primary melanoma of the esophagus (16), while the argyrophilic-positive endocrine cells are the potential progenitors of the esophageal small cell carcinoma (15).

Stratum intermedium and stratum superficialis are composed of cells derived from the basal stratum that become more flattened with pyknotic nuclei. These cells may present processes and desmosomal junctions that become fewer and more simplified superficially (17). Compared with the basal cells, the cells in the stratum intermedium and superficialis are rich in glycogen (18).

The second sublayer forming the mucosa is represented by lamina propria, a thin connective tissue structure containing vascular structures and mucous secreting glands.

The third sublayer of the mucosa is muscularis mucosa. This is a thin layer of longitudinally, irregularly arranged smooth muscle fibers and delicate elastic fibers (19). The muscularis mucosa extends through the entire esophagus and continues into the rest of the GI tract, being much thinner in the proximal part of the esophagus than in its distal part (20) (see Figure 2.4). At the pharyngeal end of the esophagus, the muscularis mucosa is represented by a few scattered smooth muscle fibers. Caudally, approaching the cardiac orifice, the muscularis mucosa forms a thick layer, so thick that sometimes it may be confused with the muscularis propria on biopsy specimens (18). The muscularis mucosa separates the lamina propria from the submucosa and retracts when it is sectioned during surgical procedures.

Submucosa

The submucosa contains loose connective tissue, as well as lymphocytes, plasma cells, nerve cells (Meissner's plexus),

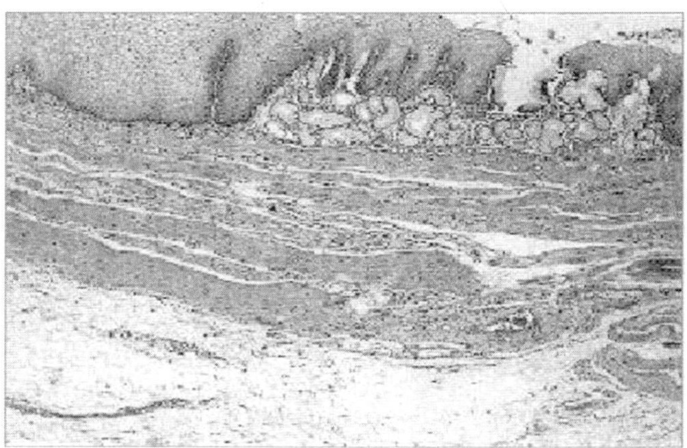

FIGURE 2.4

Histologic specimen of the distal esophagus. The mucosal layer of the gastroesophageal junction is characterized by a muscularis mucosae that is thicker than the muscularis mucosae of the more proximal esophagus. Note also the esophageal cardial-type gland situated above the muscularis mucosae. (Printed with permission from *Histology for Pathologists*, Stephen S. Sternberg, 1992, Raven Press Ltd.)

a vascular network (Heller's plexus), and submucosal glands. The esophageal submucosal glands are considered to be a continuation of the glands in the oropharynx. They are small racemose glands (18) of the mucous type more concentrated in the upper and lower regions. Their secretion is important in esophageal clearance and tissue resistance to acid (21). The post-obstructive inflammation of the glandular ducts can result in intramucosal pseudodiverticulosis (22).

Muscularis Propria

The muscularis propria is responsible for motor function. The upper 5% to 33% is composed exclusively of striated type of muscle, and the distal 33% is composed of smooth muscle. In between there is a mixture of both, called the transition zone. Functionally the transition zone can be observed with manometry as a region where there is no significant contraction amplitude during a peristaltic contraction that travels down the body of the esophagus (23). Despite the presence of two different muscle types, they function as a whole unit. Between the longitudinal and circular muscular layers, at this level, Auerbach's plexus is found. Different pathologic conditions usually affect only one muscular layer, as in sclerodema and achalasia when only the circular layer is involved (18).

Adventitia

The adventitia is an external fibrous layer that covers the esophagus, connecting it with neighboring structures. It is composed of loose connective tissue and contains small vessels, lymphatic channels, and nerve fibers providing a support role. The esophagus does not have a serosal layer except under the diaphragm level where it is formed by the peritoneum (19).

VASCULARIZATION

Arteries

The rich arterial supply of the esophagus is segmental (Figure 2.5). The cervical esophagus is supplied with branches of the left and right superior and inferior thyroid arteries. These branches travel anteriorly towards the lateral aspect of the esophagus and they anastomose on the anterior and posterior esophageal walls. Rarely, the cervical esophagus can be vascularized with branches originating from thyroideaima artery, common carotid arteries, and subclavian arteries.

The thoracic esophagus is supplied by paired esophageal branches from the tracheobronchic arteries. The later ones emerge from the caudal aspect of the aortic arch and are 1 to 2.5 mm in diameter. They course anteriorly and give off branches to the trachea and esophagus. This region of the esophagus is also supplied by unpaired esophageal branches of about 1.5 to 2 mm that arise at variable locations directly from the anterior wall of the aorta and that travel to the posterior aspect of the esophageal wall (10).

The intra-abdominal esophagus is supplied with branches from the left gastric artery. These vessels travel upward on the anterior aspect of the cardia, and they give off periesophageal tributaries before entering in the muscular wall (2). The posterior aspect of the abdominal esophagus is supplied by branches of the fundal arteries derived from the splenic artery.

The esophagus vascular system is mainly formed from branches of arteries that supply some other organs, but a dedicated vasculature to the esophagus is less developed. The vessels dip in the esophageal wall creating a network in the submucosa and mucosa, offering an "excellent blood supply" (24).

The vasculature of the esophagus determines a number of surgical particularities. During the pull-through esophagectomy without thoracotomy for excising cancer or tumors, the blood loss is moderate, making this procedure relatively safe (25,26). Usually if bleeding occurs it is a consequence of the intratumoral or tumoral adhesions hemorrhage.

Veins

The venous system of the esophagus has two main divisions: the intrinsic division, located in the submucosa, and the extrinsic division, located outside the esophagus (see Figure 2.6). The extrinsic division drains blood into larger blood vessels.

The intrinsic venous system is composed of a parallel network located in the esophageal submucosa coursing the whole length of the esophagus (27). Kitano and colleagues (28) described in detail the intrinsic venous system in the lower part of the esophagus, close to the GEJ (Figure 2.7). Using resin casting, this group identified 4 distinct layers forming the intrinsic esophageal venous plexus: (a) intraepithelial channels, running centrifugally from the epithelium and draining in the superficial venous plexus with a mean diameter of 0.043 mm, (b) superficial venous plexus located in the mucosa, right below the epithelium, and continuing with a similar plexus at the gastric level (mean diameter = 0.188 mm), (c) deep intrinsic veins, having a higher caliber and draining the blood from the superficial venous plexus (mean diameter = 0.442), (d) Adventitial veins, located more peripherally in the adventitia and also having a higher caliber (mean diameter = 0.452 mm). The

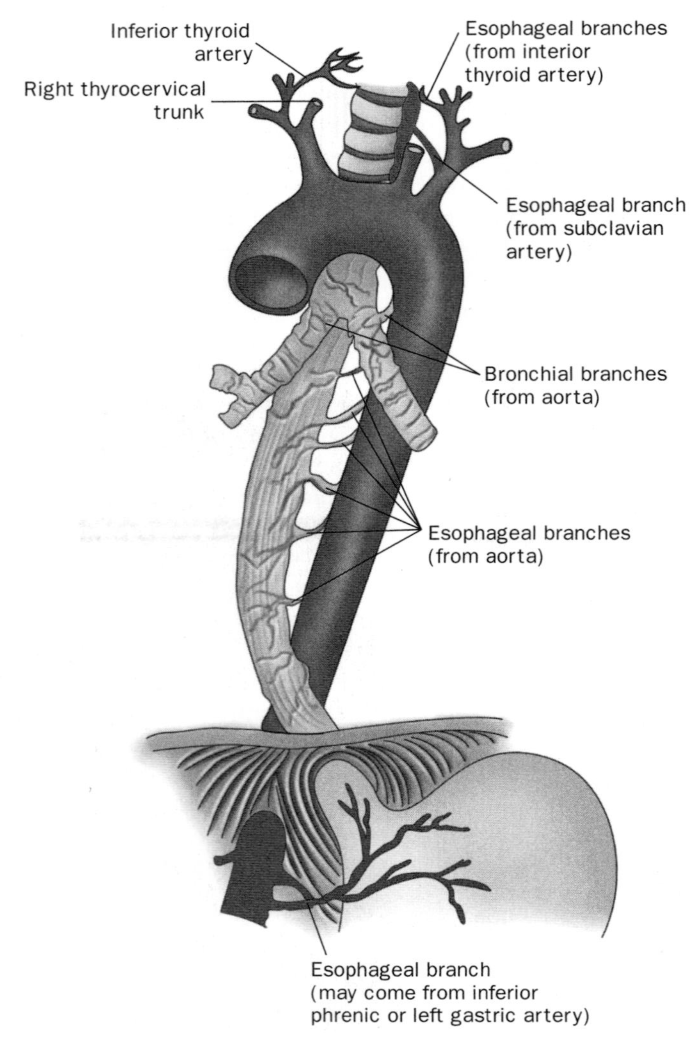

NOTE: 1) because the esophagus is an elongated organ extending from the neck to the abdomen, it receives arterial blood from at least three sources:

a) **in the neck:** most frequently from the **inferior thyroid branch** of the **thyrocervical trunk,** but it may also come directly from the subclavian, or vertebral arteries or from the costocervical trunk,

b) **in the thorax;** multiple **esophageal branches** that come directly from the aorta,

c) **in the abdomen:** from the **inferior phrenic artery** or the **left gastric artery.**

2) these vessels anastomose with each other in the substance of the esophagus.

FIGURE 2.5

Arterial system of the esophagus.

adventitial veins collect the blood from the deep intrinsic veins through perforating veins that span the muscularis propria layer.

The intrinsic esophageal plexus is of a particular clinical interest because it makes the connection between the portal and the caval venous systems, both of which are highly involved in the pathology of the esophageal varices. The esophageal varices occur mainly in conditions that complicate with portal hypertension, such as cirrhosis, schistosomiasis, portal vein thrombosis, and that rarely occur in the absence of portal hypertension (i.e., superior vena cava) (29).

The patients with portal hypertension present a specific anatomic pathology. The main changes appear at the level of the deep venous layer that transform into tortuous variceal structures (28). Esophageal varices that form as a backflow pressure accumulation may frequently bleed when the intravenous pressure passes over 12 mmHg (30).

The extrinsic venous system of the esophagus drains in large vessels: The upper esophagus blood drains in azygos and hemiazygos veins, the mid and low esophagus drain in tributaries of the portal system such as left gastric vein or splenic vein.

Of high surgical interest, the tumors originating in the mid-esophagus have a high propensity to invade the azygos vein. If the tumor presents with adhesions, there is a significant chance that during surgical maneuvers such as blunt pull-through dissection, the azygos vein can be damaged, causing fatal bleeding (2).

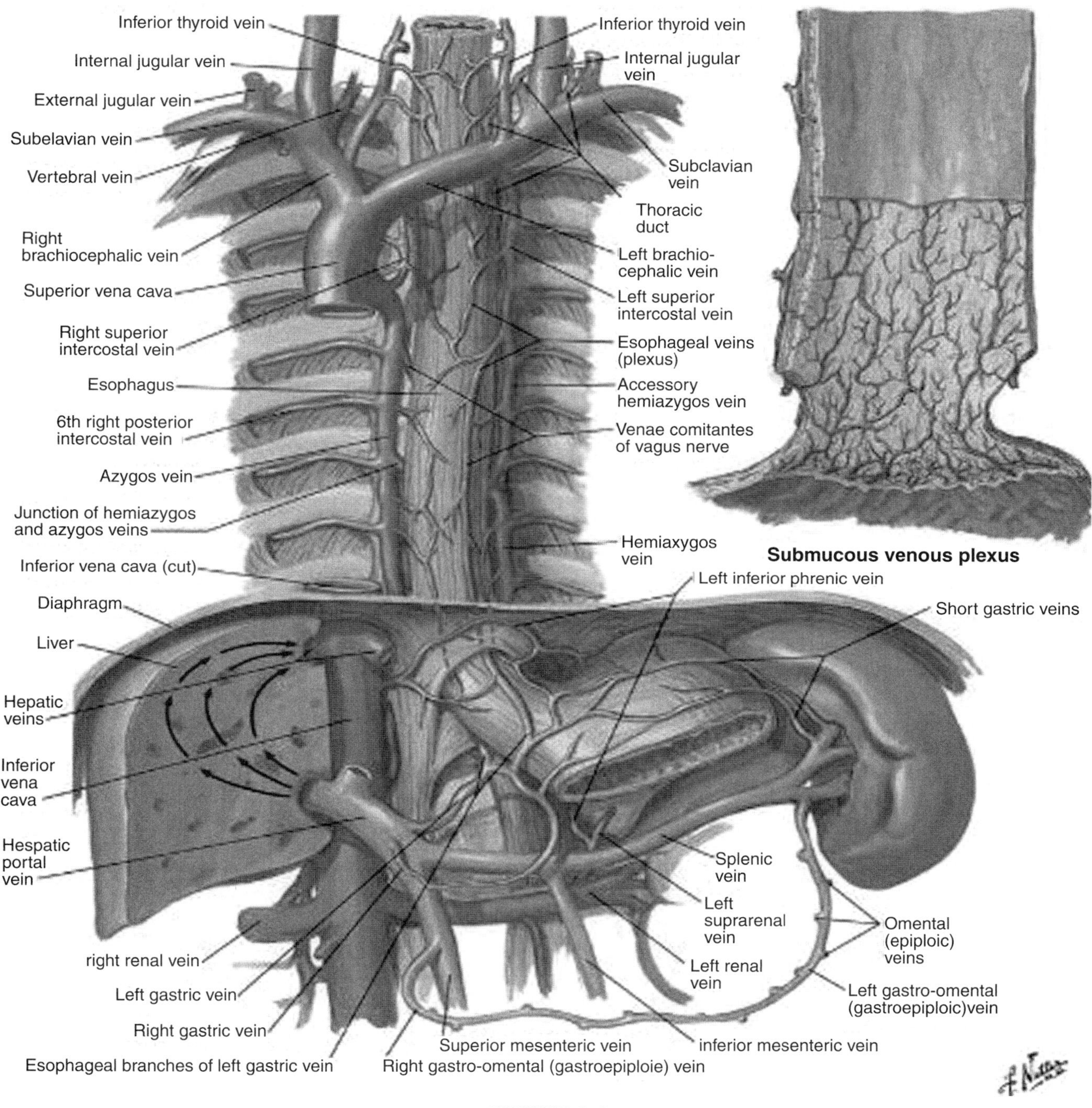

FIGURE 2.6

Venous system of the esophagus.

Lymphatic System of the Esophagus

Lymphatic drainage in the esophagus consists of two systems: the lymph channels and lymph nodules (Figure 2.8).

The lymph channels begin in the esophageal tissue space as a network of endothelial channels (20–30 μm) or as blind endothelial sacculations (40–60 μm) (31) (Figure 2.9). The location of the lymphatic capillary origin is not

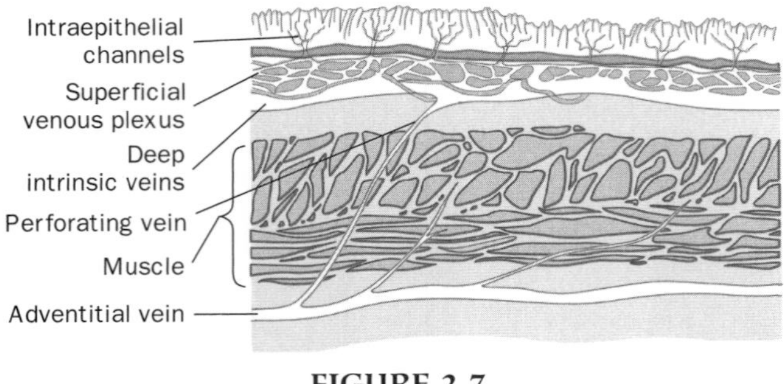

FIGURE 2.7

Diagram of the venous drainage of the esophagus.

known precisely. Some authors propose that precapillary spaces exist in the lamina mucosa, but others contend that there is an absence of true lymphatic capillaries in the upper and middle levels of the lamina mucosa (32). Electron microscopic studies show anastomotic lymph capillaries in the lower mucosal levels and small lymphatic vessels in the submucosa.

From this level fluid, colloid material, cell debris, microorganisms, and sometimes tumor cells are taken and drained into collecting lymph channels (100–200 μm) that continue through the esophageal muscular coat and are distributed parallel to the long axis of the esophagus. Paired semilunar valves within the collecting channels determine the direction of flow. The collecting lymph channels merge into small trunks that open into the regional lymph nodes.

The lymphatic drainage of the esophagus differs in the anatomic regions of the esophagus. Lymphatic flow patterns can predict potential regions of tumoral invasion. The lymphatics from the proximal third of the esophagus drain into the deep cervical lymph nodes (first station) and afterward in the thoracic duct. Some studies show that carcinoma of the cervical esophagus may involve the paratracheal lymph nodes as well (33). The lymphatics from the middle third of the esophagus drain into the superior and inferior mediastinal lymph nodes. Fujita et al. reported that the right paracardiac, periesophageal, and lesser curvature nodes were the most frequent involved in the thoracic esophageal cancer (34). Another study (35) found consistently that extramural lymphatic vessels from the middle and lower part of the esophagus drain into bifurcational nodes. The lower third of the esophagus drains into lymphatic vessels that follow the course of the left gastric artery and ultimately reach the gastric and celiac lymph nodes. Saito and colleagues (35) reported a high variability regarding the patterns of drainage, and a very rigorous structured description is challenging. Traditionally, the lymph that forms above the tracheal bifurcation was thought to drain into the thoracic duct (2) (Figure 2.10), while the lymph originating under the bifurcation was believed to drain in through the celiac and gastric lymph nodes directly in the cisterna chyli. The region around the bifurcation may present with a bidirectional lymph flow, which would explain how the lymph nodes located superiorly to carina can be invaded by tumors originating in the lower esophageal third. In pathological conditions such as tumor invasion, blockage of the lymphatic ducts, or incompetence of the valves, the lymphatic flow may deviate from the normal, and collateral lymphatic circulation may develop (2).

The longitudinal lymphatic network located in the submucosa was thought to provide easier access than the penetrating channels that drain the lymph outside the esophagus. This anatomic particularity may explain the longitudinal, intramural invasion seen in the early stages of the esophageal tumors (36). The poor lymph network in the mucosa makes this region less prone for invasion. Absence or small malignant lesions in the mucosa may be accompanied by extended submucosal tumors (2). The lymphatic flow in the longitudinal plexus of the esophagus may also explain the high postoperative recurrence because resection with the tumor-free margin does not guarantee the total removal of a tumor that can spread at the submucosal level (2).

INNERVATION OF THE ESOPHAGUS

The esophagus, like the rest of the viscera, receives dual motor and sensory innervation supplied by two divisions of the autonomic system: the sympathetic and parasympathetic systems (Figure 2.11).

The Sympathetic System

The afferent system collects the information from the wall of the esophagus using sensorial structures such as osmoreceptors, chemoreceptors, thermoreceptors, and mechanoreceptors (37). The afferent fibers are dendrites of the unipolar neurons located in the dorsal root ganglion in the thoracic spine (T1–T10). These neurons will synapse with the preganglionic neurons located in the latero-intermedial grey horns from the thoracic spine. The axons of preganglionic neurons leave the spine on the ventral root, and they synapse with neurons in the sympathetic paravertebral chain at the same level, or they can travel upward or downward to synapse with neurons at different levels. The axons of these neurons are myelinated and form the white ramicommunicantes.

The multipolarganglionic neurons are located in the sympathetic trunk, in the proximity of the spine, against the costal ends and posterior to the costal pleura (38).

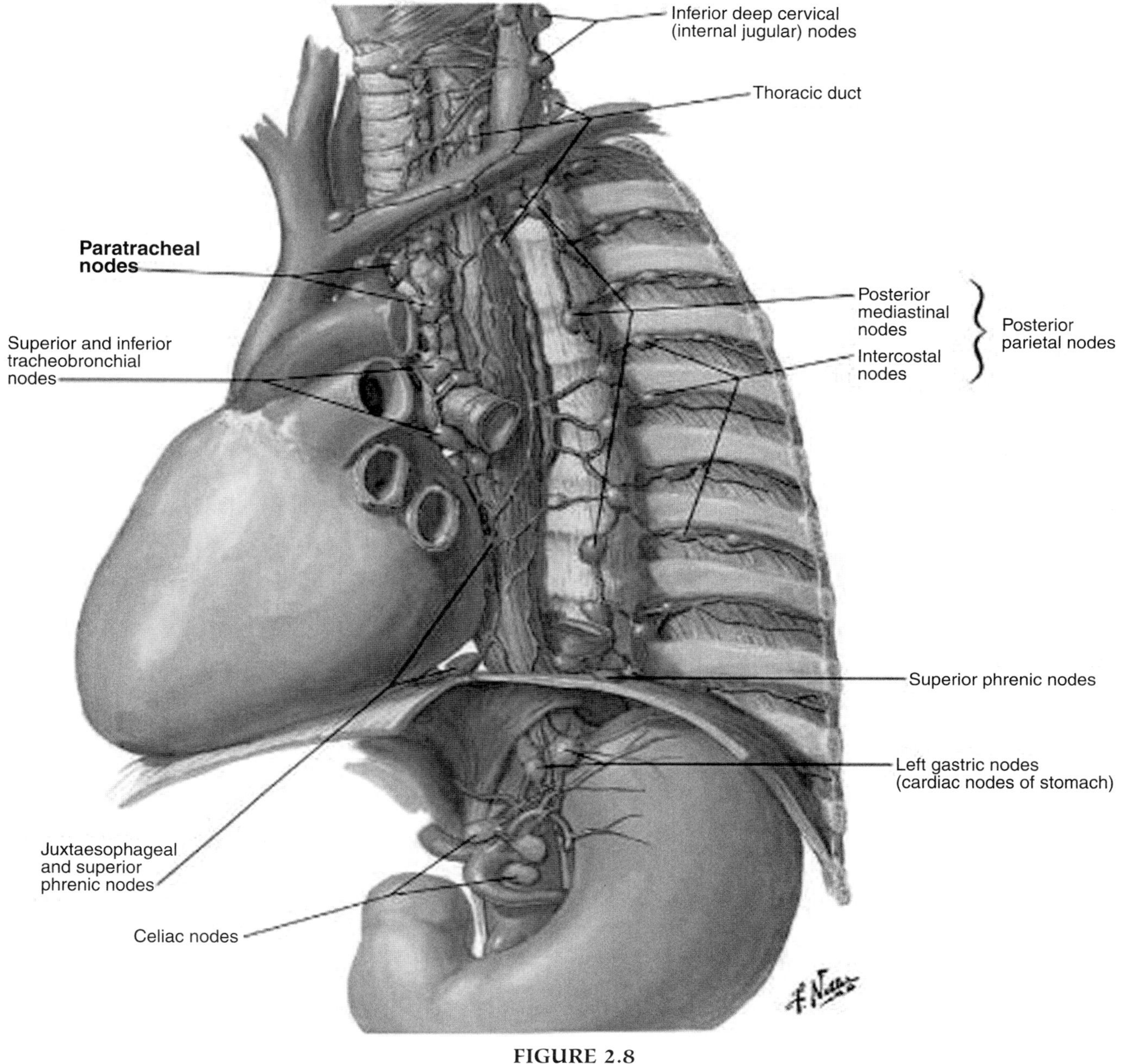

FIGURE 2.8

Lymphatic system of the esophagus.

The rami emerging from the second to the fifth ganglia form the posterior pulmonary plexus or the deep part of the cardiac plexus. These plexuses can generate small branches that distribute to the proximal esophagus (2).

The preganglionic fibers deriving from T5 to T9 merge and form the greater splanchnic nerve that descends obliquely in the proximity of the thoracic vertebral bodies and perforates the ipsilateral diaphragmatic crus on its way to the celiac ganglion. Postganglionic fibers from the celiac ganglion distribute as well to the esophagus and thereby supply sympathetic innervation (38).

The postganglionic fibers influence the activity of the target end organs, glands, muscles, and enteric nervous system. Throughout these pathways, the sympathetic

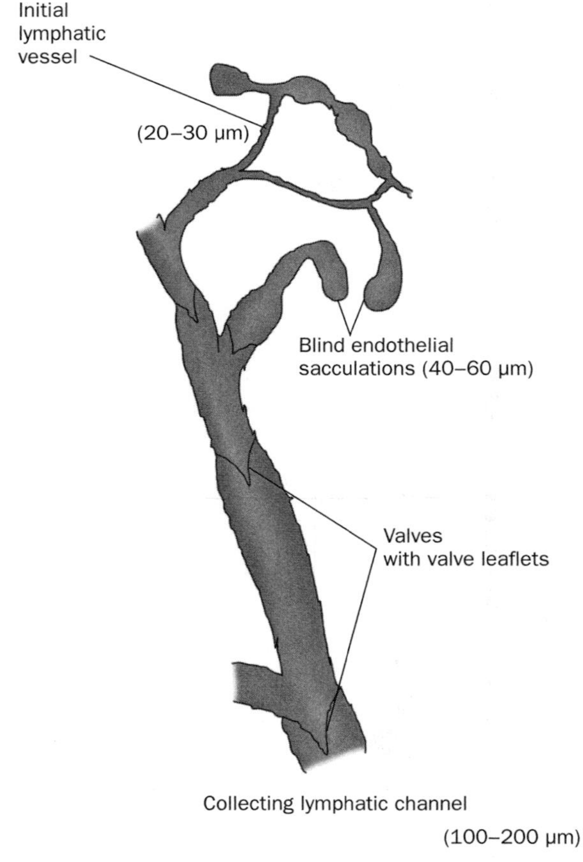

FIGURE 2.9

Initial lymphatic network, reconstructed from mesentery preparation. Most likely, this pattern is similar to that of the esophagus. This image was published in *Esophageal Surgery*, 2nd Ed., F. Griffith Pearson, Page 15, Copyright Churchill Livingstone (2002).

system generates specific activities such as relaxation of the muscular wall with depression of the peristalsis (38,39) and increase of the lower esophageal sphincter tonus (40).

The sensorial information from the esophageal wall is also transmitted ascending toward supraspinal and cortical centers, where it is interpreted as sensation. Pain, temperature, and visceroceptive information can be transmitted via lamina I Rexed and spinothalamic pathways in the ventromedial nucleus of the thalamus, projecting to the insular cortex (41,42). The information is transmitted through pathways containing numerous small interneurons in the laminae VII and X Rexed.

The sympathetic outflow of the neurons from the lateral horn in the spine is also controlled by substantial input from multiple supraspinal structures. Using transneuronal-tracing techniques with pseudorabies virus, identification of these specific supraspinal structures is possible. After injection of the pseudorabies virus in the celiac and stellate ganglia, 5 regions were labeled: (a) ventromedial medulla, (b) rostralventrolateral medulla, (c) caudalraphe nuclei, (d) A5 noradrenergic cell group, and (e) paraventricular nucleus of the hypothalamus (43).

The Parasympathetic System

The parasympathetic system at the esophageal level is mainly represented by the fibers of the vagus nerve. The sensory, afferent fibers of the parasympathetic system are mainly part of the vagus nerve. These fibers are dendritic ends of unipolar neurons located mainly in the nodose (inferior) vagal ganglion and represent approximately 80% of the vagal trunk (44). The sensory neurons within the nodose ganglion have a topographic layout suggested by Collman et al. (45). Using retrograde immunohistochemic techniques, Neuhuber demonstrated that the vagal afferents that supply mucosa and muscularis propria in the cervical esophagus have different origins. The afferent innervation of the muscularis propria originates in nodose ganglion, while the fibers supplying the mucosal layer originate mainly from petrosal and jugular ganglion (46). These observations are in agreement with some experiments that demonstrate different patterns of stimulation. The vagal afferents from the submucosa respond mainly to mechanical distention, while the afferents in the mucosa respond to various chemical and intralumninal stimulation (44). The parasympathetic afferents from the esophagus on their way to the sensory ganglion gather and form the superior laryngeal nerve (SLN). The SLN courses along the pharynx, posterior and medial to the internal carotid artery, dividing into internal and external branches. After piercing the inferior constrictor muscle, the internal SLN ascends and gives off branches supplying the sensory of the esophagus, especially on the left side (38).

The axons of the primary neurons that supply sensation of the esophagus terminate in different nuclei of the brain stem. The vagal afferents from the proximal striated esophagus project in a specific region on the medial aspect of the solitary tract called the central subnucleus. The afferents from the smooth muscled part of the esophagus project in the vicinity of the central subnucleus (47,48).

The striated and smooth parts of the esophagus are supplied with efferent fibers of different origins. The nervous fibers innervating the striated esophagus originate from the rostral part of the nucleus ambiguous (49). This structure is connected to the ipsilateral central subnucleus of the solitary tract by medullary interneurons. The efferent parasympathetic fibers going to the distal smooth muscled esophagus originate in the medial part of the dorsal nucleus, the largest parasympathetic structure in the brain stem (38). From the dorsal nucleus, the

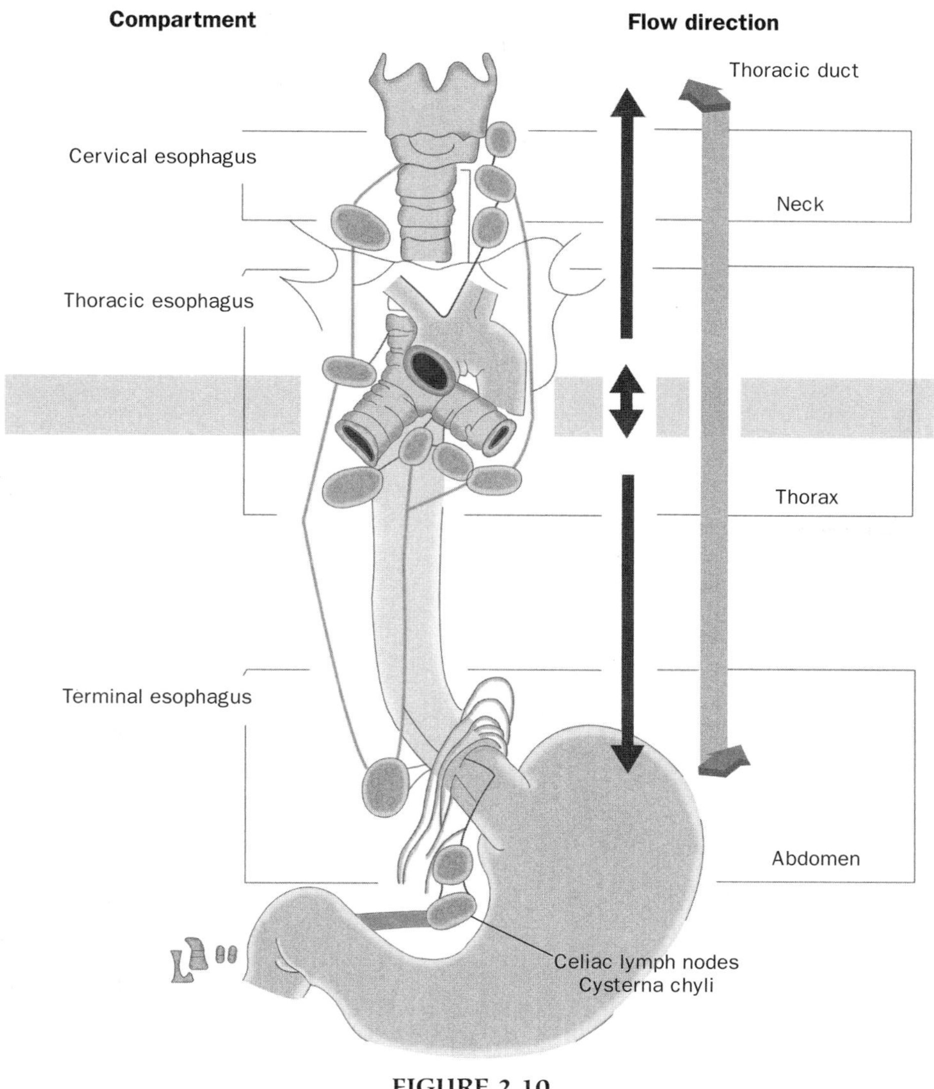

FIGURE 2.10

Concept of lymphatic pathways. The lymphatic system of the esophagus presents a bidirectional flow at the tracheal bifurcation. This feature is consistent with clinical observations. The knowledge of lymph flow and the corresponding lymph node distribution is essential in understanding potential spread of malignancy. This image was published in *Esophageal Surgery*, 2nd Ed., F. Griffith Pearson, Page 17, Copyright Churchill Livingstone (2002).

efferent fibers merge and form the main trunk of the vagus nerve that travels through the jugular foramen. The right vagus nerve courses down on the posterior aspect of the right bronchus and hilum and divides into anterior and posterior subdivision. The posterior subdivision unites with the sympathetic fibers forming the right posterior pulmonary plexus. This plexus will generate in its caudal part rami that innervate the esophagus. These rami join similar rami coming from the left side to form the anterior esophageal plexus. This plexus continues down along the anterior surface of the esophagus and courses through the diaphragmatic hiatus (38).

At the proximal part of the esophagus at the pharyngeal-esophageal junction, the efferent innervation is supplied with fibers from the recurrent right and left laryngeal nerves. These nerves originate from the vagus nerve curving backwards and upward around the subclavian artery on the right side respectively, around the aortic arch on the left side. In the ascending segments, these nerves travel in the groove formed between trachea and esophagus, and they give off esophageal branches that participate in the esophageal plexus (38). The parasympathetic efferent fibers regulate the activity of the esophageal muscle by increasing

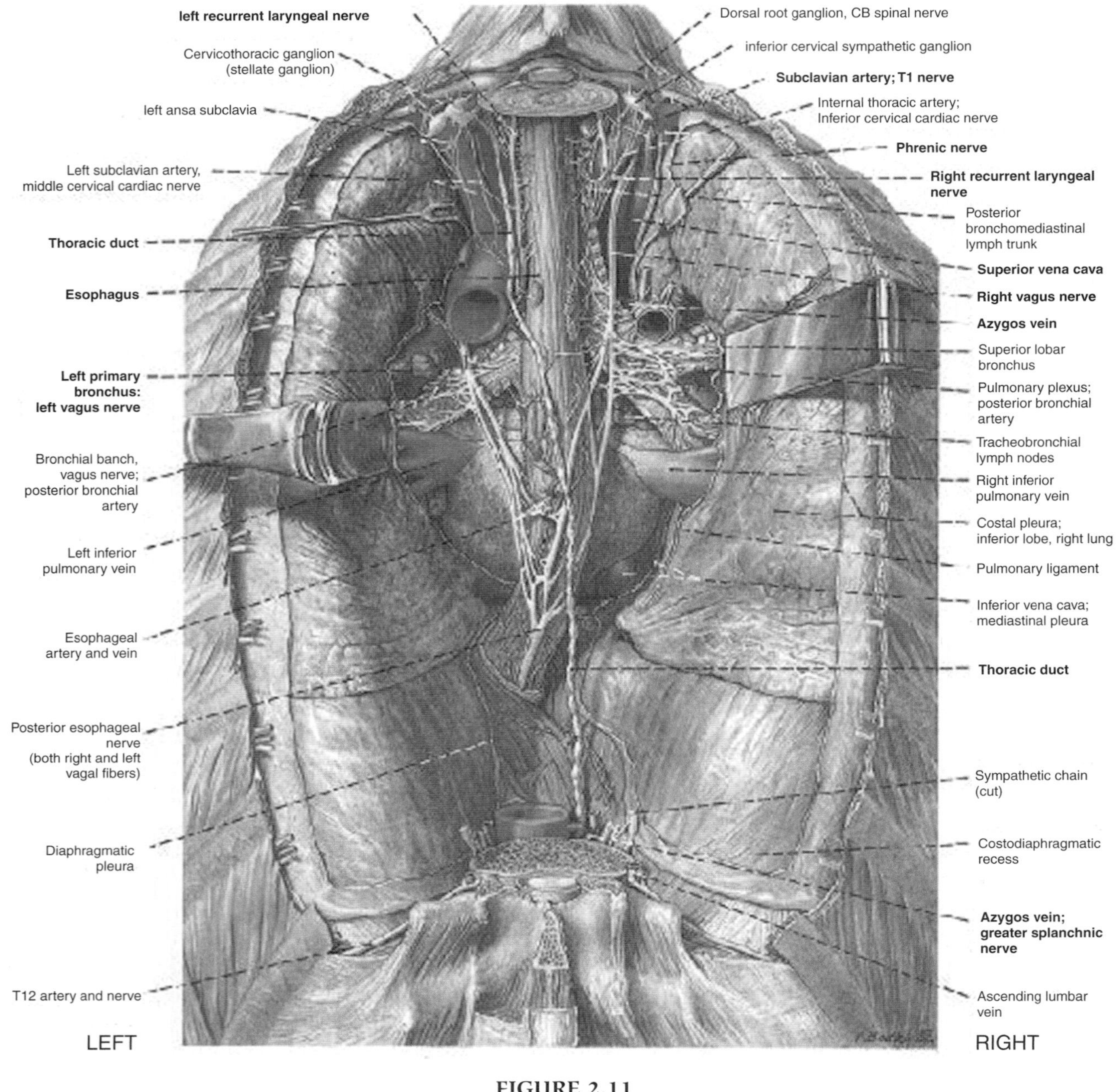

FIGURE 2.11

Posterior cutaway view of the intrathoracic esophagus in anatomic position.

peristalsis, decreasing pressure in the LES, and increasing secretory activity.

Similar to the sympathetic system, the activity of the parasympathetic system is tonically regulated by supraspinal centers, such as hypothalamus and cortical areas. Positron-emission tomography (PET) and functional Magnetic Resonance Imaging (fMRI) have been used to map the central nervous system projections from the esophagus. Esophageal stimulation at the subliminal and liminal levels is sensed peripherally and transmitted to the brain for further processing and modulation. Esophageal sensory innervation is carried by the vagus nerve to the nodose ganglion and projects through the brainstem, through the thalamus, to terminate in the cortex (45,50). Regions that are activated by esophageal stimulation include the secondary sensory and motor cortex, parieto-occipital cortex, anterior and posterior cingulate cortex, prefrontal cortical cortex, and the insula (51).

Enteric Nervous System

Similar to other segments of the gastrointestinal tract, the esophagus has its own neural systems composed of flat networks in the muscular layers that form the myenteric and submucous enteric plexuses (52,53). The thin nerve fibers and numerous ganglia of the intramural myenteric and submucosal plexuses provide the intrinsic innervation of the esophagus. The ganglia that lie between the longitudinal and the circular layers of the tunica muscularis form the myenteric or Auerbach's plexus, whereas those that lie in the submucosa form the submucous or Meissner's plexus. In the smooth muscled esophagus, the neurons of the myenteric plexus relay between the vagus and the smooth muscle, acting as postganglionic neurons. From here, short motor axons from the ganglia penetrate and innervate the muscle layers (54). The two intrinsic nervous plexuses have different roles: Auerbach's plexus regulates contraction of the outer muscle layers, whereas Meissner's plexus regulates secretion and the peristaltic contractions of the muscularis mucosae.

The neuromuscular activity is regulated by cellular entities within the circular muscular layer of the esophagus: interstitial cells of Cajal (ICC) that form gap junctions with the adjacent smooth muscle cells and play a regulatory role in the neurotransmission.

The recurrent laryngeal nerves and the superior laryngeal nerves have a significant clinical importance. Because of their length and specific location, they can be easily injured during the esophageal resections and goiter operations. These injuries cause a variety of temporary or permanent motor and sensory disfunctions such as hoarseness, aspiration issues related to respiratory, or swallowing failure (2).

References

1. Castell DO, Richter JE. *The Esophagus*. 3rd ed. Philadelphia: Lippincott, Williams, & Wilkens; 1999.
2. Pearson G, Cooper J, Deslauriers J. *Esophageal Surgery*. Second Edition, 2002.
3. Sobotta J, Putz R, Pabst R. *Atlas der Anatomie des Menschen, English version*.13th ed. Philadelphia: Lippincott, Williams, & Wilkens; 2001.
4. Eliska O. Phreno-oesophageal membrane and its role in the development of hiatal hernia. *ActaAnat (Basel)*. 1973;86(1):137–150.
5. Sivarao DV, Goyal RK. Functional anatomy and physiology of the upper esophageal sphincter. *Am J Med*. 2000;108Suppl 4a:27S–37S.
6. Achkar E. Zenker's diverticulum. *Dig Dis*. 1998;16(3):144–151.
7. Gerhardt D, et al. Human upper esophageal sphincter pressure profile. *Am J Physiol*. 1980;239(1):G49–52.
8. Lang IM, Shaker R. Anatomy and physiology of the upper esophageal sphincter. *Am J Med*. 1997;103(5A):50S–55S.
9. Kumoi K, Ohtsuki N, Teramoto Y. Pharyngo-esophageal diverticulum arising from Laimer's triangle. *Eur Arch Otorhinolaryngol*. 2001;258(4):184–187.
10. Liebermann-Meffert D, Allgower M, Schmid P, et al. Muscular equivalent of the lower esophageal sphincter. *Gastroenterology*. 1979;76(1):31–38.
11. Delattre JF, Avisse C, Marcus C, et al. Functional anatomy of the gastroesophageal junction. *Surg Clin North Am*. 2000;80(1):241–260.
12. Preiksaitis HG, Diamant NE. Regional differences in cholinergic activity of muscle fibers from the human gastroesophageal junction. *Am J Physiol*. 1997;272(6 Pt 1): G1321–1327.
13. Mittal RK, Balaban DH. The esophagogastric junction. *N Engl J Med*. 1997;336(13):924–932.
14. Boyce H, Boyce G. Esophagus: anatomy and structureal anomalies. In : *Textbook of Gastroenterology*. Yamada T, Alpers DH, Kaplowitz N, Laine L, Owyang C, Powell DW, eds. 4th ed. Philadelphia, PA: Lippincot William & Wilkins; 2003:vol. 1:1148–1165.
15. De La Pava S, et al. Melanosis of the esophagus. *Cancer*. 1963;16:48–50.
16. DiCostanzo DP, Urmacher C. Primary malignant melanoma of the esophagus. *Am J SurgPathol*. 1987;11(1):46–52.
17. Hopwood D, Logan KR, Bouchier IA. The electron microscopy of normal human oesophageal epithelium. *Virchows Arch B Cell Pathol*. 1978;26(4):345–358.
18. Sternberg S. *Histology for Pathologists*. 2nd ed. New York: Raven Press; 1997.
19. Borysenko M, Beringer T. *Functional Histology*. 3rd ed. Boston: Little, Brown; 1989.
20. Christensen J, Wingate DL, Gregory RA. *A Guide to Gastrointestinal Motility*. Bristol: John Wright & Sons Ltd; 1983.
21. Long JD, Orlando RC. Esophageal submucosal glands: structure and function. *Am J Gastroenterol*. 1999;94(10):2818–2824.
22. Medeiros LJ, Doos WG, Balogh K. Esophageal intramural pseudodiverticulosis: a report of two cases with analysis of similar, less extensive changes in "normal" autopsy esophagi. *Hum Pathol*. 1988;19(8):928–931.
23. Ghosh SK, Janiak P, Schwizer W, et al. Physiology of the esophageal pressure transition zone: separate contraction waves above and below. *Am J Physiol Gastrointest Liver Physiol*. 2005;290(3):568–576.
24. Williams DB, Payne WS. Observations on esophageal blood supply. *Mayo Clin Proc*. 1982;57(7):448–453.
25. Akiyama H. Surgery for carcinoma of the esophagus. *Curr Probl Surg*. 1980;17(2):53–120.
26. Orringer MB, Orringer JS. Esophagectomy without thoracotomy: a dangerous operation? *J Thorac Cardiovasc Surg*. 1983;85(1):72–80.
27. Vianna A, Hayes PC, Moscoso G, et al. Normal venous circulation of the gastroesophageal junction. A route to understanding varices. *Gastroenterology*. 1987;93(4):876–889.
28. Kitano S, Terblanche J, Kahn D, et al. Venous anatomy of the loweroesophagus in portal hypertension: practical implications. *Br J Surg*. 1986;73(7):525–531.
29. Pashankar D, Jamieson DH, Israel DM. Downhill esophageal varices. *J Pediatr Gastroenterol Nutr*. 1999;29(3):360–362.
30. Dell'era A, Bosch J. Review article: the relevance of portal pressure and other risk factors in acute gastro-oesophagealvariceal bleeding. *Aliment Pharmacol Ther*. 2004;20 Suppl 3:8–15; discussion 16–17.
31. Long J, Orlando R. Anatomy, histology, embryology, and developmental abnormalities of the esophagus. In: *Gastrointestinal and Liver Diseases*, Feldman M, Fieldman LS, Sleisenger MH, eds. Philadelphia, PA: W. S. Saunders; 2002:551–560.
32. Zuidema GD. *Shackelford's Surgery of the Alimentary Tract*. , Philadelphia, PA: W. S. Saunders; 1996: I- Esophagus:1–35.
33. Timon CV, Toner M, Conlon BJ. Paratracheal lymph node involvement in advanced cancer of the larynx, hypopharynx, and cervical esophagus. *Laryngoscope*. 2003;113(9):1595–1599.
34. Fujita H, Kakegawa T, Yamana H, et al. Lymph node metastasis and recurrence in patients with a carcinoma of the thoracic esophagus who underwent three-field dissection. *World J Surg*. 1994;18(2):266–272.
35. Saito H, Sato T, Miyazaki M. Extramural lymphatic drainage from the thoracic esophagus based on minute cadaveric dissections: fundamentals for the sentinel node navigation surgery for the thoracic esophageal cancers. *Surg Radiol Anat*. 2007;29(7):531–542.
36. Lehnert T, Erlandson RA, Decosse JJ. Lymph and blood capillaries of the human gastric mucosa. A morphologic basis for metastasis in early gastric carcinoma. *Gastroenterology*. 1985;89(5):939–950.
37. Goyal R, Sivarao D. Functional anatomy and physiology of swallowing and esophageal motility. In: Catell OD, Richter JE. *The Esophagus*. 3rd ed. Philadelphia: Lippincott-Raven; 1999:23.
38. Bannister LH, Berry MM, Collins P. *Gray's Anatomy*. 38th ed. Boston: Harcourt; 1995.
39. Robertson D. *Primer on the Autonomic Nervous System*. 2nd ed. Boston: Academic Press; 2004.
40. DiMarino AJ, Cohen S. The adrenergic control of lower esophageal sphincter function. An experimental model of denervation supersensitivity. *J Clin Invest*. 1973;52(9):2264–2271.
41. Saper CB. The central autonomic nervous system: conscious visceral perception and autonomic pattern generation. *Annu Rev Neurosci*. 2002;25:433–469.
42. Craig AD. An ascending general homeostatic afferent pathway originating in lamina I. *Prog Brain Res*. 1996;107:225–242.
43. Strack AM, Sawyer WB, Hughes JH, et al. A general pattern of CNS innervation of the sympathetic outflow demonstrated by transneuronalpseudorabies viral infections. *Brain Res*. 1989;491(1):156–162.
44. Goyal RK, Hirano I. The enteric nervous system. *N Engl J Med*. 1996;334(17):1106–1115.
45. Collman PI, Tremblay L, Diamant NE. The distribution of spinal and vagal sensory neurons that innervate the esophagus of the cat. *Gastroenterology*. 1992;103(3):817–822.

46. Wank M, Neuhuber WL. Local differences in vagal afferent innervation of the rat esophagus are reflected by neurochemical differences at the level of the sensory ganglia and by different brainstem projections. *J Comp Neurol.* 2001;435(1):41–59.
47. Altschuler SM, Bao XM, Bieger D, et al. Viscerotopic representation of the upper alimentary tract in the rat: sensory ganglia and nuclei of the solitary and spinal trigeminal tracts. *J Comp Neurol.* 1989;283(2):248–268.
48. Cunningham ET, Sawchenko PE. Central neural control of esophageal motility: a review. *Dysphagia.* 1990;5(1):35–51.
49. Holstege C, Graveland G, Bijker-Biemond C, et al. Location of motoneurons innervating soft palate, pharynx and upper esophagus. Anatomical evidence for a possible swallowing center in the pontine reticular formation. An HRP and autoradiographical tracing study. *Brain Behav Evol.* 1983;23(1–2):47–62.
50. Paintal AS. Vagal afferent fibres. *Ergeb Physiol.* 1963;52:74–156.
51. Kern MK, Birn RM, Jaradeh S, et al. Identification and characterization of cerebral cortical response to esophageal mucosal acid exposure and distention. *Gastroenterology.* 1998;115(6):1353–1362.
52. Christensen J, Robison BA. Anatomy of the myenteric plexus of the opossum esophagus. *Gastroenterology.* 1982;83(5):1033–1042.
53. Christensen J, Rick GA, Robison BA, et al. Arrangement of the myenteric plexus throughout the gastrointestinal tract of the opossum. *Gastroenterology.* 1983;85(4):890–899.
54. Gabella G. Innervation of the gastrointestinal tract. *Int Rev Cytol.* 1979;59:129–193.

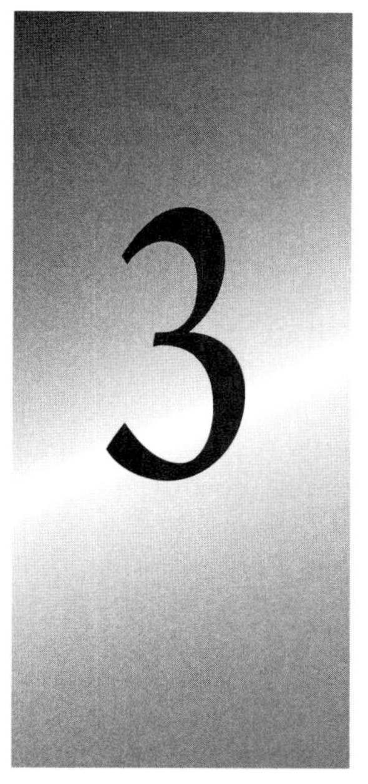

3 The Biology of Epithelial Esophageal Cancer

Eric S. Weiss
Avedis Meneshian
Malcolm V. Brock

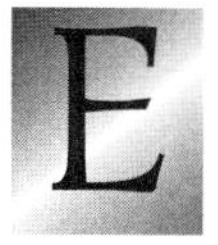

Epithelial cancers of the esophagus are commonly codified into 2 main histolopathologic groups, squamous cell cancer and adenocarcinoma. It is now widely appreciated that these 2 distinct histologies identify 2 very different disease processes. Appreciating some of these differences, as a brief introduction, sheds some light on the complex interaction between environmental influences and biology at play in these 2 very different entities.

Squamous cell cancer occurs predominantly in the developing world, especially in a wide expansive region stretching from northern Iran to north central China, the so-called esophageal cancer belt (1). Esophageal adenocarcinoma, on the other hand, is largely a disease of Western nations, especially of North America and Western Europe. In the countries where esophageal adenocarcinoma is prevalent, there has been a rapid increase in overall incidence of this disease since the mid-1970s that has outpaced the incidences of all other solid malignancies (2) (Figure 3.1).

The incidence of esophageal squamous cell carcinoma, however, even in the cancer belt has decreased or remained constant (3). Even within the same geographical regions, different ethnic groups have very different incidences of esophageal squamous cell and adenocarcinoma. In Scotland, for example, there is a higher rate of squamous cell compared to the rate observed in England and Ireland (4). Similarly in the United States, African Americans have appreciably lower rates of esophageal adenocarcinoma and significantly higher rates of squamous cell cancer than in the Caucasian population (5).

Squamous cell more often is associated with those populations with lower socioeconomic status and more frequent consumption of alcohol, tobacco, hot tea, low fruit and vegetable intake, as well as malnutrition, while esophageal adenocarcinoma has been linked to higher socioeconomic classes, obesity, and chronic gastroesophageal reflux disease (GERD). There is an unexplained gender disparity in patients affected with the two types of esophageal cancer. With squamous cell cancer, the male to female ratio is about 2:1 or 3:1, whereas the male to female ratio in adenocarcinoma is often 7:1 (1). Localization of squamous cancers in the mid- to upper esophagus is far more frequent than that of adenocarcinoma that is found predominantly in the distal third of the esophagus or at the gastroesophageal junction. This discrepancy in tumor localization necessitates different treatment strategies, especially with respect to eligibility of patients for complete surgical resection.

Many of the reasons for these various differences between the two types of esophageal cancer are unknown. Indisputably, environmental influences, such as the high nitrosamine content in the soil in countries of the esophageal belt and the persistent exposure to tobacco carcinogens (nicotine-specific nitrosamines) of

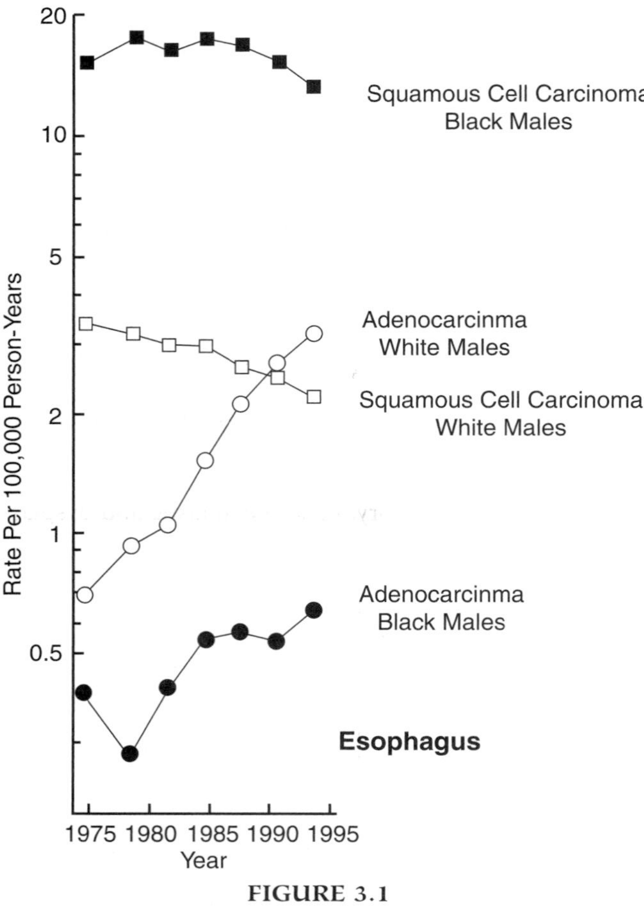

FIGURE 3.1

Esophageal cancer, SEER, 1974–1994. From DeVesa SS, Blot WJ, Fraumeni Jr JF. *Cancer*. 1998;83:2049–2053.

patients in other areas may contribute similarly to carcinogenesis. But at the same time, these similar environmental influences can give rise to tumors with separate and distinct biologies. In this chapter, we will review what is known of these tumor biologies.

Since the advent and completion of the human genome project, there has been a dizzying proliferation of science devoted to the molecular and cellular mechanisms of malignancy. Our knowledge of genetic, and now epigenetic abnormalities, expands exponentially with each passing year. This has resulted in a large scientific literature concerned with tumorigenesis at the cellular level. Topics related to tumorigenesis include: oncogenes, tumor suppressor genes, repair genes, cell cycle regulators, transcription factors, growth factors, hormones, cytokines, cyclins, anti-apoptotic genes, and so on. Changes in genes in the germline result in hereditary predisposition to cancer, while abnormalities in single somatic cells contribute to sporatic malignancies. As Hanahan and Weinberg point out, the complex cast of factors all contribute to establishing the six distinguishing phenotypes of cancer—autonomous growth, resistance to antiproliferative signals, avoidance of apoptosis, unregulated replication, promotion of angiogenesis, and propensity for local as well as distant invasion/dissemination (6).

As the number of discovered genes continues to expand with novel molecular techniques, it becomes increasingly clear that focusing on and having a salient understanding of the oncogenic networks or signal transduction pathways in which these individual genes operate to produce cancer is critical. Vogelstein and Kinzler argue that not only are the number of these oncogenic pathways far fewer than the multitudes of current as well as yet to be discovered genes, but also within these networks there are multiple ways to achieve the same effect (7). In the p53 pathway, for example, most commonly this tumor suppressor gene is rendered dysfunctional through a point mutation that limits its capacity to bind to its target. But functional inactivation of this pathway can be achieved with a non-mutated, biochemically active p53 by disruptions of other components of the pathway, such as the amplication of the MDM2 gene, or the infection of DNA tumor viruses through their gene products that bind to and inactivate p53 (7). In fact, it is well known that in the Rb pathway, only 1 of 4 genes is exclusively mutated at any one time, and the resulting functional effect of each mutation is exactly the same (8–12).

Figure 3.2 depicts an overview of the major cancer gene pathways (7). In these major pathways, there is much redundancy and cross talk both within the networks as well as between them, and in fact, many genes appear to be important in more than one pathway (7). In this chapter, we will discuss the molecular alterations inherent in squamous cell and adenocarcinoma esophageal cancer, with special emphasis on the impact of the disturbance on these networks.

ESOPHAGEAL ADENOCARCINOMA

The Barrett's-Metaplasia-Carcinoma Sequence

First described in 1950, Barrett's esophagus is defined as the replacement, or metaplasia, of the normal esophageal squamous mucosa with a columnar epithelium containing goblet cells (13) (Figure 3.3). In the ensuing 50 years, a great deal has been learned about this clinical entity, its pathogenesis, and its relation to the development of esophageal adenocarcinoma. The condition most commonly arises in the setting of chronic GERD, where repeated mucosal injury is thought to stimulate the progression of intestinal metaplasia. It has been hypothesized that this ectopic columnar epithelium predisposes patients to the

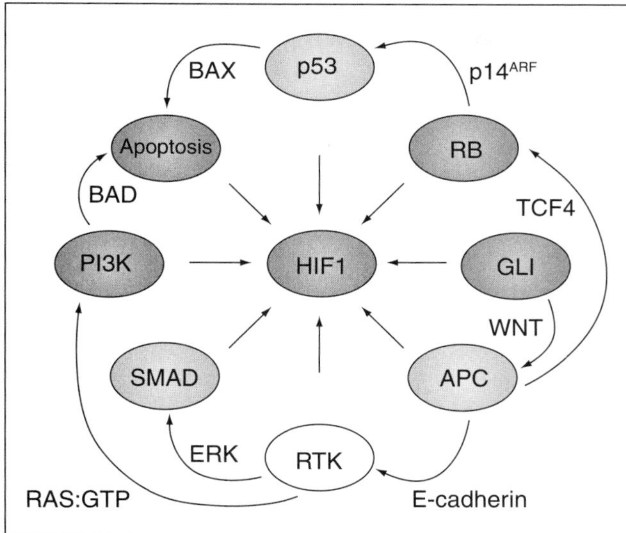

Key: HIF1—Hypoxia-inducible Transcription Factor 1 Pathway
RB—Retinoblastoma Pathway
GLI—Glioma-associated Oncogene Pathway
APC—Adenomatous polyposis coli or WNT (Wingless and Integration1) pathway
RTK—Receptor Tyrosine Kinase Pathway
SMAD Pathway
PI3K—Phophoinositide 3-Kinase Pathway
Adopted from Vogelstein & Kinsler

FIGURE 3.2

Overview of the main cancer gene pathways.

development of progressive dysplastic changes and, ultimately, adenocarcinoma. In fact, Barrett's esophagus is considered to be a premalignant condition, which carries nearly a 100-fold increased risk for esophageal cancer as compared with the general population (14).

In the Western world, up to 20% of the general population reports symptoms consistent with GERD (15). Moreover, it is estimated that the prevalence of Barrett's esophagus in the general population has grown nearly 4-fold in the last few decades, which likely reflects a combination of a changing disease prevalence and improved diagnostic capability with the increased use of flexible upper endoscopy. Simultaneously, there has been a steady rise in the incidence of esophageal adenocarcinoma, particularly at the esophagogastric junction, and in the United States and Western Europe, esophageal adenocarcinoma has supplanted squamous cancer as the most common primary esophageal epithelial malignancy. Nevertheless, it remains unclear whether the rising incidence of esophageal adenocarcinoma is specifically related to the perceived increased incidence of GERD and Barrett's esophagus in the general population. Moreover as the risk of developing esophageal adenocarcinoma in patients with documented Barrett's esophagus is only 0.5% per year (16), and the prognosis for patients with invasive cancer remains poor, it would be ideal to find a screening strategy that might identify the small number of patients with Barrett's esophagus who will go on to develop esophageal adenocarcinoma, thereby affording the opportunity for earlier detection and curative therapies.

A clearer understanding of the relationships between GERD, Barrett's esophagus, and the development of esophageal adenocarcinoma is beginning to emerge as the details of the underlying biological changes become elucidated. There is growing evidence that Barrett's epithelium can progress sequentially through a metaplasia-dysplasia-carcinoma type sequence, although this sequence and its genetic, as well as epigenetic, underpinnings are far from being completely understood. Several lines of early evidence support this theory. First, metaplastic and dysplastic epithelia are frequently found adjacent to one another within pathologic specimens. Second, the progression from metaplasia to low-grade dysplasia, then high-grade dysplasia, and finally invasive adenocarcinoma has been observed serially and temporally in individual patients who are surveyed endoscopically (17). Moreover, 30% of esophagectomy specimens collected from patients who undergo resection for high-grade dysplasia alone are found incidentally to harbor foci of invasive carcinoma within the dysplastic regions.

The clinical progression from metaplasia to dysplasia to carcinoma has been studied extensively in an attempt to better elucidate its molecular and genetic underpinnings, and the molecular pathogenesis of Barrett's esophagus and esophageal adenocarcinoma have been found to include the accumulation of multiple molecular alterations over time. These alterations may affect various aspects of carcinogenesis, including cell cycle regulation and proliferation, aneuploidy, telomerase activity, growth factors, and epigenetic modifications. Moreover, these changes may affect both somatic and stem cell populations, thereby opening broader avenues for research and potential therapeutics. In recent years, the application of concepts learned from developmental pathways has provided a novel basis for investigation of the shift in the esophageal mucosa from its original squamous to the columnar-lined epithelium seen in intestinal metaplasia, with growing evidence to suggest that pluripotent stem cells may be driven toward novel epithelial differentiation as a result of altered developmental pathway signaling.

Molecular Alterations in Barrett's Metaplasia

A number of novel developmental pathway alterations have been found in regions of Barrett's metaplasia as compared with normal regions of esophageal mucosa.

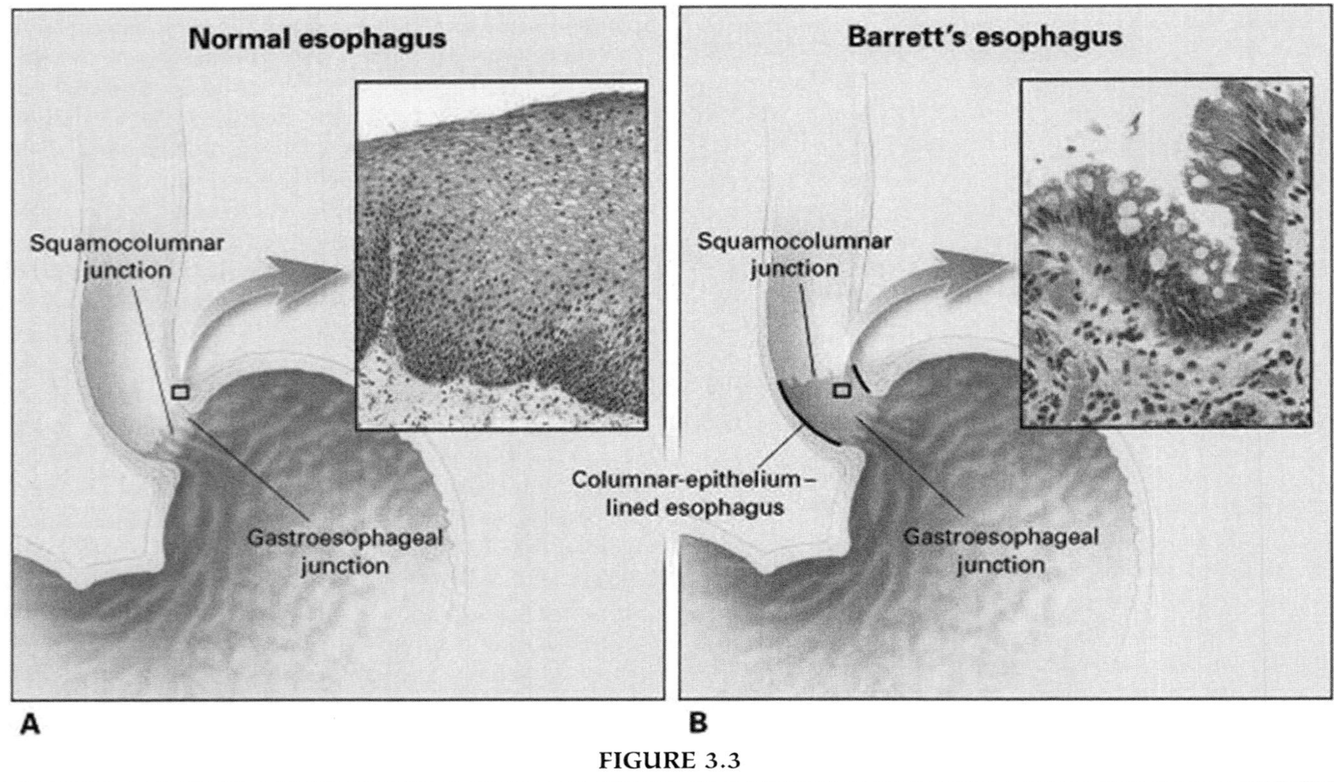

FIGURE 3.3

Histopathology of Barrett's esophagus. From Spechler SJ. *New Eng J Med*. 2002;346:836–842.

For example, CDX1 and CDX2 are homeobox proteins that play major roles in the development of the intestinal epithelium in utero. In mice, CDX2 expression is high in the proximal intestine (including the esophagus) and decreases distally along the small bowel, whereas CDX1 expression is high in the distal intestine and less so proximally, with considerable overlap in the mid-intestine (18). It has been hypothesized that such developmentally important genes might drive the transformation of the normally squamous esophageal epithelium into a more intestinal-type columnar epithelium during the clinical development of Barrett's esophagus. For example, the repeated injury posed by GERD to the distal esophageal mucosa might activate the ectopic overexpression of CDX1, which then triggers a transformation into the more distal intestinal phenotype. In support of this hypothesis, it has been found that CDX1 mRNA and protein expression are detectable in human samples of Barrett's metaplasia, but not in the normal distal esophageal squamous mucosa (19). Moreover, both conjugated bile salts and the inflammatory cytokines tumor necrosis factor-α (TNF-α) and interleukin 1b (IL-1b) were found to increase CDX2 mRNA expression in vitro through NF-κB signaling (20), the overexpression of which synergizes with CDX1 in inducing and maintaining the more distal intestinal phenotype. Furthermore, CDX2 protein and mRNA overexpression has been documented in Barrett's esophagus and esophageal adenocarcinoma epithelia, but not in patients with gastric-type (proximal) metaplasia or those with GERD without Barrett's changes (21). This overexpression reiterates the notion that alterations in the expression of these developmental regulatory proteins may trigger a change in the phenotype of the epithelial cell, possibly by driving the differentiation of pluripotent stem-cell precursors.

Molecular Changes in the Metaplasia-Dysplasia-Carcinoma Sequence

In the esophagus, the progression from dysplasia to invasive adenocarcinoma in the setting of Barrett's esophagus is a multistep process that probably takes many years to develop (22). The process is driven by genomic instability and the evolution of clones of cells with accumulated genetic errors that carry selection advantage and allow successive clonal expansion. Successive accumulation of chromosomal aberrations, such as aneuploidy and loss of heterozygosity (LOH), specific genetic alterations, and epigenetic abnormalities of tumor suppressor genes, characterize this process of malignant transformation. We will briefly explore some examples of these genomic changes in the context of esophageal adenocarcinoma.

Cell Cycle and Proliferation

Regulatory genes that have been implicated in the development of esophageal adenocarcinoma include cyclin D1 and p16. Overexpression of cyclin D1, or inactivation of p16, results in the hyperphosphorylation of the retinoblastoma protein Rb (which controls the normal transition between the G1 phase of the cell cycle and phase G0 or S), thereby inactivating Rb and stimulating cellular proliferation. Defects in p16 (via LOH, mutation, or methylation) are very prevalent in Barrett's mucosa and appear to occur very early on in the transformation process (23–25). Cyclin D1 overexpression has been documented in Barrett's esophagus and esophageal adenocarcinoma, and one prospective study has found that patients with Barrett's metaplasia and cyclin D1 overexpression were at increased risk for invasive cancer when compared with patients in whom its expression was normal (26). Although a number of such studies documenting hyperproliferation in the setting of Barrett's esophagus exist, no specific findings have proven predictive of the progression to cancer.

Telomerase

Telomeres are fragments of non-coding DNA repeats that protect the ends of chromosomes from degradation. As cells replicate, short segments of these telomeres are lost with each cell division until telomeres become too short to protect the chromosomes, thereby triggering growth arrest and the prevention of further cell division. Human cancers take advantage of this regulatory mechanism by reactivating the telomerase enzyme that stabilizes the telomeres and maintains the proliferative potential of malignant cells. In one study, telomerase activity was detected in 100% of esophageal adenocarcinoma specimens but not in normal esophageal mucosa, and a graded yet pronounced increase in activity was seen in the setting of low-grade versus high-grade dysplasia (27).

Aneuploidy

In Barrett's epithelium, it has been documented that abnormalities in DNA ploidy are associated with the progression to dysplasia. In one study, patients with Barrett's esophagus and no dysplasia or low-grade dysplasia had a 5-year cumulative incidence of cancer of 28% if aneuploidy or tetraploidy was documented by flow cytometry, whereas no patient with normal cytometric results developed invasive cancer (28). Using flow cytometry in conjunction with histology, the authors of the study have suggested increased endoscopic surveillance in patients who are high risk on the basis of abnormalities in ploidy (28).

Apoptosis

The p53 protein prevents cells with DNA damage from dividing, and activates the apoptosis pathway, thereby preventing the propagation of cells with such alterations. Disruption of native p53 function inhibits apoptosis and thereby allows the expansion of abnormal cell populations over time. Lesions in p53 have been documented in 85%–95% of esophageal adenocarcinomas, but almost never in normal esophageal tissues from the same patients. Moreover, their prevalence increases significantly with advancing histologic grades of dysplasia (29–32). In one study, LOH at the p53 locus was a strong and significant predictor for the progression to esophageal adenocarcinoma, with a relative risk of 16 in patients with this abnormality as compared to those without (33).

Invasion

Cadherins are a family of cell adhesion molecules essential to the maintenance of intercellular connections, cell polarity, and cellular differentiation, and thereby play a role in the invasiveness of cancer cells. Germline mutations of the E-cadherin gene (CDH1) have been found to be a causative agent in familial gastric cancer (34–36). It has been documented that the expression of E-cadherin is significantly lower in patients with Barrett's esophagus compared with patients with the normal esophageal epithelium, and further reduction of its expression is observed as the metaplasia-dysplasia-carcinoma sequence progresses (37). These findings suggest that E-cadherin may serve as a tumor suppressor early in the process of carcinogenesis in esophageal adenocarcinoma.

Along with decreasing E-cadherin expression in metaplastic tissue, loss of its associated membranous β-catenin expression and an increase in cytoplasmic and nuclear β-catenin localization has been observed in esophageal cancer (37). Free cytoplasmic β-catenin binds to nuclear transcription factors and promotes transcription of many target genes, including several oncogenes such as c-myc and cyclin D1, and thus promotes oncogenesis.

Furthermore, TNF-α, an inflammatory cytokine that can be detected in many cancer cells, can downregulate the expression of E-cadherin at a transcription level (38). In Barrett's metaplasia the expression of epithelial TNF-α increases with the progression from metaplasia to dysplasia to carcinoma (39).

Cyclooxygenase-2

Cyclooxygenase-2 (COX-2) is normally found in the kidney and brain, but in other tissues, its expression is inducible and rises during inflammation, wound healing, and neoplastic growth. COX-2 and its product prostaglandin E2 (PGE2) appear to be implicated in carcinogenesis because they prolong the survival of abnormal cells, which favors the accumulation of genetic changes. They reduce apoptosis and cell adhesion, increase cell proliferation, promote angiogenesis and invasion, and make cancer cells resistant to the host immune response (40). Although COX-2 is expressed in the normal esophagus, its expression is significantly increased in Barrett's esophagus and even more so in high grade dysplasia and esophageal adenocarcinoma (41–43). Some authors have suggested that COX-2 expression might be of prognostic value in esophageal adenocarcinoma, as patients with high COX-2 expression are more likely to develop distant metastases and local recurrence and have significantly reduced survival rates when compared to those with low expression (41). These findings have led to the consideration of COX-2 inhibitors as a potential chemotherapeutic alternative for patients with esophageal adenocarcinoma.

Epigenetic Abnormalities

Recently, there has been an explosion of research activity and resultant scientific knowledge in the role of epigenetic changes occurring during carcinogenesis. Epigenetics refers to alterations in patterns of gene expression that take place without any modification of the underlying primary DNA sequence. In general, our current understanding of epigenetic processes during tumorigenesis is limited largely to regional DNA hypermethylation and alterations in the chromatin components of DNA packaging. Since these modifications are heritable, they are able to be conveyed from one generation to another during replication of somatic cells, and thus have potential importance for the early diagnosis, prognosis, and even treatment of many malignancies.

DNA promoter region hypermethylation occurs mostly at CpG sites in the genome and is catalyzed by a family of 3 active DNA methyltransferases that transfer a methyl group from S-adenosyl-methionine to cytosine to form 5-methylcytosine (Figure 3.4). Tumor suppressor genes, genes that suppress metastasis and angiogenesis, as well as DNA repair genes are often targets for this transcriptional inactivation. DNA hypermethylation, and its associated effect on gene inactivation, have been widely studied in the molecular events leading to progression from Barrett's metaplasia to frank esophageal adenocarcinoma. The risk progression to esophageal adenocarcinoma in a patient under surveillance with Barrett's dysplasia is only 1 per 250 patient-years, or 0.5% per year (16,44). It is thought that epigenetic biomarkers, such as DNA hypermethylation, may streamline endoscopic surveillance and improve the risk stratification of patients with Barrett's metaplasia. This would enable better prediction of patient progression to high grade Barrett's dysplasia or esophageal adenocarcinoma. In addition, the longtime existence of a drug, 5-azacytidine, which irreversibly inhibits the aforementioned DNA methyltransferases, makes the therapeutic potential of reversing DNA hypermethylation enticing for clinical exploitation (45).

Methylation of CpG-island in many cancer types seems to represent possible early, preneoplastic epigenetic events. Hypermethylation of p16 was one of the first genes implicated in the progression of Barrett's esophagus to malignancy with 38% of premalignant and malignant lesions demonstrating this abnormality (46). Meltzer et al. identified p16 along with 7 other genes (p16, APC, TIMP3, RUNX3, CRBP1, RIZ1, HPP1) to be frequently methylated in both Barrett's esophagus as well as esophageal adenocarcinoma, but not in normal esophagus (47). Using 4 of these genes (p16, TIMP3, RUNX3, HPP1), Meltzer showed significant differences in DNA methylation prevalences between those patients who progressed from Barrett's metaplasia to frank esophageal adenocarcinoma and those who did not (47). Importantly, in this study, DNA methylation distinguished progressors within 2 years of their progression to adenocarcinoma but was unable to predict progression more than 2 years before adenocarcinoma diagnosis (47).

In contrast to colon cancer, where point mutations of p16 are frequent, this gene is rarely mutated in esophageal adenocarcinoma. Instead, DNA methylation predominates as the primary mechanism of gene inactivation. Eads et al. observed frequent DNA methylation in many esophageal cancer specimens with infrequent DNA methylation in normal esophagus from the same patients (% tumor vs. % normal specimens): p16 (41% vs. 0%), ESR1 (86% vs. 0%), MYOD1 (45% vs.0%), TIMP3 (86% vs. 19%), APC (68% vs. 3%), and CALCA (50% vs. 13%) (25,46).

Although prognostic biomarkers will be covered more thoroughly elsewhere in the text, it is worth noting that epigenetic markers are being considered to be possible prognostic markers in patients with esophageal adenocarcinoma. A recent study at Johns Hopkins found patients whose tumors had >50% of a 4 gene profile methylated had both significantly poorer survival ($P < 0.04$) and earlier tumor recurrence ($P < 0.05$) than those without methylation (48). Moreover, multivariate analysis suggested that methylation status was a more powerful predictors of survival (HR 2.7 [1.14–6.45; 95% confidence interval]) and tumor recurrence (HR2.5

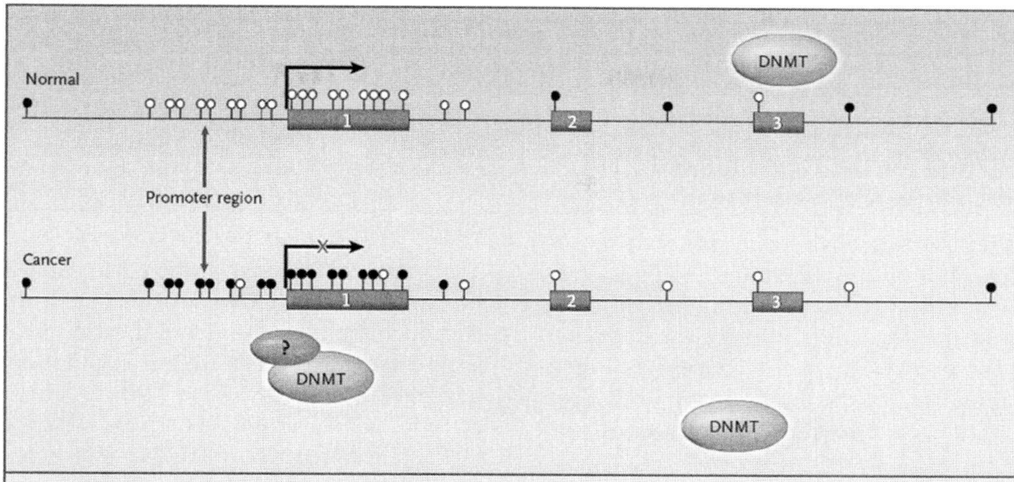

Distribution of CpG Dinucleotide in the Human Genome and Differences in Methylation Patterns between Normal Cells and Tumor Cells.

In most of the mammalian genome, which is depicted here as exons 1, 2, and 3 of a sample gene (boxes 1, 2, and 3), introns of the gene (line between the exons), and regions outside the gene, the CpG dinucleotide has been depleted during evolution, as shown by the small number of such sites (circles). Small regions of DNA, approximately 0.5 to 4.0 kb in size, harbor the expected number of CpG sites and are termed CpG islands. Most of these are associated with promoter regions of approximately half the genes in the genome (numerous circles surrounding and within exon 1 of the sample gene). In normal cells, most CpG sites outside of CpG islands are methylated (black circles), whereas most CpG-island sites in gene promoters are unmethylated (white circles). This methylated state in the bulk of the genome may help suppress unwanted transcription, whereas the unmethylated state of the CpG islands in gene promoters permits active gene transcription (arrow in upper panel). In cancer cells, the DNA-methylation and chromatin patterns are shifted. Many CpG sites in the bulk of the genome and in coding regions of genes, which should be methylated, become unmethylated, and a growing list of genes have been identified as having abnormal methylation of promoters containing CpG islands, with associated transcriptional silencing (red X at the transcription start site). Although there are possible explanations and findings from ongoing investigations, it is not known why the DNA-methylating enzymes fail to methylate where they normally would and which of these enzymes are mediating the abnormal methylation of CpG islands in promoters.

FIGURE 3.4

DNA Promoter hypermethylation (45).

[1.11–5.6[) than age (HR 2.03 and 1.96, respectively) or stage (HR 1.48 and 1.67, respectively) (48).

Stem Cells

In 2002, Seery based a model for understanding esophageal stem cell populations upon lessons learned from epidermal stem cell studies (49). In reviewing one of the existing hypotheses of the development of Barrett's esophagus that suggests that preformed tubuloalveolar gland elements in the squamous mucosa of the esophagus may be the origin of Barrett's metaplasia, Seery surmised it might instead be that the differentiation program of keratinocytes can be modified by GERD to induce columnar differentiation. He noted that GERD can trigger a similar metaplastic change in the esophagus of rats (50) that do not have preexisting glandular structures in the esophagus.

SQUAMOUS ESOPHAGEAL CANCER BIOLOGY

In stark contrast to adenocarcinoma of the esophagus, squamous cell carcinoma (SCC) is characterized by different molecular mechanisms and consequently by different risk factors. In general, squamous cell carcinoma is primarily due to chronic irritation of esophageal squamous epithelium. In this section, we will review risk factors for squamous cell carcinoma and the molecular mechanisms underlying both premalignant and malignant change.

Epidemiology of Squamous Cell Carcinoma of the Esophagus

Esophageal SCC has a distinct incidence and epidemiologic pattern from adenocarcinoma. As mentioned previously, the incidence of esophageal adenocarcinoma is on the rise in the United States and in other Western countries (51,52). By contrast, the incidence of SCC has been steadily declining since the 1970s. Although in the United States African American males have a much higher incidence of SCC when compared to whites, the incidence in this population is declining as well (53). In contrast, in Eastern countries (China in particular), the majority of esophageal cancers are SCC, and there is no increase in the incidence of adenocarcinoma. These trends point toward fundamental differences in pathogenic mechanisms associated with the development of these distinct malignancies.

Risk Factors for the Development of Squamous Cell Carcinoma

Although the exact mechanisms responsible for the formation of SCC formation are unknown, epithelial tumors frequently arise as a result of chronic irritation of a mucosal layer. In this regard, esophageal cancer is no different. There are several known risk factors, including tobacco and alcohol use, for the development of SCC of the esophagus. Many relate to chronic irritation of the esophagus.

Tobacco and Alcohol Use

Chronic use of tobacco has been definitively shown to be associated with the development of SCC (54,55). This effect persists whether one smokes cigarettes or uses smokeless tobacco products. This effect appears to be most correlated with SCC, as the effect of smoking on adenocarcinoma is less certain. Alcohol is also strongly correlated with the development of esophageal SCC (56,57). Both tobacco use and alcohol consumption contribute to the development of SCC in a dose-dependent manner. Additionally, cessation leads to a decrease in the risk of cancer development (58).

Diet

Because of the unequal distribution of esophageal cancer types worldwide, speculation that differences in diet contribute to pathogenesis have garnered significant interest. Specifically postulated have been that diets high in starch and low in fiber contribute to the development of SCC of the esophagus (59). There have been further reports of fungal contaminants (so-called mycotoxins) that may contribute to the development of SCC (60). Perhaps the most intriguing notions dealing with dietary habits and SCC focus on the intake of foods containing nitrates and nitrosamines. Because tumorigenesis has been observed with nitrosamine administration in animal models, nitrosamines have been postulated to be associated with the development of cancer in humans (61). Nitrosamines are found in a variety of foods including smoked and cured meats, pickled foods, and foods with added malt such as beer or whiskey (61). Nitrosamines are found to a much greater extent in Asian foods (62), which may explain why a greater percentage of Asians develop SCC of the esophagus. Interestingly, nitrosamines are endogenously produced in the human body from nitrates. Nitrates are found, to a large extent, in vegetables and water. It is interesting that nitrosating enzymes in the human body are produced in response to chronic inflammation, and thus, nitrate intake might be more harmful in the setting of other chronic irritants to the esophagus such as smoking or chronic alcohol consumption.

Achalasia

Much controversy exists when discussing the incidence of SCC of the esophagus in patients with previous achalasia. Although some studies have shown correlation between the two diseases (63), many population-based studies have now pointed to an increased risk of esophageal cancer with achalasia (64,65). There is strong evidence that SCC predominates over adenocarcinoma among patients with achalasia who develop esophageal cancer. A widely held belief is that esophageal cancer developing from achalasia carries a worse prognosis as compared to other esophageal cancer. Studies of patients with achalasia and esophageal cancer appear to have similar prognoses to those who develop esophageal cancer with no achalasia, and thus it appears that this notion is false (64).

Other Factors

The risk of SCC also increases with any chronic irritant, such as lye ingestion or radiation therapy. Plummer-Vinson syndrome (a disorder of iron deficiency, dysphagia, esophageal webs) is a known risk factor; and similar to other cancers, a history of previous squamous cell cancer is a risk factor as well (58).

Precursor Lesions for Squamous Cell Carcinoma

The World Health Organization (WHO) has classified esophageal dysplasia as a precancerous lesion containing cytologic and structural abnormalities (66). For squamous cells of the esophagus, it has been traditional to use the terms *mild*, *moderate*, and *severe* to describe degrees of dysplasia (67,68); however, most pathologists agree that there is a clear divide in disease severity between mild and moderate dysplasia compared to severe, and consequently use the terms *low-grade* and *high-grade* to describe levels of dysplasia (69). It is noteworthy that carcinoma in situ is a variant of high-grade dysplasia and additionally, both dysplasia and carcinoma in situ imply a lack of lymph node involvement and lack of invasion beyond the epithelial layer.

Descriptive Features

Studies of patients with squamous cell dysplasia of the esophagus receiving endoscopy have demonstrated a wide variety of clinical features (70). Specifically, dysplasia can be friable with erythema or can present as nodularity, erosions, or flat lesions. In some cases, small white plaques or patches are visible. Dysplasia is, fortunately, rarely visually normal (only 2% in a series of 398 patients by Dawsey et al.) (70). Interestingly, areas of mucosal dysplasia are visually highlighted with the use of iodine, a technique that can aid in diagnosis (71). Dysplastic areas tend not to pick up iodine staining due to a loss of glycogen in the dysplastic mucosa (68). Despite these diagnostic aids, biopsies are, at this time, the only proven way to identify mucosal dysplasia reliably.

Pathology

Transitions from dysplasia to nondysplasia are often easily noted on esophageal biopsy. This is because the nuclear enlargement, hyperchromasia, mitotic increases. and pleomorphism are all pronounced in specimens of esophageal dysplasia (68). In general, dysplastic cells invade from the superficial to deep layers of epithelium. Dysplasia is graded by the degree of epithelial involvement. In general, mild and moderate dysplasia occupy less than 50% of the epithelium, while severe occupies greater than 50% of the epithelium (72). Carcinoma in situ involves the full thickness of epithelium but does not invade beyond the epithelial layer.

Progression to Invasive Cancer

Squamous cell carcinoma of the esophagus appears to develop through a series of changes from dysplasia to invasive carcinoma. Studies examining esophageal resection specimens have observed areas of high- and low-grade dysplasia present in addition to invasive carcinoma (70,73) The molecular mechanisms leading to this progression will be the subject of the next section.

Molecular Alterations in Squamous Cell Carcinoma

Overview of Oncogenic Mechanisms

Seminal work by a multitude of investigators has revealed that unlike diseases caused by a single mutation (e.g., cystic fibrosis), tumorigenesis is the result of mutations or epigenetic changes in many different genes and molecular pathways (74). Invasive cancer is thus the result of the deleterious effects of many abnormalities. Fortunately, genes can be categorized into distinct varieties of alterations each with unique mechanisms of tumorigenesis. Specifically, as stated earlier, one can broadly divide genes responsible for tumor formation into oncogenes, tumor suppressor genes, and genes responsible for DNA stability (74).

Oncogenes refer to genes that when mutated, result in activation, leading to cellular proliferation or the allowance of selective growth as compared to other cells. Tumor suppressor genes, by contrast, result in reduced activity of a gene and are important for ceasing cellular proliferation. Finally, genes involved in stability regulate DNA maintenance and repair. When alterations in these genes occur, normal mechanisms responsible for DNA repair are altered, leading to a resultant increase in genetic alterations.

Cancer Characteristics

Alterations in these key genetic pathways lead to many of the key characteristic features of all cancer cells. As summarized by Hanahan and Weinberg (75), cancer cells: (a) have self-sufficiency in growth, (b) are self-replicative, (c) are insensitive to antigrowth signals, (c) avoid apoptosis, and (d) have angiogenic capabilities with the ability to invade tissue. Like all malignancies, investigations of squamous cell carcinoma genetic alterations have focused on genes that fall into one of the broad categories of tumorigenesis and produce these specific properties inherent to all malignant tumors (76). The following section does not attempt to provide an exhaustive review of all genetic alterations that have been identified for SCC, but rather focuses on a few examples in important mechanistic categories.

Role of Oncogenes

As previously mentioned, oncogene mutations result in active proliferation of cells. Notable examples include *ras* and *c-myc*. In contrast to tumor suppressor genes (discussed subsequently), there are few examples of identified oncogenes in the pathogenesis of squamous cell esophageal cancer. Examples in human esophageal SCC include the murine double minute 2 (MDM2) gene, which can bind to and inhibit p53, leading to cellular proliferation (77), and the erythroblastosis virus oncogene homolog 2 (ETS2), which has proliferative properties (78).

Tumor Suppressor Genes

Tumor suppressor gene abnormalities have been readily identified for esophageal SCC. In general, tumor suppressor genes provide antiproliferative signals for cells. Mutations include missense mutations, deletions or insertions, and promoter methylation rendering a nonfunctional protein product. Classic examples of tumor suppressor genes include Rb and p53, and several studies have provided examples of mutations in both of these genes early in the pathogenesis of esophageal

SCC (79–82). Relating to this pathway of tumorigenesis includes antiapoptotic signaling. The BCL-2 gene is important for prevention of apoptosis. Additional p53 has antiapoptotic mechanisms. Mutations in these genes have been shown in esophageal SCC to lead to abnormal proliferation (82).

Additional Genetic Alterations

Additional genes of interest for SCC include those involved in cell signaling, cell cycle regulation, and signal transduction (83,84). Additional important genetic alterations including upregulation of telomerase contributing to cell replication, upregulation of vascular endothelial growth factor (VEGF) leading to angiogenesis, and alterations in E and beta cadherin genes leading to abnormal cellular attachments have been observed in adenocarcinoma of the esophagus, but thus far have not been demonstrated in esophageal SCC (86).

Epigenetic Abnormalities in Squamous Cell Carcinoma of the Esophagus

A second important mechanism in the development of neoplasm involves the acquisition of epigenetic changes. Specifically, DNA promoter methylation leads to the inactivation of genes involved in tumor suppression and cell cycle regulation. Furthermore, epigenetic silencing of transcription factors can result in a loss of gene expression as well (85). In SCC of the esophagus, epigenetic alterations appear to play an important roll as well. Guo and colleagues examined methylation in the promoter regions of 8 common methylated genes in samples of esophageal SCC. This group demonstrated along the transition from dysplasia to neoplasm; epigenetic changes occur and are important mediators of tumorigenesis (86). In this study, p16 showed the highest level of methylation. Similarly, Ishii and colleagues have shown degrees of methylation specimens of esophageal SCC including background epithelium. In these specimens, transitioning from background epithelium through intraepithelial neoplasm to invasive carcinoma was associated with increasing degrees of DNA methylation (87). These findings confirmed the results of Guo's study that epigenetic changes define the transition from normal epithelium to invasive carcinoma. Finally, CDX2 (mentioned earlier as being overexpressed in esophageal adenocarcinoma) has been found to be epigenetically silenced in esophageal squamous cancers (88).

Genomics and Gene Microarrays

The development of the gene microarray by Brown and colleagues has provided a powerful tool for investigation of large-scale changes in gene expression associated with malignancies (89). Microarray technology makes it possible to analyze simultaneously gene expression for tens of thousands of genes. Typically, RNA is isolated from cells of interest and reversibly transcribed to cDNA probes. These probes are placed on a microarray with thousands of cDNA strands cloned from known human genes. Using imaging technology, active genes from the RNA sample are identified. This type of technology is leading the way to the identification of several genes involved in the pathogenesis of many tumors including esophageal SCC (90–92). Beyond the notion of using microarrays to identify new genes and gene pathways important in tumorigenesis, the applications of this technology are wide reaching. Specific possible applications include examination of cancer biology at various stages of cancer progression (92), examination of differences between different types of esophageal cancer (93), and correlation with responses to adjuvant chemotherapy (94).

Proteomics of Squamous Cell Esophageal Carcinoma

The term *proteomics* refers to the study of the protein composition cell or body tissue. It also encompasses posttranslational changes that occur following protein genesis. Protein profiles of tumor cells can be obtained and readily compared to normal cell lines. Furthermore, cellular or serum profiles for patients with tumor burden can be compared to serum from normal individuals without tumor. In this way, differentially produced proteins can be isolated, identified, and described for tumors of interest (76). Because proteomics studies the functional components of the cell (unlike genomics, which studies potential protein products), the data obtained from proteomic strategies are very powerful for predicting phenotypic changes. Proteomics has perhaps its most useful application in the development of biomarkers for diagnosis and prognosis. A useful biomarker is present and easily identified in an accessible body material such as blood or serum and predicts the magnitude of illness with a high sensitivity. Although proteomic strategies have not been widely employed for esophageal SCC, Zhang and colleagues have identified that differential expression of clusterin (a glycoprotein) is downregulated in esophageal SCC (95). Using strategies of this nature, important proteins for SCC will be identified to aid in diagnosis and prognosis.

Future Directions in Treatment: Gene Therapy for Squamous Cell Carcinoma

In addition to surgical resection, multimodality treatment has garnered favor among many oncologists in order to improve responses to traditional therapy such as chemotherapy, radiation, and surgical resection. Because p53 mutations are so common in both adeno and squamous cell esophageal carcinoma (96,97), attention has focused p53 as a potential target for esophageal cancer gene therapy (98). In fact, in preclinical animal studies (99,100), as well as phase I clinical safety studies, adenoviral p53 gene transfer has been successfully applied for lung cancer therapy (101,102). Based on these preliminary results, Japanese investigators have conducted a phase II clinical trial enrolling 10 patients and investigating the use of an adenoviral mediated p53 gene delivery to patients with advanced (T3 with multiple lymph node metastasis and T4) esophageal squamous cell carcinoma (103). Although 9 of 10 patients ultimately died, the drug was well tolerated with few adverse side effects attributable to the therapy. One patient in particular showed no tumor progression 24 months following p53 gene administration and is still alive 65 months following treatment. These encouraging results suggest that targeted molecular treatment strategies are feasible and may hold promise for the treatment of esophageal cancer.

In summary, in both esophageal adenocarcinoma and squamous cell, the separate biology of tumors produce an aggressive, virulent malignancy. Coupled by the location of a rich network of lymphatics in the esophageal submucosa, the result is rapid metastatic spread and a poor, overall 5-year survival rate for patients. Clearly, an effective, systemic therapy is sorely needed. Understanding the molecular pathways inherent in these two cancers could lead to appropriate pharmacologic intervention.

References

1. Stewart BW *World Cancer Report*. Lyon, France: International Agency for Research on Cancer; 2003.
2. Blot WJ, Devesa SS, et al. Rising incidence of adenocarcinoma of the esophagus and gastric cardia. *JAMA*. 1991;265(10):1287–1289.
3. Mosavi-Jarrahi A, Mohagheghi MA. Epidemiology of esophageal cancer in the high-risk population of Iran. *Asian Pac J Cancer Prev.* 2006;7(3):375–380.
4. Corley DA, Buffler PA. Oesophageal and gastric cardia adenocarcinomas: analysis of regional variation using the Cancer Incidence in Five Continents database. *Int J Epidemiol.* 2001;30(6):1415–1425.
5. Brown LM, Devesa SS. Epidemiologic trends in esophageal and gastric cancer in the United States. *Surg Oncol Clin N Am.* 2002;11(2):235–256.
6. Hanahan D, Weinberg RA. The hallmarks of cancer. *Cell.* 2000;100(1):57–70.
7. Vogelstein B, Kinzler KW. Cancer genes and the pathways they control. *Nat Med.* 2004;10(8):789–799.
8. Classon M, Kennedy BK, et al. Opposing roles of pRB and p107 in adipocyte differentiation. *Proc Natl Acad Sci U S A.* 2000;97(20):10826–10831.
9. Classon M, Harlow E. The retinoblastoma tumour suppressor in development and cancer. *Nat Rev Cancer.* 2002;2(12):910–917.
10. Ichimura K, K., Bolin MB, et al. Deregulation of the p14ARF/MDM2/p53 pathway is a prerequisite for human astrocytic gliomas with G1-S transition control gene abnormalities. *Cancer Res.* 2000;60(2):417–424.
11. Ortega S, Malumbres M, et al. Cyclin D-dependent kinases, INK4 inhibitors and cancer. *Biochim Biophys Acta.* 2002;1602(1):73–87.
12. Sherr CJ. The Pezcoller lecture: cancer cell cycles revisited. *Cancer Res.* 2000;60(14):3689–3695.
13. Barrett NR. Chronic peptic ulcer of the oesophagus and 'oesophagitis'. *Br J Surg.* 1950;38(150):175–182.
14. Cameron AJ, Lomboy CT, et al. Adenocarcinoma of the esophagogastric junction and Barrett's esophagus. *Gastroenterology.* 1995;109(5):1541–1546.
15. Dent J, El-Serag HB, et al. Epidemiology of gastro-oesophageal reflux disease: a systematic review. *Gut* 2005;54(5):710–717.
16. Shaheen NJ, Crosby MA, et al. Is there publication bias in the reporting of cancer risk in Barrett's esophagus? *Gastroenterology* 2000;119(2):333–338.
17. Hameeteman W, Tytgat GN, et al. Barrett's esophagus: development of dysplasia and adenocarcinoma. *Gastroenterology.* 1989;96(5 Pt 1):1249–1256.
18. Silberg DG, Swain GP, et al. Cdx1 and cdx2 expression during intestinal development. *Gastroenterology.* 2000;119(4):961–971.
19. Wong NA, Wilding J, et al. CDX1 is an important molecular mediator of Barrett's metaplasia. *Proc Natl Acad Sci U S A.* 2005;102(21):7565–7570.
20. Kazumori H, Ishihara S, et al. Bile acids directly augment caudal related homeobox gene Cdx2 expression in oesophageal keratinocytes in Barrett's epithelium. *Gut.* 2006;55(1):16–25.
21. Moons LM, Bax DA,, et al. The homeodomain protein CDX2 is an early marker of Barrett's oesophagus. *J Clin Pathol.* 2004;57(10):1063–1068.
22. Jankowski JA, Wright NA, et al. Molecular evolution of the metaplasia-dysplasia-adenocarcinoma sequence in the esophagus. *Am J Pathol.* 1999;154(4):965–973.
23. Arber N, Lightdale C, et al. Increased expression of the cyclin D1 gene in Barrett's esophagus. *Cancer Epidemiol Biomarkers Prev.* 1996;5(6):457–459.
24. Bian YS, Osterheld MC, et al. (2002). p16 inactivation by methylation of the CDKN2A promoter occurs early during neoplastic progression in Barrett's esophagus. *Gastroenterology* 122(4): 1113–1121.
25. Eads CA, Lord RV, et al. Fields of aberrant CpG island hypermethylation in Barrett's esophagus and associated adenocarcinoma. *Cancer Res.* 2000;60(18):5021–5026.
26. Herbst JJ, Berenson MM, et al. Cell proliferation in esophageal columnar epithelium (Barrett's esophagus). *Gastroenterology.* 1978;75(4):683–687.
27. Morales CP, Burdick JS, et al. In situ hybridization for telomerase RNA in routine cytologic brushings for the diagnosis of pancreaticobiliary malignancies. *Gastrointest Endosc.* 1998;48(4):402–405.
28. Reid BJ, Levine DS, et al. Predictors of progression to cancer in Barrett's esophagus: baseline histology and flow cytometry identify low- and high-risk patient subsets. *Am J Gastroenterol.* 2000;95(7):1669–1676.
29. Barrett MT, Sanchez CA, et al. Evolution of neoplastic cell lineages in Barrett oesophagus. *Nat Genet.* 1999;22(1):106–109.
30. Campomenosi P, Conio M, et al. p53 is frequently mutated in Barrett's metaplasia of the intestinal type. *Cancer Epidemiol Biomarkers Prev.* 1996;5(7):559–565.
31. Kubba AK, Poole NA, et al. Role of p53 assessment in management of Barrett's esophagus. *Dig Dis Sci.* 1999;44(4):659–667.
32. Muzeau F, Flejou JF, et al. Profile of p53 mutations and abnormal expression of p53 protein in 2 forms of esophageal cancer. *Gastroenterol Clin Biol.* 1996;20(5):430–437.
33. Reid BJ, Prevo LJ, et al. Predictors of progression in Barrett's esophagus II: baseline 17p (p53) loss of heterozygosity identifies a patient subset at increased risk for neoplastic progression. *Am J Gastroenterol.* 2001;96(10):2839–2848.
34. Guilford P, Hopkins J, et al. E-cadherin germline mutations in familial gastric cancer. *Nature.* 1998;392(6674):402–405.
35. Richards FM, McKee SA, et al. Germline E-cadherin gene (CDH1) mutations predispose to familial gastric cancer and colorectal cancer. *Hum Mol Genet.* 1999;8(4):607–610.
36. Swami S, Kumble S, et al. E-cadherin expression in gastroesophageal reflux disease, Barrett's esophagus, and esophageal adenocarcinoma: an immunohistochemical and immunoblot study. *Am J Gastroenterol.* 1995;90(10):1808–1813.
37. Bailey T, Biddlestone L, et al. Altered cadherin and catenin complexes in the Barrett's esophagus-dysplasia-adenocarcinoma sequence: correlation with disease progression and dedifferentiation. *Am J Pathol.* 1998;152(1):135–144.
38. Tselepis C, Perry I, et al. Tumour necrosis factor-alpha in Barrett's oesophagus: a potential novel mechanism of action. *Oncogene.* 2002;21(39):6071–6081.
39. Thun MJ, Henley SJ, et al. Nonsteroidal anti-inflammatory drugs as anticancer agents: mechanistic, pharmacologic, and clinical issues. *J Natl Cancer Inst.* 2002;94(4):252–266.
40. Wilson KT, Fu S, et al. Increased expression of inducible nitric oxide synthase and cyclooxygenase-2 in Barrett's esophagus and associated adenocarcinomas. *Cancer Res.* 1998;58(14):2929–2934.
41. Buskens CJ, Van Rees BP, et al. Prognostic significance of elevated cyclooxygenase 2 expression in patients with adenocarcinoma of the esophagus. *Gastroenterology.* 2002;122(7):1800–1807.
42. Morris CD, Armstrong GR, et al. Cyclooxygenase-2 expression in the Barrett's metaplasia-dysplasia-adenocarcinoma sequence. *Am J Gastroenterol.* 2001;96(4):990–996.
43. Shirvani VN, Ouatu-Lascar R, et al. Cyclooxygenase 2 expression in Barrett's esophagus and adenocarcinoma: ex vivo induction by bile salts and acid exposure. *Gastroenterology.* 2000;118(3):487–496.
44. Krishnadath KK, Reid BJ, et al. Biomarkers in Barrett esophagus. *Mayo Clin Proc.* 2001;76(4):438–446.
45. Herman JG, Baylin SB. Gene silencing in cancer in association with promoter hypermethylation. *N Engl J Med.* 2003;349(21):2042–2054.

46. Eads CA, Lord RV, et al. Epigenetic patterns in the progression of esophageal adenocarcinoma. *Cancer Res.* 2001;61(8):3410–3418.
47. Schulmann K, Sterian A, et al. Inactivation of p16, RUNX3, and HPP1 occurs early in Barrett's-associated neoplastic progression and predicts progression risk. *Oncogene.* 2005;24(25):4138–4148.
48. Brock MV, Gou M, et al. Prognostic importance of promoter hypermethylation of multiple genes in esophageal adenocarcinoma. *Clin Cancer Res.* 2003;9(8):2912–2919.
49. Seery JP. Stem cells of the oesophageal epithelium. *J Cell Sci.* 2002;115(Pt 9):1783–1789.
50. Pera M, Brito MJ, et al. Duodenal-content reflux esophagitis induces the development of glandular metaplasia and adenosquamous carcinoma in rats. *Carcinogenesis.* 2000;21(8):1587–1591.
51. Hesketh PJ, Clapp RW, Doos WG, et al. The increasing frequency of adenocarcinoma of the esophagus. *Cancer.* 1989;64(2):526–530.
52. Yang PC, Davis S. Incidence of cancer of the esophagus in the US by histologic type. *Cancer.* 1988;61(3):612–617.
53. Younes M, Henson DE, Ertan A, et al. Incidence and survival trends of esophageal carcinoma in the United States: racial and gender differences by histological type. *Scand J Gastroenterol.* 2002;37(12):1359–1365.
54. Choi SY, Kahyo H. Effect of cigarette smoking and alcohol consumption in the aetiology of cancer of the oral cavity, pharynx and larynx. *Int J Epidemiol.* 1991;20(4):878–885.
55. Newcomb PA, Carbone PP. The health consequences of smoking: cancer. *Med Clin North Am.* 1992;76(2):305–331.
56. Adami HO, McLaughlin JK, Hsing AW, et al. Alcoholism and cancer risk: a population-based cohort study. *Cancer Causes Control.* 1992;3(5):419–425.
57. Kato I, Nomura AM, Stemmermann GN, et al. Prospective study of the association of alcohol with cancer of the upper aerodigestive tract and other sites. *Cancer Causes Control.* 1992;3(2):145–151.
58. Meneshian AaH, RF. Surgical management of esophageal cancer. In: Yuh D, Vricella LA, Baumgartner WA, eds. *The Johns Hopkins Manual of Cardiothoracic Surgery.* 1st ed. New York: McGraw Hill; 2007:273–294.
59. Ghadirian P, Ekoe JM, Thouez JP. Food habits and esophageal cancer: an overview. *Cancer Detect Prev.* 1992;16(3):163–168.
60. Liu GT, Qian YZ, Zhang P, et al. Etiological role of Alternaria alternata in human esophageal cancer. *Chin Med J.* 1992;105(5):394–400.
61. Jakszyn P, Gonzalez CA. Nitrosamine and related food intake and gastric and oesophageal cancer risk: a systematic review of the epidemiological evidence. *World J Gastroenterol.* 2006;12(27):4296–4303.
62. Hotchkiss JH. Preformed N-nitroso compounds in foods and beverages. *Cancer Surveys.* 1989;8(2):295–321.
63. Chuong JJ, DuBovik S, McCallum RW. Achalasia as a risk factor for esophageal carcinoma. A reappraisal. *Dig Dis Sci.* 1984;29(12):1105–1108.
64. Brucher BL, Stein HJ, Bartels H, et al. Achalasia and esophageal cancer: incidence, prevalence, and prognosis. *World J Surg.* 2001;25(6):745–749.
65. Sandler RS, Nyren O, Ekbom A, et al. The risk of esophageal cancer in patients with achalasia. A population-based study. *JAMA.* 1995;274(17):1359–1362.
66. Watanabe HJ Jr, Sobin LH, World Health Organization. *International Histological Classification of Tumours: Histological Typing of Oesophageal and Gastric Tumours.* 2nd ed. New York: Springer-Verlag; 1990.
67. Kuwano H, Baba K, Ikebe M, et al. Histopathology of early esophageal carcinoma and squamous epithelial dysplasia. *Hepato-gastroenterology.* 1993;40(3):222–225.
68. Shimizu M, Ban S, Odze RD. Squamous dysplasia and other precursor lesions related to esophageal squamous cell carcinoma. *Gastroenterol Clin North Am.* 2007;36(4):797–811, v–vi.
69. Schlemper RJ, Dawsey SM, Itabashi M, et al. Differences in diagnostic criteria for esophageal squamous cell carcinoma between Japanese and Western pathologists. *Cancer.* 2000;88(5):996–1006.
70. Dawsey SM, Wang GQ, Weinstein WM, et al. Squamous dysplasia and early esophageal cancer in the Linxian region of China: distinctive endoscopic lesions. *Gastroenterology.* 1993;105(5):1333–1340.
71. Dawsey SM, Fleischer DE, Wang GQ, et al. Mucosal iodine staining improves endoscopic visualization of squamous dysplasia and squamous cell carcinoma of the esophagus in Linxian, China. *Cancer.* 1998;83(2):220–231.
72. Saeki H, Kimura Y, Ito S, et al. Biologic and clinical significance of squamous epithelial dysplasia of the esophagus. *Surgery.* 2002;131(1 Suppl):S22–27.
73. Kuwano H, Matsuda H, Matsuoka H, et al. Intra-epithelial carcinoma concomitant with esophageal squamous cell carcinoma. *Cancer.* 1987;59(4):783–787.
74. Vogelstein B, Kinzler KW. Cancer genes and the pathways they control. *Nat Med.* 2004;10(8):789–799.
75. Hanahan D, Weinberg RA. The hallmarks of cancer. *Cell.* 2000;100(1):57–70.
76. Kwong KF. Molecular biology of esophageal cancer in the genomics era. *Surg Clin North Am.* 2005;85(3):539–553.
77. Shibagaki I, Tanaka H, Shimada Y, et al. p53 mutation, murine double minute 2 amplification, and human papillomavirus infection are frequently involved but not associated with each other in esophageal squamous cell carcinoma. *Clin Cancer Res.* 1995;1(7):769–773.
78. Li X, Lu JY, Zhao LQ, et al. Overexpression of ETS2 in human esophageal squamous cell carcinoma. *World J Gastroenterol.* 2003;9(2):205–208.
79. Mathew R, Arora S, Khanna R, et al. Alterations in p53 and pRb pathways and their prognostic significance in oesophageal cancer. *Eur J Cancer.* 2002;38(6):832–841.
80. Mathew R, Arora S, Khanna R, et al. Alterations in cyclin D1 expression in esophageal squamous cell carcinoma in the Indian population. *J Cancer Res Clin Oncol.* 2001;127(4):251–257.
81. Busatto G, Shiao YH, Parenti AR, et al. p16/CDKN2 alterations and pRb expression in oesophageal squamous carcinoma. *Mol Pathol.* 1998;51(2):80–84.
82. Parenti AR, Rugge M, Shiao YH, et al. bcl-2 and p53 immunophenotypes in pre-invasive, early and advanced oesophageal squamous cancer. *Histopathology.* 1997;31(5):430–435.
83. Liu Y, Wang HX, Lu N, et al. Translocation of annexin I from cellular membrane to the nuclear membrane in human esophageal squamous cell carcinoma. *World J Gastroenterol.* 2003;9(4):645–649.
84. Paweletz CP, Ornstein DK, Roth MJ, et al. Loss of annexin 1 correlates with early onset of tumorigenesis in esophageal and prostate carcinoma. *Cancer Res.* 2000;60(22):6293–6297.
85. Douglas DB, Akiyama Y, Carraway H, et al. Hypermethylation of a small CpGuanine-rich region correlates with loss of activator protein-2alpha expression during progression of breast cancer. *Cancer Res.* 2004;64(5):1611–1620.
86. Guo M, Ren J, House MG, et al. Accumulation of promoter methylation suggests epigenetic progression in squamous cell carcinoma of the esophagus. *Clin Cancer Res.* 2006;12(15):4515–4522.
87. Ishii T, Murakami J, Notohara K, et al. Oesophageal squamous cell carcinoma may develop within a background of accumulating DNA methylation in normal and dysplastic mucosa. *Gut.* 2007;56(1):13–19.
88. Guo M, House M, Suzuki H, et al. Epigenetic silencing of CDX2 is a feature of squamous esophageal cancer. *Int J of Cancer.* 2007;121(6):1219–1226.
89. Brown PO, Botstein D. Exploring the new world of the genome with DNA microarrays. *Nat Genet.* 1999;21(1 Suppl):33–37.
90. Lu J, Liu Z, Xiong M, et al. Gene expression profile changes in initiation and progression of squamous cell carcinoma of esophagus. *Int J Cancer.* 2001;91(3):288–294.
91. Feber A, Xi L, Luketich JD, et al. MicroRNA expression profiles of esophageal cancer. *J Thorac Cardiovasc Surg.* 2008;135(2):255–260; discussion 260.
92. Zhou J, Zhao LQ, Xiong MM, et al. Gene expression profiles at different stages of human esophageal squamous cell carcinoma. *World J Gastroenterol.* 2003;9(1):9–15.
93. Greenawalt DM, Duong C, Smyth GK, et al. Gene expression profiling of esophageal cancer: comparative analysis of Barrett's esophagus, adenocarcinoma, and squamous cell carcinoma. *Int J Cancer.* 2007;120(9):1914–1921.
94. Kihara C, Tsunoda T, Tanaka T, et al. Prediction of sensitivity of esophageal tumors to adjuvant chemotherapy by cDNA microarray analysis of gene-expression profiles. *Cancer Res.* 2001;61(17):6474–6479.
95. Zhang LY, Ying WT, Mao YS, et al. Loss of clusterin both in serum and tissue correlate with the tumorigenesis of esophageal squamous cell carcinoma via proteomics approaches. *World J Gastroenterol.* 2003;(4):650–654.
96. Bennett WP, Hollstein MC, Metcalf RA, et al. p53 mutation and protein accumulation during multistage human esophageal carcinogenesis. *Cancer Res.* 1992;52(21):6092–6097.
97. Hollstein MC, Metcalf RA, Welsh JA, et al. Frequent mutation of the p53 gene in human esophageal cancer. *Proc Natl Acad Sci U S A.* 1990;87(24):9958–9961.
98. Shimada H, Matsushita K, Tagawa M. Recent advances in esophageal cancer gene therapy. *Ann Thorac Cardiovasc Surg.* 2008;14(1):3–8.
99. Fujiwara T, Cai DW, Georges RN, et al. Therapeutic effect of a retroviral wild-type p53 expression vector in an orthotopic lung cancer model. *J Natl Cancer Inst.* 1994;86(19):1458–1462.
100. Wills KN, Maneval DC, Menzel P, et al. Development and characterization of recombinant adenoviruses encoding human p53 for gene therapy of cancer. *Hum Gene Ther.* 1994;5(9):1079–1088.
101. Nemunaitis J, Swisher SG, Timmons T, et al. Adenovirus-mediated p53 gene transfer in sequence with cisplatin to tumors of patients with non-small-cell lung cancer. *J Clin Oncol.* 2000;18(3):609–622.
102. Schuler M, Herrmann R, De Greve JL, et al. Adenovirus-mediated wild-type p53 gene transfer in patients receiving chemotherapy for advanced non-small-cell lung cancer: results of a multicenter phase II study. *J Clin Oncol.* 2001;19(6):1750–1758.
103. Shimada H, Matsubara H, Shiratori T, et al. Phase I/II adenoviral p53 gene therapy for chemoradiation resistant advanced esophageal squamous cell carcinoma. *Cancer Sci.* 2006;97(6):554–561.

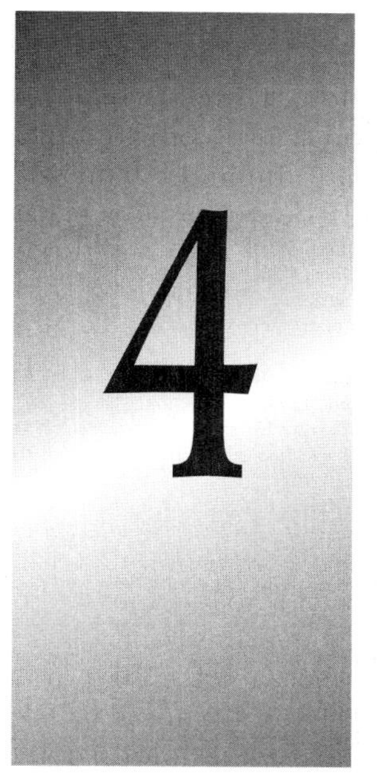

The Biology of Mesenchymal Esophageal Tumors

Billy R. Ballard

Mesenchymal tumors of the esophagus are less common than epithelial neoplasms of the esophagus. A review of the histology of the esophagus provides the tissues in the esophagus that are possible sources of mesenchymal neoplasms (Figure 4.1). Unlike the muscle bundles of stomach and intestines, which have both circular and longitudinal arrangements, the muscularis mucosa is composed of smooth muscle bundles orientated longitudinally. The muscularis mucosa becomes thicker as it proceeds distally, and at the gastroesophageal junction, the esophageal muscularis mucosa is thicker than that of the stomach and can be mistaken for muscularis propria (1). A short length (approximately 5%) of the proximal muscularis is composed of striated muscle (2). The muscularis propria is composed predominantly of smooth muscle (2) (Figure 4.2). Despite the presence of the two different muscle types, the predominant tumors of the muscularis propria are leiomyomas and leiomyosarcomas (3).

The esophagus, as with the rest of the GI tract, has an intrinsic innovation system, which contains ganglion cells in the submucosa (Meissner's plexus) and between the circular and longitudinal muscle layers (Auerbach's plexus) (Figure 4.3). The plexus are less well developed in the esophagus than in the remainder of the GI tract, and the density of neurons increases progressively toward the stomach (4). Tumors of neural origin are rare in the GI tract. Kwon et al. reviewed 53 schwannomas of 4 previously reported series and only 2 cases were of arose in the esophagus (5).

Interstitial cells of Cajal (ICC) are widely distributed within the submucosa, intramuscular, and intermuscular layers associated with the terminal networks of sympathetic nerves. The ICC in the esophagus are concentrated in the distal one-third in close association with smooth muscles as well as in the middle one-third associated with both smooth and striated muscles (3,6). Gastrointestinal stromal tumors (GISTs), including those of the esophagus, originate from ICC cells. The most common mesenchymal GI tract tumors are GISTs, except in the esophagus, where benign leiomyomas are more frequent (3).

The 3 most common mesenchymal neoplasms of the esophagus are leiomyomas, GISTs, and leiomyosarcomas (3,7). Leiomyomas are rare elsewhere in the GI tract, but are the most common esophageal mesenchymal neoplasm (3,7).

LEIOMYOMAS

Leiomyomas constitute 71% of stromal/smooth muscle tumors of the esophagus with a male to female ratio of 2:1. The lesions occur earlier in men with a mean age of 33 years and 44 in females. The presenting clinical symptoms include dysphagia, esophageal ulceration, and chest pain. The distal esophagus is the most common site of this lesion. Grossly, the lesions range from 1 to 18 cm in maximum diameter (mean 5 cm) and on section they were lobulated, gray-white, and firm with a whirled surface. Histologic examination showed a low to moderate cellularity composed of bundles of interlacing spindle-shaped smooth muscle cells with bland elongated cigar-shaped nuclei and infrequent mitoses and abundant eosinophilic cytoplasm (3,9) (Figure 4.4). Immunohistochemical examination showed all cases tested were positive for muscle markers, including smooth muscle antigen (SMA) and desmin. All of the lesions tested were negative for CD34 and CD117, GIST cell markers, and S-100 protein, a neural tumor marker (3,8). Long-term follow-up of diagnosed lesions is unnecessary, as benign leiomyomas show no tumor-related mortality (3,8,9).

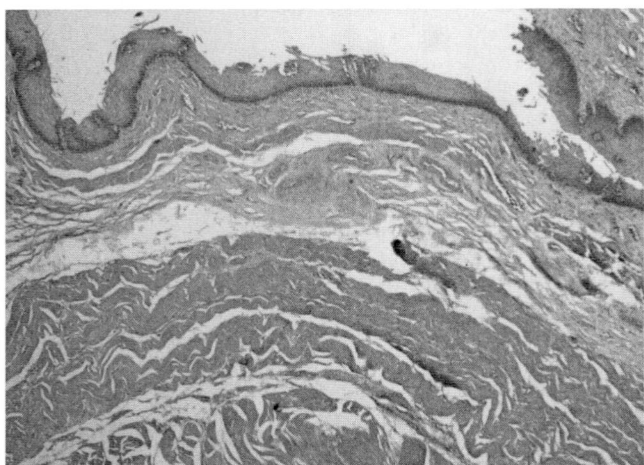

FIGURE 4.1

Mid-esophagus. The esophageal mucosa showing the surface epithelium, lamina propria, and lower muscularis propria (4X).

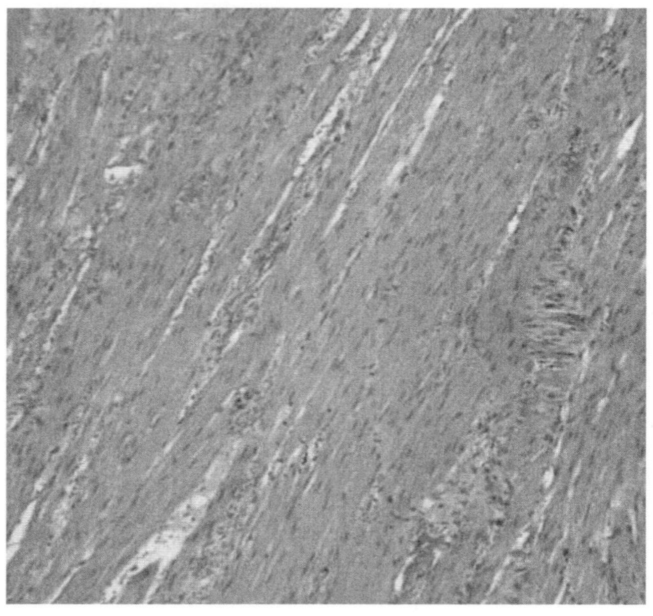

FIGURE 4.2

Muscularis propria. Fascicles of smooth muscle cells.

LEIOMYOSARCOMAS

Leiomyosarcomas are rare neoplasms of the esophagus and constitute the smallest group of mesenchymal

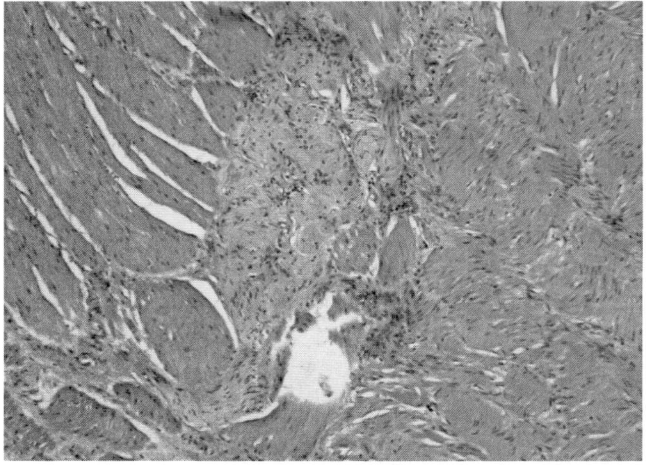

FIGURE 4.3

Auerbach's plexus found between the 2 muscle layers.

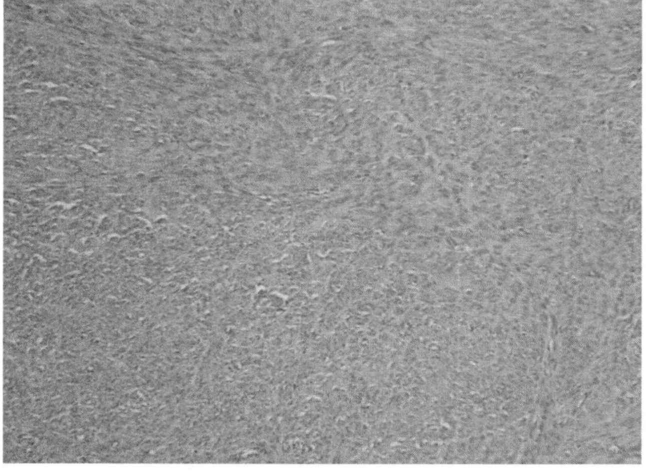

FIGURE 4.4

Leiomyoma composed of bundles and fascicles of smooth muscle cells in longitudinal and perpendicular planes.

esophageal neoplasms. This lesion occurs in an older age group and is more common in men. The lesions are large (9–16 cm), and the lesion is lethal, with patients dying from their disease within 1 to 24 months. Histologically, leiomyosarcomas are composed of fascicles of blunt-end spindle cells with moderated to marked pleomorphism, high mitotic activity, more than 5 mitoses per 50 HPFs. Immunohistochemically, the lesions show global positivity for desmin and SMA. The lesions are universally negative for CD 117 and S-100 protein (3,8).

SCHWANNOMAS

Schwannomas are rare GI tract neoplasms. Of 191 GI mesenchymal tumors reviewed by Kwon et al. (5), only 12 cases exhibited morphologic and immunohistochemical features of GI schwannomas as described by Daimaru et al. (10). Of these 12 cases, only 1 originated from the esophagus. The patient was a 70-year-old female that presented with dysphagia and chest pain. The lesion was 6 cm, well circumscribed, but not encapsulated, rubbery to firm, yellow-white to tan, glistening, and the cut surface was trabeculated. Microscopic examination revealed a lymphoid cuff in the surrounding non-neoplastic tissue, including mucosa, submucosa, muscle, and subserosa. The neoplasm was composed of broad bundles, interlacing fascicles of whorls of elongated cells with spindle-shaped, tapered, and somewhat wavy nuclei with evenly distributed chromatin, indistinct nuclei, and absent or rare mitoses. The immunohistochemical reactions for vimentin, S-100 protein, GFAP were diffusely and strongly positive, NSE was variably positive, and CD117 (c-kit), CD34, desmin, SMA, neurofilament, CD56, and synaptophysin were negative.

GASTROINTESTINAL STROMAL TUMORS

Formerly classified as smooth muscle tumors of the GI tract, leiomyomas, leiomyosarcomas, and GISTs were thought to be neoplasms of smooth muscle origin. Electron microscope studies showed inconsistent smooth muscle differentiation (11). Mazur and Clark introduced the term *stromal tumor* to distinguish this neoplasm as a clinicalopathologic entity based on mounting morphologic evidence that these lesions did not exhibit exclusive features of smooth muscle neoplasms (12). During the past decade, ultrastructural and immunohistochemical findings resulted in GIST being defined as a biologically distinctive tumor type, different from smooth muscle (leiomyomas and leiomyosarcomas) and neural (schwannomas) tumors of the GI tract.

The origin of GISTs is believed to be ICC or their stem cell–like precursors (13,14). The ICC have features of GI autonomic nervous system and smooth muscle cells and regulate the motility and autonomic nerve function (15,16). The ICC are Kit protein and Kit-ligand (stem cell factor) positive cells, and are located around the myenteric plexus and in the muscularis propria throughout the GI tract. Furthermore, they include a subset of multipotential stem-like cells that can develop into smooth muscle cells if Kit signaling is disrupted (17).

The c-kit protein, also known as CD117, is a highly sensitive and specific marker for GISTs that differentiates them from other GI mesenchymal tumors such as leiomyomas, which do not express CD117 (18,19). The c-kit proto-oncogene is located on the long arm of chromosome 4 and encodes a 145 kD transmembrane receptor with internal tyrosine kinase activity (20).

The immunohistochemical expression of the proto-oncogene *c-kit* (KIT protein or CD117) is the essential marker for confirmation of the diagnosis of GIST regardless of location (21). In addition to the expression of CD117 (Figures 4.5 and 4.6), approximately 60% to 70% of GISTs express CD34, a sialylated transmembrane glycoprotein and a hematopoietic progenitor cell antigen found in mesenchymal cells; however, the degree and rate of occurrence may vary with the site of the lesion. Esophageal GISTs (Figures 4.7 and 4.8) are consistently CD34 positive (95%–100%) (18,19). All of the esophageal GISTs studied by Miettinen displayed consistent expression of CD117 and CD34 (3).

Interstitial cells of Cajal GI pacemaker cells that control gut motility are characterized by immunophenotypic CD117 positivity and ultrastructural resemblance to GIST (14). In addition, GISTs have features in common with the myenteric plexus subtype of ICC,

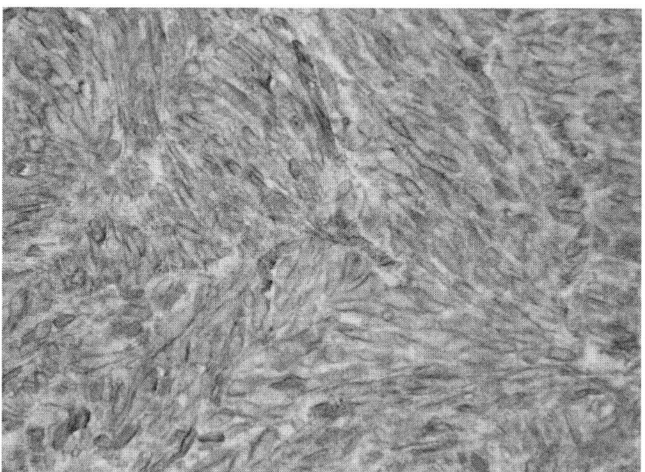

FIGURE 4.5

Gastrointestinal stromal tumor, spindle cell type, intense CD117 (c-Kit) membrane and cytoplasmisc immunohistochemical reactivity.

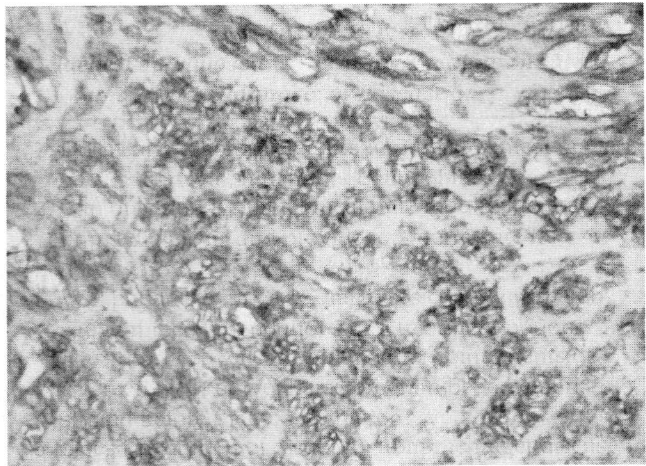

FIGURE 4.6

Gastrointestinal stromal tumor, epithelioid type, with intense CD117 (c-kit) membrane and cytoplasmic immunohistochemical reactivity.

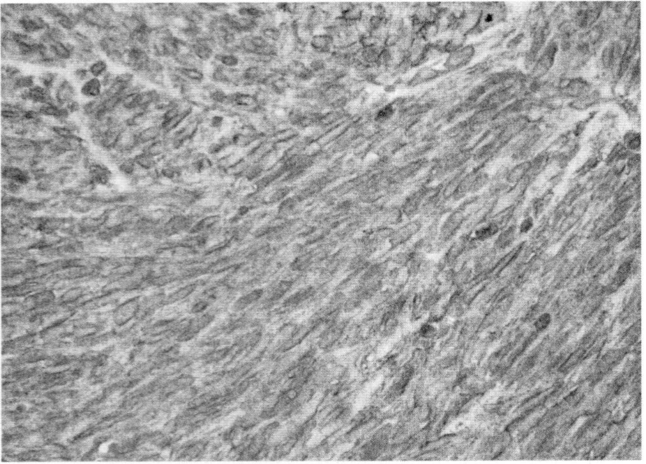

FIGURE 4.7

Gastrointestinal stromal tumor, spindle cell type, intense CD34 membrane and cytoplasmic immunohistochemical reactivity.

including the expression of CD34, embryonic smooth muscle myosin heavy chain, and the intermediate filament nestin (22,23). The immunohistochemical highlighting of ICC cells with CD117, the antibody to KIT, assisted in the discovery that this proto-oncogene is strongly expressed in most GISTs (14,21). This discovery substantiated the hypothesis that GISTs arise from or share a common stem cell with the ICC, and provided a new, more sensitive and specific marker for the diagnosis of GIST.

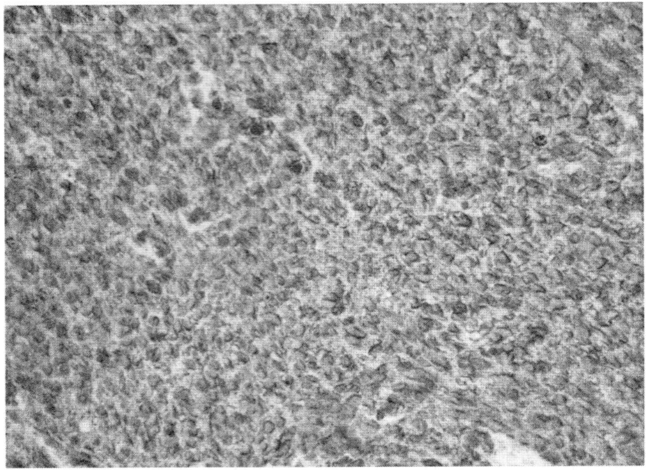

FIGURE 4.8

Gastrointestinal stromal tumor, epithelioid type, with intense CD34 membrane and cytoplasmic immunohistochemical reactivity.

Clinically, GISTs are the most common mesenchymal tumors of the GI tract and arise in all sites but predominantly in the stomach (60%) and small intestine (25%), but also occur in the rectum (5%) and esophagus (2%). Miettinen et al. identified 17 esophageal stromal tumors among 68 esophageal mesenchymal tumors (25%) (3). The lesions were more common in men (76%) with an age range from 49 to 75 years and a mean age of 63 years. The presenting symptoms include dysphagia, odynophagis, weight loss, dyspepsia, retrosternal chest pain, or hematemesis. The lesions were most frequently located in the distal esophagus and ranged from 2.6 to 25 cm in maximum diameter (mean 8 cm). Grossly, the tumors may have a thin capsule-like periphery. On section, they are pink-tan, with a soft or fish flesh–like consistency (Figure 4.9). Focal areas of necrosis and central calcification may be present.

Histologically, GISTs fall into 1 of 3 categories: spindle cell type (70%) (Figures 4.10 and 4.11), epithelioid (20%), (Figure 4.12), or mixed (Figure 4.13). Approximately 5% of lesions show a variably prominent myxoid stroma, and only a significant minority of cases (<2% to 3%) show cytologic pleomorphism.

Spindle cell GISTs are composed of relatively uniform eosinophilic cells arranged in short fascicles or whorls (Figures 4.5, 4.6, 4.10, and 4.11). The tumor cells have a paler eosinophilic cytoplasm than smooth muscle neoplasms, often with a fibrillary, syncytial appearance (i.e., with indistinct cell margins). Nuclei are uniform and more ovoid and shorter than those of smooth muscle and often with vesicular chromatin. Conspicuous juxanucelar cytoplasmic vacuoles are present in up to

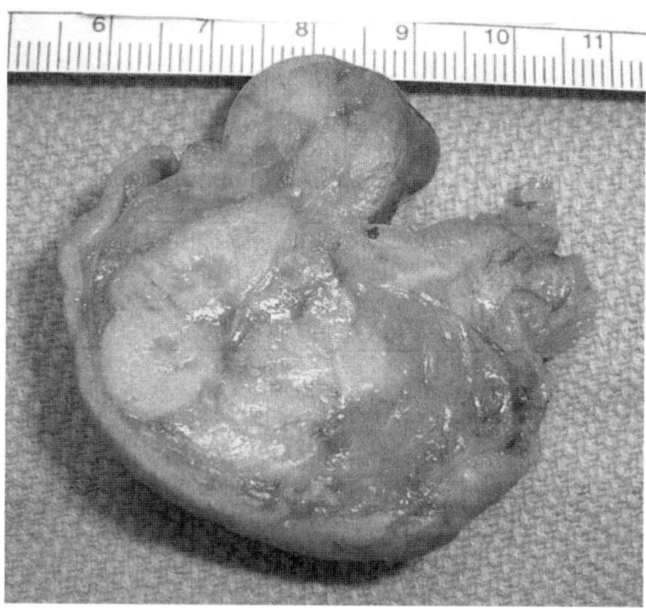

FIGURE 4.9

Gastrointestinal stromal tumor, well-circumscribed, smooth glistening, pink-white cut surface.

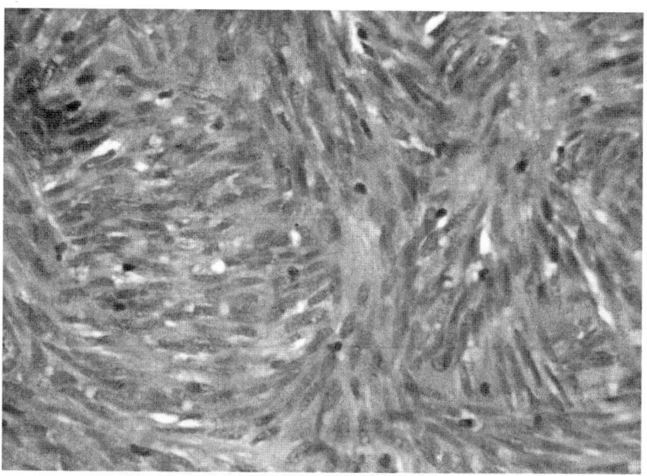

FIGURE 4.11

Gastrointestinal stromal tumor, spindle cell type, composed of hypercellular relatively uniform eosinophilic cells arranged in short fascicles or whorls. The cytoplasm of the tumor cells is paler than that of smooth muscle cells. There is often a fibrillary, syncytial appearance with indistinct margins. The nuclei are uniform and shorter, ovoid and blunted compared to smooth muscle nuclei. Chromatin is occasionally vesicular with insignificant nuclear atypia and mitotic activity (H&E 40X).

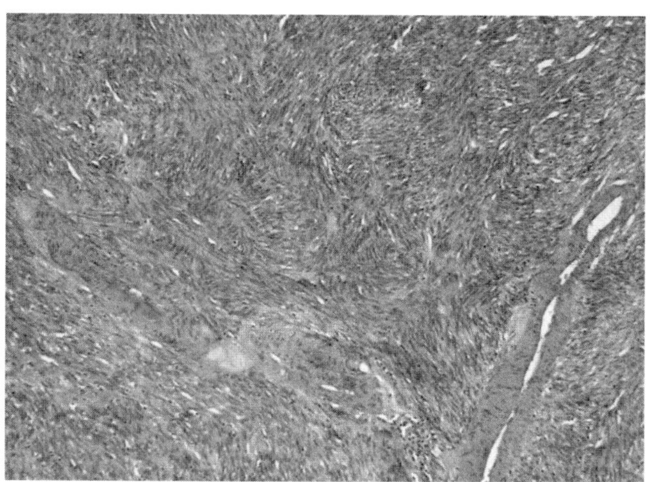

FIGURE 4.10

Gastrointestinal stromal tumor, spindle cell type, composed of hypercellular relatively uniform eosinophilic cells arranged in short fascicles or whorls. The cytoplasm of the tumor cells is paler than that of smooth muscle cells. There is often a fibrillary, syncytial appearance with indistinct margins (10X).

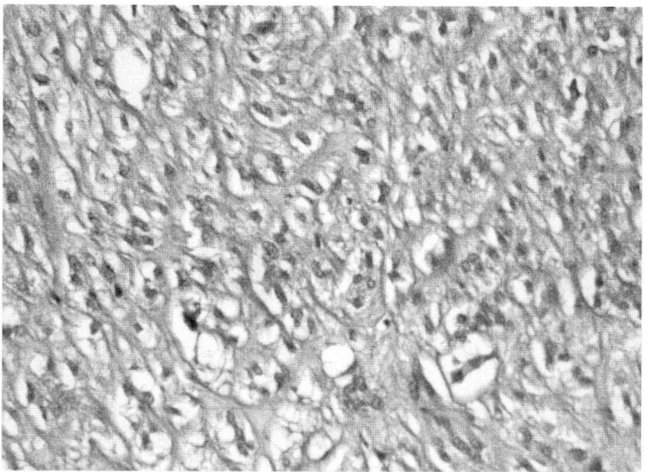

FIGURE 4.12

Gastrointestinal stromal tumor, epithelioid type, composed of round to oval cells with variably to clear cytoplasm. The clear cytoplasm is often retracted and eosinophilic (simulating inclusions) adjacent to or surrounding tumor nuclei. The nuclei are uniform to slightly pleomorphic, round to oval with vesicular chromatin and an occasional nested architecture (40X).

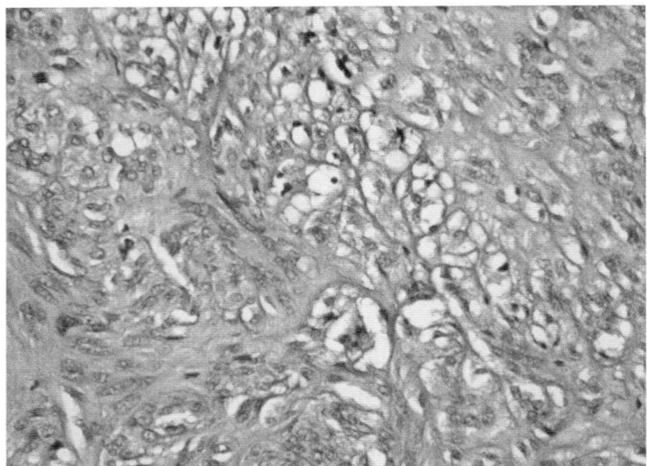

FIGURE 4.13

Gastrointestinal stromal tumor, mixed cell type, this lesion shows a combination of both spindle cell and epithelioid cells.

5% of all cases. Stromal collagen is uncommon, but delicate thin-walled vessels may be prominent, and stromal hemorrhage is a common feature of these tumors (21).

Epithelioid GISTs (Figures 4.6, 4.8, and 4.12) are composed of rounded cells with variably eosinophilic or clear cytoplasm. In cases with clear cytoplasm, often-retracted eosinophilic cytoplasm (simulating inclusions) can be seen around or adjacent to the tumor cell nuclei. Epithelioid lesions, similar to spindle cell lesions, tend to have uniform round-to-oval nuclei with vesicular chromatin, and this subset of tumors shows a nested architecture more often than spindle cell cases, enhancing the risk of confusion with an epithelial or melanocytic neoplasm. Lesions of mixed cell type may exhibit an abrupt transition between spindle cells and epithelioid areas (requiring careful and adequate sampling to assure all patterns are included) or may have a complex commingling of theses cell types throughout, leading to an intermediate ovoid cytologic appearance (21).

The most widely agreed upon and examined morphologic criteria for evaluating the biologic potential of GISTs are tumor size and mitotic activity; the latter is usually expressed per 50 high power fields (HPFs) (x40) (totaling 5 mm^2) (19,24,25). Since size and mitotic rate parameters are universally accepted as an indication of potential biological behavior, they should be recorded for all GISTs and included in the final pathology report (26). Other features of biological potential include degree of necrosis, cellularity, nuclear pleomorphism, nuclear cytoplasm ratio, mucosal invasion, and ulceration (11). A tumor size greater than 5 cm is associated with a high risk of metastasis or recurrence, and a mitotic count of greater than 5 mitoses per 50 HPFs is considered to be associated with a malignant behavior (27,28).

A study by Miettinen and colleagues (3) of esophageal GISTs showed a follow-up of 16 of 17 cases (94%), 9 patients died of their disease. All patients with tumors greater than 10 cm died of disease, whereas none of the patients with tumors smaller than 5 cm died of disease. Most of the tumors were histologically malignant with more than 5 mitoses per 50 HPFs. Fifty-nine percent of the patients (10 of 17) died of disease, with a median survival of 27 months. In this study, 1 patient died of their disease when the tumor showed only 5 mitoses per 50 HPFs, indicating that low mitotic rate does not assure benign behavior (27,28).

SUMMARY

Mesenchymal tumors of the esophagus are infrequent. The most common mesenchymal tumors of the esophagus are leiomyomas and GISTs. Leiomyosarcomas and schwannomas occur in the esophagus; they are, however, rare. The leiomyoma is the most common mesenchymal tumor of the esophagus, constituting 71%. Leiomyomas are rare elsewhere in the GI tract. Many tumors formerly classified as smooth muscle tumors, leiomyomas and leiomyosarcomas of the GI tract thought to be of smooth muscle origin were of ICC origin. Electron microscopic and immunohistochemical studies of this group of lesions confirm ICC as the cell of origin of the group of tumors, thus the name *gastrointestinal stromal tumor*. Based on clinical, morphologic, and cytologic criteria, GISTs occur in both benign and malignant forms.

References

1. Goyal RK. Columnar cell-lined (Barrett's) esophagus: a histological prospective. In: Spechler SJ, Goyal RK, eds. *Barrett's Esophagus Pathophysiology, Diagnosis and Management*. New York: Elsevier; 1985;1–18.
2. Meyer GW, Austin RM, Brady CE III, et al. Muscle anatomy of the human esophagus. *J Clin Gastroenterol.* 1986;8:131–134.
3. Miettinen M, Sarlomo-Rikala M, Sobin LH, et al. Esophageal stromal tumor. a clinicopathologic, immunohistochemical, and molecular genetic study of 17 cases and comparison with esophageal leiomyomas and leiomyosarcomas. *Am J Surg Pathol.* 2000;24:211–222.
4. Netter FH. *Atlas of Human Anatomy*. 3rd ed. St. Louis: ICDH Learning/Elsevier; 2003.
5. Kwon MS, Lee SS, Ahn GH. Schwannomas of the gastrointestinal tract: clinicopathological features of 12 cases including a case of esophageal tumor compared with those of gastrointestinal stromal tumors and leiomyomas of the gastrointestinal tract. *Pathol Res Pract.* 2002;198:605–613.
6. Faussone-Pellegrini MS, Cortesini C. Ultrastructure of striated muscle fibers in the middle third of the human esophagus. *Histol Histopathology*. 1986;1:119–128.
7. Zhu X, Zhang X-Q, Li BM, et al. Esophageal mesenchymal tumors: endoscopic, pathology and immunohistochemistry. *World J Gastroenterol.* 2007;13:768–773.
8. Klaase JM, Hulscher JB, Offerhaus GJ, et al. Surgery for unusual histopathologic variants of esophageal neoplasms: a report of 23 cases with emphasis on histologic characteristics. *Annals Surgical Oncol.* 2003;10:261–267.

9. Punpale A, et al. Leiomyoma of esophagus. *Ann Thoracic Cardivasc Surg.* 2007;13:78–78.
10. Daimaru Y, Kido H, Hashimoto H, et al. Benign schwannomas of the gastrointestinal tract: a clinicopathologic and immunohistochemical study. *Hum Pathol.* 1988;19:257–264.
11. Franquemont DW. Differentiation and risk assessment of gastrointestinal stromal tumors. *Am J Clin Pathol.* 1995;103:41–47.
12. Mazur MT, Clark HB. Gastric stromal tumors. Reappraisal of histogenesis. *Am J Surg Pathol.* 1983;7:507–519.
13. Hirosta S, Isozaki K, Moriyama Y, et al. Gain-of-function mutations of c-kit in human gastrointestinal stromal tumors. *Science.* 1998;279:577–580.
14. Kindblom LG, Remotti HE, Aldengorg F, et al. Gastrointestinal pacemaker cell tumor (GIPACT): gastrointestinal stromal tumors show phenotypic characteristics of the interstitial cells of Cajal. *Am J Pathol.* 1998;152;1259–1269.
15. Maeda H, Yamagata, A, Nishikawa S, et al. Requirement of c-kit for development of intestinal pacemaker system. *Development.* 1992;1116:369–375.
16. Huizinga JD, Thuneberg L, Kluppel M, et al. W/kit gene required for interstitial cells of Cajal and for intestinal pace maker activity. *Nature.* 1993;373:347–349.
17. Torihashi, S, Nishi K, Tokutomi Y, et al. Blockade of Kit signaling induced transdifferentiation on interstitial cells of Cajal to a smooth muscle phenotype. *Gastroenterology.* 1999;17:140–148.
18. Sarlomo-Rikala M, Kovatich AJ, Barusevicus A, et al. CD117: a sensitive marker for gastrointestinal tumors that is more specific than CD34. *Mod Pathol.* 1998;11:728–734.
19. Miettinen M, Sobin LH, Sarlomo-Rikala M. Immunohistochemical spectrum of GISTs at different sites and their differential diagnosis with a reference to CD117 (KIT). *Mod Pathol.* 2000;13:1134–1142.
20. Vliagoftis H, Worobec AS, Metcalfe DD. The protooncogene c-kit and c-dit ligand in human disease. *J Allergy Clin Immunol.* 1997;100:435–440.
21. Fletcher CD, Berman JJ, Corless C, et al. Diagnosis of gastrointestinal stromal tumor: a consensus approach. *Intl J Surg Pathol.* 2002;10:81–89.
22. Sakural S, Fukasawa T, Chong JM, et al. Embryonic form of smooth muscle myosin heavy chain (SMemb/MHCB) in gastrointestinal stromal tumor and interstitial cells of Cajal. *Am J Pathol.* 1999;154:23–28.
23. Tsujimura T, Makiishi-Shimobayashi C, Lundkvist J, et al. Expression of the intermediate filament nestin in gastrointestinal stromal tumors and interstitial cells of Cajal. *Am J Pathol.* 2001;158:817–823.
24. Miettinen M, El-Rifai W, Sobin LH, et al. Evaluation for malignancy and prognosis of gastrointestinal stromal tumors: a review. *Hum Pathol.* 2002;33:478–483.
25. Miettinen M, Sobin LH, Lasota J. Gastrointestinal stromal tumors of the stomach: a Clinicopathologic, immunohistochemical, an molecular genetic studies of 1765 cases with long-term follow-up. *Am J Surg Pathol.* 2005;29:52–68.
26. Miettinen M, Makhlouf HR, Sobin LH, et al. Gastrointestinal stromal tumors (GISTs) of the jejunum and ileum: a clinicopathologic, immunohistochemical and molecular genetic study of 906 cases, prior to imatinib with long-term follow-up. *Am J Surg Pathol.* 2006;30:477–489.
27. Miettinen M, Lasota J. Gastrointestinal stromal tumors review on morphology, molecular pathology, and differential diagnosis. *Arch Pathol Lab Med.* 2006;130:1466–1478.
28. DeMatteo RP, Lewis JJ, Leung D, et al. Two hundred gastrointestinal stromal tumors. Recurrence patterns and prognostic factors for survival. *Ann Surg.* 2000;231:51–58.

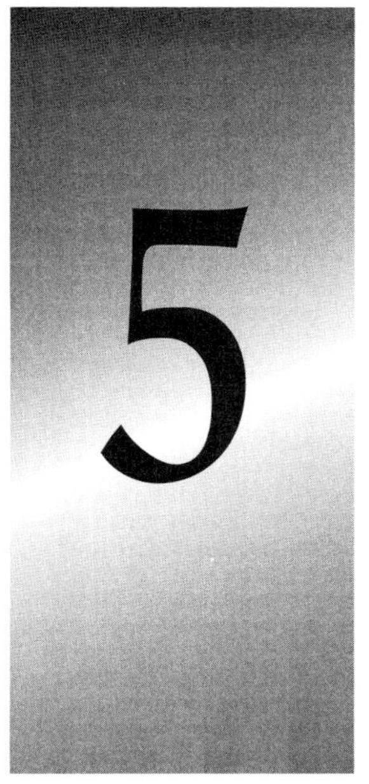

5 Barrett's Esophagus: Epidemiology and Pathogenesis

Daniel S. Oh
Tom Ryan DeMeester

The condition termed *Barrett's esophagus* is defined by the presence of both endoscopic and histologic findings: First, a columnar-lined segment of the esophagus proximal to the gastroesophageal junction must be visible on endoscopy, and second, biopsies of this segment must show goblet cells within cardiac mucosa. Although this definition appears relatively straightforward, it is the end result of many decades of confusion and controversy, and the topic is still subject to much debate.

The concept of intestinal metaplasia of the distal esophagus is a modern phenomenon. It was not well described in anatomical or medical texts until the mid-20th century, when Allison reported, in 1948, the presence of a "heterotopic gastric mucosa membrane in the oesophagus" (1). In 1950, Barrett proposed the concept that an organ should be defined by its epithelium, and since the esophagus, by this definition, ends at the squamocolumnar junction, the tubular columnar lined structure in the chest below the squamolumnar junction should be considered a tubularized stomach (2). In 1953, Allison challenged this concept by further describing the entity of an "esophagus lined with gastric mucous membrane" (3). A few years later, Barrett came into agreement with Allison and considered the columnar lining of the esophagus to actually represent abnormal esophageal mucosa (4). Allison's persuasive arguments were that the "intrathoracic tubular stomach" showed no evidence of a peritoneal covering, the musculature of the tube was that of normal esophagus, there were islands of squamous epithelium existing within the columnar epithelium, there were no oxyntic cells within the columnar epithelium or gastric mucous glands in the mucosa, and typical esophageal submucosal glands were present under the columnar epithelium. By these arguments the concept of a columnar lined esophagus began to crystallize, although at that time there were no histologic criteria used to define Barrett's esophagus.

The true etiology of the columnar lined esophagus unfolded over the next 50 years as its association with gastroesophageal reflux disease (GERD) became more firmly established (5). In 1961, Hayward introduced the concept that reflux-induced injury to the normal squamous epithelium of the esophagus could result in replacement of the distal esophagus with a columnar "junctional epithelium," which in modern terminology is termed *cardiac mucosa* (6). He hypothesized that this columnar metaplasia developed in order to provide better resistance to the acidic gastric contents bathing the lower esophagus than that provided by normal squamous mucosa. As this hypothesis was embraced, it became critical to define what was the normal epithelial histology at the junction between the esophagus and stomach. Hayward opined that the distal 1–2 centimeters of the esophagus was normally lined with junctional or cardiac mucosa. This led to a modification of the definition of a columnar lined esophagus by requiring the length of columnar epithelium to be 3 cm or greater to make the diagnosis (6). The metaplastic nature of this esophageal columnar lining was confirmed by Bremner et al. in 1970, who showed in a canine model that a denuded segment of distal esophagus in the presence of acid gastric juice regenerated as de novo columnar epithelium, and not from the migration of adjacent gastric epithelium (7).

Clarification of the epithelial histology of Barrett's esophagus started with the work of Paull et al., who reported in 1976 the presence of 3 different types of epithelium found in the columnar lined esophagus (8). They showed that the epithelial columnar lining could be junctional (cardiac), fundic (oxyntocardiac), or specialized (intestinalized cardiac) types. These investigators established for the first time that the columnar epithelium was not normal gastric mucosa, and they introduced the concept of intestinalized cardiac epithelium could be found within the columnar segment. Further studies in the late 1970s established that a columnar lined esophagus containing intestinal metaplasia had a malignant potential, which led to the emphasis of this histologic finding (9–11). In the 1980s, the histologic finding of intestinal metaplasia within the columnar lined esophagus (albeit when 3 cm or greater in length) became established as the definition of Barrett's esophagus.

As endoscopic evaluation of the esophagus became more commonplace and more sophisticated during the 1900s, it was recognized that normal individuals without GERD do not have a 2 cm columnar lined segment of distal esophagus, and that the normal esophagus is composed of squamous mucosa all the way down to the rugal folds of the stomach (12). It was also appreciated that any length of intestinal metaplasia of the distal esophagus was premalignant, and the 3 cm requirement for defining Barrett's esophagus was abandoned. Thus, the modern definition of Barrett's esophagus today is a columnar lined segment of esophagus of any length visible on endoscopy with a biopsy showing intestinal metaplasia. Despite this clarification, some residual terminology has persisted regarding the length of the intestinalized columnar segment in that it is still commonplace to make the distinction between short segment Barrett's (<3 cm) and long segment Barrett's (≥3 cm). Nevertheless, both short and long segment Barrett's are considered pathologic and premalignant. Controversy exists, however, over the significance of intestinal metaplasia at an endoscopically normal appearing gastroesophageal junction. This finding, termed *cardia intestinal metaplasia* (CIM) is currently considered a separate entity from Barrett's esophagus although there are increasing data that indicate that the pathogenesis of CIM is similar to reflux-induced Barrett's (13).

PATHOGENESIS

The pathogenesis of Barrett's esophagus is currently hypothesized to be a 2-step process—columnarization of the injured distal esophagus with cardiac mucosa followed by the formation of goblet cells or intestinal metaplasia (Figure 5.1). It is unclear how long this process takes, as it is uncommon for a clinician to follow a reflux patient with cardiac mucosa for a long enough period of time and frequently enough with extensive biopsies to identify the development of goblet cells. There is one unique clinical setting in which this can be observed in an accelerated process. Some individuals who have undergone an esophagectomy and are reconstructed with a gastric pull-up have been noted by many investigators to develop columnar mucosa in the remnant cervical esophagus above the anastomosis. In some, this change was followed by the development of intestinal metaplasia (14–18). Since the cardia was resected in these patients, it is likely that this process represents an exaggerated course of events seen in patients with Barrett's. The composition of the refluxate in these patients has been shown to be similar to that in patients with Barrett's esophagus, with exposure of the normal squamous epithelium to a combination of acid and bile. In this setting, the 2-step process of intestinalization of the esophagus occurs in a predictable course and has been observed to occur over 5 to 10 years (14).

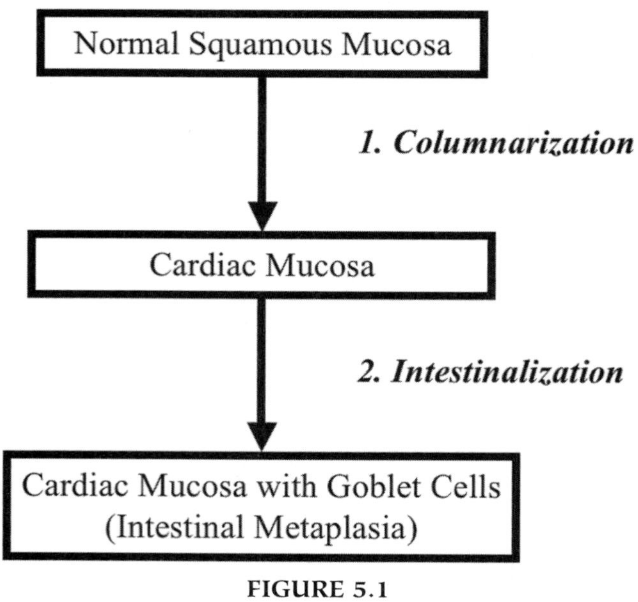

FIGURE 5.1

Overview of the 2-step development of Barrett's esophagus.

STEP 1: COLUMNARIZATION OF THE ESOPHAGUS

In discussing the columnarization of the distal esophagus, one must first define the normal gastroesophageal junction, a topic of controversy in itself. Most commonly, this is defined endoscopically where the rugal folds of the stomach transition to the flattened appearance of the tubular esophagus. In the normal state, this location also corresponds with the squamocolumnar junction, where the salmon-red mucosa of the stomach transitions to the pearly white mucosa of the esophagus. Microscopically, this represents the transition from normal squamous esophageal epithelium to the oxyntic mucosa of the stomach (19).

The pathogenesis of Barrett's esophagus begins with injury to the normal squamous epithelium of the distal esophagus. Initially, this is thought to be secondary to repeated distension of the stomach with fatty meals of large volume that results in effacement of the lower esophageal sphincter and exposure of the distal esophageal squamous epithelium to caustic gastric juice (Figure 5.2) (20). This physiologic phenomenon has been well demonstrated by Fletcher et al., who showed that the intrasphinteric portion of the lower esophagus can unfold almost 2 cm in normal volunteers as the stomach distends (21). This portion of the lower esophagus subsequently becomes exposed to an unbuffered acid pocket that floats on a lipid layer after consumption of a fatty meal, resulting in injury to the squamous epithelium. The surface of the epithelium is damaged and causes a proliferative response observed on microscopy as basal cell hyperplasia and loss of surface cornified epithelial cells giving the impression of papillary elongation. Continuing inflammatory injury in this area of the lower esophagus can cause permanent loss of the musculature of the lower esophageal sphincter, resulting in a mechanically defective and incompetent lower esophageal sphincter of short length and low resting pressure. With further loss of the gastroesophageal barrier, GERD can explode into the esophagus with resultant injury to progressively greater lengths of the squamous mucosa. This process continues up to a level where the luminal pH no longer causes epithelial injury. Endoscopically, this injury can be seen as erosive esophagitis, ranging from a subtle irritation to circumferential loss of the superficial mucosa.

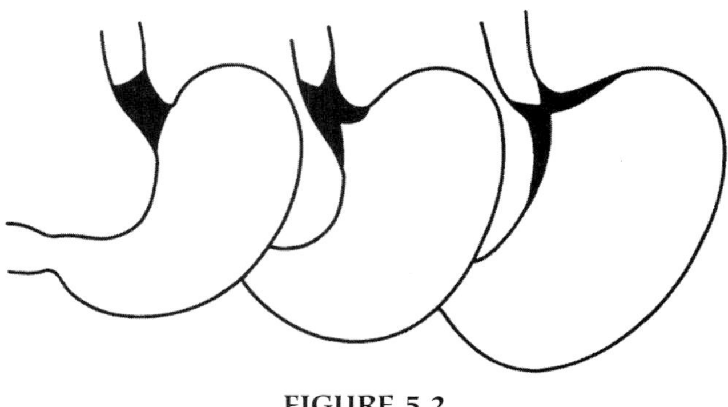

FIGURE 5.2

Gastric distention resulting in unfolding of the lower esophageal sphincter and exposure of squamous mucosa to gastric juice.

Injury to the squamous epithelium of the esophagus can be observed with the electron microscopy prior to the microscopic and endoscopic changes. Tobey et al. have shown that exposure of esophageal squamous epithelium to acid can result in dilated intercellular spaces, gaps that allow diffusion of molecules up to 20 kD in size through the multilayered squamous epithelium (22). It is hypothesized that these intercellular gaps have 2 consequences. First, they allow acidic fluid to permeate into the epithelial layer where nerve endings reside and give the sensation of heartburn. Second, these intercellular gaps may expose gastrointestinal stem cells to a luminal factor that stimulates differentiation into a columnar cell type. It is perhaps by this mechanism that a genetic switch occurs in the gastrointestinal stem cells that leads to columnarization of the esophagus. The identification of this culprit molecule and its exact mechanism remain unknown; however, the events resemble a reversion to the fetal esophagus in which a fetal columnar epithelium is present. Further research into the pathogenesis of fetal esophageal development may eventually shed light on this process (5).

The resulting columnar metaplasia that develops in a previous squamous-lined esophagus appears as a layer of mucous secreting columnar cells termed *cardiac mucosa*. This is a truly metaplastic epithelium, for it does not exist at birth. It is a highly specific mucosa that arises to replace injured squamous epithelium and is believed to be an adaptive response to better tolerate exposure to refluxing gastric juice (19). As would be predicted by the events leading to its formation, cardiac mucosa arises between the normal oxyntic mucosa of the stomach and the uninjured squamous mucosa of the esophagus. In the majority of cases, this process occurs in individuals who do not yet have bothersome symptoms of GERD, and as Chandrasoma and DeMeester point out, this process at a microscopic level may be as ubiquitous as anthracosis in the lungs or atherosclerosis in the arteries (5). The formation of cardiac mucosa represents the first step in the pathogenesis of Barrett's esophagus; however, in most asymptomatic individuals, the length of this columnar esophagus is quite small, usually less than 1 mm, and progresses only slightly further with age (19). Initially, this process can be conceptualized as reflux disease confined to the sphincter (23). However, as the lower esophageal sphincter deteriorates with worsening injury and inflammation, acid exposure increases more proximally in the esophagus, correlating with longer segments of cardiac mucosal metaplasia (20,24).

STEP 2: INTESTINALIZATION OF CARDIAC MUCOSA

Once metaplastic cardiac mucosa has developed in areas of injured squamous epithelium, there are divergent differentiation pathways that may result (Figure 5.3) (5). First, cardiac mucosa can remain cardiac mucosa, initially in the form of foveoli or, more commonly, stabilizing as glandular mucosa. Second, cardiac mucosa may form parietal cells within it and become oxyntocardiac mucosa. Finally, cardiac mucosa may develop goblet cells and become intestinalized cardiac mucosa. This heterogeneity of the columnar lined esophagus was first described by Paull et al. and has since been confirmed by others (8). Chandrasoma et al. have demonstrated that the gastrointestinal stem cells within cardiac mucosa that give rise to these different types of epithelium are sequestered in deep foveolar pits or in the neck of glandular units of cardiac mucosa (5). Presumably, the fate of cardiac mucosa to remain pure cardiac mucosa or give rise to parietal cells or goblet cells is due to different genetic signals to the stem cells driven by a specific intraluminal milieu of the esophageal lumen.

Although the specific genetic signaling pathways involved in the transformation of squamous mucosa to cardiac mucosa are not known, genes involved in the formation of parietal cells and goblet cells have been identified. In gastric fundic mucosa differentiation, the sonic hedgehog gene (SHH) has been shown to be critical in the differentiation and maintaining oxyntic mucosa (25–27). In the normal gastrointestinal tract, SHH is expressed in significant amounts only in the gastric fundus and body and appears to be directly responsible for the formation of oxyntic glands containing parietal cells. Presumably, activation of this genetic signal is also responsible for the differentiation of cardiac mucosa to oxyntocardiac mucosa. Preliminary work appears to confirm this hypothesis, and in long segment Barrett's esophagus the SHH gene has the highest expression distally near the stomach (where oxytocardiac mucosa exists) and lowest expression proximally (where intestinal metaplasia exists) (28).

The genetic signaling pathway involved in intestinal differentiation appears to be driven by a different gene, CDX2. This gene is critical for the differentiation and maintenance of normal intestinal epithelium from the duodenum to the rectum (29,30). It is not expressed in the normal foregut except in the setting of intestinal metaplasia (31–33). During the pathogenesis of Barrett's esophagus, CDX2 expression is low in cardiac and oxyntocardiac mucosa, but a 16-fold increase in expression occurs once goblet cells begin to appear (34). Further, within long segment Barrett's, a gene expression gradient of CDX2 exists, with the highest expression in the proximal end, corresponding histologically to where the goblet cell density is highest, and the lowest expression in the distal end close to the stomach where the goblet cell density is the lowest (28,35). Thus the gene expression patterns of SHH and CDX2 are inversely related within the columnar lined esophagus; this indicates that differentiation into intestinal metaplasia and oxyntocardiac mucosa are mutually exclusive processes (Figure 5.4).

Corresponding to the observed gene expression gradients of SHH and CDX2, the differentiation of cardiac mucosa within a segment of columnar lined esophagus into the 3 possible epithelia does not appear random. Intestinal metaplasia always develops at the proximal extent near the squamocolumnar junction, whereas cardiac and oxyntocardiac mucosa occur at the

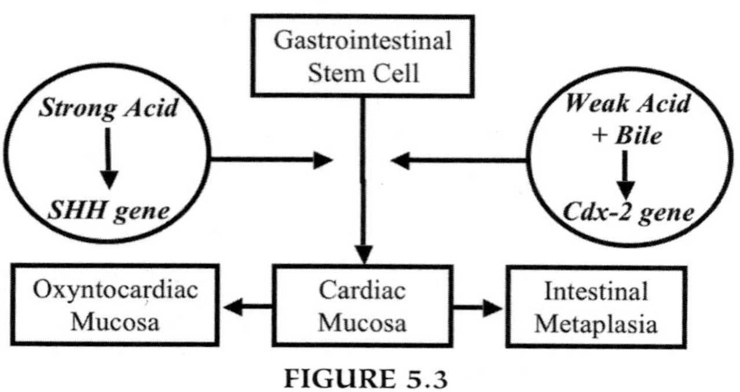

FIGURE 5.3

The different pathways of differentiation within the columnar lined esophagus.

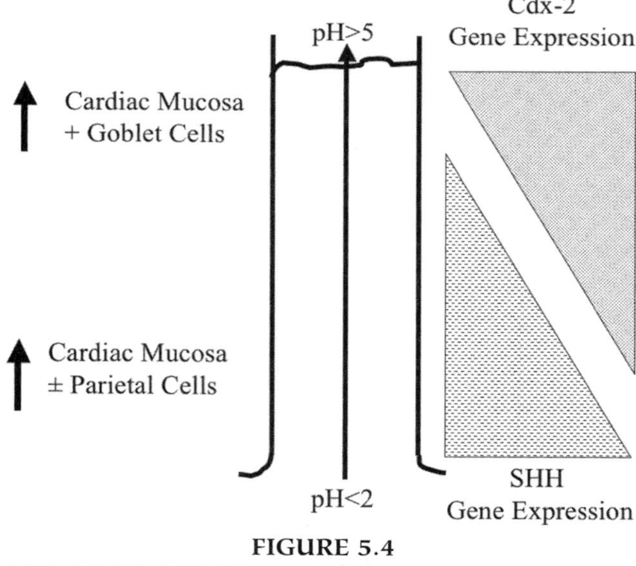

FIGURE 5.4

Heterogeneity of histology and gene expression in the columnar lined esophagus.

distal extent near the gastroesophageal junction (8,36). Although the specific stimuli that direct expression of SHH and CDX2 to lead to this pattern of differentiation has not yet been fully elucidated, there is emerging evidence that the interplay between bile acids and the pH in the esophageal lumen and cellular environment plays a critical role in determining which gene becomes activated (5) (Figure 5.4).

Clinical and experimental evidence strongly supports the role of bile acids in the pathogenesis of intestinalization. In vitro studies have demonstrated that CDX2 upregulation occurs in cells directly stimulated by exposure to bile acids, and this laboratory work is corroborated by clinical experience (37). In a multivariate analysis of over 400 patients being evaluated for GERD, Campos et al. found that the strongest predictor for the presence of Barrett's esophagus is abnormal exposure of the distal esophagus to bile (38). Another clinical study has shown that compared to acid exposure alone, the additional exposure to bile with acid increases the risk of Barrett's esophagus over 300% (39). Interlinked to bile exposure is also the pH of the esophageal lumen and the intracellular environment, specifically the relationship to the pKa of the bile acids to the pH of the environment in which they exist (40–43). In patients with gastroesophageal reflux, there is in the esophageal lumen a pH gradient between a pH of <2 in the stomach to a pH of 5 to 6 in the upper esophagus. This is due to the mixture of the refluxed gastric juice with swallowed saliva (34,43). When the pH of the luminal milieu is above the pKa of bile acids (≥6), bile acids dissociate into salts and cannot cross the cell membrane. In contrast, when the pH is well below their pKa (<3), bile acids precipitate and also cannot cross the cell membrane. It is only when the pKa is near the pH of a weak acid, that is a pH of 3 to 5, that bile acids are nonpolar and soluble, allowing them to cross the cell membrane and presumably activate CDX2 to drive intestinal metaplasia. Thus the highest expression of CDX2 and greatest concentration of goblet cells in a columnar lined esophagus occurs at the proximal portion of the Barrett's segment (28,36). At this level, the luminal pH is between 3 and 5, the optimal range for bile acid to enter the cell. As for the specific factors contributing to SHH expression and differentiation of cardiac-oxyntic mucosa, there is evidence pH appears to play a critical role in its transcription as well, with more expression in an acidic environment (44). Further, the pattern of exposure to these factors may have an influence. For example, Fitzgerald et al. have demonstrated in cell culture experiments that continuous versus pulsatile exposure to acid can affect cell proliferation and differentiation (45).

CONCLUSION

In the normal gastroesophageal junction, the squamous lined esophagus abuts the oxyntic columnar epithelium of the fundus of the stomach. The formation of Barrett's esophagus in this setting is a 2-step process: replacement of the squamous cells with mucous secreting columnar cells and acquisition of goblets cells pathognomonic for intestinalization. With repeated and prolonged episodes of gastric distention, exposure of the intersphincteric mucosa of the lower esophageal sphincter to gastric juice results in injury to the squamous epithelium, and the injured cells are replaced with cardiac mucosa. The inflammatory injury results also in the loss of the lower esophageal sphincter in a distal to proximal direction and a creeping carditis up to a level in the esophagus at which the luminal pH no longer causes epithelial injury. Columnarization of the esophagus is subsequently followed by the formation of goblet cells within cardiac mucosa to complete the intestinal metaplasia process. A key gene responsible for this intestinal differentiation is CDX2, a gene involved in maintenance of intestinal mucosa in the adult gastrointestinal tract that is not expressed in the normal foregut. Clinical and empiric evidence have shown that an interplay between pH and bile acids plays a profound role in the activation of CDX2 and the formation of Barrett's esophagus.

References

1. Allison PR. Peptic ulcer of the esophagus. *Thorax*. 1948;3:20–42.
2. Barrett NR. Chronic peptic ulcer of the oesophagus and "oesophagitis." *Br J Surg*. 1950;38:175–182.
3. Allison PR, Johnstone AS. The oesophagus lined with gastric mucous membrane. *Thorax*. 1953;8:87–101.
4. Barrett NR. The lower esophagus lined by columnar epithelium. *Surgery*. 1957;41:881–894.
5. Chandrasoma PT, DeMeester TR. *GERD: Reflux to Esophageal Adenocarcinoma*. San Diego: Elsevier; 2006.
6. Hayward J. The lower end of the esophagus. *Thorax*. 1961;16:36–41.
7. Bremner CG, Lynch VP, Ellis FH Jr. Barrett's esophagus: congenital or acquired? An experimental study of esophageal mucosal regeneration in the dog. *Surgery*. 1970;68(1):209–216.
8. Paull A, Trier JS, Dalton MD, et al. The histologic spectrum of Barrett's esophagus. *N Engl J Med*. 1976;295(9):476–480.
9. Haggitt RC, Tryzelaar J, Ellis FH, et al. Adenocarcinoma complicating columnar epithelium-lined (Barrett's) esophagus. *Am J Clin Pathol*. 1978;70(1):1–5.
10. Reid BJ, Weinstein WM. Barrett's and adenocarcinoma. *Annu Rev Med*. 1987;38:477–492.
11. Skinner DB, Walther BC, Riddell RH, et al. Barrett's esophagus. Comparison of benign and malignant cases. *Ann Surg*. 1983;198(4):554–565.
12. DeMeester SR, DeMeester TR. Columnar mucosa and intestinal metaplasia of the esophagus: fifty years of controversy. *Ann Surg*. 2000;231(3):303–321.
13. DeMeester SR, Wickramasinghe KS, Lord RVN, et al. Cytokeratin and DAS-1 immunostaining reveal similarities among cardiac mucosa, CIM, and Barrett's esophagus. *Am J Gastroenterol*. 2002;97(10):2514–2523.
14. Oberg S, Johansson J, Wenner J, et al. Metaplastic columnar mucosa in the cervical esophagus after esophagectomy. *Ann Surg*. 2002;235(3):338–345.
15. Lord RVN, Wickramasinghe K, Johansson JJ, et al. Cardiac mucosa in the remnant esophagus after esophagectomy is an acquired epithelium with Barrett's-like features. *Surgery*. 2004;136(3):633–640.

16. Lindahl H, Rintala R, Sariola H, et al. Cervical Barrett's esophagus: a common complication of gastric tube reconstruction. *J Pediatr Surg.* 1990;25(4):446–448.
17. O'Riordan JM, Tucker ON, Byrne PJ, et al. Factors influencing the development of Barrett's epithelium in the esophageal remnant postesophagectomy . *Am J Gastroenterol.* 2004;99(2):205–211.
18. Dresner SM, Griffin SM, Wayman J, et al. Human model of duodenogastro-oesophageal reflux in the development of Barrett's metaplasia . *Br J Surg.* 2003;90(9):1120–1128.
19. Chandrasoma PT, Der R, Ma Y, et al. Histology of the gastroesophageal junction: an autopsy study . *Am J Surg Pathol.* 2000;24(3):402–409.
20. DeMeester TR, Ireland AP. Gastric pathology as an initiator and potentiator of gastroesophageal reflux disease. *Dis Esoph.* 1997;10:1–8.
21. Fletcher J, Wirz A, Young J, et al. Unbuffered highly acidic gastric juice exists at the gastroesophageal junction after a meal. *Gastroenterology.* 2001;121(4):775–783.
22. Tobey NA, Hosseini SS, Argote CM, et al. Dilated intercellular spaces and shunt permeability in nonerosive acid-damaged esophageal epithelium. *Am J Gastroenterol.* 2004;99(1):13–22.
23. Theisen J, Oberg S, Peters JH, et al. Gastro-esophageal reflux disease confined to the sphincter. *Dis Esophagus.* 2001;14(3–4):235–238.
24. Csendes A, Maluenda F, Braghetto I, et al. Location of the lower oesophageal sphincter and the squamous columnar mucosal junction in 109 healthy controls and 778 patients with different degrees of endoscopic oesophagitis. *Gut.* 1993;34(1):21–27.
25. van den Brink GR, Hardwick JC, Tytgat GN, et al. Sonic hedgehog regulates gastric gland morphogenesis in man and mouse. *Gastroenterology.* 2001;121(2):317–328.
26. Silberg DG, Kaestner KH. Morphogenesis and maintenance of the gastric epithelium: a role for sonic hedgehog? *Gastroenterology.* 2001;121(2):485–487.
27. van den Brink GR, Hardwick JCH, Nielsen C, et al. Sonic hedgehog expression correlates with fundic gland differentiation in the adult gastrointestinal tract. *Gut.* 2002;51(5):628–633.
28. Oh DS, DeMeester SR, Mori R, et al. Cdx-2 and Sonic Hedgehog gene expression in the proximal, middle, and distal regions of columnar mucosa in long segment Barrett's esophagus. *Gastroenterology.* 2008;134(4)Supplement 1:A442–443.
29. Suh E, Traber PG. An intestine-specific homeobox gene regulates proliferation and differentiation. *Mol Cell Biol.* 1996;16(2):619–625.
30. Silberg DG, Swain GP, Suh ER, et al. Cdx1 and cdx2 expression during intestinal development. *Gastroenterology.* 2000;119(4):961–971.
31. Silberg DG, Sullivan J, Kang E, et al. Cdx2 ectopic expression induces gastric intestinal metaplasia in transgenic mice. *Gastroenterology.* 2002;122(3):689–696.
32. Eda A, Osawa H, Satoh K, et al. Aberrant expression of CDX2 in Barrett's epithelium and inflammatory esophageal mucosa. *J Gastroenterol.* 2003;38(1):14–22.
33. Groisman GM, Amar M, Meir A. Expression of the intestinal marker Cdx2 in the columnar-lined esophagus with and without intestinal (Barrett's) metaplasia. *Mod Pathol.* 2004;17(10):1282–1288.
34. Vallbohmer D, DeMeester SR, Peters JH, et al. Cdx-2 expression in squamous and metaplastic columnar epithelia of the esophagus. *Dis Esophagus.* 2006;19(4):260–266.
35. Theodorou D, Streets C, Chandrasoma P, et al. Comparison of the pH and intestinal metaplasia density across long segment Barrett's esophagus. *Gastroenterology.* 2002;122:A51.
36. Chandrasoma PT, Der R, Dalton P, et al. Distribution and significance of epithelial types in columnar-lined esophagus. *Am J Surg Pathol.* 2001;25(9):1188–1193.
37. Kazumori H, Ishihara S, Rumi MAK, et al. Bile acids directly augment caudal related homeobox gene Cdx2 expression in oesophageal keratinocytes in Barrett's epithelium. *Gut.* 2006;55(1):16–25.
38. Campos GM, DeMeester SR, Peters JH, et al. Predictive factors of Barrett esophagus: multivariate analysis of 502 patients with gastroesophageal reflux disease. *Arch Surg.* 2001;136(11):1267–1273.
39. Oh DS, Hagen JA, Fein M, et al. Impact of reflux composition on mucosal injury and esophageal function. *J Gastrointest Surg.* 2006;10(6):787–797.
40. Harmon JW, Johnson LF, Maydonovitch CL. Effects of acid and bile salts on the rabbit esophageal mucosa. *Dig Dis Sci.* 1981;26(1):65–72.
41. Schweitzer EJ, Bass BL, Batzri S, et al. Bile acid accumulation by rabbit esophageal mucosa. *Dig Dis Sci.* 1986;31(10):1105–1113.
42. Lillemoe KD, Gadacz TR, Harmon JW. Bile absorption occurs during disruption of the esophageal mucosal barrier. *J Surg Res.* 1983;35(1):57–62.
43. DeMeester TR, Peters JH, Bremner CG, et al. Biology of gastroesophageal reflux disease: pathophysiology relating to medical and surgical treatment. *Annu Rev Med.* 1999;50:469–506.
44. Dimmler A, Brabletz T, Hlubek F, et al. Transcription of sonic hedgehog, a potential factor for gastric morphogenesis and gastric mucosa maintenance, is up-regulated in acidic conditions. *Lab Invest.* 2003;83(12):1829–1837.
45. Fitzgerald RC, Omary MB, Triadafilopoulos G. Dynamic effects of acid on Barrett's esophagus. An ex vivo proliferation and differentiation model. *J Clin Invest.* 1996;98(9):2120–2128.

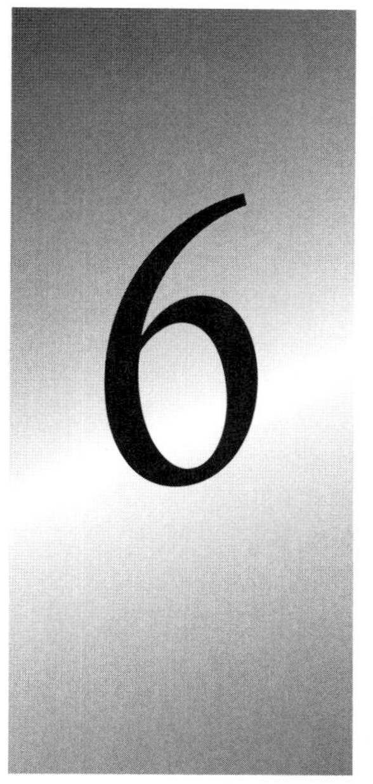

Barrett's Esophagus: Molecular Biology

Patrick I. McConnell
Blair A. Jobe

Adenocarcinoma of the esophagus that arises in the setting of Barrett's esophagus is thought to develop as part of the metaplasia–dysplasia–carcinoma sequence (Figure 6.1). This multistep process leading to the development of esophageal cancer involves genetic events that result in key abnormalities of cell cycle regulation, growth factor regulation, and intercellular adhesion mechanisms (1,2). Although high-grade dysplasia of Barrett's esophagus is generally considered a precursor to invasive carcinoma, the endoscopic as well as histopathologic recognition of this lesion can be difficult. There is no one event nor an exact sequence of changes leading from Barrett's metaplasia to adenocarcinoma rather an accumulation of these changes that seemingly is essential for cancer development. Furthermore, a surveillance program based on current concepts of risk cannot have an impact on mortality from esophageal adenocarcinoma (3,4). To be effective, it will be necessary for surveillance programs to utilize more than just basic histology; perhaps molecular markers can be for the identification of those who are most at risk of progression to adenocarcinoma.

Other malignancies have inherited highly penetrant mutations in key cancer susceptibility genes that are used to target those patients and their families needing premalignant therapy (e.g., familial adenoma polyposis syndrome; APC gene); however, progress in developing predictive biomarkers based on common somatic genetic abnormalities in "at-risk" tissues has not been as successful. In theory, neoplasia progresses by clonal evolution in which genetic instability generates variants on which natural selection acts, resulting in waves of clonal expansion, generation of new variants, and further selection (5). Therefore, early markers and those accumulated combinations of events heralding a more aggressive phenotype of metaplasia and low-grade dysplasia may help identify those patients most in need of early therapeutic strategies or at the very least more appropriate surveillance.

CELL OF ORIGIN?

The metaplastic conversion of the esophageal squamous epithelium to a columnar-lined epithelium could arise from 2 potential types of cells. The more classical teaching was that differentiated cells underwent *transdifferentiation*. Alternatively, metaplasia may develop from the conversion of a *stem* or *pluripotent cell*, meaning a cell with the capacity for unlimited or prolonged self-renewal (6,7). The origin of such a cell is not known—that is, whether the cell originates from the organ itself (interbasal layer of the epithelium between the papillae) (8,9) or from circulating pluripotent stem cells and after repopulating sites of

A

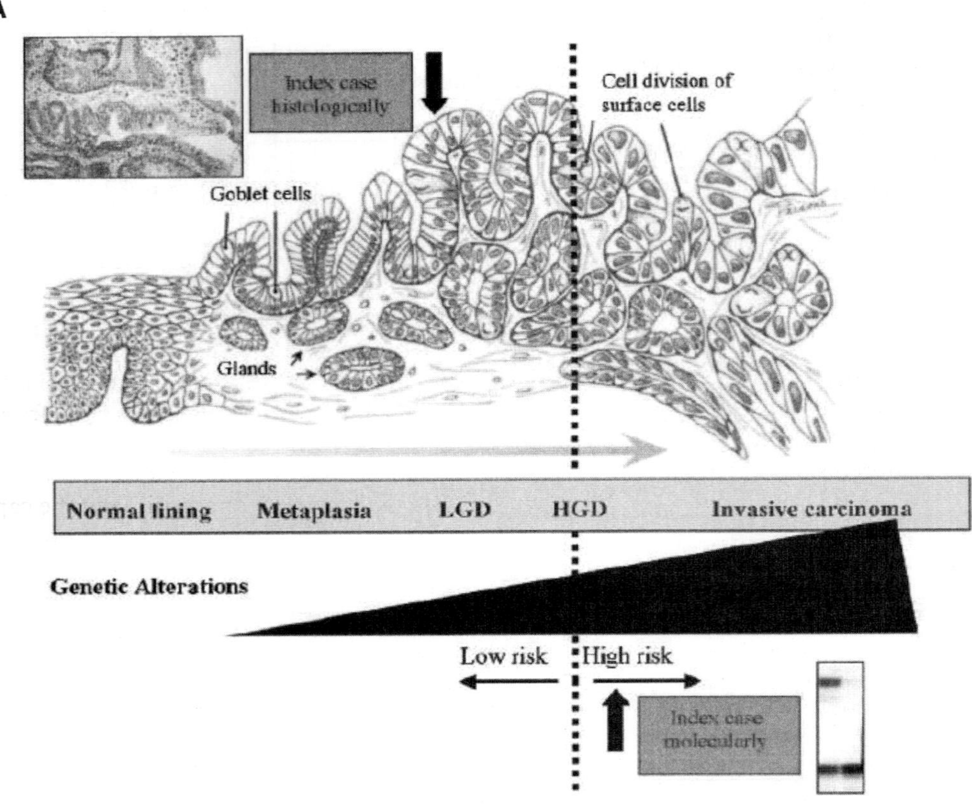

B

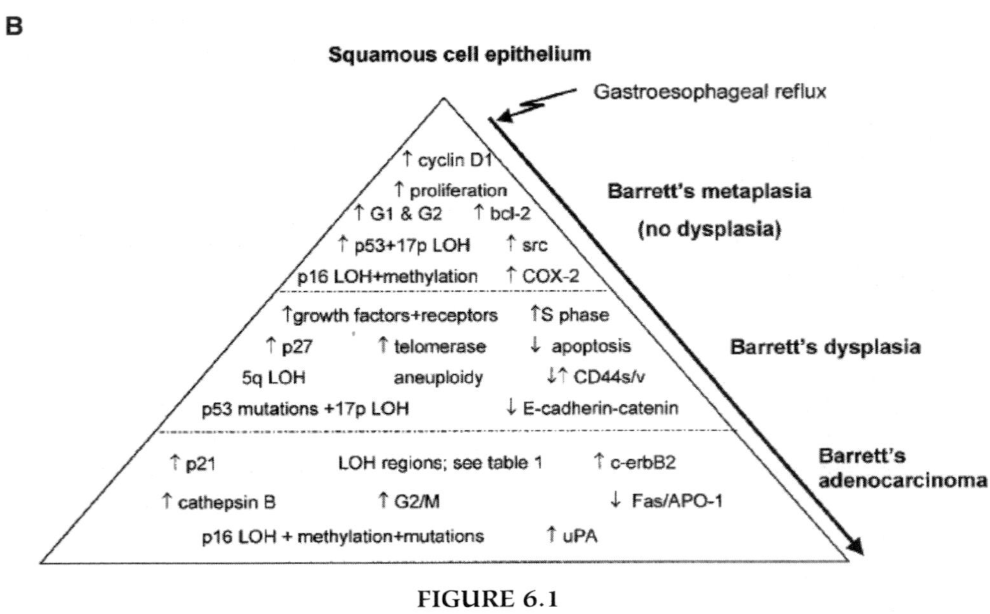

FIGURE 6.1

The accumulation of genetic defects leads to the development of esophageal adenocarcinoma through the metaplasia-dysplasia-carcinoma sequence. (A) Koppert LB, Wijnhoven BP, van Dekken H, et al. The molecular biology of esophageal adenocarcinoma. *J Surg Oncol.* 2005;92(3):169–190. (B) Wijnhoven BP, Tilanus HW, Dinjens WNM. Molecular biology of Barrett's adenocarcinoma. *Ann Surg.* 2001;(233)3:322–337.

inflammation and injury could theoretically undergo metaplastic changes. Houghton et al. recently showed that bone marrow-derived cells might represent a potential source of epithelial cancers (10,11). Working with mice infected by a Helicobacter strain, they found that these bone marrow–derived cells were able to home, repopulate the chronically inflamed gastric mucosa, and contribute over time to metaplasia, dysplasia, and cancer development. Though no animal or human studies have demonstrated the presence of esophageal tumors arising directly from circulating stem cells, parallels to the finding of Houghton in mice with gastric cancer exist—such as a known correlation of esophageal cancer with the chronicity and severity inflammation (12,13). Stem cell homing and differentiation will undoubtedly be an intense area of study and potential progress in the diagnosis and therapy for Barrett's esophagus during the next decade, particularly if key events can be documented in metaplastic tissues that lead to tumorigenesis.

CLASSIFICATION OF MOLECULAR ALTERATIONS IN BARRETT'S

It is generally accepted that some of the many somatic mutations that accumulate over time can be found only in the patient's tumor tissue. This would include epigenetic alterations like methylation of DNA sequences that through a multistep process silences the gene eventually resulting in cellular transformation and carcinogenesis (14). All of which leads the cell toward genomic instability and rendering the cell independent of regulated proliferation, apoptosis, and the capacity to metastasize,

TABLE 6.1
Categories of Genes Involved in Tumorigenesis

Gene type	Normal function	How altered	Abnormal function	Examples in BE/EA
Proto-oncogenes	These are dominant genes that act in signal transduction from extracellular stimuli to the nucleus and in regulation of gene expression. They also have a role in cell proliferation or inhibition of apoptosis.	• Mutation • Amplification • Translocation	Converted to oncogenes with unregulated, constitutive activity. This results in excessive stimulation of cell proliferation or prevention of apoptosis contributing to tumor formation	*Growth factors* • EGF,TGF-α (EGFR) • C-erbB2 (late event) • TGF-β (LOH 18q21) *Oncogenes* • src
Tumor suppressor genes	Normal recessive cellular genes that primarily are involved in cell proliferation, apoptosis, cell adhesion, and gene expression regulation.	*Genetic alteration:* • Mutation • Deletion of all or part of gene *Epigenetic alteration* • Promoter methylation (silencing)	Because these are recessive genes, both gene copies need to be inactivated for tumorigenesis via proliferation or prevention of apoptosis.	• p53 + 17p LOH • p16 • Rb • APC (EA &BE with HGD not BE) • ? FHIT
Mismatch repair genes	Genetic stability is assured by proper DNA repair via these normally functioning genes.	Contractions/expansions of short repeat sequences (micro satellites) can be found in these genes.	The mismatch repair deficiency leads to a genome-wide accumulation of mutations and specifically to proto-oncogenes and tumor suppressor genes.	• PMS1 & PMS2 • MLH1, MSH2 & MSH6 • MBD4 (MED1)
Mitotic checkpoint genes	Regulate cellular mitosis, assuring chromosomal stability and that a correct number of chromosomes are replicated in cell division.	Inactivation via mutation of at least one copy having a dominant-negative effect	Inactivation of mitotic check point genes results in chromosomal instability and an abnormal chromosome number (aneuploidy).	• Cyclin D1 (early) • p27 (down regulated) • p21 (down regulated)

Abbreviations: BE = Barrett's esophagus/metaplasia; EA = esophageal adenocarcinoma; LOH = loss of heterozygosity.

though the number of mutations needed to transform or destabilize a cell is debatable and potentially infinite—at least in variety of site mutations (15,16). Overall, genetic instability leads to either chromosomal mutations or microsatellite instability in 4 basic types of genes that contribute toward tumorigenesis: proto-oncogenes, tumor suppressor genes, mismatch repair genes, and mitotic checkpoint genes (Table 6.1).

Early Molecular Events

Phenotype Signals

Barrett's epithelium is characterized by the presence of goblet cells and the expression of intestinal markers such as MUC2, alkaline phosphatase, villin, and sucrase isomaltase (17–19). Barrett's metaplasia may result from change in the activation status of a gene as a result of repetitive injury to that of an alternative phenotype. CDX1 and CDX2 are homeobox proteins that have integral roles in the development of normal intestinal epithelium and therefore may be important transcription factors in the development of metaplastic epithelium in the esophagus (17,18,20). CDX2 expression arises in the proximal intestine and declines distally, whereas CDX1 expression arises in the distal intestine with overlap in the midgut (21). It is possible that injurious agents present in GERD activate ectopic expression of CDX1 through NF-κ signaling which, in turn, initiates the development of the intestinal phenotype. Wong et al. (22) found CDX1 mRNA and protein expression in all samples of Barrett's metaplasia, but not in normal esophageal squamous or gastric body epithelia. The presence of CDX2 protein and mRNA has also been shown in Barrett's metaplasia cells of the intestinal type in squamous epithelium of a proportion of patients with Barrett's metaplasia, and in esophageal adenocarcinoma (20,23). Furthermore, several inflammatory cytokines through NF-κB signaling are implicated in Barrett's progression in patients, and these same cytokines, as well as conjugated bile salts, were also found to increase CDX2 mRNA expression *in vitro* through NF-κB signaling (24,25).

Cell Cycle and Proliferation

Cell cycle regulatory genes known to be implicated in esophageal adenocarcinoma development include p16 (CDK inhibitor) and cyclin D1(CD1). Inactivation of p16 located on chromosome 9p or the overexpression of CD1 promote hyperphosphorylation of the retinoblastoma protein (Rb); phosphorylation inactivates Rb and stimulates proliferation via the cell cycle and the transition between phase G1 to S (Figure 6.2) (26). In organized epithelia, downregulation of CD1 expression is necessary for ordered differentiation—preventing unchecked proliferation (27). Hyperproliferation has been consistently observed in Barrett's metaplasia by many assays, including immunohistochemistry staining for division markers such as proliferating cell nuclear antigen (PCNA) and Ki67, and flow cytometry for DNA content (28–31). In Barrett's esophagus, CD1 has been proposed as an earlier or end-point biomarker for cancer development because histochemically assessed cyclin D1 overexpression has been documented in Barrett's esophagus and esophageal adenocarcinoma (32). Prospective analysis has shown that Barrett's metaplasia patients with cyclin D1 overexpression were at increased risk of cancer development compared to patients in whom this expression was normal (32).

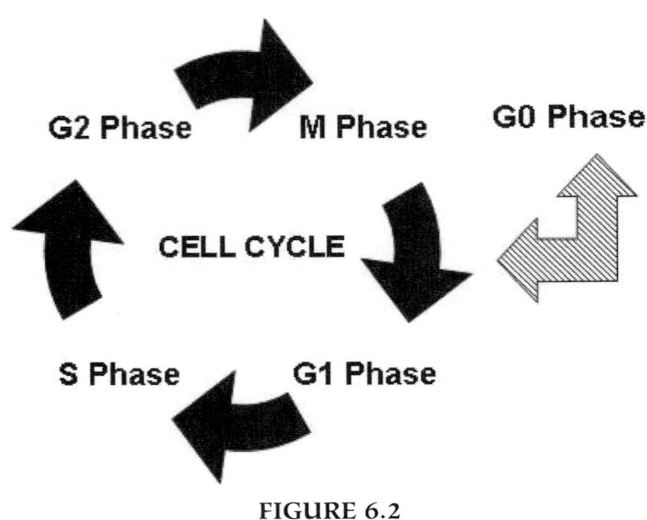

FIGURE 6.2

Cell cycle regulatory genes known to be implicated in esophageal adenocarcinoma development.

CDK Inhibitors (p16 and p27)

Due to a loss of control over the cell cycle, most notably through p16 lesions, a selection bias is conferred to a cell resulting in clonal expansion thus permitting the affected cells to grow and spread within Barrett's segments. Subsequently, these clones accumulate further genetic abnormalities that confer proliferative and survival advantage over normal cells and progress to esophageal adenocarcinoma (5,33). Many alterations of p16 are commonly observed in Barrett's metaplasia and include loss of heterozygosity, sequence mutation, and methylation of the promoter (29,34,35). Because the inactivation of 1 allele occurs in 85% to 90% of patients, the prognostic significance of p16 is not likely to be too important, but its presence in metaplastic tissues maybe an important early marker (33,36,37).

Similarly, over 80% of esophageal adenocarcinoma demonstrates low protein levels of another CDK inhibitor and tumor suppressor gene, p27, paradoxically despite increased mRNA, potentially through posttranscriptional regulation of the gene (38). That is, for p27 to arrest the cell cycle it must be localized to the nucleus while at least 50% of high-grade dysplasia (HGD) reported by Singh et al. (38) had cytoplasmic localization of the protein. This loss of localized staining for p27 correlated with higher histologic grade, depth of invasion, lymph node metastasis, and shorter survival. Therefore for p27 to be a valuable marker, one must understand its localization and posttranslational status—adding another layer of complexity to any diagnostic schema (i.e., in situ hybridization).

Cyclooxygenase-2

As alluded to before, inflammation, proliferation, and mutagenesis go hand in hand. Cyclooxygenase-2 (COX-2) is an enzyme normally found in the kidney and brain with inducible expression in most other tissues, including the esophagus, during inflammation in response to interleukins, cytokines, hormones, growth factors, and tumor promoters (13,39). Prostaglandins (PGE2) are implicated in carcinogenesis because they prolong the survival of abnormal cells by inhibiting apoptosis, but accumulated genetic changes result. Prostaglandins also directly increase cell proliferation while promoting angiogenesis and invasion and can induce tumor resistance to localized host immune responses (40).

Expression of COX-2 in the distal esophagus has been shown to be highly correlative with the amount of acid exposure based on pH monitoring, and though, the normal esophagus demonstrates COX-2 expression, its expression was found to be significantly increased in Barrett's metaplasia and even more in HGD and esophageal adenocarcinoma (41–43). Expression of COX-2 might be of prognostic value in esophageal adenocarcinoma as the COX-2 immunoreactivity in cancer tissues showed that patients with high COX-2 expression were more likely to develop distant metastases and local recurrence and had significantly reduced survival rates when compared to those with low expression (44). Recent data also suggest that COX-2 may be an early marker associated with reflux that can regress toward normal after reflux surgery (43). Together, these data illustrate how chronic inflammation can contribute to the carcinogenesis process in the gastrointestinal tract, but the prognostic value of overexpression of COX-2 in Barrett's metaplasia has not been documented in prospective studies (45). To this end, the ASPECT Trial, a phase III randomized study of aspirin and esomeprazole chemoprevention in Barrett's metaplasia, is a European, multicenter, randomized controlled trial of low- or high-dose esomeprazole with or without low-dose aspirin that should help elucidate the utility of COX-2 chemoprevention strategies in halting the progression toward cancer (46,47).

Progression of Dysplasia

Avoiding Apoptosis

The Bcl-2 family of proto-oncogenes blocks apoptosis (48). It was found to be increased in reflux esophagitis, nondysplastic Barrett's and low-grade dysplastic Barrett's epithelium, but low or virtually absent in high-grade dysplasia and carcinomas (49–51). It has been proposed that an apoptotic balance must be upset for transformation of metaplasia to adenocarcinoma, such that the cell switches toward an antiapoptotic phenotype due to increased Bcl-xl and decreased Bax expression (51,52). Inhibition of apoptosis by overexpression of Bcl-2 protein occurs mainly early in the neoplastic progression and later diminishes perhaps due to loss of normal cellular processes as tumor cells take on more mutations. Therefore, as malignancy appears, cells acquire other ways of avoiding apoptosis (i.e., p53—see later this section). For example, Bcl-xl expression demonstrated early progression in the metaplasia to low-grade to high-grade dysplasia sequence without further expression in adenocarcinoma (27%, 60%, 71%, and 59%, respectively) (53), and loss of expression was associated with poor survival (52).

Telomere shortening characterizes the normal, albeit limited life span of somatic cells as compared to cells that are not subject to replicative senescence like germ line cells and stem cells. Telomerase is a ribonucleoprotein enzyme complex that restores and maintains telomere length by the addition of telomeric sequences to chromosome ends. Telomerase activation is associated with increased expression of the telomere reverse transcriptase catalytic subunit (hTERT) that has been shown to be upregulated in Barrett's metaplasia, dysplasia, and adenocarcinoma, as compared to normal tissue (54). Although the prognostic significance of this has been contested (55), the majority of esophageal adenocarcinomas and high-grade dysplasia biopsies contained high levels of telomerase RNA, the greatest increase occurred during the transition from low- to high-grade dysplasia (56).

The tumor suppressor gene p53 has several critical functions within the cell, the most important is its role in signaling cells for repair or apoptosis, the so-called guardian of the genome (57). The p53 gene at chromosome 17p13 encodes a protein that monitors the integrity of the genome and halts cell cycle progression at G1 (via p21) if the genome is damaged, allowing time for DNA repair. When DNA damage occurs and p53 is functioning correctly, it leads to cell cycle arrest to allow for DNA repair or apoptosis if the damage is excessive (tetraploidy and aneuploidy—see next section). Loss or a mutation of p53 is probably the most common single genetic change in all cancers, including esophageal adenocarcinoma (31,58,59). Loss of heterozygosity of the p53 locus has been found in 75%–80% of esophageal adenocarcinomas as well as in 79% of patients with high-grade dysplasia, 42% of low-grade dysplasia, and 14% of Barrett's metaplasia (31). Mutations of p53 were found in 29%–66% of patients with Barrett's metaplasia and low-grade dysplasia and in 40–88% with high-grade dysplasia/adenocarcinoma31,60. 17p loss of heterozygosity analysis performed on endoscopic biopsies identified patients with Barrett's esophagus at risk of neoplastic progression within surveillance programs; therefore, it could supplement histology in determining the frequency that surveillance endoscopy should be performed (31,61,62). Reid et al. (31) found patients with p53 loss of heterozygosity to be at increased risk for progression to adenocarcinoma, high-grade dysplasia, increased 4N, and aneuploidy. In conclusion, there is clear evidence that p53 gene alterations are early and frequent events associated with malignant transformation of Barrett's esophagus.

Loss of Heterozygosity and Aneuploidy

As discussed above, loss of heterozygosity is a strong and significant predictor of progression to esophageal cancer as well as to surrogate endpoints, including increased 4N, aneuploidy, and high-grade dysplasia, in Barrett's esophagus. The chromosomal regions most commonly lost in the early stages of the M-D-A progression are 5q (APC), 9p (p16), 13q (Rb), 17p (p53) and 18q (DCC) (61,63,64). Increased tetraploid DNA and aneuploid DNA content detected by flow cytometry reflect abnormal proliferative capacity (30). In Barrett's epithelium, chromosome number abnormalities are associated with progression to dysplasia and rarely occur in normal tissue. Its predictive value has been extensively studied by the Seattle group, who have shown in prospective studies that tetraploidy is a strong and significant predictor of progression to aneuploidy, dysplasia, and cancer (29–31). The 5-year cumulative incidence of cancer was 28% in patients with Barrett's metaplasia with either aneuploidy or tetraploidy, compared to 0% in those with normal cytometric results. Based on these results, the Seattle group has included flow cytometry analysis in its assessment protocol of Barrett's esophagus patients and offers annual endoscopic surveillance to those with cytometry abnormalities detected, even if no HGD is present.

The most consistent numerical chromosomal abnormalities found in early cytogenetic studies of dysplastic Barrett's mucosa and adenocarcinoma comprised a loss of the Y-chromosome, in 31%–93% of tumors (65–67). Frequent structural rearrangements in esophageal adenocarcinomas were found in the 1p, 3q, 11p-13, and 22p regions. Doak et al. (68) showed chromosome 4 and 8 hyperploidy to represent the earliest and most common alterations identified using tissue from endoscopic cytology brushings (metaplasia 89% and 71%, low-grade dysplasia 90% and 75%, high-grade dysplasia 88% and 100%, carcinoma 100% and 100% respectively). Croft et al. (69) also found certain chromosome changes to be absent in low-grade dysplastic lesions, whereas a large amount of widespread instability was present in high dysplastic lesions (chromosome 4 amplification) and adenocarcinomas (with chromosome 8 amplified most frequently).

Later Alterations: Invasion and Metastases

Cell to Cell Adhesion Genes

Reduced cell–cell adhesion promotes growth of epithelial cells as contact inhibition of proliferation is lost. A potential crucial step toward invasion and metastases involves dysregulation of cell adhesion molecules. The cadherins, E-cadherin-catenin complex (E-cadherin), belong to a family of calcium-dependent cell adhesion molecules that form part of the adherens junction complex providing tight adhesions between epithelial cells. One of the earliest recognized molecular events in the progression of Barrett's esophagus to cancer was that E-cadherin expression was reduced in both Barrett's esophagus and esophageal adenocarcinoma and correlated with a greater frequency of lymph node metastasis and worse prognosis (70,71). Epigenetic silencing by aberrant methylation of the E-cadherin promoter seems to be a common cause of inactivation in adenocarcinomas, more so than gene mutation (72). Another component of the adherens junction complex, b-catenin, is known to have an important role in cell-signaling (73). The b-catenin protein can translocate to the nucleus, where it complexes with the transcription regulator proteins to activate transcription of oncogenes including c-myc and cyclin D1. However, oncogene activation is limited by the normal function of the APC gene product that normally targets b-catenin for degradation (74). Nuclear and cytoplasmic instead of membranous b-catenin localization has been described to occur frequently in esophageal adenocarcinomas (75,76).

The CD44 gene produces a variety of glycosylated cell surface proteins that are involved in cell–cell adhesion and matrix interactions. Several reports have focused on the expression of certain splice variants of this large 20 exon gene in esophageal adenocarcinoma. CD44V6 was detected by immunohistochemistry in up to 63% of adenocarcinomas and was associated with more aggressive pathological features (77,78).

The cysteine protease cathepsin B (CTSB) gene codes for a lysosomal enzyme that has been shown to be both overexpressed and to exhibit altered localization in cancers (79). Overexpression or altered localization of CTSB is thought to result in degradation of the basement membrane facilitating tumor invasion and metastasis. Characterization of CTSB in esophageal adenocarcinomas demonstrated that it was amplified and overexpressed (80,81). Other mechanisms (posttranslational) in addition to gene amplification may be important with regard to CTSB because gene amplification and mRNA expression were found in less than 25% of tumors, while protein staining was detected in 75% of tumors (82). These data support an important role for CTSB gene amplification and CTSB protein overexpression in invasive esophageal cancers.

CONCLUSION

The dramatic increase in esophageal adenocarcinoma incidence over the last few decades has stimulated research interest in the earliest molecular phases of its development. The most important genetic events in the neoplastic progression of Barrett's metaplasia concern loss of p16 and p53 (17p loss of heterozygosity), but also loss of APC, Rb, and DCC with aneuploidy less likely to be directive but nonetheless an important marker. Most importantly, no single genetic marker is sufficient to enable prediction of which patient will or will not develop cancer in the setting of Barrett's metaplasia. Although dysplasia has been the traditional risk factor and its presence is an indication for more vigilant surveillance and perhaps for ablative therapies, prospective studies on the prognostic significance of dysplasia, particularly low-grade dysplasia, have brought conflicting results. Perhaps combinations of markers will lead to a further differentiation in the prediction of neoplastic risk with presymptomatic intervention and individualized treatment as the ideal standard.

References

1. Jankowski JA, Harrison RF, Perry I, et al. Barrett's metaplasia. *Lancet.* 2000;356(9247):2079–2085.
2. Perry I, Tselepis C, Hoyland J, et al. Reduced cadherin/catenin complex expression in celiac disease can be reproduced in vitro by cytokine stimulation. *Lab Invest.* 1999;79(12):1489–1499.
3. Quera R, O'Sullivan K, Quigley EM. Surveillance in Barrett's oesophagus: will a strategy focused on a high-risk group reduce mortality from oesophageal adenocarcinoma? *Endoscopy.* 2006;38(2):162–169.
4. Sharma P, Wani S, Bansal A. The quest for intestinal metaplasia—is it worth the effort? *Am J Gastroenterol.* 2007;102(6):1162–1165.
5. Maley CC, Galipeau PC, Li X, et al. The combination of genetic instability and clonal expansion predicts progression to esophageal adenocarcinoma. *Cancer Res.* 2004;64(20):7629–7633.
6. Bapat SA. Evolution of cancer stem cells. *Semin Cancer Biol.* 2007;17(3):204–213.
7. Schier S, Wright NA. Stem cell relationships and the origin of gastrointestinal cancer. *Oncology.* 2005;69 Suppl 1:9–13.
8. Seery JP. Stem cells of the oesophageal epithelium. *J Cell Sci.* 2002;115(Pt 9):1783–1789.
9. Yu WY, Slack JM, Tosh D. Conversion of columnar to stratified squamous epithelium in the developing mouse oesophagus. *Dev Biol.* 2005;284(1):157–170.
10. Houghton J, Stoicov C, Nomura S, et al. Gastric cancer originating from bone marrow-derived cells. *Science.* 2004;306(5701):1568–1571.
11. Houghton J, Wang TC. Helicobacter pylori and gastric cancer: a new paradigm for inflammation-associated epithelial cancers. *Gastroenterology.* 2005;128(6):1567–1578.
12. Lambert R, Hainaut P, Parkin DM. Premalignant lesions of the esophagogastric mucosa. *Semin Oncol.* 2004;31(4):498–512.
13. Ling FC, Baldus SE, Khochfar J, et al. Association of COX-2 expression with corresponding active and chronic inflammatory reactions in Barrett's metaplasia and progression to cancer. *Histopathology.* 2007;50(2):203–209.
14. Clement G, Braunschweig R, Pasquier N, et al. Methylation of APC, TIMP3, and TERT: a new predictive marker to distinguish Barrett's oesophagus patients at risk for malignant transformation. *J Pathol.* 2006;208(1):100–107.
15. Lengauer C, Kinzler KW, Vogelstein B. Genetic instabilities in human cancers. *Nature.* 1998;396(6712):643–649.
16. Renan MJ. How many mutations are required for tumorigenesis? Implications from human cancer data. *Mol Carcinog.* 1993;7(3):139–146.
17. Kerkhof M, Bax DA, Moons LM, et al. Does CDX2 expression predict Barrett's metaplasia in oesophageal columnar epithelium without goblet cells? *Aliment Pharmacol Ther.* 2006;24(11–12):1613–1621.
18. Steininger H, Pfofe DA, Muller H, et al. Expression of CDX2 and MUC2 in Barrett's mucosa. *Pathol Res Pract.* 2005;201(8–9):573–577.
19. Chinyama CN, Marshall RE, Owen WJ, et al. Expression of MUC1 and MUC2 mucin gene products in Barrett's metaplasia, dysplasia and adenocarcinoma: an immunopathological study with clinical correlation. *Histopathology.* 1999;35(6):517–524.
20. Phillips RW, Frierson HF, Jr., Moskaluk CA. Cdx2 as a marker of epithelial intestinal differentiation in the esophagus. *Am J Surg Pathol.* 2003;27(11):1442–1447.
21. Silberg DG, Swain GP, Suh ER, et al. Cdx1 and cdx2 expression during intestinal development. *Gastroenterology.* 2000;119(4):961–971.
22. Wong NA, Wilding J, Bartlett S, et al. CDX1 is an important molecular mediator of Barrett's metaplasia. *Proc Natl Acad Sci U S A.* 2005;102(21):7565–7570.
23. Eda A, Osawa H, Yanaka I, et al. Expression of homeobox gene CDX2 precedes that of CDX1 during the progression of intestinal metaplasia. *J Gastroenterol.* 2002;37(2):94–100.
24. O'Riordan JM, Abdel-latif MM, Ravi N, et al. Proinflammatory cytokine and nuclear factor kappa-B expression along the inflammation-metaplasia-dysplasia-adenocarcinoma sequence in the esophagus. *Am J Gastroenterol.* 2005;100(6):1257–1264.
25. Kazumori H, Ishihara S, Rumi MA, et al. Bile acids directly augment caudal related homeobox gene Cdx2 expression in oesophageal keratinocytes in Barrett's epithelium. *Gut.* 2006;55(1):16–25.
26. Shapiro GI, Edwards CD, Rollins BJ. The physiology of p16(INK4A)-mediated G1 proliferative arrest. *Cell Biochem Biophys.* 2000;33(2):189–197.
27. Zhang P. The cell cycle and development: redundant roles of cell cycle regulators. *Curr Opin Cell Biol.* 1999;11(6):655–662.
28. Haggitt RC, Reid BJ, Rabinovitch PS, et al. Barrett's esophagus. Correlation between mucin histochemistry, flow cytometry, and histologic diagnosis for predicting increased cancer risk. *Am J Pathol.* 1988;131(1):53–61.
29. Rabinovitch PS, Longton G, Blount PL, et al. Predictors of progression in Barrett's esophagus III: baseline flow cytometric variables. *Am J Gastroenterol.* 2001;96(11):3071–3083.
30. Reid BJ, Levine DS, Longton G, et al Predictors of progression to cancer in Barrett's esophagus: baseline histology and flow cytometry identify low- and high-risk patient subsets. *Am J Gastroenterol.* 2000;95(7):1669–1676.
31. Reid BJ, Prevo LJ, Galipeau PC, et al. Predictors of progression in Barrett's esophagus II: baseline 17p (p53) loss of heterozygosity identifies a patient subset at increased risk for neoplastic progression. *Am J Gastroenterol.* 2001;96(10):2839–2848.
32. Bani-Hani K, Martin IG, Hardie LJ, et al. Prospective study of cyclin D1 overexpression in Barrett's esophagus: association with increased risk of adenocarcinoma. *J Natl Cancer Inst.* 2000;92(16):1316–1321.
33. Wong DJ, Paulson TG, Prevo LJ, et al. p16(INK4a) lesions are common, early abnormalities that undergo clonal expansion in Barrett's metaplastic epithelium. *Cancer Res.* 2001;61(22):8284–8289.
34. Bian YS, Osterheld MC, Fontolliet C, et al. p16 inactivation by methylation of the CDKN2A promoter occurs early during neoplastic progression in Barrett's esophagus. *Gastroenterology.* 2002;122(4):1113–1121.
35. Schulmann K, Sterian A, Berki A, et al. Inactivation of p16, RUNX3, and HPP1 occurs early in Barrett's-associated neoplastic progression and predicts progression risk. *Oncogene.* 2005;24(25):4138–4148.
36. Eads CA, Lord RV, Kurumboor SK, et al. Fields of aberrant CpG island hypermethylation in Barrett's esophagus and associated adenocarcinoma. *Cancer Res.* 2000;60(18):5021–5026.
37. Fahmy M, Skacel M, Gramlich TL, et al. Chromosomal gains and genomic loss of p53 and p16 genes in Barrett's esophagus detected by fluorescence in situ hybridization of cytology specimens. *Mod Pathol.* 2004;17(5):588–596.
38. Singh SP, Lipman J, Goldman H, et al. Loss or altered subcellular localization of p27 in Barrett's associated adenocarcinoma. *Cancer Res.*1998;58(8):1730–1735.
39. Buskens CJ, Sivula A, van Rees BP, et al. Comparison of cyclooxygenase 2 expression in adenocarcinomas of the gastric cardia and distal oesophagus. *Gut.* 2003;52(12):1678–1683.
40. Wilson KT, Fu S, Ramanujam KS, et al. Increased expression of inducible nitric oxide synthase and cyclooxygenase-2 in Barrett's esophagus and associated adenocarcinomas. *Cancer Res.* 1998;58(14):2929–2934.

41. Lagorce C, Paraf F, Vidaud D, et al. Cyclooxygenase-2 is expressed frequently and early in Barrett's oesophagus and associated adenocarcinoma. *Histopathology.* 2003;42(5):457–465.
42. Lurje G, Vallbohmer D, Collet PH, et al. COX-2 mRNA expression is significantly increased in acid-exposed compared to nonexposed squamous epithelium in gastroesophageal reflux disease. *J Gastrointest Surg.* 2007;11(9):1105–1111.
43. Vallbohmer D, DeMeester SR, Oh DS, et al. Antireflux surgery normalizes cyclooxygenase-2 expression in squamous epithelium of the distal esophagus. *Am J Gastroenterol.* 2006;101(7):1458–1466.
44. Buskens CJ, Van Rees BP, Sivula A, et al. Prognostic significance of elevated cyclooxygenase 2 expression in patients with adenocarcinoma of the esophagus. *Gastroenterology.* 2002;122(7):1800–1807.
45. Buttar NS, Wang KK, Anderson MA, et al. The effect of selective cyclooxygenase-2 inhibition in Barrett's esophagus epithelium: an in vitro study. *J Natl Cancer Inst.* 2002;94(6):422–429.
46. Leedham S, Jankowski J. The evidence base of proton pump inhibitor chemopreventative agents in Barrett's esophagus—the good, the bad, and the flawed! *Am J Gastroenterol.* 2007;102(1):21–23.
47. Robertson EV, Jankowski JA. Genetics of gastroesophageal cancer: paradigms, paradoxes, and prognostic utility. *Am J Gastroenterol.* 2008 Feb;103(2):443–449.
48. Reed JC, Doctor KS, Godzik A. The domains of apoptosis: a genomics perspective. *Sci STKE.* 2004;2004(239):re9.
49. Chatelain D, Flejou JF. High-grade dysplasia and superficial adenocarcinoma in Barrett's esophagus: histological mapping and expression of p53, p21 and Bcl-2 oncoproteins. *Virchows Arch.* 2003;442(1):18–24.
50. Rioux-Leclercq N, Turlin B, et al. Analysis of Ki-67, p53 and Bcl-2 expression in the dysplasia-carcinoma sequence of Barrett's esophagus. *Oncol Rep.* 1999;6(4):877–882.
51. van der Woude CJ, Jansen PL, Tiebosch AT, et al. Expression of apoptosis-related proteins in Barrett's metaplasia-dysplasia-carcinoma sequence: a switch to a more resistant phenotype. *Hum Pathol.* 2002;33(7):686–692.
52. Raouf AA, Evoy DA, Carton E, et al. Loss of Bcl-2 expression in Barrett's dysplasia and adenocarcinoma is associated with tumor progression and worse survival but not with response to neoadjuvant chemoradiation. *Dis Esophagus.* 2003;16(1):17–23.
53. Iravani S, Zhang HQ, Yuan ZQ, et al. Modification of insulin-like growth factor 1 receptor, c-Src, and Bcl-XL protein expression during the progression of Barrett's neoplasia. *Hum Pathol.* 2003;34(10):975–982.
54. Lord RV, Salonga D, Danenberg KD, et al. Telomerase reverse transcriptase expression is increased early in the Barrett's metaplasia, dysplasia, adenocarcinoma sequence. *J Gastrointest Surg.* 2000;4(2):135–142.
55. Barclay JY, Morris A, Nwokolo CU. Telomerase, hTERT and splice variants in Barrett's oesophagus and oesophageal adenocarcinoma. *Eur J Gastroenterol Hepatol.* 2005;17(2):221–227.
56. Morales CP, Lee EL, Shay JW. In situ hybridization for the detection of telomerase RNA in the progression from Barrett's esophagus to esophageal adenocarcinoma. *Cancer.* 1998;83(4):652–659.
57. Koppert LB, Wijnhoven BP, van Dekken H, et al. The molecular biology of esophageal adenocarcinoma. *J Surg Oncol.* 2005;92(3):169–190.
58. Hamelin R, Flejou JF, Muzeau F, et al. TP53 gene mutations and p53 protein immunoreactivity in malignant and premalignant Barrett's esophagus. *Gastroenterology.* 1994;107(4):1012–1018.
59. Prevo LJ, Sanchez CA, Galipeau PC, et al. p53-mutant clones and field effects in Barrett's esophagus. *Cancer Res.* 1999;59(19):4784–4787.
60. Bian YS, Osterheld MC, Bosman FT, et al. p53 gene mutation and protein accumulation during neoplastic progression in Barrett's esophagus. *Mod Pathol.* 2001;14(5):397–403.
61. Dolan K, Morris AI, Gosney JR, et al. Loss of heterozygosity on chromosome 17p predicts neoplastic progression in Barrett's esophagus. *J Gastroenterol Hepatol.* 2003;18(6):683–689.
62. Dolan K, Walker SJ, Gosney J, et al. TP53 mutations in malignant and premalignant Barrett's esophagus. *Dis Esophagus.* 2003;16(2):83–89.
63. Dolan K, Garde J, Walker SJ, et al. LOH at the sites of the DCC, APC, and TP53 tumor suppressor genes occurs in Barrett's metaplasia and dysplasia adjacent to adenocarcinoma of the esophagus. *Hum Pathol.* 1999;30(12):1508–1514.
64. Suspiro A, Pereira AD, Afonso A, et al. Losses of heterozygosity on chromosomes 9p and 17p are frequent events in Barrett's metaplasia not associated with dysplasia or adenocarcinoma. *Am J Gastroenterol.* 2003;98(4):728–734.
65. Garewal HS, Sampliner R, Liu Y, et al. Chromosomal rearrangements in Barrett's esophagus. A premalignant lesion of esophageal adenocarcinoma. *Cancer Genet Cytogenet.* 1989;42(2):281–286.
66. Krishnadath KK, Tilanus HW, Alers JC, et al. Detection of genetic changes in Barrett's adenocarcinoma and Barrett's esophagus by DNA in situ hybridization and immunohistochemistry. *Cytometry.* 1994;15(2):176–184.
67. Raskind WH, Norwood T, Levine DS, et al. Persistent clonal areas and clonal expansion in Barrett's esophagus. *Cancer Res.* 1992;52(10):2946–2950.
68. Doak SH, Jenkins GJ, Parry EM, et al. Chromosome 4 hyperploidy represents an early genetic aberration in premalignant Barrett's oesophagus. *Gut.* 2003;52(5):623–628.
69. Croft J, Parry EM, Jenkins GJ, et al. Analysis of the premalignant stages of Barrett's oesophagus through to adenocarcinoma by comparative genomic hybridization. *Eur J Gastroenterol Hepatol.* 2002;14(11):1179–1186.
70. Bailey T, Biddlestone L, Shepherd N, et al. Altered cadherin and catenin complexes in the Barrett's esophagus-dysplasia-adenocarcinoma sequence: correlation with disease progression and dedifferentiation. *Am J Pathol.* 1998;152(1):135–144.
71. Swami S, Kumble S, Triadafilopoulos G. E-cadherin expression in gastroesophageal reflux disease, Barrett's esophagus, and esophageal adenocarcinoma: an immunohistochemical and immunoblot study. *Am J Gastroenterol.* 1995;90(10):1808–1813.
72. Wijnhoven BP, de Both NJ, van Dekken H, et al. E-cadherin gene mutations are rare in adenocarcinomas of the oesophagus. *Br J Cancer.* 1999;80(10):1652–1657.
73. Morin PJ. Beta-catenin signaling and cancer. *Bioessays.* 1999;21(12):1021–1030.
74. Clement G, Braunschweig R, Pasquier N, et al. Alterations of the Wnt signaling pathway during the neoplastic progression of Barrett's esophagus. *Oncogene.* 2006;25(21):3084–3092.
75. Bian YS, Osterheld MC, Bosman FT, et al. Nuclear accumulation of beta-catenin is a common and early event during neoplastic progression of Barrett esophagus. *Am J Clin Pathol.* 2000;114(4):583–590.
76. Osterheld MC, Bian YS, Bosman FT, et al. Beta-catenin expression and its association with prognostic factors in adenocarcinoma developed in Barrett esophagus. *Am J Clin Pathol.* 2002;117(3):451–456.
77. Bottger TC, Youssef V, Dutkowski P, et al. Expression of CD44 variant proteins in adenocarcinoma of Barrett's esophagus and its relation to prognosis. *Cancer.* 1998;83(6):1074–1080.
78. Lagorce-Pages C, Paraf F, Dubois S, et al. Expression of CD44 in premalignant and malignant Barrett's oesophagus. *Histopathology.* 1998;32(1):7–14.
79. Keppler D, Sameni M, Moin K, et al. Tumor progression and angiogenesis: cathepsin B & Co. *Biochem Cell Biol.* 1996;74(6):799–810.
80. Altorjay A, Paal B, Sohar N, et al. Significance and prognostic value of lysosomal enzyme activities measured in surgically operated adenocarcinomas of the gastroesophageal junction and squamous cell carcinomas of the lower third of esophagus. *World J Gastroenterol.* 2005;11(37):5751–5756.
81. Hughes SJ, Glover TW, Zhu XX, et al. A novel amplicon at 8p22–23 results in overexpression of cathepsin B in esophageal adenocarcinoma. *Proc Natl Acad Sci U S A.* 1998;95(21):12410–12415.
82. Lin L, Aggarwal S, Glover TW, et al. A minimal critical region of the 8p22–23 amplicon in esophageal adenocarcinomas defined using sequence tagged site-amplification mapping and quantitative polymerase chain reaction includes the GATA-4 gene. *Cancer Res.* 2000 Mar 1;60(5):1341–7.

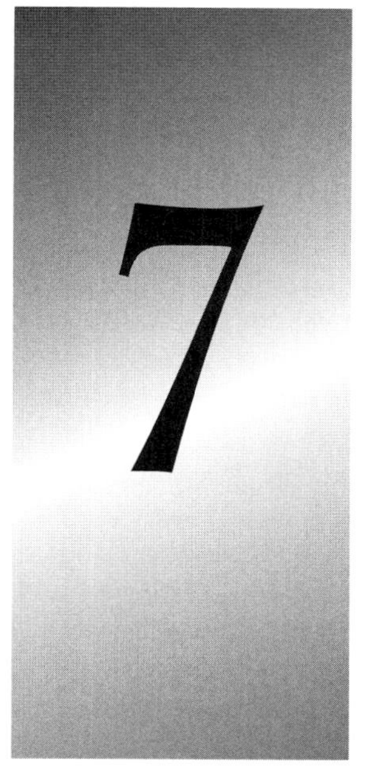

7 Barrett's Esophagus: Preclinical Models for Investigation

Xiaoxin Chen
Chung S. Yang

Animal models are great tools for research on human diseases. An ideal animal model should recapitulate the disease in humans in etiology, pathogenesis, and molecular features. Animals should be reasonably easy to maintain, be of sufficient size to provide enough samples for analysis, be affordable, and survive long enough for experimental observation. It is expected that any single model system has its limitations, or there is no perfect animal model. Therefore, multiple models are desired to meet the needs of various research on mechanism, prevention, and therapy of the disease in humans. These principles apply to the case of animal models of Barrett's esophagus (BE) and esophageal adenocarcinoma (EAC). Readers are encouraged to refer to recent review articles on this subject (1–3).

SELECTION OF ANIMAL SPECIES

The human esophagus is covered with non-keratinized stratified squamous epithelium containing submucosal glands. Histology of the esophagus is a critical issue to consider for developing an animal model of BE. Most commonly used laboratory animals have stratified squamous epithelium in the esophagus, except zebrafish. Two histologic features need to be taken into consideration: submucosal glands and the keratinization status of the squamous epithelium. Submucosal glands normally secrete mucus for protection of the epithelium against gastroesophageal reflux. Studies on both human tissues and animal models have suggested that the neck of submucosal glands may contain so-called esophageal stem cells, which may be a cellular origin of BE (4). Keratinization indicates terminal differentiation necessary for protection of the esophagus from mechanical and chemical injuries.

Rodents, especially rats (e.g., Sprague-Dawley, F344, Wistar), are the most commonly used animals to study BE and EAC. This is mainly because surgery on the rat esophagus is relatively easy to perform. Rats are highly susceptible to BE and EAC induced by reflux of small intestinal contents, or combined reflux of both gastric and small intestinal contents. Reflux of gastric contents alone has never been reported to induce BE in rats. Nevertheless, the histologic structure and pathology of the rat esophagus are dissimilar to those of the human esophagus in the following aspects: (a) there are no submucosal glands in the rat esophagus; (b) there is marked keratinization in the squamous epithelium of the rat esophagus; (c) the normal rat esophagus often shows endophytic epithelial ingrowths that invade the lamina propria of the mucosa but never extend through it, and should not be regarded as precancerous lesions; (d) esophageal papilloma is frequently seen in the rat, but rarely in humans; and (e) rat esophageal carcinomas almost never metastasize (5).

The mouse esophagus is very similar to the rat esophagus in histology. The major advantage of mice is the potential of genetic modifications for mechanistic studies. However, the mouse esophagus may respond to gastroesophageal reflux and carcinogens in a different way than the rat esophagus (6,7). Therefore, caution should be taken when a rat model is translated into a mouse model of BE.

Dogs, cats, pigs, rabbits, and opossums have been used to study mechanism and therapy of gastroesophageal reflux disease (GERD) and BE. These animals have non-keratinized stratified squamous epithelium in their esophagi. Dogs, pigs, raccoons, guinea pigs, and opossums also have submucosal glands (8). Despite anatomic differences from humans, dogs and pigs are very similar to humans in gastrointestinal physiology. They have been used extensively as gastrointestinal models for nutritional studies. Pigs, especially miniature pigs, may be even better model animals than dogs because of closer anatomic similarities to humans, better acceptance by the public, and lower cost of maintenance. In large animals, disease progression can be monitored by endoscopy and biopsy. Their esophagi are big enough to provide multiple samples for pathologic and molecular analysis. Moreover, gastroesophageal reflux and hiatal hernia are seen in dogs and cats (9,10). Pigs also suffer from GERD and stress ulceration of the esophagus (11). Even metaplastic columnar esophageal epithelium has been reported in cats as a complication of GERD (12).

Different strains of the same species may vary significantly in their susceptibility to BE induced by reflux surgery and/or genetic manipulations. This is especially true when mice are used for model development.

SELECTION OF EXPERIMENTAL METHODS

Genetic modifications have not yet successfully induced BE in animals. Esophagus-specific transgenic overexpression of CDX2, an intestinal transcription factor, failed to produce intestinal metaplasia in the mouse esophagus according to Dr. Anil Rustgi (University of Pennsylvania, personal communication).

Surgery is still the most commonly used method for creating reflux of gastric and/or small intestinal contents into the esophagus. Various surgical procedures and modifications have been designed to induce GERD, BE, and EAC by gastric reflux, small intestinal reflux (bile reflux and pancreatic reflux), or combined reflux. Although rats were used in most previous studies, mice and large animals are also suitable for surgery. Nitrosamines (e.g., methyl-n-amylnitrosamine, 2,6-dimethylnitrosomorpholine, methylbenzylnitrosamine, diethylnitrosamine), or medications (e.g., pentagastrin) can be combined with surgery to enhance carcinogenesis. However, nitrosamines alone tend to induce esophageal squamous cell carcinoma (ESCC), not EAC. A combination of reflux surgery and nitrosamine produces ESCC, EAC, and adenosquamous carcinomas (13,14). Interestingly, dietary zinc deficiency induces glandular metaplasia in the mouse esophagus (15). Although no goblet cells are present, it does suggest that zinc may play a critical role in transdifferentiation of esophageal epithelial cells.

Esophageal mucosal stripping in dogs induces regeneration of squamous epithelium only. However, creation of gastroesophageal reflux and stimulation of acid secretion in addition to mucosal stripping predominantly induces regeneration of columnar epithelium. Continuity of the regenerated columnar epithelium with ducts of submucosal glands suggests the submucosal gland as the cellular origin (16,17). Anti-reflux surgery and antacid therapy with Omeprazole allow regeneration of squamous islands in columnar epithelium (17). Unfortunately, goblet cells, which are diagnostic of BE, are not observed in these studies. Nevertheless, this procedure has the potential of inducing BE in the dog esophagus after a long period of reflux, or when used in combination with other procedures.

Esophagoduodenostomy (also called *esophagoduodenal anastomosis* (EDA)) in rats was developed by Dr. Tom DeMeester's group (University of Southern California) (13). At 22 weeks after surgery, EDA itself produced EAC in 7% rats and benign diffuse papillomatosis in 50% rats, but did not induce ESCC. Addition of a nitrosamine increased the incidences of both ESCC (~40%) and EAC (~30%). Most rat tumors showed both ESCC and EAC with nests of cells producing keratin in one area and mucin in another. Only a small percentage of tumors were pure, well-differentiated EAC (14,18). When we adapted this model in our lab (19), rats developed BE, BE with dysplasia, and EAC at a low incidence rate (~10%). However, when iron (50 mg Fe/kg/month, i.p.) was administered to the animals to alleviate the postoperative iron-deficiency anemia, the incidence of EAC dramatically increased to 73% at 30 weeks after surgery. Similar to EDA, esophagojejunostomy also induces BE and EAC in rats and mice.

We further modified the EDA procedure by making an anastomosis between the gastroesophageal junction and the duodenum. This procedure, known as *esophagogastroduodenal anastomosis* (EGDA), produces BE and EAC in rats without major nutritional complications and severe large-area esophagitis, which are unwanted effects of the EDA procedure (20). Compared with the other procedures, EGDA has several advantages: (a) it allows food to pass through the normal alimentary tract, and the EGDA rats have normal stomach function and normal nutritional status; (b) there is substantial reflux of both gastric and duodenal contents into the esophagus; and (c) recirculation of bile through the stomach raises the antral pH, thus resulting in gastrin release by the antral G cells. Gastrin is known to have a trophic effect on the gastrointestinal epithelium by encouraging the growth of esophageal carcinoma.

Duodeno-forestomach reflux may also induce BE without disturbance to the anti-reflux mechanism of the lower esophagus. Miwa et al. observed an incidence ESCC of 18% rats at 50 weeks after the surgery. Although they did not observe any EAC, the authors suggested that EAC might appear if the esophagus was exposed to refluxate for a longer period of time (21). Pancreaticoesophageal reflux procedures and bilio-esophageal reflux procedures were designed to examine the effects of pancreatic juice or bile on rat esophagus, respectively (22–24). It appears that pancreatic juice is carcinogenic, while bile exerts a co-carcinogenic effect when combined with pancreatic juice.

Several other procedures have also been reported to produce reflux in animals, e.g., Wendel cardioplasty, pyloplasty, gastrectomy, cardiectomy. These procedures may be combined with procedures, such as Roux-en-Y reconstruction, to manipulate the reflux constituents in the esophagus (25,26).

Recently, 2 interesting procedures have been reported in the literature: external esophageal perfusion and heterotropic transplantation (27,28). In the perfusion model, rat esophagus was cannulated at the upper esophagus and connected to a subcutaneous osmotic micropump to perfuse the esophageal lumen with bile and/or acid. In the transplantation model, a piece of rat esophagus was transplanted into the stomach or the duodenum to induce transdifferentiation into the gastric or duodenal phenotype. Because of their unique features, these newly developed procedures hold promises in studying mechanism of BE.

RAT MODEL

Pathologic phenotypes of rat surgical models are similar to each other. We have systematically compared the phenotype of the rat EGDA model to human BE and EAC (29). At week 40 after EGDA, BE, dysplasia, and EAC were found in 53.5%, 34.9%, and 25.6%, of 43 rats, respectively. Iron supplementation (4 mg Fe/kg/week, i.p.) greatly promoted esophageal lesions and increased the tumor incidence to 53.7%. Careful characterization has demonstrated that rat EGDA model mimics human carcinogenesis in 3 consecutive histopathologic stages (Figure 7.1):

1. Inflammation stage: Normal esophageal squamous epithelium develops GERD as a result of chronic reflux. At this stage, the esophageal epithelium is covered by squamous epithelium which expresses squamous differentiation markers.
2. Metaplasia/precancerous stage: Squamous epithelial cells undertake intestinal metaplasia to develop multilayered epithelium and BE. At this transition stage, esophageal epithelial cells start to lose squamous differentiation markers, and begin to express columnar differentiation markers. The esophageal epithelium consists of a mixture of squamous epithelial cells and columnar epithelial cells.
3. Dysplasia/cancer stage: Columnar epithelial cells become dysplastic, and finally develop adenocarcinoma.

Multilayered epithelium consists of 4 to 8 layers of cells that show squamous differentiation in the basal portion and columnar differentiation in the superficial layers at the neo-squamocolumnar junction, and occasionally in the mid-esophagus.

The occurrence of intestinal metaplasia, which is defined by the presence of goblet cells in the esophagus, characterizes BE. Multilayered epithelium and BE in rats resemble the lesions in human BE in morphology, mucin features, and expression of differentiation markers (keratin 7, keratin 20, Das-1, villin and trefoil factor 1). Invasive EAC in EGDA rat is observed as well-differentiated mucinous adenocarcinoma. Both in rat and human BE and EAC, p53, c-myc, and cyclooxygenase 2 are overexpressed. These similarities make the EGDA rats a useful model of human BE and EAC.

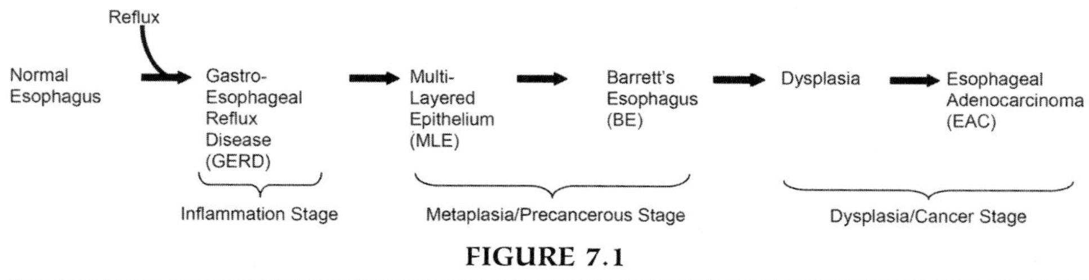

FIGURE 7.1

Pathologic progression of esophageal adenocarcinogenesis in the rat EGDA model.

Many studies have been conducted with rat surgical models by us and others to understand the mechanism, prevention, and therapy of BE and EAC. Small intestinal contents are believed to be the primary causative factor, in conjunction with gastric contents (26,30). Using *lacI* transgenic rats and the EDA model, bile reflux was found to generate gene mutations mainly at the CpG dinucleotides in the form of C to T or G to A transitions. This pattern of gene mutation is similar to *p53* mutations in human EAC (31). Dietary or tobacco carcinogens, iron supplementation, high-fat diet, antacid therapy, and certain intestinal microflora may modulate the disease process in rats (19,20,26,32–36). Accumulation of p53 and gene overexpression (e.g., cyclin D1, inducible nitric oxide synthase, cyclooxygenase 2, microsomal prostaglandin E synthase 1, prostaglandin E receptors, 5-lipoxygenase, leukotriene A4 hydrolase, and EGFR/ErbB2) are associated with the progression of the disease (25,29,37–43). Gene microarray studies have identified altered expression of many genes in rat tumor, upregulation of the DNA damage pathway and the interleukin 6 signaling pathway, and downregulation of the DNA mismatch repair pathway (44–47). Using proteomic technique, we have reported overexpression of proteins (e.g., glucose-regulated protein 94) in rat tumor in a way similar to human cancer (48).

Oxidative stress and aberrant arachidonic acid metabolism are critical in the development of EAC, and agents targeting these pathways have chemoprevention effects on the development of rat tumor (14,39–41,48–54). Other agents, such as difluoromethylornithine, nordihydroguaiaretic acid, curcumin, superoxide dismutase, thioproline, and combinations of different agents have also shown more or less chemopreventive effects on rat EAC (39,41,55–57). Biliary diversion for rats with surgically induced BE prevents the development of EAC, although it does not lead to regression of BE. It suggested that bile reflux is a major promoting factor of carcinogenesis and may be a factor to deal with for treatment of BE and prevention of EAC (58).

In order to further understand the mechanism of BE, we have recently examined the expression patterns of transcription factors and differentiation markers of squamous epithelium and columnar epithelium on serial paraffin sections of rat esophagi with immunohistochemistry. Several transcription factors and differentiation markers of squamous epithelium (p63, Sox2, K14, K4, loricrin) are found to be expressed in the squamous epithelial cells, but progressively lost during intestinal metaplasia. Meanwhile, several other transcription factors and differentiation markers of columnar epithelium (CDX1, CDX2, GATA4, HNF1α, and villin) appear in columnar epithelial cells, and eventually fully expressed in BE. Consistent with these findings in the rat model, similar expression patterns of these transcription factors and differentiation markers are observed during intestinal metaplasia in human esophageal biopsy samples (unpublished data). These data suggest that squamous de-differentiation and columnar differentiation may be the mechanism of intestinal metaplasia of the esophagus in rats. Pluripotent stem cells in the esophageal squamous epithelium are very likely a cellular origin of intestinal metaplasia (59) (Figure 7.2).

MOUSE MODEL

Mouse models of BE may offer great advantages over the rat models. Many genetically modified mouse lines are readily available for investigating the functional roles of specific genes in the development of BE. Experiments with mice are likely more economic than those with rats and large animals.

Esophagojejunostomy has been used in mice to induce BE and EAC (7). In Swiss-Webster mice, surgery alone induced BE in 42% of mice at 19 weeks after surgery. When combined with a nitrosamine, it induced BE in 20% of mice. It was surprising that carcinogen treatment alone induced BE in 12.5% of mice. Some animals developed EAC, ESCC, or adenosquamous carcinoma. Significant promotion of BE and EAC by loss of *p27* was observed using this model in *p27*$^{-/-}$ mice 60. Flavopiridol, a cyclin-dependent kinase inhibitor, had preventive effects on both BE and EAC in this model (61).

With this procedure in mice, loss of *p53* seemed to enhance carcinogenesis (62), although this study was inconclusive because of the small number of animals used. We performed EGDA on *p53-/-* mice. However, 28 of 32 operated mice died within 20 weeks after surgery and most within 8 weeks, due to spontaneous lymphomas or sarcomas. All of the 4 mice that survived 20 weeks after surgery developed visible tumors (63).

Several other mouse lines with genetic defects have been tested, such as *APC*$^{Min/+}$ mice, *iNOS* knockout mice, *COX-2* knockout mice, and *arginase* knockout mice (personal communications). In a recent study, we performed EGDA with or without gastrectomy on wild-type, *p53*^{A135V} transgenic, and *INK4a/Arf*$^{+/-}$ A/J mice. After surgery, some mice were further treated with Omeprazole or intraperitoneal iron supplementation for 20, 40, or 80 weeks. To our surprise, none of these mice developed EAC, and many developed ESCC instead. Consistent with this observation, only scattered mucinous cells were observed in the squamous epithelium of mouse esophagus, but not the multilayered epithelium or full-blown BE that was reported in the rats, *p53*$^{-/-}$ C57BL mice, and wild-type or *p27*$^{-/-}$ Swiss-Webster mice. This experiment suggests that genetic background may play a critical role in developing BE and EAC in mice.

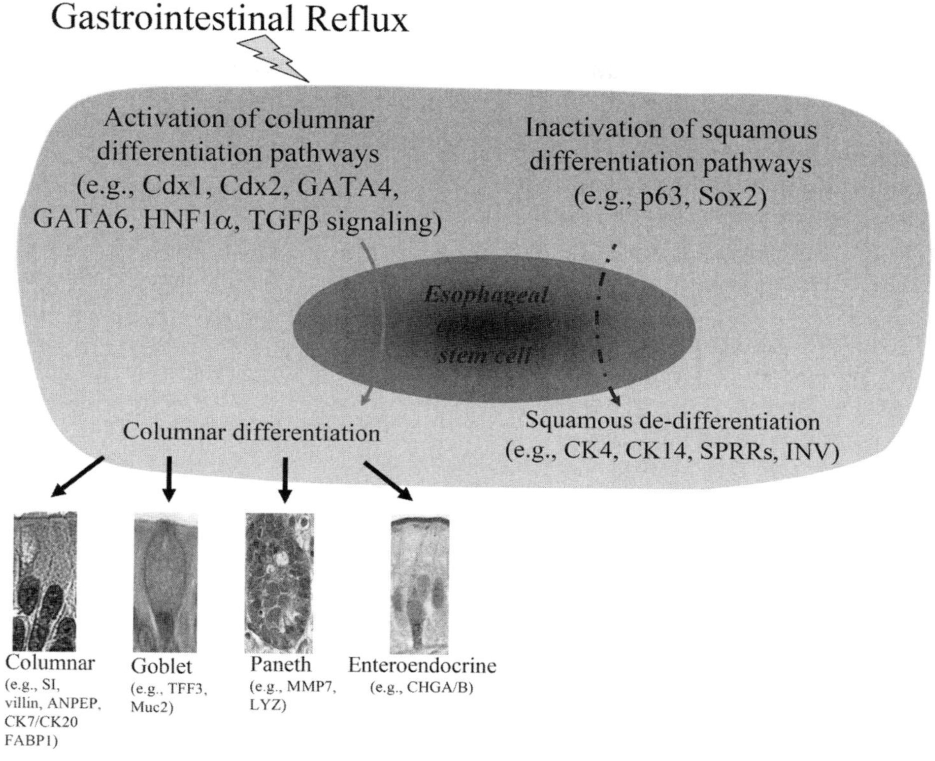

FIGURE 7.2

Proposed mechanism of intestinal metaplasia of the esophagus in the EGDA rats. When esophageal epithelial stem cells are stimulated by refluxate, the squamous differentiation pathway may be inactivated through loss of expression of some critical transcription factors. Meanwhile, the columnar differentiation pathway may be activated through gain of expression of intestinal transcription factors. In the presence of hyperproliferation and chronic inflammation, these molecular events may lead to squamous de-differentiation (i.e., loss of squamous differentiation markers [e.g., keratin 4, keratin 14, SPRRs, involucrin]), and columnar differentiation (i.e., gain of columnar differentiation markers). Once metaplasia is initiated in stem cells, it tends to undergo clonal expansion and finally develops histological intestinal metaplasia consisting of four major cell lineages with specific differentiation markers. Similar mechanism may apply to human BE.

Several issues need to be considered: (a) early death due to genetic defects, such as spontaneous tumor development of $p53^{-/-}$ mice and renal insufficiency of $COX\text{-}2^{-/-}$ mice, may not allow long-term studies; (b) mouse surgery is technically challenging because of the small size of the mouse esophagus; (c) certain genetically modified strains do not breed well, and it may take a long period of time to breed compound mutant mice.

Although a genetic mouse model of BE is currently not available yet, it is still highly feasible if the genetic background and target genes are properly selected. It is known that embryonic esophageal epithelium of $p63^{-/-}$ mice appear columnar containing both ciliated and goblet-like cells (64). A murine transgenic model introducing E1A/E1B under the control of the mouse mammary tumor virus-long terminal repeat promoter developed adenocarcinoma at the squamocolumnar junction in the foregut (65). Several relatively esophagus-specific promoters have been reported in the literature: keratin 5, keratin 6A, and keratin 14 promoters (basal cells) (66–68); ED-L2 promoter (parabasal and basal cells) (69); tamoxifen- and tetracycline-inducible systems (68,70); and *cre-lox* system driven by constitutive or inducible K14 promoters (66,71). These genetic tools will certainly help us develop a mouse model of BE.

CANINE MODEL

Cardioplasty, mucosal stripping, and other reflux procedures with dogs have been reported in the literature (16,17,25,72,73). None of these studies provided solid evidence of goblet cells in the esophagus, except one recent long-term study (25). Cardiectomy and total gastrectomy plus esophagojejunostomy were performed on dogs to induce gastric reflux and small intestinal reflux, respectively. With endoscopy, BE was detected between 18 and 39 months after cardiectomy, low-grade dysplasia between 42 and 69 months, high-grade dysplasia at 57 months, and adenocarcinoma at 63 months. For those with small intestinal reflux, BE was observed between 21 and 36 months, low-grade dysplasia between 48 and 63 months, high-grade dysplasia at 60 months, and adenocarcinoma at 66 months. Notably, these 2 cases of EAC were reported as glandular adenocarcinoma, the commonly seen form of human EAC, whereas most rat and mouse EAC are mucinous adenocarcinoma that is less commonly seen in humans. To our knowledge, this is the first study showing dogs may develop a full spectrum of pathology leading to EAC when exposed to either gastric reflux or small intestinal reflux alone for a long period of time. Further studies are needed to confirm these findings and explore the underlying mechanisms.

FUTURE PERSPECTIVES

Genetic mouse models of BE need to be developed. Such models will be very useful in studying the mechanism of BE. Since stem cells have long been hypothesized as the cellular origin of BE, recent research on esophageal stem cells has caught attention in this field (74). Mouse models will definitely help us understand how stem cells may transdifferentiate into multiple lineages of specialized columnar epithelium when stimulated by chronic gastroesophageal reflux.

When histologic and physiologic resemblance to humans is considered, a model with miniature pigs may offer many advantages over other species. Pigs are also well suited for genetic modifications. A lentiviral vector containing the human keratin 14 promoter was able to drive expression of transgenes in pig skin, and probably also in the esophagus (75). A pig model of BE will be extremely valuable for experimental therapy of BE and EAC.

Combination of genetic modifications and surgery may not only produce models of BE and EAC, but also allow us to study gene-environment interactions. Animal models may help us explain why some patients with GERD are more susceptible to BE than the others, and why white males are more likely to develop BE and EAC than black males.

References

1. Chen X, Yang CS. Esophageal adenocrcinoma: a review and perspectives on the mechanism of carcinogenesis and chemoprevention. *Carcinogenesis.* 2001;22:1119–1129.
2. Koak Y, Winslet M. Changing role of in vivo models in columnar-lined lower esophagus. *Dis Esophagus.* 2002;15:271–277.
3. Pera M, Pera M. Experimental Barrett's esophagus and the origin of intestinal metaplasia. *Chest Surg Clin N Am.* 2002;12:25–37.
4. Jankowski JA. Barrett's metaplasia. *Lancet.* 2000;356:2079–2085.
5. Pozharisski KM. Tumors of the esophagus. In: Turusov VS, Mohr U, eds. *Pathology of Tumors in Laboratory Animals.* Lyon: International Agency for Research on Cancer; 1990:109–129.
6. Fong LY, Magee PN. Dietary zinc deficiency enhances esophageal cell proliferation and N-nitrosomethylbenzylamine (NMBA)-induced esophageal tumor incidence in C57BL/6 mouse. *Cancer Lett.* 1999;143:63–69.
7. Xu X, LoCicero J III, Macri E, et al. Barrett's esophagus and associated adenocarcinoma in a mouse surgical model. *J Surg Res.* 2000;88:120–124.
8. Long JD, Orlando RC. Esophageal submucosal glands: structure and function. *Am J Gastroenterol.* 1999;94:2818–2824.
9. Lorinson D, Bright RM. Long-term outcome of medical and surgical treatment of hiatal hernias in dogs and cats: 27 cases (1978–1996). *J Am Vet Med Assoc.* 1998;213:381–384.
10. Callan MB, Washabau RJ, Saunders HM, et al. Congenital esophageal hiatal hernia in the Chinese shar-pei dog. *J Vet Intern Med.* 1993;7:210–215.
11. Christie KN, Thomson C, Hopwood D. A comparison of membrane enzymes of human and pig oesophagus; the pig oesophagus is a good model for studies of the gullet in man. *Histochem J.* 1995;27:231–239.
12. Gualtieri M, Olivero D. Reflux esophagitis in three cats associated with metaplastic columnar esophageal epithelium. *J Am Anim Hosp Assoc.* 2006;42:65–70.
13. Attwood SE, Smyrk TC, DeMeester TR, et al. Duodenoesophageal reflux and the development of esophageal adenocarcinoma in rats. *Surgery.* 1992;111:503–510.
14. Pera M, Cardesa A, Bombi JA, et al. Influence of esophagojejunostomy on the induction of adenocarcinoma of the distal esophagus in Sprague-Dawley rats by subcutaneous injection of 2,6-dimethylnitrosomorpholine. *Cancer Res.* 1989;49:6803–6808.
15. Fong LY, Ishii H, Nguyen VT, et al. p53 deficiency accelerates induction and progression of esophageal and forestomach tumors in zinc-deficient mice. *Cancer Res.* 2003;63:186–195.
16. Gillen P, Keeling P, Byrne PJ, et al. Experimental columnar metaplasia in the canine oesophagus. *Br J Surg.* 1988;75:113–115.
17. Li H, Walsh TN, O'Dowd G, et al. Mechanisms of columnar metaplasia and squamous regeneration in experimental Barrett's esophagus. *Surgery.* 1994;115:176–181.
18. Clark GW, Smyrk TC, Mirvish SS, et al. Effect of gastroduodenal juice and dietary fat on the development of Barrett's esophagus and esophageal neoplasia: an experimental rat model. *Ann Surg Oncol.* 1994;1:252–261.
19. Goldstein SR, Yang GY, Curtis SK, et al. Development of esophageal metaplasia and adenocarcinoma in a rat surgical model without the use of a carcinogen. *Carcinogenesis.* 1997;18:2265–2270.
20. Chen X, Yang G, Ding WY, et al. Esophagogastroduodenal anastomosis model for esophageal adenocarcinogenesis in rats and enhancement by iron overload. *Carcinogenesis.* 1999;20:1801–1807.
21. Miwa K, Segawa M, Takano Y, et al. Induction of oesophageal and forestomach carcinomas in rats by reflux of duodenal contents. *Br J Cancer.* 1994;70:185–189.
22. Clemente G, Manni R, Vecchio FM, et al. Effect of different fractions of alkaline reflux on the gastric stump and the esophagus: an experimental research on pigs. *J Surg Res.* 1990;48:121–126.
23. Pera M, Trastek VF, Carpenter HA, et al. Influence of pancreatic and biliary reflux on the development of esophageal carcinoma. *Ann Thorac Surg.* 1993;55:1386–1392; discussion 1392–1393.
24. Lambert R. Relative importance of biliary and pancreatic secretions in the genesis of esophagitis in rats. *Am J Dig Dis.* 1962;7:1026–1033.
25. Kawaura Y, Tatsuzawa Y, Wakabayashi T, et al. Immunohistochemical study of p53, c-erbB-2, and PCNA in barrett's esophagus with dysplasia and adenocarcinoma arising from experimental acid or alkaline reflux model. *J Gastroenterol.* 2001;36:595–600.
26. Mirvish SS. Studies on experimental animals involving surgical procedures and/or nitrosamine treatment related to the etiology of esophageal adenocarcinoma. *Cancer Lett.* 1997;117:161–174.

27. Li Y, Wo JM, Ellis S, Ray MB, et al. A novel external esophageal perfusion model for reflux esophageal injury. *Dig Dis Sci*. 2006;51:527–532.
28. Watanabe H, Kinoshita K, Katayama M, et al. Acquisition of a gastric or duodenal phenotype on heterotropic transplantation of esophagus and bladder tissues in F344 rats. *J Exp Clin Cancer Res*. 2003;22:619–622.
29. Su Y, Chen X, Klein M, et al. Phenotype of columnar-lined esophagus in rats with esophagogastroduodenal anastomosis: similarity to human Barrett's esophagus. *Lab Invest*. 2004;84:753–765.
30. al-Kasspooles M, Moore JH, Orringer MB, et al. Amplification and over-expression of the EGFR and erbB-2 genes in human esophageal adenocarcinomas. *Int J Cancer*. 1993;54:213–219.
31. Theisen J, Peters JH, Fein M, et al. The mutagenic potential of duodenoesophageal reflux. *Ann Surg*. 2005;241:63–68.
32. Fein M, Fuchs KH, DeMeester TR, et al. Evaluation of the intestinal microflora in the rat model for esophageal adenocarcinoma. *Dis Esophagus*. 2000;13:39–43.
33. Miwa K, Hattori T, Miyazaki I. Duodenogastric reflux and foregut carcinogenesis. *Cancer*. 1995;75:1426–1432.
34. Moore KH, Barry P, Burn J, et al. Adenocarcinoma of the rat esophagus in the presence of a proton pump inhibitor: a pilot study. *Dis Esophagus*. 2001;14:17–22.
35. Ireland AP, Peters JH, Smyrk TC, et al. Gastric juice protects against the development of esophageal adenocarcinoma in the rat. *Ann Surg*. 1996;224:358–370; discussion 370–371.
36. Clark GWB, Smyrk TC, Mirvish SS, et al. Effect of gastroduodenal juice and dietary fat on the development of Barrett's esophagus and esophageal neoplasia: an experimental rat model. *Ann Surg Oncol*. 1994;1(3):252–261.
37. Pera M, Fernandez PL, Palacin A, et al. Expression of cyclin D1 and p53 and its correlation with proliferative activity in the spectrum of esophageal carcinomas induced after duodenal content reflux and 2,6-dimethylnitrosomorpholine administration in rats. *Carcinogenesis*. 2001;22:271–277.
38. Fujiwara Y, Higuchi K, Takashima T, et al. Increased expression of epidermal growth factor receptors in basal cell hyperplasia of the oesophagus after acid reflux oesophagitis in rats. *Alimentary Pharmacol Ther*. 2002;16 Suppl 2:52–58.
39. Chen X, Li N, Wang S, et al. Aberrant arachidonic acid metabolism in esophageal adenocarcinogenesis, and the effects of sulindac, nordihydroguaiaretic acid, and alpha-difluoromethylornithine on tumorigenesis in a rat surgical model. *Carcinogenesis*. 2002;23:2095–2102.
40. Chen X, Li N, Wang S, et al. Leukotriene A4 hydrolase in rat and human esophageal adenocarcinomas and inhibitory effects of bestatin. *J Natl Cancer Inst*. 2003;95:1053–1061.
41. Chen X, Wang S, Wu N, et al. Overexpression of 5-lipoxygenase in rat and human esophageal adenocarcinoma and inhibitory effects of Zileuton and Celecoxib on carcinogenesis. *Clin Cancer Res*. 2004;10:6703–6709.
42. Hayakawa T, Fujiwara Y, Hamaguchi M, et al. Roles of cyclooxygenase 2 and microsomal prostaglandin E synthase 1 in rat acid reflux oesophagitis. *Gut*. 2006;55:450–456.
43. Jang TJ, Min SK, Bae JD, et al. Expression of cyclooxygenase 2, microsomal prostaglandin E synthase 1, and EP receptors is increased in rat oesophageal squamous cell dysplasia and Barrett's metaplasia induced by duodenal contents reflux. *Gut*. 2004;53:27–33.
44. Bonde P, Gao D, Chen L, et al. Duodenal reflux leads to down regulation of DNA mismatch repair pathway in an animal model of esophageal cancer. *Ann Thorac Surg*. 2007;83:433–440; discussion 440.
45. Bonde P, Sui G, Dhara S, et al. Cytogenetic characterization and gene expression profiling in the rat reflux-induced esophageal tumor model. *J Thorac Cardiovasc Surg*. 2007;133:763–769.
46. Naito Y, Kuroda M, Uchiyama K, et al. Inflammatory response of esophageal epithelium in combined-type esophagitis in rats: a transcriptome analysis. *Int J Mol Med*. 2006;18:821–828.
47. Cheng P, Gong J, Wang T, et al. Gene expression in rats with Barrett's esophagus and esophageal adenocarcinoma induced by gastroduodenoesophageal reflux. *World J Gastroenterol*. 2005;11:5117–5122.
48. Chen X, Ding Y, Liu CG, et al. Overexpression of glucose-regulated protein 94 (Grp94) in esophageal adenocarcinomas of a rat surgical model and humans. *Carcinogenesis*. 2002;23:123–130.
49. Goldstein SR, Yang G-Y, Chen X, et al. Studies of iron deposits, inducible nitric oxide synthase and nitrotyrosine in a rat model for esophageal adenocarcinoma. *Carcinogenesis*. 1998;19:1445–1449.
50. Lee JS, Oh TY, Ahn BO, et al. Involvement of oxidative stress in experimentally induced reflux esophagitis and Barrett's esophagus: clue for the chemoprevention of esophageal carcinoma by antioxidants. *Mutat Res*. 2001;480–481:189–200.
51. Chen X, Ding YW, Yang G, et al. Oxidative damage in an esophageal adenocarcinoma model with rats. *Carcinogenesis*. 2000;21:257–263.
52. Chen X, Mikhail SS, Ding YW, et al. Effects of vitamin E and selenium supplementation on esophageal adenocarcinogenesis in a surgical model with rats. *Carcinogenesis*. 2000;21:1531–1536.
53. Buttar NS, Wang KK, Leontovich O, et al. Chemoprevention of esophageal adenocarcinoma by COX-2 inhibitors in an animal model of Barrett's esophagus. *Gastroenterology*. 2002;122:1101–1112.
54. Oyama K, Fujimura T, Ninomiya I, et al. A COX-2 inhibitor prevents the esophageal inflammation-metaplasia-adenocarcinoma sequence in rats. *Carcinogenesis*. 2005;26:565–570.
55. Piazuelo E, Cebrian C, Escartin A, et al. Superoxide dismutase prevents development of adenocarcinoma in a rat model of Barrett's esophagus. *World J Gastroenterol*. 2005;11:7436–7443.
56. Martin RC, Liu Q, Wo JM, et al. Chemoprevention of carcinogenic progression to esophageal adenocarcinoma by the manganese superoxide dismutase supplementation. *Clin Cancer Res*. 2007;13:5176–5182.
57. Kumagai H, Mukaisho K, Sugihara H, et al. Thioproline inhibits development of esophageal adenocarcinoma induced by gastroduodenal reflux in rats. *Carcinogenesis*. 2004;25:723–727.
58. Nishijima K, Miwa K, Miyashita T, et al. Impact of the biliary diversion procedure on carcinogenesis in Barrett's esophagus surgically induced by duodenoesophageal reflux in rats. *Ann Surg*. 2004;240:57–67.
59. Miyashita T, Ohta T, Fujimura T, et al. Duodenal juice stimulates oesophageal stem cells to induce Barrett's oesophagus and oesophageal adenocarcinoma in rats. *Oncol Rep*. 2006;15:1469–1475.
60. Ellis FH Jr, Xu X, Kulke MH, et al. Malignant transformation of the esophageal mucosa is enhanced in p27 knockout mice. *J Thorac Cardiovasc Surg*. 2001;122:809–814.
61. Lechpammer M, Xu X, Ellis FH, et al. Flavopiridol reduces malignant transformation of the esophageal mucosa in p27 knockout mice. *Oncogene*. 2005;24:1683–1688.
62. Fein M, Peters JH, Baril N, et al. Loss of function of Trp53, but not Apc, leads to the development of esophageal adenocarcinoma in mice with jejunoesophageal reflux. *J Surg Res*. 1999;83:48–55.
63. Chen X, Samer M, Chen W, et al. Loss of p53 gene increases the incidence of esophageal adenocarcinoma in a surgical model using p53 knockout mice. *Proc Am Assoc Cancer Res*. 2001;42:A4067.
64. Yang A, Schweitzer R, Sun D, et al. p63 is essential for regenerative proliferation in limb, craniofacial and epithelial development. *Nature*. 1999;398:714–718.
65. Duncan MD, Tihan T, Donovan DM, et al. Esophagogastric adenocarcinoma in an E1A/E1B transgenic model involves p53 disruption. *J Gastrointest Surg*. 2000;4:290–297.
66. Jonkers J, Meuwissen R, van der Gulden H, et al. Synergistic tumor suppressor activity of BRCA2 and p53 in a conditional mouse model for breast cancer. *Nat Genet*. 2001;29:418–425.
67. Vassar R, Rosenberg M, Ross S, et al. Tissue-specific and differentiation-specific expression of a human K14 keratin gene in transgenic mice. *Proc Natl Acad Sci U S A*. 1989;86:1563–1567.
68. Xie W, Chow LT, Paterson AJ, et al. Conditional expression of the ErbB2 oncogene elicits reversible hyperplasia in stratified epithelia and up-regulation of TGFalpha expression in transgenic mice. *Oncogene*. 1999;18:3593–3607.
69. Opitz OG, Harada H, Suliman Y, et al. A mouse model of human oral-esophageal cancer. *J Clin Invest*. 2002;110:761–769.
70. Stratis A, Pasparakis M, Markur D, et al. Localized inflammatory skin disease following inducible ablation of I kappa B kinase 2 in murine epidermis. *J Invest Dermatol*. 2006;126:614–620.
71. Vasioukhin V, Degenstein L, Wise B, et al. The magical touch: genome targeting in epidermal stem cells induced by tamoxifen application to mouse skin. *Proc Natl Acad Sci U S A*. 1999;96:8551–8556.
72. Bremner CG, Lynch VP, Ellis FH Jr. Barrett's esophagus: congenital or required. *Surgery*. 1970;68:209–216.
73. Evander A, Little AG, Riddell RH, et al. Composition of the refluxed material determines the degree of reflux esophagitis in the dog. *Gastroenterology*. 1987;93:280–286.
74. Seery JP. Stem cells of the oesophageal epithelium. *J Cell Sci*. 2002;115:1783–1789.
75. Hofmann A, Kessler B, Ewerling S, et al. Efficient transgenesis in farm animals by lentiviral vectors. *EMBO Rep*. 2003;4:1054–1060.

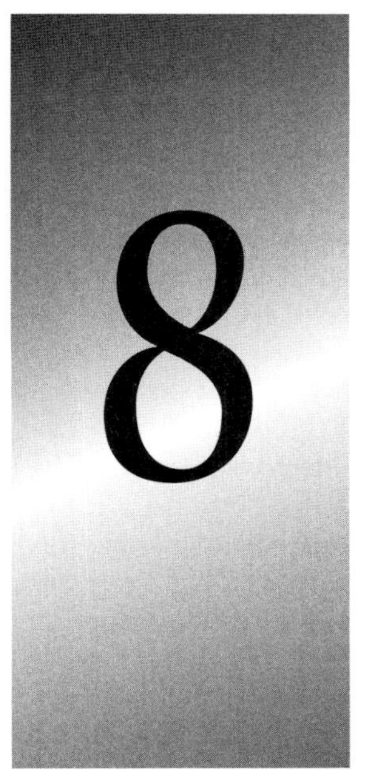

Barrett's Esophagus: Screening and Surveillance

Richard Sampliner

Barrett's esophagus (BE) is a change in the lining of the distal esophagus seen at endoscopy and documented to have intestinal metaplasia (IM) by biopsy (1). This definition has evolved over the last 30 years from extensive columnar lining, to columnar lining proximal to the manometric lower esophageal sphincter (LES), to 3 cm of columnar lining or any IM above the LES. The definition is critical for case detection when embarking on screening and/or surveillance. It implies the need for endoscopists to identify the apparent columnar lining in the esophagus and to biopsy it to determine the presence of the necessary histologic criterion of goblet cells of IM (2).

The major definitional controversy is whether IM is necessary for the definition of BE. The fact that IM harbors the vast majority of dysplasia and esophageal adenocarcinoma (EAC) (3) argues for this criterion. Given the general awareness of the cancer risk of BE, engendering unnecessary concern on the patient's part is to be avoided if no IM is present. It is also appropriate to avoid the increased financial burden for insurance in the United States when this label is unnecessarily applied (4). Erosive esophagitis can be mistaken for columnar lining. Additionally, a columnar lined esophagus lacking IM will often yield IM on subsequent endoscopic biopsies (5), confirming the diagnosis. So this methodologic issue of controversy may be resolved over time for an individual patient or by future endoscopic technology with refinements in our ability to recognize IM by patterns at high resolution endoscopy (see Chapter 17) (6).

SCREENING FOR BE

Who

The highest risk patients for EAC identify those most likely to have BE—male, Caucasian, older (7), with long-standing reflux symptoms (Table 8.1). The specific criteria for age and duration of reflux are not evidence based. Although the yield of BE is highest in the above patients, many people with BE do not fit these criteria. Females, people of color, and especially people without reflux symptoms experience BE. Other than by impractical universal screening of adults, we have no current way to identify BE in the asymptomatic. About 40% of population determined BE patients are asymptomatic (8). If BE could be identified without endoscopy, less targeted screening would be more feasible. Esophageal capsule endoscopy offers a technique to identify patients likely to have BE, but the current sensitivity, 67%–77%, is not adequate (9, 10). Additionally, the cost of the capsule is a barrier to wider usage. Other emerging non-endoscopic screening tests (sponge immunocytology for detection of minichromosome maintenance protein [2]) do not yet have the necessary sensitivity and specificity (11).

TABLE 8.1
Risk Factors for Barrett's Esophagus

Male
Caucasian
Older - ? specific age
Long-standing GERD - ? specific duration
Visceral adiposity - ? specific measure

Epidemiologic evidence suggests abdominal obesity is a risk factor for BE. Case control studies document that visceral adipose tissue (OR 1.5), waist to hip ratio (OR 2.4), and abdominal circumference (OR 2.2) are associated with BE (12–14). But this does not provide a specific criterion to identify people with BE.

Can we increase the yield of finding BE at the time of endoscopy by defining pre-endoscopic criteria? In a Veterans Affairs medical center, independent predictions of BE by multivariate logistic regression (88 patients with BE, 88 with GERD) were age >40, heartburn or acid regurgitation, and heartburn more than once a week (15). In a logistic regression analysis of 517 GERD patients, significant predictors of BE were male gender, heartburn, nocturnal pain, odynophagia, and dysphagia (99 with BE and 418 with GERD) (16). A screening nomogram for BE had a sensitivity of 77% and specificity of 63%. Another Veterans study found no symptoms predictive of BE comparing 235 BE patients to 306 with erosive esophagitis (17). Eight gastrointestinal (GI) departments in Italy found GERD symptoms of more than 13 years duration were a risk factor for BE (149 BE and 143 esophagitis) (18). Finally, after eliminating BE patients undergoing surveillance, in 1011 adults undergoing endoscopy only the duration of acid regurgitation for more than 5 years was associated with BE (OR 7.86 [95% CI 1.61–38.4]) (19). At a sensitivity of 80%, the model for BE had a specificity of 57%; at a specificity of 80%, the sensitivity was 62%. The only risk factors in common in positive studies was heartburn.

LIMITATIONS OF SCREENING

Pre-endoscopic criteria to predict BE are not validated. There are no prospective trials to document the impact of screening. Screening makes intuitive sense and analyses have demonstrated the cost-effectiveness of screening in relation to what society is willing to spend (see Chapter 9) (20).

In the future, screening will be more feasible when high-risk groups for BE can be identified and the initial phase of screening is less expensive and more sensitive.

SURVEILLANCE

Who

Patients with documented BE who have an expected survival of greater than 5 years and agree to interval endoscopy are candidates for surveillance. It is not reasonable to undertake surveillance in frail elderly patients or in those with life-limiting comorbidity (21). When the only treatment of high-grade dysplasia (HGD) and early EAC was esophagectomy, candidates for surveillance had to be able and willing to undergo major surgery. With the availability and documented impact of endoscopic therapy (22), the latter is no longer true. The ideal selection of BE patients for surveillance would include risk stratification. We know males, Caucasians, and patients with longer segment BE have a greater risk of EAC. However, the precise criteria are not evidence based. The current biologic marker used to determine surveillance intervals is the grade of dysplasia (Table 8.2). Dysplasia is the first step in the neoplastic process. It is an unequivocal change in the cellular characteristics of the glands in the BE that involve the crypts as well as the surface epithelium.

When no dysplasia has been documented with systematic biopsies—4-quadrant every 2 cm—on 2 endoscopies over 1 year, the interval of endoscopy can be extended to 3 to 5 years. When low-grade dysplasia (LGD) is found, confirmation by an expert pathologist is necessary. The prevalence and incidence of LGD is higher than that of HGD and EAC. In a large multicenter cohort of patients with documented BE, the prevalence of LGD was 7.3% and annual incidence 4.3% (23). Frequency of endoscopy in surveillance tends to be driven by LGD, and the greatest variability in histologic interpretation is found in LGD cases. A study of the economic impact of the diagnosis of dysplasia

TABLE 8.2
Grade of Dysplasia and Surveillance

Dysplasia	Endoscopy (EGD)
None	• 2 EGDs with biopsy in 1 year • Every 3–5 years
Low grade	• Highest grade on repeat EGD in 6 months with expert pathologist confirmation • Yearly until no dysplasia x2
High grade	• Endoscopic resection for mucosal irregularity. Repeat EGD in 3 months. Expert pathologist confirmation • 3-month surveillance or individualized intervention

estimated that 61% of endoscopies are performed because of the "transient" dysplasia—dysplasia not persistent at 24 months of follow-up (24). When dysplasia is categorized into 4 clinically relevant groups, the interobserver agreement is only moderate (kappa = 0.46) (25). This confirmation of the diagnosis is an effort to focus surveillance on high-risk patients—the more pathologists who agree on LGD, the greater the risk of neoplastic progression (26). This finding suggests that when more pathologists agree, changes are present that can be discriminated from normal. The natural history of LGD is highly variable, but BE patients with LGD should undergo an additional EGD in 6 months to exclude a worse lesion in the esophagus. Thereafter, once-yearly endoscopy can be done until no dysplasia is found on 2 consecutive endoscopies.

The finding of HGD, documented by an expert GI pathologist, warrants a repeat endoscopy within 3 months to exclude the presence of concomitant (synchronous) EAC. Any mucosal irregularities should undergo endoscopic resection to ensure the absence of EAC. Endoscopic resection provides the opportunity to evaluate a large piece (usually 1 cm) of tissue, which includes the submucosa. This enables actual T staging. With the confirmation of HGD, the next step is intensive surveillance (endoscopies every 3 months for 1 year) or individualized intervention. The threshold for therapeutic endoscopic intervention in BE is HGD. The options of esophagectomy, intensive surveillance, and endoscopic ablative therapy need to be carefully considered by the patient. Patient and institutional issues factor into the complex network of decision making. The patient's lesion—the length of the segment of BE—the stage of the EAC, age, comorbidity, and aversion to surgery, and/or cancer are involved in tailoring the therapy. The institutional factors include the volume of esophagectomy and expertise in staging techniques (EUS, CT, PET scanning) and endoscopic therapy.

LIMITATIONS OF SURVEILLANCE

There is no randomized trial documenting the efficacy of surveillance in improving the outcome of EAC in patients with BE. Dysplasia is an imprecise biomarker with major limitations in the variability of pathology interpretation. Additionally, even with the recommended biopsy protocols, only a fraction of the surface area of the Barrett's segment is sampled. Therefore, sampling error remains a problem. Risk stratification for EAC is not precise or accurate. Patients have to be adherent to a program of regular endoscopic evaluation for advanced neoplasia, which can be a rigorous endeavor.

CONCLUSION

Both screening and surveillance are de facto practiced in the United States. Although not necessarily evidence based and not supported by prospective trials, it would be worthwhile to use the best information to rationalize, if not standardize, our practice. Clues are present concerning the high-risk patients for both BE and EAC. We can look forward to results of ongoing research to enhance our recognition of high risk patients—molecular markers, for instance. Further technologic developments of non-endoscopic detection of probable BE can also be anticipated.

References

1. Sampliner RE, Practice Parameters Committee ACG. Updated guidelines for the diagnosis, surveillance, and therapy of Barrett's esophagus. *Am J Gastroenterol.* 2002;97:1888–1895.
2. Weinstein WM, Ippoliti AF. The diagnosis of Barrett's esophagus: goblets, goblets, goblets. *Gastrointest Endosc.* 1996;44:91–96.
3. Hamilton SR, Smith RRL. The relationship between columnar epithelial dysplasia and invasive adenocarcinoma arising in Barrett's esophagus. *Am J Clin Pathol.* 1987;87:301–312.
4. Shaheen NJ, Dulai GS, Ascher B, et al. Effect of a new diagnosis of Barrett's esophagus on insurance status. *Am J Gastro.* 2005;100:577–580.
5. Oberg S, Johansson J, Wenner J, et al. Endoscopic surveillance of columnar-lined esophagus: frequency of intestinal metaplasia detection and impact of antireflux surgery. *Ann Surg.* 2001;234:619–626.
6. Kara MA, Peters FP, Rosmolen WD, et al. High resolution endoscopy plus chromoendoscopy or narrow band imaging in Barrett's esophagus: a prospective randomized crossover study. *Endoscopy.* 2005;37:929–936.
7. Blot W, Devesa SS, Kneller RW, et al. Rising incidence of adenocarcinoma of the esophagus and gastric cardia. *JAMA.* 1991;265(10):1287–1289.
8. Ronkainen J, Aro P, Storskrubb T, et al. Prevalence of Barrett's esophagus in the general population: an endoscopic study. *Gastroenterology.* 2005;129:1825–1831.
9. Sharma P, Wani R, Rastojg A, et al. The diagnostic accuracy of wireless capsule endoscopy for the detection of Barrett's esophagus. *Am J Gastro.* 2007;102:1–8.
10. Lin O, Schembre DB, Kozarek R, et al. Blinded comparison of esophageal capsule endoscopy versus conventional endoscopy for diagnosis of Barrett's esophagus in patients with chronic gastroesophageal reflux. *Gastrintest Endosc.* 2007;65(4):577–583.
11. Lao-Siriex P, Rous B, O'Donovan M, et al. Non-endoscopic immunocytological screening test for Barrett's esophagus. *Gut.* 2007:1033–1034.
12. El-Serag HB, Kvapil P, Hacken-Bitar J, et al. Abdominal obesity and the risk of Barrett's esophagus. *Am J Gastro.* 2005;100:2151–2156.
13. Edelstein ZR, Farrow DC, Bronner MP, et al. Central adiposity and risk of Barrett's esophagus. *Gastroenterology.* 2007;133:403–411.
14. Corley DA, Kubo A, Levin TR, et al. Abdominal obesity and body mass index as risk factors for Barrett's esophagus. *Gastroenterology.* 2007;133:34–41.
15. Eloubeide MA, Provenzale D. Clinical and demographic predictors of Barrett's esophagus among patients with gastroesophageal reflux disease. *J Clin Gastroenterol.* 2001;33(4):306–309.
16. Gerson LB, Edson R, Lavori PW, et al. Use of a simple symptom questionnaire to predict Barrett's esophagus in patients with symptoms of gastroesophageal reflux. *Am J Gastroenterol.* 2001;96:2005–2012.
17. Avidan B, Sonnenberg A, Schnell TG, et al. There are no reliable symptoms for erosive oesophagitis and Barrett's oesophagus: endoscopic diagnosis is still essential. *Aliment Pharmacol.* 2002;16:735–742.
18. Conio M, Filiberti R, Blanchi S, et al. Risk factors for Barrett's esophagus: a case-control study. *Int J Cancer.* 2002;97:225–29.
19. Locke III GR, Zinsmeister AR, Talley NJ. Can symptoms predict endoscopic findings in GERD? *Gastrintest Endosc.* 2003;58:661–670.
20. Inadomi JM, Sampliner RE, Lagergren J, et al. Screening and surveillance for Barrett's esophagus in high-risk groups: a cost-utility analysis. *Ann Intern Med.* 2003;138(3):176–186.

21. Gross GP, McAvay GJ, Krumholz HM, et al. The effect of age and chronic illness on life expectancy after a diagnosis of colorectal cancer: implications for screening. *Ann Intern Med.* 2006;145:646–653.
22. Prasad GA, Wang KK, Buttar NS, et al. Long term survival following endoscopic and surgical treatment of high grade dysplasia in Barrett's esophagus. *Gastroenterology.* 2007;132:1226–1233.
23. Sharma P, Dent J, Armstrong D, et al. The development and validation of an endoscopic grading system for Barrett's esophagus: the Prague C & M criteria. *Gastroenterology.* 2006;131:1392–1399.
24. Ofman JJ, Lewin K, Ramers C, et al. The economic impact of the diagnosis of dysplasia in Barrett's esophagus. *Am J Gastroenterol.* 2000;95:2946–2952.
25. Montgomery E, Bronner MP, Goldblum JR, et al. Reproducibility of the diagnosis of dysplasia in Barrett's esophagus: a reaffirmation. *Hum Pathol.* 2001;32:368–378.
26. Skacel M, Petras R, Gramlich TL, et al. The diagnosis of low-grade dysplasia in Barrett's esophagus and its implications for disease progression. *Am J Gastroenterol.* 2000;95:3383–3387.

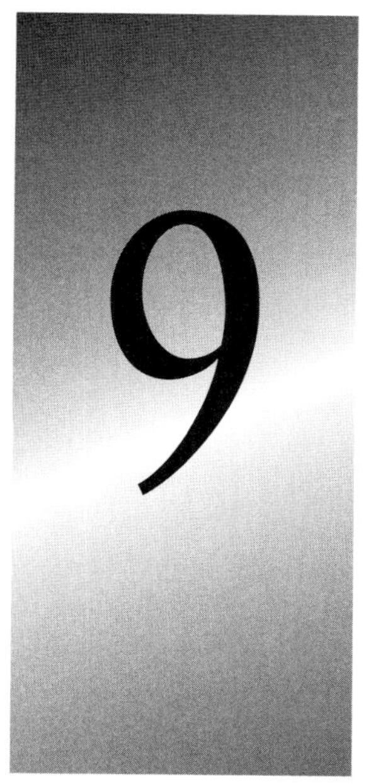

Barrett's Esophagus: Models for Cost-Effective Screening and Surveillance

Jonathan Hata
Aurora Pryor

Esophageal carcinoma is one of the most increasingly prevalent and highly lethal cancers in the United States and Europe. While the increasing incidence of esophageal cancer is between 4% and 10% per year, the 5-year survival rate may be as low as 10%. Of the approximately 14,000 new cases of esophageal cancer each year, over 50% represent the adenocarcinoma variant. The development of esophageal carcinoma is thought to be a histologic progression from metaplasia and low-grade dysplasia to high-grade dysplasia and invasive cancer. Barrett's esophagus (BE) is the abnormal finding of intestinal metaplasia in the distal esophageal mucosa and is a well-characterized premalignant precursor of esophageal adenocarcinoma (EAC). Thought to result from chronic gastroesophageal reflux disease (GERD), BE carries a 30–50 fold risk of developing EAC (1). Although debated, the incidence of EAC in patients with known BE (termed *incident cases*) may be as high as 0.5% per year. The association of GERD with BE and eventual progression to EAC represents a potential target for an effective cancer screening program.

Screening for BE and subsequent surveillance of afflicted patients has been proposed as a way to improve early detection of EAC and increase overall survival. The traditional cornerstone of these efforts is upper endoscopy with biopsies of the gastroesophageal junction and esophageal mucosa. Over the past decade, this practice has been endorsed by gastroenterologists and other health care providers, despite a lack of direct evidence supporting its efficacy or cost-effectiveness (2). While the ultimate goal of any screening and surveillance program is to decrease morbidity and mortality from disease, such techniques must also be evaluated from a cost-effective perspective in a health care environment of increasing expenditures and limited access to services. The purpose of this chapter is to review and summarize the available data on screening and surveillance of BE from this point of view.

DEFINITION OF COST-EFFECTIVENESS

To begin any discussion of *cost-effectiveness*, several key terms must be clarified. In general, the overall *effectiveness* of a medical screening or surveillance program is its total benefit to society, which for many diseases is measured in terms of *patient life-years saved*. Obviously, this outcome measure is heavily influenced not only by the validity of the intervention itself but also by many other factors such as disease prevalence and virulence. As noted in a recent review by Shaheen et al., specific criteria have been described to help guide an evaluation of any proposed screening or surveillance program (Table 9.1) (3,4). While answers to these basic

TABLE 9.1
Sackett's Proposed Criteria for Seeking an Early Diagnosis of Disease

1. Does early diagnosis lead to improved clinical outcomes (survival, function, quality of life)?
2. Can one manage the clinical time required to confirm a diagnosis and provide long-term care for those who screen positive?
3. Will patients with early diagnoses comply with subsequent recommendations and treatment options?
4. Has the effectiveness of individual components of a screening or surveillance program been demonstrated before their combination?
5. Does the burden of disability from the target disease warrant action?
6. Are the costs, accuracy, and acceptability of the screening test adequate?

questions determine a program's overall effectiveness, they also comprise the baseline set of assumptions for any subsequent calculation of cost-effectiveness. This concept combines an intervention's overall benefit to society with the financial cost required to produce such a benefit. In other words, determining the cost-effectiveness of an intervention requires a comparison to the cost of not performing that same intervention. A common unit of measurement in cost-effectiveness calculations is the *incremental cost-effectiveness ratio*, which is the cost difference between 2 strategies (usually intervention versus no intervention) divided by the gain in life expectancy. This typically yields a calculated unit reported as a monetary amount per life-year saved. In order to interpret this calculated value in the larger context of a health care system, it is useful to compare the incremental cost-effectiveness ratio of the intervention in question to that of other widely accepted and practiced interventions. Ultimately, cost-effectiveness is simply a value judgment on the part of the decision maker (either patient, physician, or policy maker) regarding their level of willingness to pay for a particular intervention. Thus, the *value* of any intervention or program in a given population is determined by a host of societal, cultural, and financial forces, and often moves the debate from medical to political arenas.

As with any derived value or outcome measure, the assessment of an intervention's cost-effectiveness is completely dependent on the primary data used in the equation. From a theoretical perspective, it is the answers to criteria such as those proposed by Sackett (Table 9.1) that provide this primary data or set of assumptions. Specifically for BE, there are no data available from randomized, controlled studies on the effectiveness of screening or surveillance. Therefore, decision-making and practice patterns have been developed based on cohort or observational studies. While providing valuable information, the data derived from these types of studies may be prone to inaccurate generalizations, bias, or other forms of methodologic error; any inaccuracies in data would ultimately call into question the reliability of subsequent cost-effectiveness calculations.

SCREENING

Regardless of the disease process, the concepts of screening and surveillance are 2 separate yet related entities. Screening is defined as the examination of a large sample of a population to detect a specific disease. In this case, upper endoscopy is performed on a selected subset of the general population in hopes of achieving earlier detection of premalignant conditions (BE or dysplasia) or adenocarcinoma. Early detection allows for more effective treatment for esophageal cancer and ultimately improves survival. In order for such a screening program to be effective, some general criteria must be met. First, a high-risk population must be identified to target initial screening efforts. In the case of BE, this population comprises patients with chronic symptoms of gastrointestinal reflux disease (GERD). Second, upper endoscopy must be able to accurately diagnose BE and dysplastic changes before their progression to adenocarcinoma. Finally, there must be potential interventions (such as mucosal resection or esophagectomy) that can be used to treat dysplastic or neoplastic changes, and result in improved survival and QOL. While a full discussion of these topics are beyond the scope of this chapter, taken together they determine the cost-effectiveness of screening for BE and esophageal cancer.

While the complete epidemiology of BE is not completely understood, there is evidence that patients with EAC found as part of a screening program have improved survival relative to those who are symptomatic. However, there are no prospective studies confirming that screening programs directly reduce overall mortality. The exact prevalence of BE is unknown, but it has been demonstrated that greater severity of GERD symptoms is associated with an increased prevalence (5,6). The current American Gastroenterological Association (AGA) guidelines for screening for BE state that "patients with chronic GERD symptoms are those most likely to have BE and should undergo upper endoscopy" (2). With 14% of the United States population suffering from chronic symptomatic GERD, even if screening were limited to patients greater than 50 years of age, an overwhelming 10 million patients would still qualify for screening endoscopy (3). However, with only 6,000 new cases of EAC diagnosed in the United States annually, such a massive screening effort would still be very low-yield. Clearly, this highlights the need for further identifying higher risk sub-populations for more targeted screening. Risk factors for BE include male gender (2:1 male to female predominance), white race, > 40 years of age, positive family history, and concomitant hiatal hernias (7). Other risk factors may include obesity and use of medications reducing lower esophageal sphincter pressure (6). As a screening tool, endoscopy is able to reliably differentiate the absence of dysplasia from the presence of high-grade dysplasia or frank cancer (>80% specificity), yet may struggle to distinguish between different grades of dysplasia (8). Finally, the requirement to act on positive results from an endoscopic screening program has far-reaching implications for any health care system. With a finding of high-grade dysplasia or EAC, subsequent esophageal resection will need to be performed in a relatively small number of patients. However, as many as 3 million Americans may be diagnosed with BE, requiring a large investment of health care resources in order to carry out future surveillance. As more data are acquired on less invasive methods for esophageal resection, surveillance may have more of an impact.

While the majority of cost-effectiveness models regarding BE include both screening and surveillance, Soni et al. performed an analysis of endoscopic screening in patients with GERD to detect BE and dysplasia (9) (Table 9.2). Using a decision-tree analysis, several key assumptions were included. Patients at age 60 underwent a single endoscopy with biopsies of abnormal epithelium. Positive biopsy findings of high-grade dysplasia or adenocarcinoma resulted in esophagectomy. Transition rates were estimated from published data and national cancer statistics, including a high specificity/sensitivity of endoscopy (90%), high prevalence of BE (10%) and high-grade dysplasia (7%) with GERD, and minimal reduction in quality of life (QOL) after esophagectomy. The costs of endoscopy and cancer care were estimated from Medicare data. Using the incremental cost-effectiveness ratio (ICER) as an outcome measure, screening endoscopy cost $24,700 per life-year saved when compared to no screening. Subsequent univariate and multivariate analysis demonstrated that this outcome is highly sensitive to assumptions about the prevalence of BE and dysplasia, ability of endoscopy to diagnose abnormalities, and health-related QOL after surgery. For instance, a small decrease of 10% in QOL following esophagectomy increases the calculated ICER to $63,000 per life-year saved, while a 16% decrease eliminates any benefit. Nevertheless, this study suggests that in the setting of favorable parameters, endosopic screening of a population (>60 yrs age) of patients with symptomatic GERD may be cost-effective. As with any screening program, further risk stratification is needed to better define those patients most at risk of harboring undiagnosed disease, thus leading to increased cost-effectiveness.

SURVEILLANCE

Surveillance is defined as the ongoing, periodic monitoring of patients considered to be at high-risk for a disease, which is often determined by prior testing (i.e., screening). In this case, surveillance involves follow-up endoscopy at scheduled intervals in patients with BE in order to detect early progression toward dysplasia or cancer. Early detection would permit early surgical or other therapeutic interventions before development of invasive cancer, thus improving survival. Although endoscopic surveillance of BE has not been definitively shown in prospective, randomized trials to decrease cancer incidence or increase life expectancy, this strategy is widely practiced. Retrospective and cohort studies have demonstrated that patients diagnosed with EAC in the setting of surveillance endoscopy have a lower stage cancer and improved survival (10–12). While promising, these types of studies may be influenced by selection, lead-time, or

TABLE 9.2
Cost-Effectiveness Models of Screening and Surveillance of Barrett's Esophagus

Study	Surveillance interval	Incidence cancer (Barrett's esophagus)	Survival (5-yr) (esophagectomy)	QOL (esophagectomy)	ICER [a] ($/life-yr gained)
Soni (2000)	n/a	7% (screening only)	23%	100%	$24,718
Provenzale (1999)	5-year	0.4%/year	22%	97%	$98,000
Sonnenberg (2002)	2-year	0.5%/year	20%	100%	$16,965
Inadomi (2003)	5-year	0.5%/year	20%	97%	$12,336

[a] Incremental cost-effectiveness ratio (compared to no screening/surveillance program)

publication bias, and may overestimate critical parameters such as the incidence of EAC in BE (13). The current recommendations are based on guidelines from the AGA and include multiple 4-quadrant biopsies performed in patients with BE at intervals determined chiefly by the presence, and histologic grade, of dysplasia (2).

As with screening, there are no prospective randomized trials studying the clinical role or cost-effectiveness of surveillance for BE. Such research would be very difficult to perform given statistical requirements for a large patient population, long-term follow-up, and standardized protocols. Instead, economic decision models have been developed to calculate the cost-effectiveness of intervention strategies (14). Perhaps the most controversial variable influencing the cost-effectiveness of surveillance of BE is its natural history. While an estimated 700,000 patients in the United States have BE, their annual estimated risk of progression to adenocarcinoma is reported to range between 0.2% and 2%, with a generally accepted incidence of 0.5% per year (13,15–17). If progression to high-grade dysplasia is included, this risk may be as high as 1.4% per year (18). As listed in Table 9.3, other important variables include the surveillance interval, cost of endoscopy, and the ability of endoscopy to accurately diagnose dysplasia and cancer. Finally, accurate data regarding the clinical outcomes, costs, and QOL after esophagectomy are necessary in order to calculate how much patients benefit from an intervention following a positive endoscopic finding. As will be discussed, varying the baseline values of any of these parameters can dramatically alter the cost-effectiveness of any proposed surveillance strategy for BE.

TABLE 9.3
Baseline Variables Most Influencing the Cost-Effectiveness of Surveillance for Barrett's Esophagus[a]

Variable	Rate or cost range	Reference
Incidence rate of adenocarcinoma per year arising from Barrett's esophagus	0.2%–2.0%	13,16,17
Starting age of surveillance endoscopy	40–60 years	43
Surveillance interval for endoscopy	1–10 years	43
Efficacy of endoscopy in preventing cancer	25%-75%	27
Cost of endoscopy	$400–$1500	25
5-year survival after esophagectomy	20%	17
Health-related quality of life after esophagectomy	83%–100%	21,25
Cost of esophagectomy for cancer or high-grade dysplasia	$21,277	25
Cost of medical care for adenocarcinoma	$44,931	25

[a]Adapted from Sonnenberg et al. *Aliment Pharmacol Ther.* 2002;16:41–50.

SURVEILLANCE COST-EFFECTIVENESS MODELS

The first cost-effectiveness analysis for surveillance of BE was published by Provenzale et al. in 1994 (19) (Table 9.2). A Markov model (20), a mathematical model used to estimate life expectancy in medical contexts, was used to construct a computer cohort simulation of 10,000 55-year-old men with BE. In the simulation, the surveillance interval was varied between 1 and 5 years, and a diagnosis of either high-grade dysplasia or adenocarcinoma resulted in esophagectomy. The analysis concluded that surveillance every 5 years resulted in an ICER of $27,400 per life-year gained. Shortening the surveillance interval to 4 years provided a greater gain in life expectancy but increased the ICER to $276,700 per life-year gained. Further analysis revealed that the 2 most important parameters influencing the analysis were the incidence of cancer and the QOL after esophagectomy.

In a follow-up study, the same authors performed a similar analysis using updated estimates for cancer risk and esophagectomy outcomes (21). In this simulation, the average annual incidence of cancer was estimated at 0.4%, while the QOL adjustment factor following surgery was 0.97. The assumed costs for endoscopy were $600, esophagectomy $23,800, and long-term cancer care $34,000 per year. Using these estimates and a surveillance interval of 5 years, the incremental cost-utility ratio (ICUR; which is the ICER adjusted for QOL) was $98,000 per life-year gained. In a sensitivity analysis, once again the incidence of cancer in BE was demonstrated to be the most important parameter. For instance, if the annual incidence of cancer was set at <0.2%, no surveillance would be preferred, as the risks of surveillance and the potential surgery would outweigh potential gains in survival or QOL. Conversely, if the incidence rate approached 2% per year, more frequent endoscopy (every 1–2 years) became cost-effective. Similarly, if operative mortality and morbidity from esophagectomy increases, less frequent surveillance is required to maintain equivalent cost-effective ratios with other accepted medical practices. For an operative mortality between 6% and 10%, surveillance every 5 years was the only strategy that increased quality-adjusted life expectancy, with an ICUR ranging from $80,000–$120,000.

Recent surgical series reporting outcomes after esophagectomy suggest that perioperative mortality rates may range from 10% to as high as 24% (22), with an associated morbidity of 50%–64% (23,24). If these outcome data are used, the calculated cost-effectiveness ratios become prohibitively high.

A computer-simulated Markov model of bi-annual surveillance was performed by Sonnenberg et al. (25) (Table 9.2). Using baseline assumptions including an adenocarcinoma incidence rate of 0.5%, a low surgical mortality rate (0%–3.5%), and a 20% 5-year survival rate, the ICER of surveillance was $16,695 per life-year saved. If either the estimated operative mortality rate was increased (to 7%) or the QOL after surgery was reduced (to 50%), the ICER recalculated to $19,488 or $33,929, respectively. Once again, sensitivity analysis demonstrated that the incidence of EAC in patients with BE and outcomes after esophagectomy were the most important determinants of cost-effectiveness. While the true 5-year survival rate following esophagectomy for EAC ranges from 15%–24% (26), the operative mortality is certainly greater than 7%, suggesting that the ICER is probably higher than reported in this analysis.

The most comprehensive cost-effectiveness model was reported by Inadomi et al., and incorporated a simulation of both screening and surveillance for BE (27) (Table 9.2). A decision analysis Markov model was created to analyze white 50-year old male patients with symptomatic GERD; the model included over 7,000 decision points encompassing the natural history of patients with GERD compared to strategies of screening and surveillance for BE, dysplasia, and cancer. This simultaneous evaluation allowed comparison of the benefit and cost of screening for prevalent EAC with that of surveillance for incident EAC. When screening and surveillance of patients with BE and evidence of dysplasia was compared to no intervention, the ICER was $10,440 per life-year saved; this amount increased to $12,336 for patients without dysplasia. Viewed from a different perspective, however, the incremental ICER was >$500,000 for surveillance in patients with BE without dysplasia compared to those with both BE and dysplasia, suggesting that such a surveillance strategy may not be cost-effective. From this, the authors concluded that the benefit obtained from screening is greater than that of surveillance, since the prevalence of EAC in patients with symptomatic GERD is greater than the subsequent annual incidence of EAC in patients with BE. An additional sensitivity analysis highlighted the importance of several key factors, including identifying groups of patients most at risk of developing EAC and quantifying the QOL of patients undergoing surveillance for BE and following surgery. Cost-effectiveness may also be improved by decreasing the costs of screening and surveillance programs through increased utilization of physician extenders or lowering the cost of endoscopy. Finally, while esophagectomy for high-grade dysplasia has been the traditional therapeutic approach, continued close surveillance (28) or less aggressive surgical options in this subgroup may also be a viable strategy, especially in light of recently published esophagectomy outcomes (22–24,26). Finally, a threshold analysis demonstrated that performing esophagectomy for both EAC and high-grade dysplasia resulted in higher survival only if the annual incidence of EAC with BE was >0.75%, and proved cost-effective (ICER <$50,000) only if this rate was >0.82%.

COMPARISON TO OTHER HEALTH CARE EXPENDITURES

Any discussion regarding cost-effectiveness of a screening or surveillance program is inadequate without a comparison to other accepted medical practices. League tables are commonly used to group and rank interventions in terms of their overall cost-effectiveness, and often form the basis of difficult health care policy decisions (14,29). As summarized in Table 9.4, screening and

TABLE 9.4
Cost-Effectiveness Comparison with Other Medical Practices

Health care interventions	Incremental cost-effectiveness ratios ($/life-year gained)	References
Screening and surveillance of Barrett's esophagus	$12,000–$98,000	2,21
Colon cancer screening	$11,000–$20,000	30,31
Breast cancer screening with annual mammography	$8,300–$57,000	17,32,33
Evaluation of chest pain	$57,700	34
Screening carotid disease (asymptomatic men)	$130,000	35
Cervical cancer screening (Pap smear every 3 yr)	$250,000	32
Heart transplantation	$160,000	36
Empiric omeprazole therapy for dyspepsia	$780,000	37

surveillance programs for BE and EAC compare favorably to similar programs for other diseases. For example, screening for colon cancer with annual fecal occult blood testing and flexible sigmoidoscopy in asymptomatic 50-year old men has an estimated ICER of $20,000 (30,31). Screening mammography for breast cancer carries an ICER ranging from $8,000 to nearly $60,000, which compares favorably with surveillance for BE in a head-to-head analysis (32,33). Commonly accepted interventions such as work-up of chest pain, screening for carotid artery stenosis, and heart transplantation may be less cost-effective, while long-term proton-pump inhibitor therapy and cervical cancer screening are even more expensive (28,34–37).

FUTURE DIRECTIONS

In the past several years, there have been several promising developments with potential to increase the cost-effectiveness of screening and surveillance of BE. Perhaps the most influential factor for improvement is a more precise identification of patient populations most at risk for developing BE and subsequent EAC. A recent study found that age > 40 years and GERD symptoms more than once per week were independent predictors of BE (7). In patients undergoing surveillance of BE, progression to high-grade dysplasia and EAC was associated with BE segment length > 2 cm, hiatal hernia > 3 cm, and the presence of any dysplasia during earlier surveillance (38). Biologic and genetic markers may also eventually prove useful in identifying higher-risk patients; however, no marker has yet emerged that is superior to histologic diagnosis of dysplasia or cancer. Novel techniques for screening and surveillance have been developed, including capsule endoscopy, brush cytology, and chromoendoscopy. When compared to traditional endoscopy, capsule endoscopy cannot obtain biopsies; however, it is less invasive, with comparable sensitivity (97%) and specificity (99%) for diagnosing BE based on visual clues (39). When analyzed using a Markov model, this technology was suggested to be equivalent in efficacy and cost-effectiveness to upper endoscopy as a screening tool (40). Techniques such as brush cytology, chromoendoscopy, and magnification endoscopy may prove more sensitive than traditional endoscopy for detecting early dysplastic changes in the esophageal mucosa, but currently may be too expensive to make them cost-effective. Finally, new therapies for treating high-grade dysplasia of the esophagus, such as endoscopic resection techniques and tissue ablative procedures may prove less costly and carry less morbidity and mortality than that associated with traditional esophagectomy (41,42). These technologies will continue to favor screening and surveillance.

CONCLUSIONS

At the recent AGA Barrett's Esophagus Workshop in 2004, a critical review of the literature covering all aspects of BE was undertaken (43). This expert panel decided that there was insufficient evidence to conclude that screening of the general public for BE was either cost-effective or significantly improved mortality in patients with EAC. Targeted screening of high-risk patients, however, may be effective in diagnosing EAC at a less-invasive stage and therefore improving survival in this selected population. Unfortunately, there is no consensus at this time regarding which patients should be viewed as "high-risk." In terms of surveillance, it is clear that upper endoscopy with multiple biopsy sites is effective for detecting potentially curable dysplastic lesions. However, a careful review of the literature calls into question any conclusion that a routine surveillance program for BE either prolongs overall survival or is proven to be cost-effective (43), especially considering the reported morbidity and mortality of esophagectomy in recent series (22–24,26). Clearly, further research is needed to better characterize the baseline parameters used in cost-effectiveness modeling, such as incidence of BE and EAC, efficacy of endoscopy, and QOL outcomes after surgery. Future development of new diagnostic technologies may prove important for improving the sensitivity and specificity of tests used in screening and surveillance for BE. Finally, less-invasive ablative techniques for esophageal dysplasia may eventually reduce the need for esophagectomy with its accompanying morbidity and mortality. Such therapeutic advances may ultimately make screening and surveillance programs for patients with BE cost-effective.

References

1. Wani S, Sharma P. The rationale for screening and surveillance of Barrett's metaplasia. *Best Pract Res Clin Gastroenterol.* 2006;20:829–842.
2. Sampliner RE, the Practice Parameters Committee of the American College of Gastroenterology. Updated guidelines for the diagnosis, surveillance, and therapy of Barrett's esophagus. *Am J Gastroenterol.* 2002;97:1888–1895.
3. Shaheen NJ, Provenzale D, Sandler RS. Upper endoscopy as a screening and surveillance tool in esophageal adenocarcinoma: a review of the evidence. *Am J Gastroenterol.* 2002;97:1319–1327.
4. Sackett D, Haynes RB, Guyatt GH, eds. *Clinical Epidemiology: A Basic Science for Clinical Medicine.* Boston: Little, Brown; 1991;153–170.
5. Sampliner RE. Epidemiology, pathophysiology, and treatment of Barrett's esophagus: reducing mortality from esophageal adenocarcinoma. *Med Clin North Amer.* 2005;89:293–312.
6. Lagergren J, Bergstrom R, Lindgren A, et al. Symptomatic gastroesophageal reflux as a risk factor for esophageal adenocarcinoma. *N Engl J Med.* 1999;340:825–831.
7. Eloubeide MA, Provenzale D. Clinical and demographic predictors of Barrett's esophagus among patients with gastroesophageal reflux disease. *J Clin Gastroenterol.* 2001;33:306–309.
8. Reid BJ, Haggitt RC, Rubin CE, et al. Observer variation in the diagnosis of dysplasia in Barrett's esophagus. *Hum Pathol.* 1988;19:166–178.

9. Soni A, Sampliner RE, Sonnenberg A. Screening for high-grade dysplasia in gastroesophageal relux disease: is it cost-effective? *Am J Gastroenterol.* 2000;95:2086–2093.
10. van Sandick JW, van Lanschot JJ, Kuiken BW, et al. Impact of endoscopic biopsy surveillance of Barrett's esophagus on pathological stage and clinical outcome of Barrett's carcinoma. *Gut.* 1998;43:216–222.
11. Corley DA, Levin TR, Habel LA, et al. Surveillance and survival in Barrett's adenocarcinomas: a population-based study. *Gastroenterology.* 2002;122:633–640.
12. Aldulaimi DM, Cox M, Nwokolo CU, et al. Barrett's surveillance is worthwhile and detects curable cancers: a prospective cohort study addressing cancer incidence, treatment outcome and survival. *Eur J Gastroenterol Hepatol.* 2005;17(9):943–950.
13. Shaheen, NJ, Crosby MA, Bozymski EM, et al. Is there publication bias in the reporting of cancer risk in Barrett's esophagus? *Gastroenterology.* 2000;119:333–338.
14. Drummond MF, O'Brien B, Stoddart GL, et al. *Methods for the Economic Evaluation of Health Care Programmes.* 2nd ed. New York: Oxford University Press; 1997:96–138, 268–272.
15. O'Connor JB, Falk GW, Richter JE. The incidence of adenocarcinoma and dysplasia in Barrett's esophagus. *Am J Gastroenterol.* 1999;94:2037–2042.
16. Spechler SF, Lee D, Ahnen D, et al. Long-term outcome of medical and surgical therapies for gastroesophageal reflux disease. *JAMA.* 2001;285:2331–2338.
17. Drewitz DJ, Sampliner RE, Garewal HS. The incidence of adenocarcinoma in Barrett's esophagus: a prospective study of 170 patients followed for 4–8 years. *Am J Gastroenterol.* 1997;92:212–215
18. Sharma P, Reker D, Falk G, et al. Progression of Barrett's esophagus to high-grade dysplasia and cancer: preliminary results of the Barrett's esophagus study trial. *Gastroenterology.* 2001;120:A16.
19. Provenzale D, Kemp JA, Sanjeev A, et al. A guide for surveillance of patients with Barrett's esophagus. *Am J Gastroenterol.* 1994;89:670–680.
20. Beck JR, Pauker SG. The Markov process in medical prognosis. *Med Decis Making.* 1983;3:419–458.
21. D, Schmitt C, Wong JB. Barrett's esophagus: a new look at surveillance based on emerging estimates of cancer risk. *Am J Gastroenterol.* 1999;94:2043–2053.
22. Dimick JB, Goodney PP, Orringer MB, Birkmeyer JD. Specialty training and mortality after esophageal cancer resection. *Ann Thorac Surg.* 2005;80:282–286.
23. Bailey SH, Bull DA, Harpole DH, et al. Outcomes after esophagectomy: a ten-year prospective cohort. *Ann Thorac Surg.* 2003;75:217–222.
24. Atkins BZ, Shah AS, Hutcheson KA, et al. Reducing hospital morbidity and mortality following esophagectomy. *Ann Thorac Surg.* 2004;78:1170–1176.
25. Sonnenberg A, Soni A, Sampliner RE. Medical decision analysis of endoscopic surveillance of Barrett's esophagus to prevent esophageal carcinoma. *Aliment Pharmacol Ther.* 2002;16:41–50.
26. Enzinger PC, Mayer RJ. Esophageal cancer. *NEJM.* 2003;349:241–252.
27. Inadomi JM, Sampliner R, Lagergren J, et al. Screening and surveillance for Barrett esophagus in high-risk groups: a cost-utility analysis. *Ann Intern Med.* 2003;138:176–186.
28. Schnell TG, Sontag SF, Chejfec G, et al. Long-term nonsurgical management of Barrett's esophagus with high-grade dysplasia. *Gastroenterology.* 2001;120:1607–1619.
29. Tengs TO, Adams ME, Pliskin JS, et al. Five-hundred life-saving interventions and their cost-effectiveness. *Risk Anal.* 1995;15:369–390.
30. Gold MR, Seigel JE, Russell LB, et al. *Cost-Effectiveness in Health and Medicine.* Oxford: Oxford University Press, 1996.
31. Sonnenberg A, Delco F, Inadomi JM. The cost-effectiveness of colonoscopy in screening for colorectal cancer. *Ann Intern Med.* 2000;133:573–584.
32. Tengs TO, Meyer G, Siegel JE, et al. Oregon's Medicaid ranking and cost-effectiveness: is there any relationship? *Med Decis Making.* 1996;2:99–107.
33. Streitz JM, Ellis FH, Tilden RL, et al. Endoscopic surveillance of Barrett's esophagus: a cost-effectiveness comparison with mammographic surveillance for breast cancer. *Am J Gastroenterol.* 1998;93:911–915.
34. Kuntz KM, Fleischmann KE, Hunink MG, et al. Cost-effectiveness of diagnostic strategies for patients with chest pain. *Ann Intern Med.* 1999;130:709–718.
35. Lee TT, Solomon NA, Heidenriech PA, et al. Cost-effectiveness of screening for carotid stenosis in asymptomatic persons. *Ann Intern Med.* 1997;126:337–346.
36. Pennock JL, Pyer, PE, Reitz BA, et al. Cardiac transplantation in perspective for the future: survival complications, rehabilitation, and cost. *J Thorac Cardiovasc Surg.* 1982;83:168–177.
37. Ebell MH, Warbasse L, Brenner C. Evaluation of the dyspeptic patient: a cost-utility study. *J Fam Pract.* 1997;44:545–555.
38. Weston AP, Badr AS, Hassan RS. Prospective multivariate analysis of clinical, endoscopic, and histological risk factors predictive of the development of Barrett's multifocal high-grade dysplasia or adenocarcinoma. *Am J Gastroenterol.* 1999;94:3413–3419.
39. Eliakim R, Sharma VK, Yassin K, et al. A prospective study of the diagnostic accuracy of PillCam ESO esophageal capsule endoscopy versus conventional upper endoscopy in patients with chronic gastroesophageal reflux diseases. *J Clin Gastroenterol.* 1997;112:1787–1797.
40. Rubenstein JH, Inadomi JM, Brill JV, et al. Cost utility of screening for Barrett's esophagus with esophageal capsule endoscopy versus conventional upper endoscopy. *Clin Gastroenterol Hepatol.* 2007;5(3):312–318.
41. Panjehpour M, Overholt BF, Haydeck JM, et al. Results of photodynamic therapy for ablation of dysplasia and early cancer in Barrett's esophagus and effect of oral steroids on stricture formation. *Am J Gastroenterol.* 2000;95:2177–2184.
42. Bergman JJ. Latest developments in the endoscopic management of gastroesophageal reflux disease and Barrett's esophagus: an overview of the year's literature. *Endoscopy.* 2006;38:122–132.
43. Sharma P, McQuaid K, Dent J, et al. A critical review of the diagnosis and management of Barrett's esophagus: the AGA Chicago workshop. *Gastroenterology.* 2004;127:310–330.

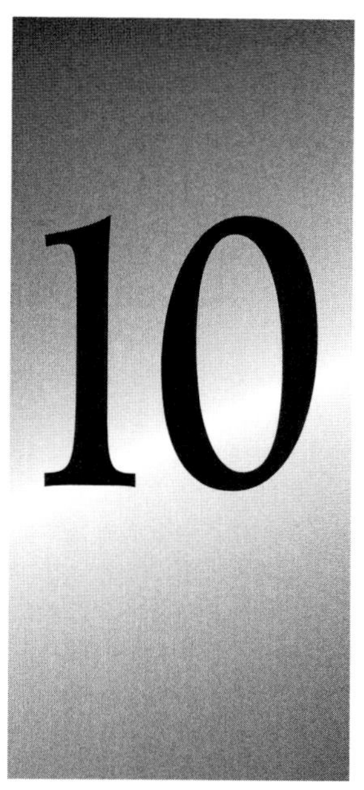

Barrett's Esophagus: Chemoprevention

George Triadafilopoulos

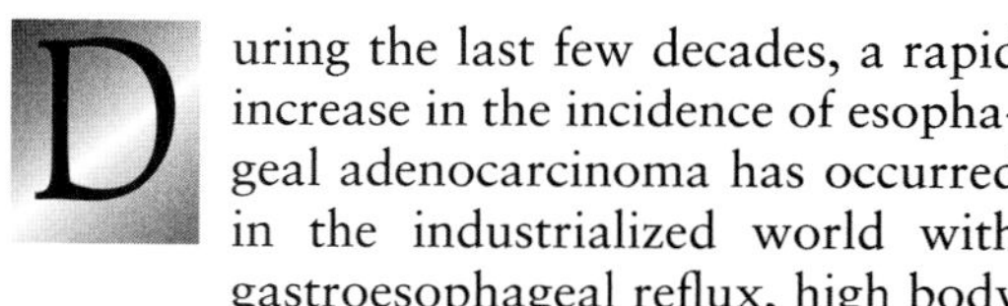

During the last few decades, a rapid increase in the incidence of esophageal adenocarcinoma has occurred in the industrialized world with gastroesophageal reflux, high body mass, male sex, Barrett's esophagus, and tobacco smoking having been identified as key risk factors. Several other potential risk factors, such as the use of medications that relax the lower esophageal sphincter, high fat diets, or diets low in nutrients from plant foods, have also been identified. In contrast, infection with *Helicobacter pylori* and the use of anti-inflammatory drugs (such as aspirin and other non-steroidal anti-inflammatory drugs, including cyclooxygenase inhibitors) have been inversely linked with the risk of esophageal adenocarcinoma (1). This rise in incidence of esophageal adenocarcinoma and the improved understanding of the epidemiology and pathophysiology of the disease has spurred robust clinical and research activity aimed at preventing cancer development through application of early screening of subjects at risk, endoscopic surveillance, and widespread use of new technologies, such as ablation and endoscopic resection before invasive cancer develops.

Cancer chemoprevention is the pharmacologic intervention that aims to intervene in pathways that lead to cancer before such cancer occurs. Esophageal cancer chemoprevention is a new field that has been mostly ignited by observational studies, showing that non-steroidal anti-inflammatory drugs (NSAIDs) are protective against esophageal adenocarcinoma, while a combination of beta-carotene, alpha-tocopherol, and selenium may protect against squamous esophageal cancer (2). Herein we review the current evidence that promotes the concept of chemoprevention of esophageal adenocarcinoma utilizing various agents either alone or in combination. However, there are no randomized clinical trials demonstrating a clear clinical benefit on chemoprevention of dysplasia and adenocarcinoma. Instead, using intermediate end-points (i.e., cellular proliferation, dysplasia rates), studies have suggested that maximal intraesophageal acid suppression with proton pump inhibition (PPI) therapy and cyclooxygenase-2 (COX-2) inhibition may be useful.

Since symptoms of gastroesophageal reflux disease (GERD) and Barrett's esophagus are the key risk factors for esophageal adenocarcinoma, the evidence has centered on patients with these conditions. Nevertheless, up to 40% of esophageal adenocarcinoma cases occur in people without prior or concurrent reflux symptoms, and future efforts should focus on chemoprevention strategies that would be applied to the general population (3). Table 10.1 outlines the specific means for chemoprevention of esophageal adenocarcinoma.

TABLE 10.1
Means for Chemoprevention of Esophageal Adenocarcinoma

Control of acid reflux for the prevention of Barrett's esophagus
Acid suppressive therapy
Control of bile reflux
Inhibition of ornithine decarboxylase
Aspirin and NSAIDs
Combination of PPI and aspirin

GENERALITIES

Barrett's esophagus, defined as endoscopically recognized and histologically proven intestinal metaplasia of the esophagus, is a 3-phase process (4). During the *initiation* phase, genetically predisposed individuals (typically white men) are exposed to clinical or occult gastroesophageal reflux, suffer esophageal squamous epithelial damage, and develop a new cell phenotype (transformation). During the *formation* phase, the new phenotype matures to short-segment (< 3cm) or long-segment (> 3cm) Barrett's esophagus and does not expand further. During the *progression* phase, low-grade dysplasia, high-grade dysplasia, or invasive cancer may occur at rates of 4.3%, 0.9%, and 0.5% per year respectively, under the influence of a cascade of molecular events leading to proliferation, increasing DNA damage and cellular aneuploidy (5). Hence, chemoprevention efforts focus on one or more of these genetic and epigenetic alterations that are involved in the progression of Barrett's esophagus to adenocarcinoma. It is important to emphasize that Barrett's esophagus progression is not geographic; that is, not associated with expansion of the length or surface of the metaplasia. Instead, progression is molecular, with increased proliferation under the influence of acid and bile reflux and associated genetic and cytometric abnormalities.

Simplistically seen, the overall risk for cancer is a function of the number of dividing metaplastic cells over time: $r = f(n / t)$. If such dividing cells are removed by biopsy or endoscopic mucosal resection, ablated by photodynamic therapy or balloon-based radiofrequency current, or their rate of cell division is suppressed or halted pharmacologically, the risk for cancer will be reduced or eliminated. This latter approach could be viewed as cancer chemoprevention.

CONTROL OF ACID REFLUX FOR THE PREVENTION OF BARRETT'S ESOPHAGUS

It is unclear why only a minority of patients with GERD develop Barrett's esophagus, but some recent in vitro evidence suggests that, damaged by acid, the esophageal squamous epithelium of such patients becomes metaplastic rather than regenerating more squamous esophageal cells (6). Evaluating the response of the extracellular regulated kinase (ERK)1/2, an enzyme involved in stimulating cell proliferation, following acid exposure of the squamous esophagus of GERD patients with and without Barrett's esophagus, Souza et al. found that baseline levels of ERK1/2 were significantly lower in the squamous mucosa of GERD patients without metaplasia and that acid exposure increased the activity of ERK1/2 in the squamous epithelium of GERD patients without but not in those with Barrett's esophagus. It is therefore possible that individuals who have high baseline levels of ERK1/2 and fail to activate this pro-proliferative pathway in response to acid exposure may be predisposed to intestinal metaplasia rather than squamous re-epithelialization. Hence, early institution of acid suppressive therapy in patients with GERD might prevent this first *formation* step in the metaplasia-dysplasia-carcinoma sequence described above. Further, it may also be possible to identify a molecular biomarker that would identify GERD patients bound to develop Barrett's esophagus and therefore select a subgroup which might benefit from endoscopic screening/surveillance or cancer chemoprevention.

Acid suppressive therapy is associated with a reduction in the eventual length of newly diagnosed Barrett's esophagus in patients with GERD (Figure 10.1). A retrospective analysis of a well-characterized large cohort of patients with Barrett's esophagus compared the length of metaplasia between patients who received acid suppressive therapy prior to their diagnosis to those who did not receive such therapy. In the same study, the authors further examined the association between prior use of acid suppressive therapy and the length of Barrett's esophagus in correlation and multivariate linear regression analyses. Of all patients, 139 (41%) had prior use of histamine-2 receptor antagonists (H2RAs), or PPIs (41 used both), and 201 (59%) used neither prior to the diagnosis of Barrett's esophagus. The mean length of Barrett's esophagus was significantly shorter in patients with prior PPI use (3.4 cm) or PPIs and H2RAs (3.1 cm) when compared to those with none of these medications (4.8 cm). In the multivariate linear regression model, the prior PPI use or either PPI or H2RAs was an independent predictor of shorter length of Barrett's esophagus (7).

This evidence suggests that early utilization of PPI therapy in patients with acid reflux symptoms would protect against the development of Barrett's metaplasia and in turn of adenocarcinoma. However, despite the over-the-counter availability and accessibility of acid suppressants and their lower costs, we have not seen an impact on the incidence of Barrett's esophagus detected on endoscopy, and the role of such therapy in averting Barrett's esophagus formation remains unclear.

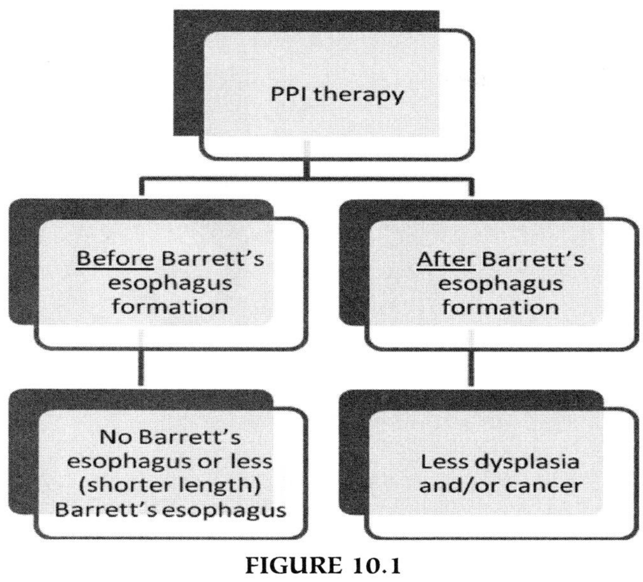

FIGURE 10.1

Possible beneficial role of PPI therapy in Barrett's esophagus chemoprevention (based on references 7 and 13).

CONTROL OF ACID REFLUX IN PATIENTS WITH ESTABLISHED BARRETT'S ESOPHAGUS FOR THE PREVENTION OF CANCER

Aggressive control of gastric acid secretion resulting in reduction or elimination of intraesophageal acid exposure has been proposed as a strategy to decrease the risk of cancer in Barrett's esophagus (Figure 10.1). This notion is based on ex vivo as well as in vivo data suggesting that intraesophageal acid suppression decreases proliferation in the metaplastic epithelium. However, prospective randomized trials using clinical endpoints (i.e., development of dysplasia or cancer, cancer mortality) are not yet available and only intermediate surrogate endpoints with unclear clinical significance have been used.

Fitzgerald et al. investigated the ex vivo effects of acid on cell differentiation (as determined by villin expression) and on cell proliferation (as determined by tritiated thymidine incorporation and proliferating cell nuclear antigen expression) (8). To mimic known physiologic conditions, endoscopic biopsies of normal esophagus, Barrett's esophagus, and duodenum were exposed, in organ culture, to acidified media (pH 3–5) either continuously, or as a 1-hour pulse and compared with exposure to pH 7.4 for up to 24 hours. Before culture, villin expression was noted in 25% of Barrett's esophagus samples, and increased after 6 or 24 hours of continuous acid to 50% or 83% of samples, respectively. Increased villin expression correlated with ultrastructural maturation of the brush border. In contrast, an acid-pulse followed by culture at pH 7.4, did not alter villin expression in Barrett's esophagus. Moreover, continuous acid exposure blocked cell proliferation in these explants, whereas, an acid-pulse enhanced cell proliferation, as compared to pH 7.4. Based on these ex vivo findings, Fitzgerald et al. proposed a model in which the diverse patterns of acid exposure in vivo may contribute to the observed heterogeneity and unpredictable progression to dysplasia and neoplasia of Barrett's esophagus (8).

Acid may contribute to carcinogenesis in Barrett's esophagus through activation of MAPK pathways. In a study by Souza et al., Barrett's adenocarcinoma cell line (SEG-1) cells were exposed to acidic media for 3 minutes, and the activities of 3 MAPKs (ERK, p38, and JNK) were determined. Proliferation was assessed using flow cytometry, and cell growth and apoptosis were assessed using cell counts and an apoptosis ELISA assay. Further, MAPK activation was studied in biopsy specimens taken from patients with Barrett's esophagus before and after esophageal perfusion for 3 minutes with 0.1N HCl. Acid-exposed SEG-1 cells exhibited a significant increase in proliferation and total cell numbers, and a significant decrease in apoptosis. These effects were preceded by a rapid increase in the activities of ERK and p38, and a delayed increase in JNK activity. The acid-induced decrease in apoptosis was abolished by inhibition of either ERK or p38. In patients, acid exposure significantly increased the activity of p38 in metaplastic tissues (9).

In another in vitro study, treatment with PPIs favorably altered the expression and DNA copy number of key cell cycle regulatory genes in paired normal and Barrett's esophagus samples. In this study, protein levels were evaluated in 60 formalin-fixed and paraffin-embedded human tissues by immunohistochemistry while DNA copy number was analyzed by Southern blot analysis in 20 fresh tissue pairs. All normal mucosal samples expressed the p27 (kip1) protein but did not exhibit nuclear staining for p16 (kip4), p21 (cip1) or cyclins D1 and E. In contrast, Barrett's metaplastic samples revealed increased expression of p16 (kip4) (74%), p21 (cip1) (89%), and cyclins D1 (43%) and E (37%) levels. p27 protein was absent in 3 cases. There was a significant correlation between p16 (kip4) and cyclin E expression, while p21 (cip1) and p27 (kip4) correlated with cyclin D1. Although DNA analysis did not reveal any amplification or deletion of these genes, acid suppression was associated with significantly lower expression levels of key cell cycle proteins (10).

Contradicting these in vivo and ex vivo studies, acid exposure has p53-mediated, antiproliferative effects in non-neoplastic Barrett's epithelial cells. In a study of the effects of acid on proliferation and apoptosis in a non-neoplastic, telomerase-immortalized Barrett's epithelial cell line, cells were treated with two 3-minute exposures to acidic media and cell growth was determined using cell counts, proliferation was studied by flow cytometry, cell viability was determined by trypan blue staining, and apoptosis was assessed by TUNEL and Annexin V. The expression levels of p53 and p21 were determined by Western blotting; p53 siRNA was used to study the effect of p53 inhibition on total cell numbers after acid exposure. Acid exposure significantly decreased total cell numbers at 24 hours without affecting either cell viability or apoptosis. Acid exposure resulted in cell cycle prolongation that was associated with greater expression of p53, but not p21. The acid-induced decrease in total cell numbers was abolished by p53 RNAi (11).

Cell proliferation and differentiation were studied in vivo in biopsy specimens of Barrett's esophagus before and after 6 months of therapy with the PPI lansoprazole at doses needed to render patients acid reflux symptom-free. Cellular proliferation (as measured by PCNA immunohistochemical staining) decreased while differentiation (as measured by villin immunoblotting) increased in the patients who exhibited normalization of esophageal acid exposure by 24-hour ambulatory pH monitoring but not in those who—despite being asymptomatic on therapy—exhibited persistently abnormal acid exposure (12). Further, a more recent study showed that patients with Barrett's esophagus treated with PPIs developed dysplasia less frequently than those treated with H2RAs, which are less effective at controlling gastric acid secretion and, in turn, intraesophageal pH (13). In this retrospective study of 236 veteran patients, 86% Caucasian and 98% male, during 1,170 patient-yr of follow-up, 56 patients developed dysplasia giving an annual incidence rate of 4.7%. Of those, 14 had high-grade dysplasia. The cumulative incidence of dysplasia was significantly lower among patients who received PPI after the diagnosis of Barrett's esophagus than in those who received no therapy or used H2RAs. Furthermore, among those on PPIs, a longer duration of use was associated with less frequent occurrence of dysplasia. In multivariate analysis, the use of PPI after the diagnosis of Barrett's esophagus was independently associated with reduced risk of dysplasia, with a hazards ratio of 0.25. Longer segments of Barrett's metaplasia and Caucasian race were other independent risk factors for developing dysplasia. Similar findings were also observed when only cases with high-grade dysplasia were analyzed (Figure 10.2).

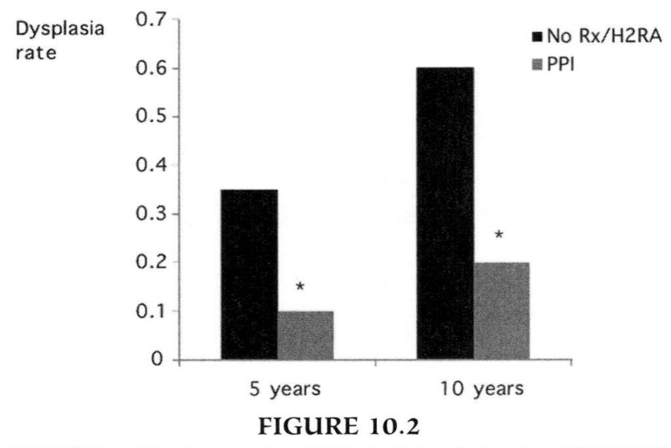

FIGURE 10.2

Dysplasia rates in patients with Barrett's esophagus treated with PPIs versus those either not receiving any treatment or receiving H2RA therapy (adapted from reference 13).

Furthermore, a significantly increased rate of cell proliferation and pro-proliferative cell cycle abnormalities have been detected in biopsies of Barrett's epithelium taken from patients treated with H2RAs compared with similar biopsies from patients treated with PPIs. In 1 randomized 2-year follow-up study, 45 patients with long-segment Barrett's esophagus were treated with either omeprazole 40 mg or ranitidine 150 mg both taken twice daily and were compared for the effect on epithelial cell proliferation (14). Biopsies were taken 3 cm above the GEJ at 0, 3, 9, and 24 months. Epithelial cell proliferation was determined by in vitro labeling with 5-bromo-2-deoxyuridine and immunohistochemistry and labeling indices for luminal and crypt epithelium were used separately. Ambulatory 24-hour esophageal monitoring was performed at 0 and 3 months. Omeprazole reduced mean acid reflux to 0.1% per 24 hours, while ranitidine to 9.4% and this was associated with a significant increase in the labeling index in ranitidine-treated patients, while in those on omeprazole it remained stable.

It should be noted that, aggressive acid suppression that goes beyond what is required to effectively control reflux symptoms and tissue healing and does not concomitantly eliminate other harmful components of the gastro-duodenal refluxate may have unfavorable consequences. A very important role of duodenal components (i.e., bile acids) in the development of Barrett's adenocarcinoma has been raised in several clinical studies. Kauer et al. showed that patients with Barrett's metaplasia have a significantly higher prevalence of abnormal intraesophageal bilirubin exposure than those with erosive or non-erosive reflux disease. In their study, the correlation of pH and bilirubin monitoring showed that the majority (87%) of esophageal bilirubin exposure occurred when the pH of the esophagus was between 4 and 7, suggesting that bile acids—the major component of duodenal juice—are capable of damaging the esophageal mucosa at a near-neutral pH (15).

In another study, Kaur et al. investigated the effect of bile salts, with or without acid, on cell proliferation in ex vivo mucosal explants. In order to mimic physiologic conditions in this study, biopsies of esophagus, Barrett's esophagus, and duodenum were exposed to a bile salt mixture, either continuously or at 1-hour pulses, and were compared with control media without bile salts (pH 7.4) for up to 24 hours. Similar experiments were also performed with acidified media (pH 3.5), combined with the bile salt mixture as 1-hour pulses. Bile salt pulses enhanced cell proliferation only in Barrett's explants without affecting cell proliferation in esophageal or duodenal epithelia. In contrast, 1-hour pulses of bile salts in combination with acid significantly inhibited proliferation in Barrett's esophagus but had no effect on esophagus or duodenum. The authors concluded that, in Barrett's esophagus explants, brief exposure to bile salts, in the absence of acid, increases proliferation, whereas exposure to a combination of bile salts and acid together inhibits proliferation (16). In order to further understand the mechanisms of acid- and bile-induced hyperproliferation in Barrett's esophagus, these researchers further investigated the release of PGE_2 in response to acid or bile salt exposure. Biopsies of esophagus, Barrett's esophagus, and duodenum were exposed to a bile salt mixture at 1-hour pulses and compared with exposure to pH 7.4 for up to 24 hours, and PGE_2 release, cyclooxygenase-2 (COX-2), and protein kinase C (PKC) expression were compared. Similar experiments were also performed with acidified media (pH 3.5) alone, in the presence or absence of a selective PKC inhibitor, and a COX-2 inhibitor. One-hour pulses of bile salts or acid significantly enhanced proliferation, COX-2 expression, and PGE_2 release in Barrett's esophagus. In contrast, the combination pulse of acid and bile salts had no such effect. Furthermore, treatment with either PKC or COX-2 inhibitors led to a dramatic decrease in PGE_2 release in Barrett's esophagus explants and a suppression of proliferation, suggesting that the acid- or bile salt-mediated hyperproliferation is related to COX-2-mediated PGE_2 release and explain, at least in part, the tumor-promoting effects of acid and bile in Barrett's metaplasia (17). Taken together, these ex vivo studies suggest that complete acid inhibition may not be beneficial unless associated by concomitant effective control of bile reflux. In contrast, if intraesophageal acid exposure is effectively controlled pharmacologically, unabated bile reflux may promote proliferation in Barrett's metaplasia and increase the risk for cancer.

Chronic PPI therapy frequently leads to elevated serum gastrin levels. Gastrin is a mitogen capable of inducing growth in both normal and malignant gastrointestinal mucosa and has been linked to increased proliferation in Barrett's biopsy specimens in vitro. Performing reverse-transcription polymerase chain reaction (RT-PCR) and northern analysis for the cholecystokinin (CCK-2) receptor on normal squamous, inflamed squamous, Barrett's metaplastic, and malignant esophageal mucosa, Haigh et al. noted that gastrin induces proliferation via the CCK-2 receptor in Barrett's mucosa. Real-time PCR quantified receptor expression in 10 patients with Barrett's esophagus showing twice the level of expression than that of 12 controls. Further, 10 nmol/L of G17 induced a 2-fold increase in [3-H]-thymidine incorporation in mucosal biopsy specimens (18). Abdalla et al. noted that biopsies from non-dysplastic Barrett's esophagus expressed increased gastrin mRNA levels compared with other epithelia. Further, gastrin significantly induced COX-2, prostaglandin E2, and cell proliferation in biopsies and cell lines. Gastrin-induced proliferation could be inhibited by inhibitors for CCK-2 and COX-2 suggesting that, during carcinogenesis, gastrin is a significant determinant of COX-2 activity levels via the CCK-2 receptor (19).

Chronic acid suppressive therapy in patients with gastroesophageal reflux disease (GERD) may induce gastric bacterial overgrowth leading to an increased amount of deconjugated bile acids and increased mucosal injury. In one study, 30 patients with GERD who were treated with omeprazole 40 mg daily for at least 3 months and 10 patients with GERD who were untreated for at least 2 weeks were studied by gastric fluid aspiration and analyzed for bacterial growth and bile acids. Eleven of the 30 patients taking omeprazole had bacterial overgrowth compared to 1 of the 10 control patients. Bacterial overgrowth only occurred when the pH was >3.8. The ratio of conjugated to unconjugated bile acids changed from 4:1 in the patients without bacterial overgrowth to 1:3 in those with bacterial growth greater than 1000/ml (20). Chronic PPIs can also result in increased production of secondary bile acids, particularly deoxycholic acid (DCA), which has been demonstrated to have a tumor-promoting capacity (see below).

The aforementioned experimental and clinical data support the concept of potent acid suppression as a chemopreventive strategy in patients with Barrett's esophagus. However, because of possibly unabated bile reflux, this approach will require proper validation by controlled, prospective clinical trials before it can be recommended for widespread long-term practice. Presently, although some groups feel that patients with Barrett's esophagus should be treated with PPIs given in doses that adequately eliminate acid reflux symptoms and heal esophagitis, others are more aggressive and (in such asymptomatic patients with Barrett's esophagus) they routinely advocate 24-hour esophageal pH monitoring while on PPI therapy to document the "normalization" of esophageal acid exposure. Although it is generally assumed that acid suppressive therapy with PPIs improves or eliminates GERD symptoms by normalizing intraesophageal pH, such normalization has been reported to happen in less than 50% of patients with Barrett's esophagus treated with PPIs and rendered asymptomatic. For example, in one study, 62 patients with GERD and 48 with Barrett's esophagus were prospectively evaluated by dual sensor 24h pH monitoring while receiving PPI therapy for complete symptom control. Only 24 (50%) patients with Barrett's esophagus normalized their intraesophageal pH profiles on PPI. Overall, as compared with patients with GERD, patients with Barrett's esophagus were more likely to have higher degree of pathologic acid reflux despite PPI therapy and exhibited less intragastric acid suppression, particularly supine, suggesting that intraesophageal and intragastric pH control are significantly more difficult to achieve in patients with Barrett's esophagus (21).

In another study to assess the efficacy of esomeprazole on symptom relief and intraesophageal and intragastric acid suppression in patients with Barrett's esophagus, all patients tolerated esomeprazole (40–80 mg/day) with good symptom control. However, 62% of these patients had abnormal intraesophageal pH profiles and significant nocturnal breakthrough despite adequate symptom control despite PPI therapy. Low nocturnal intragastric pH correlated highly with nocturnal intraesophageal acid reflux, and there was a relative failure of nocturnal intragastric acid control with esomeprazole. These authors concluded that for an antisecretory treatment aimed at chemoprevention of esophageal adenocarcinoma to be effective, higher PPI dosing confirmed by pH monitoring may be necessary (22).

Since patients with Barrett's esophagus may continue to have abnormal esophageal acid exposure despite PPI therapy, Wani et al. evaluated esophageal acid exposure in a large Barrett's esophagus population treated with twice daily PPIs and determined clinical factors predicting normalization of intraesophageal pH on therapy. In this study, 34 of the Barrett's esophagus patients (73.9%) had a normal pH study and 12 patients (26.1%) had an abnormal result. The authors found no significant differences between patients with a normal and abnormal 24h pH result with respect to age, Barrett's esophagus length, hiatal hernia size, and presence of *H. pylori* infection; hence, such factors cannot be used to predict persistent abnormal intraesophageal pH on PPI (23).

Nevertheless, PPIs have been shown to decrease the bile component of the refluxate. Using a spectrophotometric technique to measure bile reflux and 24-hour esophageal pH monitoring, 4 groups were studied: healthy subjects, reflux patients, patients with Barrett's esophagus, and patients with esophageal symptoms after partial gastrectomy. Such simultaneous 24-hour pH and bile monitoring of distal esophagus found a close association ($r = 0.78$) between intraesophageal acid exposure and duodeno-gastroesophageal reflux. The use of omeprazole (20 mg twice daily) normalized both acid reflux and duodeno-gastroesophageal reflux suggesting that aggressive acid suppression markedly decreases both (24).

CONTROL OF BILE REFLUX IN PATIENTS WITH ESTABLISHED BARRETT'S ESOPHAGUS FOR THE PREVENTION OF CANCER

The molecular mechanisms by which bile acids promote the development of esophageal adenocarcinoma are still largely unknown and have not been fully investigated. Combined pH and bilirubin monitoring and esophageal aspiration studies in humans suggest a combined role for bile acids, particularly taurine-conjugated bile acids, in causing esophageal mucosal injury. Animal model experiments have also shown that duodenal juice alone may induce Barrett's esophagus and cancer. Likewise, ex vivo studies with biopsies from patients with Barrett's esophagus have shown increased proliferation and COX-2 expression after a pulsed exposure to acid or conjugated bile acids, but not if acid and bile acids are combined (25).

Unconjugated bile acids induce CREB and AP-1-dependent COX-2 expression in Barrett's esophagus and adenocarcinoma through ROS-mediated activation of PI3K/AKT and ERK1/2. The secondary bile acid, DCA, is one of the commonly refluxed bile acids that causes chromosome damage and induces human p53 gene mutations at both neutral and acidic pH. Since it can induce DNA damage at neutral pH, suppressing the acidity of the refluxate will not completely remove its carcinogenic potential. The genotoxicity of DCA is, however, reactive oxygen species (ROS) dependent, hence anti-oxidant supplementation in addition to acid suppression may block DCA-driven carcinogenesis in Barrett's patients (26).

The oral administration of ursodeoxycholic acid (UDCA) decreases plasma and biliary endogenous bile acid concentrations while UDCA itself is found in high concentrations in these compartments (27). It is unclear if the reduction in endogenous bile acid concentration is induced by competition for intestinal absorption of endogenous bile acids or if there is increased hepatic clearance of endogenous bile acids. The endogenous bile acids have greater detergent activity and are therefore more cytotoxic than UDCA. Thus, such UDCA-induced decrease in endogenous bile acids in the gastroduodenal refluxate could have a favorable chemopreventive role in patients with Barrett's esophagus. A small, open pilot study, however, failed to show a significant reduction in cellular proliferation or PGE2 decrease in biopsies of patients treated with UDCA (unpublished observations). The use of bile acid-binding agents, such as cholestyramine, cholestipol, or sucralfate has not been studied.

Because it controls both acid and bile reflux, antireflux surgery (fundoplication) has been proposed as more effective than antisecretory therapy for preventing cancer in Barrett's esophagus (28). For example, 2 small, uncontrolled studies found fewer cases of dysplasia and cancer among patients with Barrett's esophagus who had undergone fundoplication than among those who had received medical treatment. McCallum et al. prospectively followed 181 patients with Barrett's esophagus: 29 who had anti-reflux surgery and 152 who were treated medically (29). Dysplasia was found in 3.4% of the surgical group after a mean follow-up of 62 months and in 19.7% of the medical group after a mean follow-up of 49 months. No patient in the surgically treated group developed adenocarcinoma, compared with 2 medically treated patients. Similarly, Katz et al. followed 102 patients with Barrett's esophagus for a mean of 4.8 years (30). By 3 years, dysplasia had developed in approximately 8% of the medically treated patients. In contrast, patients treated by anti-reflux surgery had a significantly reduced risk of developing dysplasia. In contrast, a randomized trial of medical versus surgical therapy of 247 veteran patients with erosive esophagitis (including 108 with Barrett's esophagus) did not show that fundoplication prevents esophageal adenocarcinoma better than medical therapy (31). In this study, during 10 to 13 years of follow-up, 4 of 165 patients (2.4%) receiving medical therapy and 1 of 82 (1.2%) who had undergone fundoplication developed esophageal adenocarcinoma, a insignificant difference due to inadequate statistical power. In another large, Swedish, population-based cohort study, patients with GERD were followed for up to 32 years. The relative risk for developing esophageal adenocarcinoma (compared with the general population) among 35,274 men who received medical anti-reflux therapy was 6.3, whereas the relative risk for 6,406 men treated with fundoplication was 14.1 (32). A recent meta-analysis also found no significant cancer-protective effect of anti-reflux surgery (33).

INHIBITION OF ORNITHINE DECARBOXYLASE

Ornithine decarboxylase (ODC) is the rate-limiting enzyme in the synthesis of polyamines that are essential for cells to progress through the cell cycle (34). Barrett's esophagus expresses higher ODC than control epithelia and such expression increases significantly with dysplasia (35–37). The ODC inhibitor DFMO has been used in clinical trials as a chemopreventive and chemotherapeutic agent, but its use has been limited by ototoxicity (38–40). In one study, low-dose (0.5 g/m2) DFMO treatment of patients with Barrett's esophagus for 6 weeks decreased the polyamine tissue content by 60% (41) but, in another study, 1 patient treated with DFMO developed irreversible ototoxicity (42).

Indirect inhibitors of ODC may also have a potential role for chemoprevention in Barrett's esophagus. For example, troglitazone, a peroxisome proliferator-activated receptor gamma (PPAR-gamma) ligand, reduces ODC activity in human esophageal adenocarcinoma cells in vitro by inhibiting cell growth and inducing apoptosis (43). In vitro treatment of a human esophageal adenocarcinoma cell line with troglitazone significantly inhibited cell growth and induced apoptosis, events which would limit the growth of neoplastic cells in vivo. Controlled clinical trials will be needed before ODC inhibitors can be recommended for cancer chemoprevention in patients with Barrett's esophagus.

ASPIRIN AND SELECTIVE OR NON-SELECTIVE NON-STEROIDAL ANTI-INFLAMMATORY DRUGS

Aspirin, as well as both selective and non-selective non-steroidal anti-inflammatory drugs (NSAIDs), all inhibitors of cyclooxygenase, have been extensively studied as potential chemopreventive agents in patients with Barrett's esophagus. Cyclooxygenase and its 2 isoforms, COX-1 and COX-2, mediate the production of prostaglandins from arachidonic acid. Whereas COX-1 is expressed constitutively in many epithelia, COX-2 expression is inducible by cytokines, growth factors, and tumor promoters, and maybe detected in many gastrointestinal premalignant and malignant epithelia (44–46). Since increased COX-2 expression promotes proliferation and decrease apoptosis in vitro, its inhibition by COX-2 inhibitors may have chemopreventive effect (47,48).

Several epidemiologic studies suggest that the use of aspirin and other NSAIDs protects against gastrointestinal neoplasia, including adenocarcinoma of the esophagus (49–52). However, the anti-neoplastic effect of NSAIDs may also be independent of COX inhibition (53,54). In a prospective study of the relation between duration, frequency, and recent use of NSAIDs and the risk of esophageal adenocarcinoma, aneuploidy, and tetraploidy in a cohort of 350 people with Barrett's esophagus followed for 20,770 person-months, NSAID use was shown to be an effective chemopreventive strategy, reducing the risk of neoplastic progression in patients with Barrett's esophagus. Compared with never users, hazard ratios for esophageal adenocarcinoma in current NSAID users was 0.32, and in former users was 0.70. The 5-year cumulative incidence of esophageal adenocarcinoma was 14.3% for never users, 9.7% for former users, and 6.6% for current NSAID users. Further, compared with never users, current NSAID users (at baseline and follow-up) had less aneuploidy and tetraploidy (55).

A systematic review with meta-analysis of observational studies evaluating the association of aspirin or NSAID use and esophageal cancer identified 9 studies

(2 cohort, 7 case control) containing 1,813 cancer cases and showed a protective association between any use of aspirin/NSAID and esophageal cancer (odds ratio [OR] = 0.57). Further, the study provided evidence for a dose effect since both intermittent (OR = 0.82) and frequent medication use were protective (OR = 0.54) with greater protection with more frequent use. Stratified by medication type, aspirin use was protective (OR = 0.5) and NSAIDs had a borderline protective association (OR = 0.75) (56).

A literature review identified 27 studies that qualitatively or quantitatively assessed COX-2 protein or gene expression in either Barrett's esophagus, dysplastic, or adenocarcinoma tissue in humans. In this study, there was general agreement that COX-2 was either absent or very weakly expressed in normal esophageal squamous mucosa, but there was considerable disagreement regarding the presence of COX-2 in Barrett's and low-grade dysplasia. All studies agreed that high-grade dysplasia and adenocarcinoma expressed COX-2 to some extent although levels varied considerably between tissue samples (57).

Sonnenberg et al. analyzed the incremental cost-effectiveness ratio (ICER) of chemoprevention—as compared with endoscopic surveillance or with no surveillance—using a Markov computer model (58). They found that under baseline conditions for all patients with Barrett's esophagus (neoplastic and non-neoplastic), the ICER of chemoprevention ranges between $12,700 and $18,500 per life-year saved. However, these cost values are sensitive to variations in the costs of chemoprevention, incidence of cancer in patients with Barrett's esophagus, and efficacy of NSAIDs in reducing the incidence of cancer, which can shift the ICER into a cost range that is prohibitively expensive. Conversely, in those patients with Barrett's esophagus and high-grade dysplasia, the ICER ranges between $3,900 and $5,000, and chemoprevention remains a cost-effective option even under rather unfavorable conditions, such as higher cost and lower efficacy of chemoprevention and lower incidence of cancer. However, chemoprevention may not be a cost-effective measure in the general population of all patients with Barrett's esophagus, depending on unknown factors such as cost and efficacy of chemoprevention as well as true incidence of cancer (58).

Although aspirin use is associated with many complications, such as gastrointestinal bleeding and hemorrhagic stroke, its use in the management of Barrett's esophagus appears to be a cost-effective strategy to prevent esophageal adenocarcinoma. A Markov Monte Carlo decision model was constructed to compare, from a societal perspective from age 55 years until death, 4 strategies for management of Barrett's esophagus: aspirin therapy, endoscopic surveillance with biopsies, both, or neither. Patients who took a daily enteric-coated aspirin were modeled to have a 50% reduction in the incidence of esophageal adenocarcinoma but could have complications related to therapy, at which point the aspirin was discontinued. Potential cardiac benefits of aspirin and its role in the chemoprevention of other cancers were not analyzed. Sensitivity analyses were performed to investigate the effects of changes in model parameters on estimated costs and effectiveness outcomes across a wide range of assumptions. Aspirin therapy was more effective and less costly than no therapy, resulting in 0.19 more quality-adjusted life years (QALYs). The combination of aspirin and endoscopic surveillance produced 0.27 more QALYs than no therapy at a cost of $13,400 more, for an associated incremental cost-effectiveness ratio of $49,600/QALY. Aspirin use in combination with endoscopic surveillance dominated endoscopic surveillance alone, resulting in 0.06 more QALYs and $11,400 less cost. These results, however, were sensitive to increasing age and to decreased benefit or delay in the chemopreventive efficacy of aspirin (59).

In Barrett's esophagus, selective COX-2 inhibitors have been used both in vivo and in vitro studies and shown to decrease proliferation and increase apoptosis in vitro in combined primary cultures of dysplastic and non-dysplastic Barrett's epithelial cells and in human esophageal adenocarcinoma cell lines (60,61). In an animal model, selective inhibition of COX-2 decreases both the development of Barrett's esophagus and the incidence of esophageal adenocarcinoma (62,63). Further, short-term treatment of patients with the selective COX-2 inhibitor rofecoxib decreases cellular proliferation in Barrett's epithelia in vivo (64).

In adenocarcinoma cells in vitro and in an animal model of Barrett's esophagus, the administration of nonselective NSAIDs induces apoptosis and decreases the risk of tumor formation (65). However, in an animal model of Barrett's esophagus, there is no significant difference in the risk of tumor formation in animals treated with MF-tricyclic (a selective COX-2 inhibitor) and sulindac (a nonselective NSAID) (66).

The effect of long-term administration of celecoxib in 100 patients with low- or high-grade Barrett's dysplasia was investigated in the Chemoprevention for Barrett's Esophagus Trial (CBET), a phase IIb multicenter randomized placebo-controlled trial. Patients were randomly assigned to treatment with 200 mg of celecoxib or placebo, both administered orally twice daily, and then stratified by grade of dysplasia. The primary outcome was the change from baseline to 48 weeks of treatment in the proportion of biopsy samples with dysplasia between the celecoxib and placebo arms. Secondary and tertiary outcomes included evaluation of changes in histology and expression levels of relevant biomarkers. After 48 weeks of treatment, no difference was observed in the median change in the proportion of biopsy samples with dysplasia or cancer between treatment groups in either the low- or high-grade dysplasia and there were no significant differences in total surface area of the Barrett's esophagus, in prostaglandin levels, in cyclooxygenase-1/2 mRNA levels, or in methylation of tumor suppressor genes p16, adenomatous polyposis coli, and E-cadherin (67). Further, the risk of cardiovascular side effects has limited the utility of the COX-2 selective agents for chemoprevention in Barrett's esophagus. However, aspirin is cardioprotective and, in conjunction with PPI therapy to treat acid reflux and prevent aspirin-induced gastrotoxicity, it could be used in patients with Barrett's esophagus (68) (see below).

COMBINATION OF PPI AND ASPIRIN

Epidemiologically, the use of NSAIDS and aspirin, most likely via inhibition of COX-2 and other inflammatory pathways, is associated with a reduction of adenocarcinoma rates (69). In a recent exploratory, multicenter, randomized, open-label, crossover study in 45 patients with Barrett's esophagus, the combined treatment of esomeprazole 40 mg twice daily and aspirin 325 mg daily significantly decreased mucosal prostaglandin E(2) content and reduced proliferating cell nuclear antigen expression (70). Combining the anti-inflammatory effects of acid suppression with aspirin, is the subject of the Aspirin Esomeprazole Chemoprevention Trial (ASPECT; http://www.digestivediseases.org/) clinical trial, which has been initiated in the United Kingdom (71). This randomized controlled trial will involve 5,000 male patients 40–75 years of age with long-segment Barrett's esophagus and will have a 2-by-2 intervention trial factorial design. The agents tested are a high-dose proton pump inhibitor (PPI) and a low-dose PPI. In addition, half of these patients will receive either low-dose aspirin or no aspirin. The follow-up will be at least 8 years long, with 2 years of initial recruitment, for a total of 10 years. Patients will receive endoscopy and biopsy examinations every 2 years. The primary end point is all-cause mortality. This trial explores the chemoprevention potential of standard (20 mg/d) versus twice daily (80 mg/d) doses of esomeprazole in conjunction with or without low-dose (300 mg) aspirin. If new dyspeptic symptoms arise, a dose reduction protocol will be used for aspirin, decreasing from 300 mg/day, then 100 mg/day, and ultimately 75 mg/day. If a gastrointestinal bleed occurs, then immediate and permanent cessation of the aspirin will occur. No washout period will be required for individuals already on aspirin or PPI to allow baseline blood tests and biopsy samples to be assessed easily.

CONCLUSIONS

Barrett's esophagus is a premalignant condition that, through a dysplasia-adenocarcinoma pathway, confers at least a 40-fold increased risk for esophageal adenocarcinoma (0.5% to 1% per year) compared with the general population. Such adenocarcinoma risk further rises to 40%–50% within 5 years for those patients with high-grade dysplasia. Currently, the only strategies available to diminish or eliminate the risk for cancer are regular surveillance endoscopy and biopsies, endoscopic thermal or photodynamic ablation, endoscopic mucosal resection or esophagectomy. Low-risk pharmacologic strategies aiming at cancer chemoprevention are needed. Both acid and bile acid reflux, through a range of molecular signaling (i.e., by COX-2, c-myc, and MAPK), initiate and propagate a cascade of events leading to neoplasia. Bile acids, present especially frequently in the refluxate of Barrett's esophagus patients, also influence the development and persistence of metaplasia. PPIs not only suppress acid but also bile reflux, cause partial regression in Barrett's esophagus length, increase cell differentiation and apoptosis, reduce proliferation and COX-2 levels, and may diminish cancer risk. However, PPI-induced symptom control is a poor guide as to adequacy of the underlying acid suppression and the correct dosage needed is unknown. Epidemiologically, the use of NSAIDS and aspirin, most likely via inhibition of COX-2 and other inflammatory pathways, is associated with a reduction of adenocarcinoma rates. Both PPIs and NSAIDs/aspirin may therefore be potential chemopreventive agents but randomized controlled trials are under way to precisely address their use because the existing data are limited. Such large clinical trials will need to have hard endpoints, like high-grade dysplasia or cancer development or mortality, as in the ASPECT trial. Currently however, aspirin, COX-2 inhibitors, and NSAIDs cannot be recommended for the prevention of esophageal adenocarcinoma. Similarly, since there is no strong evidence of a preventive effect of medical or surgical antireflux therapy with regard to cancer risk, such therapy cannot be recommended.

References

1. Lagergren J. Etiology and risk factors for oesophageal adenocarcinoma: possibilities for chemoprophylaxis? *Best Pract Res Clin Gastroenterol.* 2006;20:803–812.
2. Grau MV, Rees JR, Baron JA. Chemoprevention in gastrointestinal cancers: current status. *Basic Clin Pharmacol Toxicol.* 2006;98:281–287.
3. Gerson LB, Shetler K, Triadafilopoulos G. Prevalence of Barrett's esophagus in asymptomatic individuals. Gastroenterology. 2002;123:636–639.
4. Triadafilopoulos G. Acid and bile reflux in Barrett's esophagus: a tale of two evils. [Editorial]. *Gastroenterology.* 2001;121:1502–1506.

5. Sharma P, Falk GW, Weston AP, et al. Dysplasia and cancer in a large multicenter cohort of patients with Barrett's esophagus. *Clin Gastroenterol Hepatol*. 2006;4:566–572.
6. Souza RF, Shewmake KL, Shen Y, et al. Differences in ERK activation in squamous mucosa in patients who have gastroesophageal reflux disease with and without Barrett's esophagus. *Am J Gastroenterol*. 2005;100:551–559.
7. El-Serag HB, Aguirre T, Kuebeler M, et al. The length of newly diagnosed Barrett's oesophagus and prior use of acid suppressive therapy. *Aliment Pharmacol Ther*. 2004;19:1255–1260.
8. Fitzgerald RC, Omary MB, Triadafilopoulos G. Dynamic effects of acid on Barrett's esophagus. An ex vivo proliferation and differentiation model. *J Clin Invest*. 1996;98:2120–2128.
9. Souza RF, Shewmake K, Terada LS, et al. Acid exposure activates the mitogen-activated protein kinase pathways in Barrett's esophagus. *Gastroenterology*. 2002;122:299–307.
10. Umansky M, Yasui W, Hallak A, et al. Proton pump inhibitors reduce cell cycle abnormalities in Barrett's esophagus. *Oncogene*. 2001;20:7987–7991.
11. Feagins LA, Zhang HY, Hormi-Carver K, et al Acid has antiproliferative effects in nonneoplastic Barrett's epithelial cells. *Am J Gastroenterol*. 2007;102:10–20.
12. Ouatu-Lascar R, Fitzgerald RC, Triadafilopoulos G. Differentiation and proliferation in Barrett's esophagus and the effects of acid suppression. *Gastroenterology*. 1999;117:327–335.
13. El Serag HB, Aguirre TV, Davis S, et al. Proton pump inhibitors are associated with reduced incidence of dysplasia in Barrett's esophagus. *Am J Gastroenterol*. 2004;99:1877–1883.
14. Peters FT, Ganesh S, Kuipers EJ, et al. Effect of elimination of acid reflux on epithelial cell proliferative activity of Barrett esophagus. *Scand J Gastroenterol*. 2000;35:1238–1244.
15. Kauer WK, Peters JH, DeMeester TR, et al. Mixed reflux of gastric and duodenal juices is more harmful to the esophagus than gastric juice alone. The need for surgical therapy re-emphasized. *Ann Surg*. 1995;222:525–531.
16. Kaur BS, Ouatu-Lascar R, Omary MB, et al. Bile salts induce or blunt cell proliferation in Barrett's esophagus in an acid-dependent fashion. *Am J Physiol Gastrointest Liver Physiol*. 2000;278(6):G1000–1009.
17. Kaur BS, Triadafilopoulos G. Acid- and bile-induced PGE(2) release and hyperproliferation in Barrett's esophagus are COX-2 and PKC-epsilon dependent. *Am J Physiol Gastrointest Liver Physiol*. 2002;283:G327–334.
18. Haigh CR, Attwood SE, Thompson DG, et al. Gastrin induces proliferation in Barrett's metaplasia through activation of the CCK2 receptor. *Gastroenterology*. 2003;124:615–625.
19. Abdalla SI, Lao-Sirieix P, Novelli MR, et al. Gastrin-induced cyclooxygenase-2 expression in Barrett's carcinogenesis. *Clin Cancer Res*. 2004;10:4784–4792.
20. Theisen J, Nehra D, Citron D, et al. Suppression of gastric acid secretion in patients with gastroesophageal reflux disease results in gastric bacterial overgrowth and deconjugation of bile acids. *J Gastrointest Surg*. 2000;4:50–54.
21. Gerson LB, Boparai V, Ullah N, et al. Oesophageal and gastric pH profiles in patients with gastro-oesophageal reflux disease and Barrett's oesophagus treated with proton pump inhibitors. *Aliment Pharmacol Ther*. 2004;20(6):637–643.
22. Yeh RW, Gerson LB, Triadafilopoulos G. Efficacy of esomeprazole in controlling reflux symptoms, intra-esophageal, and intra-gastric pH in patients with Barrett's esophagus. *Dis Esophagus*. 2003;16:193–198.
23. Wani S, Sampliner RE, Weston AP, et al. Lack of predictors of normalization of oesophageal acid exposure in Barrett's oesophagus. *Aliment Pharmacol Ther*. 2005;22:627–633.
24. Champion G, Richter JE, Vaezi MF, et al. Duodenogastroesophageal reflux: relationship to pH and importance in Barrett's esophagus. *Gastroenterology*. 1994;107:747–754.
25. Sital RR, Kusters JG, De Rooij FW, et al. Bile acids and Barrett's oesophagus: a sine qua non or coincidence? *Scand J Gastroenterol Suppl*. 2006;243:11–17.
26. Jenkins GJ, D'Souza FR, Suzen SH, et al. Deoxycholic acid at neutral and acid pH is genotoxic to oesophageal cells through the induction of ROS: The potential role of anti-oxidants in Barrett's oesophagus. *Carcinogenesis*. 2007;28:136–142.
27. Lazaridis KN, Gores GJ, Lindor KD. Ursodeoxycholic acid 'mechanisms of action and clinical use in hepatobiliary disorders'. *J Hepatol*. 2001;35:134–146.
28. DeMeester SR, DeMeester TR. Columnar mucosa and intestinal metaplasia of the esophagus: fifty years of controversy. *Ann Surg*. 2000;231:303–321.
29. McCallum R, Polepalle S, Davenport K, et al. Role of anti-reflux surgery against dysplasia in Barrett's esophagus. *Gastroenterology*. 1991;100:A121.
30. Katz D, Rothstein R, Schned A, et al. The development of dysplasia and adenocarcinoma during endoscopic surveillance of Barrett's esophagus. *Am J Gastroenterol*. 1998;93:536–541.
31. Spechler SJ, Lee E, Ahnen D, et al. Long-term outcome of medical and surgical therapies for gastroesophageal reflux disease: follow-up of a randomized controlled trial. *JAMA*. 2001;285:2331–2338.
32. Ye W, Chow WH, Lagergren J, et al. Risk of adenocarcinomas of the esophagus and gastric cardia in patients with gastroesophageal reflux diseases and after antireflux surgery. *Gastroenterology*. 2001;121:1286–1293.
33. Corey KE, Schmitz SM, Shaheen NJ. Does a surgical antireflux procedure decrease the incidence of esophageal adenocarcinoma in Barrett's esophagus? A meta-analysis. *Am J Gastroenterol*. 2003;98:2390–2394.
34. Fong LY, Pegg AE, Magee PN. Alpha-difluoromethylornithine inhibits N-nitrosomethylbenzylamine-induced esophageal carcinogenesis in zinc-deficient rats: effects on esophageal cell proliferation and apoptosis. *Cancer Res*. 1998;58:5380–5388.
35. Garewal HS, Gerner EW, Sampliner RE, et al. Ornithine decarboxylase and polyamine levels in columnar upper gastrointestinal mucosae in patients with Barrett's esophagus. *Cancer Res*. 1988;48:3288–3291.
36. Gray MR, Wallace HM, Goulding H, et al. Mucosal polyamine metabolism in the columnar lined oesophagus. *Gut*. 1993;34:584–587.
37. Garewal HS, Sampliner R, Gerner E, et al. Ornithine decarboxylase activity in Barrett's esophagus: a potential marker for dysplasia. *Gastroenterology*. 1988;94:819–821.
38. Verma AK. Inhibition of tumor promotion by DL-alpha-difluoromethylornithine, a specific irreversible inhibitor of ornithine decarboxylase. *Basic Life Sci*. 1990;52:195–204.
39. Meyskens FL Jr, Gerner EW, Emerson S, et al. Effect of alpha-difluoromethylornithine on rectal mucosal levels of polyamines in a randomized, double-blinded trial for colon cancer prevention. *J Natl Cancer Inst*. 1998;90:1212–1218.
40. Meyskens FL Jr, Gerner EW. Development of difluoromethylornithine (DFMO) as a chemoprevention agent. *Clin Cancer Res*. 1999;5:945–951.
41. Garewal HS, Sampliner RE, Fennerty MB. Chemopreventive studies in Barrett's esophagus: a model premalignant lesion for esophageal adenocarcinoma. *J Natl Cancer Inst Monogr*. 1992;51–54.
42. Lao CD, Backoff P, Shotland LI, et al. Irreversible ototoxicity associated with difluoromethylornithine. *Cancer Epidemiol Biomarkers Prev*. 2004;13:1250–1252.
43. Takashima T, Fujiwara Y, Higuchi K, et al. PPAR-gamma ligands inhibit growth of human esophageal adenocarcinoma cells through induction of apoptosis, cell cycle arrest and reduction of ornithine decarboxylase activity. *Int J Oncol*. 2001;19:465–471.
44. Eberhart CE, Coffey RJ, Radhika A, et al. Up-regulation of cyclooxygenase 2 gene expression in human colorectal adenomas and adenocarcinomas. *Gastroenterology*. 1994;107:1183–1188.
45. Tucker ON, Dannenberg AJ, Yang EK, et al. Cyclooxygenase-2 expression is upregulated in human pancreatic cancer. *Cancer Res*. 1999;59:987–990.
46. Steinbach G, Lynch PM, Phillips RK, et al. The effect of celecoxib, a cyclooxygenase-2 inhibitor, in familial adenomatous polyposis. *N Engl J Med*. 2000;342:1946–1952.
47. Ding XZ, Tong WG, Adrian TE. Blockade of cyclooxygenase-2 inhibits proliferation and induces apoptosis in human pancreatic cancer cells. *Anticancer Res*. 2000;20:2625–2631.
48. Kawamori T, Rao CV, Seibert K, et al. Chemopreventive activity of celecoxib, a specific cyclooxygenase-2 inhibitor, against colon carcinogenesis. *Cancer Res*. 1998;58:409–412.
49. Giardiello FM, Hamilton SR, Krush AJ, et al. Treatment of colonic and rectal adenomas with sulindac in familial adenomatous polyposis. *N Engl J Med*. 1993;328:1313–1316.
50. Thun MJ, Namboodiri MM, Calle EE, et al. Aspirin use and risk of fatal cancer. *Cancer Res*. 1993;53:1322–1327.
51. Farrow DC, Vaughan TL, Hansten PD, et al. Use of aspirin and other nonsteroidal anti-inflammatory drugs and risk of esophageal and gastric cancer. *Cancer Epidemiol Biomarkers Prev*. 1998;7:97–102.
52. Greenberg ER, Baron JA, Freeman DHJ, et al. Reduced risk of large-bowel adenomas among aspirin users. The Polyp Prevention Study Group. *J Natl Cancer Inst*. 1993;85:912–916.
53. Molina MA, Sitja-Arnau M, Lemoine MG, et al. Increased cyclooxygenase-2 expression in human pancreatic carcinomas and cell lines: growth inhibition by non-steroidal anti-inflammatory drugs. *Cancer Res*. 1999;59:4356–4362.
54. Piazza GA, Rahm AL, Krutzsch M, et al. Antineoplastic drugs sulindac sulfide and sulfone inhibit cell growth by inducing apoptosis. *Cancer Res*. 1995;55:3110–3116.
55. Vaughan TL, Dong LM, Blount PL, et al. Non-steroidal anti-inflammatory drugs and risk of neoplastic progression in Barrett's oesophagus: a prospective study. *Lancet Oncol*. 2005;6:945–952.
56. Corley DA, Kerlikowske K, Verma R, et al. Protective association of aspirin/NSAIDs and esophageal cancer: a systematic review and meta-analysis. *Gastroenterology*. 2003;124:47–56.
57. Mehta S, Boddy A, Johnson IT, et al. Systematic review: cyclo-oxygenase-2 in human oesophageal adenocarcinogenesis. *Aliment Pharmacol Ther*. 2006;24:1321–1331.
58. Sonnenberg A, Fennerty MB. Medical decision analysis of chemoprevention against esophageal adenocarcinoma. *Gastroenterology*. 2003;124:1758–1766.
59. Hur C, Nishioka NS, Gazelle GS. Cost-effectiveness of aspirin chemoprevention for Barrett's esophagus. *J Natl Cancer Inst*. 2004;96:316–325.
60. Souza RF, Shewmake K, Beer D.G., et al. Selective inhibition of cyclooxygenase-2 suppresses growth and induces apoptosis in human esophageal adenocarcinoma cells. *Cancer Res*. 2000;60:5767–5772.
61. Buttar NS, Wang KK, Anderson MA, et al. The effect of selective cyclooxygenase-2 inhibition in Barrett's esophagus epithelium: an in vitro study. *J Natl Cancer Inst*. 2002;94:422–429.
62. Buttar NS, Wang KK, Leontovich O, et al. Chemoprevention of esophageal adenocarcinoma by COX-2 inhibitors in an animal model of Barrett's esophagus. *Gastroenterology*. 2002;122:1101–1112.
63. Oyama K, Fujimura T, Ninomiya I, et al. A COX-2 inhibitor prevents the esophageal inflammation-metaplasia-adenocarcinoma sequence in rats. *Carcinogenesis*. 2005;26:565–570.
64. Kaur BS, Khamnehei N, Iravani M, et al. Rofecoxib inhibits cyclooxygenase 2 expression and activity and reduces cell proliferation in Barrett's esophagus. *Gastroenterology*. 2002;123:60–67.
65. Aggarwal S, Taneja N, Lin L, et al. Indomethacin-induced apoptosis in esophageal adenocarcinoma cells involves upregulation of Bax and translocation of mitochondrial cytochrome C independent of COX-2 expression. *Neoplasia*. 2000;2:346–356.

66. Buttar NS, Wang KK, Leontovich O, et al. Chemoprevention of esophageal adenocarcinoma by COX-2 inhibitors in an animal model of Barrett's esophagus *Gastroenterology*. 2002;122:1101–1112.
67. Heath EI, Canto MI, Piantadosi S, et al. Chemoprevention for Barrett's Esophagus Trial Research Group. Secondary chemoprevention of Barrett's esophagus with celecoxib: results of a randomized trial. *J Natl Cancer Inst*. 2007;99:545–557.
68. Raj A, Jankowski J. Acid suppression and chemoprevention in Barrett's oesophagus. *Dig Dis*. 2004;22:171–180.
69. Jankowski JA, Anderson M. Review article: management of oesophageal adenocarcinoma—control of acid, bile and inflammation in intervention strategies for Barrett's oesophagus. *Aliment Pharmacol Ther*. 2004 ;20(Suppl 5):71–80.
70. Triadafilopoulos G, Kaur B, Sood S, et al. Effects of esomeprazole combined with aspirin or rofecoxib on prostaglandin E2 production in patients with Barrett's esophagus. *Aliment Pharmacol Ther*. 2006;23:997–1005.
71. Leedham S, Jankowski J. The evidence base of proton pump inhibitor chemopreventative agents in Barrett's esophagus—the good, the bad, and the flawed. *Am J Gastroenterol*. 2007;102:21–23.

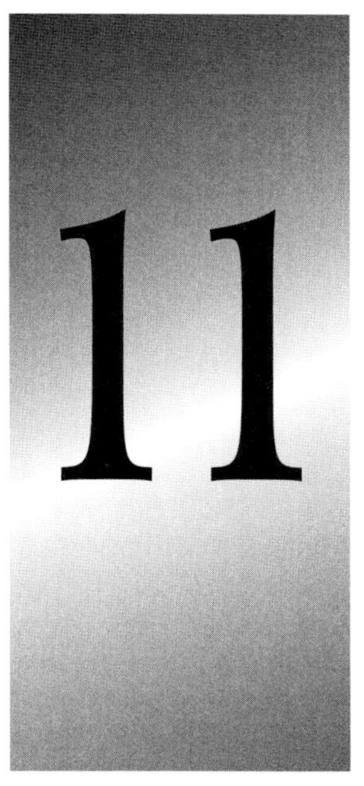

11 Epidemiology of Esophageal Cancer: Molecular

David W. Cescon
Jessica Patricia Hopkins
Penelope A. Bradbury
Darren Tse
Geoffrey Liu

Genetic polymorphisms are common inherited variations in the genetic code, typically defined as comprising at least 1% of the population of interest. They exert their effects through a high prevalence (i.e., common) but low penetrance (i.e., small amount of effect per polymorphism) genetic model. Among the most common genetic variations are single nucleotide polymorphisms (SNPs), which are single nucleotide substitutions in the genetic code (Figure 11.1). Some of these SNPs will lead to changes in the amino acid sequence (known as exonic non-synonymous SNPs), while many others do not change the sequence (synonymous SNPs), or sit in regions of the gene that are not transcribed. SNPs located in non-coding regions (e.g., splice sites, promoter regions, transcriptional binding sites, untranslated regions adjacent to a gene, etc.) can exert an effect through indirect gene or protein regulatory effects. With an estimated 1–3 million SNPs in the human genome, deciphering which SNP affects specific risks or outcomes of esophageal cancer is overwhelming. In addition, there are other common genetic variations that include microsatellite variations, insertions, and deletions. Microsatellite polymorphisms typically involve repeated sequences that vary according to the number of sequence repetitions. For example, CACACACACA or $(CA)_5$ is a dinucleotide repeat, and in the case of an intron 1 *EGFR* gene polymorphism, individuals can have between 14 and 23 repeats—or $(CA)_{14}$ to $(CA)_{23}$. Insertions/deletions may be of only one or a few base pairs but can be as large as that of an entire gene, as in the case of the glutathione s-transferases, *GSTM1* and *GSTT1* deletions. Recently, genetic variations consisting of duplication or deletion of thousands of bases have been described and termed *copy number variants*. Most of the existing literature has focused on single nucleotide polymorphisms, insertions, deletions, and microsatellites.

Genetic factors can affect both the risk and prognosis of cancer (Figure 11.1). The genetic factors may be tumor-specific (such as somatic p53 mutation) or inherited/germline (e.g., germline *p53* mutation in Li-Fraumeni syndrome). A variety of pathways are involved in both esophageal carcinogenesis and prognosis (Figure 11.2), and for each pathway, human genetic variation exists that can alter the efficiency or effectiveness of that pathway or pathways. The development of most cancers involves the interaction of genetic and environmental factors. In esophageal cancer, the known risk factors are distinct by histology: for squamous cell cancers (ESCCs), the risk factors include tobacco and alcohol exposure and physical trauma to the esophagus; for adenocarcinoma (EAC), the risk factors include tobacco exposure, obesity, gastroesophageal reflux disease,

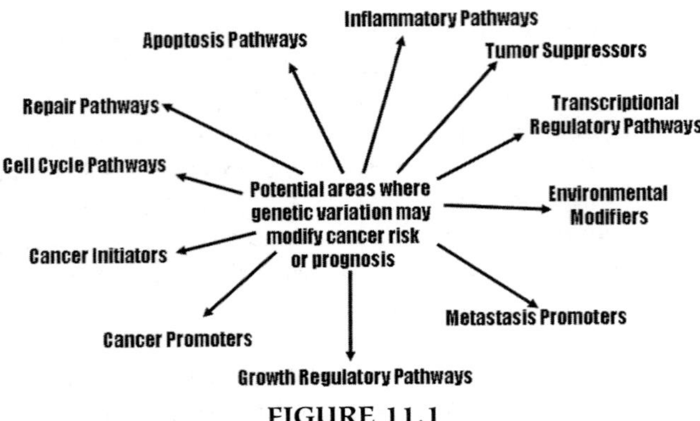

FIGURE 11.1

Examples of pathways involved in esophageal cancer risk and outcomes. Within each pathway, genetic variation can modify risk and outcomes.

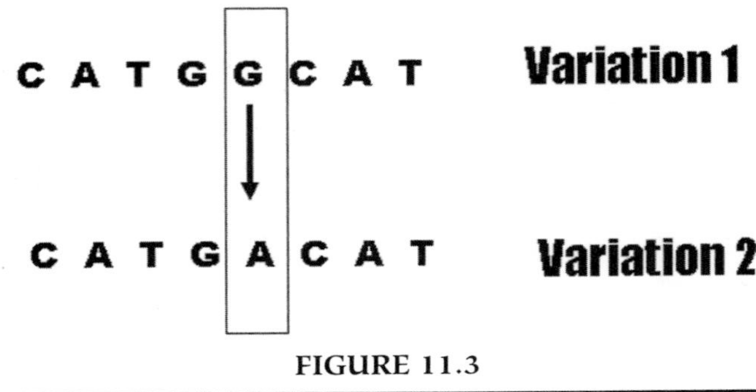

FIGURE 11.3

Single nucleotide polymorphisms (SNPs). SNPs are single nucleotide substitutions in the genetic code. In the example shown, most individuals have 2 copies (alleles) of genetic variation 1 (the wildtype genotype) in their DNA, but a minority of patients have 1 or 2 copies of variation 2 (heterozygous and homozygous variant genotypes, respectively).

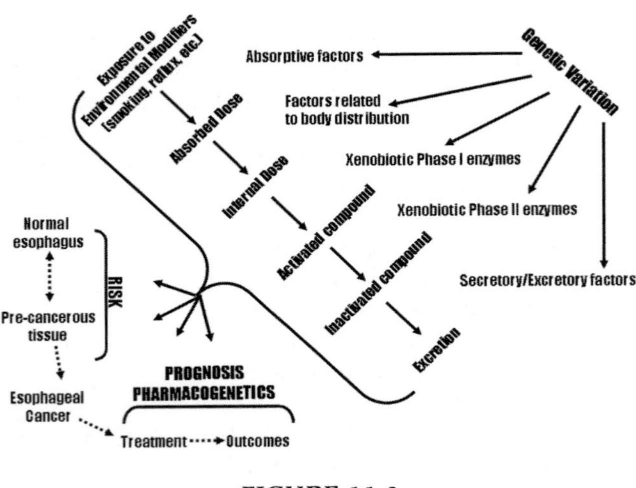

FIGURE 11.2

Gene-environmental interactions in esophageal cancer risk and prognosis. Genetic variation in a variety of factors can alter the exposure of environmental factors that affect esophageal cancer risk and prognosis. When these genetic factors are modifying the effects of drugs on treatment outcomes, it is known as a pharmacogenetic factor.

and the presence of a pre-neoplastic lesion, Barrett's esophagus. Gene-environment interaction has been the cornerstone of molecular epidemiologic research in the past three decades. Figure 11.3 illustrates how these interactions can affect both risk and prognosis of disease. Thus, molecular epidemiology is the study of *inherited* (not tumor specific) human genetic variations in the risk or prognosis of esophageal cancer, either by itself or in conjunction with environmental factors.

Molecular and genetic factors can also affect disease outcome. These factors may be prognostic, reflecting an association between the factor and the metastatic potential or aggressiveness of the cancer, which enables the identification of patients requiring additional treatment. It is predictive and may aid the selection of the most beneficial treatment modality. Molecular prognostic factors have been identified in lung, breast, colon, and ovarian cancers, among many others (1).

This chapter will focus on 2 common themes: (a) the current state of the literature on genetic polymorphisms and esophageal cancer risk and prognosis; and (b) where the future lies in these areas of active research. The separate role of genetic polymorphisms in ESCC and EAC risk will be discussed first, followed by the role of genetic polymorphisms in the prognosis of these cancers. We will also focus on methodologic issues, since the field is still emerging in the post-genome era.

GENETIC POLYMORPHISMS AND RISK OF ESOPHAGEAL CANCER

Familial Susceptibility to Esophageal Cancer

Esophageal cancer is typically considered a sporadic disease. However, familial clusters have been found, and there is an increased risk of esophageal cancer in individuals with a family history of esophageal cancer (both ESCC and EAC) (2,3). Further, familial association of the risk factors of esophageal cancer, particularly gastroesophageal reflux disease and Barrett's esophagus are also associated with elevated risks of EAC (4,5). These data suggest a familial susceptibility in a proportion of individuals who develop esophageal cancers, arguing for the evaluation of genetic factors in esophageal cancer risk.

Genetic Polymorphisms and Esophageal Cancer Risk

Interest in, and progress toward, defining the genetic contribution to susceptibility of complex diseases has increased substantially with the development of tools for high-volume, low-cost genetic analysis, and the availability of detailed genomic information accumulated through the Human Genome Project and its offshoots (6–8). An understanding of the molecular epidemiology of esophageal cancer risk would enable 2 major advances in the management of this disease: (a) the identification of genetically susceptible groups that could be targeted for risk-reduction, screening or chemoprevention strategies; and (b) an improved understanding of the biologic basis of esophageal cancer, which could inform the rational development of novel therapeutic strategies.

Much attention has been devoted recently to large-scale genome-wide association studies that have identified putative risk alleles or loci in an ever-expanding array of conditions. These studies generally are conducted under the umbrella of international consortia, which permit the collection of large cohorts of affected individuals, necessary to achieve the statistical power these designs demand (9,10). In contrast, the published literature on genetic risk factors in esophageal cancer consists primarily of small, case-control studies that investigate the impact of genetic polymorphisms in a small number of candidate genes. These studies have been the subject of a recent review, which identified 100 publications and 3 meta-analyses (11), the vast majority of which focused on Asian populations. Given the distinct epidemiology and pathogenesis of the 2 major histologic subtypes of EAC and ESCC, most research into the genetic factors associated with this disease has analyzed these histologies separately. Approximately 90% of the published studies have focused on ESCC.

Genetic Polymorphisms and Squamous Cell Carcinoma Risk

To date, most studies of the molecular epidemiology of ESCC risk have focused on individuals in areas of high incidence, primarily in China and Japan. Based on an understanding of the environmental factors (including smoking, alcohol consumption, exposure to nitrosamines, and dietary deficiencies in specific micronutrients) known or believed to contribute to the development of ESCC, investigations of the genetic susceptibility to this disease have concentrated on genetic polymorphisms involved in pathways that may modify the effects of these exposures. Enzymes include those responsible for carcinogen detoxification: Phase I (activation pathways of the Cytochrome P450 [*CYP*] family) (12–25), and Phase II (deactivation enzymes such as the glutathione s-transferase [*GST*] family) (12–15,17–23,25–29), NAD(P)H: quinine oxidoreductase 1 (*NQO1*) (30–35), microsomal epoxide hydrolase (*mEH*) (36,37), alcohol metabolism (aldehyde dehydrogenase [*ALDH2*] and alcohol dehydrogenase [*ADH2*]) (12,26,38–44), and folate metabolism (thymidylate synthase [*TS*] [45–47] and methylenetetrahydrofolate reductase [*MTHFR*] [45,48–51]). Another group of candidates that has been considered includes genes involved in cell cycle control, DNA repair, and apoptosis (i.e., *p5329* [52–57]; cyclin D1 [*CCND1*] [58,59]; nucleotide excision repair [NER] genes [60–63]; base excision repair [BER] genes [44,60,61,64–68]; and others), which are critical to the cellular response to damage from carcinogen exposure and are known to contribute to the susceptibility to other cancers.

The results of these studies are summarized in Table 11.1. Few genes have been demonstrated consistently to be associated with susceptibility to ESCC. A polymorphism in aldehyde dehydrogenase (*ALDH2*), the gene responsible for elimination of acetaldehyde produced in the metabolism of alcohol, confers the greatest increase in ESCC risk, with an odds ratio (OR) of 3.2 for the *ALDH2 *1/*2* heterozygous genotype (38). This polymorphism, common in East Asians but rare in other populations, codes for an inactive enzyme that results in elevated serum acetaldehyde levels after consumption of alcohol and is associated with a flushing reaction. This polymorphism is an excellent example of a gene-environment interaction, whereby the increased risk it confers is strongly dependent on the amount of alcohol consumed. Interestingly, the homozygous *2/*2 variant is associated with a lower risk of ESCC, which has been attributed to the intolerance to alcohol that this genotype imparts.

Genetic Polymorphisms and Esophageal Adenocarcinoma Risk

While much has been written about the classic epidemiology and rapidly increasing incidence of EAC, comparatively little has been published on its molecular epidemiology. In contrast to the large number of studies involving ESCC, fewer than 20 studies assessing roughly 2 dozen genetic polymorphisms in adenocarcinoma have been reported. In keeping with the epidemiology of EAC, these studies have included mostly North American and European Caucasians. The number of cases in the majority of these studies has been very small, with most involving fewer than 50 individuals (the smallest involving only 9 patients) (69,70). Only recently have studies with larger cohorts (up to 203 cases) been published (71). As with squamous cell carcinoma, the polymorphisms chosen for study have included genes involved in DNA repair, cell cycle control, and carcinogen metabolism. Results of these

TABLE 11.1
Polymorphic Genes [a] Associated with Esophageal Squamous Cell Carcinoma Susceptibility (11).

	Mostly positive studies	Positive & negative studies	Mostly negative studies		Single, unreplicated positive study	
Phase I enzymes	*CYP1A1*		*CYP2E1*		*CYP3A5*	
Phase II enzymes	*NQO1*	*SULT1A1* *NAT2*	*GSTM1* *GSTT1*	*GSTP1* *mEH*	*GSTM3*	
DNA repair/ Cell cycle/ Apoptosis		*p53* *p73* *XRCC1* *XPD*	*XRCC1* *hOGG1* *L-Myc* *CCND1*		*Fas* *Fas-L* *MDM2*	*ECRG2* *ECRG1* *p21*
Other	*ALDH2* *ADH2* *MTHFR*	*TS*	*MTHFR*		*MTRR* *12-LOX* *COX-2* *BRCA2* *Mitochondrial DNA* *MMP7*	*MMP2* *SHMT1* *TAP2* *LMP7* *androgen receptor*

[a] For some genes, more than one SNP has been evaluated.

studies are summarized in Table 11.2: *XPC* and *XPD* are DNA repair genes; Cyclin D1 and *p73* are cell cycle/*p53* pathway genes; *GSTT1, GSTP1,* and *GSTM3* are Phase II enzymes. The lack of consistency and conflicting results among studies that have examined the same genetic polymorphisms is notable. While this may reflect differences between the populations studied, it is more likely a reflection of the small sample sizes examined in earlier studies, and the consequent high rate of false positive and false negative results that this generates. A number of genetic polymorphisms have been reported to show no association with EAC susceptibility, though many of these studies lack the statistical power to detect such an association (Table 11.3) (21,69,70,72,73).

Future Directions

The goal of identifying the genetic factors associated with the risk of esophageal cancer will best be achieved through the conduct of suitably large cohort studies that consider and adjust for possible confounders, employ rigorous statistical methods including adjustment for multiple hypotheses testing, and ensure adequate statistical power to detect the associations of interest. Consensus guidelines for the design and reporting of such studies have been developed recently, and should contribute to the advancement of this field of research reporting (74). As with all investigations of this nature, replication of results in independent validation cohorts is critical, and publication of methodologically sound negative findings is important. Much work remains to be performed to identify the interactions between genetic polymorphisms and environmental exposures, and to investigate the importance of gene-gene interactions among risk alleles. One avenue, recently attempted on a pilot scale in esophageal cancer, to assess many genetic polymorphisms concurrently involves the application of DNA micro-arrays or "SNP chips." This powerful technology, which can evaluate from several hundred to even a million SNPs, enables the consideration of complex gene-gene interactions and holds much promise, though study design and statistical issues discussed above are still of paramount importance in ensuring the validity of this high-throughput method.

Identification of novel alleles and confirmation of previously suggested esophageal cancer risk alleles is sure to occur at an increasing pace as this field matures. Once confirmed, the application of genetic risk factors to interventional screening or chemoprevention studies in a prospective, randomized fashion can be considered definitively to assess their role in clinical practice.

GENETIC POLYMORPHISMS AND ESOPHAGEAL CANCER PROGNOSIS

Research into the association between germline polymorphic variants, and either survival or toxicity outcomes in EAC and ESCC, is an emerging field of study.

TABLE 11.2
Polymorphic Genes [a] Associated with Esophageal Adenocarcinoma Susceptibility

Gene	Polymorphism	Genotype/effect	Ethnicity	Country	Evidence[b]
XPC	Intron 9 Poly AT insertion	Homozygous insertion ↑	Caucasian	Canada	Single study (n=56) (86)
XPD	*Lys751Gln*	*Gln/-* ↑, *Gln/Gln* ↓	Caucasian	Canada, United States, Sweden	Conflicting (61,86)
Cyclin D1	*G870A*	*A/A* ↑	Caucasian	Canada, Germany	Weak (72,73)
P73	*5'UTR G4A + C14T*	*AT/AT* ↓	Caucasian	Ireland	Single study (n=59) (87)
GSTT1	Deletion (*1->*2)	**2/*2* ↓	Caucasian	Canada, France	Weak (15,21,88)
GSTP1	*Ile104Val*	*-/Val* ↑	Caucasian	Canada, Netherlands, United Kingdom, France	Weak (15,18,21,71,88)
GSTM3	**A→*B*	*-/*B* ↑	Indian	India	Single study (n=9) (70)
NQO1	*C609T*	*T/-* ↑, *T/T* ↓, null	Caucasian	Germany, United Kingdom	Conflicting (89–91)
ADH3	**1→*2*	*1/1* ↑	Caucasian	United States	Single study (n=114) (92)

[a] For some genes, more than one SNP has been evaluated.
[b] Weak = positive result in single study and multiple studies with negative results; Conflicting = positive results in multiple studies but with conflicting definitions of at-risk allele; Single study = unreplicated data. For single studies, number of cases shown in parentheses.

Current research is attempting to identify candidate genes that can be tested in methodologically rigorous validation studies. The ultimate goal is to create prognostic models incorporating genetic and clinical data, which will inform management and prognosis of patients with esophageal cancer.

Outcome studies are of interest in esophageal cancer because overall survival remains poor despite treatment, and the morbidity and consequences resulting from treatment (including disfigurement, dysphagia, and reduced quality of life [75]) remain significant. Polymorphic variants have the potential to contribute to the identification of those individuals who would benefit most from treatment, thus maximizing survival outcomes while minimizing toxicity. Outcomes of clinical interest include overall survival, disease/progression-free survival, response to treatment, and early and late toxicity caused by chemotherapy and/or radiotherapy. However, different outcomes may require evaluation of different polymorphic variants, since the relevant associated genetic pathways may be distinct. Conversely, variants from a single pathway may affect survival and toxicity in opposite ways. For instance, nucleotide excision DNA repair pathway genes conferring improved DNA repair capacity are thought to play a role in resistance to cisplatin-based chemotherapy in non-small cell lung cancer (76) and ovarian cancer (77). In contrast, the same DNA repair pathway genes may have a role in predicting outcomes such as toxicity, where improved DNA repair capacity may reduce toxic side effects of platinum agents.

Current State of Literature

The current literature is limited to a handful of studies (Table 11.4). Histologic subtypes studied were generally divided along ethnic lines, with adenocarcinoma being studied primarily in Caucasians and squamous cell carcinoma being studied primarily in Asians. Study types were limited to case series or cohort studies of modest size. Although most studies reported overall survival and disease-free survival (47,78–84), 2 reported intermediate end-points, such as response to treatment (80,83). Often, the selection of polymorphic variants was based on previous information from cancer risk studies or hypothesized functional pathways. Polymorphic variants of interest represented a number of different pathways, including DNA repair (e.g., *XRCC1*) (83) and xenobiotic metabolism (e.g., *GSTT1, GSTM1*) (78,84), among others. Pharmacogenetic pathway analyses have focused primarily on either the folate pathway because of the common use of 5-fluorouracil in the treatment of this cancer

TABLE 11.3
Other Polymorphisms Reported with No Demonstrated Associations with Adenocarcinoma Risk

Pathway	Gene	Polymorphism
Cell cycle	*p53*	*p53 Arg72Pro* (93)
	p16	*p16 3' UTR C540G (rs11515)* (73)
	Murine double minute oncogene	*MDM2 -T309G* (55)
DNA repair	Xeroderma pigmentosum group C	*XPC Lys939Gln* (61)
	Xeroderma pigmentosum group D	*XPD Arg156Arg* *XPD Asp312Asn* (61,94)
	X-ray repair cross complimenting protein	*XRCC1 Arg194Trp* *XRCC1 Arg399Gln* *XRCC1 Thr241Met* *XRCC3 Thr241Met* (61,86)
Xenobiotic metabolism	Cytochrome P450	*CYP 2E1 c2/c1* *CYP 1A1 Ile462Val* (15,21,95)
	Microsomal epoxide hydrolase	*mEH His113Tyr* *mEH His139Arg* (21,88)
	Glutathione peroxidase	*GPX2 intron 1 A/G (rs4902346)* *GPX2 intron 1 C/T (rs2737844)* (71)
	Glutathione s-transferase	*GSTM1 deletion* (15,21,88)
	Manganese superoxide dismutase	*SOD2 Ala16Val* *SOD2 intron 4 A/G (rs3798215)* *SOD2 3' UTR (rs1967802)* (71)

(particularly genetic polymorphisms of thymidylate synthase [*TS*] [47,78,80,82,83] and methylenetetrahydrofolate reductase [*MTHFR*] [80,83], or polymorphisms of the glutathione s-transferase and DNA repair pathways because of the common use of cisplatin chemotherapy to treat these tumors [83,84]). Overall, no consistent pattern of results has emerged. A few polymorphic variants of other pathways (*IL-1ß, L-Myc, IL-6*) have also been evaluated in very small studies (79,81,83). Wu et al. reported a prognostic association with the polymorphic variant of the gene coding for the multidrug resistant protein *MDR1* (83). Independent replication of these results has not yet been performed.

Future Directions

Currently, genotypic information is not used in the management of esophageal cancer. In order for the translation from clinical science to clinical practice to occur, future studies will need to improve in design methodology, statistical analysis, and reporting. Polymorphism-outcomes association studies suffer from a lack of thorough reporting (74) and fail to include important information such as a description of the source population, inclusion/exclusion criteria, follow-up time/losses-to-follow-up, and complete clinical data for other important prognostic factors. As such, multivariate analyses are necessary as they provide more information about the role of polymorphic variants within the larger clinical context and can take gene-gene and gene-environment interactions into account. However, special attention should be given to adjustment for multiple comparisons when testing multiple genes and outcomes; otherwise, there is a high probability of false positive results (85). Researchers should also consider polymorphic variants that have been previously studied but yielded negative results, as many studies are underpowered, leading to a high probability of falsely negative results.

Once candidate genes have been identified, validation should take place. Two reasonable options for polymorphism validation studies exist: (a) a multistage validation approach and (b) controlled trials.

Multistage Validation Approach

A case series or small cohort study can represent the first stage of the multistage validation approach. Statistically significant polymorphisms from these initial studies can

TABLE 11.4
Genetic Polymorphisms and Esophageal Cancer Outcomes

Study	Gene	Polymorphism	Results
Okuno et al. (squamous) Japan (n=31) (78)	*TS* *GSTP1*	*TSER/6bp del 3' UTR* *Ile105Val*	Two or 3 homozygous variants of *TSER, 6bp del 3'UTR,* and *Ile-105Val* had better prognosis
Shibuta et al. (squamous) Japan (n=65) (79)	*L-myc*	Intron 2 long/short	Short allele had poorer prognosis
Sarbia et al. (squamous) Europe (n=68) (80)	*MTHFR*	*C677T*	No prognostic significance
	TS	*TSER*	No prognostic significance
	MTR	*A2756G*	*A/G* & *G/G* more responsive to chemoradiation
Deans et al. (adeno) United Kingdom (n=56) (81)	*IL-1ß*	511	Not significant
	IL-6	174	*C/C* had reduced survival
Liao et al. (adeno) United States (n=146) (82)	*TS*	6bp del 3'*UTR*	Deletion had non-significant improved prognosis
Wu et al. (83% adeno) United States (n=210) (83)	*MTHFR*	A429C C222T	*G/A* & *A/A* had better prognosis and combined variants had better prognosis
	TS and MTR	Multiple	"at-risk" allele combos had worse prognosis
	MDR1	*C3435T*	*C/C* & *C/T* had improved prognosis
	NER genes	9 SNPs	Decreasing number of "at-risk" alleles had better prognosis
	XRCC1	*Arg399Gln*	*A/A* & *G/A* had worse prognosis
Lee et al. (squamous) Taiwan (n=233) (84)	*GSTT1*	deletion	No prognostic significance
	GSTM1	deletion	No prognostic significance
	GSTP1	*Ile105Val*	*Ile/Val* & *Val/Val* had worse prognosis
Zhang et al (squamous). China (n=465) (47)	*TS* *TS*	*TSER* *G/C in TSER*	*2R/3G (vs 3R/3R)* genotype had 11-fold increase in lymph node metastasis in ESCC patients
	TS	6bp del 3'*UTR*	No prognostic significance

be tested in a larger validation cohort study. Subsequent sequential validation cohorts consist of groups of patients who are relatively homogeneous as a group and similar in characteristics to the original study participants. With each stage, the number of polymorphic variants being tested decreases, since each validation cohort acts as an additional filter for false-positive results. Care must be taken to ensure complete collection of important clinical prognostic factors. When planned carefully to answer a specific question, validation cohorts may represent a higher level of evidence than case series or small single cohort studies.

Controlled Trials

Ideally, researchers would like to perform controlled trials. To date, no controlled trials have been performed in this field. Generally, controlled studies are methodologically difficult to design and more expensive to implement. One of the largest barriers to this is the requirement of large numbers of participants, which is often not feasible in esophageal cancer studies. However, controlled trials have an advantage over validation cohorts by balancing known and unknown confounding factors and could be useful for ultimate validation as well as implementation into clinical practice.

SUMMARY

In general, the literature describing the role of germline polymorphic variants in outcomes represents a new burgeoning research area, though many published examples to date suffer from methodologic problems: The reporting often lacks information on the source population, there is a lack of statistical adjustment for multiple comparisons, and studies are generally underpowered. There is also inadequate consideration and documentation of environmental factors that may confound risk results. In addition, publication bias may exist leading to underrepresentation of negative results in the published literature. Finally, for risk studies pertaining to ESCC, the external validity of reported findings is limited by the heavy focus on isolated populations with very high disease incidence. In these special populations, distinct genetic and environmental risk factors may exist that lack relevance in other groups. However, this is an emerging field, and information from these initial studies can help to identify candidate genes to test in future larger and validative studies.

The mapping of the entire human genome has advanced this field in quantum leaps. A new series of larger, comprehensive, multistage test and validation studies involving multiple replication patient populations that are well characterized will likely be available in the next few years. The information gleaned from these studies should yield good candidates for the development of future interventional studies designed to identify strategies to clinically exploit this genetic information. The ultimate goal of this research is to improve our understanding of esophageal cancer, its treatment and prognosis, with a more practical goal of utilizing these polymorphic data to better stratify at-risk individuals and better classify individuals who already have this disease.

References

1. Liu G, Zhou W, Wang Z, et al. Incorporating molecular oncology in prognosis. In: Gospodarowicz MK, O'Sullivan B, Sobin L, eds. *Prognostic Factors in Cancer*. 3rd ed. Hoboken, NJ: Wiley and Sons; 2006:79–94.
2. Hu N, Goldstein AM, Albert PS, et al. Evidence for a familial esophageal cancer susceptibility gene on chromosome 13. *Cancer Epidemiol Biomarkers Prev*. 2003;12:1112–1115.
3. Ji J, Hemminki K. Familial risk for esophageal cancer: an updated epidemiologic study from Sweden. *Clin Gastroenterol Hepatol*. 2006;4:840–845.
4. Chak A, Ochs-Balcom H, Falk G, et al. Familiality in Barrett's esophagus, adenocarcinoma of the esophagus, and adenocarcinoma of the gastroesophageal junction. *Cancer Epidemiol Biomarkers Prev*. 2006;15:1668–1673.
5. Akbari MR, Malekzadeh R, Nasrollahzadeh D, et al. Familial risks of esophageal cancer among the Turkmen population of the Caspian littoral of Iran. *Int J Cancer*. 2006;119:1047–1051.
6. Gudmundsson J, Sulem P, Manolescu A, et al. Genome-wide association study identifies a second prostate cancer susceptibility variant at 8q24. *Nat Genet*. 2007;39:631–637.
7. Sladek R, Rocheleau G, Rung J, et al. A genome-wide association study identifies novel risk loci for type 2 diabetes. *Nature*. 2007;445:881–885.
8. Saxena R, Voight BF, Lyssenko V, et al. Genome-wide association analysis identifies loci for type 2 diabetes and triglyceride levels. *Science*. 2007;316:1331–1336.
9. Easton DF, Pooley KA, Dunning AM, et al. Genome-wide association study identifies novel breast cancer susceptibility loci. *Nature*. 2007;447:1087–1093.
10. Gudmundsson J, Sulem P, Steinthorsdottir V, et al. Two variants on chromosome 17 confer prostate cancer risk, and the one in TCF2 protects against type 2 diabetes. *Nat Genet*. 2007;39:977–983.
11. Hiyama T, Yoshihara M, Tanaka S, et al. Genetic polymorphisms and esophageal cancer risk. *Int J Cancer*. 2007;121:1643–1658.
12. Hori H, Kawano T, Endo M, et al. Genetic polymorphisms of tobacco- and alcohol-related metabolizing enzymes and human esophageal squamous cell carcinoma susceptibility. *J Clin Gastroenterol*. 1997;25:568–575.
13. Morita S, Yano M, Shiozaki H, et al. CYP1A1, CYP2E1 and GSTM1 polymorphisms are not associated with susceptibility to squamous-cell carcinoma of the esophagus. *Int J Cancer*. 1997;71:192–195.
14. Shao G, Su Y, Huang G, et al. Relationship between CYP1A1, GSTM1 genetic polymorphisms and susceptibility to esophageal squamous cell carcinoma [in]. *Zhonghua Liu Xing Bing Xue Za Zhi* [Chinese]. 2000;21:420–423.
15. Abbas A, Delvinquiere K, Lechevrel M, et al. GSTM1, GSTT1, GSTP1 and CYP1A1 genetic polymorphisms and susceptibility to esophageal cancer in a French population: different pattern of squamous cell carcinoma and adenocarcinoma. *World J Gastroenterol*. 2004;10:3389–3393.
16. Wu MT, Lee JM, Wu DC, et al. Genetic polymorphisms of cytochrome P4501A1 and oesophageal squamous-cell carcinoma in Taiwan. *Br J Cancer*. 2002;87:529–532.
17. Wang LD, Zheng S, Liu B, et al. CYP1A1, GSTs and mEH polymorphisms and susceptibility to esophageal carcinoma: study of population from a high- incidence area in north China. *World J Gastroenterol*. 2003;9:1394–1397.
18. van Lieshout EM, Roelofs HM, Dekker S, et al. Polymorphic expression of the glutathione S-transferase P1 gene and its susceptibility to Barrett's esophagus and esophageal carcinoma. *Cancer Res*. 1999;59:586–589.
19. Nimura Y, Yokoyama S, Fujimori M, et al. Genotyping of the CYP1A1 and GSTM1 genes in esophageal carcinoma patients with special reference to smoking. *Cancer*. 1997;80:852–857.
20. Wang AH, Sun CS, Li LS, et al. Relationship of tobacco smoking CYP1A1 GSTM1 gene polymorphism and esophageal cancer in Xi'an. *World J Gastroenterol*. 2002;8:49–53.
21. Casson AG, Zheng Z, Chiasson D, et al. Associations between genetic polymorphisms of Phase I and II metabolizing enzymes, p53 and susceptibility to esophageal adenocarcinoma. *Cancer Detect Prev*. 2003;27:139–146.
22. Lin DX, Tang YM, Peng Q, et al. Susceptibility to esophageal cancer and genetic polymorphisms in glutathione S-transferases T1, P1, and M1 and cytochrome P450 2E1. *Cancer Epidemiol Biomarkers Prev*. 1998;7:1013–1018.
23. Tan W, Song N, Wang GQ, et al. Impact of genetic polymorphisms in cytochrome P450 2E1 and glutathione S-transferases M1, T1, and P1 on susceptibility to esophageal cancer among high-risk individuals in China. *Cancer Epidemiol Biomarkers Prev*. 2000;9:551–556.
24. Gao C, Takezaki T, Wu J, et al. Interaction between cytochrome P-450 2E1 polymorphisms and environmental factors with risk of esophageal and stomach cancers in Chinese. *Cancer Epidemiol Biomarkers Prev*. 2002;11:29–34.
25. Yang CX, Matsuo K, Wang ZM, et al. Phase I/II enzyme gene polymorphisms and esophageal cancer risk: a meta-analysis of the literature. *World J Gastroenterol*. 2005;11:2531–2538.
26. Yokoyama A, Kato H, Yokoyama T, et al. Genetic polymorphisms of alcohol and aldehyde dehydrogenases and glutathione S-transferase M1 and drinking, smoking, and diet in Japanese men with esophageal squamous cell carcinoma. *Carcinogenesis*. 2002;23:1851–1859.
27. Gao CM, Takezaki T, Wu JZ, et al. Glutathione-S-transferases M1 (GSTM1) and GSTT1 genotype, smoking, consumption of alcohol and tea and risk of esophageal and stomach cancers: a case-control study of a high-incidence area in Jiangsu Province, China. *Cancer Lett*. 2002;188:95–102.
28. Morita S, Yano M, Tsujinaka T, et al. Association between genetic polymorphisms of glutathione S-transferase P1 and N-acetyltransferase 2 and susceptibility to squamous-cell carcinoma of the esophagus. *Int J Cancer*. 1998;79:517–520.

29. Lee JM, Lee YC, Yang SY, et al. Genetic polymorphisms of p53 and GSTP1, but not NAT2, are associated with susceptibility to squamous-cell carcinoma of the esophagus. *Int J Cancer.* 2000;89:458–464.
30. Zhang WC, Yin LH, Pu YP, et al. Relationship between quinone oxidoreductase1 gene ns-cSNP and genetic susceptibility of esophageal cancer [in]. *Zhonghua Yu Fang Yi Xue Za Zhi* [Chinese]. 2006;40:324–327.
31. Li Y, Zhang JH, Guo W, et al. Polymorphism of NAD(P)H dehydrogenase (quinone) 1 (NQO1) C 609 T and risk of esophageal neoplasm [in]. *Zhonghua Liu Xing Bing Xue Za Zhi* [Chinese]. 2004;25:731.
32. Zhang JH, Li Y, Wang R, et al. The NAD(P)H: quinone oxidoreductase 1 C609T polymorphism and susceptibility to esophageal cancer [in]. *Zhonghua Yi Xue Yi Chuan Xue Za Zhi* [Chinese]. 2003;20:544–6.
33. Zhang JH, Li Y, Wang R, et al. NQO1 C609T polymorphism associated with esophageal cancer and gastric cardiac carcinoma in North China. *World J Gastroenterol.* 2003;9:1390–1393.
34. Zhang J, Schulz WA, Li Y, et al. Association of NAD(P)H: quinone oxidoreductase 1 (NQO1) C609T polymorphism with esophageal squamous cell carcinoma in a German Caucasian and a northern Chinese population. *Carcinogenesis.* 2003;24:905–909.
35. Hamajima N, Matsuo K, Iwata H, et al. NAD(P)H: quinone oxidoreductase 1 (NQO1) C609T polymorphism and the risk of eight cancers for Japanese. *Int J Clin Oncol.* 2002;7:103–108.
36. Zhang JH, Jin X, Li Y, et al. Epoxide hydrolase Tyr113His polymorphism is not associated with susceptibility to esophageal squamous cell carcinoma in population of North China. *World J Gastroenterol.* 2003;9:2654–2657.
37. Lin YC, Wu DC, Lee JM, et al. The association between microsomal epoxide hydrolase genotypes and esophageal squamous-cell-carcinoma in Taiwan: interaction between areca chewing and smoking. *Cancer Lett.* 2006;237:281–288.
38. Lewis SJ, Smith GD. Alcohol, ALDH2, and esophageal cancer: a meta-analysis which illustrates the potentials and limitations of a Mendelian randomization approach. *Cancer Epidemiol Biomarkers Prev.* 2005;14:1967–1971.
39. Yokoyama A, Muramatsu T, Omori T, et al. Alcohol and aldehyde dehydrogenase gene polymorphisms and oropharyngolaryngeal, esophageal and stomach cancers in Japanese alcoholics. *Carcinogenesis.* 2001;22:433–439.
40. Boonyaphiphat P, Thongsuksai P, Sriplung H, et al. Lifestyle habits and genetic susceptibility and the risk of esophageal cancer in the Thai population. *Cancer Lett.* 2002;186:193–199.
41. Itoga S, Nomura F, Makino Y, et al. Tandem repeat polymorphism of the CYP2E1 gene: an association study with esophageal cancer and lung cancer. *Alcohol Clin Exp Res.* 2002;26:15S–19S.
42. Wu CF, Wu DC, Hsu HK, et al. Relationship between genetic polymorphisms of alcohol and aldehyde dehydrogenases and esophageal squamous cell carcinoma risk in males. *World J Gastroenterol.* 2005;11:5103–5108.
43. Chen YJ, Chen C, Wu DC, et al. Interactive effects of lifetime alcohol consumption and alcohol and aldehyde dehydrogenase polymorphisms on esophageal cancer risks. *Int J Cancer.* 2006;119:2827–28231.
44. Cai L, You NC, Lu H, et al. Dietary selenium intake, aldehyde dehydrogenase-2 and X-ray repair cross-complementing 1 genetic polymorphisms, and the risk of esophageal squamous cell carcinoma. *Cancer.* 2006;106:2345–2354.
45. Wang LD, Guo RF, Fan ZM, et al. Association of methylenetetrahydrofolate reductase and thymidylate synthase promoter polymorphisms with genetic susceptibility to esophageal and cardia cancer in a Chinese high-risk population. *Dis Esophagus.* 2005;18:177–184.
46. Tan W, Miao X, Wang L, et al. Significant increase in risk of gastroesophageal cancer is associated with interaction between promoter polymorphisms in thymidylate synthase and serum folate status. *Carcinogenesis.* 2005;26:1430–1435.
47. Zhang J, Cui Y, Kuang G, et al. Association of the thymidylate synthase polymorphisms with esophageal squamous cell carcinoma and gastric cardiac adenocarcinoma. *Carcinogenesis.* 2004;25:2479–2485.
48. Song C, Xing D, Tan W, et al. Methylenetetrahydrofolate reductase polymorphisms increase risk of esophageal squamous cell carcinoma in a Chinese population. *Cancer Res.* 2001;61:3272–3275.
49. Stolzenberg-Solomon RZ, Qiao YL, et al. Esophageal and gastric cardia cancer risk and folate- and vitamin B(12)-related polymorphisms in Linxian, China. *Cancer Epidemiol Biomarkers Prev.* 2003;12:1222–1226.
50. Zhang J, Zotz RB, Li Y, et al. Methylenetetrahydrofolate reductase C677T polymorphism and predisposition towards esophageal squamous cell carcinoma in a German Caucasian and a northern Chinese population. *J Cancer Res Clin Oncol.* 2004;130:574–580.
51. Larsson SC, Giovannucci E, Wolk A. Folate intake, MTHFR polymorphisms, and risk of esophageal, gastric, and pancreatic cancer: a meta-analysis. *Gastroenterology.* 2006;131:1271–1283.
52. Cai L, Mu LN, Lu H, et al. Dietary selenium intake and genetic polymorphisms of the GSTP1 and p53 genes on the risk of esophageal squamous cell carcinoma. *Cancer Epidemiol Biomarkers Prev.* 2006;15:294–300.
53. Peixoto Guimaraes D, Hsin Lu S, et al. Absence of association between HPV DNA, TP53 codon 72 polymorphism, and risk of oesophageal cancer in a high-risk area of China. *Cancer Lett.* 2001;162:231–25.
54. Zhang L, Xing D, He Z, Lin D. p53 gene codon 72 polymorphism and susceptibility to esophageal squamous cell carcinoma in a Chinese population [in]. *Zhonghua Yi Xue Yi Chuan Xue Za Zhi* [Chinese]. 2002;19:10–3.
55. Hong Y, Miao X, Zhang X, et al. The role of P53 and MDM2 polymorphisms in the risk of esophageal squamous cell carcinoma. *Cancer Res.* 2005;65:9582–9587.
56. Vos M, Adams CH, Victor TC, et al. Polymorphisms and mutations found in the regions flanking exons 5 to 8 of the TP53 gene in a population at high risk for esophageal cancer in South Africa. *Cancer Genet Cytogenet.* 2003;140:23–30.
57. Hu N, Li WJ, Su H, et al. Common genetic variants of TP53 and BRCA2 in esophageal cancer patients and healthy individuals from low and high risk areas of northern China. *Cancer Detect Prev.* 2003;27:132–138.
58. Yu C, Lu W, Tan W, et al. Lack of association between CCND1 G870A polymorphism and risk of esophageal squamous cell carcinoma. *Cancer Epidemiol Biomarkers Prev.* 2003;12:176.
59. Zhang J, Li Y, Wang R, et al. Association of cyclin D1 (G870A) polymorphism with susceptibility to esophageal and gastric cardiac carcinoma in a northern Chinese population. *Int J Cancer.* 2003;105:281–284.
60. Xing D, Qi J, Miao X, et al. Polymorphisms of DNA repair genes XRCC1 and XPD and their associations with risk of esophageal squamous cell carcinoma in a Chinese population. *Int J Cancer.* 2002;100:600–605.
61. Ye W, Kumar R, Bacova G, et al. The XPD 751Gln allele is associated with an increased risk for esophageal adenocarcinoma: a population-based case-control study in Sweden. *Carcinogenesis.* 2006;27:1835–1841.
62. Yu HP, Wang XL, Sun X, et al. Polymorphisms in the DNA repair gene XPD and susceptibility to esophageal squamous cell carcinoma. *Cancer Genet Cytogenet.* 2004;154:10–15.
63. Cui Y, Morgenstern H, Greenland S, et al. Polymorphism of Xeroderma Pigmentosum group G and the risk of lung cancer and squamous cell carcinomas of the oropharynx, larynx and esophagus. *Int J Cancer.* 2006;118:714–720.
64. Hao B, Wang H, Zhou K, et al. Identification of genetic variants in base excision repair pathway and their associations with risk of esophageal squamous cell carcinoma. *Cancer Res.* 2004;64:4378–4384.
65. Ratnasinghe LD, Abnet C, Qiao YL, et al. Polymorphisms of XRCC1 and risk of esophageal and gastric cardia cancer. *Cancer Lett.* 2004;216:157–164.
66. Yu HP, Zhang XY, Wang XL, et al. DNA repair gene XRCC1 polymorphisms, smoking, and esophageal cancer risk. *Cancer Detect Prev.* 2004;28:194–199.
67. Xing DY, Tan W, Song N, et al. Ser326Cys polymorphism in hOGG1 gene and risk of esophageal cancer in a Chinese population. *Int J Cancer.* 2001;95:140–143.
68. Lee JM, Lee YC, Yang SY, et al. Genetic polymorphisms of XRCC1 and risk of the esophageal cancer. *Int J Cancer.* 2001;95:240–246.
69. Jain M, Kumar S, Rastogi N, et al. GSTT1, GSTM1 and GSTP1 genetic polymorphisms and interaction with tobacco, alcohol and occupational exposure in esophageal cancer patients from North India. *Cancer Lett.* 2006;242:60–67.
70. Jain M, Kumar S, Lal P, et al. Role of GSTM3 polymorphism in the risk of developing esophageal cancer. *Cancer Epidemiol Biomarkers Prev.* 2007;16:178–181.
71. Murphy SJ, Hughes AE, Patterson CC, et al. A population-based association study of SNPs of GSTP1, MnSOD, GPX2 and Barrett's esophagus and esophageal adenocarcinoma. *Carcinogenesis.* 2007;28:1323–1328.
72. Casson AG, Zheng Z, Evans SC, et al. Cyclin D1 polymorphism (G870A) and risk for esophageal adenocarcinoma. *Cancer.* 2005;104:730–739.
73. Geddert H, Kiel S, Zotz RB, et al. Polymorphism of p16 INK4A and cyclin D1 in adenocarcinomas of the upper gastrointestinal tract. *J Cancer Res Clin Oncol.* 2005;131:803–808.
74. Chanock SJ, Manolio T, Boehnke M, et al. Replicating genotype-phenotype associations. *Nature.* 2007;447:655–660.
75. Kleinberg L, Forastiere AA. Chemoradiation in the management of esophageal cancer. *J Clin Oncol.* 2007;25:4110–4117.
76. Rosell R, Taron M, Barnadas A, et al. Nucleotide excision repair pathways involved in Cisplatin resistance in non-small-cell lung cancer. *Cancer Control.* 2003;10:297–305.
77. Selvakumaran M, Pisarcik DA, Bao R, et al. Enhanced cisplatin cytotoxicity by disturbing the nucleotide excision repair pathway in ovarian cancer cell lines. *Cancer Res.* 2003;63:1311–1316.
78. Okuno T, Tamura T, Yamamori M, et al. Favorable genetic polymorphisms predictive of clinical outcome of chemoradiotherapy for stage II/III esophageal squamous cell carcinoma in Japanese. *Am J Clin Oncol.* 2007;30:252–257.
79. Shibuta K, Inoue H, Sato K, et al. L-myc restriction fragment length polymorphism in Japanese patients with esophageal cancer. *Jpn J Cancer Res.* 2000;91:199–203.
80. Sarbia M, Stahl M, von Weyhern C, et al. The prognostic significance of genetic polymorphisms (Methylenetetrahydrofolate Reductase C677T, Methionine Synthase A2756G, Thymidilate Synthase tandem repeat polymorphism) in multimodally treated oesophageal squamous cell carcinoma. *Br J Cancer.* 2006;94:203–207.
81. Deans DA, Wigmore SJ, Gilmour H, et al. Elevated tumour interleukin-1beta is associated with systemic inflammation: a marker of reduced survival in gastro-oesophageal cancer. *Br J Cancer.* 2006;95:1568–1575.
82. Liao Z, Liu H, Swisher SG, et al. Polymorphism at the 3'-UTR of the thymidylate synthase gene: a potential predictor for outcomes in Caucasian patients with esophageal adenocarcinoma treated with preoperative chemoradiation. *Int J Radiat Oncol Biol Phys.* 2006;64:700–708.
83. Wu X, Gu J, Wu TT, et al. Genetic variations in radiation and chemotherapy drug action pathways predict clinical outcomes in esophageal cancer. *J Clin Oncol.* 2006;24:3789–3798.
84. Lee JM, Wu MT, Lee YC, et al. Association of GSTP1 polymorphism and survival for esophageal cancer. *Clin Cancer Res.* 2005;11:4749–4753.
85. Hunter DJ, Kraft P. Drinking from the fire hose—statistical issues in genomewide association studies. *N Engl J Med.* 2007;357:436–439.

86. Casson AG, Zheng Z, Evans SC, et al. Polymorphisms in DNA repair genes in the molecular pathogenesis of esophageal (Barrett) adenocarcinoma. *Carcinogenesis.* 2005;26:1536–1541.
87. Ryan BM, McManus R, Daly JS, et al. A common p73 polymorphism is associated with a reduced incidence of oesophageal carcinoma. *Br J Cancer.* 2001;85:1499–1503.
88. Casson AG, Zheng Z, Porter GA, et al. Genetic polymorphisms of microsomal epoxide hydroxylase and glutathione S-transferases M1, T1 and P1, interactions with smoking, and risk for esophageal (Barrett) adenocarcinoma. *Cancer Detect Prev.* 2006;30:423–431.
89. Sarbia M, Bitzer M, Siegel D, et al. Association between NAD(P)H: quinone oxidoreductase 1 (NQ01) inactivating C609T polymorphism and adenocarcinoma of the upper gastrointestinal tract. *Int J Cancer.* 2003;107:381–386.
90. von Rahden BH, Stein HJ, Langer R, et al. C609T polymorphism of the NAD(P)H: quinone oxidoreductase I gene does not significantly affect susceptibility for esophageal adenocarcinoma. *Int J Cancer.* 2005;113:506–508.
91. di Martino E, Hardie LJ, Wild CP, et al. The NAD(P)H:quinone oxidoreductase I C609T polymorphism modifies the risk of Barrett esophagus and esophageal adenocarcinoma. *Genet Med.* 2007;9:341–347.
92. Terry MB, Gammon MD, Zhang FF, et al. Alcohol dehydrogenase 3 and risk of esophageal and gastric adenocarcinomas. *Cancer Causes Control.* 2007;18:1039–1046.
93. Hamajima N, Matsuo K, Suzuki T, et al. No associations of p73 G4C14-to-A4T14 at exon 2 and p53 Arg72Pro polymorphisms with the risk of digestive tract cancers in Japanese. *Cancer Lett.* 2002;181:81–85.
94. Liu G, Zhou W, Yeap BY, et al. XRCC1 and XPD polymorphisms and esophageal adenocarcinoma risk. *Carcinogenesis.* 2007;28:1254–1258.
95. Lucas D, Menez C, Floch F, et al. Cytochromes P4502E1 and P4501A1 genotypes and susceptibility to cirrhosis or upper aerodigestive tract cancer in alcoholic Caucasians. *Alcohol Clin Exp Res.* 1996;20:1033–1037.

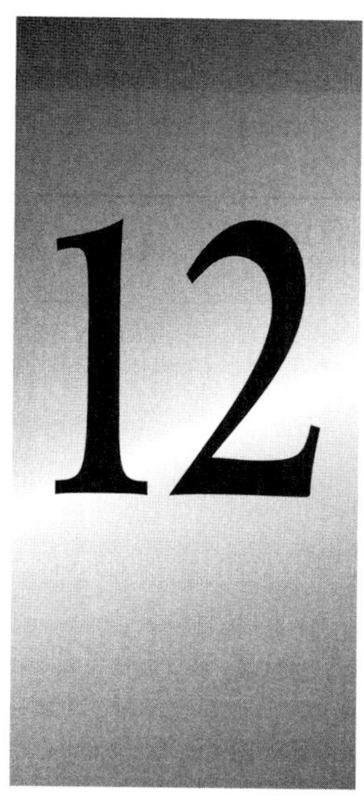

Epidemiology and Risk of Esophageal Cancer: Clinical

Linda Morris Brown
Susan S. Devesa

This chapter reviews the epidemiology of esophageal cancer and its 2 major histologic types, squamous cell carcinoma (SCC) and adenocarcinoma (AC). Although patients with either of the tumors share a poor prognosis, the cancers have rather distinct epidemiologic profiles. Herein we review the descriptive patterns of both tumors, along with known and suspected risk or protective factors. Because AC comprised only a small fraction of esophageal cancers until recently, most epidemiologic studies of esophageal cancer did not distinguish histologic types and results largely reflect the risk factors for SCC. However, special attention has recently centered on AC in view of the rapidly rising incidence rates of this tumor.

DEMOGRAPHIC CHARACTERISTICS

Mortality Patterns and Trends

Globally, esophageal cancer is the sixth most common cause of cancer death (261,162 deaths among men; 124,730 deaths among women) (1). Fatality rates are high, so that global estimates of age-standardized rates per 100,000 are generally comparable for incidence (11.5 for men, 4.7 for women) and mortality (9.9 for men, 3.9 for women) (1). The most recent estimates of global cancer incidence indicate that esophageal cancer is the eighth most frequent cancer in the world (315,394 cases in men; 146,723 cases in women) (1). Esophageal cancer is known for its marked variation by geographic region, ethnicity, and gender. Some of the highest mortality rates in both men and women occur in the so-called Asian esophageal cancer belt, an area not covered by population-based tumor registries that stretches from northern Iran and central Asia (including Turkmenistan and Kazakhstan) into northern and western China. Other high-rate areas are found in southern and eastern Africa.

In the United States, esophageal cancer accounts for only 1% of all diagnosed cancers; however, it is the seventh leading cause of death from cancer among men (2). According to estimates provided by the American Cancer Society, approximately 11,250 men and 3,030 women are expected to die from esophageal cancer in the United States during 2008 (2).

Based on data from the National Center for Health Statistics, 1950–2004, mortality rates for esophageal cancer almost doubled among non-whites between 1950 and 1984, reaching a high of 16.1/100,000 among non-white men and 4.0/100,000 among non-white women (Figure 12.1). However, since 1985 rates have decreased steadily, with rates for nonwhite men and women falling to 8.1/100,000 and 2.4/100,000, respectively, in

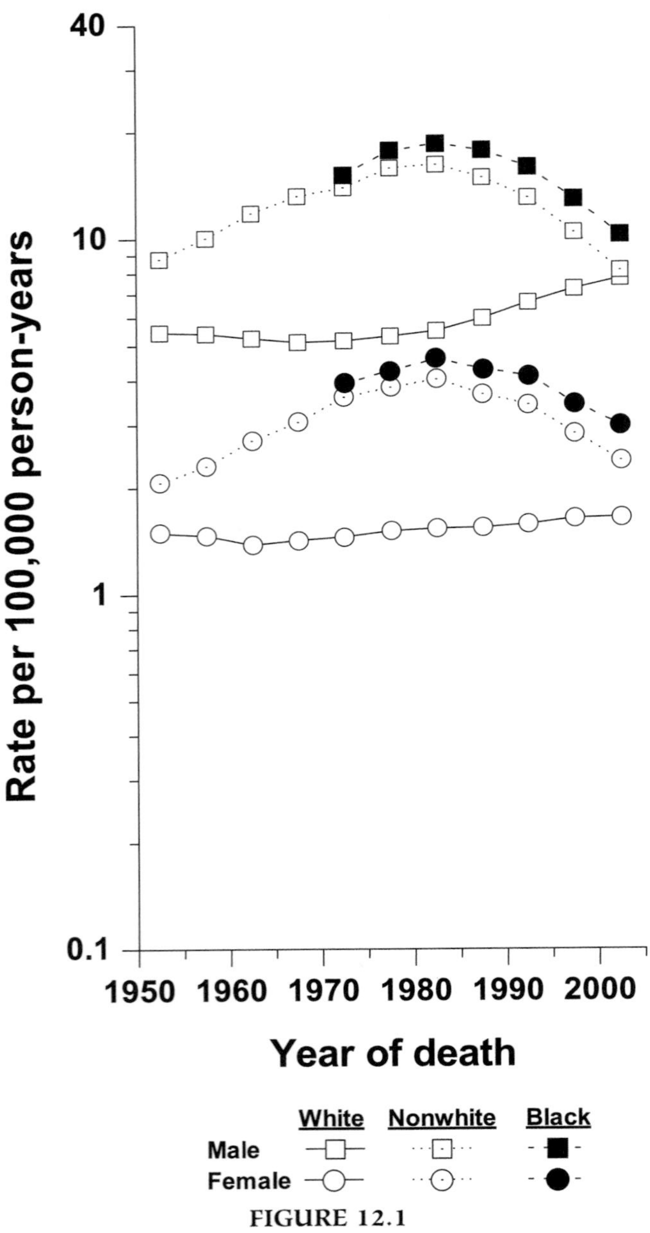

FIGURE 12.1

Trends in esophageal cancer mortality rates (per 100,000 person-years, age-standardized to the 2000 U.S. population) in the United States by race and sex, 1950–2004. Data from the Surveillance, Epidemiology, and End Results (SEER) Program of the National Cancer Institute (www.seer.cancer.gov) SEER*Stat Database: Mortality—Cancer, Total U.S. (1950–2004), National Cancer Institute, DCCPS, Surveillance Research Program, Cancer Statistics Branch, released March 2007. Underlying mortality data provided by NCHS (www.cdc.gov/nchs).

2000–2004. Among whites, mortality rates changed little during 1950–1984; rates have risen notably since 1985 among men, but not women. Mortality rates for white men and women in 2000–2004 were 7.7/100,000 and 1.6/100,000, respectively. Rates specific for blacks, available since the early 1970s, are higher than rates for all nonwhites combined.

Incidence Patterns and Trends

International differences in esophageal cancer incidence rates are striking (Figure 12.2) (3). Based on updated data available on the International Agency for Research on Cancer (IARC) website (http://www.iarc.fr/), recent esophageal cancer rates varied 7-fold among males, from 18 in Calvados, France, to 2.5 in Israel. Recent rates among females varied over 20-fold, from 6.6 in India to 0.3 in Spain. Male to female rate ratios varied from less than 2 in India and China to more than 6 in Japan, Italy, and Calvados, France, and to more than 10 in Spain; Bas-Rhin, France; and Slovakia. Rates in all populations rose consistently with age.

Among men, rates declined by 24%–60% over most of the time period in U.S. blacks, France, Italy, India, China, and Singapore; increased by 20%–98% in U.S. whites, Australia, Scotland, England, Denmark, and Norway; and more than doubled in Slovakia. Although rates among females tended to fluctuate more over time due to the smaller number of cases, similar to males, rates decreased 27%–65% in U.S. blacks, India, China, and Singapore, whereas they rose 21%–83% in Scotland, England, Denmark, Norway, and Slovakia.

These divergent incidence trends and patterns reflect the changing frequencies of SCC and AC in these populations. Rates of SCC, which tend to be higher in developing countries and U.S. blacks, appear to be falling, whereas AC rates, which tend to be higher in more developed countries and in U.S. whites, have been steadily increasing (4). Examples of these trends are presented in Figure 12.3, which demonstrates the impact of changing rates of SCC and AC on total esophageal cancer rates among U.S. black and white men and women in the 9 Surveillance, Epidemiology, and End Results (SEER) registries over the time period 1973–1976 to 2001–2004, as well as the marked differences in cell type distribution by race (5).

Total esophageal cancer incidence rates among U.S. blacks peaked at 21.7 in 1977–1980 and then began a marked decline, reaching 10.0 in 2001–2004, whereas rates among white men increased from 5.8 in 1973–1976 to 8.4 in 2001–2004. Rates among white women remained around 2 over the several decades, but they declined among black women since the early 1980s. The dramatic decrease in total esophageal cancer rates for black men was driven by the concurrent 57% drop in rates for SCC (from 19.1 in 1981–1984 to 8.2 in 2001–2004). Rates of SCC also decreased 50%,

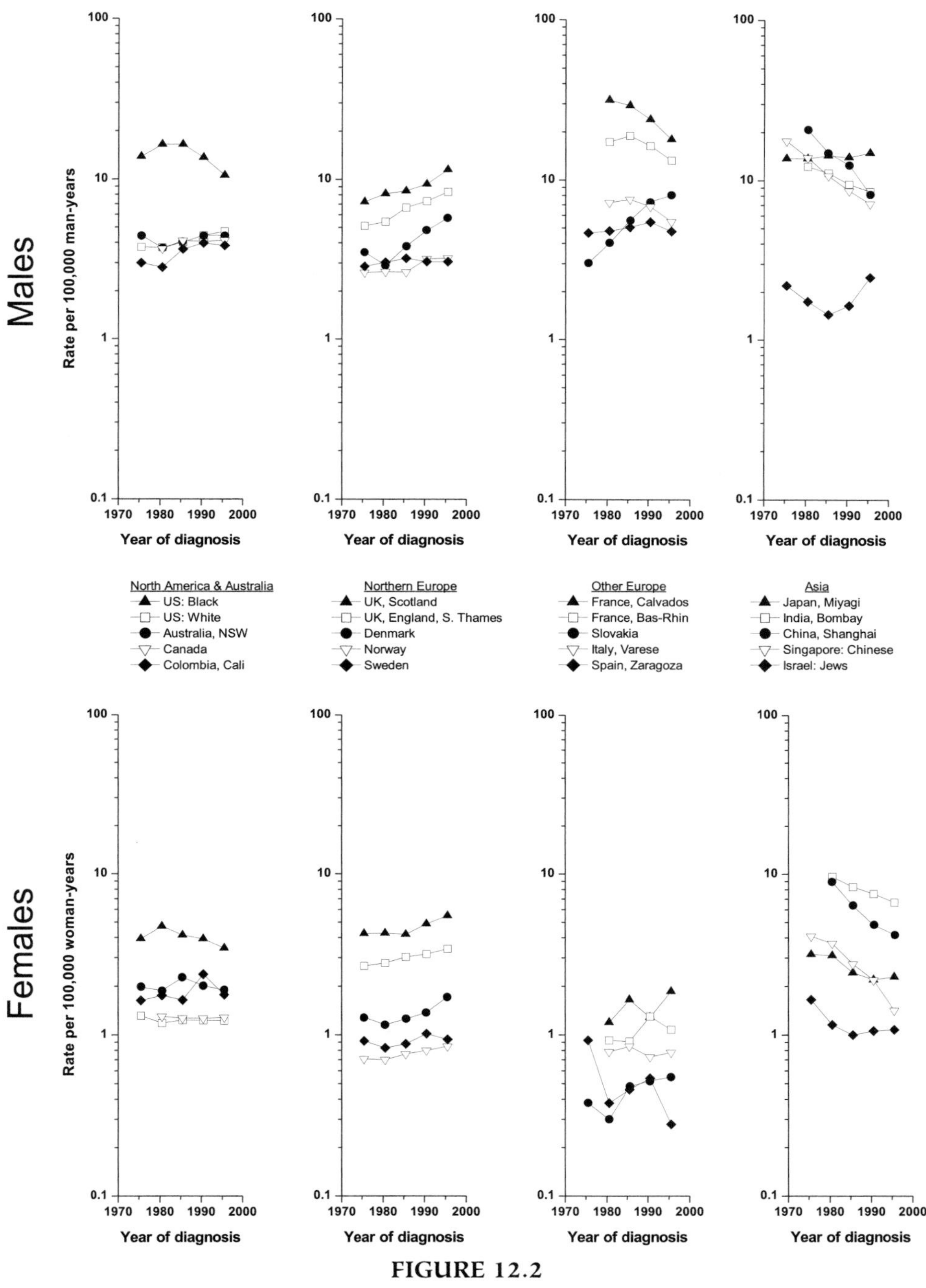

FIGURE 12.2

International trends in esophageal cancer incidence rates (per 100,000 person-years, age-standardized to the world population) by geographic area, registry, and sex, circa 1973–1977 to 1993–1997. Adapted from updated data available at http://www.iarc.fr/.

48%, and 35% among white males, black females, and white females, respectively. In contrast, the increase in total esophageal cancer rates for white men reflects the dramatic increase of over 600% in the incidence of AC (from 0.8 in 1973–1976 to 5.7 in 2001–2004). With the decreases in SCC and the increases in AC, the AC rate among white men surpassed that for SCC during the late 1980s. In addition, AC rates rose over 400% among white women. Rates of AC among black men more than doubled; however, the rates of SCC remain considerably higher. Rates of AC among black females were more variable since they were based on the fewest number of cases. During 2001–2004, AC, SCC, and other histologies accounted for 61.6%, 31.0%, and

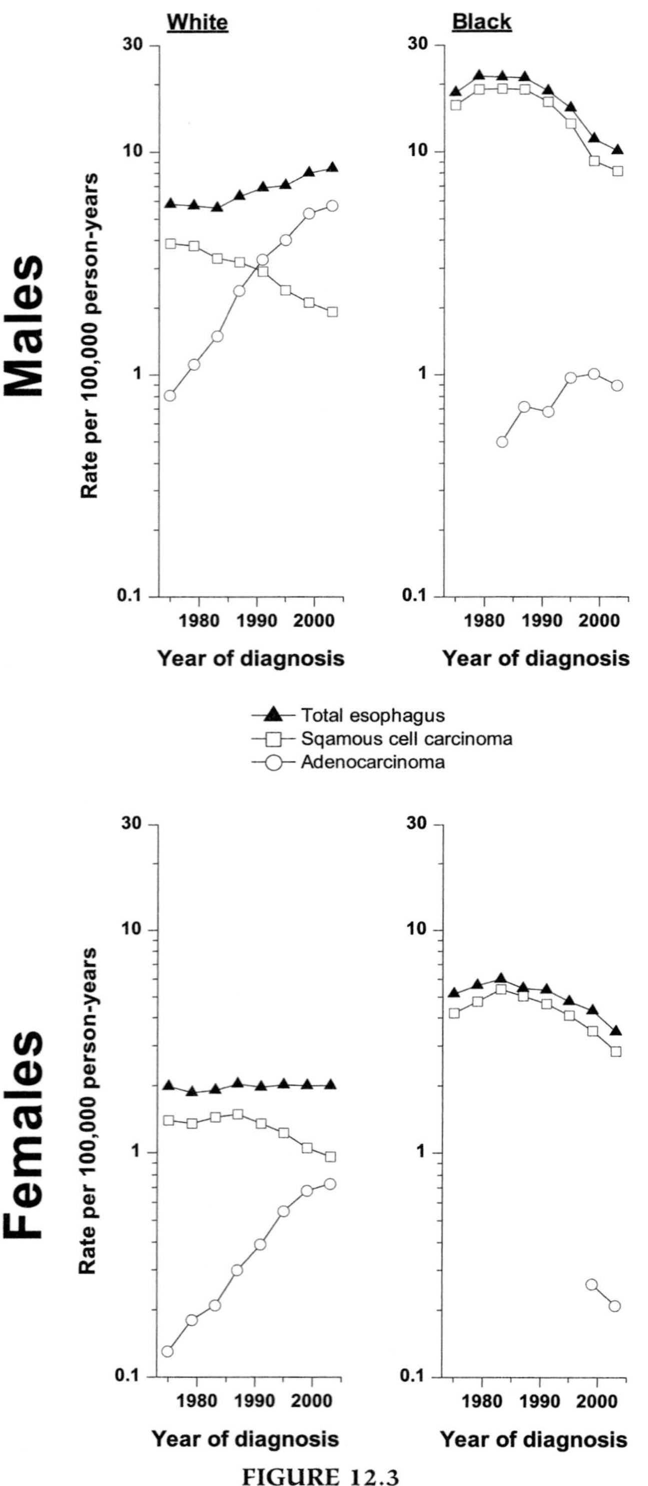

FIGURE 12.3

Trends in esophageal cancer incidence rates (per 100,000 person-years, age-standardized to the 2000 U.S. population) in 9 SEER areas in the United States by histologic cell type, race and sex, 1973–1976 to 2001–2004. Data from the Surveillance, Epidemiology, and End Results (SEER) Program of the National Cancer Institute (www.seer.cancer.gov)

FIGURE 12.3 (*continued*)

SEER*Stat Database: Incidence—SEER 9 Regs Limited-Use, Nov 2006 Sub (1973–2004)—Linked To County Attributes—Total U.S., 1969–2004 Counties, National Cancer Institute, DCCPS, Surveillance Research Program, Cancer Statistics Branch, released April 2007, based on the November 2006 submission.

7.5% of esophageal cancer among whites and 11.6%, 82.7%, and 5.6% among blacks, respectively (6).

Esophageal cancer incidence rates in the 17 SEER registries by race/ethnicity and gender during 2001–2005 are presented in Table 12.1. Among both males and females, rates were highest for blacks and lowest for Asian/Pacific Islanders. Rates were higher for males than for females among all race/ethnicity groups (7).

U.S. Survival Patterns

Presented in Table 12.2 are survival data for patients diagnosed with esophageal cancer during 1975–2004 in 9 SEER population-based cancer registries (7). Although survival among patients diagnosed with esophageal cancer is poor for all race-gender groups, marked improvements in the 5-year relative survival rates have occurred

TABLE 12.1
Age-Adjusted Esophageal Cancer SEER Incidence Rates [a] 2001–2005 by Race/Ethnicity and Gender (7) [b]

Race/ethnicity	Total	Male	Female
All races	4.6	7.8	2.0
White	4.6	8.0	1.9
Black	5.9	9.9	3.0
Asian/Pacific Islander	2.4	4.0	1.2
American Indian/ Alaska Native [c]	4.4	7.1	2.0
Hispanic [d]	3.1	5.5	1.2

[a] Rates per 100,000 person-years, age-adjusted to the 2000 U.S. standard.
[b] Based on November 2007 SEER data submission, posted to the SEER website, 2008, from 17 population-based registries: San Francisco, San Jose-Monterey, Los Angeles, other California, Connecticut, Detroit, Hawaii, Iowa, New Mexico, Seattle, Utah, Atlanta, Alaska Native Registry, Rural Georgia, Kentucky, Louisiana, and New Jersey.
[c] Based on the CHSDA (Contract Health Service Delivery Area) counties.
[d] Excludes data from the Alaska Native Registry and Kentucky.

TABLE 12.2
Esophageal Cancer 5-Year Relative Survival Rates, 1975–2004, by Diagnosis Year, Gender, and Race (7) [a]

	All races		White		Black	
Year of diagnosis	**Male**	**Female**	**Male**	**Female**	**Male**	**Female**
1975–1979	4.3%	6.6%	5.1%	6.2%	2.2%	6.8%
1985–1989	9.5%	10.6%	10.8%	10.5%	6.7%	10.3%
1996–2004	16.4%	18.9%	17.6%	19.7%	9.0%	15.6%

[a] Based on November 2007 SEER data submission, posted to the SEER website, 2008. Based on data from 9 population-based registries: San Francisco, Connecticut, Detroit, Hawaii, Iowa, New Mexico, Seattle, Utah, and Atlanta. Rates are based on follow-up of patients through 2005.

over the past three decades. The 5-year relative survival rates for those diagnosed during 1996–2004 were 17.6% for white males, 19.7% for white females, 9.0% for black males, and 15.6% for black females. Survival rates for SCC and AC are similar (data not shown), and there is a strong decreasing gradient in patient survival with increasing extent of disease. For total esophageal cancer, the 5-year relative survival rates, 1996–2004, ranged from 34.4% for localized, to 17.1% for regional, to 2.8% for distant, and 11.6% for unstaged disease at diagnosis (7).

ETIOLOGIC FACTORS

The established or suspected risk or protective factors for SCC and AC are listed in Table 12.3 and explained in greater detail below.

Tobacco

Squamous Cell Carcinoma

Tobacco use, regardless of form, is a major risk factor for esophageal cancer in most parts of the world. Several case-control studies have reported strong positive dose-response effects with duration and/or intensity of cigarette smoking (8–13). In most studies evaluating the effect of quitting smoking, a 50% reduction in risk has been seen for ex-smokers compared with current smokers, along with an inverse effect with time since stopped smoking (8,13,14). Smoking has been associated with esophageal cancer risk among nondrinkers, supporting an independent effect of tobacco smoke on the esophageal epithelium (13,15). In some studies, pipe smokers have shown a higher risk of esophageal cancer than smokers of commercial cigarettes, perhaps because pipe tobacco condensates are swallowed, allowing tobacco carcinogens to have direct contact with the esophagus (13). In case-control studies in the United States, the percentage of SCC attributable to ever smoking has ranged from 57% to 65% (16,17). In several studies from South America, the risks of esophageal cancer for use of black (air-cured) tobacco were 2-fold or more higher than those for blond (flue-cured) tobacco (13). Elevated risks have also been reported for hand-rolled cigarettes, which have a higher tar content than commercial cigarettes (13). Case-control studies in India and Taiwan identified bidi smoking (a native cigarette of coarse tobacco in a dry temburni leaf), pan chewing (a mixture of betel leaf, sliced areca nut, and aqueous shell lime), and betel quid chewing (areca nut chewing with a piece of Piper betle inflorescence, which contains approximately 15 mg/g of the animal carcinogen safrole) as major risk factors for esophageal cancer (10,12,13,18).

Adenocarcinoma

Although smoking is a less potent cause of AC than SCC, cigarette smoking, especially heavy/long-term smoking, is a significant risk factor for AC in most of the world (13,19–21). Although results are inconsistent, quitting smoking appears to attenuate risks for AC somewhat (22). It has been suggested that changes in the constituents of tobacco smoke or the introduction of filtered cigarettes might have differentially affected rates of SCC and AC (23). The percentage of AC attributable to ever use of cigarettes was recently estimated at 40% and 58%, based on U.S. case-control and cohort data, respectively (16,22).

Alcohol

Squamous Cell Carcinoma

There are clear-cut epidemiologic data indicating that alcoholic beverages are a major cause of SCC, particularly

TABLE 12.3
Risk and Protective Factors for Esophageal Cancers by Histologic Cell Type

Factors	Squamous cell carcinoma	Adenocarcinoma
Tobacco use	+++	++
Alcohol use	+++	+
Dietary deficiencies	++	0
Obesity/high Body Mass Index (BMI)	--	+++
High fruit and vegetable intake	++	++
Hot food and beverages	++	0
Gastroesophageal reflux disease	0	+++
Barrett's esophagus	0	+++
Helicobacter pylori prevalence	+/-	-
Human papilloma virus	+	0
Aspirin/NSAID[a] use	--	--
Other medical conditions	++	0
Poverty/low socioeconomic status	++	+
Radiotherapy	++	++
Occupational exposures	+	0

Abbreviation: [a]NSAID = non-steroidal anti-inflammatory drugs.
Risk factor: +++ (strong and well documented); ++ (medium); + (weak/not well documented)
Protective factor: --- (strong and well documented); -- (medium); - (weak/not well documented)
No documented relationship: 0

in Western populations (12). Strong dose-response relationships for ethanol consumption, after adjustment for smoking, have been demonstrated in many case-control and cohort studies in the United States, Europe, South America, Asia, and South Africa (8,10,12,13,24). However, alcohol drinking has not been shown to be a risk factor in some developing countries with exceptionally high rates of SCC, including rural parts of Africa, Iran, and China (13,25). In the United States, the percentage of SCC attributable to alcohol intake has been estimated to range from 72% to 82% (16,17).

In case-control studies in Italy, Hong Kong, and South America, the dose-response gradients for alcohol consumption remained strong when analyses were restricted to lifelong nonsmokers (13). However, other measures of exposure such as duration and age started drinking have not shown significant gradients in risk (13). Years since stopping drinking did not affect the risk of esophageal cancer in France or Argentina but did in Hong Kong, Paraguay, and Taiwan (12,13).

Variability in risks by type of alcoholic beverage may reflect culturally or economically determined drinking habits. Generally, the beverage most strongly associated with the risk of esophageal cancer has been the one most frequently consumed by the study population (13). For example, in most studies, the risk was greatest among users of hard liquor. However, wine was most strongly implicated in a region of Italy where wine is the major contributor to ethanol intake, and moonshine (home-brewed) whiskey was implicated in a high-risk area of coastal South Carolina (13). In addition, consumption of apple brandy, home-brewed rum, *aguardiente* (a local spirit), and *shochu* has been associated with excess risk of esophageal cancer in France, Puerto Rico, Paraguay, and Japan, respectively (13).

Although alcohol is strongly related to risk of esophageal cancer, the components or mechanisms responsible for its carcinogenicity have not been identified. Findings of studies conducted in Italy and Switzerland have supported the notion that subjects who drank alcohol outside meals (i.e., not with food) regardless of level were at greater risk of SCC than subjects who drank only with meals, possibly because of the more rapid absorption of alcohol (26). The results of several studies suggest that concentrated liquor is associated with higher risk than diluted liquor because of local effects on tissue (13). While certain kinds of alcoholic beverages, including beer and whiskey, may contain compounds that are carcinogenic, findings suggest that the risk of SCC is associated with alcohol per se, rather than with the presence of contaminants, flavoring compounds, or additives that may vary among types of beverages (13). Acetaldehyde, a metabolite of alcohol and a recognized animal carcinogen, may play a critical role in the mechanism by which alcohol causes esophageal cancer (13).

Adenocarcinoma

Although several earlier case-control studies suggested a modest association between alcohol intake and risk of AC, more recent studies found no association with any measure of alcohol intake or type of beverage (13,19,20,22).

Alcohol-Tobacco Interactions

Squamous Cell Carcinoma

In Western Europe and North America, 80%–90% of the risk of SCC has been attributed to alcohol and tobacco use (13,17). Alcohol and tobacco appear to act independently, with the importance of each factor depending on the baseline characteristics of the population under study. In most studies, heavy consumers of both alcohol and tobacco have the highest risk of esophageal cancer, often consistent with multiplicative interaction (8,12,13).

Diet and Nutrition

Body Mass Index (BMI), Food Groups, and Nutrients

Squamous Cell Carcinoma

Dietary insufficiencies appear to contribute to the varying incidence of SCC around the world (13). High-risk populations for SCC are frequently malnourished, and risk tends to increase as BMI decreases (11,13,24,27).

A protective effect of fruit and vegetable consumption, especially those eaten raw, is supported by a large quantity of epidemiologic data from around the world (13,28–30). Fruits and vegetables contain a variety of micronutrients and other dietary components with potential anticarcinogenic effects. The population attributable risk for low fruit and vegetable intake has been estimated to range from 29% to 44% in U.S. case-control studies (16,17).

A number of case-control studies have suggested a protective effect of vitamin C from supplements and food sources (13,31–33). Vitamin C blocks the endogenous formation of N-nitroso compounds, which are suspected factors in the etiology of esophageal cancer in some high-risk areas of the world (13).

Case-control studies that have attempted to evaluate other food groups and nutrients have found an elevated risk associated with high consumption of retinol, dietary cholesterol, animal protein, polyunsaturated fat/linoleic acid, total fat, and vitamin B12, while alpha- and beta-carotene, beta-crytoxantin, lycopene, folate, vitamin E, vitamin B6, zinc, selenium, and flavonoids generally appeared to be protective (13,31–40).

Some case-control studies of SCC have reported elevated risks associated with consumption of barbequed or fried meats, possibly due to the formation of heterocyclic amines during cooking (13). In addition, the higher risks associated with red meat (especially cured or processed meat); pickled vegetables; salted fish; and moldy breads, rice, and cereals suggest an effect of N-nitroso compounds or their precursors (nitrates and amines) (13,28,30,41). A protective effect of frequent consumption of fish high in polyunsaturated omega-3 essential fatty acids has also been reported (13,30).

It has been difficult to disentangle the influence of dietary and nutritional factors from the potent effects of alcohol and tobacco on the risk of esophageal cancer. In particular, heavy consumption of alcoholic beverages can interfere with the consumption and utilization of a variety of nutrients, including vitamins A, C, D, the B vitamins, zinc, and protein (13). Also, since poor nutrition is a risk factor for esophageal cancer, it is conceivable that alcohol increases risk, in part, by reducing nutrient intake. In addition, smokers appear to have lower intake of several nutrients including vitamin C than nonsmokers (13).

Adenocarcinoma

In contrast to SCC, where high-risk populations are generally poorly nourished, AC risk tends to rise as BMI increases, with subjects in the highest quartile of BMI having 3–7 times the risk of subjects in the lowest quartile (13,21,27,42,43). The mechanism by which obesity affects the risk of AC is unclear (21), although it may be linked to the predisposition of obese individuals to develop gastroesophageal reflux disease (GERD) (13). Whatever the process, it seems likely that obesity contributes to the upward trend in AC, in view of the sharply increasing prevalence of individuals classified as overweight and/or obese in the United States (44). The percentage of AC attributable to the highest vs. the lowest quartile of BMI was recently estimated at 21% in a U.S. case-control study (16).

Various foods, food groups, and nutrients have been associated with risk of AC, but most consistent is a protective effect of consumption of fruits and vegetables as well as fiber (13). In the United States, the percentage of AC attributable to low consumption of fruits and vegetables was recently estimated at 15% (16).

Nutrients that may be protective against AC include antioxidants (vitamin C, vitamin E, and beta-carotene), vitamin B6, vitamin B12, and folate (13,36,40,45). Animal-based foods (total meat, processed meat, red meat) and associated macronutrients (e.g., total fat, saturated fat, total protein, animal protein, and cholesterol) have been associated with elevated risk in some studies (13,46).

Hot Food and Beverages

Squamous Cell Carcinoma

Although consumption of green tea at normal temperatures has been associated with a reduced risk of esophageal cancer (13,28), drinking tea, including green tea, at exceptionally hot temperatures appears to increase SCC (13). Excess risks have also been associated with consumption of burning hot soup, gruel, porridge, and other beverages, suggesting a role for thermal injury to the esophagus (13,28,41).

Consumption of hot alcoholic beverages, especially hot Calvados, was associated with elevated risks of esophageal cancer in France; declines in that formerly widespread habit likely contributed to the downward trend in incidence in western France (13). In high-risk areas of South America, chronic thermal injury from mate, a local tea prepared as an infusion of the herb *Ilex paraguayenis* and usually drunk very hot, has been linked to esophageal cancer (13,24,47). Based on the South American data, an IARC working group concluded in 1991 that "hot mate drinking is probably carcinogenic to humans" (48). In Uruguay, the percentage of SCC due to consumption of mate was estimated at 53% (47).

Medical Conditions and Medications

Gastroesophageal Reflux Disease (GERD) and Helicobacter pylori

Squamous Cell Carcinoma

Helicobacter pylori (H. pylori) infection, especially with CagA+ strains, has been associated with an increased risk of SCC in some studies and a protective effect in others (49–51). The discrepancy may result from the interplay of *H. pylori* infection and atrophic gastritis (52). *H. pylori* infection appears to be associated with an increased risk of SCC when it induces atrophic gastritis but a decreased risk when it induces an antral-predominant, non-atrophic gastritis (52).

Adenocarcinoma

Significant 2-fold or greater risks of AC have been associated with the presence of GERD, a major risk factor that predisposes the esophagus to Barrett's esophagus, a precursor lesion for AC (13,21,53). It has been hypothesized that use of lower esophageal sphincter-relaxing (LES) drugs such as anticholinergic agents, may promote GERD and thus contribute to the risk of AC (13). An elevated risk with LES drug use was observed in a Norwegian case-control study (20) but not in most other studies (13,54).

Several but not all case-control studies found that infection with CagA+ strains of *H. pylori* was associated with a reduced AC risk (13,51,55–57). Further investigations are needed to determine whether the decreasing prevalence of *H. pylori* infection may contribute in some way to the upward trend for AC.

Human Papilloma Virus

Squamous Cell Carcinoma

Human papilloma virus (HPV) (particularly HPV-16 and HPV-18) is an oncogenic virus that appears to play an etiologic role in some high risk areas with an exceptionally high incidence of esophageal cancer, such as China, Iran, South Africa, and South America (13,58–65). However, HPV does not appear to be related to the risk of SCC in the United Kingdom and North America (13).

Other Medical Conditions

Squamous Cell Carcinoma

Elevated risks of esophageal cancer have been reported with certain medical conditions, such as pernicious anemia, achalasia, some autoimmune diseases, gastrectomy, and chemical injuries to the esophagus (13). In clinical and case-control studies, a high risk of SCC has been reported in association with tylosis, a dominantly inherited disorder characterized by palmar and plantar keratoses (PPK) and often accompanied by esophageal hyperkeratosis (13,66). It has been suggested that a hereditary predisposition may cause both PPK and SCC (66). Some studies have indicated a familial tendency for esophageal cancer, although it is difficult to distinguish genetic from environmental factors (11,13,67). A striking excess risk of SCC has been demonstrated following other tumors of the upper aerodigestive tract that share major risk factors (alcohol and tobacco) and may share genetic mechanisms (13).

Aspirin and Non-Steroidal Anti-Inflammatory Drugs (NSAIDs)

Squamous Cell Carcinoma

Use of aspirin and other NSAIDs has been associated with reduced risk of SCC in most epidemiologic studies (13,20,68)

Adenocarcinoma

Use of aspirin and other NSAIDs, COX-2 inhibitors, and corticosteroids have been associated with a reduced risk of AC in some but not all studies (20,54,69,70). There is a suggestion that recent use may be more important than long-term use and might protect against development of AC in people with Barrett's esophagus (68,71).

Socioeconomic Status

Squamous Cell Carcinoma

The highest rates of SCC are generally found in areas of the world where the population is impoverished. Within various populations, the risk of esophageal cancer is greatest among those with the lowest socioeconomic status (SES), whether measured by income, education, or occupation (11,13,30,47). In addition, increased risks have been reported for single compared with married men (13). Low SES is obviously a surrogate for a set of lifestyle and other environmental factors (e.g., poor housing, unemployment or workplace hazards, limited access to medical care, stress, poor nutrition, exposure to infectious agents), some of which may affect susceptibility to environmental carcinogens (13).

Adenocarcinoma

Low SES based on income, education, and occupation has been related to excess risk of AC (13,19,72), although the effect is less pronounced than for SCC. This differential is consistent with studies reporting a higher percentage of AC cases in professional/skilled occupations as compared with SCC cases (13).

Radiation

Squamous Cell Carcinoma

Ionizing radiation has been linked to esophageal cancer, particularly among patients irradiated for ankylosing spondylitis and for breast cancer (13,73–76). In one study, postmastectomy radiation therapy was associated with greater than a 2-fold risk of SCC, whereas no significant increase in risk was associated with lower-dose postlumpectomy radiation therapy (75). In addition, increased risk was restricted to SCCs in the upper and middle thirds of the esophagus. Significant excesses of esophageal cancer risk also have been reported among A-bomb survivors in Japan (13).

Adenocarcinoma

In a study based on U.S. SEER data, no significant risk of AC was found following either postmastectomy or postlumpectomy radiation (75).

Occupation and Industry

Squamous Cell Carcinoma

Esophageal cancer is not usually considered to be an occupational disease, although elevated risks have been reported for several exposures. Presented below are some of the more consistent findings.

Excesses reported among Swedish brewery workers and Norwegian and Swedish hotel and restaurant workers are likely due to their higher intake of alcohol or tobacco or to exposure to passive smoking (13,77). The lower risk of esophageal cancer generally reported among farmers appears to be related to their lower intake of alcohol compared with the general population (13,78).

Increased risks of esophageal cancer have been observed among chimney sweeps, printers, metal workers exposed to metalworking fluids, metal polishers and platers, dry cleaners, gas station attendants, vulcanization and other rubber industry workers, asphalt workers, automobile manufacturing workers, and textile finishers and dyers exposed to fumes from incomplete combustion of organic material or to perchloroethylene (PCE) and other chemical solvents and detergents (13,79). Excess risks of esophageal cancer have been reported among workers exposed to silica and metal dust, and among concrete and construction workers (13,77,78). The association between asbestos exposure and esophageal cancer is unclear, as increased risks have been reported in some but not all studies (13,80).

Adenocarcinoma

Although a few associations between employment and AC have been noted (e.g., construction workers exposed to asbestos and cement dust, and health services workers), occupational exposures are thought to play only a minor etiologic role (81,82). Occupational physical activity was associated with a modest protective effect in a recent U.S. case-control study (83).

Impact of Risk Factors in the United States

Squamous Cell Carcinoma

In a U.S. case-control study, moderate/heavy levels of alcohol intake, use of tobacco, infrequent consumption of raw fruits and vegetables, and low income were found to account for over 98% of the SCC among both black and white men (17). It is likely that declines in the prevalence of smoking since the 1960s, especially among men, may have contributed to the downward trends reported for this cancer.

Adenocarcinoma

In another U.S. case-control study, use of tobacco, high BMI, infrequent consumption of fruits and vegetables, and GERD were found to account for almost 82% of the AC among white men and 51% among white women (16). Data emerging from recent studies suggest that the relationship with obesity may account for part of the upward trend in AC incidence. Obesity increases the incidence of GERD and its progression to Barrett's esophagus, the main precursor of AC.

References

1. Ferlay J, Bray F, Pisani P, et al. *GLOBOCAN 2002: Cancer Incidence, Mortality and Prevalence Worldwide*. IARC Cancer Base No.5 [version 2.0]. 2004. Lyon, France, IARC.
2. Jemal A, Siegel R, Ward E, et al. Cancer statistics, 2008. *CA Cancer J Clin*. 2008;58:71–96.
3. Parkin DM, Whelan SL, Ferlay J, et al. *Cancer Incidence in Five Continents, Vol. IV to VIII*. Cancer Base No 7, Lyon, France: IARC; 2005.
4. Brown LM, Devesa SS, Chow W-H. Incidence of adenocarcinoma of the esophagus among white Americans by sex, stage, and age. *J Natl Cancer Inst*. 2008;100:1184–1187.
5. Ries LAG, Melbert D, Krapcho M, et al, eds. *SEER Cancer Statistics Review, 1975–2004*. Bethesda, MD: National Cancer Institute; 2007.
6. Surveillance, Epidemiology, and End Results (SEER) Program (www.seer.cancer.gov) SEER*Stat Database: Incidence—SEER 9 Regs Limited-USE, Nov 2006 Sub (1973–2004)—Linked to County Attributes—Total U.S., 1969–2004 Counties, National Cancer Institute, DCCPS, Surveillance Research Program, Cancer Statistics Branch, released April 2007, based on the November 2006 submission.
7. Ries LAG, Melbert D, Krapcho M, et al, eds. *SEER Cancer Statistics Review, 1975–2005*. Bethesda, MD: National Cancer Institute; 2008.
8. Hashibe M, Boffetta P, Janout V, et al. Esophageal cancer in Central and Eastern Europe: tobacco and alcohol. *Int J Cancer*. 2007;120:1518–1522.
9. Jiang JM, Zeng XJ, Chen JS, et al. Smoking and mortality from esophageal cancer in China: a large case-control study of 19,734 male esophageal cancer deaths and 104,846 living spouse controls. *Int J Cancer*. 2006;119:1427–1432.
10. Wu IC, Lu CY, Kuo FC, et al. Interaction between cigarette, alcohol and betel nut use on esophageal cancer risk in Taiwan. *Eur J Clin Invest*. 2006;36:236–241.
11. Wu M, Zhao JK, Hu XS, et al. Association of smoking, alcohol drinking and dietary factors with esophageal cancer in high- and low-risk areas of Jiangsu Province, China. *World J Gastroenterol*. 2006;12:1686–1693.
12. Lee CH, Lee JM, Wu DC, et al. Independent and combined effects of alcohol intake, tobacco smoking and betel quid chewing on the risk of esophageal cancer in Taiwan. *Int J Cancer*. 2005;113:475–482.
13. Brown LM, Devesa SS, Fraumeni JF Jr. Epidemiology of esophageal cancer. In: Posner MC, Vokes EE, Weichselbaum RR, eds. *Cancer of the Upper Gastrointestinal Tract*. Hamilton / London: BC Decker; 2002:1–21.
14. Bosetti C, Franceschi S, Levi F, et al. Smoking and drinking cessation and the risk of oesophageal cancer. *Br J Cancer*. 2000;83:689–691.
15. Lee CH, Wu DC, Lee JM, et al. Carcinogenetic impact of alcohol intake on squamous cell carcinoma risk of the oesophagus in relation to tobacco smoking. *Eur J Cancer*. 2007;43:1188–1199.
16. Engel LS, Chow WH, Vaughan TL, et al. Population attributable risks of esophageal and gastric cancers. *J Natl Cancer Inst*. 2003;95:1404–1413.
17. Brown LM, Hoover R, Silverman D, et al. Excess incidence of squamous cell esophageal cancer among U.S. Black men: role of social class and other risk factors. *Am J Epidemiol*. 2001;153:114–122.
18. Wu MT, Wu DC, Hsu HK, et al. Constituents of areca chewing related to esophageal cancer risk in Taiwanese men. *Dis Esophagus*. 2004;17:257–259.
19. de Jonge PJ, Steyerberg EW, Kuipers EJ, et al. Risk factors for the development of esophageal adenocarcinoma in Barrett's esophagus. *Am J Gastroenterol*. 2006;101:1421–1429.
20. Ranka S, Gee JM, Johnson IT, et al. Non-steroidal anti-inflammatory drugs, lower oesophageal sphincter-relaxing drugs and oesophageal cancer. A case-control study. *Digestion*. 2006;74:109–115.
21. Whiteman DC, Sadeghi S, Pandeya N, et al. Combined effects of obesity, acid reflux and smoking of the risk of adenocarcinomas of the oesophague. *Gut*. 2008;57:173–180.
22. Freedman ND, Abnet CC, Leitzmann MF, et al. A prospective study of tobacco, alcohol, and the risk of esophageal and gastric cancer subtypes. *Am J Epidemiol*. 2007;165:1424–1433.
23. Cockburn MG, Wu AH, Bernstein L. Etiologic clues from the similarity of histology-specific trends in esophageal and lung cancers. *Cancer Causes Control*. 2005;16:1065–1074.
24. De Stefani E, Boffetta P, Deneo-Pellegrini H, et al. The role of vegetable and fruit consumption in the aetiology of squamous cell carcinoma of the oesophagus: a case-control study in Uruguay. *Int J Cancer*. 2005;116:130–135.
25. Alcbari MR, Malekzadeh R, Nasrollahzadeh D, et al. Familial risks of esophageal cancer among the Turkmen population of the Caspian littoral of Iran. *Int J Cancer*. 2006;119:1047–1051.
26. Dal ML, La VC, Polesel J, et al. Alcohol drinking outside meals and cancers of the upper aero-digestive tract. *Int J Cancer*. 2002;102:435–437.
27. Ryan AM, Rowley SP, Fitzgerald AP, et al. Adenocarcinoma of the oesophagus and gastric cardia: male preponderance in association with obesity. *Eur J Cancer*. 2006;42:1151–1158.
28. Hung HC, Huang MC, Lee JM, et al. Association between diet and esophageal cancer in Taiwan. *J Gastroenterol Hepatol*. 2004;19:632–637.
29. Bosetti C, Gallus S, Trichopoulou A, et al. Influence of the Mediterranean diet on the risk of cancers of the upper aerodigestive tract. *Cancer Epidemiol Biomarkers Prev*. 2003;12:1091–1094.
30. De Stefani E, Deneo-Pellegrini H, Ronco AL, et al. Food groups and risk of squamous cell carcinoma of the oesophagus: a case-control study in Uruguay. *Br J Cancer*. 2003;89:1209–1214.
31. De Stefani E, Ronco AL, Boffetta P, et al. Nutrient intake and risk of squamous cell carcinoma of the esophagus: a case-control study in Uruguay. *Nutr Cancer*. 2006;56:149–157.
32. Bollschweiler E, Wolfgarten E, Nowroth T, et al. Vitamin intake and risk of subtypes of esophageal cancer in Germany. *J Cancer Res Clin Oncol*. 2002;128:575–580.
33. Franceschi S, Bidoli E, Negri E, et al. Role of macronutrients, vitamins and minerals in the aetiology of squamous-cell carcinoma of the oesophagus. *Int J Cancer*. 2000;86:626–631.
34. Rossi M, Garavello W, Talamini R, et al. Flavonoids and risk of squamous cell esophageal cancer. *Int J Cancer*. 2007;120:1560–1564.
35. Galeone C, Pelucchi C, Levi F, et al. Folate intake and squamous-cell carcinoma of the oesophagus in Italian and Swiss men. *Ann Oncol*. 2006;17:521–525.
36. Larsson SC, Giovannucci E, Wolk A. Folate intake, MTHFR polymorphisms, and risk of esophageal, gastric, and pancreatic cancer: a meta-analysis. *Gastroenterology*. 2006;131:1271–1283.
37. Lu H, Cai L, Mu LN, et al. Dietary mineral and trace element intake and squamous cell carcinoma of the esophagus in a Chinese population. *Nutr Cancer*. 2006;55:63–70.
38. Abnet CC, Lai B, Qiao YL, et al. Zinc concentration in esophageal biopsy specimens measured by x-ray fluorescence and esophageal cancer risk. *J Natl Cancer Inst*. 2005;97:301–306.
39. De Stefani E, Oreggia F, Boffetta P, et al. Tomatoes, tomato-rich foods, lycopene and cancer of the upper aerodigestive tract: a case-control in Uruguay. *Oral Oncol*. 2000;36:47–53.
40. Terry P, Lagergren J, Ye W, et al. Antioxidants and cancers of the esophagus and gastric cardia. *Int J Cancer*. 2000;87:750–754.
41. Wang JM, Xu B, Rao JY, et al. Diet habits, alcohol drinking, tobacco smoking, green tea drinking, and the risk of esophageal squamous cell carcinoma in the Chinese population. *Eur J Gastroenterol Hepatol*. 2007;19:171–176.
42. Merry AH, Schouten LJ, Goldbohm RA, et al. Body mass index, height and risk of adenocarcinoma of the oesophagus and gastric cardia: a prospective cohort study. *Gut*. 2007;56:1503–1511.
43. Kubo A, Corley DA. Body mass index and adenocarcinomas of the esophagus or gastric cardia: a systematic review and meta-analysis. *Cancer Epidemiol Biomarkers Prev*. 2006;15:872–878.
44. Brown LM, Devesa SS. Epidemiologic trends in esophageal and gastric cancer in the United States. *Surg Oncol Clin N Am*. 2002;11:235–256.
45. Kubo A, Corley DA. Meta-Analysis of Antioxidant Intake and the Risk of Esophageal and Gastric Cardia Adenocarcinoma. *Am J Gastroenterol*. 2007;102:2323–2330.
46. Gonzalez CA, Jakszyn P, Pera G, et al. Meat intake and risk of stomach and esophageal adenocarcinoma within the European Prospective Investigation Into Cancer and Nutrition (EPIC). *J Natl Cancer Inst*. 2006;98:345–354.
47. Sewram V, De SE, Brennan P, et al. Mate consumption and the risk of squamous cell esophageal cancer in Uruguay. *Cancer Epidemiol Biomarkers Prev*. 2003;12:508–513.
48. International Agency for Research on Cancer. *IARC Monographs on the Evaluation of Carcinogenic Risks to Humans. Coffee, Tea, Mate, Methylxanthines and Methylglyoxal* (Vol. 51). Lyon, France: World Health Organization, International Agency for Research on Cancer; 1991:273–287.
49. Kamangar F, Qiao YL, Blaser MJ, et al. Helicobacter pylori and oesophageal and gastric cancers in a prospective study in China. *Br J Cancer*. 2007;96:172–176.
50. Wu DC, Wu IC, Lee JM, et al. Helicobacter pylori infection: a protective factor for esophageal squamous cell carcinoma in a Taiwanese population. *Am J Gastroenterol*. 2005;100:588–593.
51. Ye W, Held M, Lagergren J, et al. *Helicobacter pylori* infection and gastric atrophy: risk of adenocarcinoma and squamous-cell carcinoma of the esophagus and adenocarcinoma of the gastric cardia. *J Natl Cancer Inst*. 2004;96:388–396.
52. McColl KE. *Helicobacter pylori* and oesophageal cancer—not always protective. *Gut*. 2007;56:457–459.

53. Lassen A, Hallas J, de Muckadell OB. Esophagitis: incidence and risk of esophageal adenocarcinoma—a population-based cohort study. *Am J Gastroenterol.* 2006;101:1193–1199.
54. Fortuny J, Johnson CC, Bohlke K, et al. Use of anti-inflammatory drugs and lower esophageal sphincter-relaxing drugs and risk of esophageal and gastric cancers. *Clin Gastroenterol Hepatol.* 2007;5:1154–1159.
55. de Martel C, Llosa AE, Farr SM, et al. Helicobacter pylori infection and the risk of development of esophageal adenocarcinoma. *J Infect Dis.* 2005;191:761–767.
56. Wu AH, Crabtree JE, Bernstein L, et al. Role of Helicobacter pylori CagA+ strains and risk of adenocarcinoma of the stomach and esophagus. *Int J Cancer.* 2003;103:815–821.
57. Henrik SJ, Forsgren A, Berglund G, et al. Helicobacter pylori infection is associated with a decreased risk of developing oesophageal neoplasms. *Helicobacter.* 2001;6:310–316.
58. Shuyama K, Castillo A, Aguayo F, et al. Human papillomavirus in high- and low-risk areas of oesophageal squamous cell carcinoma in China. *Br J Cancer.* 2007;96:1554–1559.
59. Far AE, Aghakhani A, Hamkar R, et al. Frequency of human papillomavirus infection in oesophageal squamous cell carcinoma in Iranian patients. *Scand J Infect Dis.* 2007;39:58–62.
60. Castillo A, Aguayo F, Koriyama C, et al. Human papillomavirus in esophageal squamous cell carcinoma in Colombia and Chile. *World J Gastroenterol.* 2006;12:6188–6192.
61. Yao PF, Li GC, Li J, et al. Evidence of human papilloma virus infection and its epidemiology in esophageal squamous cell carcinoma. *World J Gastroenterol.* 2006;12:1352–1355.
62. Qi ZL, Huo X, Xu XJ, et al. Relationship between HPV16/18 E6 and 53, 21WAF1, MDM2, Ki67 and cyclin D1 expression in esophageal squamous cell carcinoma: comparative study by using tissue microarray technology. *Exp Oncol.* 2006;28:235–240.
63. Matsha T, Erasmus R, Kafuko AB, et al. Human papillomavirus associated with oesophageal cancer. *J Clin Pathol.* 2002;55:587–590.
64. Syrjanen KJ. HPV infections and oesophageal cancer. *J Clin Pathol.* 2002; 55:721–728.
65. Chang F, Syrjanen S, Shen Q, et al. Human papillomavirus involvement in esophageal carcinogenesis in the high-incidence area of China. A study of 700 cases by screening and type-specific in situ hybridization. *Scand J Gastroenterol.* 2000;35:123–130.
66. Ilhan M, Erbaydar T, Akdeniz N, et al. Palmoplantar keratoderma is associated with esophagus squamous cell cancer in Van region of Turkey: a case control study. *BMC Cancer.* 2005;5:90.
67. Garavello W, Negri E, Talamini R, et al. Family history of cancer, its combination with smoking and drinking, and risk of squamous cell carcinoma of the esophagus. *Cancer Epidemiol Biomarkers Prev.* 2005;14:1390–1393.
68. Jayaprakash V, Menezes RJ, Javle MM, et al. Regular aspirin use and esophageal cancer risk. *Int J Cancer.* 2006;119:202–207.
69. Anderson LA, Johnston BT, Watson RG, et al. Nonsteroidal anti-inflammatory drugs and the esophageal inflammation-metaplasia-adenocarcinoma sequence. *Cancer Res.* 2006;66:4975–4982.
70. Lindblad M, Lagergren J, Garcia Rodriguez LA. Nonsteroidal anti-inflammatory drugs and risk of esophageal and gastric cancer. *Cancer Epidemiol Biomarkers Prev.* 2005;14:444–450.
71. Vaughan TL, Dong LM, Blount PL, et al. Non-steroidal anti-inflammatory drugs and risk of neoplastic progression in Barrett's oesophagus: a prospective study. *Lancet Oncol.* 2005;6:945–952.
72. Jansson C, Johansson AL, Nyren O, et al. Socioeconomic factors and risk of esophageal adenocarcinoma: a nationwide Swedish case-control study. *Cancer Epidemiol Biomarkers Prev.* 2005;14:1754–1761.
73. Brown LM, Chen BE, Pfeiffer RM, et al. Risk of second non-hematological malignancies among 376,825 breast cancer survivors. *Breast Cancer Res Treat.* 2007;106:439–451.
74. Mellemkjaer L, Friis S, Olsen JH, et al. Risk of second cancer among women with breast cancer. *Int J Cancer.* 2006;118:2285–2292.
75. Zablotska LB, Chak A, Das A, et al. Increased risk of squamous cell esophageal cancer after adjuvant radiation therapy for primary breast cancer. *Am J Epidemiol.* 2005;161:330–337.
76. Scholl B, Reis ED, Zouhair A, et al. Esophageal cancer as second primary tumor after breast cancer radiotherapy. *Am J Surg.* 2001;182:476–480.
77. Jansson C, Plato N, Johansson AL, et al. Airborne occupational exposures and risk of oesophageal and cardia adenocarcinoma. *Occup Environ Med.* 2006;63:107–112.
78. Cucino C, Sonnenberg A. Occupational mortality from squamous cell carcinoma of the esophagus in the United States during 1991–1996. *Dig Dis Sci.* 2002;47:568–572.
79. Kuzmickiene I, Didziapetris R, Stukonis M. Cancer incidence in the workers cohort of textile manufacturing factory in Alytus, Lithuania. *J Occup Environ Med.* 2004;46:147–153.
80. Parent ME, Siemiatycki J, Fritschi L. Workplace exposures and oesophageal cancer. *Occup Environ Med.* 2000;57:325–334.
81. Jansson C, Johansson AL, Bergdahl IA, et al. Occupational exposures and risk of esophageal and gastric cardia cancers among male Swedish construction workers. *Cancer Causes Control.* 2005;16:755–764.
82. Engel LS, Vaughan TL, Gammon MD, et al. Occupation and risk of esophageal and gastric cardia adenocarcinoma. *Am J Ind Med.* 2002;42:11–22.
83. Vigen C, Bernstein L, Wu AH. Occupational physical activity and risk of adenocarcinomas of the esophagus and stomach. *Int J Cancer.* 2006;118:1004–1009.

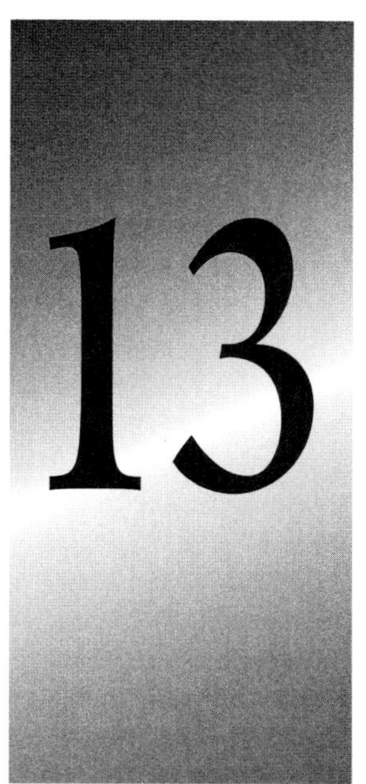

Pathology of Barrett's Esophagus and Esophageal Neoplasms

Gregorio Chejfec
Elizabeth Louise Wiley
Stephen Sontag

HISTOLOGIC ASPECTS AND DEFINITIONS

The presence of islands of columnar epithelium amidst the esophageal squamous mucosa was described by investigators in early publications. It was Norman R. Barrett, however, who investigated in depth the esophageal mucosa in hundreds of specimens, finally concluding that foci of columnar epithelium could regularly be found in the esophagus in 3 circumstances: (a) in hiatal hernia, (b) as true ectopic mucosa, and (c) as an extension of the esophagogastric junction. In his last paper, presented at the Mayo Clinic in 1957, he speculated that these islands represented a failure of the embryonic lining of the esophagus to achieve maturity (congenital origin). In his last remark, however, he emphasized that chronic gastroesophageal reflux could also pay a role (1). Subsequent publications described 3 types of epithelia in these islands: (a) fundic glands, (b) cardiac-type glands, and (c) "specialized" (intestinal) epithelium (2). Currently only the presence of specialized epithelium, namely goblet cells, is considered essential to diagnose Barrett's esophagus (3). The types of intestinal metaplasia present in Barrett's esophagus are either type II, where the glands are a mixture of gastric foveolar type and goblet cells, or type III, consisting only of goblet cells (Figure 13.1). Both types are considered incomplete intestinal metaplasia. Rarely, type I complete intestinal metaplasia, containing Paneth and absorptive cells, is present in Barrett's esophagus. The mucin present in goblet cells is Alcian blue (pH 2.5) positive and consists of sialomucins and sulfomucins, with the former predominating (Figures 13.2 and 13.3).

Alcian blue positivity has been observed in columnar cells lacking goblet cell morphology, leading some investigators to diagnose Barrett's esophagus (4), but currently is not considered as Barrett's epithelium.

Islands of columnar epithelium containing fundic or intestinal glands are found occasionally in the cervical esophagus ("inlet patches"); these are not considered Barrett's esophagus, although adenocarcinomas may arise in them.

Fundic or cardiac type glands are considered to be part of the normal esophageal mucosa in the distal 3 cm of esophagus, within the lower esophageal sphincter (LES) area. This area lies immediately above the squamocolumnar junction (Z line—SQC), which does not necessarily coincide with the gastroesophageal junction (GEJ) or muscular GEJ (5). If fundic epithelium is found proximal to 3 cm above the SCJ, it most likely represents a hiatal hernia. In general, however, columnar epithelium present above 3 cm from the SCJ usually contains metaplastic intestinal epithelium, although it may be mixed with cardiac-type epithelium.

The prevalence of Barrett's esophagus has been estimated to be 10% of the patients with gastroesophageal

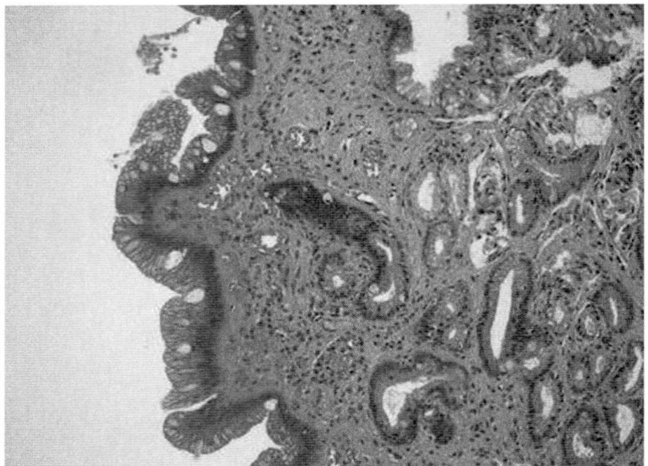

FIGURE 13.1

Low-power view of columnar lined esophageal mucosa with "specialized" (intestinal) epithelium.

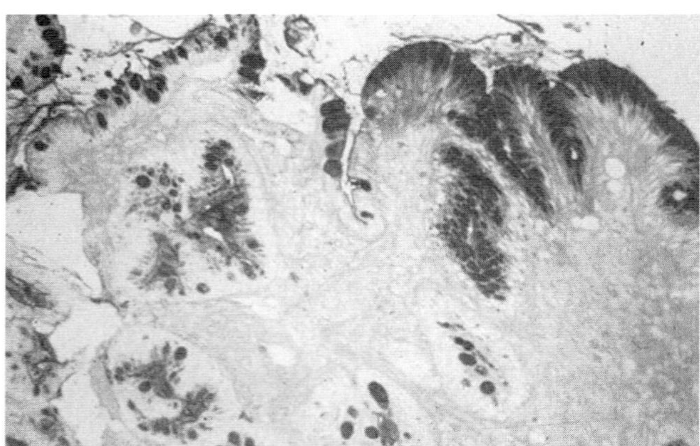

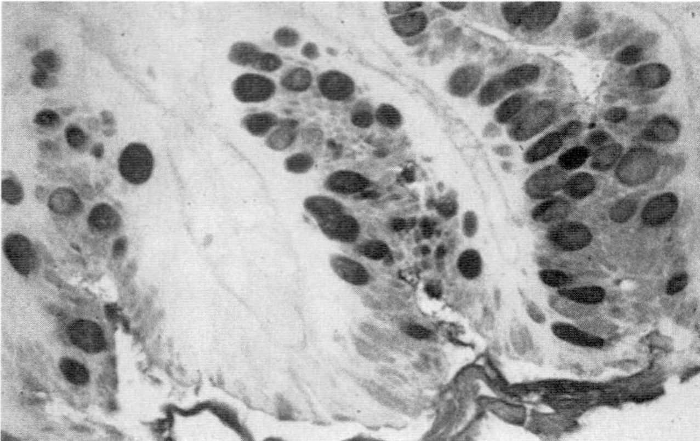

FIGURE 13.2

Lower-power view of gastric and intestinal type epithelia at squamocolumnar junction (PAS-Alcian blue x 100).

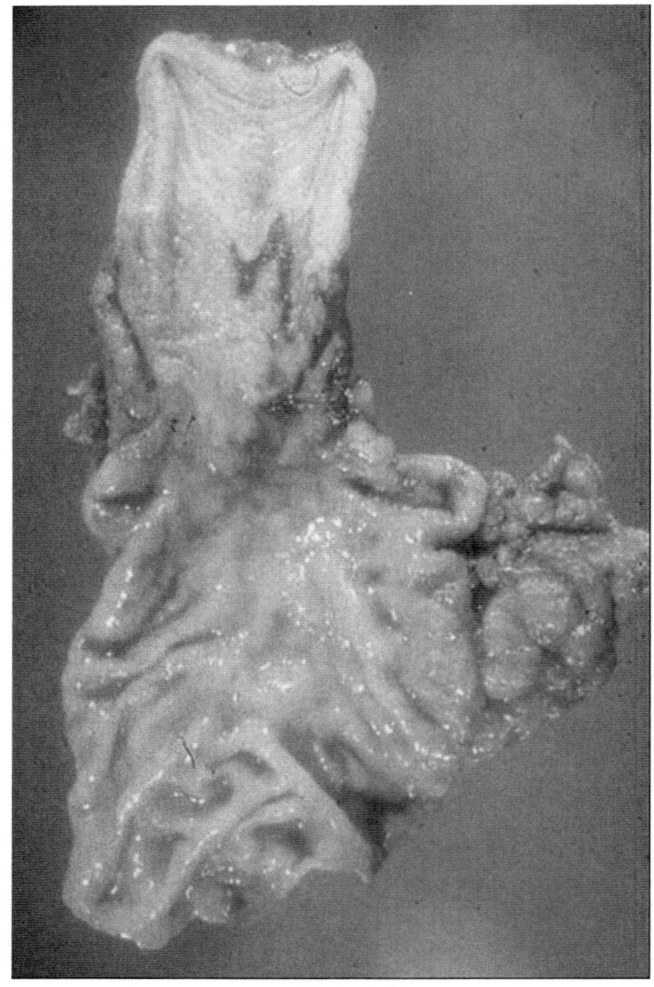

FIGURE 13.3

High-power view of goblet cells containing sulfomucins (high iron diamine stain x 400).

reflux referred for endoscopy (6). The true frequency may be much higher, up to 20% (7).

Currently the diagnosis of Barrett's esophagus requires that a clear endoscopic finding of red, velvety appearing mucosa accompanies the histologic finding of goblet cells, according to the American College of Gastroenterology (8) (Figure 13.4).

Barrett's esophagus is a disorder found mainly in white middle-aged males with chronic gastroesophageal reflux disease (GERD); it is extremely infrequent in African Americans, where it was reported with a prevalence of 3.5% (9). It also occurs in children, also as a result of GERD, although its frequency in this population is unknown (10). The mechanisms leading to GERD include the presence of hiatal hernia, lower esophageal sphincter (LED) dysfunction, gastric hypersecretion, and duodenal gastric reflux (11).

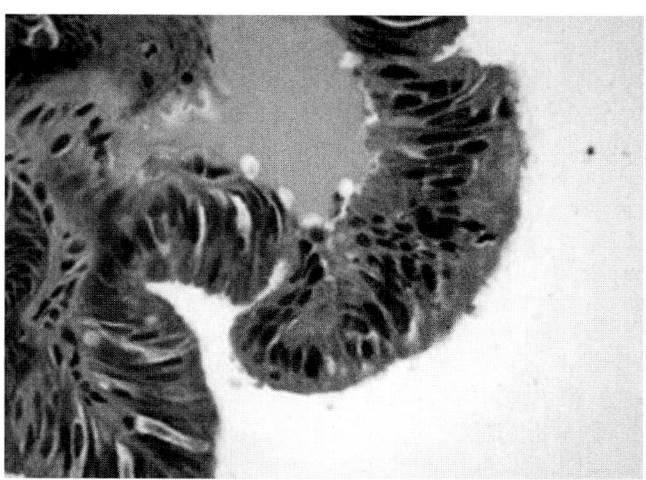

FIGURE 13.4

Partial esophagogastrectomy showing the replacement of squamous mucosa by glandular type in the lower esophagus.

Dysplasias

Barrett's esophagus is a preneoplastic disorder, thus a marker for the development of esophageal adenocarcinoma (12). The progression of columnar epithelium to malignancy is the result of sequential events from metaplasia to dysplasia to adenocarcinoma.

The term *dysplasia* was coined by Ober in 1949, cited by Papanicolau, to describe the neoplastic transformation of the uterine cervix squamous mucosa confined to the epithelium. The same year, Warren and Sommers used the term to describe similar changes occurring in the colon in long-standing ulcerative colitis.

In 1967, Morson reported the use of rectal biopsy to control cancer in ulcerative colitis. Subsequently, a group of gastrointestinal pathologists, members of the "Committee on Dysplasia," established a classification of dysplasia in inflammatory bowel disease (13). The classification established 3 categories: negative for dysplasia, indefinite for dysplasia, and positive for dysplasia. Positive cases were subclassified as low- or high-grade dysplasia.

This classification has been similarly used in Barrett's esophagus. The microscopic features that are important in the diagnosis of dysplasia are: (a) alterations in glandular architecture, (b) cytologic changes, (c) surface maturation, and (d) inflammation with erosions or ulcers. Surface maturation refers to the decrease in size of the nuclei reaching the surface and the presence of regularly interspersed goblet cells, replicating normal colonic epithelium.

CLASSIFICATION

Negative for dysplasia: The glandular architecture and cellular morphology are normal, but the basal portion of the glands shows regenerative (reactive) activity. There is nuclear enlargement, pleomorphism, hyperchromasia and stratification. The surface, however, displays smaller nuclei (mature) with smooth contours, less intensity of staining, and absence of stratification.

Indefinite for dysplasia: Glandular architecture and cytologic changes are either intact or may be slightly abnormal. Changes are more pronounced when there are marked inflammatory changes, erosions or ulcerations, and frequent mitoses. In indefinite without inflammation, there are similar features without active mitotic rate. The classification is also used when there is no visible intact surface to evaluate.

Low-grade dysplasia: Crypt architecture is usually preserved, or it may show slight distortion. The nuclei are enlarged, hyperchromatic, pleomorphic, and crowded. Abnormal mitoses may be present. Goblet cells are decreased. The stratification of nuclei does not reach the apical surface of the cells. The abnormalities are present in the basal portion of the glands and extend to the surface (Figure 13.5).

High-grade dysplasia: There is marked architectural distortion of glands, with branching and lateral budding. The nuclear changes are similar to those in low-grade, but in high-grade, the nuclear stratification is more pronounced on the surface and there is loss of nuclear polarity. The surface may have a villiform appearance. When intraglandular bridging occurs ("cribriform pattern"), it indicates an intramucosal carcinoma. The goblet cell population is markedly depleted, if not

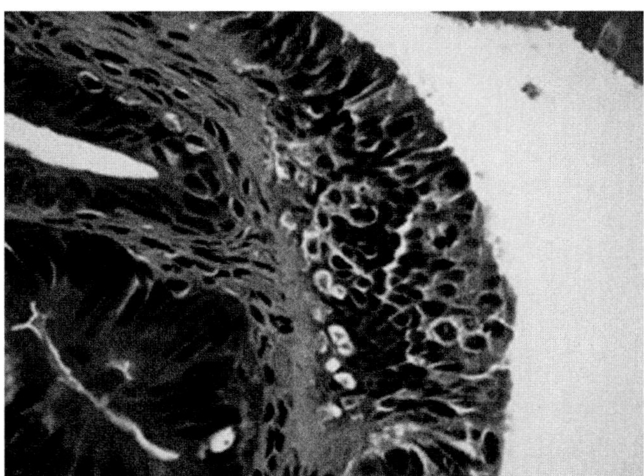

FIGURE 13.5

High-power view of low-grade dysplasia (H&E x 400).

absent. Some of the goblet cells may be dystrophic, where the mucus droplet is not in contact with the luminal surface (Figure 13.6) (see Table 13.1).

INTERPRETATION OF DYSPLASIA

The dysplastic changes observed in Barrett's esophagus are not exactly of a single type that would permit clear-cut separation of the different types. It usually displays features encompassing the entire spectrum of abnormalities. Thus a great deal of subjectivity is involved in arriving at a diagnosis (14). In an effort to overcome discrepancies in interpretation of biopsies, a group of gastrointestinal pathologists examined a number of biopsy specimens; they concluded that there was a high degree of intra- and interobserver variability in low-grade dysplasia. On the other hand, there was nearly 80% agreement in high-grade dysplasia (15). The study revealed a blurring in the boundaries between grades, particularly between indefinite and low-grade dysplasia. As a consequence many pathologists currently combine those 2 stages into a 1.

Recently, another study confirmed the much higher agreement among pathologists in the diagnosis of high-grade dysplasia and intramucosal carcinoma (16).

Another problem in establishing the diagnosis of dysplasia is related to sampling. Since dysplasia is not endoscopically apparent, sampling must take this fact into consideration. Most protocols recommend 4 quadrant biopsies at intervals of 2 cm or less throughout the endoscopically visible Barrett's mucosa.

Although complications arising from using jumbo forceps are not greater than smaller ones, many endoscopists are reluctant to use the jumbo size. It is controversial whether there is a discrepancy in the diagnostic yield of both approaches.

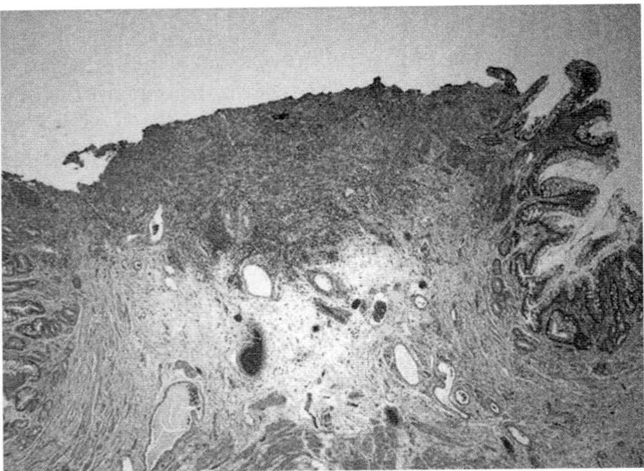

FIGURE 13.6

High-power view of high-grade dysplasia) (H&E x 400).

TABLE 13.1
Morphologic Characteristics of Dysplasia

	Indefinite for dysplasia	Low-grade dysplasia	High-grade dysplasia
Glandular distortion	– Absent	+ Mild distortion	++ / +++ Branching and lateral budding—may have cribriform areas
Nuclear enlargement	– / +	+ / ++	++ / +++
Nuclear hyperchromasia	– / +	– / +	++ / +++
Nuclear crowding / stratification	– / +	++	++ / +++
Loss of nuclear polarity	– / +	– / +	++ / +++
Surface maturation	++	– / +	–
Goblet cells	++ / +++	– / +	–
Inflammation	+ / +++	+	–
Mitotic activity	+	+ / ++ Abnormal mitoses may be present	+++ Up to luminal surface Abnormal mitoses

A final consideration is the orientation of the specimen in order to examine luminal surface, which is critical for the diagnosis. Best results are obtained by orienting the specimen in the endoscopy suite, rather than in the histology laboratories at the time of embedding into paraffin block (17).

FOLLOW-UP OF BARRETT'S ESOPHAGUS

The recommendations from the American College of Gastroenterology are as follows (8):

Low-grade: repeat yearly until no dysplasia.
High-grade: repeat every 3 months; sample adequately to exclude cancer.

Confirmation of HGD by another pathologist with expertise in gastrointestinal pathology is highly recommended.

Ancillary Techniques for Barrett's Dysplasia

A number of techniques have been proposed to supplement the microscopic impression. None of them, however, have been proven to be superior to the histologic examination. Among them flow cytometry seems to be most promising. Several consecutive studies showed prevalence of DNA aneuploidy and elevated S fraction, which correlated with histologic severity (18). Another study of 62 patients correlated histology and flow cytometry; 9 of 13 patients with aneuploidy eventually developed high-grade dysplasia or carcinoma in a follow-up of 34 months. None of the 42 patients without aneuploidy progressed to HGD or carcinoma (16). In contrast, another study found no definite correlation between HGD and flow cytometric abnormalities (19).

Other screening techniques include the analysis of goblet cell mucus by histochemistry to demonstrate sulfomucins (20); immunohistochemistry to detect p53 overexpression (21) and c-erb B2, H-ras, C-myc, TGF alpha, EGF (22,23).

None of these techniques, however, have been found to be of clinical utility.

ADENOCARCINOMA

Invasion through the basement membrane into the lamina propria is difficult to diagnose in its early phase. There may be effacement of the stroma and a syncitial growth pattern in small clusters; occasionally single cells can be identified. Later on, desmoplasia develops, especially when the muscularis mucosa is penetrated and the tumor cells reach the submucosa (Figure 13.7).

Invasive adenocarcinoma of the esophagus was reported to develop in 50%–60% of patients within 3–5 years of a diagnosis of high-grade dysplasia; overall, 10% of all patients with Barrett's esophagus developed adenocarcinoma. This number, however, is questionable since it includes both prevalent and incident adenocarcinomas. The real risk for patients with Barrett's esophagus to develop cancer is most likely 2.5%–3%. The risk factors for development of cancer are the same as in Barrett's esophagus: middle-aged white males. Smoking and alcohol consumption are not significant factors; obesity may play a role.

The most common location of tumors is in the distal third of the esophagus. Grossly they appear as firm, white masses; the adjacent Barrett's mucosa is salmon color with velvety appearance (Figure 13.8). Microscopically

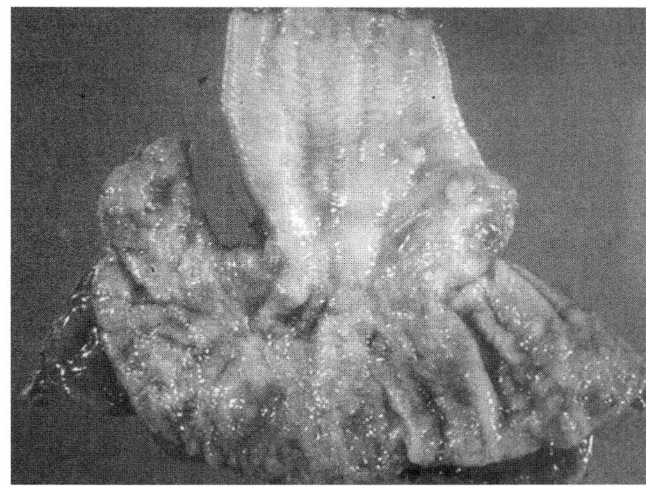

FIGURE 13.7

Low-power view of adenocarcinoma in mucosa and submucosa (H&E x 100).

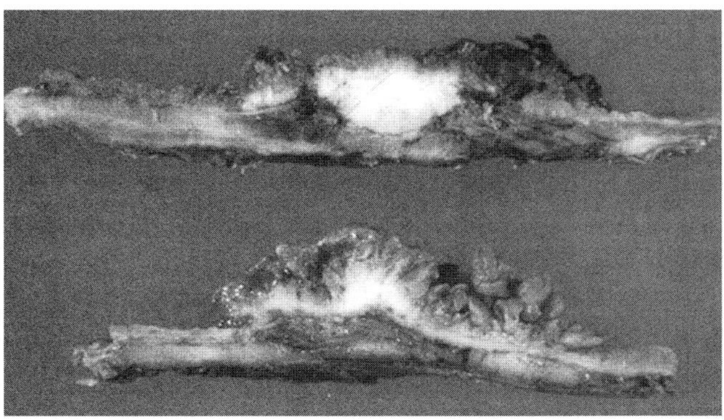

FIGURE 13.8

Polypoid adenocarcinoma at gastroesophageal junction.

they may have a papillary or tubular growth. Neuroendocrine or Paneth cells are present in some tumors. The majority of adenocarcinomas are either moderate or well differentiated. A linitis plastica-like growth pattern was reported (24). Small subsets of adenosquamous, adenoid cystic, mucoepidermoid, and spindle cell types have also been reported.

Esophagectomy is the treatment of choice, preceded by neoadjuvant chemotherapy and radiotherapy. The prognosis is poor in stages T2 and beyond. Tumors in stage T1 have a good prognosis (see below).

MANAGEMENT OF DYSPLASIAS AND CARCINOMAS

Our Experience

During the past 25 years, we have diagnosed and followed a cohort of 1,556 patients with Barrett's esophagus through an organized surveillance program at Hines Veterans Affairs Hospital, Hines, Illinois. Of the 1,156 patients, 483 had Barrett's metaplasia, 976 had indefinite/low-grade dysplasia, and 97 had high-grade dysplasia. The protocol was in accordance with the standards of the American College of Gastroenterology (see above section on the follow-up of Barrett's esophagus) (8). Of the 97 with high-grade dysplasia, 34 were prevalent (diagnosed at first endoscopy or within 1 year after first endoscopy) and 46 were incident (developed after 1 year of first endoscopy). There were a total of 22 adenocarcinomas; 5 were prevalent and 17 were incident adenocarcinomas. Of the 17 incident adenocarcinomas, 9 were cured by surgery or ablation therapy. Seven patients died of non-Barrett's related causes and 1 died of adenocarcinoma of the esophagus with metastases. This last patient moved out of state after the diagnosis was made and was lost to follow-up for 10 years, when he returned with generalized metastases. Of the other 80 cases of high-grade dysplasia, 52 are alive and continue their follow-up. Twenty-eight patients with high-grade dysplasia died of non Barrett's-related causes.

In conclusion, the incidence of carcinoma developing in this cohort was 12%, with a prevalence of 3.7%. A smaller number of patients with similar findings was reported in 2001 (25). We conclude that the majority of patients with Barrett's esophagus follow a benign course; furthermore, adenocarcinomas arising in Barrett's esophagus in a surveillance program can be cured by surgery or ablation procedures.

References

1. Barrett NR. The lower esophagus lined by columnar epithelium. *Surgery*. 1957;41:881–894.
2. Paull A, Trier JS, Dalton MD, et al. The histologic spectrum of Barrett's esophagus. *N Engl J Med*. 1976; 295:476–480.
3. Chejfec G. Atypias, dysplasias, and neoplasias of the esophagus and stomach. *Semin Diagn Pathol*. 1985;2:31–41.
4. McArdle JE, Levin KJ, Randall G. Distribution of dysplasia and early invasive carcinoma in Barrett's esophagus. *Hum Pathol*. 1992;23:479–482.
5. Weinstein W, Van Deventer G, et al. A histologic evaluation of Barrett's esophagus using a standardized endoscopic biopsy protocol [abstract]. *Gastroenterol*. 1984;86:1296.
6. Winters C, Spurling TJ, Chobanian SJ, et al. Barrett's esophagus. A prevalent occult complication of gastroesophageal reflux disease. *Gastroenterol*. 1987;92:118–124.
7. Cameron AJ, Zansmeister AR, Ballard DJ, et al. Prevalence of columnar-lined (Barrett's) esophagus. *Gastroenterol*. 1992;98:654–661.
8. Sampliner RE. Practice Parameters Committee of the American College of Gastroenterology Updated Guidelines for the diagnosis, surveillance and therapy of Barrett's Esophagus. *Am J Gastroenterol*. 2002;97:1888–1895.
9. Montgomery EA. Barrett's esophagus and esophageal neoplasia. In: *Biopsy Interpretation of the Gastrointestinal Tract Mucosa*. Philadelphia: Lippincott, Williams & Wilkins; 2006: 37–70.
10. Hassal E. Barrett's esophagus: new definitions and approaches in children. *J Pediatr Gastroenterol*. 1993;15:345–364.
11. Der R, Tsao-Wei DD, DeMeéster T, et al. Carditis: a manifestation of gastroesophageal reflux disease. *Am J Surg Pathol*. 2001;25:245–252.
12. Chejfec G, Schnell T, Sontag S. Barrett's Esophagus: a preneoplastic disorder [editorial]. *Am J Clin Path*. 1992;98:5–7.
13. Riddell RH, Goldman H, Ransohoff DF, et al. Dysplasia in inflammatory bowel disease: standardized classification with provisional clinical implications. *Hum Pathol*. 1983;14:931–968.
14. Reid BJ, Haggett RC, Rubin CE, et al. Observer variation in the diagnosis of dysplasia in Barrett's esophagus. *Hum Pathol*. 1988;19:166–178.
15. Montgomery E, Bronner MP, Goldblum JR, et al. Reproducibility of the diagnosis of dysplasia in Barrett's esophagus: a reaffirmation. *Hum Pathol*. 2001;32:368–378.
16. Reid BJ, Levine DS, Longton G, et al. Predictors of progression to cancer in Barrett's esophagus: baseline histology and flow cytometry identify low and high risk patient subsets. *Am J Gastroenterol*. 2000;95:1669–1676.
17. Haggett RC. Barrett's esophagus, dysplasia and adenocarcinoma. *Hum Pathol*. 1994;25:982–993.
18. Reid BJ, Haggett RC, Rubin CE, et al. Flow cytometry complements histology in detecting patients at risk for Barrett's adenocarcinoma. *Gastroenterol*. 1987;93:1–11.
19. Fennerty MB, Sampliner RE, Way D. Discordance between flow cytometric abnormalities and dysplasia in Barrett's esophagus. *Gastroenterol*. 1989;97:815–820.
20. Haggett RC, Reid BJ, Rubin CE, et al. Barrett's esophagus: correlation between mucin histochemistry, flow cytometry and histologic diagnosis for predicting increased cancer risk. *Am J Pathol*. 1988;131:53–61.
21. Younes M, Lebovitz RM, Lechago LV. P53 protein accumulation in Barrett's metaplasia, dysplasia and carcinoma. A follow up study. *Gastroenterol*. 1993;105:1637–1642.
22. Abelatef OMA, Chandler FW, Mills LR, et al. Differential expression of C-myc and H-RAS oncogenes in Barrett's epithelium. *Arch Pathol Lab Med*, 1991;115:880–885.
23. Jankowski J, Hopwood D, Wormsely KG. Flow cytometric analysis of growth-regulatory peptides and their receptors in Barrett's esophagus and adenocarcinoma. *Scand J Gastroenterol*. 1992;27:147–154.
24. Chejfec G, Jablokow V, Gould V. Linitis plastica carcinoma of the esophagus. *Cancer*. 1983;51:2139–2143.
25. Schnell T, Sontag S, Chejfec G, et al. Long term nonsurgical management of Barrett's esophagus with high-grade dysplasia. *Gastroenterol*. 2001;120:1607–1619.

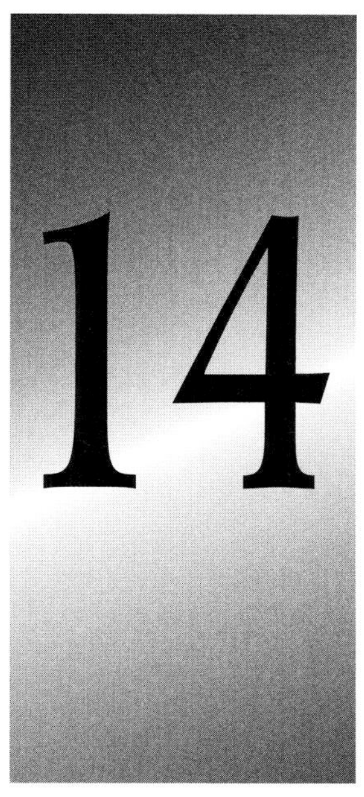

The Link Between Esophageal Cancer and Morbid Obesity

Robert W. O'Rourke

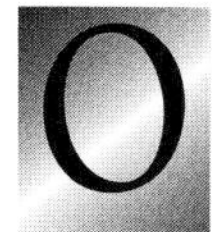

Obesity is a worldwide epidemic with significant impact on public health. Obesity is defined as a body mass index (BMI; weight [kg]/height [m]^2) greater than 30, while the term *morbid obesity* is generally applied to patients who meet NIH consensus criteria for surgical therapy, which include BMI> = 40, or BMI> = 35 with a serious comorbidity of obesity (NIH conference 1991). Increased adipose tissue mass is the sine qua non of obesity and has detrimental effects on virtually all physiologic systems. Obesity is therefore an important risk factor for multiple comorbid disease processes. Cancer ranks among these, as a large body of literature demonstrates that obesity has important effects on anti-tumor immunity and is associated with an increased risk of most cancers (1–3). Animal models of caloric restriction are associated with reduced incidences of cancer (4), further supporting a link between mechanisms that regulate carcinogenesis and weight. Appropriate preventive and interventional management of cancer of all types must therefore include consideration of body weight. Obesity is associated with an increased risk of esophageal adenocarcinoma and its predecessors, gastroesophageal reflux disease (GERD) and Barrett's esophagus, and is therefore an important factor to consider in the evaluation of the patient with or at risk for esophageal cancer.

OBESITY AND ESOPHAGEAL CANCER

Due to its low incidence, population-based studies and meta-analyses have become important tools for the study of associations between esophageal cancer and putative risk factors such as obesity. As a whole, this literature demonstrates a strong association between obesity and esophageal adenocarcinoma with a dose-dependent effect of increasing BMI on odds ratios for developing disease, which range from 2 to 8 at the extremes of BMI (Table 14.1). Some studies distinguish between tumors of the distal esophageal and gastric cardia, and taken together, these data suggest that while obesity is also a risk factor for adenocarcinoma of the cardia, associated odds ratios are generally lower than for adenocarcinoma of the distal esophagus, suggesting different mechanisms of disease pathogenesis. The prevalences of obesity and esophageal adenocarcinoma have increased in parallel over the past 3 decades, but a causal relationship between obesity and esophageal adenocarcinoma remains unproven. Other potential mitigating factors have also increased in prevalence over the same time period, most notably the use of effective antacid therapy and an increasingly high-fat, low-fiber diet. The precise mechanisms underlying the relationship between obesity and esophageal adenocarcinoma remain unknown and are the focus of the following discussion, but these

TABLE 14.1
Obesity and Esophageal Adenocarcinoma

Author	Location	Study design	OR for esophageal cancer	OR for cardia cancer	n (cancer or case subject or total population studied)
Brown et al. 1995	U.S.	National population-based case-control cancer registry interview	3.1	N/A	174
Vaughan et al. 1995	U.S.	Population-based Washington state SEER cancer registry database	1.6–2.5	0.8–1.6	298
Lagergren et al. 1999	Sweden	National population-based case-control	2.2–7.6	0.9–2.3	189
Veugelers et al. 2003	Canada	Case control, single center	4.7	N/A	57
Engel et al. 2003	U.S.	State-based (NJ, CT, WA) population-based case-control	5.4–21.3	0.9–12.9	293
Kubo et al. 2006	N/A	Meta-analysis	2.2	1.5	2,488
Ryan et al. 2006	Ireland	Case control, single center	4.3–11.3	3.5	760
Hampel et al. 2007	N/A	Meta-analysis	1.5–2.8	N/A	N/A

Odds ratios are a range from lowest to highest risk, and methods of calculation vary depending on stratification method (e.g., quartiles, deciles, etc.), referent group (lean vs. less obese), and adjusted confounders. Subject number (n) is reported as number of cases or total population depending on study design.

associations are certainly multifactorial, and variables in addition to obesity clearly play a role in the development of esophageal cancer.

In contrast to the strong association between obesity and esophageal adenocarcinoma, most studies demonstrate either no such association (5,6) or in some cases, an inverse correlation (7) between adiposity and squamous cell carcinoma of the esophagus. Indirect support for a lack of a causal association between these entities is provided by the observation that worldwide, the incidence of squamous cell carcinoma of the esophagus is stable or decreasing (8,9), despite the dramatic rise in the prevalence of obesity. Consistent with these observations, squamous cell carcinoma of the esophagus may be more strongly associated with tobacco use, which is also decreasing in prevalence (10). Also of interest but of unknown significance, histologic prevalence trends between adenocarcinoma and squamous cell carcinoma of the lung over the last few decades are similar to those associated with esophageal cancer. It is postulated that similar as yet unknown epidemiologic trends may underlie these phenomena (9). This chapter will discuss the putative mechanisms underlying the association between obesity and esophageal cancer.

GASTROESOPHAGEAL REFLUX DISEASE

Obesity is a risk factor for gastroesophageal reflux disease (GERD), which is in turn a primary risk factor for esophageal adenocarcinoma. The association between obesity and esophageal cancer may be related to GERD. It is important to understand the complexities of the relationship between GERD and esophageal adenocarcinoma in order to fully appreciate the role of obesity in these disease processes. A detailed discussion of the relationship between GERD, Barrett's esophagus, and esophageal adenocarcinoma is beyond the scope of this chapter and is addressed elsewhere in this book. In brief, strong epidemiologic evidence identifies GERD as a principal risk factor for the development of esophageal adenocarcinoma and Barrett's esophagus as an intermediate premalignant precursor (11). Despite this evidence, a direct casual link between GERD and esophageal cancer, while strongly suspected, has not been definitively established. Proving such an intuitive and biologically plausible association has been difficult for a number of reasons, including the low overall prevalence of esophageal adenocarcinoma, the inaccuracies of symptomatic assessment and paucity of objective diagnostic testing for GERD in large population-based studies, and the increasing variety of currently available testing methods that define GERD. In addition, GERD is a diverse disease that encompasses both acid and non-acid reflux, degrees of severity, and periods of remission and exacerbation. Not surprisingly, conflicting epidemiologic trends suggest a complex and multifactorial relationship between GERD and esophageal adenocarcinoma. For example, while adenocarcinoma of the esophagus has a strong male and Caucasian predominance, only weak gender and ethnicity predispositions exist for GERD (12–14). In addition, the increased prevalence of both GERD and esophageal adenocarcinoma appear to have begun simultaneously, a finding inconsistent with the long latency period between initiation and development of cancer. Despite these inconsistencies, however, a preponderance of data support the hypothesis that GERD is indeed an important risk factor for esophageal adenocarcinoma. Three large population-based case-control studies demonstrate severity and duration of GERD to be associated with increasing risk of esophageal adenocarcinoma in a dose-dependent fashion (6,15,16).

The relationship between obesity and GERD is similarly complex. Despite conflicting data (17,18) and a long history of debate, the majority of literature (19–23), including large recent studies (24,25) and a comprehensive meta-analysis (26), confirm that obesity is an independent risk factor for GERD and that increasing BMI has a dose-dependent effect on the likelihood and severity of symptomatic GERD (Table 14.2). Obesity also appears to be associated with an increased risk of erosive esophagitis and Barrett's esophagus (27,28), although these relationships have been more difficult to establish given their relatively lower prevalence and requirement for endoscopic diagnosis. Most of the literature addressing the relationship between GERD and obesity study BMI. Of interest, at least 2 studies identify waist circumference, often used as a surrogate for visceral adiposity, as a risk factor for Barrett's esophagus independent of BMI (29). These data not only underscore the weakness of relying on a single measure of obesity, in this case BMI, as a determinant of risk but also suggest the possibility that visceral adiposity may be a more specific predictor of obesity-related esophageal disease when compared to subcutaneous adiposity. Indeed, the mechanic effects of increased visceral adipose tissue mass on the anti-reflux mechanism are commonly proposed

TABLE 14.2
Obesity and GERD

Author	Location	Study design	OR for GERD	n (obese or case subjects, or total population studied)
Locke et al. 1999	Minnesota, U.S.	Cross-sectional state-based survey	2.8	1,524
Ruhl et al. 1999	U.S.	National population-based case-control	1.2 per 5 BMI points	12,349
Lagergren et al. 2000	Sweden	National population-based case-control	0.99–1.03 (not significant)	820
Nilsson et al. 2003	Sweden	National population-based case-control	3.3–6.3	3,113
El-Serag et al. 2005	VA employees, Texas, U.S.	Cross-sectional survey	2.5	453
Jacobson et al. 2006	U.S.	National population-based case-control	2.2–2.9	10,545
Hampel et al. 2007	N/A	Meta-analysis	1.4–1.9	N/A

Odds ratios are a range from lowest to highest risk, and methods of calculation vary depending on stratification method (e.g., quartiles, deciles, etc.), referent group (lean vs. less obese), and adjusted confounders. Subject number (n) is reported as number of cases or total population depending on study design.

as a mechanism underlying the association between obesity and GERD. Detailed manometric study of obese humans demonstrates increased intragastric pressures and gastroesophageal pressure gradients with increasing BMI (30), suggestive of greater mechanical stress on the lower esophageal sphincter (LES) and the anti-reflux mechanism as a whole. Nonetheless, obese humans demonstrate a wide range of functional disorders of the esophageal body and LES. Elevated LES pressure is among the most common abnormalities of LES function in obese humans (31), but a subset of obese patients demonstrates decreased LES pressure (32). Obesity also appears to be a risk factor for disorders of esophageal body motility that may contribute to GERD. These include nutcracker esophagus, diffuse esophageal spasm, and non-specific esophageal motility disorders, which are present at a higher prevalence in obese subjects (21,33,34). Finally, the importance of hiatal hernia in obesity-related GERD is emphasized by data that show that the risk of GERD in obese subjects is increased only in those with hiatal hernia (35). It is currently unknown whether elevated LES pressure and subtle disorders of esophageal body motility represent an early compensatory response to mechanical stress on the antireflux mechanism from increased intra-abdominal pressure that precede subsequent LES failure and more marked disorders of esophageal body function, but such a theory is plausible. At the least, these findings suggest a spectrum of effects of obesity on LES and esophageal body function.

Despite these observations, the effects of obesity on intra-abdominal and intragastric pressures are relatively modest (19), and other mechanisms likely also underlie the association between esophageal adenocarcinoma and obesity. Visceral adipose tissue manifests differences in metabolism and inflammation compared to subcutaneous adipose tissue and may influence GERD and esophageal cancer through related systemic effects on LES and esophageal function independent of mechanical effects (29). Epidemiologic evidence suggests that other factors in addition to GERD play a role in the development of esophageal cancer in the obese. Obesity is a relatively weak risk factor for GERD, with an odds ratio of approximately 1.5, in contrast to its much stronger effect on the development of esophageal adenocarcinoma, with odds ratios ranging from 2 to 9 (26). Furthermore, obesity is a risk factor for esophageal cancer independent of GERD (6,16). These observations suggest that mechanisms in addition to GERD play a role in the evolution of esophageal cancer in the obese patient.

DIET

Dietary habits associated with obesity may also contribute to the pathogenesis of esophageal cancer. Obesity is generally associated with a high calorie diet. Accurate measures of dietary constituents in the general population are notoriously difficult and prone to significant recall bias, but in general, obesity is associated with a diet that consists of a higher than average percentages of calories from fats and simple sugars, and a lower than average intake of complex carbohydrates and dietary fiber (36,37). Obesity is associated with and increased prevalence of specific micronutrient deficiencies as well, including vitamin D (38–40), folate, B6 (41), B12 (42), and selenium (43). The mechanisms underlying these deficiencies in obesity are not completely understood. Certainly, dietary habits likely contribute, but increased adipose tissue mass and its physiologic sequelae may also contribute to perpetuating specific deficiencies, and data from animal models suggest that specific micronutrients may reciprocally affect the degree and distribution of adiposity (44). The significance of these observations in humans remains unknown.

Dietary macro- and micronutrient intake patterns associated with obesity have been linked to many types of cancer, including esophageal. Two large population-based case-control studies, one from the United States (45) and another from Sweden (46), studied the effects of dietary constituents on esophageal and cardia cancers. Increased dietary fiber intake was associated with a decreased risk of adenoncarcinoma of both the distal esophagus and gastric cardia in both studies, while decreased fiber intake was associated with an increased risk of squamous cell carcinoma of the esophagus only in the U.S. study (45,47). The United States–based study also identified high dietary cholesterol, animal protein, and vitamin B12 as risk factors for adenocarcinoma the esophagus and cardia as well as squamous cell carcinoma of the esophagus, while plant-based diets were associated with lower risk of these cancers (45). With respect to micronutrients, increased intake of vitamins C, E, B6, folate, and β-carotene were associated with lower rates of both adenocarcinoma and squamous cell carcinoma of the distal esophagus, but not cardia cancer (45,48). Others have independently identified associations between esophageal cancer and these and other micronutrients, including iron, zinc, niacin, selenium, and vitamin A, all of which impart a protective effect that appears to be stronger for esophageal adenocarcinoma than squamous cell carcinoma (49–52). Finally, a prospective study of micronutrient supplementation in over 29,000 adults performed in Linxian China over a 5-year period demonstrated reduced rates of esophageal and gastric cancer in patients receiving supplemental β-carotene, vitamin E, and selenium (53). The variability in associations between specific nutrients and specific cancers among these trials speaks to the broad heterogeneity of the patient populations studied, as well as the effects of multiple potential confounders. Complex statistical analyses are required to reduce the effect of such confounders and these study design challenges limit the conclusions that can be drawn from such data. Nevertheless, the literature as a whole suggests that diets derived primarily from animal products are associated with increased risk of esophageal cancer, while diets derived primarily from plant sources are associated with reduced risk. These effects appear to apply to both adenocarcinoma and squamous cell carcinoma, but the associations are stronger for the former. Much further research will be necessary to fully clarify the effects of specific nutrients on cancer risk and the role of obesity in contributing to these associations.

The mechanisms underlying the effects of specific dietary constituents on the pathogenesis of esophageal cancer are unknown. At least with respect to adenocarcinoma, macro- and micronutrients may act via direct effects on lower esophageal sphincter function and gastric acid secretion that contribute directly to GERD. High vitamin C intake has been shown to have a protective effect on the development of GERD independent of its effect on cancer risk (49), while dietary fat appears to increase distal esophageal acid exposure (54), possibly by increasing gastric acid secretion (55). Despite this latter observation, however, others have shown no direct correlation between dietary fat and GERD (21,22,56), despite the presence of a correlation between obesity and GERD, casting doubt on increased dietary fat intake as the explanation for the association between obesity and GERD. Dietary constituents have also been shown to directly affect basic cellular functions that contribute to carcinogenesis. Vitamin E has been shown to inhibit tumor growth in vitro (57), and B-vitamins have been implicated in DNA repair mechanisms and lymphocyte function (58–60). With respect to esophageal cancer, in vitro studies demonstrate that vitamin C enhances the sensitivity of esophageal cancer cells to chemotherapy in vitro (61), while vitamin A suppresses proliferation of esophageal squamous cell carcinoma cell lines (62). At least 1 study, however, demonstrates that dietary factors, including diets low in fats and high in fruits and vegetables, do not impact on biomarkers of cell proliferation in Barrett's esophagus (63), although the effects of these dietary factors in frank cancer remain unknown. The literature implicating dietary constituents in GERD, Barrett's esophagus, and cancer is complex and fraught with potential confounders. A challenge moving forward will be to identify specific mechanisms that underlie the effects of dietary constituents on the pathogenesis of these disease processes.

INFLAMMATION

One of the most important realizations regarding obesity over the past decade is that increased adiposity has profound effects on basic mechanisms of immunity and inflammation. Obesity in both animals and humans appears to be associated with a state of chronic, systemic, low-grade inflammation characterized by elevated serum inflammatory cytokine levels as well as phenotypic and functional abnormalities in a broad range of lymphocyte subsets (5,64–73). Chronic inflammation has important effects on fundamental cellular processes that may contribute to increased cell turnover, mutagenesis, and carcinogenesis. Inflammatory mediators are dysregulated in numerous cancers, with increased activation of NFκB, toll-like receptors, and other critical regulators of innate and adaptive immunity (74,75). Strong clinical evidence similarly supports a role for chronic inflammation in the pathogenesis of cancer, as chronic inflammatory diseases including inflammatory bowel disease, hepatitis, primary sclerosing cholangitis, and pancreatitis are associated with increased incidences of cancer of involved organs (76,77). Barrett's esophagus is the premalignant inflammatory precursor of esophageal adenocarcinoma, and many of the same mediators implicated in chronic systemic inflammation in obesity are also implicated in Barrett's esophagus and esophageal adenocarcinoma, which demonstrate upregulation of IL-8, IL1β, and NFκB as esophageal mucosal cells transition from normal to metaplasia to frank adenocarcinoma (78). Studies in both animals and humans implicate cyclo-oxygenase 2, an important mediator of inflammation, in the development of esophageal cancer (79). Furthermore, the chronic use of anti-inflammatory drugs, including aspirin, is associated with a reduced the risk of esophageal cancer in humans (80), although whether this association is causal is unknown. Despite these and other uncertainties, it is clear that inflammation is an important underlying mechanism in the development of esophageal cancer and may explain its association with obesity.

Much attention has recently focused on tissue macrophages as potential effectors of inflammation in obesity. Increased macrophage infiltration of adipose tissue has been described in obese mice and humans and specific subpopulations of tissue macrophages with heightened inflammatory responses have been identified in adipose tissue of obese but not lean mice. These data are particularly relevant in light of the increasing importance attributed to tumor-associated macrophages in regulating cancer immunity and tumor adaptation. Tumor-associated macrophages play an important role in anti-tumor immunity and tumors in turn evolve to express factors which downregulate macrophage immune function as a protective response (81,82). The few data that study macrophages in esophageal cancer have focused on squamous cell carcinoma. Investigators have demonstrated increased tumor-associated macrophages in squamous cell tumors of the esophagus relative to normal esophageal mucosa (83), and furthermore, upregulation of matrix metalloprotease expression (84), macrophage products that may play a role in regulating tumor invasion. Others have correlated expression of macrophage migration inhibitory factor (MIF) in esophageal squamous cell carcinoma with tumor progression and lymph node metastases (85), and linked MIF expression to both bile acid exposure and inflammation (86). These data suggest that common mechanisms of inflammation within macrophages may underlie both obesity and esophageal cancer. Therapy designed to manipulate tumor-associated macrophages phenotype and function holds promise for the treatment of esophageal as well as other types of cancer.

One of the most exciting aspects of the study of systemic inflammation in obesity is increasing evidence that suggests that chronic inflammation is an important causative factor in the pathogenesis of many important comorbidities of obesity in addition to cancer, including diabetes, atherosclerosis, and steatohepatitis (87–94). Aberrations in inflammation and immunity therefore likely underlie many serious comorbidities of obesity in addition to esophageal cancer. Therapy directed at underlying defects in inflammation in obesity therefore has the potential to treat not only esophageal cancer but other cancers and nonmalignant comorbid diseases as well.

ADIPOKINES

Adipose tissue, far from being simply a storage depot for triglycerides, is a biologically active organ that is comprised not only of adipocytes but a stromovascular cell fraction that consists of lymphocytes, endothelial cells, pre-adipocytes, and other cell types. Adipose tissue is a rich source of cytokines, hormones, and other signaling mediators, among them the adipokines, a broad family of proteins with diverse functions that are expressed primarily but not exclusively in adipose tissue. Leptin, a 16kDa protein that acts on receptors in hypothalamic neurons to affect satiety, is the best studied of the adipokines. Like many adipokines, leptin has a broad array of functions in addition to its role in regulating body weight, including effects on immune, endocrine, and reproductive systems. In these capacities, leptin regulates fundamental cellular processes, including proliferation, apoptosis, angiogenesis (95), as well as inflammatory and adaptive immune responses (96–99). Other adipokines are also dysregulated in obesity, including ghrelin, adiponectin, and resistin, all of which have also been implicated in the regulation of immune and inflammatory function.

Clinical evidence implicating adipokines in the pathogenesis cancer is conflicting and complex. Serum leptin levels are elevated in the vast majority of obese humans, likely secondary to increased adipose tissue mass, which is the primary source of leptin in vivo. Epidemiologic evidence demonstrates that elevated serum leptin levels correlate directly with an increased risk of prostate (100), breast (101), renal cell (102), and hematologic malignancies (103), but inversely with risk of hepatocellular carcinoma (104) and advanced gastric and colon cancers (105,106). Low serum levels of the adipokine adiponectin, expression of which is downregulated in obesity, are associated with an increased risk of breast cancer (107), and exogenous adiponectin inhibits tumor growth and angiogenesis in animal models (108). Aberrations in serum levels of ghrelin, an orexigenic hormone secreted by gastric mucosa, have been associated with gastric and colon cancer, although whether this relationship is causal or instead related to the effects of cancer on gastric mucosal ghrelin expression is unknown (109). Finally, elevated serum levels of the adipokine resistin have been linked to lymphoma (103).

Few data specifically address the role of adipokines in esophageal cancer. Leptin independently induces proliferation of a number of different types of tumor cell lines in vitro, including esophageal adenocarcinoma and Barrett's esophagus cell lines (87,110). Furthermore, leptin enhances the proliferative effects of acid on an esophageal adenocarcinoma cell line (111). Only scattered reports study the role of other adipokines in esophageal cancer. Elevated serum levels of ghrelin are associated with decreased risk of developing esophageal adenocarcinoma in obese subjects (112), and ghrelin secreting cells are absent from esophageal adenocarcinoma tumors, but present in surrounding gastric mucosa (113). The role of adipokines in the pathogenesis of esophageal cancer remains poorly defined and therefore fertile ground for future study.

INSULIN RESISTANCE AND DIABETES

Insulin resistance and type II diabetes mellitus are strongly linked to overweight and obesity, and diabetes is an independent risk factor for multiple types of cancer, including colon, renal, hepatocellular, and others (114–116). The mechanisms underlying the association between diabetes and cancer are unknown. Chronic inflammation contributes to the pathogenesis of diabetes and may explain its association with cancer. Of interest, many of the same mediators implicated in systemic inflammation in obesity, including TNF-α and IL-6, directly induce insulin resistance in a variety of cell types (117,118) and have also been implicated in the pathogenesis of cancer (119). In addition, specific mediators of glucose homeostasis that are upregulated in diabetes, such as insulin-like growth factor-1, have been identified as promoters of carcinogenesis (120). Few data address the association between esophageal cancer and diabetes. A single nested case control study using data culled from an administrative database demonstrated no association between diabetes and esophageal adenocarcinoma or cardia cancer, although this study had numerous limitations inherent to its design (121). Despite this negative finding, therefore, further research will be necessary to define the relationship between esophageal cancer and diabetes.

ESTROGEN

Adipose tissue is one of the few in vivo tissue depots that express estrogen aromatase and is therefore a primary source of estrogen in both men and postmenopausal women. Serum estrogen levels are elevated in obesity (122), and consistent with this observation, obesity has been identified as an independent risk factor for estrogen-sensitive breast cancers (123). While estrogen has also been shown to induce cancer in other hormone-dependent organs, including prostate, testicle, uterus, and ovary, its role in regulating carcinogenesis in other organ systems, including the esophagus, is less well defined. Estrogen receptor is expressed in a majority of esophageal adenocarcinomas (124), and estrogen inhibits in vitro proliferation of esophageal adenocarcinoma and squamous cell carcinoma cell lines (125–127). Furthermore, estrogen has been implicated in the pathogenesis of gastroesophageal reflux disease: female gender and hormone therapy are associated with an increase likelihood of GERD symptoms (24). Despite these observations, however, clinical evidence for a role for estrogen in esophageal cancer is lacking. One study demonstrated no difference in esophageal cancer rates among multiparous compared with nulliparous women (128), while in another population-based study, there was no difference in esophageal cancer rates between patients with prostate cancer treated with long-term estrogen therapy compared with the general population (129). In a single study, breast feeding, which reduces estrogen exposure, was protective for esophageal adenocarcinoma, however, suggesting a potential role for estrogen in cancer risk (130). The precise role of sex hormones in esophageal cancer therefore remains unclear.

TREATMENT CONSIDERATIONS IN OBESE PATIENTS

Sparse data specifically address outcomes in obese subjects treated for esophageal cancer. At least 2 single-center studies reported no increased overall morbidity and mortality associated with esophagectomy in obese, although blood loss and the need for partial sternotomy to provide access to the cervical esophagus may be greater (131,132). Underscoring this latter observation, in one study, recurrent laryngeal nerve injury was more common in obese subjects, likely related to difficulty in cervical exposure (131). The addition of neoadjuvant therapy to surgery may increase risk disproportionately in obese patients. One study demonstrated a 4-fold increase in perioperative morbidity after preoperative chemoradiotherapy followed by surgery for treatment of gastric and gastroesophageal adenocarcinomas in patients with a BMI greater than 25 compared to those with a BMI less than 25 (133). Further study of clinical outcomes will be necessary to accurately risk stratify patients undergoing treatment for esophageal cancer based body weight.

CONCLUSION

Obesity clearly plays an important role in cancers of all types. Data addressing its role in esophageal cancer are sparse, in a large part because of the rarity of this cancer subtype. Nonetheless, obesity has pleiotropic effects on the pathogenesis of esophageal cancer, especially adenocarcinoma, and certainly acts through multiple mechanisms. The study of the basic mechanisms of obesity's effects on carcinogenesis, including the role of diet, inflammation, adipokines, macrophage function, and other possible mediators, has the potential to yield important insights that will guide development of therapy directed towards a wide range of benign and malignant disease processes, including esophageal cancer.

References

1. Calle EE, Rodriguez C, Walker-Thurmond K, et al. Overweight, obesity, and mortality from cancer in a prospectively studied cohort of U.S. Adults. *NEJM*. 2004;348(17):1625–1638.
2. Carroll K. Obesity as a risk factor for certain types of cancer. *Lipids*. 1998;33:1055–1059.
3. Bergstrom A, Pisani P, Tenet V, et al. Overweight as an avoidable cause of cancer in Europe. *Int J Cancer*. 2001;91:421–430.
4. Hursting SD, Lavigne JA, Berrigan D, et al. Calorie restriction, aging, and cancer prevention: mechanisms of action and applicability to humans. *Annu Rev Med*. 2003;54:131–152.
5. Engeli S, Feldpausch M, Gorzelniak K, et al.. Association between adiponectin and mediators of inflammation in obese women. *Diabetes*. 2003;52(4):942–947.
6. Chow WH, Blot WJ, Vaughan TL, et al. Body mass index and risk of adenocarcinomas of the esophagus and gastric cardia. *J Natl Cancer Inst*. 1998;90:150–155.
7. Vaughan TL, Davis S, Kristal A, et al. Obesity, alcohol, and tobacco as risk factors for cancers of the esophagus and gastric cardia: adenocarcinoma vs. squamous cell carcinoma. *Cancer Epidemiol Biomarkers Prev*. 1995;4:85–92.
8. Hansen S, Wiig JN, Giercksky KE, et al. Esophageal and gastric carcinoma in Norway 1958–1992: incidence time trend variability according to morphological subtypes and organ subsites. *Int J Cancer*. 1997;71(3):340–344.

9. Cockburn MG, Wu AH, Bernstein L. Etiologic clues from the similarity of histology-specific trends in esophageal and lung cancers. *Cancer Causes Control*. 2005;16(9): 1065–1074.
10. Fernandes ML, Seow A, Chan YH, et al. Opposing trends in incidence of esophageal squamous cell carcinoma and adenocarcinoma in a multi-ethnic Asian country. *Am J Gastroenterol*. 2006;101(7):1430–1436.
11. Fitzgerald RC. Molecular basis of Barrett's oesophagus and oesophageal adenocarcinoma. *Gut*. 2006;55(12):1810–1820.
12. Bollschweiler E, Wolfgarten E, Gutschow C, et al. Demographic variations in the rising incidence of esophageal adenocarcinoma in white males. *Cancer*. 2001;92: 549–555.
13. Cook MB, Wild CP, Forman D. A systematic review and meta-analysis of the sex ratio for Barrett's esophagus, erosive reflux disease, and nonerosive reflux disease. *Am J Epidemiol*. 2005;162(11):1050–1061.
14. Nilsson M, Johnsen R, Ye W, et al. Prevalence of gastro-oesophageal reflux symptoms and the influence of age and sex. *Scand J Gastroenterol*. 2004;39:1040–1045.
15. Wu A, Wan P, Bernstein L. A multiethnic population based study of smoking, alcohol and body size and risk of adenocarcinoma of the stomach and esophagus (United States). *Cancer Causes Control*. 2001;12:721–732.
16. Lagergren J, Bergstrom R, Nyren O. Association between body mass and adenocarcinoma of the esophagus and gastric cardia. *Ann Intern Med*. 1999;130:883–890.
17. Lundell L, Ruth M, Sandberg N, et al. Does massive obesity promote abnormal gastroesophageal reflux? *Dig Dis Sci*. 1995;40(8):1632–1635.
18. Lagergren J, Bergstrom R, Nyren O. No relation between body mass and gastro-oesophageal reflux symptoms in a Swedish population based study. *Gut*. 2000;47(1):26–29.
19. El-Serag HB, Graham DY, Satia JA, et al. Obesity is an independent risk factor for GERD symptoms and erosive esophagitis. *Am J Gastroenterol*. 2005;100:1243–1250.
20. Locke GR, Talley NJ, Fett SL, et al. Risk factors associated with symptoms of gastroesophageal reflux. *Am J Med*. 1999;106(6):642–649.
21. Suter M, Dorta G, Giusti V, et al. Gastro-esophageal reflux and esophageal motility disorders in morbidly obese patients. *Obes Surg*. 2004;14(7):959–966.
22. Ruhl CE, Everhart JE. Overweight but not high dietary fat intake increases risk of gastroesophageal reflux disease hospitalization: the NHANES I Epidemiologic Followup Study. First National Health and Nutrition Examination Survey. *Ann Epidemiol*. 1999;9:424–435.
23. Wajed SA, Streets CG, Bremner CG, et al. Elevated body mass disrupts the barrier to gastroesophageal reflux. *Arch Surg*. 2001;136(9):1014–1018.
24. Nilsson M, Johnsen R, Ye W, et al. Obesity and estrogen as risk factors for symptomatic gastroesophageal reflux. *JAMA*. 2003;290:66–72.
25. Jacobson BC, Somers SC, Fuchs CS, et al. Body-mass index and symptoms of gastroesophageal reflux in women. *N Engl J Med*. 2006;354:2340–2348.
26. Hampel H, Abraham NS, El-Serag HB. Meta-analysis: obesity and the risk for gastroesophageal reflux disease and its complications. *Ann Intern Med*. 2005;143(3):199–211.
27. Edelstein ZR, Farrow DC, Bronner MP, et al. Central adiposity and risk of Barrett's esophagus. *Gastroenterology*. 2007;133(2):403–411.
28. Smith KJ, O'Brien SM, Smithers BM, et al. Interactions among smoking, obesity, and symptoms of acid reflux in Barrett's esophagus. *Cancer Epidemiol Biomarkers Prev*. 2005;14:2481–2486.
29. Corley DA, Kubo A, Levin TR, et al. Abdominal obesity and body mass index as risk factors for Barrett's esophagus. *Gastroenterology*. 2007;133(1):34–41.
30. Pandolfino JE, El-Serag HB, Zhang Q, et al. Obesity: a challenge to esophagogastric junction integrity. *Gastroenterology*. 2006;130(3):639–649.
31. Herbella FA, Sweet MP, Tedesco P, et al. Gastroesophageal reflux disease and obesity. Pathophysiology and implications for treatment. *J Gastrointest Surg*. 2007;11(3):286–290.
32. Koppman JS, Poggi L, Szomstein S, et al. Esophageal motility disorders in the morbidly obese population. *Surg Endosc*. 2007;21(5):761–764.
33. Hong D, Khajanchee YS, Pereira N, et al. Manometric abnormalities and gastroesophageal reflux disease in the morbidly obese. *Obes Surg*. 2004;14(6):744–749.
34. Jaffin BW, Knoepflmacher P, Greenstein R. High prevalence of asymptomatic esophageal motility disorders among morbidly obese patients. *Obes Surg*. 1999;9(4):390–395.
35. Wilson LJ, Ma W, Hirschowitz BI. Association of obesity with hiatal hernia and esophagitis. *Am J Gastroenterol*. 1999;94:2840–2844.
36. Murakami K, Sasaki S, Okubo H, et al. Dietary fiber intake, dietary glycemic index and load, and body mass index: a cross-sectional study of 3931 Japanese women aged 18–20 years. *Eur J Clin Nutr*. 2007;61(8):986–995.
37. Karnehed N, Tynelius P, Heitmann BL, et al. Physical activity, diet and gene-environment interactions in relation to body mass index and waist circumference: the Swedish young male twins study. *Public Health Nutr*. 2006;9(7):851–858.
38. Yanoff LB, Parikh SJ, Spitalnik A, et al. The prevalence of hypovitaminosis D and secondary hyperparathyroidism in obese Black Americans. *Clin Endocrinol (Oxf)*. 2006;64(5):523–529.
39. Linnebur SA, Vondracek SF, Griend JP, et al. Prevalence of vitamin D insufficiency in elderly ambulatory outpatients in Denver, Colorado. *Am J Geriatr Pharmacother*. 2007;5(1):1–8.
40. Carlin AM, Rao DS, Meslemani AM, et al. Prevalence of vitamin D depletion among morbidly obese patients seeking gastric bypass surgery. *Surg Obes Relat Dis*. 2006;2(2):98–103.
41. Tungtrongchitr R, Pongpaew P, Tongboonchoo C, et al. Serum homocysteine, B12 and folic acid concentration in Thai overweight and obese subjects. *Int J Vitam Nutr Res*. 2003;73(1):8–14.
42. Pinhas-Hamiel O, Doron-Panush N, Reichman B, et al. Obese children and adolescents: a risk group for low vitamin B12 concentration. *Arch Pediatr Adolesc Med*. 2006;160(9):933–936.
43. Arnaud J, Bertrais S, Roussel AM, et al. Serum selenium determinants in French adults: the SU.VI.M.AX study. *Br J Nutr*. 2006;95(2):313–320.
44. Ribot J, Felipe F, Bonet ML, et al. Changes of adiposity in response to vitamin A status correlate with changes of PPAR gamma 2 expression. *Obes Res*. 2001;9(8):500–509.
45. Mayne ST, Risch HA, Dubrow R, et al. Nutrient intake and risk of subtypes of esophageal and gastric cancer. *Cancer Epidemiol Biomarkers Prev*. 2001;10(10):1055–1062.
46. Terry P, Lagergren J, Ye W, Nyren O, et al. Antioxidants and cancers of the esophagus and gastric cardia. *Int J Cancer.*. 2000;87(5):750–754.
47. Terry P, Lagergren J, Ye W, et al. Inverse association between intake of cereal fiber and risk of gastric cardia cancer. *Gastroenterology*. 2001;120(2):387–391.
48. Terry P, Lagergren J, Wolk A, et al. Reflux-inducing dietary factors and risk of adenocarcinoma of the esophagus and gastric cardia. *Nutr Cancer*. 2000;38(2):186–191.
49. Veugelers PJ, Porter GA, et al. Obesity and lifestyle risk factors for gastroesophageal reflux disease, Barrett esophagus and esophageal adenocarcinoma. *Dis Esophagus*. 2006;19(5):321–328.
50. Tzonou A, Lipworth L, Garidou A, et al. Diet and risk of esophageal cancer by histologic type in a low-risk population. *Int J Cancer.*. 1996;68(3):300–304.
51. Mark SD, Qiao YL, Dawsey SM, et al. Prospective study of serum selenium levels and incident esophageal and gastric cancers. *J Natl Cancer Inst.*. 2000;92(21):1753–1763.
52. Zhang ZF, Kurtz RC, Yu GP, et al. Adenocarcinomas of the esophagus and gastric cardia: the role of diet. *Nutr Cancer*. 1997;27(3):298–309.
53. Blot WJ, Li JY, Taylor PR, et al. Nutrition intervention trials in Linxian, China: supplementation with specific vitamin/mineral combinations, cancer incidence, and disease-specific mortality in the general population. *J Natl Cancer Inst*. 1993;85(18):1483–1492.
54. Fox M, Barr C, Nolan S, et al. The effects of dietary fat and calorie density on esophageal acid exposure and reflux symptoms. *Clin Gastroenterol Hepatol*. 2007;5(4):439–444.
55. Sammon AM, Alderson D. Diet, reflux and the development of squamous cell carcinoma of the oesophagus in Africa. *Br J Surg*. 1998;85(7):891–896.
56. Nandurkar S, Locke GR III, Fett S, et al. Relationship between body mass index, diet, exercise and gastro-oesophageal reflux symptoms in a community. *Aliment Pharmacol Ther*. 2004;20:497–505.
57. Das S. Vitamin E in the genesis and prevention of cancer. *Acta Oncol*. 1994;33(6):615–619.
58. Folkers K. Relevance of the biosynthesis of coenzyme Q10 and of the four bases of DNA as a rationale for the molecular causes of cancer and a therapy. *Biochem Biophys Res Commun*. 1996;224(2):358–361.
59. Folkers K, Morita M, McRee J Jr. The activities of coenzyme Q10 and vitamin B6 for immune responses. *Biochem Biophys Res Commun*. 1993;193(1):88–92.
60. Jacobson EL, Dame AJ, Pyrek JS, et al. Evaluating the role of niacin in human carcinogenesis. *Biochimie*. 1995;77(5):394–398.
61. Abdel-Latif MM, Raouf AA, Sabra K, et al. Vitamin C enhances chemosensitization of esophageal cancer cells in vitro. *J Chemother*. 2005;17(5):539–549.
62. Muller A, Nakagawa H, Rustgi AK. Retinoic acid and N-(4-hydroxy-phenyl) retinamide suppress growth of esophageal squamous carcinoma cell lines. *Cancer Lett*. 1997;113(1–2):95–101.
63. Kristal AR, Blount PL, Schenk JM, et al. Low-fat, high fruit and vegetable diets and weight loss do not affect biomarkers of cellular proliferation in Barrett esophagus. *Cancer Epidemiol Biomarkers Prev*. 2005;14(10):2377–2383.
64. Festa A, D'Agostino R Jr, Williams K, et al. The relation of body fat mass and distribution to markers of chronic inflammation. *Int J Obes Relat Metab Disord*. 2001;25(10):1407–1415.
65. Festa A, D'Agostino R Jr, Tracy RP, et al. Elevated levels of acute-phase proteins and plasminogen activator inhibitor-1 predict the development of type 2 diabetes. *Diabetes*. 2002;51(4):1131–1137.
66. Meier CA, Bobbioni E, Gabay C, et al. IL-1 receptor antagonist serum levels are increased in human obesity: a possible link to the resistance to leptin? *J Clin Endocrinol Metab*. 2002;87:1184–1188.
67. Bastard JP, Jardel C, Bruckert E, et al. Elevated levels of IL-6 are reduced in serum and subcutaneous adipose tissue of obese women after weight loss. *J Clin Endo Met*. 2000;85:3338–3342.
68. Somm E, Cettour-Rose P, Asensio C, et al. Interleukin-1 receptor antagonist is upregulated during diet-induced obesity and regulates insulin sensitivity in rodents. *Diabetologia*. 2006;49:387–393.
69. O'Rourke RW, Kay T, Lyle EA, et al. Alterations in cytokine expression in peripheral blood lymphocytes in obesity. *Clin Exp Immunol*. 2006;146(1):39–46.
70. O'Rourke RW, Kay T, Scholz M, et al. Alterations in T-cell subset frequency in peripheral blood in obesity. *Obes Surg*. 2005:15(10):1463–1468.
71. Chandra RK, Au B. Spleen hemolytic plaque-forming cell response and generation of cytotoxic cells in genetically obese (C57Bl/6J ob/ob) mice. *Int Arch Allergy Appl Immunol*. 1980;62:94–98.
72. Cottam, DR, Schaefer P, Shaftan G, et al. Effect of surgically-induced weight loss on leukocyte indicators of chronic inflammation in morbid obesity. *Obes Surg*. 2002;12(3):335–342.
73. Cottam DR, Schaefer PA, Shaftan GW, et al. Dysfunctional immune-privilege in morbid obesity: implications and effect of gastric bypass surgery. *Obes Surg*. 2003;13(1):49–57.
74. Chen R, Alvero AB, Silasi DA, et al. Inflammation, cancer and chemoresistance: taking advantage of the toll-like receptor signaling pathway. *Am J Reprod Immunol*. 2007;57(2):93–107.

75. Escarcega RO, Fuentes-Alexandro S, Garcia-Carrasco M, et al. The transcription factor nuclear factor-kappa B and cancer. *Clin Oncol (R Coll Radiol)*. 2007;19(2):154–161.
76. Huang C, Lichtenstein DR. Pancreatic and biliary tract disorders in inflammatory bowel disease. *Gastrointest Endosc Clin N Am*. 2002;12(3):535–559.
77. Jackson L, Evers BM. Chronic inflammation and pathogenesis of GI and pancreatic cancers. *Cancer Treat Res*. 2006;130:39–65.
78. Fitzgerald RC, Abdalla S, Onwuegbusi BA, et al. Inflammatory gradient in Barrett's oesophagus: implications for disease complications. *Gut*. 2002;51(3):316–322.
79. Dannenberg AJ, Altorki NK, Boyle JO, et al. Inhibition of cyclooxygenase-2: an approach to preventing cancer of the upper aerodigestive tract. *Ann N Y Acad Sci*. 2001;952:109–115.
80. Farrow DC, Vaughan TL, Hansten PD, et al. Use of aspirin and other nonsteroidal anti-inflammatory drugs and risk of esophageal and gastric cancer. *Cancer Epidemiol Biomarkers Prev*. 1998;7(2):97–102.
81. Saccani A, Schioppa T, Porta C, et al. p50 nuclear factor-kappaB overexpression in tumor-associated macrophages inhibits M1 inflammatory responses and antitumor resistance. *Cancer Res*. 2006;66(23):11432–11440.
82. Porta C, Subhra Kumar B, Larghi P, et al. Tumor promotion by tumor-associated macrophages. *Adv Exp Med Biol*. 2007;604:67–86.
83. Guo SJ, Lin DM, Li J, et al. Tumor-associated macrophages and CD3-zeta expression of tumor-infiltrating lymphocytes in human esophageal squamous-cell carcinoma. *Dis Esophagus*. 2007;20(2):107–116.
84. Ding Y, Shimada Y, Gorrin-Rivas MJ, et al. Clinicopathological significance of human macrophage metalloelastase expression in esophageal squamous cell carcinoma. *Oncology*. 2002;63(4):378–384.
85. Ren Y, Law S, Huang X, et al. Macrophage migration inhibitory factor stimulates angiogenic factor expression and correlates with differentiation and lymph node status in patients with esophageal squamous cell carcinoma. *Ann Surg*. 2005;242(1):55–63.
86. Xia HH, Zhang ST, Lam SK, et al. Expression of macrophage migration inhibitory factor in esophageal squamous cell carcinoma and effects of bile acids and NSAIDs. *Carcinogenesis*. 2005;26(1):11–15.
87. Ogunwobi O, Mutungi G, Beales IL. Leptin stimulates proliferation and inhibits apoptosis in Barrett's esophageal adenocarcinoma cells by cyclooxygenase-2-dependent, prostaglandin-E2-mediated transactivation of the epidermal growth factor receptor and c-Jun NH2-terminal kinase activation. *Endocrinology*. 2006; 147(9):4505–4516.
88. Yuan M, Konstantopoulos N, Lee J, et al. Reversal of obesity- and diet-induced insulin resistance with salicylates or targeted disruption of Ikkbeta. *Science*. 2001;293:1673–1677.
89. Liuzzo G, Goronzy JJ, Yang H, et al. Monoclonal T-cell proliferation and plaque instability in acute coronary syndromes. *Circulation*. 2000;101(25):2883–2888.
90. Schonbeck U, Mach F, Sukhova GK, et al. CD40 ligation induces tissue factor expression in human vascular smooth muscle cells. *Am J Pathol*. 2000;156:7–14.
91. Reardon CA, Getz GS. Mouse models of atherosclerosis. *Curr Opin Lipidol*. 2001;12:167–173.
92. Michelsen KS, Wong MH, Shah PK, et al. Lack of TLR-4 or Myd88 reduces atherosclerosis and alters plaque phenotype in mice deficient in apolipoprotein E. *Proc Natl Acad Sci USA*. 2004;101:10679–10684.
93. Li G, Hangoc G, Broxmeyer HE. Interleukin-10 in combination with M-CSF and IL-4 contributes to development of the rare population of CD14+CD16++ cells derived from human monocytes. *Biochem Biophys Res Commun*. 2004;322(2):637–643.
94. Diehl AM. Nonalcoholic steatosis and steatohepatitis IV. Nonalcoholic fatty liver disease abnormalities in macrophage function and cytokines. *Am J Physiol Gastrointest Liver Physiol*. 2002;282(1):G1–5.
95. Gonzalez RR, Cherfils S, Escobar M, et al. Leptin signaling promotes the growth of mammary tumors and increases the expression of vascular endothelial growth factor (VEGF) and its receptor type two (VEGF-R2). *J Biol Chem*. 2006;281(36):26320–26328.
96. Lord G, Matarese G, Howard J, et al. Leptin inhibits anti-CD3-driven proliferation of T-cells but enhances production of proinflammatory cytokines. *J Leuk Biol*. 2002;72:330.
97. Lord G, Matarese G, Howard J, et al. Leptin Modulates T-cell immune response and reverses starvation-induced immunosuppression. *Nature*. 1998;394:897–901.
98. Fujita Y, Murakami M, Ogawa Y, et al. Leptin inhibits stress-induced apoptosis of T lymphocytes. *Clin Exp Immunol*. 2002;128:21–26.
99. Santos-Alvarez J, Goberna R, Sánchez-Margalet V. Human leptin stimulates proliferation and activation of human circulating monocytes. *Cell Immunol*. 1999;194:6–11.
100. Chang S, Hursting SD, Contois JH, et al. Leptin and prostate cancer. *Prostate*. 2001;46(1):62–67.
101. Han C, Zhang HT, Du L, et al. Serum levels of leptin, insulin, and lipids in relation to breast cancer in china. *Endocrine*. 2005;26(1):19–24.
102. Horiguchi A, Sumitomo M, Asakuma J, et al. Increased serum leptin levels and over expression of leptin receptors are associated with the invasion and progression of renal cell carcinoma. *J Urol*. 2006;176(4, pt 1):1631–1635.
103. Pamuk GE, Demir M, Harmandar F, et al. Leptin and resistin levels in serum of patients with hematologic malignancies: correlation with clinical characteristics. *Exp Oncol*. 2006;28(3):241–244.
104. Ataseven H, Bahcecioglu IH, Kuzu N, et al. The levels of ghrelin, leptin, TNF-a, and IL-6 in liver cirrhosis and hepatocellular carcinoma due to HBV and HDV infection. *Mediators Inflamm*. 2006(4):78380.
105. Dulger H, Alici S, Sekeroglu MR, et al. Serum levels of leptin and proinflammatory cytokines in patients with gastrointestinal cancer. *Int J Clin Pract*. 2004;58(6):545–549.
106. Bolukbas FF, Kilic H, Bolukbas C, et al. Serum leptin concentration and advanced gastrointestinal cancers: a case controlled study. *BMC Cancer*. 2004;4:29.
107. Mantzoros C, Petridou E, Dessypris N, et al.Adiponectin and breast cancer risk. *J Clin Endocrinol Metab*. 2004;89:1102–1107.
108. Brakenhielm E, Veitonmaki N, Cao R, et al. Adiponectin- induced antiangiogenesis and antitumor activity involve caspase-mediated endothelial cell apoptosis. *Proc Natl Acad Sci USA*. 2004;101:2476–2481.
109. Huang Q, Fan YZ, Ge BJ, et al. Circulating ghrelin in patients with gastric or colorectal cancer. *Dig Dis Sci*. 2007;52(3):803–809.
110. Somasundar P, Riggs D, Jackson B, et al. Leptin stimulates esophageal adenocarcinoma growth by nonapoptotic mechanisms. *Am J Surg*. 2003;186(5):575–578.
111. Beales IL, Ogunwobi OO. Leptin synergistically enhances the anti-apoptotic and growth-promoting effects of acid in OE33 oesophageal adenocarcinoma cells in culture. *Mol Cell Endocrinol*. 2007;274(1-2):60–68.
112. de Martel C, Haggerty TD, Corley DA, et al. Serum ghrelin levels and risk of subsequent adenocarcinoma of the esophagus. *Am J Gastroenterol.*. 2007;102(6):1166–1172.
113. Mottershead M, Karteris E, Barclay JY, et al. Immunohistochemical and quantitative mRNA assessment of ghrelin expression in gastric and oesophageal adenocarcinoma. *J Clin Pathol*. 2007;60(4):405–409.
114. Schoen RE, Tangen CM, Kuller LH, et al. Increased blood glucose and insulin, body size, and incident colorectal cancer. *J Natl Cancer Inst*. 1999;91:1147–1154.
115. Yang YX, Hennessy S, Lewis JD. Insulin therapy and colorectal cancer risk among type 2 diabetes mellitus patients. *Gastroenterology*. 2004;127:1044–1050.
116. Davila JA, Morgan RO, Shaib Y, et al. Diabetes increases the risk of hepatocellular carcinoma in the United States: a population based case control study. *Gut*. 2005;54:533–539.
117. De Taeye BM, Novitskaya T, McGuinness OP, et al. Macrophage TNF-{alpha} contributes to insulin resistance and hepatic steatosis in diet-induced obesity. *Am J Physiol Endocrinol Metab*. 2007;293(3):E713–725.
118. Leclercq IA, Da Silva Morais A, Schroyen B, et al. Insulin resistance in hepatocytes and sinusoidal liver cells: mechanisms and consequences. *J Hepatol*. 2007;47(1):142–156.
119. Aggarwal BB, Shishodia S, Sandur SK, et al. Inflammation and cancer: how hot is the link? *Biochem Pharmacol*. 2006;72(11):1605–1621.
120. Kaaks R, Lukanova A. Energy balance and cancer: the role of insulin and insulin-like growth factor-I. *Proc Nutr Soc*. 2001;60:91–106.
121. Rubenstein JH, Davis J, Marrero JA, et al. Relationship between diabetes mellitus and adenocarcinoma of the oesophagus and gastric cardia. *Aliment Pharmacol Ther*. 2005;22(3):267–271.
122. Olson MB, Shaw LJ, Kaizar EE, et al. Obesity distribution and reproductive hormone levels in women: a report from the NHLBI-sponsored WISE Study. *J Womens Health (Larchmt)*. 2006;15(7):836–842.
123. Key TJ, Appleby PN, Reeves GK, et al. Significance of macrophage chemoattractant protein-1 expression and macrophage infiltration in squamous cell carcinoma of the esophagus. *Am J Gastroenterol.*. 2004;99(9):1667–1674.
124. Liu L, Chirala M, Younes M. Expression of estrogen receptor-beta isoforms in Barrett's metaplasia, dysplasia and esophageal adenocarcinoma. *Anticancer Res*. 2004;24(5A):2919–2924.
125. Ueo H, Matsuoka H, Sugimachi K, et al. Inhibitory effects of estrogen on the growth of a human esophageal carcinoma cell line. *Cancer Res*. 1990;50(22):7212–7215.
126. Utsumi Y, Nakamura T, Nagasue N, et al. Effect of 17 beta-estradiol on the growth of an estrogen receptor-positive human esophageal carcinoma cell line. *Cancer*. 1991;67(9):2284–2289.
127. Matsuoka H, Sugimachi K, Ueo H, et al. Sex hormone response of a newly established squamous cell line derived from clinical esophageal carcinoma. *Cancer Res*. 1987;47(15):4134–4140.
128. Lagergren J, Jansson C. Sex hormones and oesophageal adenocarcinoma: influence of childbearing? *Br J Cancer*. 2005;93(8):859–861.
129. Lagergren J, Nyren O. Do sex hormones play a role in the etiology of esophageal adenocarcinoma? A new hypothesis tested in a population-based cohort of prostate cancer patients. *Cancer Epidemiol Biomarkers Prev*. 1998;7(10):913–915.
130. Cheng KK, Sharp L, McKinney PA, et al. A case–control study of oesophageal adenocarcinoma in women: a preventable disease. *Br J Cancer*. 2000;83:127–132
131. Scipione CN, Chang AC, Pickens A, et al. Transhiatal esophagectomy in the profoundly obese: implications and experience. *Ann Thorac Surg*. 2007;84(2):376–382.
132. Morgan MA, Lewis WG, Hopper AN, et al. Prognostic significance of body mass indices for patients undergoing esophagectomy for cancer. *Dis Esophagus*. 2007;20(1):29–35.
133. Fujitani K, Ajani JA, Crane CH, et al. Impact of induction chemotherapy and preoperative chemoradiotherapy on operative morbidity and mortality in patients with locoregional adenocarcinoma of the stomach or gastroesophageal junction. *Ann Surg Oncol*. 2007;14(4):1305–1311.

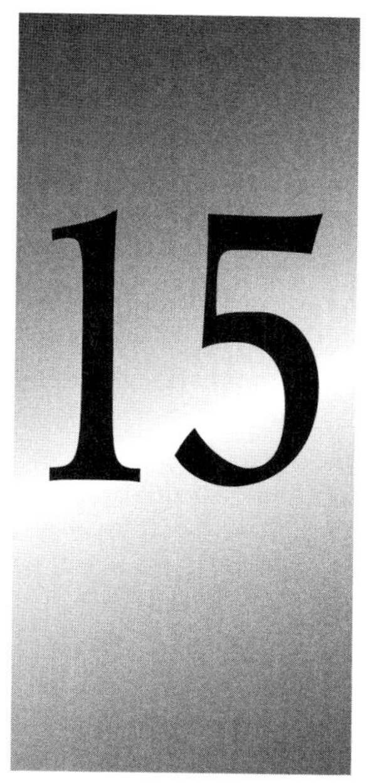

The Relationship Between *Helicobacter Pylori* and Barrett's Esophagus

Attila Dubecz
Jeffrey H. Peters

The possible pathogenic role of helical-shaped bacteria found in gastric fluids was first suggested in the late 19th century by the Polish scientist Walery Jaworski of the University of Krakow (1). Luck and Seth reported in 1924 that the human stomach exhibits abundant urease activity that disappears following antibiotic treatment (2). It was the publication of 2 Australian scientists in 1983 that convincingly demonstrated the pathogenic role of *Helicobacter pylori (H. pylori)* (3). These pioneering studies of Barry Marshall and Robin Warren from Perth included self experiments and were later awarded the Nobel Prize. Since this "rediscovery" of *Helicobacter pylori* (then called *Campylobacter pyloridis*) as an important pathogenic bacterium colonizing the human stomach, it has been linked to a number of foregut diseases, most prominently peptic ulcer disease and MALT lymphoma. In fact, a unit of the World Health Organization, the International Agency for Research on Cancer, classifies *H. pylori* as a class I human carcinogen (4).

Interest has recently arisen in the well-documented observation of an inverse correlation between *H. pylori* infection and the prevalence of GERD, Barrett's esophagus, and esophageal adenocarcinoma. Many have suggested the hypothesis that *H. pylori* alters the gastric biology in a fashion that is protective toward GERD and its complications, and that the eradication of *H. pylori* in developed countries has contributed to the rise in the prevalence of GERD and Barrett's esophagus. Blaser argues that as the evidence shows that *H. pylori* has been part of microbial flora since the evolution of human race (5), there must be equilibrium between the host and *H. pylori*, with both benefits and costs of the colonization (6). On the other hand, many authors agree with Graham, who states that "the only good *Helicobacter pylori* is a dead *Helicobacter pylori*" (7).

BACTERIOLOGY AND EPIDEMIOLOGY

Helicobacter pylori is a 3.5 x 0.5 micron-sized, spiral-shaped, microaerophilic, gram negative bacterium with 4–6 flagellae. It is capable of forming biofilms and in hostile environments, coccoid forms of Helicobacter have been observed. Biochemically, it is characterized by the production of urease, catalase, and oxidase, with urease likely important for bacterial survival in the gastric milieu (8).

Simulation of human ancestral genetic patterns suggest that modern humans were infected with *H. pylori* prior to their migration 58,000 years ago from East Africa (6). This hypothesis makes Helicobacter infection one of the oldest chronic bacterial infections of the human race. More than the half of the world's population is infected. It affects all age groups and races. In developed countries, serologic evidence of *H. pylori* infection is unusual in early childhood, but increases steadily with age, reaching over 50% after the age 60. Contrary to suggestions that the incidence has an even distribution during the life period, new evidence shows that even in developed countries, the prevalence of infection in any given age group reflects bacterial acquisition during childhood (9,10). The majority of the population acquires the infection before the age of 10. The risk of *H. pylori* infection correlates with one's socioeconomic environment, the number of siblings, the number of cohabitants in a room, and the presence or absence of running water (11,12). Most children in developing countries acquire *H. pylori* before the age of 10 and more than 80% of adults are infected before age 50. Improved sanitation in the second half of the 19th century initiated a continuous decline in prevalence of *H. pylori* in the United States, ultimately resulting in a greatly reduced overall prevalence of *H. pylori* (13).

The exact route of *H. pylori* acquisition is not entirely clear, but most authors agree that fecal-oral and oral-oral transmission is most likely (14). *Helicobacter pylori* is found in contaminated water supplies in endemic areas, and the bacterium can be cultured from stool samples. There is little evidence regarding oral transmission. Gastroenterologists have higher prevalence of infection compared to control population (15), but dentists and oral hygienists, who are presumed to have a similar occupational exposure, do not (16). Twin studies suggest the presence of a genetic risk of *H. pylori* infection, but twins raised together have higher concordance of infection than twins raised separately, further highlighting the importance of the childhood socioeconomic environment in *H. pylori* acquisition (17,18). Reacquisition rate after cure is rare (around 2%/year) in both children and adults (19).

PATHOPHYSIOLOGY

Bacterial Factors

Helicobacter pylori is highly adapted to the gastric environment, with an array of capabilities that aid colonization of gastric mucosa. It has also been shown that the genome of *H. pylori* is continuously changing, importing DNA of other colonizing strains during chronic infection (20,21). Bacteria bind to mucosal epithelial cells by adhesion molecules of the Hop (Helicobacter outer membrane protein) family, the 3 most important of which are BabA, OipA, and SabA. The best characterized adhesin molecule BabA binds to Lewis B blood group antigen on the host cell (22).

Urease activity is considered one of the most important virulence factors. The hydrolysis of urea produces ammonia, which neutralizes gastric acid in the local environment of the bacterium promoting the organism's survival. Despite this, the role of urease has been questioned recently. Mine et al. showed that urease-negative Helicobacter are able to induce gastritis in an animal model (23). More than half of all *H. pylori* strains express a 95kD vacuolating cytotoxin, VacA. This secreted exotoxin inserts itself into the cell membrane, forming a voltage-depending channel, releasing bicarbonate and anions and acting like a passive urea transporter, increasing the permeability of the gastric epithelium to urea, creating a favorable environment for *H. pylori* infection. Furthermore, VacA targets mitochondria causing apoptosis in affected cells (24,25).

The genome of most *H. pylori* strains include a cag pathogenicity island (cagPAI), a 37kb fragment containing 29 genes that encode a protein channel functioning to inject several proteins, including the 120 kD CagA protein into the host cell. The function of cagA remains unclear; it is not cytotoxic, but is antigenic and can be detected serologically. The clinical significance of cagA is supported by the fact that more than 90% of peptic ulcer patients are infected with cagA+ *H. pylori*, compared with 64.6% of patients with functional dyspepsia (26). The effect of cagA positivity on gastric cancer risk is still debated. Parsonnet et al. found that subjects infected with cagA+ *H. pylori* had 5.8-fold increased risk of developing gastric cancer (27). In contrast, Lu, Yamaoka, and Graham found that *H. pylori* infection alone is associated with the development of gastric cancer, but neither CagA nor VacA seropositivity added additional risk (28). A 2001 meta-analysis of case-control studies concluded that presence of CagA was an independent risk factor for noncardia gastric cancer (29).

Host Responses

Helicobacter pylori induces a significant inflammatory and immune response in the affected host, resulting in persistent inflammation in virtually all infected subjects. Since the bacterium rarely, if ever, invades the gastroduodenal mucosal layer, host response is triggered by its adhesion to host cells (25). The infected mucosa has elevated levels of cytokines (IL-1, IL-2, IL-6, IL8, TNFα), among which IL-8 activates neutrophil leukocytes (30). CagA+ strains induce enhanced IL-8 levels (31). *Helicobacter pylori* activates a vigorous systemic and mucosal humoral response that doesn't lead to eradication, but contributes to tissue damage. Many infected patients have antibodies directed against the H+/K+ ATPase of gastric parietal cells (32). Recent research shows that host genetic factors that affect interleukin-1-beta, a powerful inhibitor of gastric acid secretion, may determine why some individuals infected with *H. pylori* develop gastric cancer while others do not. Interleukin-1 gene cluster polymorphisms suspected of enhancing production of interleukin-1-beta are associated with an increased risk of both hypochlorydia induced by *H. pylori* and gastric cancer (33).

HELICOBACTER PYLORI AND GASTROESOPHAGEAL REFLUX DISEASE

The relationship between *H. Pylori* and GERD has been of interest for decades. The observation that gastric mucosal atrophy was less frequent in patients with reflux esophagitis was made well before the *H. pylori* era (34). More recent epidemiologic studies have revealed a remarkable inverse relationship between *H. pylori* eradication in the population and the increase in GERD and its complications (35). Over the period from 1970 to 1995, the incidence of both duodenal ulcer compared to erosive esophagitis and distal gastric cancer compared to gastric cardia cancer display strikingly opposing time-trends. It has been postulated that changes in *H. pylori* infection among the population may be a primary reason for these observations, and that *H. pylori*-induced chronic corpus gastritis may in some way protect against the development of GERD and its malignant transformation (35).

Further evidence of an inverse relationship between *H. pylori* and gastroesophageal reflux comes from clinical observations of their association. The emergence of new onset GERD symptoms following *H. pylori* eradication, first reported by Schütze in 1995 (36), led to the hypothesis of a possible protective effect of *H. pylori* colonization. A detailed report by Labenz et al. in 1997 added further evidence to this theory (37). In a case control study of 460 duodenal ulcer patients, new onset GERD symptoms were significantly higher in patients who had successful *H. pylori* eradication than in those with persisting infection. A number of subsequent studies have raised doubts as to whether a true relationship exists (Table 15.1) (39).

TABLE 15.1
Worsening of GERD Symptoms Related to* Helicobacter pylori *Status 4 Weeks After Completion Therapy (32)

H. pylori status	Worsening	No worsening	OR (95% CI)
Eradication (n=269)	20 (7.4%)	249 (92.6%)	0.47 (0.24–0.917.4%)
Persistence (n=137)	20 (14.6%)	117 (85.4.%)	p=0.02

Raghunath et al. reviewed the available evidence via a meta-analysis published in 2003. The data showed an average prevalence of *H. pylori* infection of 38.2% in GERD patients compared to 49.5% in non-GERD controls ($p<0.001$). They concluded that geographic location is a strong contributor to the heterogeneity of the data, probably the result of wide variations in the baseline prevalence of *H. pylori* infection. Studies from the Far East, where baseline *H. pylori* infection is high, report a lower prevalence of Helicobacter infection in reflux patients than the studies conducted in Europe or North America, where the baseline *H. pylori* prevalence is low (38). A recent analysis of 8 double-blind prospective studies concluded that on average, *H. pylori* eradication does not lead to development of new-onset GERD or worsening of symptoms of pre-existing GERD. Despite the confusion, it is likely that a relationship exists between the eradication of *H. pylori* from the population and the raising incidence of gastroesophageal reflux (39).

The difficulty in proving a relationship between *H. pylori* and GERD is almost certainly due in part to the complex biology of variable *H. pylori* infection patterns in any individual patient. The final result of an *H. pylori* infection of gastric acid secretion depends on the pattern of gastritis resulting from chronic infection. For example, antrum predominant gastritis affects somatostatin, producing antral D cells resulting in less feedback inhibition of gastrin and increased intraluminal acid. This pattern explains the common observation of increased gastrin levels in some *H. pylori* infected subjects. Corpus gastritis, on the other hand, is characterized by decreased intraluminal acid secretion subsequent to the release of TNF alpha and IL-1 beta stimulated by local inflammation and ultimately mucosal atrophy. Thus it seems logical that eradication of *H. pylori* infection in patients with antral predominant gastritis would improve GERD symptoms, while *H. pylori* treatment in corpus predominant gastritis would worsen existing GERD or unmask reflux esophagitis in previously asymptomatic susceptible patients, thus showing a protective effect.

Helicobacter pylori eradication is clearly indicated in patients with duodenal ulcer patients, but early evidence suggests that eradication might worsen GERD, resulting in resistance toward eradication in the non-ulcer population. Since antral-predominant Helicobacter-induced gastritis is associated with increased gastric acid secretion, and thus an increased risk for developing GERD and duodenal ulcer disease, one might suppose both conditions improve after eradication. The systematic review of 27 studies by Raghunath et al. alluded to above reached this conclusion (38).

Further support for the benefits of *H. pylori* eradication in GERD patients as opposed to its potential detrimental effects come from the observation that without eradication, PPI and H2 blocker treatment in *H. pylori* positive patients causes worsening of corpus gastritis (40). This is not seen in GERD patients not taking proton pump inhibitors (PPI) as, for example, after Nissen-fundoplication (41). Interestingly, Peetsalu et al. recently reported less antral gastritis and a higher prevalence of chronic active corpus gastritis with or without mucosal atrophy in patients 14 years after truncal vagotomy (42). These data lead to the suggestion that acid "protects" against "proximal-migration" of the *H. pylori* infection (Helicobacter-induced antral gastritis turning into corpus dominant gastritis) and the recommendation that *H. pylori* treatment is indeed indicated in *H. pylori* positive GERD patients who require chronic antisecretory medications (43).

We can conclude that the prevalence of *H. pylori* infection in patients with GERD is lower than non-GERD control populations and that there is likely an inverse epidemiologic relationship between GERD and *H. pylori*. Eradication does not affect the success of PPI treatment in GERD in Western populations, and *H. pylori* testing and subsequent treatment should be considered in GERD patients receiving long-term maintenance treatment with PPIs (44).

BARRETT'S ESOPHAGUS

Helicobacter pylori is not found in esophageal squamous or native intestinal mucosa, nor has it been reported to colonize the specialized intestinal type epithelium characteristic of Barrett's esophagus (45). Interestingly, it can be identified in areas of gastric-type metaplasia found in a columnar segment in patients with a columnar lined esophagus (CLE) (46,47). When present in the CLE, it is invariably detected in the gastric mucosa also. Consequently, the association between *H. pylori* and Barrett's esophagus is based upon the presence of *H. pylori* in the stomach, not in the normal or metaplastic esophageal mucosa.

The relationship of Barrett's esophagus to gastric *H. pylori* colonization is debated, although most studies show an even stronger inverse relationship than that of GERD alone. Bowrey et al. reported an *H. pylori* prevalence of 27% in patients with Barrett's esophagus, compared to 41% in healthy control subjects (48). Werdmuller and Loffield also found significantly lower *H. pylori* infection rates in Barrett's than non-Barrett's patients (23% vs. 51%), whereas Loffeld reported very high rates (62%) in a retrospective analysis of 107 consecutive patients with CLE (49,50). Blaser et al. found no statistic difference between patients with and without Barrett's using serologic testing for *H. pylori* (40% vs. 39%) (51).

The conflicting findings in Barrett's may be due to the presence or absence of the cagA+ marker, which has been postulated to be necessary for the protective effect. Vicari et al. reported a prevalence of cagA+ *H. pylori* infection in 13.3% of Barrett's, 36.7% of GERD, and 43% of control subjects (52). The reason for this possible protective effect is the severe pangastritis and decreased gastric acid production associated with cagA+ *H. pylori* infection, although Peters et al. reported that *H. pylori* status does not influence 24 hour esophageal pH measurements (53).

ESOPHAGEAL ADENOCARCINOMA

The incidence of adenocarcinoma of the esophagus has increased dramatically in the past 20 years, outpacing any other cancer (54). This change is among the most remarkable alterations in human cancer biology ever observed. Why it has occurred remains unknown, although the clear inverse relationship of the decrease in *H. pylori* infection in developed countries (9) and the increase in adenocarcinoma of the esophagus and cardia certainly raise the suspicion that they may be true cause and effect. Recent epidemiologic studies have reported a strong negative association between the presence of *H. pylori* infection and the risk of esophageal adenocarcinoma. Ye et al., studying patients in Sweden, found a significant inverse relation between Helicobacter infection and esophageal adenocarcinoma. *Helicobacter pylori* infection was statistically significantly associated with a reduced risk for esophageal adenocarcinoma (for HP-CSA antibodies, odds ratio [OR] = 0.3, 95% confidence interval [CI] = 0.2 to 0.6; for CagA antibodies, OR = 0.5, 95% CI = 0.3 to 0.8; for both, OR = 0.2, 95% CI = 0.1 to 0.5). But interestingly, gastric atrophy, measured by the serum level of pepsinogen I, was not associated with the risk for esophageal adenocarcinoma (OR = 1.1, 95% CI = 0.5 to 2.5). Serum CagA antibodies and gastric atrophy were associated with an increased risk for esophageal squamous-cell carcinoma (OR = 2.1, 95% CI = 1.1 to 4.0, and OR = 4.3, 95% CI = 1.9 to 9.6, respectively) (55).

In a large multicenter case-control trial conducted by the National Cancer Institute, Chow et al. found no difference in the overall prevalence of *H. pylori* infection in patients with esophageal adenocarcinoma but did find that infection with cagA+ strains significantly reduced the risk of developing esophageal adenocarcinoma with an odds ratio of 0.4 (56). Others have failed to show a significant relationship between cagA+ *H. pylori* status and esophageal adenocarcinoma (57), including a population based, case-control study by Engel et al. that found that esophageal adenocarcinoma could be linked to smoking, obesity, and reflux disease but not *H. pylori* infection (58).

Hirota et al. reported a significant relationship of *H. pylori* infection to the histologic precursors stages of esophageal adenocarcinoma. Dysplasia or cancer

TABLE 15.2
Prevalence of Helicobacter in Different Esophageal Pathologies (60)

	GERD control (n=217)	Barrett's esophagus (n=208)	Barrett's LGD/ IND (n=47)	Barrett's HGD (n=14)	Barrett's carcinoma (n=20)	p value (ANOVA)
H. pylori prevalence	44.2%	35.1%	36.2%	14.3%	15.0%	0.001

was noted in 31% of LSBE, 10% of SSBE, and 6.4% of EGJ-SIM patients. *Helicobacter pylori* infection was observed in 2.5% of LSBE, 4.7% of SSBE, and 21.3% of EGJ-SIM patients, a significant inverse relationship (59). Confirming these findings, Weston et al. prospectively investigated the prevalence of gastric *H. pylori* infection and the development of dysplasia or cancer in 219 patients with nondysplastic Barrett's esophagus at entry. *Helicobacter pylori* infection was present in 44% of non-Barrett's GERD controls, 35% of patients developing low-grade dysplasia, 15% of those developing with high-grade dysplasia, and in none of 145 of individuals with esophageal adenocarcinoma (Table 15.2) (60). Similarly, Wright et al. reported a 34% vs. 17% difference between prevalence of Helicobacter infection in patients with non-dysplastic Barrett's vs. those with dysplasia or adenocarcinoma (61).

The possible pathophysiologic reasons of these associations are not yet clear. Apoptosis induced by cagA+ Helicobacter in Barrett's adenocarcinoma cell lines has been reported (62). The fact that *H. pylori* does not directly colonize Barrett's epithelium suggests that a direct effect is unlikely, and that its influence on the contents, pH, and chemistry of the gastroesophageal reflux is more relevant.

Based on the evidence discussed above, the risk of eradicating *H. pylori* in otherwise asymptomatic patients with chronic gastritis seems to outweigh the possible benefits. The impact of *H. pylori* on the development of gastric cancer must be remembered, however. Nakajima and Hattori estimated that the annual incidence of gastric cancer developing from *H. pylori*-induced chronic gastritis will always be higher (5.8 x at least) than that of esophageal cancer potentially aggravated by *H. pylori* eradication (63). Anand and Graham, in a similar study, suggested even higher (10–60x) relative risks (64). Whether this hold true in populations at low risk for gastric adenocarcinoma, such as Caucasian men, and at high risk for esophageal adenocarcinoma is unclear.

SUMMARY

The association of *H. pylori* and upper gastrointestinal diseases is overwhelming. In addition to its well-known effects on gastric disease, it is likely linked to esophageal pathology as well. Evolutionary hypotheses assume, and the majority of available epidemiologic data show, that the decline of *H. pylori* infection is one of the reasons behind the increasing incidence of GERD-related diseases including esophageal and cardia adenocarcinoma in the Western world. This inverse relationship is strongest between *H. pylori* and esophageal adenocarcinoma although significant evidence relates *H. pylori* and the development of Barrett's esophagus and GERD. Further investigation is needed to clarify the underlying mechanisms. We can conclude that the risks of chronic Helicobacter infection clearly outweigh the possible protective effects and, as such, based on available data, eradication is indicated.

References

1. Konturek JW. Discovery by Jaworski of Helicobacter pylori and its pathogenetic role in peptic ulcer, gastritis and gastric cancer. *J Physiol Pharmacol.* 2003;54 Suppl 3:23–41.
2. Luck JM, Seth TN. Gastric urease. *Biochem J.* 1924;18:1227–1231.
3. Marshall BJ, Warren JR. Unidentified curved bacilli in the stomach of patients with gastritis and peptic ulceration. *Lancet.* 1984;1:1311–1315.
4. IARC Monographs Volume 61. *Schistosomes, Liver Flukes and Helicobacter pylori.* Lyon, France: IARC; 1994.
5. Blaser MJ. Hypothesis: the changing relationships of Helicobacter pylori and humans: implications for health and disease. *J Infect Dis.* 1999;179:1523–1530.
6. Linz B, Balloux F, Moodley Y, et al. An African origin for the intimate association between humans and Helicobacter pylori. *Nature.* 2007;445:915–918.
7. Graham DY. The only good Helicobacter pylori is a dead Helicobacter pylori. *Lancet.* 1997;350:70–72.
8. Correa P, Houghton J. Carcinogenesis of Helicobacter pylori. *Gastroenterology.* 2007;133:659–672.
9. Parsonnet J. The incidence of Helicobacter pylori infection. *Aliment Pharmacol Ther.* 1995;9 Suppl 2:45–51.
10. Rowland M, Daly L, Vaughan M, et al. Age-specific incidence of Helicobacter pylori. *Gastroenterology.* 2006;130:65,72,211.
11. Ford AC, Forman D, Bailey AG, et al. Effect of sibling number in the household and birth order on prevalence of Helicobacter pylori: a cross-sectional study. *Int J Epidemiol.* 2007;36(6):1327–1333.
12. Webb PM, Knight T, Greaves S, et al. Relation between infection with Helicobacter pylori and living conditions in childhood: evidence for person to person transmission in early life. *BMJ.* 1994;308:750–753.
13. Rupnow MF, Shachter RD, Owens DK, et al. A dynamic transmission model for predicting trends in Helicobacter pylori and associated diseases in the United States. *Emerg Infect Dis.* 2000;6:228–237.
14. Parsonnet J, Shmuely H, Haggerty T. Fecal and oral shedding of Helicobacter pylori from healthy infected adults. *JAMA.* 1999;282:2240–2245.
15. Hunt RH, Sumanac K, Huang JQ. Review article: should we kill or should we save Helicobacter pylori? *Aliment Pharmacol Ther.* 2001;15 Suppl 1:51–59.
16. Malaty HM, Evans DJ Jr, Abramovitch K, et al. Helicobacter pylori infection in dental workers: a seroepidemiology study. *Am J Gastroenterol.* 1992;87:1728–1731.

17. Malaty HM, Graham DY, Isaksson I, et al. Co-twin study of the effect of environment and dietary elements on acquisition of Helicobacter pylori infection. *Am J Epidemiol.* 1998;148:793–797.
18. Malaty HM, Engstrand L, Pedersen NL, et al. Helicobacter pylori infection: genetic and environmental influences. A study of twins. *Ann Intern Med.* 1994;120:982–986.
19. Borody TJ, Andrews P, Mancuso N, et al. Helicobacter pylori reinfection rate, in patients with cured duodenal ulcer. *Am J Gastroenterol.* 1994;89:529–532.
20. Falush D, Kraft C, Taylor NS, et al. Recombination and mutation during long-term gastric colonization by Helicobacter pylori: estimates of clock rates, recombination size, and minimal age. *Proc Natl Acad Sci U S A.* 2001;98:15056–15061.
21. Suerbaum S, Smith JM, Bapumia K, et al. Free recombination within Helicobacter pylori. *Proc Natl Acad Sci U S A.* 1998;95:12619–12624.
22. Guruge JL, Falk PG, Lorenz RG, et al. Epithelial attachment alters the outcome of Helicobacter pylori infection. *Proc Natl Acad Sci U S A.* 1998;95:3925–3930.
23. Mine T, Muraoka H, Saika T, et al. Characteristics of a clinical isolate of urease-negative Helicobacter pylori and its ability to induce gastric ulcers in Mongolian gerbils. *Helicobacter.* 2005;10:125–131.
24. Peek RM. Pathogenesis of Helicobacter pylori infection. *Springer Semin Immunopathol.* 2005;27:197–215.
25. Suerbaum S, Michetti P. Helicobacter pylori infection. *N Engl J Med.* 2002;347:1175–1186.
26. Weel JF, van der Hulst RW, Gerrits Y, et al. The interrelationship between cytotoxin-associated gene A, vacuolating cytotoxin, and Helicobacter pylori-related diseases. *J Infect Dis.* 1996;173:1171–1175.
27. Parsonnet J, Friedman GD, Vandersteen DP, et al. Helicobacter pylori infection and the risk of gastric carcinoma. *N Engl J Med.* 1991;325:1127–1131.
28. Lu H, Yamaoka Y, Graham DY. Helicobacter pylori virulence factors: facts and fantasies. *Curr Opin Gastroenterol.* 2005;21:653–659.
29. Helicobacter and Cancer Collaborative Group. Gastric cancer and Helicobacter pylori: a combined analysis of 12 case control studies nested within prospective cohorts. *Gut.* 2001;49:347–353.
30. Yamaoka Y, Kita M, Kodama T, et al. Induction of various cytokines and development of severe mucosal inflammation by cagA gene positive Helicobacter pylori strains. *Gut.* 1997;41:442–451.
31. Keates S, Keates AC, Warny M, et al. Differential activation of mitogen-activated protein kinases in AGS gastric epithelial cells by cag+ and cag- Helicobacter pylori. *J Immunol.* 1999;163:5552–5559.
32. Negrini R, Savio A, Appelmelk BJ. Autoantibodies to gastric mucosa in Helicobacter pylori infection. *Helicobacter.* 1997;2 Suppl 1:S13–16.
33. El-Omar EM, Carrington M, Chow WH, et al. Interleukin-1 polymorphisms associated with increased risk of gastric cancer. *Nature.* 2000;404:398–402.
34. Hongo M. Reflux esophagitis and Helicobacter pylori: East and West. *J Gastroenterol.* 2004;39:909–910.
35. el-Serag HB, Sonnenberg A. Opposing time trends of peptic ulcer and reflux disease. *Gut.* 1998;43:327–333.
36. Schütze K, Hentschel E, Dragosics B, et al. Helicobacter pylori reinfection with identical organisms: transmission by the patients' spouses. *Gut.* 1995;36:831–833.
37. Labenz J, Blum AL, Bayerdorffer E, et al. Curing Helicobacter pylori infection in patients with duodenal ulcer may provoke reflux esophagitis. *Gastroenterology.* 1997;112:1442–1447.
38. Raghunath A, Hungin APS, Wooff D, et al. Prevalence of Helicobacter pylori in patients with gastro-oesophageal reflux disease: systematic review. *BMJ.* 2003;326:737–744.
39. Laine L, Sugg J. Effect of Helicobacter pylori eradication on development of erosive esophagitis and gastroesophageal reflux disease symptoms: a post hoc analysis of eight double blind prospective studies. *Am J Gastroenterol.* 2002;97:2992–2997.
40. Meining A, Kiel G, Stolte M. Changes in Helicobacter pylori-induced gastritis in the antrum and corpus during and after 12 months of treatment with ranitidine and lansoprazole in patients with duodenal ulcer disease. *Aliment Pharmacol Ther.* 1998;12:735–740.
41. Kuipers EJ, Lundell L, Klinkenberg-Knol EC, et al. Atrophic gastritis and Helicobacter pylori infection in patients with reflux esophagitis treated with omeprazole or fundoplication. *N Engl J Med.* 1996;334:1018–1022.
42. Peetsalu M, Valle J, Harkonen M, et al. Changes in the histology and function of gastric mucosa and in Helicobacter pylori colonization during a long-term follow-up period after vagotomy in duodenal ulcer patients. *Hepatogastroenterology.* 2005;52:785–791.
43. Kuipers EJ, Nelis GF, Klinkenberg-Knol EC, et al. Cure of Helicobacter pylori infection in patients with reflux oesophagitis treated with long term omeprazole reverses gastritis without exacerbation of reflux disease: results of a randomised controlled trial. *Gut.* 2004;53:12–20.
44. Malfertheiner P, Megraud F, O'Morain C, et al. Current concepts in the management of Helicobacter pylori infection: the Maastricht III Consensus Report. *Gut.* 2007;56:772–781.
45. Pei Z, Bini EJ, Yang L, et al. Bacterial biota in the human distal esophagus. *Proc Natl Acad Sci U S A.* 2004;101:4250–4255.
46. Ricaurte O, Flejou JF, Vissuzaine C, et al. Helicobacter pylori infection in patients with Barrett's oesophagus: a prospective immunohistochemical study. *J Clin Pathol.* 1996;49:176–177.
47. Henihan RD, Stuart RC, Nolan N, et al. Barrett's esophagus and the presence of Helicobacter pylori. *Am J Gastroenterol.* 1998;93:542–546.
48. Bowrey DJ, Williams GT, Clark GW. Interactions between Helicobacter pylori and gastroesophageal reflux disease. *Dis Esophagus.* 1998;11:203–209.
49. Werdmuller BF, Loffeld RJ. Helicobacter pylori infection has no role in the pathogenesis of reflux esophagitis. *Dig Dis Sci.* 1997;42:103–105.
50. Loffeld RJ, Ten Tije BJ, Arends JW. Prevalence and significance of Helicobacter pylori in patients with Barrett's esophagus. *Am J Gastroenterol.* 1992;87:1598–1600.
51. Blaser MJ, Perez-Perez GI, Lindenbaum J, et al. Association of infection due to Helicobacter pylori with specific upper gastrointestinal pathology. *Rev Infect Dis.* 1991;13 Suppl 8:S704–708.
52. Vicari JJ, Peek RM, Falk GW, et al. The seroprevalence of cagA-positive Helicobacter pylori strains in the spectrum of gastroesophageal reflux disease. *Gastroenterology.* 1998;115:50–57.
53. Peters FT, Kuipers EJ, Ganesh S, et al. The influence of Helicobacter pylori on oesophageal acid exposure in GERD during acid suppressive therapy. *Aliment Pharmacol Ther.* 1999;13:921–926.
54. Blot WJ, Devesa SS, Kneller RW, et al. Rising incidence of adenocarcinoma of the esophagus and gastric cardia. *JAMA.* 1991;265:1287–1289.
55. Ye W, Held M, Lagergren J, et al. Helicobacter pylori infection and gastric atrophy: risk of adenocarcinoma and squamous-cell carcinoma of the esophagus and adenocarcinoma of the gastric cardia. *J Natl Cancer Inst.* 2004;96:388–396.
56. Chow WH, Blaser MJ, Blot WJ, et al. An inverse relation between cagA+ strains of Helicobacter pylori infection and risk of esophageal and gastric cardia adenocarcinoma. *Cancer Res.* 1998;58:588–690.
57. Wu AH, Crabtree JE, Bernstein L, et al. Role of Helicobacter pylori CagA+ strains and risk of adenocarcinoma of the stomach and esophagus. *Int J Cancer.* 2003;103:815–821.
58. Engel LS, Chow WH, Vaughan TL, et al. Population attributable risks of esophageal and gastric cancers. *J Natl Cancer Inst.* 2003;95:1404–1413.
59. Hirota WK, Loughney TM, Lazas DJ, et al. Specialized intestinal metaplasia, dysplasia, and cancer of the esophagus and esophagogastric junction: prevalence and clinical data. *Gastroenterology.* 1999;116:277–285.
60. Weston AP, Badr AS, Topalovski M, et al. Prospective evaluation of the prevalence of gastric Helicobacter pylori infection in patients with GERD, Barrett's esophagus, Barrett's dysplasia, and Barrett's adenocarcinoma. *Am J Gastroenterol.* 2000;95:387–394.
61. Wright TA, Myskow M, Kingsnorth AN. Helicobacter pylori colonization of Barrett's esophagus and its progression to cancer. *Dis Esophagus.* 1997;10:196–200.
62. Jones AD, Bacon KD, Jobe BA, et al. Helicobacter pylori induces apoptosis in Barrett's-derived esophageal adenocarcinoma cells. *J Gastrointest Surg.* 2003;7:68–76.
63. Nakajima S, Hattori T. Oesophageal adenocarcinoma or gastric cancer with or without eradication of Helicobacter pylori infection in chronic atrophic gastritis patients: a hypothetical opinion from a systematic review. *Aliment Pharmacol Ther.* 2004;20 Suppl 1:54–61.
64. Anand BS, Graham DY. Ulcer and gastritis. *Endoscopy.* 1999;31:215–225.
65. Ahmed N, Sechi LA. Helicobacter pylori and gastroduodenal pathology: New threats of the old friend. *Ann Clin Microbiol Antimicrob.* 2005;4:1.

16 Ethnic Disparities in Cancer of the Esophagus

Allan Pickens

Annually, approximately 400,000 people are diagnosed with esophageal cancer worldwide, and more than 350,000 people die of this malignancy each year. This makes esophageal cancer the eighth most common cancer and the sixth most common cause of cancer mortality. The prognosis of esophageal cancer is poor, and 5-year survival rates are less than 10% (1). Surgical resection is the treatment of choice when the aim is to cure local and regional disease. Chemotherapy and radiation therapy, either neoadjuvant or adjuvant, may improve prognosis. The increasing frequency and high mortality of esophageal malignancy provides a compelling argument for the detailed evaluation of risk.

The epidemiology of esophageal cancer may provide key evidence for understanding the etiology and pathogenesis of this devastating cancer. The epidemiology of esophageal cancer is characterized by distinctly higher incidence in certain geographic locations and in specific races. Disparities have been noted in many cancers with respect to race, but there are striking epidemiologic differences when analyzing esophageal cancer. These differences in epidemiology are further delineated by histologic subtype of esophageal cancer.

Squamous cell carcinoma and adenocarcinoma are the most common histologic subtypes of esophageal cancer (2). Both histologic subtypes have very different biologic and epidemiologic profiles. Consequently, esophageal squamous cell carcinoma and esophageal adenocarcinoma must be viewed as separate disease entities. Squamous cell carcinoma occurs primarily in the middle third of the esophagus, while adenocarcinoma predominately occurs in the lower third of the esophagus (3). Squamous cell carcinoma remains the most common histologic subtype of esophageal cancer worldwide, and its incidence has remained relatively stable. However, the incidence of primary esophageal adenocarcinoma has increased at a rate exceeding any other cancer. Esophageal adenocarcinoma has a reported incidence increase of over 350% over the past 2 decades (4).

There are particular geographic differences in esophageal cancer. Areas of particularly high incidence of esophageal squamous cell carcinoma (expressed as crude incidence per 100,000) are as follows: China (21 per 100,000), South America (13 per 100,000), western Europe (11 per 100,000), southern Africa (10 per 100,000), Japan (9 per 100,000), and the former Soviet Union (8 per 100,000) (1,2) (Table 16.1). Within each of these broad geographic areas are identifiable smaller regions in which the incidence may be 10 to 50 times higher. Such regions include central and northern China, southern Thailand, northern Italy, mountainous regions of Japan, costal parts of Iran, and certain

TABLE 16.1
Geographic Regions with High Incidence of Esophageal Cancer According to Esophageal Cancer Cell Type[a]

Squamous cell		Adenocarcinoma	
China	21	United States	5.00
South America	13	Scotland	4.26
Western Euro	11	Sweden	1.99
South Africa	10	Finland	1.52
Japan	9	Denmark	1.32
Former Soviet Union	8	Canada	1.26

[a]The esophageal cancer incidence is expressed as crude cases per 100,000 people.

TABLE 16.2
Risk Factors According to Esophageal Cancer Cell Type

Squamous cell	Adenocarcinoma
Low income	Barrett's esophagus
Alcohol	Obesity
Smoking	Alcohol
Diet	Smoking
Cultural practices	
Infection	
Intrinsic esophageal diseases	

French provinces. In the United States, high incidence areas are the District of Columbia and the coastal regions of southern states. Similarly, esophageal adenocarcinoma exhibits certain geographic predilections. Developed countries in Europe and North America have higher incidence rates of esophageal adenocarcinoma. The incidence of esophageal adenocarcinoma has been rising in northern Europe (Sweden, Denmark, Norway), western Europe (England, Wales, Scotland), central Europe (Switzerland), and southern Europe (Italy). In North America, the United States and Canada have had the highest incidence rates for esophageal adenocarcinoma. Geographic areas of high prevalence must be identified to encourage early diagnostic testing and assessment of epidemiologic factors contributing to the increased incidence.

The incidence rates for both major histologic subtypes of esophageal cancer is extremely low under age 40, but both rise with each increasing decade of age. The male-to-female ratio for adenocarcinoma varies among age-groups but peaks during the fifth decade of life. The male-to-female ratio of squamous cell carcinoma remains relatively even throughout life (3).

Population-based case-control studies suggest few clinical conditions and modifiable risk factors that account for the majority of esophageal cancer; thus, there are limited opportunities for interventions to reverse the rapidly rising incidence of esophageal cancer. Risk factors for both common histologic cell types are listed in Table 16.2. A large majority, nearly 90%, of esophageal squamous cell carcinoma can be accounted for by smoking, alcohol consumption, or low consumption of fruits and vegetables. Approximately 79% of esophageal adenocarcinoma can be attributed to obesity, gastroesophageal reflux, smoking and alcohol consumption (5,6).

Squamous cell carcinoma of the esophagus is the most common form of esophageal cancer worldwide. Case control studies have identified risk factors for esophageal squamous cell carcinoma, including moderate/heavy alcohol intake, smoking, infrequent consumption of raw fruit and vegetables, cultural practices, infection, intrinsic esophageal disease, and low economic status. Heavy drinkers of hard liquor (>35 drinks per week) have significantly higher risk. The relationship between smoking and esophageal squamous cell cancer is less clear. The highest relative risk is present when cigarette smoking is combined with heavy hard liquor consumption. This observation implies synergy between chemical mutagens in tobacco and alcoholic drinks (2). Several nutritional surveys of high-incidence regions have suggested that diets rich in carbohydrates and low in protein, green vegetables, and fruit were associated with the development of esophageal squamous cell carcinoma. Deficiencies of certain vitamins and minerals may also contribute (vitamin A, vitamin C, zinc) (7). Infection (human papilloma virus) and intrinsic esophageal diseases (tylosis, Plummer-Vinson syndrome, achalasia, diverticula, stricture, radiation injury) produce esophageal mucosal changes that result in increased incidence of esophageal squamous cell carcinoma (8).

There has been a rapid increase in the incidence of adenocarcinoma of the esophagus in the United States and Europe. The annual rate of esophageal adenocarcinoma rose from 0.7 per 100,000 to 3.2 per 100,000 over 2 decades, reflecting an increase of greater than 350% (4). Adenocarcinoma is now equal to the rate of squamous cell esophageal cancer in many developed countries. The exact reason for the surge in esophageal adenocarcinoma incidence is unknown. The steady population of alcohol consumers and the declining number of cigarette smokers make these 2 factors less important when searching for a cause of the adenocarcinoma surge. Numerous speculations exist. Increasing awareness of gastroesophageal reflux and more aggressive surveillance of Barrett's esophagus is believed to contribute to the rise in esophageal adenocarcinoma. In addition, obesity may be an important factor behind the changing incidence. Numerous studies show a concurrent increase in the prevalence of obesity in the United States and other developed countries (9). Two recent case-control studies have examined body mass index (BMI) as a risk factor for esophageal adenocarcinoma and found increased risk in the highest quartile. One study reports a 3-fold increase in the risk for esophageal adenocarcinoma among persons with BMI in the highest quartile. Overall, 59.3% of adenocarcinoma cases had a BMI over the median value of the controls (26.2 kg/m^2 for males and 25.4 kg/m^2 for females) (9,10). This is worrisome, considering reports of an annual increase in BMI of 0.6% for men and 1% for women in the United States between 1980 and 1987 (9). The similar increase in obesity observed in the United States is consistent with the increase in adenocarcinoma of the esophagus. In contrast, an inverse relationship between BMI and risk of esophageal squamous cell carcinoma was documented (9). The physiologic rationale is that increased abdominal girth promotes gastroesophageal reflux. Reflux, in turn, is a known risk factor for Barrett's esophagus. Barrett's esophagus is metaplastic change of esophageal mucosa to "intestine-like" columnar epithelium. Patients with Barrett's esophagus have a 30- to 40-fold increased risk of developing adenocarcinoma; thus, Barrett's mucosa should be considered a premalignant lesion. Nevertheless, most patients with esophageal adenocarcinoma do not have a previous diagnosis of Barrett's esophagus. The prevalence rates of Barrett's esophagus of 10% for the symptomatic population and less than 1% for the asymptomatic general population do not entirely account for the recent dramatic increase in esophageal adenocarcinoma. In addition, there is no clear evidence that either medical or surgical treatment of reflux or Barrett's esophagus can prevent the development of esophageal adenocarcinoma (2).

Cultural factors play a role in health behaviors, attitudes toward illness, and belief in modern medicine versus alternative medicine. Over the past decade, there has been increasing awareness of cancer disparities by race. Numerous programs have been formed to help eliminate the unequal burden of cancer among racial and ethnic minorities and the medically underserved. Such programs are listed in Table 16.3. The elimination of disparities is defined as a reduction in cancer incidence and mortality in conjunction with an increase in cancer survival among socioeconomically disadvantaged people to levels comparable to the general population (5). The presence of such programs represents progress in understanding and addressing disparities; however, these efforts can be only partially effective in the absence of equal access to high-quality medical care.

TABLE 16.3
National Programs Evaluating Racial and Ethnic Disparities in Cancer

Program	Sponsor
National Center on Minority Health and Health Disparities	National Institutes of Health
Center to Reduce Cancer Health Disparities	National Cancer Institute
Special Populations Networks for Cancer Awareness, Research and Training	National Cancer Institute
Surveillance, Epidemiology, and End Results	National Cancer Institute
Racial and Ethnic Approaches to Community Health	Centers for Disease Control and Prevention

The National Cancer Institute's Surveillance, Epidemiology, and End Results Program provides data on cancer incidence, mortality, stage at diagnosis, and survival for whites and African Americans since 1975 and for Hispanic/Latino, American Indian/Alaskan, and Asian/Pacific Islander populations since 1992. African Americans have the highest death rate for all cancer sites combined and from individual malignancies of the lung, colon, female breast, prostate, and cervix in comparison to all racial and ethnic groups in the United States. The death rate from cancer among African American males is 1.4 times higher than that among white males; for African American females, it is 1.2 times higher (5). The disparity in death rate from all cancers combined between African American and white males widened from 1975 until the early 1990s. A similar, although smaller, divergence occurred in death rates between African American and white women (5).

Esophageal cancer disproportionately affects certain ethnic groups and races. Esophageal cancer was reported as the fourth leading cause of cancer death in African Americans (11). The incidence of esophageal squamous cell carcinoma is more than 5-fold higher among African Americans (16.8 per 100,000) than among whites (3 per 100,000) in the United States (12). In contrast, esophageal adenocarcinoma is 4-fold more prevalent in whites than in African Americans. Recent data from cancer registries in the United States indicate that the rate of esophageal cancer among white males tripled between 1976 and 1990 (Figure 16.1). White men constituted 82% of all cases of esophageal adenocarcinoma (13). Although the incidence of esophageal

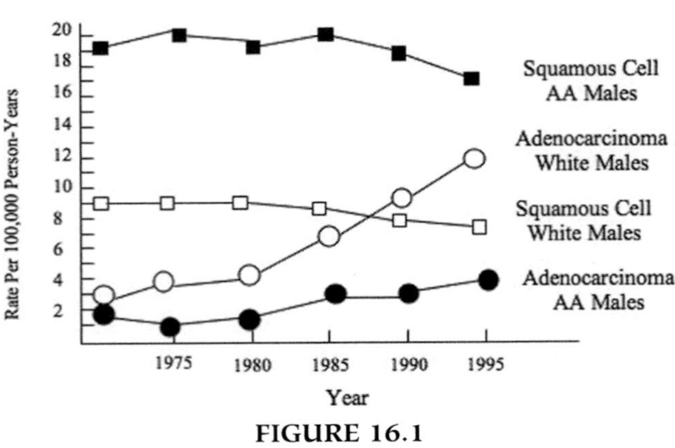

FIGURE 16.1

Incidence of esophageal carcinoma by race and cell type. ▪ = squamous cell in African American males; ◦ = adenocarcinoma in white males; □ = squamous cell in white males; • = adenocarcinoma in African American males.

adenocarcinoma among African American males and among both African American and white females is substantially lower than it is among white males, it does appear that the incidence among these groups is also rising rapidly. The Asian/Pacific Islander (API) population have different incidence patterns of esophageal cancer. When comparing cancer registries representing over 80% of the API population of both men and women in the United States, greater than 75% of esophageal cancer cases among API were squamous cell carcinomas. Overall, the total prevalence of esophageal adenocarcinoma was lower among API than among both genders of whites and African Americans (14). Such extreme racial disparity must be analyzed to identify risk factors and points of intervention.

Esophageal cancer treatment patterns may differ by medically relevant choices such as age and comorbidity, but treatment may also differ depending on nonmedical characteristics such as geographic region, socioeconomic status, sex, and race. These differences in treatment have been shown to account for differences in survival. The extent of variation in treatment and outcomes is not well known, and the mechanisms underlying the selective use of cancer treatment are still poorly understood. There have been studies of esophageal cancer patients to evaluate disparities in the rates of referral to a specialist (surgeon, radiation oncologist, or medical oncologist) and actual utilization of various forms of treatment according to race. In a large study of primary esophageal cancer, most patients were treated by a surgeon (77%) and closely followed by a medical oncologist or radiation oncologist (64% and 63%, respectively) (15). Surgery was performed in 43% of patients, 55% received radiation therapy, and 39% received chemotherapy. Substantial racial disparities were found for surgery. Only 25% of African American patients underwent resection, whereas 46% of white patients had resections. There were no significant differences in the use of radiation therapy or chemotherapy in terms of race (15).

Racial disparity in cancer survival has generally revealed a lower survival for African American patients than white patients, despite controlling for confounding variables such as age, sex, clinical factors, insurance status, and socioeconomic status. For esophageal cancer, the 5-year survival is 9% for African Americans and 13% for whites, according to the National Cancer Institute's Surveillance, Epidemiology, and End Results Program. This survival difference was present despite similar rates of distant spread (26% distant spread for African Americans and 25% distant spread for whites (11). The survival disparity can be attributed largely to differences in treatment received. Postulated explanations for the racial variation in patient treatment and outcome include differences in severity of disease, unmeasured coexisting conditions, cultural differences in attitudes toward procedures and medical care, and systematic bias. Referring physicians and treating specialists must ensure that biases and barriers to care do not deprive any patient of the best medical care.

Opportunities to reduce cancer disparity range from primary prevention to palliative care. The prevalence of underlying risk factors for some cancers differs among racial and ethnic groups. Modifiable esophageal cancer risk factors that vary by race include smoking, physical activity, and obesity. Some disparities result from targeted promotions and advertising directed at certain ethnic groups. Much of the excess incidence of cancer in African Americans has been attributed to lower socioeconomic status. Socioeconomic class appears to be an independent risk factor, and the risk is highest for those with annual incomes less than $10,000 (12). The percentage of African Americans living below this poverty level was reportedly higher than the percentage of whites. According to the 2002 U.S. census, 24% of African Americans, 21% Hispanics, 10% API, and 8% whites were below the poverty level (5). Lack of individual socioeconomic status data for most esophageal cancer patients prevents comparison of significant populations. The exact link between low socioeconomic status and esophageal cancer is unclear. Low socioeconomic class is a source for lifestyle and environmental factors, including poor housing, workplace hazards, limited health care access, poor nutritional status, and exposure to infectious agents.

The importance of genetic factors in the etiology of esophageal cancer is uncertain. According to studies performed in the United States and Sweden, the occurrence of esophageal cancer among first-degree relatives did not increase the risk of squamous cell carcinoma or adenocarcinoma of the esophagus. Neither were there any significant associations with familial occurrence of other gastrointestinal tumors (16). Heredity did not appear to contribute importantly to the occurrence of esophageal cancer of any histologic type in these studies. In contrast, several epidemiologic studies of endemic areas of China have demonstrated excess risk of esophageal cancer (mainly squamous cell carcinoma) among members of families with a history of such cancers (17). Confounding by family-specific environmental or lifestyle factors may explain these associations.

The epidemiologic factors that contribute to an individual's susceptibility to esophageal cancer are likely multifactorial. It also appears that risk factors influence histologic subtypes of esophageal cancer differently. Exposure to environmental factors contributes to the prevalence of squamous cell carcinoma worldwide. The short time frame over which the incidence of esophageal adenocarcinoma has increased in numerous populations provides strong argument for environmental factors as etiologic agents. These environmental factors likely interact with genetic characteristics to define an individual's susceptibility. Race certainly influences both environment and genetics. The short survival of esophageal cancer patients makes epidemiologic analysis difficult. Nevertheless, a better understanding of the epidemiology of esophageal cancer is crucial to the implementation of effective screening, treatment, and prevention strategies for esophageal cancer.

References

1. Vizcaino AP, Moreno V, Lambert R, et al. Time trends incidence of both major types of esophageal carcinomas in selected countries. *Int J Cancer.* 2002;99:860–868.
2. Pearson FG, Cooper JD, Deslauriers J, et al. *Thoracic Surgery.* Philadelphia, PA: Churchill Livingstone; 2002.
3. Yang PC, Davis S. Incidence of cancer of the esophagus in the US by histologic type. *Cancer.* 1988;61:612–617.
4. Devesa SS, Blott WJ, Fraumeni JF Jr. Changing patterns in the incidence of esophageal and gastric carcinoma in the United States. *Cancer.* 1998;83:2049–2053.
5. Ward E, Jemal A, Cokkinides V, et al. Cancer disparities by race/ethnicity and socioeconomic status. *CA Cancer J Clin.* 2004;54:78–93.
6. Engel LS, Chow W, Vaughan TL, et al. Population attributable risks for esophageal and gastric cancers. *J Natl Cancer Inst.* 2003;95:1404–1413.
7. Hu J, Nyren O, Wolk A, et al. Risk factors for oesophageal cancer in northeast China. *Int J Cancer.* 1994;57:38–46.
8. Suzuk L, Noffsinger AE, Hui YZ, et al. Detection of human papillomavirus in esophageal squamous cell carcinoma. *Cancer.* 1996;78:704–710.
9. Vaughan T, Davis S, Kristal A, et al. Obesity, alcohol, and tobacco as risk factors for cancers of the esophagus and gastric cardia: adenocarcinoma versus squamous cell carcinoma. *Cancer Epidemiol Biomarkers Prev.* 1995;4:85–92.
10. Wong A, Fitgerald R. Epidemiologic risk factors for Barrett's esophagus and associated adenocarcinoma. *Clin Gastroenterol Hepatol.* 2005;3:1–10.
11. Dominitz JA, Maynard C, Billingsley DG, et al. Race, treatment, and survival of veterans with cancer of the distal esophagus and gastric cardia. *Med Care.* 2002;40(suppl):I14–I26.
12. Brown LM, Hoover R, Silverman D, et al. Excess incidence of squamous cell esophageal cancer among US black men: role of social class and other risk factors. *Am J Epidemiol.* 2001;153:114–122.
13. El-Serag HB, Mason AC, Petersen N, et al. Epidemiological differences between adenocarcinoma of the oesophagus and adenocarcinoma of the gastric cardia in the USA. *Gut.* 2002;50:368–372.
14. Wu X, Chen VW, Ruiz B, et al. Incidence of esophageal and gastric carcinomas among American Asians/Pacific Islanders, whites, and blacks. *Cancer.* 2006;106:683–692.
15. Steyerberg EW, Neville B, Weeks JC, et al. Referral patterns, treatment choices, and outcomes in locoregional esophageal cancer: a population based analysis of elderly patients. *J Clin Oncol.* 2007;25:2389–2396.
16. Lagergren J, Ye W, Lindgren A, et al. Heredity and risk of cancer of the esophagus and gastric cardia. *Cancer Epidemiol, Biomarkers Prev.* 2000;9:757–760.
17. Hu J, Nyren O, Wolk A, et al. Risk factors for oesophageal cancer in northeast China. *Int J Cancer.* 1994;57:38–46.

II

IMAGING AND STAGING

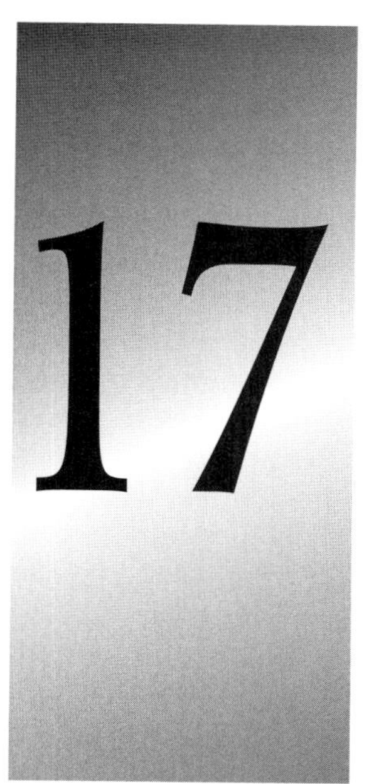

State of the Art in Esophageal Imaging: Endoscopic Technology and Evaluation of Esophageal Mucosa

Michael J. Pollack
Amitabh Chak
Ananya Das

Barrett's esophagus (BE) is a pathologic condition in which the normal stratified squamous cells that line the esophagus are replaced by metaplastic specialized intestinal-type epithelium. Its clinical relevance lies in its potential to progress from metaplastic through dysplastic stages into adenocarcinoma of the esophagus. The past 3 decades have seen a dramatic increase in the incidence of esophageal adenocarcinoma. Strategies to monitor this potential transformation are limited by the fact that only 0.5% to 1 % of all patients with BE develop adenocarcinoma annually. The majority of patients with BE do not progress even to a dysplastic stage. However, the poor prognosis associated with symptomatic adenocarcinoma has stimulated great efforts to detect BE, understand its dysplastic progression to cancer, and develop effective interventions to prevent this progression.

Practice guidelines recommend endoscopic surveillance of patients with BE in an attempt to detect cancer at an early, potentially curable stage. Current surveillance techniques utilize standard white-light endoscopes and random large particle "jumbo" biopsies obtained at 2-cm intervals in a 4-quadrant fashion, the so-called Seattle protocol. This recommended technique of endoscopic surveillance contains several shortcomings. The protocol is labor intensive, and many endoscopists do not follow the protocol. The strategy of random undirected biopsies is also subject to sampling error. Dysplasia and even early adenocarcinoma are multifocal and patchy. They are virtually indistinguishable from nondysplastic BE using white-light endoscopy and therefore may easily be missed on random biopsy. While high-resolution imaging using high-quality charge-coupled devices (CCDs) may increase the sensitivity of white-light endoscopy for detecting subtle mucosal abnormalities (1), early dysplastic changes are not always discernable as grossly visible mucosal abnormalities.

One of the difficulties in identifying dyplastic foci in BE is the large esophageal surface area that must be examined. Therefore, significant efforts have been made to improve the overall yield when performing endoscopic surveillance for dysplasia by utilizing a variety of novel endoscopic techniques. In general, imaging methods with higher resolution that provide greater tissue detail or histologic information are difficult, if not impossible, to apply in scanning an entire segment of BE. Lower-resolution methods can usually be used to image the entire esophagus but are less reliable in distinguishing dysplastic from nondysplastic epithelium. The ideal imaging technique would have the following characteristics: high sensitivity for dysplasia, moderate specificity not affected by inflammation, the ability to scan a wide area in real time, high interobserver agreement, ability to localize dysplastic areas for biopsy, and nonprohibitive cost. No single currently available imaging method has all these criteria or even several of these criteria. However, the development of new endoscopic imaging techniques has opened exciting avenues in the area of Barrett's research with the potential to improve on surveillance and treatment strategies that constitute the current standard of care. In the future, we may find that the combination of various imaging methods provides the best management algorithm.

ENDOSCOPIC IMAGING METHODS

Chromoendoscopy

Chromoendoscopy refers to the application of contrast stains to the mucosa at endoscopy such that surface patterns are highlighted. Chromoendoscopy using absorptive stains (methylene blue, cresyl violet, Lugol's solution), contrast stains (indigo carmine), and reactive stains (Congo red) has been described. Methylene blue (MB)-based chromoendoscopy, the most common form of chromoendoscopy, involves the direct application of MB to the mucosa, which is avidly absorbed by intestinal-type epithelium. Therefore, application of MB results in staining of Barrett's epithelium with sparing of nonintestinal columnar and squamous epithelium (Figure 17.1). Furthermore, dysplastic Barrett's epithelium stains less than BE without dysplasia because of the paucity of goblet cells in the setting of dysplasia. Therefore, areas of BE with dysplasia may be more evident on chromoendoscopy using MB.

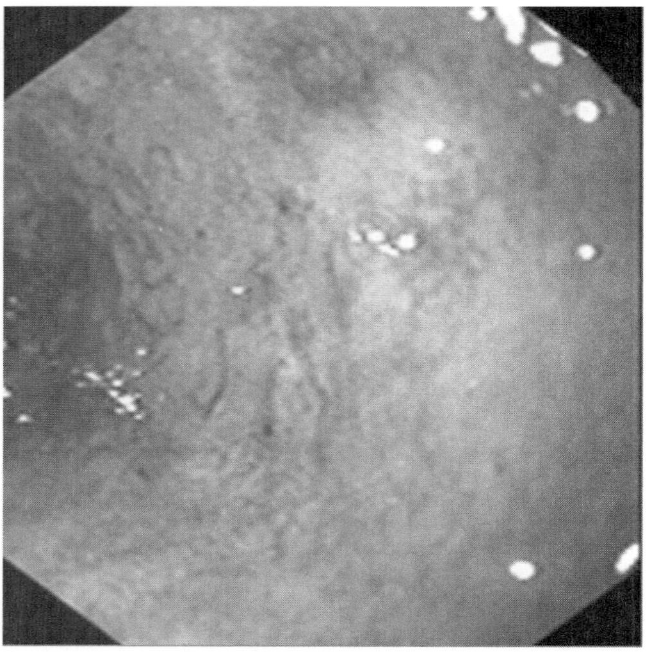

FIGURE 17.1

Methylene blue staining of Barrett's esophagus.

The technique of chromoendoscopy using MB involves clearance of surface mucus in the esophagus by flushing with 10% N-acetylcysteine. Subsequently, 0.5% MB is applied to the esophageal mucosa using an endoscopic spray catheter. After a 2-minute staining period, excess MB is cleared by flushing with sterile water. In reported studies, the sensitivity and specificity of chromoendoscopy-targeted biopsy in detection of specialized columnar epithelium varies from 53% to 98% and 32% to 97%, respectively (2). In detecting dysplasia in patients with BE, the yield of chromoendoscopy-guided biopsy compared to random biopsy is even more variable. Some of the discrepancies in the reported accuracy of MB-based chromoendoscopy could be related to variations in the technique of chromoendoscopy and intra- and interobserver variations. The pattern of mucosal staining with MB appears to be important with focal areas of decreased stain intensity and/or increased stain heterogeneity being associated with areas with higher grades of dysplastic changes (3). High-magnification endoscopes have been used to improve the yield of chromoendoscopy, but in a recent prospective multicenter study, the yield of high-magnification chromoendoscopy was similar to the technique of random biopsy in this setting (4). Chromoendoscopy is often cumbersome, time consuming, and potentially toxic with MB being implicated in oxidative DNA damage (5). Another important limitation is its inability to highlight the subepithelial capillary network, which is often distorted in the vicinity of superficial neoplasia. The MB chromoendoscopy technique has not been adopted widely, and recent studies have suggested that MB chromoendoscopy is likely of limited benefit in BE surveillance.

Unlike MB, indigo carmine is simply a contrast agent that accentuates mucosal surface patterns. Indigo carmine is applied during endoscopy using a typical endoscopic spray catheter, after clearing of surface mucus with a water, saline, or N-acetylcysteine flush. The use of a cap fitted at the endoscope tip has been described to stabilize high-magnification images and image areas of interest. Sharma et al. (6) have investigated the surface patterns in BE using magnification chromoendoscopy with indigo carmine. In their study of 80 patients with BE, 3 distinct surface patterns were appreciated: ridged/villous, circular, and irregular/distorted. The ridged/villous pattern, which has a cerebriform appearance, and circular pattern, which has uniform circular or oval areas, were observed in nondysplastic BE and in low-grade dysplasia. The irregular/distorted pattern was observed in high-grade dysplasia (HGD) with a 100% sensitivity and specificity.

Narrowband Imaging

Until recently, endoscopic systems exclusively used visible white light with wavelengths ranging from approximately 400 to 800 nm for illumination during endoscopic imaging of the gastrointestinal mucosa (Figure 17.2). Recent advances in endoscopic imaging have led to the use of narrowband imaging (NBI) for visualization of the esophageal mucosa. In NBI, optical interference filters are placed in front of a sequential red-green-blue illumination system for narrowing the spectral bandwidths; the depth of light penetration into the tissue is dependent on its wavelength, and the blue component of white light, which is preferentially enhanced during NBI, penetrates only superficially, highlighting the superficial capillary network and also the mucosal pit patterns (Figure 17.3). Reports have indicated the utility of NBI, particularly in combination with high-resolution magnification endoscopy in improving the detection of specialized columnar epithelium and also dysplastic epithelium in patients with BE, and the yield is at least comparable to that of conventional chromoendoscopy (7–9). In a randomized crossover controlled trial, indigo carmine chromoendoscopy and NBI were comparable as adjuncts to high-resolution endoscopy in detecting early neoplasia in patients with BE (10). A recently introduced multispectral endoscopic imaging technique based on postprocessing of digital endoscopic images by spectral estimation also has been shown to improve visualization of the subepithelial capillary network and may be comparable or superior to conventional chromoendoscopy (11).

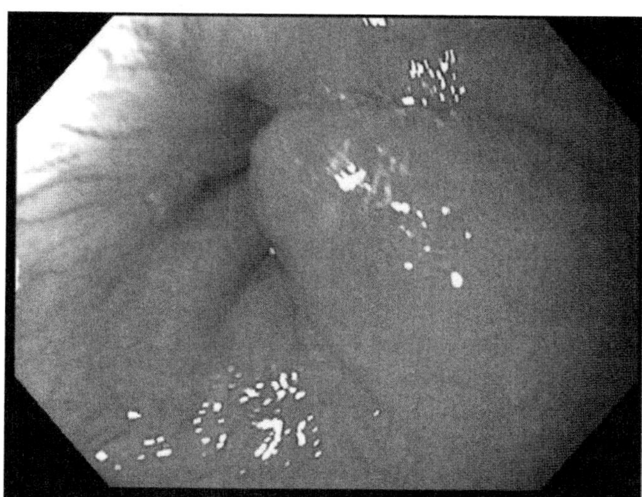

FIGURE 17.2

Barrett's esophagus with high-grade dysplasia on standard white-light video-endoscopy.

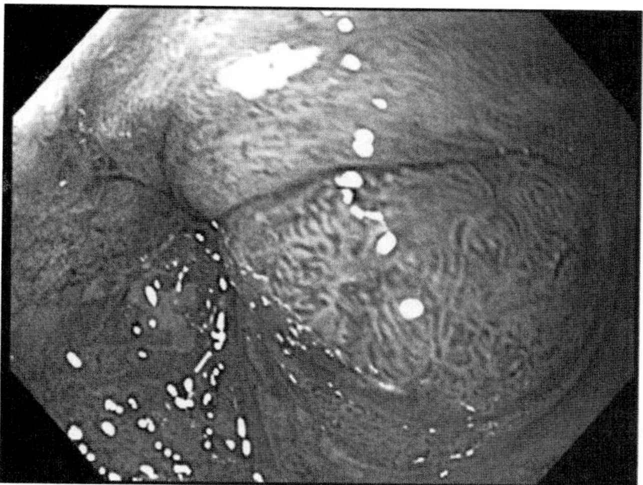

FIGURE 17.3

The same area with narrowband imaging. An irregular/distorted mucosal pattern is apparent in an area of high-grade dysplasia.

Autofluorescence

Fluorescence is the process in which certain molecules, termed fluorophores, absorb light energy and reach an excited state. From the excited state, fluorophores return to the ground state and, in that process, emit light of a longer wavelength than the light that produced the excited state. Emitted light within the visible light spectrum accounts for the optical phenomenon of fluorescence. The use of fluorescence for imaging may be based on endogenous fluorophores, such as NADH or collagen, or the use of exogenously supplied fluorophores, such as porfimer sodium or the fluorescent dye fluorescein. The exploitation of endogenous fluorophores in biologic tissue for imaging is termed autofluorescence (12). Variations in molecular composition and tissue microstructure lead to differences in fluorescence, thereby creating the potential for distinguishing neoplastic from nonneoplastic tissue. Prototype endoscopes that make use of this technology have been developed. Additional tissue characteristics based on red and green light reflectance have also been incorporated to improve the image production algorithm. The application of the concept of autofluorescence using the endoscope as the source of excitation light waves has been termed light-induced fluorescence endoscopy (LIFE).

Early fiber-optic endoscopy technology that incorporated LIFE found that inflammation as well as dysplasia leads to increased autofluorescence. The autofluorescence signal is also quite weak and difficult to identify, limiting the applicability of this technology for BE surveillance. The use of intravenous or topical fluorophores such as 5-aminolevulinic acid improved the performance of LIFE but still not to a level where it could be applied clinically (13). Kara et al. (14) compared autofluorescence-targeted biopsies with random 4-quadrant biopsies in 50 patients presenting for BE surveillance. Using a fiber-optic endoscope with the LIFE II autofluorescence system (Xillix Corp, British Columbia, Canada), the investigators found that the use of LIFE-targeted biopsies did not improve the detection of HGD and adenocarcinoma over standard white-light endoscopy with the Seattle protocol.

The value of autofluorescence endoscopy in the detection of dysplasia in BE has been improved by the development of new autofluorescence-reflectance imaging (AFI) techniques that utilize CCD endoscopes and imaging algorithms that also incorporate red/green reflectance. Investigators from Amsterdam used this prototype combined AFI system (Olympus, Inc., Tokyo, Japan). Nondysplastic BE appears green with this system, and suspected dysplastic BE appears blue/violet (Figures 17.4 and 17.5) (15). The video image is much clearer than the older fiber-optic system. In this initial unblinded pilot study, the investigators compared the rate of detection of HGD in all-comers being evaluated with BE using AFI-guided biopsies and random 4-quadrant biopsies. In 60 patients, AFI-guided biopsies increased the detection rate of HGD or adenocarcinoma from 23% to 33%. The positive predictive value of AFI-suspicious areas was 49%, while the negative predictive value was 89%.

The same investigators from Amsterdam performed a subsequent study of 20 patients with known BE with

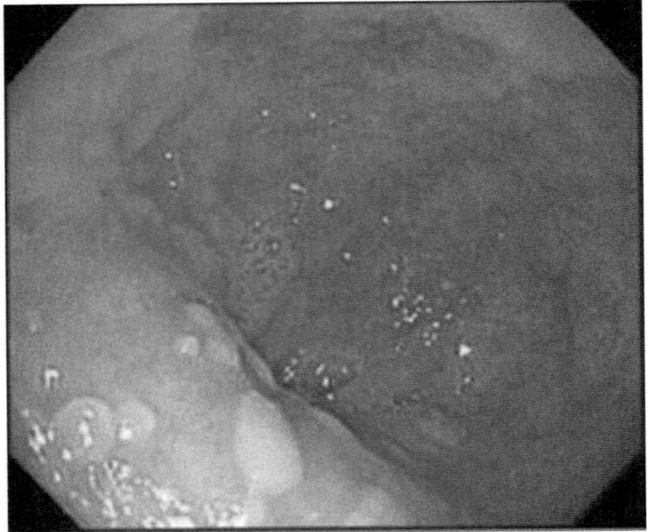

FIGURE 17.4

Barrett's esophagus with standard white-light video-endoscopy.

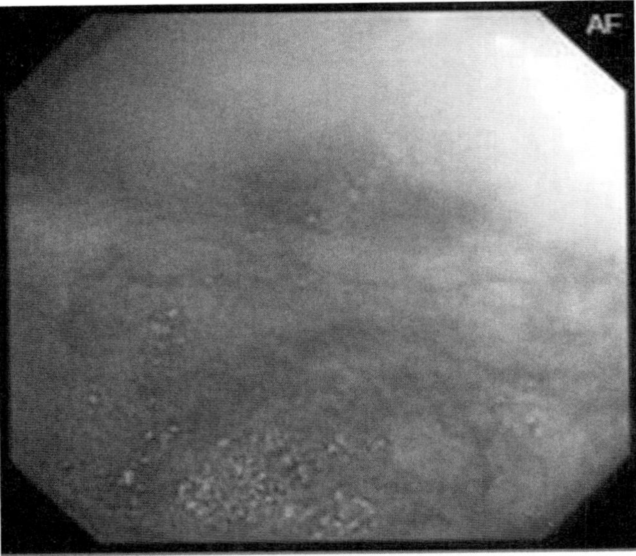

FIGURE 17.5

The same area with autofluorescence imaging. Nondyplastic Barrett's esophagus appears green, while high-grade dysplasia appears violet.

high-grade dysplasia. Suspicious areas were identified as purple areas using AFI (16). NBI examination was then performed to determine whether these areas had inflammatory or dysplastic features. Biopsies obtained from all suspicious areas were used to determine the accuracy of histologic prediction based on combined AFI and NBI. They found that the false-positive rate of AFI alone for predicting dysplasia was 40%. Additional interpretation of NBI following AFI imaging reduced false positivity to 10%. This "proof of principle" study suggests that perhaps a combination of novel imaging methods will be necessary for sensitive detection of dysplasia while maintaining reasonable specificity.

Unlike NBI, which is more of a "focal" technique, AFI is a "global" technique that can be used to scan the entire segment of BE. However, early data also show that AFI lacks the sensitivity and specificity to warrant routine use in guiding endoscopic surveillance. As AFI instruments continue to evolve, these parameters are likely to improve. The combination of 2 novel (17) imaging techniques such as AFI and NBI may ultimately prove to be an effective way of detecting dysplastic BE, although the expense of combining multiple imaging technologies might make this approach cost prohibitive.

Optical Coherence Tomography

Optical coherence tomography (OCT) is an imaging technology that allows imaging of biologic tissues to the micrometer scale (18). OCT performs imaging by sending an optical beam of infrared light into the tissues and then measures the reflected or backscattered intensity and depth of the light from various layers, planes, structures, and cell membranes within the tissues. It is conceptually analogous to B-mode ultrasound, except that OCT uses light waves rather than sound waves. Light waves derived from a low-coherence light source are delivered to an optical-fiber splitter that sends half the light to the area to be imaged and the other half to a reference mirror. By a process termed interferometry, the backscattered light from tissue and the time delay between reflected light waves from tissue and the reference mirror are processed (19–21). The resulting image is a 2-dimensional tomogram with a resolution of 1 to 15 microns and scanning depth of 1 to 3 mm. This permits examination of not just the gastrointestinal wall layers but also microstructures and possible cellular features within these wall layers. OCT is able to image dysplastic epithelium within a segment of BE. OCT uses optical fiber technology allowing for incorporation into a catheter-probe design that can be passed through an endoscope channel. Although the resolution of OCT is not quite at the level of histopathology, the aim of OCT imaging, in contrast to chromoendoscopy, NBI, and AFI, is to produce images that provide some degree of histologic detail. In this context, OCT not only can differentiate Barrett's epithelium from squamous epithelium and detect villous/crypt architecture, but also has the potential to differentiate nondysplastic BE from dysplastic BE.

Studies in the colon polyp model were initially used to determine the OCT characteristics of dysplasia—loss of tissue organization and reduced light scattering that have since been applied to the esophagus (22). In the normal esophagus, several distinct layers are clearly visualized: a relatively homogeneous epithelium, a high backscattering lamina propria, a low scattering muscularis mucosa, a high scattering submucosa, and a low scattering and thick muscularis propria (Figure 17.6) (23). In contrast, the uniformly layered structure is disrupted in BE and multiple crypt and gland-like structures are seen as pockets of low backscattering (Figures 17.7 and 17.8). Using these criteria in a double-blinded, prospective study of 33 patients with BE, Isenberg et al. (24) found that OCT had a sensitivity and specificity of 68% and 82%, respectively, for detecting dysplasia in BE. Another study by Evans et al. (25) using analogous criteria found that OCT could be used to distinguish BE from nonmetaplastic epithelium at the squamocolumnar junction. The currently available endoscopic OCT probes do not have the capability of providing images at the nuclear level and are applicable only for research purposes. However, ongoing development of these devices with improved resolution is likely to increase the diagnostic accuracy of OCT in BE.

Light-Scattering Spectroscopy

The scatter of light after interacting with tissue can help in identifying cellular characteristics because nuclei are the major organelles that cause scatter. Light-scattering spectroscopy is a variant of reflectance spectroscopy,

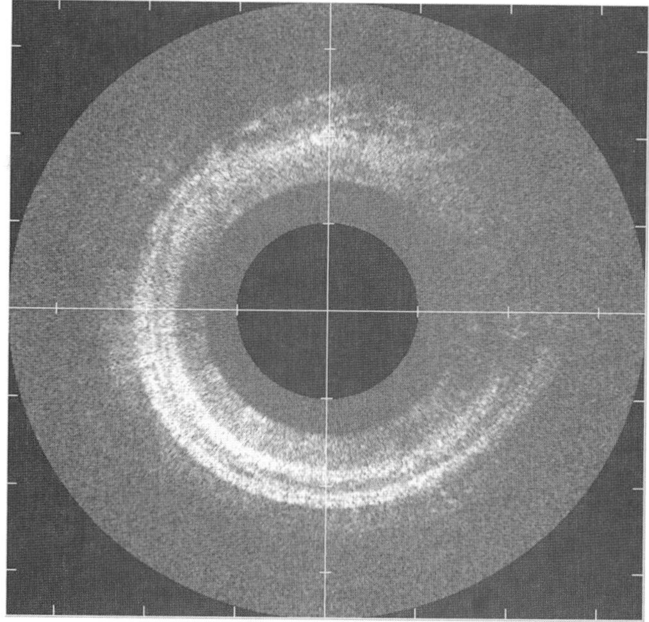

FIGURE 17.6

Optical coherence tomography image of a normal esophagus.

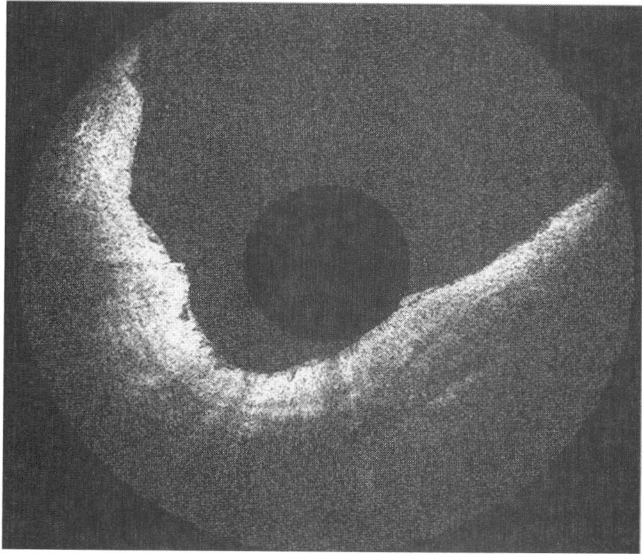

FIGURE 17.7

Optical coherence tomography image of Barrett's esophagus. Villous surface pattern is apparent.

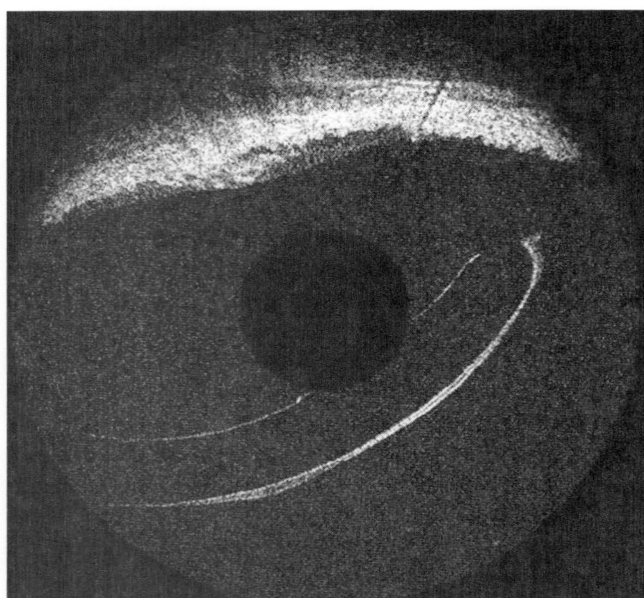

FIGURE 17.8

Optical coherence tomography image of Barrett's esophagus with high-grade dysplasia characterized by loss of tissue organization.

which examines the spectrum of multiply scattered light. It provides information about the size and density of epithelial nuclei. In vitro studies show that the composite measurements of the spectrum based on the size and clustering of the scattering particle could differentiate dysplastic Barrett's epithelium from normal epithelium with a high sensitivity and specificity (26). The processing of data with this technology is not yet rapid enough for real-time endoscopic use, and it remains a focal technique that has not been tested in the clinical setting.

Confocal Endomicroscopy

The technique of fluorescence-aided confocal endomicroscopy has been recently introduced, allowing real-time in vivo microscopy of the mucosal layer of the gastrointestinal tract and perhaps increasing detection of early neoplasia by enabling "smart," guided biopsies (27). During confocal endomicroscopy, an argon ion laser with an excitation wavelength of 488 nm emerging from the confocal unit at the tip of the endoscope is focused on the tissue, applied fluorescent material is excited by the incident laser light, and the emitted fluorescing light is exclusively detected by the confocal unit at an exactly defined horizontal level, thus producing a microscopic image of the tissue at the focal point with an optical slice thickness of 7 micrometers, lateral resolution of 0.7 micrometer, and sampling area of 450 by 450 micrometers. The image data are collected at scanning rates varying from 0.8/s to 1.6/s and the range of depth of imaging (z-axis) from 0 to 250 micrometers. The confocal endomicroscope can be used as standard video-endoscope with biopsy capabilities, and recently a miniprobe-based confocal endomicroscopic imaging system also has become commercially available. From initial reports of this technology, it appears that unlike any other endoscopic technique, confocal endomicroscopy can provide a real-time diagnosis of specialized columnar epithelium in areas of columnar-lined epithelium by identifying the pathognomic goblet cells (Figure 17.9). Potentially, this technique could identify neoplastic lesions in BE and have important implications for endoscopic therapy in BE patients. In a report of 63 patients of BE undergoing confocal endomicroscopy with histopathologic correlation, Barrett's epithelium, with its villous, dark, regular, cylindrical epithelial cells with characteristic goblets cells appearing as dark spots in the single-cell layer of the columnar-lined epithelium, could be easily identified. The typical appearance of Barrett's epithelium was readily distinguishable from gastric type epithelium, which is often seen in areas of columnar-lined epithelium and is characterized by round glandular openings and a cobblestone appearance. In addition to identification of areas of intestinal metaplasia, high-grade intraepithelial neoplasia could

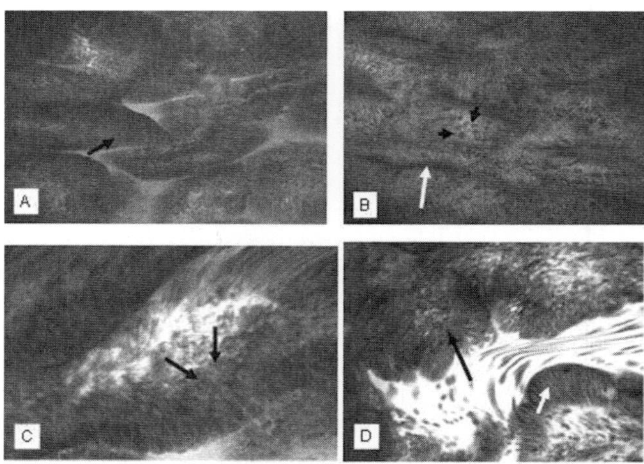

FIGURE 17.9

(A) Columnar epithelium with (dark arrow) without goblet cells. (B) Goblet cells (black arrow) and narrow lumen of a Barrett's gland (white arrow). (C) Features of high-grade dysplasia with loss of basal border (black arrows) of dysplastic cells. (D) Disorganized architecture of the gland consistent with invasive cancer (black arrow); white arrow shows a nondysplastic Barrett's gland with single-layered thin columnar epithelium.

also be identified by presence of irregular, dark, polygonal cells without a regular basal border and also by presence of an irregular capillary network in the mucosa, particularly in the deeper parts. Overall, the accuracy in identifying intestinal metaplasia in this exploratory study was reported as 97%, and the accuracy in identifying Barrett's associated neoplastic changes was also very high (28).

Given the initial reports of high accuracy of the technique of confocal endomicroscopy, it will be important to evaluate this technique in a controlled blinded fashion and compare the yield of confocal endomicroscopy guided biopsy with that of the established technique of 4-quadrant random biopsy in identifying intestinal metaplasia and early neoplasia in these patients. It is conceivable that this optical technique could even replace histologic biopsy. However, the difficulty with this microscopic technique remains the inability to examine the entire esophagus. Since it can examine only small areas, it will be subject to the same sampling error that is associated with random biopsies. It will be able to identify HGD or early cancer only if there is a morphologic finding that directs the endoscopist to image the affected area. Interpretation of confocal images will also require endoscopists to be trained in interpretation of histopathology.

Endocytoscopy

Another novel technique based on flexible catheter probe equipped with an ultra-high-magnifying video-endoscope, known as the endocytoscope, has been recently introduced. With this technique, individual cells or nuclei can be visualized in a real-time fashion with a fixed magnification of 450 times or 1,125 times in a sampling area of 300 by 300 micrometers. Although the initial reports of this technology are exciting, its clinical utility remains questionable (29,30).

CONCLUSION

Identification of the ideal endoscopic method for surveillance of BE and detection of dysplasia remains an elusive goal. Whether recent advances in endoscopic imaging such as NBI, OCT, and AFI will complement or replace some of the older methods of mucosal enhancement such as chromoendoscopy from a clinically practical standpoint is uncertain. What is clear is that the more sophisticated techniques such as OCT, confocal endomicroscopy, light-scattering spectroscopy, and endocytoscopy, which produce higher-resolution images, inevitably narrow the endoscopic "field of view," making these techniques difficult to use in scanning an entire segment of BE. In the future, combining techniques that can scan a large region and then focus in on suspicious areas for targeted biopsies may be an attractive approach. Of course, a novel imaging method will succeed only if it is not prohibitively expensive and can be mastered by practicing endoscopists.

References

1. Bruno MJ. Magnification endoscopy, high resolution endoscopy, and chromoscopy: towards a better optical diagnosis. *Gut.* 2003;52(suppl 4):iv7–iv11.
2. Canto MI, Kalloo A. Chromoendoscopy for Barrett's esophagus in the twenty-first century: to stain or not to stain? *Gastrointest Endosc.* 2006;64(2):200–205.
3. Canto MI, Setrakian S, Willis JE, et al. Methylene blue staining of dysplastic and nondysplastic Barrett's esophagus: an in vivo and ex vivo study. *Endoscopy.* 2001;33(5):391–400.
4. Sharma P, Marcon N, Wani S, et al. Non-biopsy detection of intestinal metaplasia and dysplasia in Barrett's esophagus: a prospective multi-center study. *Endoscopy.* 2006;38(12):1206–1212.
5. Olliver JR, Wild CP, Sahay P, et al. Chromoendoscopy with methylene blue and associated oxidative DNA damage in Barrett's esophagus. *Lancet.* 2003;362(9381):373–374.
6. Sharma P, Weston AP, Topalovski M, et al. Magnification chromoendoscopy for the detection of intestinal metaplasia and dysplasia in Barrett's oesophagus. *Gut.* 2003;52:24–27.
7. Tajiri H, Ikegami M, Urashima M, et al. Usefulness of magnifying endoscopy with narrow band imaging for the detection of specialized intestinal metaplasia in columnar-lined esophagus and Barrett's adenocarcinoma. *Gastrointest Endosc.* 2007;65(1):36–46.
8. Higbee A, Hall S, Weston A. The utility of a novel narrow band imaging endoscopy system in patients with Barrett's esophagus. *Gastrointest Endosc.* 2006;64(2):167–175.
9. Anagnostopoulos GK, Yao K, Kaye P, et al. Novelendoscopic observation in Barrett's oesophagus using high resolution magnification endoscopy and narrow band imaging. *Aliment Pharmacol Ther.* 2007;26(3):501–507.
10. Kara MA, Peters FP, Rosmolen WD, et al. High-resolution endoscopy plus chromoendoscopy or narrow-band imaging in Barrett's esophagus: a prospective randomized crossover study. *Endoscopy.* 2005;37(10):929–936.
11. Pohl J, May A, Rabenstein T, et al. Comparison of computed virtual chromoendoscopy and conventional chromoendoscopy with acetic acid for detection of neoplasia in Barrett's esophagus. *Endoscopy.* 2007;39(7):594–598.
12. Kara MA, Bergman JJ. Autofluorescence imaging and narrow-band imaging for the detection of early neoplasia in patients with Barrett's esophagus. *Endoscopy.* 2006;38:627–631.
13. Messmann H, Knuchel R, Baumler W, et al. Endoscopic fluorescence detection of dysplasia in patients with Barrett's esophagus, ulcerative colitis, or adenomatous polyps after 5-aminolevulinic acid-induced protoporphyrin IX sensitization. *Gastrointest Endosc.* 1999;49:97–101.
14. Kara MA, Smits ME, Rosmolen WD, et al. A randomized crossover study comparing light-induced fluorescence endoscopy with standard videoendoscopy for the detection of early neoplasia in Barrett's esophagus. *Gastrointest Endosc.* 2005;61:671–678.
15. Kara MA, Peters FP, ten Kate FJ, et al. Endoscopic video autofluorescence imaging may improve the detection of early neoplasia in patients with Barrett's esophagus. *Gastrointest Endosc.* 2005;61:679–685.
16. Kara MA, Peters FP, Fockens P, et al. Endoscopic video-autofluoroescence imaging followed by narrow band imaging for detecting early neoplasia in Barrett's esophagus. *Gastrointest Endosc.* 2006;64:176–185.
17. Borovicka J, Fischer J, Neuweiler J, et al. Autofluorescence endoscopy in surveillance of Barrett's esophagus: a multicenter randomized trial on diagnostic efficacy. *Endoscopy.* 2006;38:867–872.
18. Huang HD, Swanson EA, Lin CP, et al. Optical coherence tomography. *Science.* 1991;254:1178–1181.
19. Chak A, Wallace MB, Poneros JM. Optical coherence tomography of Barrett's esophagus. *Endoscopy.* 2005;37:587–590.
20. Li XD, Boppart SA, Van Dam, J et al. Optical coherence tomography: advanced technology for the endoscopic imaging of Barrett's esophagus. *Endoscopy.* 2000;32:921–930.
21. Evans JA, Nishioka NS. The use of optical coherence tomography in screening and surveillance of Barrett's esophagus. *Clin Gastroenterol Hepatol.* 2005;3:S8–S11.

22. Pfau PR, Sivak MV, Chak A, et al. Criteria for the diagnosis of dysplasia by endoscopic optical coherence tomography. *Gastrointest Endosc.* 2003;59:196–202.
23. Sivak MV Jr, Kobayashi K, Izatt JA, et al. High-resolution endoscopic imaging of the GI tract using optical coherence tomography. *Gastrointest Endosc.* 2000;51:474–479.
24. Isenberg G, Sivak MV, Chak A, et al. Accuracy of endoscopic optical coherence tomography in the detection of dysplasia in Barrett's esophagus: a prospective, double-blinded study. *Gastrointest Endosc.* 2005;62:825–831.
25. Evans JA, Nishioka NS. The use of optical coherence tomography in screening and surveillance of Barrett's esophagus. *Clin Gastroenterol Hepatol.* 2005;3:S8–S11.
26. Wallace MB, Perelman LT, Backman V, et al. Endoscopic detection of dysplasia in patients with Barrett's esophagus using light-scattering spectroscopy. *Gastroenterology.* 2000;119(3):677–682.
27. Hoffman A, Goetz M, Vieth M, et al. Confocal laser endomicroscopy: technical status and current indications. *Endoscopy.* 2006;38(12):1275–1283.
28. Kiesslich R, Gossner L, Goetz M, et al. In vivo histology of Barrett's esophagus and associated neoplasia by confocal laser endomicroscopy. *Clin Gastroenterol Hepatol.* 2006;4:979–987.
29. Koch M, Khalifa A, Papanikolaou IS, et al. Evaluation of endocytoscopy in the surveillance of patients with Barrett's esophagus. *Endoscopy.* 2007;39(6):492–496.
30. Fujishiro M, Takubo K, Sato Y, et al. Potential and present limitation of endocytoscopy in the diagnosis of esophageal squamous-cell carcinoma: a multicenter ex vivo pilot study. *Gastrointest Endosc.* 2007;66(3):551–555.

18 Esophageal Imaging: Anatomic

Gregory G. Ginsberg

This chapter details endoscopic and endoscopic ultrasound (EUS) imaging and staging of esophageal tumors including squamous cell carcinoma (SCCA), adenocarcinoma (ADCA), and subepithelial neoplasms. Enhanced endoscopic imaging and endoscopic mucosal resection contributions are detailed elsewhere, as are complimentary cross-sectional imaging, positron-emission tomography, and clinical staging.

ENDOSCOPY IN SUSPECTED ESOPHAGEAL CANCER

Flexible endoscopy is indicated in suspected esophageal carcinoma. Endoscopy allows direct visualization of the esophagus as well as tissue sampling to confirm the diagnosis. Endoscopy may also facilitate initial relief of dysphagia in that dilation can be performed at the time of diagnosis.

Endoscopy allows accurate characterization of the tumor's configuration, length, and localization. These features may provide clues as to the histopathology (Figures 18.1 and 18.2). SCCA are more apt to occur in the upper and middle thirds of the esophagus, and ADCA are more apt to occur in the lower third and at the level of the esophagogastric junction (EGJ). However, both SCCA and ADCA may be found continuously or discontinuously throughout the esophagus. SCCA of the esophagus is an aggressively invasive tumor, and esophagorespiratory fistulas occur more commonly because of direct tumor extension.

Advanced lesions typically appear endophytic as polypoid, fungating, or ulcerated masses. Lesions may be eccentric or circumferential. Coincident Barrett's appearing epithelium may be recognizable associated with ADCA, but in advanced lesions the tumor will have overtaken any preexisting Barrett's esophagus (BE), and as such no associated BE will be recognizable. Otherwise, there are no particularly distinguishing morphologic features to distinguish advanced SCCA from ADCA based on endoscopic imaging alone. In many instances, it is difficult or impossible to categorize ADCA involving the EGJ as a primary gastric cardia cancer extending proximally versus true a EGJ ADCA versus a lower esophageal ADCA extending distally. Occasionally, this difficulty with designation may vex treatment decision making.

Standard endoscopic forceps biopsy typically yields the histopathologic diagnosis. Brush cytology may be used as a complementary technique to enhance the yield in establishing a diagnosis. Biopsy procedures should be directed at nonnecrotic-appearing areas. At least 6 biopsy samples should be obtained to yield an accuracy approaching 100% (1). Both tumor types

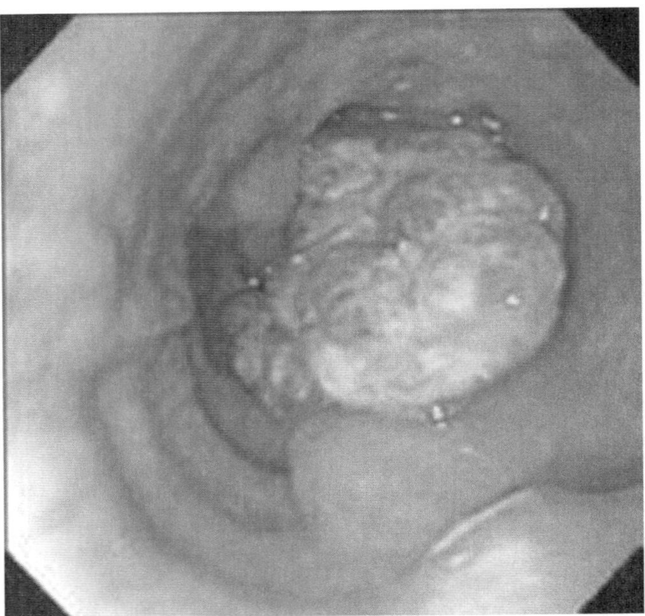

FIGURE 18.1

Endoscopic image of an esophageal squamous cell carcinoma of the mid-esophagus arising from a background of otherwise normal-appearing esophageal mucosa.

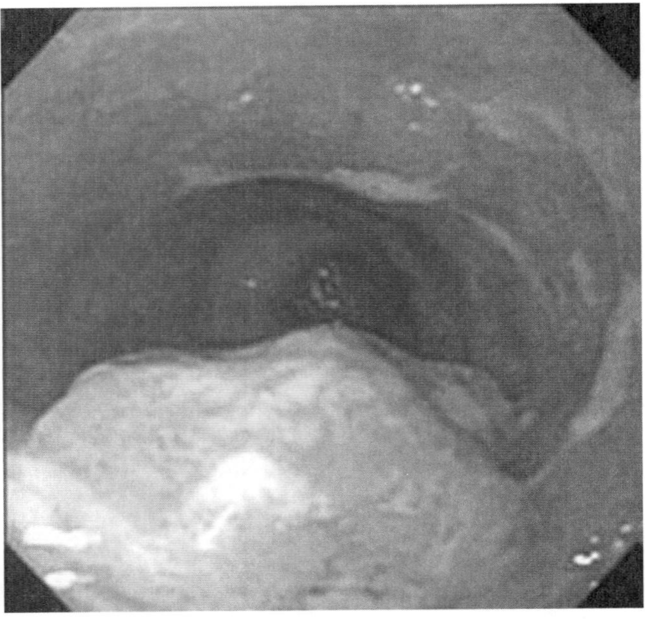

FIGURE 18.2

Endoscopic image of esophageal adenocarcinoma in the mid-esophagus arising at the proximal aspect of long-segment Barrett's metaplasia.

may also exhibit an infiltrative submucosal spreading process with no appreciable intraluminal mass. These submucosal spreading tumors undermine histopathologically normal-appearing epithelium. Tumors that show these characteristics may defy a histologic diagnosis by endoscopic biopsy forceps tissue sampling. When this is suspected, EUS-guided fine-needle aspiration (FNA) may be considered to clarify and confirm the diagnosis. Undermining submucosal carcinomas at the EGJ may mimic achalasia and as such is termed *pseudoachalasia.*

In contrast to advanced lesions, early cancers are more likely to be asymptomatic. Screening, surveillance, and serendipitous endoscopy may permit the diagnosis of intramucosal and superficial submucosal cancers. Not surprisingly, these early cancers have better prognoses compared to advanced cancers and may by amenable to curative nonoperative therapies. While screening and surveillance in BE and state-of-the-art esophageal mucosal imaging are covered elsewhere in this book, the following observations regarding early SCCA are offered for completeness. Dysplastic squamous mucosa may appear normal; flat, raised, or depressed; nodular; or pale or erythematous or as an erosion or plaque. When screening is performed endoscopically, visual inspection to identify pathology is the first step. If dysplasia or cancer is endoscopically recognizable, these lesions can be targeted directly. If there are no visible lesions, then a large number of systematic biopsies should be taken. Early detection of SCCA may be enhanced by vital staining with diluted Lugol's solution delivered endoscopically through a spray catheter. Lugol's solution is rapidly taken up by normal squamous mucosa, in contrast to dysplastic or malignant squamous epithelium, which remains unstained (Figure 18.3). This technique may also be applied to detect the extent of mucosal surface involvement when endoscopic therapy is being contemplated for macroscopically recognized lesions. Tissue sampling from the unstained areas confirms the presence and extent of mucosal involvement.

ENDOSCOPIC ULTRASOUND IN ESOPHAGEAL CANCER

To image into and through the luminal digestive tract, EUS incorporates flexible endoscopy and high-frequency ultrasound. It enables the endosonographer to evaluate the wall layer pattern of the esophagus and to detect the presence of regional and celiac lymph nodes. EUS-guided FNA permits directed tissue sampling of subdiaphragmatic and mediastinal lymph nodes. EUS is used for staging esophageal cancer and in the evaluation and management of patients with BE and high-grade dysplasia (HGD).

EUS is available in an endoscope-based system and a catheter-based system. The endoscope-based systems

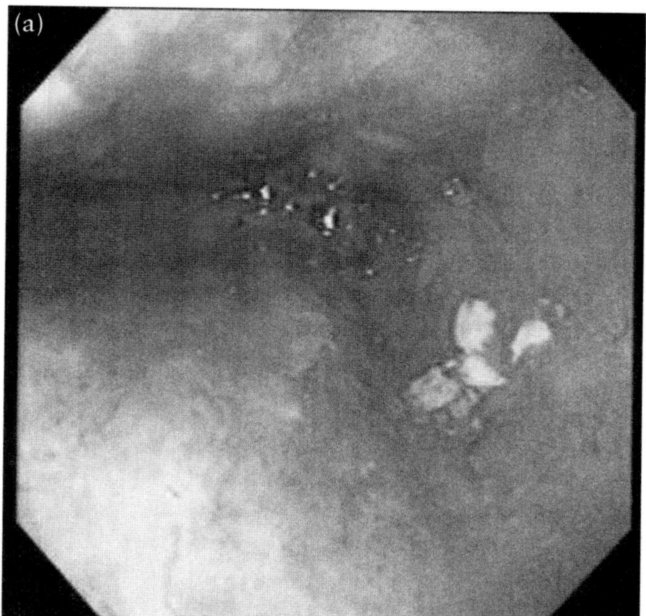

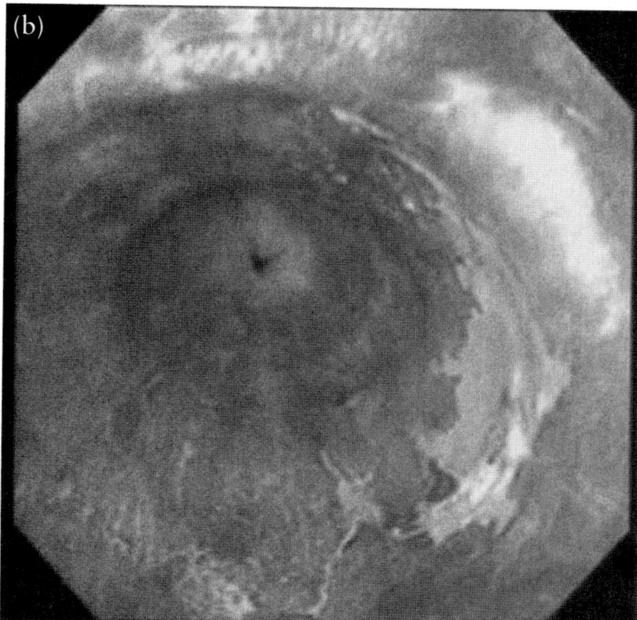

FIGURE 18.3

The unstained image on the left (a) shows only slightly nodular esophageal mucosa. Biopsies had demonstrated squamous cell carcinoma in situ. After Lugol's staining, the image on the right (b) demonstrates broad areas of unstained mucosa, directing targeted sampling or endoscopic resection.

are divided into radial and linear array scanning systems. The radial echoendoscope uses a mechanically rotated transducer to generate a real-time 360-degree cross-sectional image perpendicular to the long axis of the instrument. Radial scanning echoendoscopes provide imaging at 5, 7.5, 12, and 20 MHz.

The linear array echoendoscope has an electronically operated transducer that produces a ~270-degree real-time image parallel to the long axis of the endoscope. The linear array echoendoscope permits FNA under direct EUS guidance. The linear array echoendoscope also has power Doppler capability, allowing confirmation of vascular structures.

High-frequency catheter ultrasound probes may be passed through the accessory channel of a forward viewing endoscope, allowing visually directed probe localization and substituting for a dedicated scope-based system. The catheter-based probes may be placed directly over a small target lesion. The probes are available as 2, 2.4, and 2.6 mm in diameter with frequencies of 12, 15, and 20 MHz. These high-frequency probes may delineate up to 7 to 9 layers within the esophageal wall but at the expense of a limited depth of penetration.

EUS more typically generates a 5-layer wall pattern of alternating hyperechogenicity (bright) and hypoechogenicity (dark) that correlates with histology (Figure 18.4). To improve acoustic coupling, scanning is performed with water immersion or with a water-filled balloon sheath over the probe.

EUS is used in the evaluation of regional lymph nodes. Mediastinal lymph nodes may be detected by EUS in disease and health. Lymph nodes appear as spheroid, ovoid, or pyramidal echogenicities. It may be difficult to differentiate between malignant and benign nodes with imaging alone. Sonographic characteristics of malignant lymph nodes include size greater than 1 cm in diameter, hypoechogenicity, and round in shape with sharp borders (2). The introduction of FNA increases the accuracy of EUS in detecting malignant nodes (3). The presence of malignant appearing lymph nodes in patients with suspected "early" cancer, based on endoscopy and computer tomography (CT) scan findings, would support operative rather than endoscopic therapy. Doppler elastography and computer analyses may enhance the EUS discrimination between benign and malignant lymph nodes (4,5).

ENDOSCOPIC ULTRASOUND STAGING OF ESOPHAGEAL CANCER

Esophageal cancer is highly lethal. The prognosis and treatment of esophageal cancer is dependent upon the

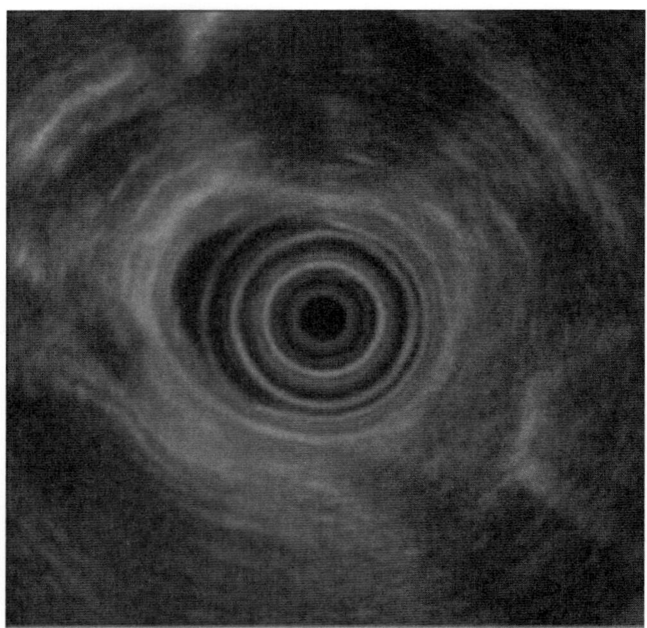

FIGURE 18.4

Esophageal endoscopic ultrasound generates a 5-layer wall pattern of alternating hyperechogenicity (bright) and hypoechogenicity (dark) that correlates with the superficial mucosa (first bright layer), deep mucosa including the muscularis mucosa (first dark layer), the submucosa (second bright layer), the muscularis propria (second dark layer), and the adventitia (third bright layer). The endoscopic ultrasound transducer is central with surrounding water-filled coupling balloon. In this image, the anechoic descending aorta is at 12:00 and azygous vein at 9:00.

stage of the disease at the time of diagnosis. The staging of esophageal carcinoma is based upon the tumor, node, and metastasis classification (detailed elsewhere in this volume) (6). The biologic behavior of advanced SCCA and ADCA are sufficiently similar to permit their coincident consideration here. Once the diagnosis of esophageal cancer is made, cross-sectional imaging should be performed to evaluate for liver and other distant lymph node metastases. CT scanning is most commonly employed. Positron-emission tomography (PET) scanning is gaining increasing acceptance for the detection of distant metastases as well. In the absence of distant metastases, EUS is recommended for local tumor and nodal staging when stage-based therapy is being considered. The T staging of esophageal ADCA is demonstrated in (Figure 18.5).

EUS more accurately determines T stage and regional lymphadenopathy as compared to other imaging modalities (7,8). Staging accuracy holds for both esophageal SCCA and ADCA. The T stage of esophageal carcinoma can help to predict the N stage. The relationship between the T stage and N stage was studied in a retrospective review of 359 patients undergoing esophagectomy for esophageal carcinoma. The prevalence of regional lymph nodes in patients with ADCA with invasion into the lamina propria and muscularis mucosa (T1 intramucosal) was 2.8%. The prevalence of regional lymph nodes increased with the depth of tumor invasion ($P < 0.0001$) (9). A comparison of CT scan, laparoscopic ultrasound, and EUS was made in a group of 36 patients for staging of esophagogastric carcinoma (7). CT scan was more accurate in locally advanced tumors (T3 and T4) when compared with EUS, 95% versus 88%, respectively. EUS performed superiorly when assessing early tumors and locoregional nodal involvement with accuracies of 62% and 72%, respectively. Distant metastases were more accurately detected with laparoscopic ultrasound (81%) compared with CT scan (72%). Another study performed by Wallace et al. (10) showed that combination imaging tests (i.e., PET with EUS/FNA or CT scan with EUS/FNA) proved to be more cost effective in a decision analysis model. EUS is also superior to CT scanning for detection of celiac lymph nodes. In a study of 62 patients, EUS was used to evaluate celiac lymph

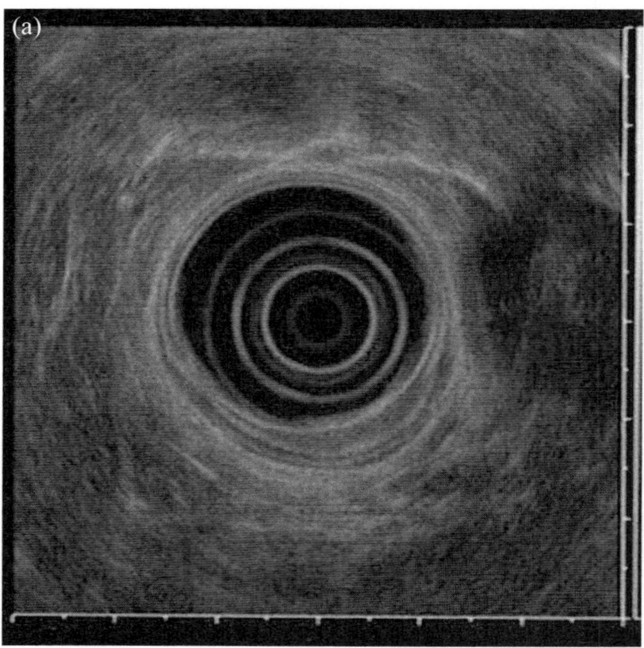

FIGURE 18.5

T1 lesions are limited to the mucosa and submucosal layers (first 3 layers) (a); T2 lesions invade into but not though the muscularis propria (fourth) layer (b); T3 lesions penetrate through the muscularis propria and into the periesophageal fat (c); T4 lesions directly invade vital surrounding structures, like the aorta, as seen here (d); and regional metastases are seen as enlarged spheroid hypoechoic periesophageal lymph nodes (e).

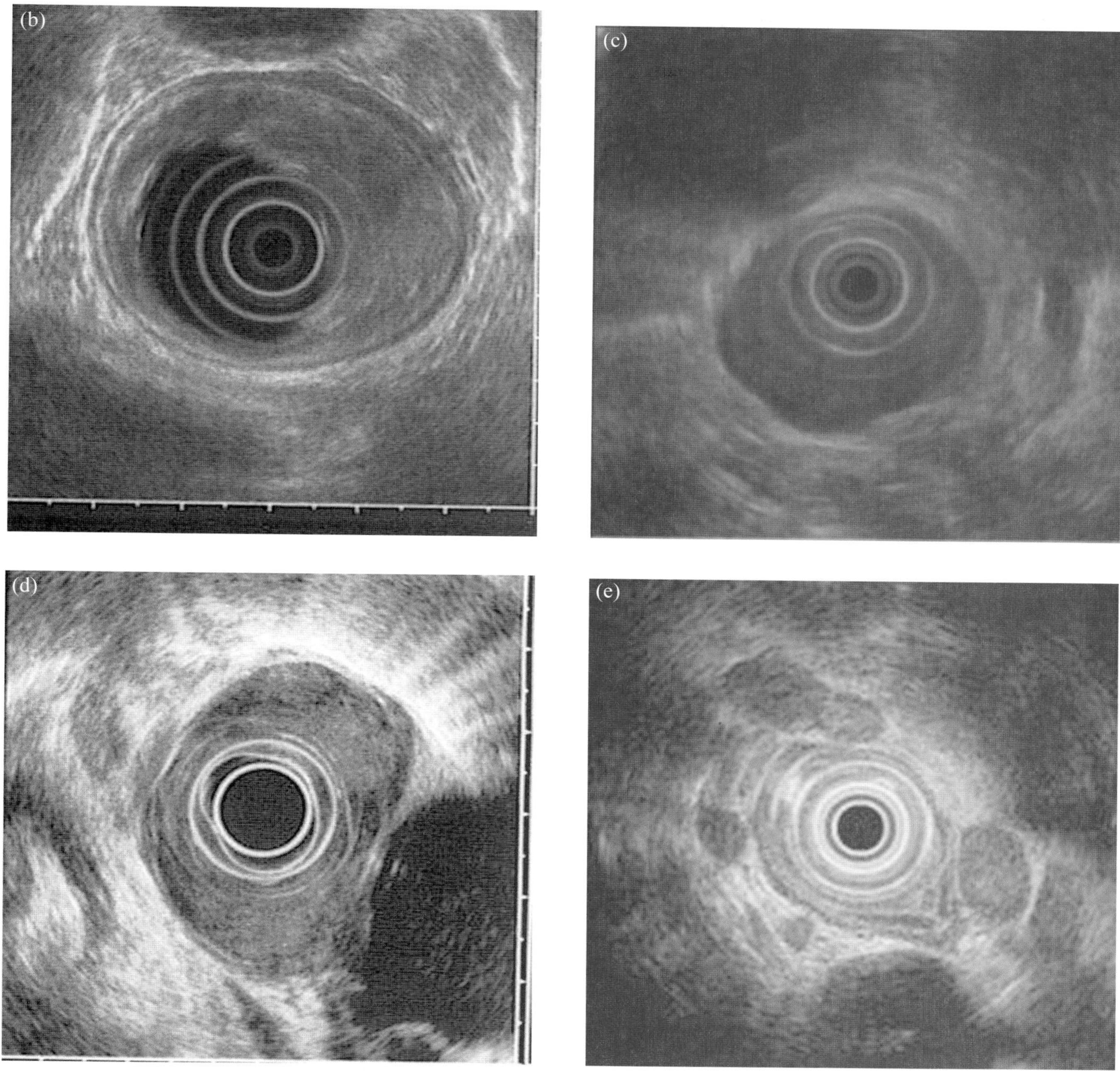

FIGURE 18.5 (*continued*)

nodes in 95% of the patients. EUS was positive in 19 patients, and CT scan was positive in 2. The sensitivity and specificity of EUS was 72% and 97%, respectively, versus 8% and 100%, respectively, for CT scan. EUS with FNA can identify patients with M1a disease (i.e., positive celiac lymphadenopathy) and therefore helps direct management (11). This more accurate staging identifies patients with advanced locoregional disease who would benefit most from preoperative neoadjuvant chemoradiation therapy (12).

IMPACT OF ENDOSCOPIC ULTRASOUND STAGING IN ESOPHAGEAL CANCER

Staging of EUS has a positive clinical impact in patients with esophageal cancer. Hiele et al. (13) analyzed the survival data of 86 patients who underwent EUS for staging of tumors of the esophagus or EGJ. A surgical resection was performed in 73 patients. Survival of patients was significantly dependent on EUS T staging

($P = 0.05$), EUS N staging ($P = 0.02$), and the presence of stenosis ($P = 0.02$). The worst prognosis was related to patients with celiac lymph node metastasis ($P = 0.0027$). In this study there was a decreased accuracy of T staging (59%). The majority of patients went to surgery, and only 1 patient had preoperative chemoradiation. Another study by Harewood et al. (14) compared the outcomes of patients diagnosed with esophageal cancer in 1998 (i.e., pre-EUS) to patients diagnosed in 2000 after EUS had become available. Tumor recurrence and survival was better in the EUS group. This study demonstrated that EUS more accurately identified patients who benefited from preoperative neoadjuvant therapy. In this study, there were 5 patients with T1 disease who had endoscopic mucosal resection (EMR) performed and therefore did not require surgery. There are now a number of studies that suggest that preoperative chemoradiation provides the best results for patients with stage II and III cancer. In this regard, it is important to identify these patients so that they receive the most appropriate care. EUS can provide more accurate staging and therefore improve patient outcome.

EUS staging in esophageal cancer also contributes to cost-effectiveness. Shumaker et al. (15) performed a retrospective review of the CORI database to identify patients who had a preoperative EUS for esophageal carcinoma. Cost analysis was done on 188 procedures. It was assumed that patients with stage I disease would go directly to surgery, while patients with stage IV disease would not have combined modality therapy. In this study group, 26% of patients were spared the combined modality therapy and that resulted in a projected cost savings. A prospective case series by Chang et al. (16) demonstrated similar findings. In this study, there was decreased cost of care by $12,340 per patient by reducing the number of thoracotomies because of improved staging. Harewood et al. (17) used a computer model to determine the cost of EUS in the staging of esophageal cancer. In this study, EUS FNA provided the least costly approach to patients with celiac lymph node involvement as compared with CT FNA and surgery. The data are dependent on the prevalence of celiac lymph nodes of 16%. These 3 studies show that there is a cost savings for patients that have EUS performed because more accurate staging permits more appropriate individualized therapy.

ENDOSCOPIC ULTRASOUND IN ESOPHAGEAL CANCER WITH STENOSIS

Concurrent luminal stenosis does not permit the echoendoscope to traverse the tumor in up to 30% of cases of esophageal cancer at presentation. In these cases, stricture dilation of up to 12 to 15 mm is required to permit passage of the EUS scope. This is compelling, as it is necessary to provide complete staging to include inspection for celiac adenopathy. When tumor stenosis is encountered, several options are available, including dilation to allow passage of the echoendoscope or the use of miniprobes or aborting the procedure with limited staging information. In that the risk of perforation accompanies dilation of malignant strictures, these options should be individualized. In an early experience, Van Dam et al. (18) reported a complication rate of 24%. In this study, the strictures were dilated up to 18 mm to accommodate larger-diameter, more primitive echoendoscopes, which may have contributed to the high complication rate. A later study performed by Pfau et al. (19) included 81 patients who required dilation to allow passage of the Olympus GF-UM-30 echoendoscope. The dilations were performed in a stepwise fashion with fixed-diameter wire-guided tapered dilation catheters or through-the-scope hydrostatic dilating balloons to about 14 mm. The majority of dilations were performed in 1 session. Immediately following dilation, the echoendoscope was able to traverse the stricture in 85.2% of patients. There were no complications. Similar results were obtained by Kallimanis et al. (20). Given these findings, and with the further reduction in EUS scope diameters, stepwise dilation can generally be safely performed to allow complete tumor and nodal staging in patients with esophageal cancer and malignant stenosis.

The use of catheter ultrasound miniprobes is another means of tumor staging in patients with a tight esophageal stricture related to tumor. The miniprobes can be passed through the accessory channel of the endoscope and through the stricture under fluoroscopic guidance. A study was carried out by Menzel et al. (21) to compare the results of the echoendoscope, GF-UM3 (Olympus, Melville, NY), plus esophagoprobe with the miniprobe. The T staging overall was more accurate with the miniprobe as compared with the echoendoscope plus esophagoprobe, 62% versus 86.8%. The miniprobe was also more accurate with regard to the presence or absence of periesophageal lymph nodes. There were no complications reported with the use of the miniprobes. However, these results have not been repeated, and most authorities perceive that high-frequency miniprobes do not provide a depth of imaging to satisfy tumor and lymph node assessment in large tumors.

ENDOSCOPIC ULTRASOUND IN BARRETT'S ESOPHAGUS

In BE, there is a thickening of the esophageal wall that can be detected by EUS (Figure 18.2). Srivastava et al.

(22) compared the esophageal wall thickness of patients with BE and those without using the Olympus EU-M3 at 12 MHz. The 15 patients with BE were split into those with dysplasia and those without. In the control group, the esophageal wall thickness was 2.6 mm, the nondysplastic BE group had a wall thickness of 3.3, and those with dysplasia measured 4.0 mm. The difference between the nondysplastic measurement and the dysplastic measurement was not statistically significant ($P < 0.01$). The only patients with esophageal wall thickness greater than 4 mm had dysplasia. There were 2 patients with a focal carcinoma with otherwise unsuspected submucosal invasion as proved on surgical pathology. Adrain et al. (23) performed a similar study with high-resolution endoluminal sonographic examination using a 20-MHz ultrasound transducer. In this series of patients, BE was identified by EUS as a second (hypoechoic) layer of the esophageal mucosa that was thicker than the first (hyperechoic) layer. All 17 patients with BE were correctly identified (100% sensitivity). Ten of the 12 controls were identified as normal (specificity 86%). This study was not able to differentiate those patients with dysplasia, but only 2 patients had dysplasia. Kinjo et al. (24) took this analysis one step further by investigating the cost-effectiveness of EUS in patients with BE. In 39 of 56 patients with BE, the esophageal wall appeared thickened as compared with controls ($P < 0.005$). Based on EUS imaging, the endosonographers could not differentiate patients with BE and no dysplasia, low-grade dysplasia, or HGD. There was a false-positive rate of 13% in detecting cancer in patients with BE and ADCA.

EUS cannot reliably differentiate between the presence and absence of dysplasia in the setting of BE. Hence, EUS is not indicated for routine screening or surveillance in patients with nondysplastic BE.

ENDOSCOPIC ULTRASOUND IN BARRETT'S ESOPHAGUS WITH DYSPLASIA

EUS may be considered in selected patients with BE and HGD because coexistent ADCA may be detected in 30% to 47% of cases (25–27). The clinical evaluation of EUS in this setting has yielded conflicting results. Falk et al. (28) performed preoperative EUS on 9 patients with HGD and intramucosal carcinoma. Four of the 6 patients with HGD were correctly diagnosed as T0. The 2 patients who were overstaged had mucosal nodularity. EUS identified tumor in only 1 of 3 patients with intramucosal carcinoma. In this small group of patients, EUS did not reliably predict the presence of intramucosal carcinoma in patients with BE and HGD. Conversely, a larger study by Scotiniotis et al. (29) reported more promising results. In 22 patients with BE and HGD or intramucosal carcinoma, preoperative EUS findings were compared to surgical pathology. The emphasis in this study was the detection of locally confined versus advanced carcinoma, specifically the presence or absence of submucosal invasion or regional lymphadenopathy. EUS accurately predicted the absence of submucosal invasion as confirmed by surgical pathology in all 16 patients who were stage Tcis or T1a. EUS correctly predicted submucosal invasion confirmed by histopathology in 5 of 6 patients (83% positive predictive value). There was 1 false-positive prediction of submucosal invasion by EUS. The specificity of T stage was 94%. EUS overstaged suspected lymphadenopathy as malignant in 4 cases (18%) but did not understage in any of the cases.

EUS of BE can change the staging that was originally predicted by esophagogastroscopy (EGD) (30). A total of 45 patients with BE with HGD had an EGD and EUS performed. Fifteen patients were suspected endoscopically to have tumor present, while 30 patients were thought to have just dysplasia. Thirty-six patients underwent surgical resection. The BE segment staging and nodal staging were accurate in the majority of patients. Six of the 30 patients not suspected of having cancer on EGD were felt to have cancer by EUS. Five of these, 83%, were found to have cancer on surgical resection. In this study, EUS helped to identify occult malignancy. These results support the use of EUS when nonoperative therapy is being considered in patients with BE with HGD and/or intramucosal carcinoma.

EUS is indicated in patients with BE with dysphagia and/or a focal nodule or stricture, as there is an increased likelihood of underlying carcinoma. Patients with a stricture or a nodule have an increased likelihood of submucosal invasion (29). There were 12 patients in the Scotiniotis study with a nodule and/or stricture. Five patients in this group had lesions that invaded into the submucosa; conversely, there was no submucosal invasion in the group with BE and no macroscopically recognizable lesions (Fisher exact test, 42% vs. 0%, $P = 0.04$). In an earlier study (28), the presence of the nodularity in BE with HGD and carcinoma resulted in overstaging of the tumor. In the Scotiniotis study, the patients were on acid-suppressive medications prior to the endoscopic examination, which may have reduced inflammation as a contributor to false-positive staging.

Endoluminal eradication therapies employing resection and/or ablation techniques are being increasingly applied to patients with HGD and early cancer. Endoscopic mucosal resection techniques allows for further histopathologic staging confirmation that compliment EUS staging in this selected patient population (31,32) (Figure 18.6).

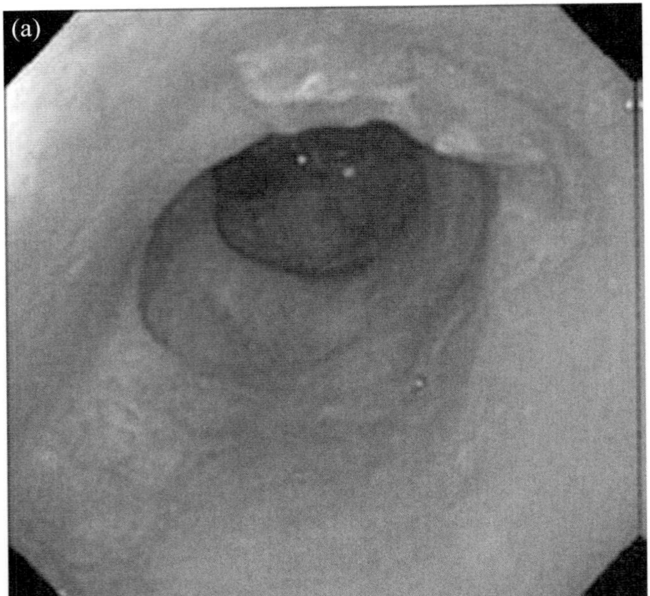

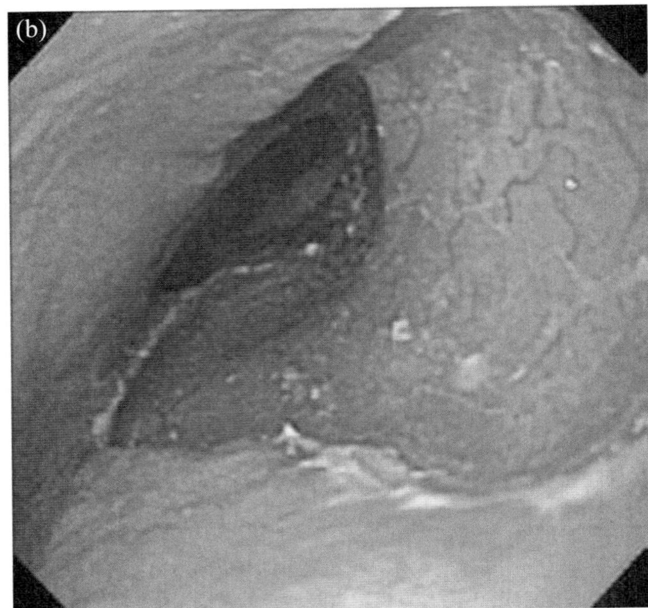

FIGURE 18.6

High-grade epithelial dysplasia was detected on forceps biopsies obtained from focal mucosal nodularity within a Barrett's segment (a). When endoscopic ultrasound identified mural thickening limited to the mucosal layers, piecemeal wide-area endoscopic resection was performed (b). Histopathology from the resected specimens confirmed moderately differentiated adenocarcinoma with invasion into but not through the muscularis mucosa.

LIMITATIONS OF ENDOSCOPIC ULTRASOUND IN BARRETT'S ESOPHAGUS AND ESOPHAGEAL CANCER

EUS is operator dependent, and as such the training and experience of the endosonographer are likely to impact EUS staging accuracy. In one study (33), interobserver agreement among experienced endosonographers was excellent for all T stages except for T2. There was good concordance for EUS stage T1, T3, and T4 lesions, but it was poor for T2 lesions. In the less experienced group of endosonographers, the agreement for T staging was poor at all stages but was satisfactory for lymph node detection.

EUS artifacts can be created by oblique scanning and balloon compression of the esophageal wall. These artifacts may result in overstaging of the tumor. Ideally, the echoendoscope should be placed perpendicular to the tissue being examined. The balloon should be inflated so as to permit acoustic coupling but not so as to compress the esophageal wall and thereby distort imaging. The anatomic configuration at the EGJ may not permit ideal transducer positioning for tumor staging of lesions that extend to and beyond that region. The tubular esophagus does not lend itself to water filling, so circumstances are encountered in which acoustic coupling cannot be ideally achieved.

OTHER EPITHELIAL AND NONEPITHELIAL TUMORS

Other Malignant Epithelial Tumors of the Esophagus

Squamous Cell Carcinoma Variants

An uncommon variant of SCCA, verrucous carcinoma, is characterized by an exophytic papillary growth (34). Carcinosarcomas (SCCA mixed with spindle cell elements) may be solitary or multiple. They are often large polypoid lesions occurring more commonly in men (35). (See Table 18.1 for classifcation of esophageal tumors.)

Small Cell Carcinoma

The esophagus is the most common extrapulmonary site of small cell carcinoma. Primary small cell carcinomas of the esophagus account for 0.8% to 4.7% of all esophageal neoplasms (36). Like SCCA, small cell tumors metastasize early and are highly lethal. Their endoscopic and EUS features are indistinguishable from SCCA.

Malignant Melanoma

Primary esophageal melanoma is rare and is estimated to account for 0.1% of esophageal tumors (37). It is

TABLE 18.1
Classification of Esophageal Tumors

Epithelial tumors	Nonepithelial tumors
Malignant	Malignant
Squamous cell carcinoma	Lymphoma
Adenocarcinoma of the esophagus	Sarcoma
Adenocarcinoma of the esophagogastric junction	Metastatic carcinoma
Verrucous carcinoma	
Carcinosarcoma	
Small cell carcinoma	
Malignant melanoma	
Benign	Benign
Squamous papilloma	Leiomyoma
Adenoma	Granular cell tumor
Inflammatory fibroid polyps	Fibrovascular tumor
	Hemangioma
	Hamartoma
	Lipoma

suspected when primary skin, ocular, and anal melanoma are ruled out. Primary esophageal melanomas begin as polypoid tumors. When they grow large and ulcerate, bleeding and odynophagia are the presenting symptoms.

Benign Epithelial Tumors of the Esophagus

Squamous Papilloma

Squamous cell papillomas (Figure 18.7) are usually small, white or pink, sessile or polypoid benign tumors that are histologically composed of finger-like projections of lamina propria covered by hyperplastic squamous epithelium (38). Mucosal biopsy or endoscopic mucosal resection is safe, diagnostic, and therapeutic. Squamous papilloma of the esophagus does not appear to predispose to esophageal cancer, and there is no apparent association with human papilloma virus.

Adenoma

True adenomatous polyps, arising within segments of esophageal or EGJ specialized intestinal metaplasia, are occasionally observed. They are benign but are considered dysplastic with malignant potential similar to that of adenomas elsewhere in the digestive tract (39). In addition, they may harbor unsuspected carcinoma. They may be sessile or pedunculated. Endoscopic management using standard snare or injection mucosectomy techniques may be curative.

Inflammatory Fibroid Polyps

Inflammatory fibroid polyps are rare in the esophagus (40,41). These nonneoplastic polyps are also called *inflammatory pseudopolyps* and *eosinophilic granulomas*. Chronic inflammation from gastroesophageal reflux disease (GERD) is thought to have a causal role. They occur in the distal esophagus or at the EGJ. Endoscopic resection yields diagnosis and cure.

Malignant Nonepithelial Tumors

Lymphoma

Lymphomatous involvement of the esophagus is generally due to extrinsic compression or direct invasion from mediastinal lymph nodes. Except in patients with acquired immunodeficiency syndrome (AIDS), the esophagus is rarely the primary site of extranodal lymphoma (42). B cell lymphoma is most common. The endoscopic appearance may be exophytic or ulcerative. Esophageal fistulas are common. When forceps biopsy is nondiagnostic, EUS-guided FNA of the mural tumor or predictably present surrounding lymphadenopathy yield the diagnosis.

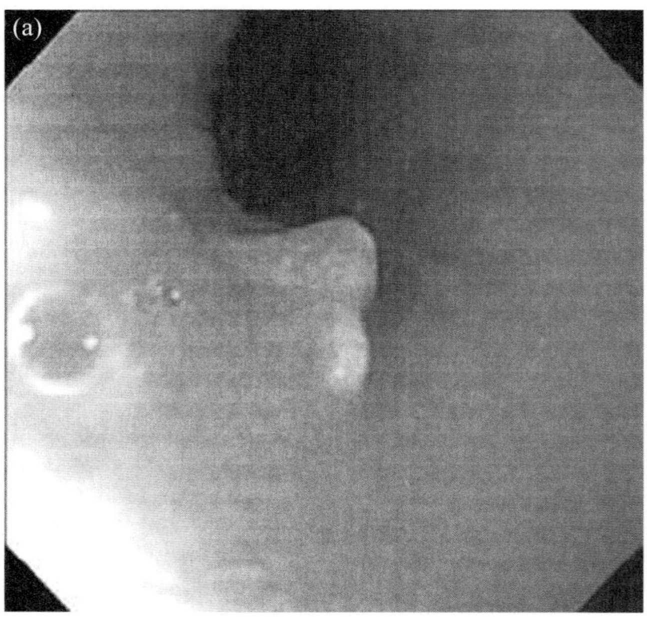

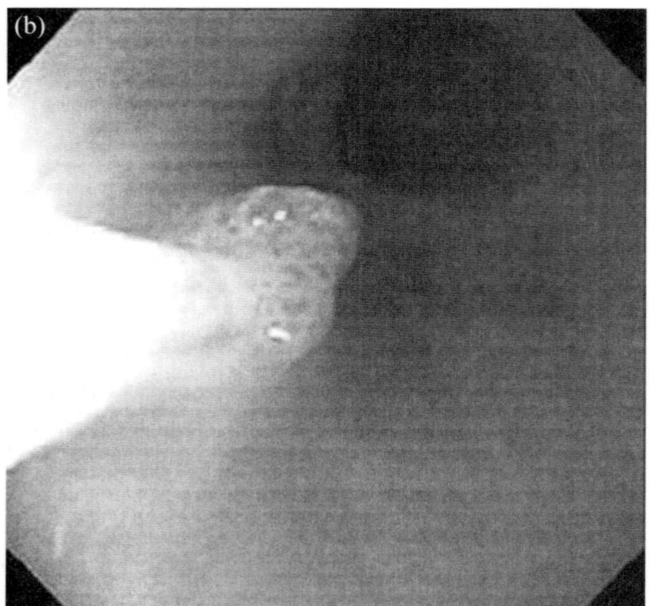

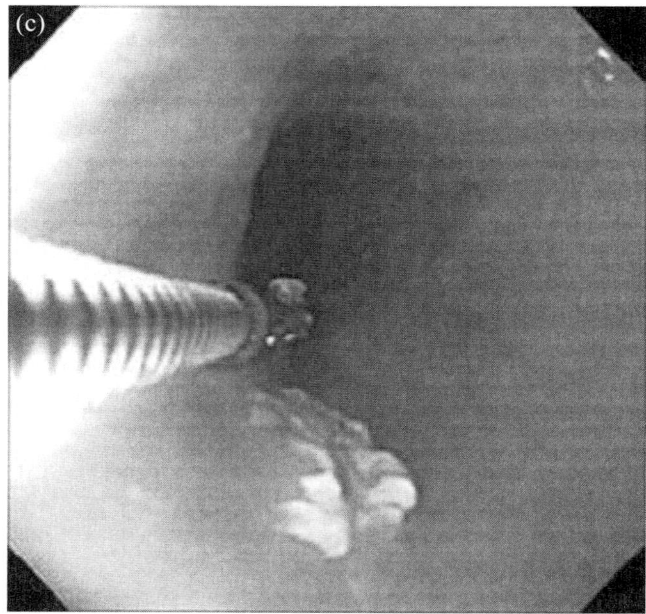

FIGURE 18.7

A typical esophageal squamous papilloma is seen in the proximal esophagus (a). Electrocautery snare resection is performed (b), and the lesion is retrieved with a grasping forceps (c).

Sarcoma

Malignant mesenchymal esophageal tumors are rare (43). About 5% of all gastrointestinal sarcomas occur in the esophagus. Leiomyosarcomas are the most common and can be difficult to distinguish from leiomyomas (see discussion later in this chapter). Other sarcomas include rhabdomyosarcoma, fibrosarcoma, fibrous histiocytoma, and choriocarcinoma. Tumor characteristics include spindle-shaped smooth muscle cells, high mitotic rates, local invasion, and, infrequently, distant metastasis. Most patients present with dysphagia. Endoscopic biopsy specimens are typically nondiagnostic, although the bite-on-bite technique may improve yield. EUS with EUS-guided FNA may contribute to diagnosis (44). Negative FNA specimens, however, cannot reliably exclude malignancy. Core biopsy using a true-cut needle may enhance histopathologic analysis.

Kaposi's sarcoma, a rare mesenchymal tumor before the AIDS epidemic, has been reported in the esophagus. Esophageal involvement is typically seen with concomitant oral and skin lesions (45). Esophageal lesions are found incidentally or during evaluation of dysphagia or odynophagia. These may mimic esophageal varices but are firm and do not bleed with biopsy forceps tissue sampling, though the diagnostic yield is suspect.

Metastatic Carcinoma

Metastatic carcinoma to the esophagus is unusual. Melanoma and breast cancer are the malignancies that most frequently metastasize to the esophagus (46). Radiographic and endoscopic studies typically demonstrate compression without disruption of the mucosa. EUS is useful in distinguishing extrinsic and intrinsic involvement and in detecting lymphadenopathy. EUS-guided FNA has proved useful in confirming the suspected diagnosis.

Benign Nonepithelial Tumors

Leiomyoma

Leiomyomas are the most common benign tumors of the esophagus (47) (Figure 18.8). Leiomyomas may occur in all parts of the esophagus; however, most (90%) are in the distal third. Most patients have a single tumor, though multiple leiomyomas may occur. Leiomyomas arise from smooth muscle cells or their precursors in the muscularis propria or less commonly in the muscularis mucosa. Most leiomyomas are endocentric (intraluminal polypoid growth). On endoscopy, the mucosa is usually intact, and the mass appears as a rounded, smooth, raised lesion protruding into the esophageal lumen. Rarely, there may be central umbilication or ulceration. Palpation with a closed tip of a biopsy forceps reveals a firm but pliable lesion. Forceps biopsies typically are nondiagnostic revealing only normal surface epithelium.

EUS is the most accurate tool for diagnosing leiomyomas and distinguishing them from other submucosal lesions (48). EUS evaluation reveals that leiomyomas typically arise from the fourth wall layer (the muscularis propria) and are hypoechoic and homogeneous and have sharply demarcated margins. Less commonly, leiomyomas arise from the muscularis mucosa within the deep mucosa, the second wall layer as seen on EUS examination. Leiomyomas arising from this layer may be amenable to endoscopic excision. Neither EUS nor FNA cytologic examination accurately distinguish benign from malignant smooth muscle tumors preoperatively.

Granular Cell Tumor

Granular cell tumors are submucosal neoplasms that are thought to originate from cells of neural origin.

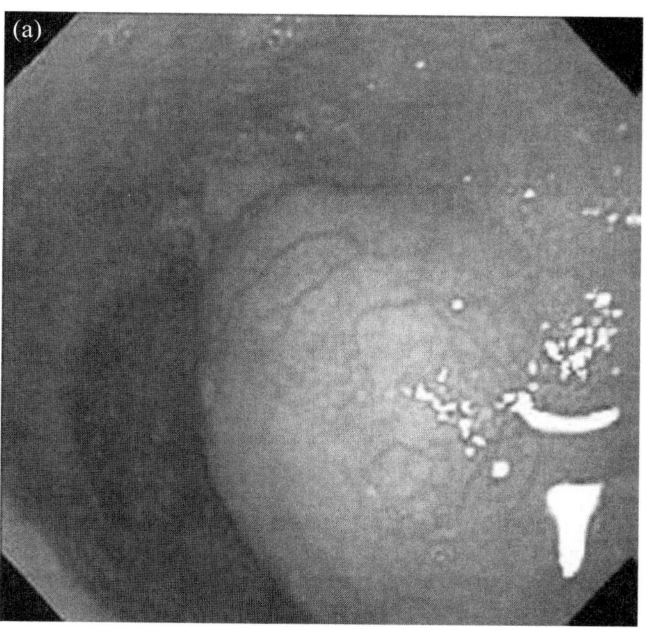

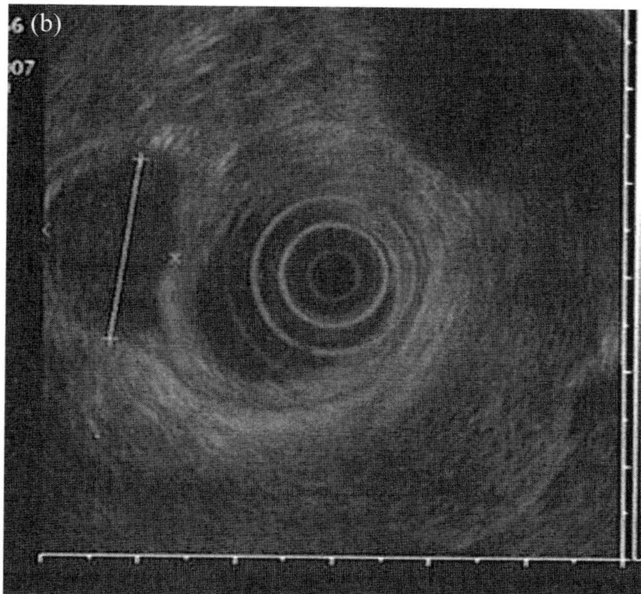

FIGURE 18.8

Endoscopic image of a subepithelial esophageal leiomyoma (a). Endoscopic ultrasound demonstrates the lesion as a smooth-margined hypoechoic mass arising from the muscularis propria layer (b).

Approximately 10% of granular cell tumors involve the gastrointestinal tract; the esophagus is the most frequent site, and most occur in the lower third (49). Endoscopically, they appear broad based, with normal overlying mucosa (Figure 18.9). Yellow-tan in color, they display a rubbery in consistency. On EUS, they are hypoechoic to isoechoic and arise within the submucosal layer. Diagnostic tissue can usually be confirmed with endoscopic biopsy samples obtained by the bite-on-bite technique. Management options include observation, endoluminal resection, and surgery. We remove 5 to 20 mm granular cell tumors using the suction-cap-ligation-snare-resection technique.

Fibrovascular Tumor

Large benign fibrovascular polyps occur most commonly on the upper third of the esophagus, near the cricopharyngeus muscle. They may contain a mixture of fibrovascular tissue, adipose cells, and stroma but are uniformly covered by squamous epithelium (50). Endoscopy is usually sufficient for diagnosis, but magnetic resonance imaging can help to determine the origin of these polyps and to plan for surgery. The latter is recommended for polyps larger than 2 cm in size. Endoscopic snare resection of fibrovascular polyps can safely be done if EUS detects no large feeding vessels in the polyp stalk. Consideration should be given to airway protection.

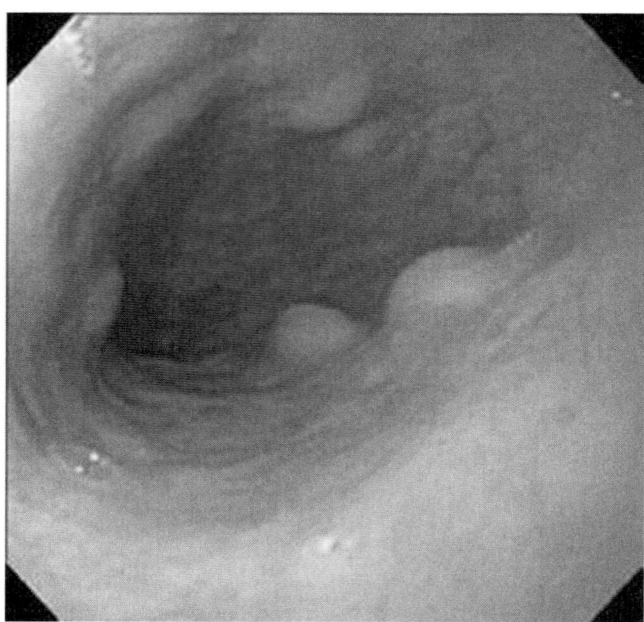

FIGURE 18.9

Typical endoscopic image of esophageal granular cell tumor (multiple in this case). They appear broad based, with normal overlying mucosa, yellow-tan in color, and display a rubbery consistency.

Hamartoma

Hamartomas of the esophagus are uncommon (51). They are frequently included in the category of fibrovascular polyps. As in other locations in the body, esophageal hamartomas are benign developmental tumors consisting of disorganized and excessive focal growth of mature normal cells. On pathologic examination, the mass can contain various elements, including cartilage, bone and bone marrow, adipose and fibrous tissue, and smooth and skeletal muscle. Esophageal hamartomas may grow to large size as long pedunculated polyps. Most occur in the upper esophagus and show obstructive symptoms and, less commonly, hematemesis. Surgical or endoscopic excision is required for symptomatic lesions.

Hemangioma

Hemangiomas represent 2% to 3% of benign esophageal tumors (52). Two types have been described: cavernous hemangiomas, which are the vast majority, and capillary hemangiomas. Hemangiomas appear nodular, are blue to red, and are soft and pliable when probed with a closed biopsy forceps (Figure 18.10). Classically, pressure from the forceps causes the lesion to blanch. Common symptoms are hemorrhage and dysphagia. Differential diagnosis should consider Kaposi's sarcoma. EUS may demonstrate venous lakes in the mucosal and submucosa (53).

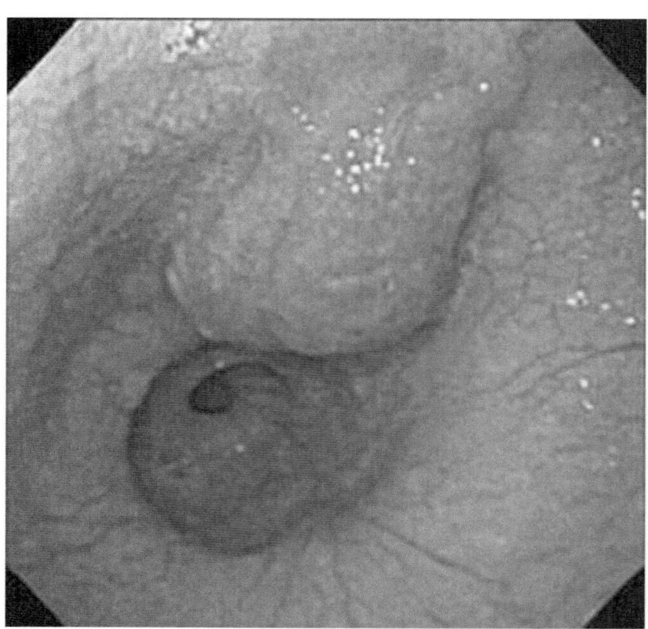

FIGURE 18.10

Esophageal hemangioma appears subepithelial, blue in color, and soft and pliable when probed with a closed biopsy forceps.

Lipoma

Esophageal lipomas are encapsulated tumors composed of well-differentiated adipose tissue generally arising in the submucosa. They are rare and most exhibit intramural morphology. However, they may become pseudopedunculated and promote obstructive symptoms. Like fibrovascular polyps, lipomas with long pedicles may produce laryngeal obstruction and asphyxiation (51). On endoscopy, lipomas classically have smooth and normal appearing overlying mucosa and a yellowish tint. Occasionally there is central ulceration and bleeding (54). When grasped with biopsy forceps, these lesions tend to "tent." When palpated with a closed biopsy forceps, they indent or "cushion." Simple biopsy specimens are often nondiagnostic, but bite-on-bite technique may yield fate cells to support the diagnosis. EUS classically reveals a homogeneous hyperechoic lesion with smooth outer margins, arising in the third wall layer (corresponding to the submucosa) (55). Because most other tumors that arise in the submucosa are hypoechoic, the EUS appearance is virtually diagnostic, provided that there are no features suggesting invasion or metastases, as in the exceedingly uncommon liposarcoma.

References

1. Graham DY, Schwartz JT, Cain GF, et al. Prospective evaluation of biopsy number in the diagnosis of esophageal and gastric carcinoma. *Gastroenterology.* 1982;82:228.
2. Catalano MF, Sivak MV Jr, Rice T. Endoscopic features predictive of lymph node metastasis. *Gastrointest Endosc.* 1994;40(4):442–446.
3. Vazquez-Sequeiros E, Wiersema MJ, Clain JE, et al. Impact of lymph node staging on therapy of esophageal carcinoma. *Gastroenterology.* 2003;125(6):1626–1633.
4. Giovannini M, Hookey LC, Bories E, et al. Endoscopic ultrasound elastography: the first step towards virtual biopsy? Preliminary results in 49 patients. *Endoscopy.* 2006;38(4):344–348.
5. Loren DE, Seghal CM, Ginsberg GG, et al. Computer-assisted analysis of lymph nodes detected by EUS in patients with esophageal carcinoma. *Gastrointest Endosc.* 2002;56:742–746.
6. Greene FL, Page DL, Fleming ID, et al, eds. American Joint Committee on Cancer. *Cancer Staging Manual.* 6th ed. New York: Springer; 2002:91–98.
7. Wakelin SJ, Deans C, Crofts TJ, et al. A comparison of computerized tomography, laparoscopic ultrasound and endoscopic ultrasound in the preoperative staging of oesophago-gastric carcinoma. *Eur J Radiol.* 2002;41(2):161–167.
8. Reed CE, Mishra G, Sahai AV, et al. Esophageal cancer staging: improved accuracy by endoscopic ultrasound of celiac lymph nodes. *Ann Thorac Surg.* 1999;67(2):319–321.
9. Rice TW, Zuccaro G Jr, Adelstein DJ, et al. Esophageal carcinoma: depth of tumor invasion is predictive of regional lymph nodes status. *Ann Thorac Surg.* 1998;65:787–792.
10. Wallace MB, Nietert PJ, Earle C, et al. An analysis of multiple staging management strategies for carcinoma of the esophagus: computed tomography, endoscopic ultrasound, positron emission tomography, and thoracoscopy/laparoscopy. *Ann Thorac Surg.* 2002;74:1026–1032.
11. Parmar KS, Zwischenberger JB, Reeves AL, et al. Clinical impact of endoscopic ultrasound-guided fine needle aspiration of celiac axis lymph nodes (M1a disease) in esophageal cancer. *Ann Thorac Surg.* 2002;73(3):916–920.
12. Lerut T, Coosemans W, De Leyn P, et al. Optimizing treatment of carcinoma of the esophagus and gastroesophageal junction. *Surg Oncol Clin N Am.* 2001;10:863–864.
13. Hiele M, De Leyn P, Schurmans P, et al. Relation between endoscopic ultrasound findings and outcome of patients with tumors of the esophagus or esophagogastric junction. *Gastrointest Endosc.* 1997;45(5):381–386.
14. Harewood GC, Kumar KS. Assessment of clinical impact of endoscopic ultrasound on esophageal cancer. *J Gastroenterol Hepatol.* 2004;19:433–439.
15. Shumaker DA, de Garmo P, Faigel DO. Potential impact of preoperative EUS on esophageal cancer management and cost. *Gastrointest Endosc.* 2002;56:391–396.
16. Chang KJ, Soetikno RM, Bastas D, et al. Impact of endoscopic ultrasound combined with fine-needle aspiration biopsy in the management of esophageal cancer. *Endoscopy.* 2003;35(11):962–966.
17. Harewood GC, Wiersema MJ. A cost analysis of endoscopic ultrasound in the evaluation of esophageal cancer. *Am J Gastroenterol.* 2002;97(2):452–458.
18. Van Dam J, Rice TW, Catalano MF, et al. High-grade malignant stricture is predictive of esophageal tumor stage. *Cancer.* 1993;71:2910–2917.
19. Pfau PR, Ginsberg GG, Lew RJ, et al. Esophageal dilation for endosonographic evaluation of malignant esophageal strictures is safe and effective. *Am J Gastroenterol.* 2000;95(10):2813–2815.
20. Kallimanis GE, Gupta PK, al-Kawas FH, et al. Endoscopic ultrasound for staging of esophageal cancer, with or without dilation, is clinically important and safe. *Gastrointest Endosc.* 1995;41(6):613–615.
21. Menzel J, Hoepffner N, Nottberg H, et al. Preoperative staging of esophageal carcinoma: miniprobe sonography versus conventional endoscopic ultrasound in a prospective histopathology verified study. *Endoscopy.* 1999;31(4):291–297.
22. Srivastava AK, Vanagunas A, Kamel P, et al. Endoscopic ultrasound in the evaluation of Barrett's esophagus: a preliminary report. *Am J Gastroenterol.* 1994;89(12):2192–2195.
23. Adrain AL, Ter HC, Cassidy MJ, et al. High-resolution endoluminal sonography is a sensitive modality for the identification of Barrett's metaplasia. *Gastrointest Endosc.* 1997;46(2):51.
24. Kinjo M, Maringhini A, Wang KK, et al. Is endoscopic ultrasound (EUS) cost effective to screen for cancer in patients with Barrett's esophagus? *Gastrointest Endosc.* 1994;40:205A.
25. Altorki NK, Sunagawa M, Little AG, et al. High-grade dysplasia in the columnar-lined esophagus. *Am J Surg.* 1991;26:1–32.
26. Cameron AJ, Carpenter HA. Barrett's esophagus, high-grade dysplasia, and early adenocarcinoma: a pathological study. *Am J Gastroenterol.* 1997;92:586–591.
27. Ferguson MK, Naunheim KS. Resection for Barrett's mucosa with high-grade dysplasia: implications for prophylactic photodynamic therapy. *J Thorac Cardiovasc Surg.* 1997;114:824–829.
28. Falk GW, Catalano MF, Sivak MV Jr, et al. Endosonography in the evaluation of patients with Barrett's esophagus and high-grade dysplasia. *Gastrointest Endosc.* 1994;40(2):207–212.
29. Scotiniotis IA, Kochman ML, Lewis JD, et al. Accuracy of EUS in the evaluation of Barrett's esophagus and high grade dysplasia or intramucosal carcinoma. *Gastrointest Endosc.* 2001;54:689–696.
30. Wang KK, Norbash A, Geller A, et al. Endoscopic ultrasonography in the assessment of Barrett's esophagus with high grade dysplasia or carcinoma. *Gastroenterology.* 1996;110(4):A611.
31. Nijhawan PK, Wang KK. Endoscopic mucosal resection for lesions with endoscopic features suggestive of malignancy and high-grade dysplasia within Barrett's esophagus. *Gastrointest Endosc.* 2000;52(3):328–332.
32. Ginsberg GG. Endoluminal therapy for Barrett's with high grade dysplasia and early esophageal adenocarcinoma. *Clin Gastroenterol Hepatol.* 2003;1:241–245.
33. Burtin P, Napoleon B, Palazzo L. Interobserver agreement in endoscopic ultrasonography staging of esophageal and cardia cancer. *Gastrointest Endosc.* 1996;43(1):20–24.
34. Devlin S, Falck V, Urbanski SJ, et al. Verrucous carcinoma of the esophagus eluding multiple sets of endoscopic biopsies and endoscopic ultrasound: a case report and review of the literature. *Can J Gastroenterol.* 2004;18(7):459–462.
35. Gal AA, Martin SE, Kernen JA, et al. Esophageal carcinoma with prominent spindle cells. *Cancer.* 1987;60:2244.
36. Yun JP, Zhang MF, Hou JH, et al. Primary small cell carcinoma of the esophagus: clinicopathological and immunohistochemical features of 21 cases. *BMC Cancer.* 2007;7:38.
37. Mikami T, Fukuda S, Shimoyama T, et al. A case of early stage primary malignant melanoma of the esophagus. *Gastrointest Endosc.* 2001;53:365–367.
38. Mosca S, Manes G, Monaco R, et al. Squamous papilloma of the esophagus: long-term follow up. *J Gastroenterol Hepatol.* 2001;16(8):857–861.
39. Fang SY, Wu CY, Chen HC, et al. Giant adenoma arising in the lower esophagus with adenocarcinoma. *Dig Dis Sci.* 2007;52(11):3181–3183.
40. Makino H, Miyashita M, Nomura T, et al. Solitary fibrous tumor of the cervical esophagus. *Dig Dis Sci.* 2007;52(9):2195–2200.
41. LiVolsi V, Perzin K. Inflammatory pseudotumors (inflammatory fibrous polyps) of the esophagus: a clinicopathologic study. *Dig Dis.* 1975;20:475–479.
42. Weeratunge CN, Bolivar HH, Anstead GM, et al. Primary esophageal lymphoma: a diagnostic challenge in acquired immunodeficiency syndrome—two case reports and review. *South Med J.* 2004;97(4):383–387.
43. Miller PR, Jackson SL, Pineau BC, et al. Radiation-induced gastrointestinal stromal sarcoma of the esophagus. *Ann Thorac Surg.* 2000;70(2):660–662.
44. Tio TL, Tytgat GNJ. Endoscopic ultrasound in analyzing periintestinal lymph node abnormality. *Scand J Gastroenterol.* 1986;21(suppl 123):158–163.
45. Connolly GM, Hawkins D, Harcourt-Webster JN, et al. Oesophageal symptoms, their causes, treatment, and prognosis in patients with the acquired immunodeficiency syndrome. *Gut.* 1989;30:1033–1038.
46. Goldberg RI, Ranis H, Stone B, et al. Dysphagia as the presenting symptoms of recurrent breast carcinoma. *Cancer.* 1987;135:1243–1245.
47. Mutrie CJ, Donahue DM, Wain JC, et al. Esophageal leiomyoma: a 40-year experience. *Ann Thorac Surg.* 2005;79(4):1122–1125.
48. Lee LS, Singhal S, Brinster CJ, et al. Current management of esophageal leiomyoma. *J Am Coll Surg.* 2004;198(1):136–146.

49. Orlowska J, Pachlewski J, Gugulski A, et al. A conservative approach to granular cell tumors of the esophagus: four case reports and literature review. *Am J Gastroenterol.* 1993;88:311–315.
50. Avezzano EA, Fleischer DE, Merida MA, et al. Giant fibrovascular polyps of the esophagus. *Am J Gastroenterol.* 1990;85:299–301.
51. Caceres M, Steeb G, Wilks SM, et al. Large pedunculated polyps originating in the esophagus and hypopharynx. *Ann Thorac Surg.* 2006;81(1):393–396.
52. Kim AW, Korst RJ, Port JL, et al. Giant cavernous hemangioma of the distal esophagus treated with esophagectomy. *J Thorac Cardiovasc Surg.* 2007;133(6):1665–1667.
53. Sogabe M, Taniki T, Fukui Y, et al. A patient with esophageal hemangioma treated by endoscopic mucosal resection: a case report and review of the literature. *J Med Invest.* 2006;53(1–2):177–182.
54. Sou S, Nomura H, Takaki Y, et al. Hemorrhagic duodenal lipoma managed by endoscopic resection. *J Gastroenterol Hepatol.* 2006;21(2):479–481.
55. Yoshikane H, Tsukamoto Y, Niwa Y, et al. The coexistence of esophageal submucosal tumor and carcinoma. *Endoscopy.* 1995;27:119–123.

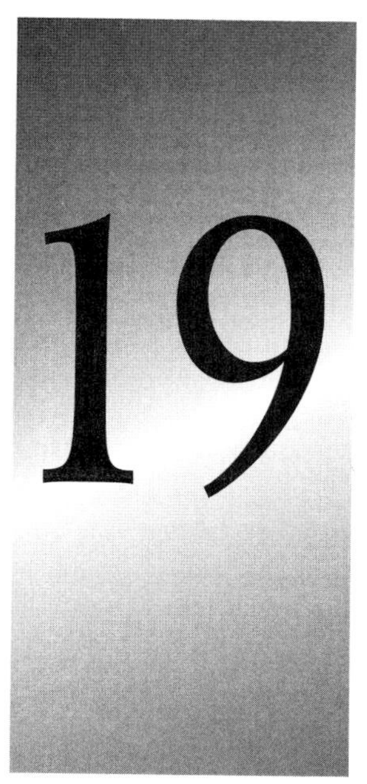

Esophageal Imaging: Functional—PET

Timothy D. Wagner
Milind Javle
Gary Y. Yang

Of the roughly 15,560 patients diagnosed with esophageal cancer annually in the United States, nearly 14,000 will succumb to the disease, yielding a death-to-incidence ratio of approximately 0.9 (1). This dismal prognosis is due in large part to patients remaining relatively asymptomatic until the disease has progressed past its early stages. Thus, the majority of patients present with locally advanced or metastatic disease (2). The management of locally advanced versus metastatic disease is vastly different, and traditionally it has been challenging to accurately stage patients into 1 of these 2 groups. In many cases, this failure to stage properly has helped lead to inappropriate management and a high rate of treatment failure even after aggressive multimodality treatment. Continuing to advance modern therapies is a worthwhile objective, but so too is improving the tools of staging to ensure that patients receive optimal therapeutic management. Complete and accurate staging allows identification of those patients who can potentially benefit from local treatment while sparing patients with distant metastases from undergoing intensive local multimodality therapy (2,3). Additionally, more precise staging can aid in the assessment of future clinical trials in esophageal cancer, where results have historically been hindered by imprecise or incomplete initial staging of patients.

IMAGING MODALITIES

Anatomic Imaging

For over a decade, endoscopic ultrasonography (EUS) and computed tomography (CT) have been mainstays of esophageal staging. The role of EUS is in evaluating the primary tumor and adjacent lymph nodes. Alone, it is used to differentiate between early and advanced primary lesions, and when used in combination with fine-needle aspiration (FNA), EUS is utilized to assess regional lymph nodes as well (2,4). EUS has shown to be most effective in assessing primary lesions with reported sensitivity of 80% to 90% and with regional nodal sensitivity in the range of 70% to 80% (2,5). Bulky esophageal lesions causing luminal obstruction limit the effectiveness of EUS, and it has little role beyond the esophagus and adjacent tissue (3). CT acts as an adjunct to EUS, providing additional information about bulky primary lesions, regional lymph node involvement, and distant metastases. The usefulness of CT in the locoregional setting is marginal, with sensitivities in the 50% range for primary staging and in the 60% to 87% range for regional nodal involvement (6).

Physiologic Imaging

The previously mentioned staging tools deliver anatomic information at a snapshot in time, while positron-emission tomography (PET) is a nuclear medicine imaging modality that evaluates physiologic and biochemical processes (7,8). Depending on the radiopharmaceutical selected, this technology has the ability to determine information regarding various metabolic processes (7). Many esophageal tumors demonstrate high levels of cellular metabolism when compared to surrounding normal tissue. These tumors have also been shown to have increased glycolysis and an increased number of glucose transporter proteins (9). In an effort to identify cells with increased metabolism, a positron-emitting radiotracer, 2-[^{18}F]fluoro-2-deoxyglucose (FDG), was developed. FDG is a glucose analogue and is transported into cells, where it is then phosphorylated to 2-[^{18}F]fluoro-2-deoxyglucose-6-phosphate (FDG-6-phosphate) in a manner mimicking glucose (Figure 19.1). Within the cell, further metabolism and breakdown of FDG-6-phosphate is limited by a relative lack of glucose phosphatase, and because it is highly polar, it cannot exit the cell (7). Secondary to high metabolic rates, many tumor cells selectively uptake FDG and trap FDG-6-phosphate intracellularly. This FDG-6-phosphate then accumulates in tumors cells following intravenous injection and provides a signal of high glycolytic tissue activity in involved areas throughout the whole body when imaged (10). While limited in some anatomic regions, like the brain and urinary tract, FDG-PET is successful in identifying malignant tumors throughout the body (11).

STAGING

Primary Site Evaluation

FDG-PET has been used in evaluating both squamous cell carcinomas (SCCs) and adenocarcinomas of the esophagus. In most cases, FDG accumulation within SCC primary tumors is relatively high, with visualization usually limited only by the size of the lesion (PET imaging devices have limited spatial resolution with lesions smaller than 5–8 mm) (12). FDG accumulation in adenocarcinoma primary tumors is more variable, however, with avidity related to various tumor characteristics (13). In many cases, non-avid tumors tend to be more mucus containing and poorly differentiated, often showing a diffuse, nonintestinal growth type (13). FDG-PET has the ability to detect primary lesions within the esophagus, but its capacity to determine stage is not nearly that of EUS, and thus its role in primary tumor evaluation in limited.

Regional Evaluation

Prognostically, overall survival (OS) is impacted by the involvement of regional lymph nodes, with worse outcomes associated with increased nodal involvement (14). Traditional anatomical imaging modalities are limited in their ability to detect nodal involvement in cases where nodes are of normal size, are enlarged because of nonmalignant conditions, or are obscured by the primary tumor. FDG-PET is useful tool in staging regional disease, especially in situations where there is some question after EUS and CT. The ability of FDG-PET to properly identify nodal disease can potentially preclude more invasive procedures, such as mediastinoscopy, that are associated with increased cost and morbidity.

Evaluating esophagectomy and lymph node dissection specimens, a study of 47 patients compared the ability FDT-PET and CT to detect regional nodal involvement (15). Sensitivity, 52% versus 15% ($P < 0.005$), was superior using FDG-PET, while accuracy, 84% versus

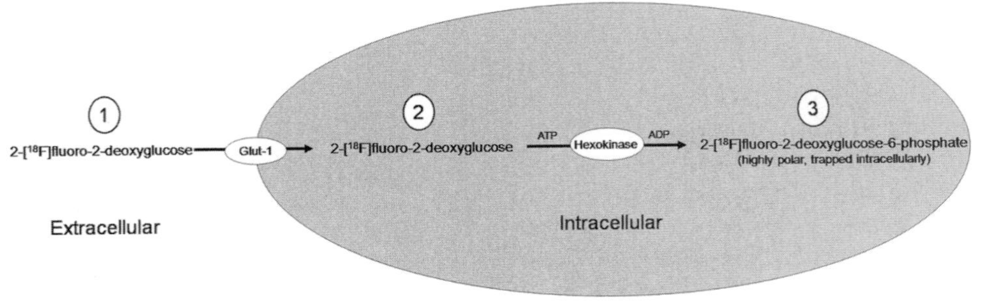

FIGURE 19.1

Cellular metabolism. Extracellular 2-[^{18}F]fluoro-2-deoxyglucose (FDG) is transported into the cell with the aid of glucose transporter proteins. Via the same pathways as glucose, it is then phosphorylated to 2-[^{18}F]fluoro-2-deoxyglucose-6-phosphate (FDG-6-phosphate). With inadequate amounts of glucose phosphatase within the cell, FDG-6-phosphate is prevented from metabolizing further. The highly polar FDG-6-phosphate is then trapped within the malignant cell.

77%, and specificity, 94% versus 97%, were similar between the 2 modalities. In comparing FDG-PET to EUS for nodal evaluation, a study of 74 esophageal cancer patients showed FDG-PET to have 33% sensitivity and 89% specificity compared to 81% sensitivity and 67% specificity for EUS (16). Meta-analysis of 12 studies evaluating the ability of FDG-PET to detect regional metastases found sensitivity of 51% (95% confidence interval [CI], 34%–69%) and specificity of 84% (95% CI, 76%–91%) (17). Limitations of FDG-PET to detect nodal involvement are small nodal size and close proximity to highly glucose-avid primary tumors that obscure the imaging (18). In these situations, EUS can provide additional useful diagnostic information for detecting regional metastases (16). Falsely positive nodes seen on FDG-PET can be secondary to inflammatory disease like sarcoidosis, appearing to represent locally advanced disease (7). Secondary to limitations of CT, EUS, and FDG-PET, nodal sampling and dissection is done during definitive surgery for both therapeutic and prognostic benefit (12).

Distant Metastatic Evaluation

Esophageal carcinoma commonly metastasizes to distant organ systems, frequently involving the liver, lungs, and nonregional lymph nodes (2). FDG-PET is an attractive modality for identifying distant metastases because the FDG can accumulate nearly anywhere a metastasis may have deposited (Figure 19.2). In a study comparing 74 patients, FDG-PET was found to have superior accuracy (82% vs. 64%, $P = 0.004$) compared to the combination of CT and EUS for detecting distant metastases (16). Among the patients staged with FDG-PET, 15% (11/71) were upstaged to metastatic (M1) disease, and another 7% (5/71) were downstaged from M1 to locoregional (M0) disease. Meta-analysis of FDG-PET in detecting M1 disease revealed a pooled sensitivity of 67% (95% CI, 58%–76%) and specificity of 97% (95% CI, 90%–100%) (17). Table 19.1 summarizes a number of studies evaluating the efficacy of FDG-PET in the detecting distant metastases.

The American College of Surgeons Oncology Group completed a prospective multi-institutional study evaluating FDG-PET in detecting metastases that preclude definitive surgery in esophageal cancer patients deemed surgical candidates after routine staging procedures (24). Recently published results of 189 evaluable patients in this study demonstrated that FDG-PET following standard clinical staging showed that nearly 5% (9/189) of patients harbored previously undetected M1 disease. These findings were then confirmed prior to resection, thereby preventing surgery. Thus, FDG-PET was demonstrated to be a noninvasive method to prevent unnecessary esphagectomies (24). Similarly, in a study of 85 patients completing neoadjuvant chemoradiation, 8% (7/85)

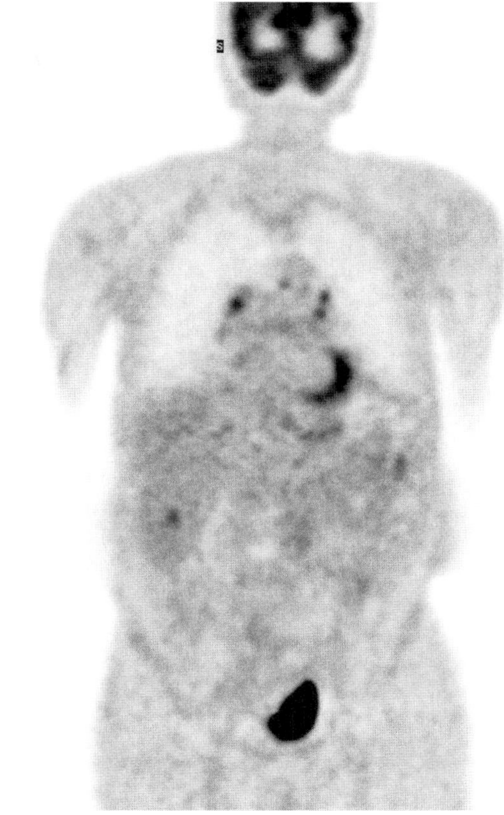

FIGURE 19.2

Distant metastases. This image demonstrates modest FDG-PET uptake in the primary tumor located in the mid-esophagus. There is also more intense uptake in the bilateral hila and a solitary intense focus of radiotracer uptake within the liver.

were diagnosed with interval distant metastases detected by postneoadjuvant treatment FDG-PET (25). Typically, distant metastases at least 1 cm in size can be detected with high sensitivity (7). It is possible to detect lesions smaller than this cutoff, provided there is high FDG uptake by the metastatic cells. Likewise, larger lesions can go undetected if there is relatively low glucose metabolism in metastatic cells. False positives, while rare, can occur when there is increased uptake caused by inflammatory processes or normal healthy tissues. Thus, biopsy confirmation of metastatic lesions detected by FDG-PET is recommended before altering patient management.

Cost-Effectiveness

While FDG-PET appears to offer additional information to conventional staging modalities, the question remains whether FDG-PET provides sufficient benefit compared to its added cost. A study by Wallace et al. (26) evaluated

TABLE 19.1
Comparison of CT and FDG-PET in the Detection of Metastatic Disease in Patients with Newly Diagnosed Esophageal Carcinoma

			CT			FDG-PET		
Study	**Number of patients**	**% With distant metastasis**	**Sensitivity (%)**	**Specificity (%)**	**Accuracy (%)**	**Sensitivity (%)**	**Specificity (%)**	**Accuracy (%)**
Kneist et al. (19)	81	35	63	11	45	38	89	52
Luketich et al. (20)	91	43	46	74	63	69	93	84*
Liberale et al. (21)	58	22	45	95	80	88*	88	88
Sihvo et al. (22)	55	35	32	97	75	53	89	76
Flamen et al. (16)	74	46	41	83	64	74	90	82*
Block et al. (23)	58	29	29	NS	NS	100	NS	NS

Abbreviations: % = percent; CT = computed tomography; FDG-PET = ^{18}F-fluoro-2-deoxyglucose positron-emission tomography; NS = not stated.
[a]Denotes statistically significant compared to CT, $P \leq 0.05$.

the cost and effectiveness of multiple different preoperative staging regimens. Six different combinations of staging evaluations were done: (a) CT alone, (b) CT and EUS with FNA, (c) CT with mediastinoscopy/laparoscopy, (d) CT and EUS with FNA and mediastinoscopy/laparoscopy, (e) CT and EUS with FNA and FDG-PET, and (f) FDG-PET and EUS with FNA. Using a third-party-payer perspective, a model was designed evaluating stage of disease, life expectancy, cost, and morbidity of the procedure. After evaluating the 6 combinations, FDG-PET and EUS with FNA was found to be a more favorable cost-effective staging procedure for third-party payers (26).

RESTAGING

Following Neoadjuvant Treatment

A combination of multimodality therapy is often the treatment of choice in localized esophageal cancer. Indeed, a recently published meta-analysis of randomized comparisons of both neoadjuvant chemoradiation and chemotherapy to surgery alone has confirmed an absolute 2-year survival benefit of 7% to 13% in favor of multimodality therapy (27). In many cases, multimodality therapy includes neoadjuvant radiation in combination with chemotherapy, followed by surgical resection. In preparation for surgical resection, neoadjuvant chemoradiation is utilized to provide distant disease control while acting on the primary tumor and regional lymph nodes. In cases where the disease is too advanced to allow for complete surgical resection or in patients with medical comorbidities, chemoradiation is used as definitive therapy. Whether following its use as definitive or neoadjuvant therapy, assessing response to chemoradiation is important for giving prognostic information and guiding further management. In esophageal cancer, response to chemoradiation is unpredictable, but lack of tumor response to therapy is considered a poor prognostic factor (28). Thus, nonresponders need to be identified early in the course of treatment in order to potentially alter their planned management and avoid the toxicity of unwarranted therapy. Static anatomic imaging modalities like EUS and CT often cannot distinguish between residual disease and posttherapy changes, thereby delaying posttherapy assessment (3). Even when anatomical imaging reveals response to therapy, there is often little or no correlation with pathological findings (29). FDG-PET is a measure of cellular metabolism and theoretically should be effective in evaluating cellular response to therapy. The accuracy of FDG-PET, EUS, and CT for assessing primary tumor response to neoadjuvant therapy was evaluated in a review of the literature (30). In this review, accuracy of assessing response was 85%, 86%, and 54% for FDG-PET, EUS, and CT, respectively. Both FDG-PET (P = 0.006) and EUS (P = 0.003) were found to be significantly more accurate than CT, while 6% of patients were not able to undergo EUS secondary due to the obstructing nature of the primary tumor (30).

Functional imaging, such as FDG-PET (Figure 19.3), serves as a promising modality for assessing response to treatment. However, questions remain regarding the optimal timing of the pre- and posttherapy scans and in determining what degree of response on FDG-PET is significant. In a study of 40 patients with tumors of the gastroesophageal junction (GEJ) receiving neoadjuvant chemotherapy, FDG-PET was performed pretreatment and 2 weeks after the start of neoadjuvant therapy (31). The response seen on FDG-PET was then compared to either endoscopic response seen several months after therapy or with pathologic response at the time of surgical excision. A majority of patients with decreased avidity by FDG-PET also had a pathologic response. Using a 35% reduction in FDG uptake measured as of standard uptake value (SUV) as a cutoff, 53% of metabolic responders had a complete or near complete pathologic response, while only 5% of those without a response by FDG-PET responded pathologically. FDG-PET was found to have a sensitivity and specificity of 93% and 95%, respectively, in predicting pathologic response to therapy. Pathologic response to neoadjuvant chemoradiation has also been studied using pre- and posttherapy FDG-PET. Flamen et al. (32) reported that FDG-PET performed before and 4 to 6 weeks after the completion of chemoradiation can accurately predict response to therapy. In this series, FDG-PET was able to predict "major pathologic response" with an accuracy of 78% and a sensitivity and specificity of 71% and 82%, respectively. Using at least 52% reduction in FDG uptake following neoadjuvant chemoradiation as a cutoff, a similar study found the sensitivity of FDG-PET to predict pathologic response to be 100%, with a sensitivity of 55% (33). In this case, the posttherapy FDG-PET was performed at 3 weeks following completion of therapy, and the relatively low specificity was felt to be related to inflammation due to chemoradiation. Table 19.2 exhibits several trials that have studied the effectiveness of FDG-PET in predicting response to neoadjuvant therapy.

When used for restaging, FDG-PET has usually been employed early after initiation of therapy or later, several weeks after completion of therapy. Different timing of the follow-up scan can yield different information (12). Shortly after the start of therapy, as seen in cases of neoadjuvant chemotherapy, FDG-PET can

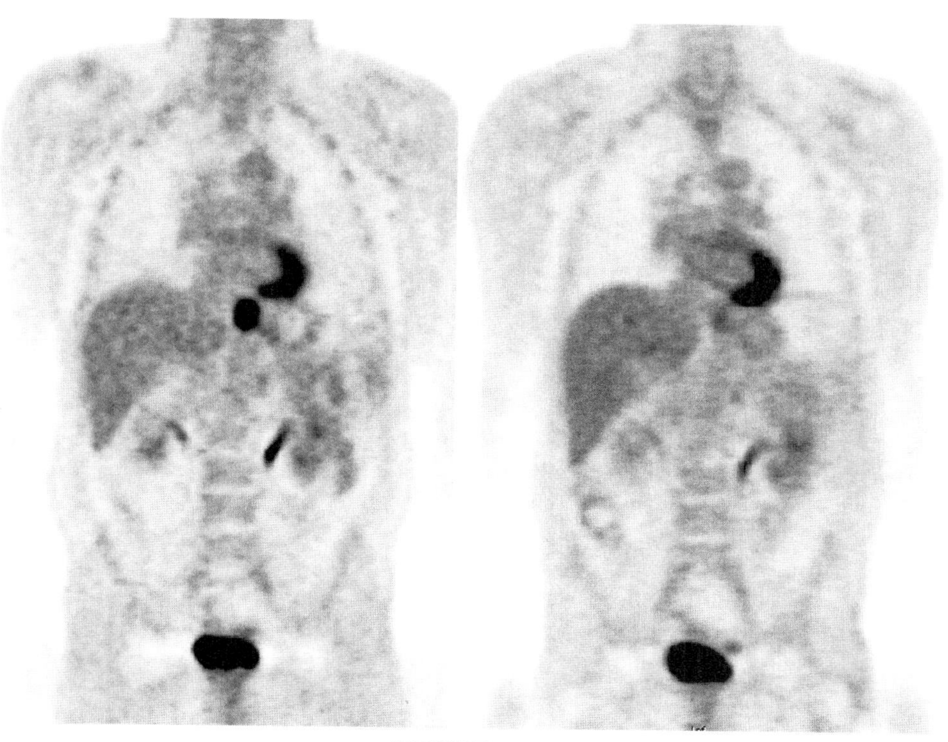

FIGURE 19.3

FDG-PET response to chemoradiation. The image on the left represents an initial staging FDG-PET for a patient with locally advanced adenocarcinoma of the distal esophagus with associated lymphadenopathy. The FDG-PET image on the right, obtained approximately 4 weeks after completion of neoadjuvant chemoradiation, shows near complete metabolic resolution of both the primary disease and regional nodal metastases.

TABLE 19.2
FDG-PET Predicting Pathologic Response and Prognosis Following Neoadjuvant Therapy for Esophageal Cancer

Study	Brücher et al. (33)	Flamen et al. (32)	Wieder et al. (34)	Weber et al. (31)	Ott et al. (35)	Port et al. (36)
Number of patients	27	36	27	40 a	65 a	62
Therapy	ChemoRT	ChemoRT	ChemoRT	Chemotherapy	Chemotherapy	Chemotherapy
Timing	3–4 wks post-treatment	4–6 wks post-treatment	2 wks after start	2 wks after start	2 wks after start	2–3 wks after start
SUV reduction threshold	52%	80%	30%	35%	35%	50%
Sensitivity (response)	100%	71%	93%	93%	80%	77.8%
Specificity (response)	55%	82%	88%	95%	78%	52.9%
Median OS (responders)	22.5 mos [b]	16.3 mos [b]	38 mos [b]	NR [b]	NR [b]	35.5 mos [b,c]
Median OS (non-responders)	8.8 mos	6.4 mos	18 mos	13 mos	18 mos	17.9 mos [c]

Abbreviations: SUV = standard uptake value; chemoRT = chemotherapy concurrently with external beam irradiation; Sensitivity = sensitivity of FDG-PET to detect pathologic response; Specificity = specificity of FDG-PET to detect pathologic response; Median OS = median overall survival; mos = months; NR = median survival not yet reached.
[a] Study evaluated patients with tumors of the gastroesophageal junction.
[b] Denotes statistically significant, $P \leq 0.05$.
[c] Represents median disease-free survival (overall survival not calculated).

assess the responsiveness of the tumor to a given therapy and whether treatment should continue as planned. In cases of neoadjuvant chemoradiation, the FDG-PET is often obtained at least a month after therapy and is used to gauge overall response and often to aid in prognosis. When setting a threshold value for response to treatment, a high response value is used in order to have a high sensitivity for detecting nonresponders, while a lower cutoff for response evaluation will have the effect of increasing sensitivity of detecting response (12). While FDG-PET has had some success in assessing disease response, it is not without its shortcomings. Many studies have identified that microscopic disease often falls below the level of detection by FDG-PET, and chemoradiation-induced inflammation and esophagitis often obscure treatment response (12,37,38). In addition, one particular study found that treatment-related esophageal ulceration frequently led to false-positive results when assessing for residual tumor (39). These posttherapy changes and normal tissue responses limit the predictive capability, making the timing of post-treatment scans important in order to maximize their value (3).

Prognostic Value

Initial FDG-PET imaging appears to hold some prognostic value as well as acting as a staging tool. One study of 89 patients found that a higher maximum SUV correlated with more poorly differentiated tumors and advanced tumor stage (40). This association with more aggressive and advanced tumors was found to be predictive of survival, with the 4-year survival among patients with a maximum SUV > 6.6 of 31%. Conversely, in those patients with a maximum SUV ≤ 6.6, 4-year survival was significantly better (89%, $P < 0.001$). The number of metabolic abnormalities detected by FDG-PET may also be of prognostic significance. In a report of 47 patients treated with neoadjuvant chemoradiation and definitive surgery, Hong et al. (41) found that patients with >1 lesion by FDG-PET had a death hazard ratio (HR) of 4.49 (reference: 1 lesion). In addition, the number of lesions detected by staging FDG-PET was significantly associated with both OS ($P = 0.02$) and disease-free survival (DFS) ($P = 0.04$).

Not only can FDG-PET evaluate response to therapy, but it appears that this degree of response is predictive of prognosis. In a series of 83 esophageal cancer patients receiving neoadjuvant chemoradiation, posttherapy SUV ≥4 predicted for a significantly worse prognosis, with a 2-year survival of 33% compared to a 60% 2-year survival in patients with SUV <4 ($P = 0.01$) (42). A recent retrospective review found that following definitive chemoradiation, posttreatment FDG-PET SUV was significantly associated with DFS ($P = 0.01$) among the 63 patients undergoing posttherapy scans (43). In a related study, 27 patients with esophageal SCC were treated with neoadjuvant chemoradiation and underwent pre- and posttreatment FDG-PET in an effort to identify the prognostic value of FDG-PET response (33). Using a 52% threshold to represent significant response, responders had a mean OS of 22.5 months, while nonresponders had a mean OS of 8.8 months. Another study of 36 patients found that median survival was significantly improved to 16.3 months in therapy responders compared to 6.4 months among nonresponders ($P = 0.05$) (32). Ott et al. (35) prospectively evaluated 65 patients with tumors of the GEJ, obtaining one FDG-PET at presentation and a follow-up FDG-PET at 2 weeks after induction of chemotherapy. Using a predetermined cutoff of 35% reduction in tracer uptake, 3-year OS among responders was doubled compared to nonresponders, 70% versus 35% ($P = 0.01$), respectively (35). Survival among metabolic responders compared to nonresponders is summarized in Table 19.2 (bottom 2 rows).

Recurrent Disease

Anatomic diagnostics are often of limited value following definitive management secondary to inaccuracies in evaluating tissue that has been altered by chemotherapy, radiation, surgery, or some combination of the 3. Distorted posttreatment anatomy can still be imaged by FDG-PET with high sensitivity for detecting both locoregional and distant recurrent disease (12). In a study utilizing FDG-PET for posttreatment restaging for 41 patients, 27% (11/41) of the patients had additional information detected due to the addition of FDG-PET (44). Of these, 12% (5/41) were diagnosed with recurrent disease after negative or equivocal findings with conventional anatomic imaging. In addition, another 12% (5/41) with recurrent local disease were diagnosed with distant recurrence by FDG-PET. In this setting, FDG-PET has the potential to detect recurrent disease earlier in its course, allowing for earlier and potentially more successful intervention (44).

CURRENT AND FUTURE PET APPLICATIONS

FDG-PET, Patient Management, and Oncologic Drug Development

The functional information provided by FDG-PET is beginning to impact not only individual patient management but also therapeutic development for future patients with esophageal cancer. FDG-PET has been shown to identify therapy response early in the course of treatment, distinguishing those patients benefiting from treatment from those for whom treatment is ineffective (31). This application of FDG-PET can potentially detect suboptimal neoadjuvant therapy that would otherwise cost patients their time and health expenses and allow for tumor proliferation and unnecessary toxicity (45). In the recently published MUNICON phase II clinical trial, patient management was dictated by restaging FDG-PET obtained 2 weeks after the initiation of neoadjuvant chemotherapy (45). Metabolic responders (≥35 reduction in SUV from initial staging FDG-PET) continued with neoadjuvant therapy, while nonresponders went directly to surgery. As predicted, metabolic responders had a significantly better OS and DFS, as this trial demonstrated the possibility of using FDG-PET response to guide therapy (45). Alternatively, with information regarding response available early in their therapy, those patients not responding to standard treatments can initiate salvage therapies sooner. Another option for patients not responding to initial chemotherapy would be to consider radiation-based definitive management (46). These high-risk patients would then be spared the morbidity of esophagectomy when surgery would be of unlikely benefit (46).

Regarding FDG-PET's role in therapy development, a reduction in tracer uptake has been significantly correlated to DFS, OS, and other end points routinely used in studying new cancer drugs (47). Based on this ability to detect response early in treatment, FDG-PET can potentially be used in drug development as a tool for predicting clinical benefit. In the proper setting, FDG-PET can be used to expedite the development of new therapies by providing information in a more timely manner than was possible in the past. Additionally, baseline FDG-PET can also be used a factor for stratification in future randomized trials (41).

PET/CT Fusion

FDG-PET has been demonstrated to provide useful physiologic information utilized for a variety of purposes in oncologic management, but the associated anatomic information it provides lacks the spatial resolution to be of much value (48). A topic of recent investigation has been the integration of functional imaging (FDG-PET) with anatomic imaging (CT). Utilizing nearly identical patient positioning and coregistration techniques, FDG-PET and CT are combined into a shared diagnostic study, with fused PET/CT images (Figure 19.4) (38,48). Ideally, this fusion will allow for more accurate localization of suspected disease and ultimately improve

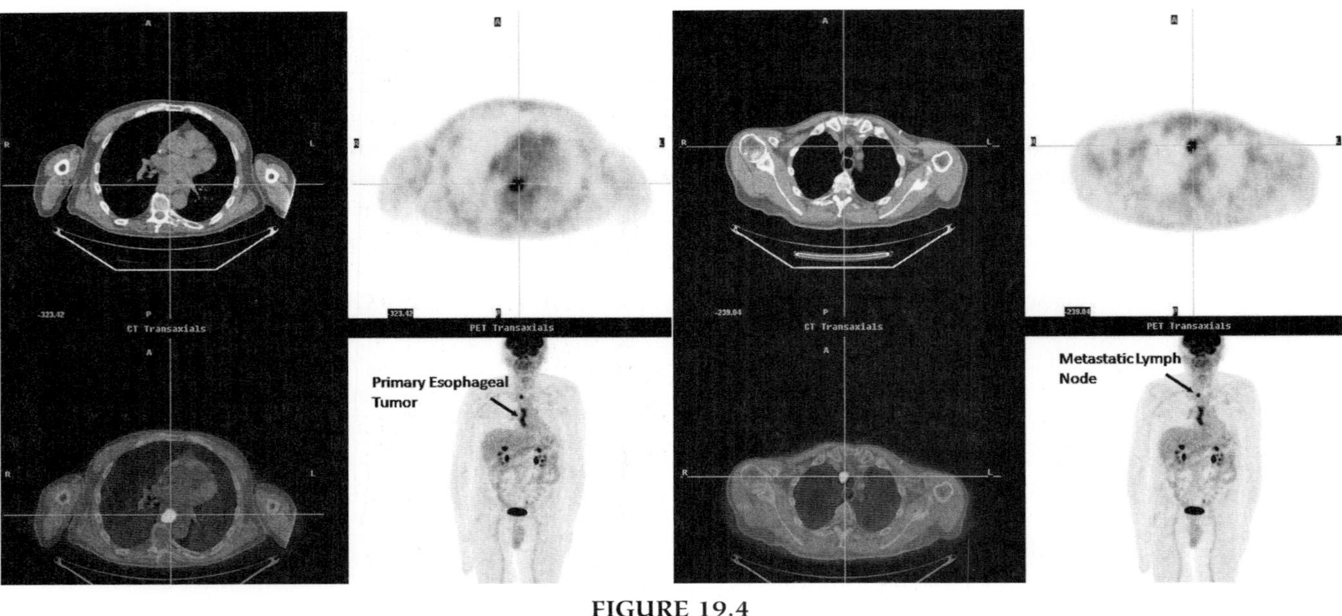

FIGURE 19.4

PET/CT assessing primary and regional nodal disease. Displayed are the primary tumor (left) and metastatic regional lymph node (right) as they appear on CT, FDG-PET, and FDG-PET/CT fusion. These images demonstrate the synergy of combining anatomic and functional imaging in esophageal cancer staging

the accuracy of cancer detection. With improved spatial resolution to evaluate scenarios like questionable nodal metastases in close proximity to the primary tumor, the combination of FDG-PET/CT should be better able to determine disease extent compared to FDG-PET alone. While PET/CT has been shown to improve initial staging in non–small cell lung cancer, recent data suggest it is beneficial in esophageal cancer as well (49,50). In a prospective study of 45 patients with SCC of the esophagus, FDG-PET/CT was compared to FDG-PET alone for the diagnosis of regional lymph node metastases. For FDG-PET/CT, the sensitivity, specificity, and accuracy for detecting pathologically involved nodes were 94%, 92%, and 92%, respectively compared to 82%, 87%, and 86% for FDG-PET alone. The superior sensitivity (P = 0.032) and accuracy (P = 0.006) for FDG-PET/CT were statistically significant (49). FDG-PET/CT is also well suited for disease restaging with its ability to simultaneously provide characteristics of tumor size and activity (7). In addition, FDG-PET/CT has a role in radiation planning, where accurate disease localization is crucial, by aiding the radiation oncologist in determining both local and regional disease extent.

Radiation Treatment Planning

FDG-PET provides additional data to the planning CT and staging EUS that should assist in designing radiation targets and allows for more conformal radiation treatment fields (Figure 19.5) (51). In a study of 34 patients, radiation planning CTs were fused FDG-hybrid PET scans, with image coregistration facilitated by the placement of fiducial markers (52). Radiation targets were first identified by planning CT and then modified by the additional PET information. The addition of PET allowed for detection of 2 patients with metastatic disease, and the gross tumor volume (GTV) was reduced in 35% (12/34) patients and increased in another 21% (7/34). The modifications by PET were considerable (≥25% of volume) in 17% (6/34) patients, and over half the treatment fields were changed to accommodate the additional information provided by the PET (52). How these changes impact outcome is unknown, but certainly accurate target delineation is critical to the success of radiation therapy. Another series of 25 patients compared FDG-PET, planning CT, and staging EUS and their ability to delineate the primary target and regional lymph nodes (34). Among this group, the mean length of the primary tumor was significantly longer (P = 0.0063) using the planning CT compared FDG-PET, which had mean tumor length similar to EUS, possibly suggesting overestimation by planning CT (53). While FDG-PET is not the final solution to the problems of radiation target identification, this study demonstrates that the additional information provided can assist with treatment planning. Recently, a prospective study of 21 patients

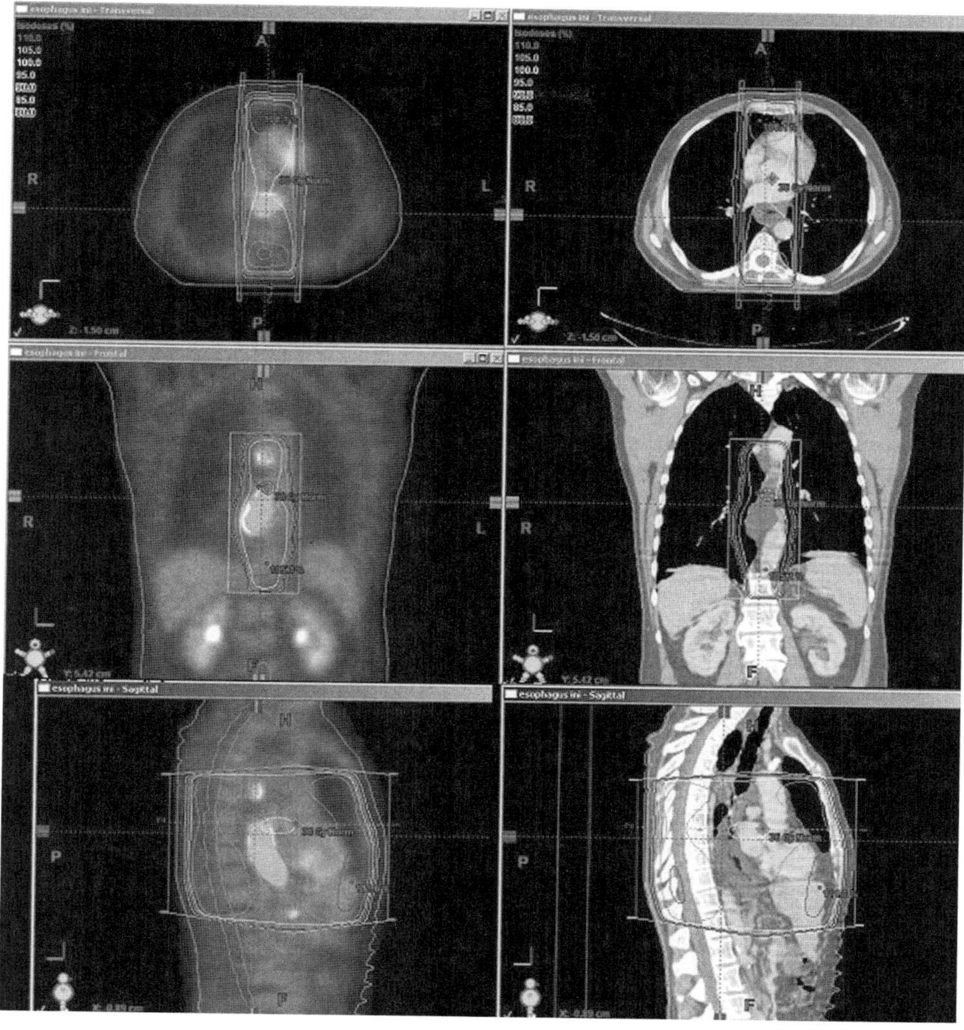

FIGURE 19.5

FDG-PET in radiation planning. A staging FDG-PET is fused with a radiation treatment planning CT to aid in the delineation of the primary tumor. The isodose lines of the treatment to be delivered are pictured on both the planning CT (right) and the FDG-PET (left) to ensure that the tumor is receiving the prescribed radiation dose.

comparing treatment planning CT versus FDG-PET/CT found that the clinical stage was altered in 38% (8/21) by the addition of FDG-PET/CT, with distant metastases detected in 4 patients and regional (N1) disease extension revealed in another 4 patients (54). Among the 16 patients who ultimately underwent radiation planning, 69% (11/16) of the GTVs planned by CT alone missed FDG-PET avid tumor. Among these cases, 31% (5/16) would have resulted in a geographic miss of the GTV during treatment, assuming that the avid disease on FDG-PET demonstrates active tumor (54). With the evolution of PET/CT and other functional/anatomical imaging modalities in development, there is going to be a continued impact on radiation planning for esophageal cancer.

Non-FDG PET

FDG-PET has been incorporated into both staging and predicting response to treatment, thus beginning to allow for individual tailoring of treatment. As a tool for measuring increased metabolic rate, FDG-PET is not specific for cancer cells and cannot make a distinction between malignant cells and highly metabolic normal cell activity or nonmalignant processes like infection (55). Also, its use in treatment response assessment is often limited by treatment-related inflammation overestimating the remainder of disease burden (56,57). Spatial constraints often make it difficult to differentiate between partial and complete response to treatment. Moreover, some esophageal tumors, primarily adenocarcinomas, do not have high metabolic uptake or uptake that is obscured by other tumor processes, thus limiting the effectiveness of FDG-PET. Fortunately, there are other biologic targets to assess besides glucose metabolism in the evaluation of malignancies, and many new radiolabeled tracers are being developed (55,58).

Choline metabolism is one such biologic process being investigated. Choline is naturally found in the body, and many organ systems utilize its metabolites in various reactions (55). In tumors, however, the only pathway for choline is incorporation into cell membrane phospholipids. Cell membrane production represents replication of tumor cells, and a measure of this membrane synthesis is representative of cell replication (55). Most commonly, ^{11}C is utilized to tag methylcholine, and because of its rapid acquisition into cells, imaging can be done within minutes (59). ^{11}C does have a short half-life; thus, ^{18}F is currently being investigated as an alternative (60). In those esophageal tumors where there is lower glucose metabolism or metabolism is obscured by other tumor cell characteristics like mucus production, radiolabeled choline has a potential role.

Another radiolabeled biologic marker showing promise in esophageal cancer is 3'-deoxy-3'-[^{1}8F]fluorothymidine (FLT). FLT-PET is able to measure tissue proliferation, as it utilizes intracellular thymidine kinase 1 (TK1) for intracellular metabolism (55,56). Once metabolized by TK1, it is incorporated into DNA synthesis and trapped in the cell (55,56). TK1 expression is related to the late G1 and S phases of the cell cycle, meaning that it is not readily produced in nondividing cells and commonly found in proliferating tumor cells. FLT-PET has shown the potential to be of value in evaluating malignant proliferation and assessing treatment response for a variety of tumors (56). Recently, FLT-PET was compared to FDG-PET for the detection of early changes in tumor proliferation after chemoradiation in esophageal carcinoma experimental models (61). In this study, FLT-PET was found to be more efficacious than FDG-PET in detecting early proliferative changes in both human SEG-1 cells and mouse SEG-1 xenografts and correlated better with histologic findings (56,61). Besides choline metabolism and amino acid/protein metabolism, there are many biologic processes that are currently under investigation as potential tools for malignant assessment. Oxygen metabolism, gene expression, angiogenesis, and apoptosis are all biologic targets that may someday play a role in esophageal cancer (55).

CONCLUSION

The ability of FDG-PET to provide functional imaging in esophageal cancer has led to its increasingly frequent and varied use. While its role in initial staging is becoming more clearly defined, its use in the postneoadjuvant setting as a tool to assess response and provide prognostic information continues to develop. In addition, its effectiveness as a routine follow-up study after definitive therapy is promising. Going forward, fusion with anatomical imaging make it an attractive tool for radiation planning, while other forms of PET may further elucidate other tumor characteristics to allow for continued optimization of therapy.

References

1. Jemal A, Siegel R, Ward E, et al. Cancer statistics, 2007. *CA J Clin.* 2007;57:43–66.
2. Enzinger PC, Mayer RJ. Esophageal cancer. *N Engl J Med.* 2003;349:2241–2252.
3. Dehdashti F, Siegel BA. Neoplasms of the esophagus and stomach. *Semin Nucl Med.* 2004;34:198–208.
4. Reed CE, Mishra G, Sahai AV, et al. Esophageal cancer staging: Improved accuracy by endoscopic ultrasound of celiac lymph nodes. *Ann Thorac Surg.* 1999;67:319–321.
5. Romagnuolo J, Scott J, Hawes RH, et al. Helical CT versus EUS fine needle aspiration for celiac nodal assessment in patients with esophageal cancer. *Gastrointest Endosc.* 2002;55:648–654.
6. Wren SM, Stijns P, Srinivas S. Positron emission tomography in the initial staging of esophageal cancer. *Arch Surg.* 2002;137:1001–1006.
7. Weber WA, Ott K. Imaging of esophageal and gastric cancer. *Semin Oncol.* 2004;31:530–541.
8. Juweid ME, Cheson BD. Positron-emission-tomography and assessment of cancer therapy. *N Engl J Med.* 2006;354:496–507.
9. Chin BB, Chang PP. Gastrointestinal malignancies evaluated with 18F-fluoro-2-deoxyglucose positron emission tomography. *Best Pract Res Clin Gastroenterol.* 2006;20:3–21.
10. Chin BB, Wahl RL. 18F-Fluoro-2-deoxyglucose positron emission tomography in the evaluation of gastrointestinal malignancies. *Gut.* 2003;52:23–29.
11. Shreve PD, Anzai Y, Wahl RL. Pitfalls in oncologic diagnosis with FDG PET imaging: physiologic and benign variants. *Radiographics.* 1999;19:61–77.
12. Flamen P. Positron emission tomography in gastric and esophageal cancer. *Curr Opin Oncol.* 2004;16:359–363.
13. Stahl A, Ott K, Weber WA, et al. FDG-PET imaging of locally advanced gastric carcinomas: correlation with endoscopic and histopathological findings. *Eur J Nucl Med Mol Imaging.* 2003;30:288–295.
14. Lerut T, Coosemans W, Decker G, et al. Cancer of the esophagus and gastro-esophageal junction: potentially curative therapies. *Surg Oncol.* 2001;10:113–122.
15. Kim K, Park SJ, Kim BT, et al. Evaluation of lymph node metastases in squamous cell carcinoma of the esophagus with positron emission tomography. *Ann Thorac Surg.* 2001;71:290–294.
16. Flamen P, Lerut A, Van Cutsem E, et al. Utility of positron emission tomography for the staging of patients with potentially operable esophageal carcinoma. *J Clin Oncol.* 2000;18:3202–3210.
17. van Westreenen HL, Westerterp M, Bossuyt PM, et al. Systematic review of the staging performance of ^{18}F-fluorodeoxyglucose positron emission tomography in esophageal cancer. *J Clin Oncol.* 2004;22:3805–3812.
18. Choi JY, Lee KH, Shim YM, et al. Improved detection of individual nodal involvement in squamous cell carcinoma of the esophagus by FDG PET. *J Nucl Med.* 2000;41:808–815.
19. Kneist W, Schreckenberger M, Bartenstein P, et al. Prospective evaluation of positron emission tomography in the preoperative staging of esophageal carcinoma. *Arch Surg.* 2004;139:1043–1049.

20. Luketich JD, Friedman DM, Weigel TL, et al. Evaluation of distant metastases in esophageal cancer: 100 consecutive positron emission tomography scans. *Ann Thorac Surg.* 1999;68:1133–1137.
21. Liberale G, Van Laethem JL, Gay F, et al. The role of PET scan in the preoperative management of oesophageal cancer. *Eur J Surg Oncol.* 2004;30:942–947.
22. Sihvo IT, Räsänen JV, Knuuti M, et al. Adenocarcinoma of the esophagus and the esophagogastric junction: positron emission tomography improves staging and prediction of survival in distant but not in locoregional disease. *J Gastrointest Surg.* 2004;8:988–996.
23. Block MI, Sundaresan SR, Patterson GA, et al. Improvement in staging of esophageal cancer with the addition of positron emission tomography. *Ann Thorac Surg.* 1997;64:770–777.
24. Meyers BF, Downey RJ, Decker PA, et al. The utility of positron emission tomography in staging of potentially operable carcinoma of the thoracic esophagus: results of the American College of Surgeons Oncology Group Z0060 trial. *J Thorac Cardiovasc Surg.* 2007;133:38–45.
25. Bruzzi JF, Swisher SG, Truong MT, et al. Detection of interval distant metastases: clinical utility of integrated CT-PET imaging in patients with esophageal carcinoma after neoadjuvant therapy. *Cancer.* 2007;109:125–134.
26. Wallace MB, Nietert PJ, Earle C, et al. An analysis of multiple staging management strategies for carcinoma of the esophagus: computed tomography, endoscopic ultrasound, positron emission tomography, and thoracoscopy/laparoscopy. *Ann Thorac Surg.* 2002;74:1026–1032.
27. Gebski V, Burmeister B, Smithers BM, et al. Survival benefits from neoadjuvant chemoradiotherapy or chemotherapy in oesophageal carcinoma: a meta-analysis. *Lancet Oncol.* 2007;8:226–234.
28. Law S, Fok M, Chow S, et al. Preoperative chemotherapy versus surgical therapy alone for squamous cell carcinoma of the esophagus: a perspective randomized trial. *J Thorac Cardiovasc Surg.* 1997;114:210–217.
29. Jones DR, Parker LA Jr, Detterbeck FC, et al. Inadequacy of computed tomography in assessing patients with esophageal carcinoma after induction chemoradiotherapy. *Cancer.* 1999;85:1026–1032.
30. Westerterp M, van Westreenen HL, Reitsma JB, et al. Esophageal cancer: CT, endoscopic US, and FDG PET for assessment of response to neoadjuvant therapy—systematic review. *Radiology.* 2005;236:841–851.
31. Weber WA, Ott K, Becker K, et al. Prediction of response to preoperative chemotherapy in adenocarcinomas of esophagogastric junction by metabolic imaging. *J Clin Oncol.* 2001;19:3058–3065.
32. Flamen P, Van Cutsem E, Lerut A, et al. Positron emission tomography for assessment of the response to induction radiochemotherapy in locally advanced oesophageal cancer. *Ann Oncol.* 2002;13:361–368.
33. Brücher BL, Weber W, Bauer M, et al. Neoadjuvant therapy of esophageal squamous cell carcinoma: response evaluation by positron emission tomography. *Ann Surg.* 2001;233:300–309.
34. Wieder HA, Brücher BL, Zimmerman F, et al. Time course of tumor metabolic activity during chemoradiotherapy of esophageal squamous cell carcinoma and response to treatment. *J Clin Oncol.* 2004;22:900–908.
35. Ott K, Weber WA, Lordick F, et al. Metabolic imaging predicts response, survival, and recurrence in adenocarcinomas of the esophagogastric junction. *J Clin Oncol.* 2006;24:4692–4698.
36. Port JL, Lee PC, Korst RJ, et al. Positron emission tomographic scanning predicts survival after induction chemotherapy for esophageal carcinoma. *Ann Thorac Surg.* 2007;84:393–400.
37. Arslan N, Miller T, Dehdashti F, et al. Evaluation of response to neoadjuvant therapy by quantitative FDG-PET in patients with esophageal cancer. *Mol Imaging Biol.* 2002;4:301–310.
38. Bar-Shalom R, Yefremov N, Guralnik L, et al. Clinical performance of PET/CT in evaluation of cancer: additional value for diagnostic imaging and patient management. *J Nucl Med.* 2003;44:1200–1209.
39. Erasmus JJ, Munden RF, Truong MT, et al. Preoperative chemo-radiation-induced ulceration in patients with esophageal cancer: a confounding factor in tumor response assessment in integrated computed tomographic-positron emission tomographic imaging. *J Thorac Oncol.* 2006;1:478–486.
40. Cerfolio RJ, Bryant AS. Maximum standardized uptake values on positron emission tomography of esophageal cancer predicts stage, tumor biology, and survival. *Ann Thorac Surg.* 2006;82:391–394.
41. Hong D, Lunagomez S, Kim EE, et al. Value of baseline positron emission tomography for predicting overall survival in patient with nonmetastatic esophageal or gastroesophageal junction carcinoma. *Cancer.* 2005;104:1620–1626.
42. Swisher SG, Erasmus J, Maish M, et al. 2-Fluoro-2-deoxy-D-glucose positron emission tomography imaging is predictive of pathologic response and survival after preoperative chemoradiation in patients with esophageal carcinoma. *Cancer.* 2004;101:1776–1785.
43. Konski AA, Cheng JD, Goldberg M, et al. Correlation of molecular response as measured by 18-FDG positron emission tomography with outcome after chemoradiotherapy in patients with esophageal carcinoma. *Int J Radiat Oncol Biol Phys.* 2007; Available online May 29, 2007 ahead of print: 1–6.
44. Flamen P, Lerut A, Van Cutsem E, et al. The utility of positron emission tomography (PET) for the diagnosis and staging of recurrent esophageal cancer. *J Thorac Cardiovasc Surg.* 2000;120:1085–1092.
45. Lordick F, Ott K, Krause BJ, et al. PET to assess early metabolic response and to guide treatment of adenocarcinoma of the oesophagogastric junction: the MUNICON phase II trial. *Lancet Oncol.* 2007;8:797–805.
46. Downey RJ, Ilson DH. PET-guided induction chemotherapy. *Lancet Oncol.* 2007;8:754–755.
47. Kelloff GJ, Hoffman JM, Johnson B, et al. Progress and promise of FDG-PET imaging for cancer patient management and oncologic drug development. *Clin Cancer Res.* 2005;11:2785–2808.
48. Erasmus JJ, Munden RF. The role of integrated computed tomography positron-emission tomography in esophageal cancer: staging and assessment of therapeutic response. *Semin Radiat Oncol.* 2006;17:29–37.
49. Yuan S, Yu Y, Chao KS, et al. Additional value of PET/CT over PET in assessment of locoregional lymph nodes in thoracic esophageal squamous cell cancer. *J Nucl Med.* 2006;47:1255–1259.
50. Lardinois D, Weder W, Hany TF. Staging of non-small-cell lung cancer with integrated positron-emission tomography and computed tomography. *N Engl J Med.* 2003;348:2500–2507.
51. Vrieze O, Haustermans K, De Wever W, et al. Is there a role for FGD-PET in radiotherapy planning in esophageal carcinoma? *Radiother Oncol.* 2004;73:269–275.
52. Mourneau-Zabotto L, Touboul E, Lerouge D, et al. Impact of CT and ^{18}F-deoxyglucose positron emission tomography image fusion for conformal radiotherapy in esophageal carcinoma. *Int J Radiat Oncol Biol Phys.* 2005;63:340–345.
53. Konski A, Doss M, Milestone B, et al. The integration of 18-fluoro-deoxy-glucose positron emission tomography and endoscopic ultrasound in the treatment-planning process for esophageal carcinoma. *Int J Radiat Oncol Biol Phys.* 2005;61:1123–1128.
54. Leong T, Everitt, Yuen K, et al. A prospective study to evaluate the impact of FDG-PET on CT-based radiotherapy treatment planning for oesophageal cancer. *Radiother Oncol.* 2006;78:254–261.
55. Groves AM, Win T, Haim SB, et al. Non-[^{1}8F]FDGPET in clinical oncology. *Lancet Oncol.* 2007:8:822–830.
56. Chao KS. 3'-deoxy-3'-^{18}F-fluorothymidine (FLT) positron emission tomography for early prediction of response to chemoradiotherapy—a clinical application model of esophageal cancer. *Semin Oncol.* 2007;34(suppl 1):S31–S36.
57. van Westreenen HL, Heeren PAM, Jager PL, et al. Pitfalls of positive findings in staging esophageal cancer with F-18-fluorodeoxyglucose positron emission tomography. *Ann Surg Oncol.* 2003;10:1100–1105.
58. Mankoff DA, Eary JF, Link JM, et al. Tumor-specific positron emission tomography imaging in patients: [18F] fluorodeoxyglucose and beyond. *Clin Cancer Res.* 2007;13:3460–3469.
59. Hara T, Kosaka N, Shinoura N, et al. PET imaging of brain tumor with [methyl-^{11}C] choline. *J Nucl Med.* 1997;38:842–847.
60. Zöphel K, Kotzeeke J. Is ^{11}C-choline the most appropriate tracer for prostate cancer? Against. *Eur J Nucl Med Mol Imaging.* 2004;31:756–759.
61. Apisarnthanarax S, Alauddin MM, Mourtada F, et al. Early detection of chemoradioresponse in esophageal carcinoma by 3'-deoxy-3'-^{3}H-fluorothymidine using preclinical tumor models. *Clin Cancer Res.* 2006;12:4590–4597.

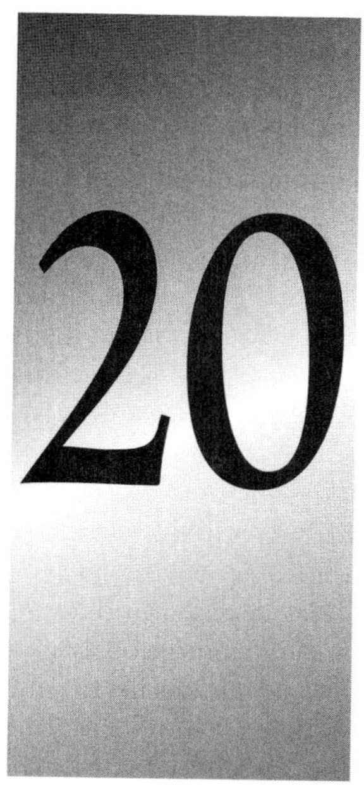

20 Esophageal Imaging: Functional—MRI

Eugene Y. Chang
Blair A. Jobe

ROLE OF FUNCTIONAL IMAGING IN ESOPHAGEAL CANCER

Despite multimodal treatment for patients with esophageal cancer, this disease carries a poor prognosis, and there is a need to improve the outcomes of therapy. One component of the efforts to optimize therapy is the use of functional esophageal imaging. Unlike anatomic modalities such as computed tomography or endoscopic ultrasound (EUS), the goal of functional imaging is to assess tumor activity independently of anatomic changes brought on by the tumor. The limitations of anatomic imaging techniques become apparent when using them to assess the response to chemoradiation. Computed tomography and endoscopic ultrasound, for example, cannot reliably discriminate between the expected postchemoradiation scarring and residual, live tumor (1–5). In contrast, functional imaging could facilitate ongoing evaluation of therapeutic effectiveness with serial scanning, potentially eliminating the need for surgery in complete responders. Additionally, it could improve the quality of palliation by stopping chemoradiation in those who progress with therapy, improve prognostication based on tumor response, facilitate the evaluation of new therapies, and enhance the quality of clinical trials. Modalities developed for functional imaging include dynamic contrast enhanced magnetic resonance imaging (DCE-MRI) and positron-emission tomography (PET) scanning (see Chapter 22).

DYNAMIC CONTRAST ENHANCED MRI

DCE-MRI has been studied as a diagnostic tool in several types of malignancy (6) and can discriminate between histologic varieties of malignancy (7). It identifies tumors on the basis of their altered vascular integrity, which result from pathologic angiogenesis (8,9). Esophageal adenocarcinoma exhibits increased expression of proangiogenic factors, including basic fibroblast growth factor and vascular endothelial growth factor (10,11). This form of malignancy is associated with greater vascularization and has a higher microvascular density compared with normal esophageal tissue and precancerous lesions (12,13). Microvascular density also differs between prechemoradiation and postchemoradiation specimens (12). It is thought that these properties form the pathologic basis on which DCE-MRI can detect esophageal adenocarcinoma and evaluate its response to chemoradiation.

In DCE-MRI, a bolus of gadolinium chelate is administered intravenously as cross-sectional magnetic resonance images of the esophagus are rapidly and repeatedly acquired. A sufficient number of images are acquired to capture the rise and decline of the signal intensity in the esophageal tissue. For each spatial point included in the scan, a time course of signal intensity is generated. This time course appears to follow reproducible patterns that have the ability to differentiate benign from malignant tissue (6–9). Although these differences may be assessed qualitatively, pharmacokinetic modeling techniques are used to characterize the differences in a quantitative fashion.

The typical method for analyzing the signal intensity time course relies on the "Tofts" model of pharmacokinetic analysis (8). This widely used model (also called the "standard model") predicts the time course using 7 parameters that describe the exchange of molecules across membranes as contrast reagent leaves the plasma. Under most implementations of this model, a curve that best fits the observed time course is generated by varying 2 parameters: a pseudo–first-order rate constant for contrast reagent transfer between plasma and the interstitial space (K^{trans}) and the volume fraction of the interstitial space (v_e). The signal intensity at the aorta is used as the arterial input function. This limited model, however, may under- or overestimate the signal intensity at various times (Figure 20.1). Nonetheless, the parameter K^{trans} has been used to discriminate between benign and malignant tissue. An image map produced by plotting K^{trans} for each anatomic point can identify malignant tissue areas of increased K^{trans} compared with the surrounding background—known as "hot spots"—in the map.

Another model, termed the "shutter-speed" model, involves a more refined pharmokinetic analysis. While the Tofts model assumes that the contrast agent is homogeneously distributed over the compartments it enters, the shutter-speed model takes into account that water exchange across the cell membrane is not infinitely fast and introduces an eighth parameter: the mean intracellular water lifetime (τ_i). These kinetics play an important role in the interpretation of DCE studies (14–16). Theoretical data simulations and experimental animal tumor models (17–19) have shown that K^{trans} and v_e can be underestimated by a factor of 2 to 3 if the kinetics of water exchange across a cell membrane are neglected. The shutter-speed model produces a much closer curve fit to the measured data (Figure 20.1) and may discriminate between malignant and benign breast disease more accurately (20). K^{trans}, v_e, and τ_i are evaluated and can be mapped pixel by pixel to generate images based on the shutter-speed model of DCE-MRI (18).

ANATOMIC IMAGING OF THE ESOPHAGUS WITH MRI

Functional data from DCE-MRI are typically coregistered with anatomic data to facilitate the interpretation of the images. The acquisition of anatomic esophageal images with MRI poses a number of technical challenges. These include the potential for artifacts due to cardiac and respiratory motion and distortion of the magnetic

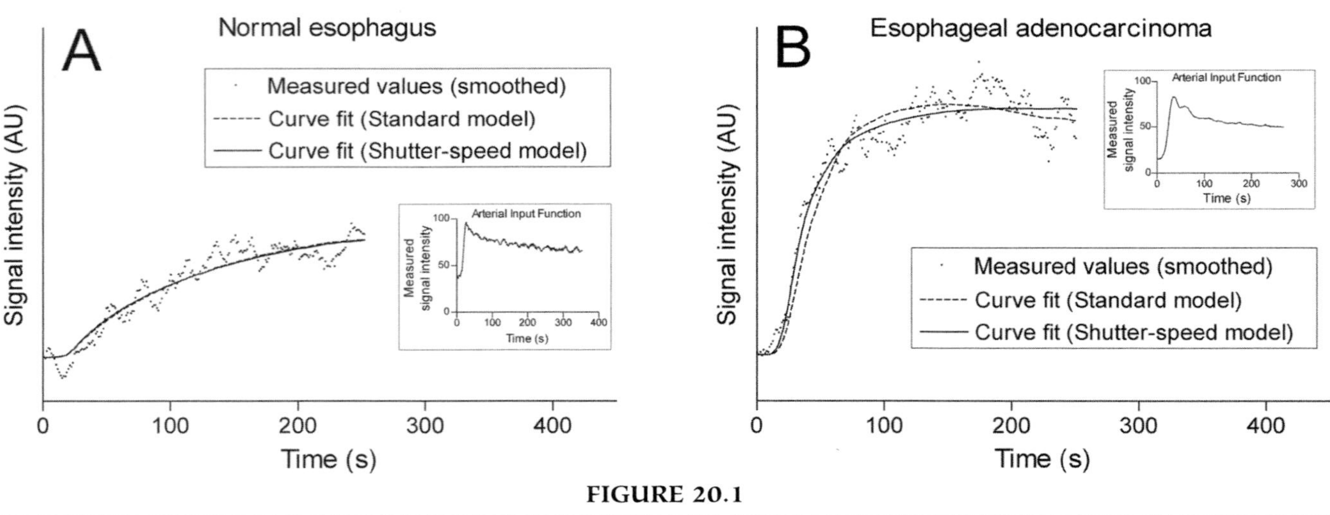

FIGURE 20.1

Time courses of signal intensity in the region of interest in normal esophageal tissue (A) and in esophageal adenocarcinoma (B). Dots denote the measured values, which have been smoothed (by averaging adjacent values) in order to illustrate trends. Dashed lines demonstrate the best-fitting curve generated using the standard model. Solid lines demonstrate the best-fitting curve generated using the shutter-speed model. Arterial input functions (insets) were measured from regions of interest on the aorta. Note the more rapid initial increase in signal intensity in esophageal adenocarcinoma, followed by a gradual decrease, suggesting greater vascular permeability in adenocarcinoma (from Chang et al. [22]).

flux lines due to the nearby presence of air-filled lungs. Furthermore, anatomic planes in the gastroesophageal junction are often indistinct on MRI, making it difficult to distinguish the distal esophagus from the surrounding tissues. Early trials of conventional MRI, however, showed that esophageal imaging is feasible. In one early study, a group demonstrated that interpretable images can be acquired with MRI, which was found to have 60% accuracy in evaluating the depth of invasion of esophageal adenocarcinoma (21). A more recent study using a 3-Tesla magnet has demonstrated that anatomic imaging of the esophagus can readily be performed using a half-Fourier single shot turbo spin echo (HASTE) protocol and that the esophagus could be identified in the coronal, sagittal, and axial planes (22) (Figure 20.2). Using T_1-weighted sagittal imaging, the entire esophagus can be scanned in under 2 seconds. The positioning of slices for image acquisition can be guided by the use of oral contrast agents, which identify the esophageal lumen. Although no product has been marketed specifically for use as an oral contrast agent in T_1-weighted MRI, it has been reported that blueberry juice is a safe, inexpensive, and readily available agent that can serve this role (23–25) (Figure 20.3) This property is related to its significant manganese content, which acts to reduce its T_1 value.

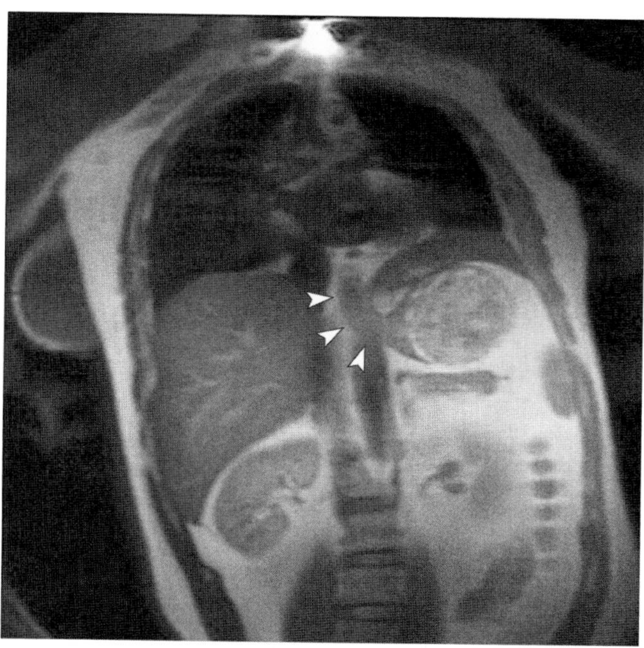

FIGURE 20.2

Anatomic images of the esophagus in the coronal section, taken with the T_2-weighted HASTE protocol (from Chang et al. [22]).

ROLE OF K^{TRANS} IN ESOPHAGEAL DCE-MRI

DCE-MRI of the esophagus poses a further challenge since it is potentially susceptible to artifacts introduced by cardiac, pulmonary, and diaphragmatic motion. These movements cause the signal intensity at a given spatial point to fluctuate, affecting the pharmacokinetic analysis. Nonetheless, DCE-MRI has been performed in a small series of patients with esophageal adenocarcinoma and compared with healthy controls.

In DCE-MRI, K^{trans} is evaluated for each spatial point in the scanned region. K^{trans} is a pseudo–first-order rate constant measuring the transfer of contrast reagent from the intravascular space to the interstitial space within the esophageal tissue. This rate constant carries particular significance since the endothelium within tumor blood vessels exhibits altered permeability with cancer angiogenesis. This enables both a more rapid transfer of contrast reagent into the interstitium and an accelerated clearance of the reagent when compared to benign tissue (6).

Using the shutter-speed model, K^{trans}, v_e, and τ_i were evaluated in the distal esophagus of study subjects after the acquisition of at least 250 time points (22). It was demonstrated that K^{trans} was 5 times greater in adenocarcinoma patients than in controls. Hot spots were seen in patients with adenocarcinoma, producing a qualitative difference in parametric maps of K^{trans} (Figure 20.4). One patient with esophageal adenocarcinoma underwent DCE-MRI before and after neoadjuvant chemoradiation. Measurements of K^{trans}, v_e, and τ_i in these hot spots demonstrated a substantial decrease in K^{trans} after chemoradiation, from 2.41 to 0.21/min. According to the size of the tumor by EUS (prechemoradiation) and the pathologic exam (postchemoradiation), this patient developed a partial response to chemoradiation. This finding suggests that DCE-MRI findings, particularly K^{trans}, show promise in gauging the response to chemoradiation. These findings demonstrate that this imaging technique is feasible and diagnostically informative in the detection of esophageal adenocarcinoma. Despite a significant amount of esophageal movement, pixel-by-pixel K^{trans} maps can be generated, suggesting that signal intensity fluctuations at any given pixel "average out" when a sufficient number of time points are sampled. Based on these characteristics, K^{trans} may prove useful for improved characterization of esophageal adenocarcinoma beyond currently available methods. K^{trans} may allow for a means of monitoring therapy and gaining a more detailed understanding of individual tumor behavior, providing what is in essence an in vivo assay of endothelial permeability.

These studies have shown that DCE-MRI has great potential to impact the treatment of esophageal adenocarcinoma by improving the ability to stage

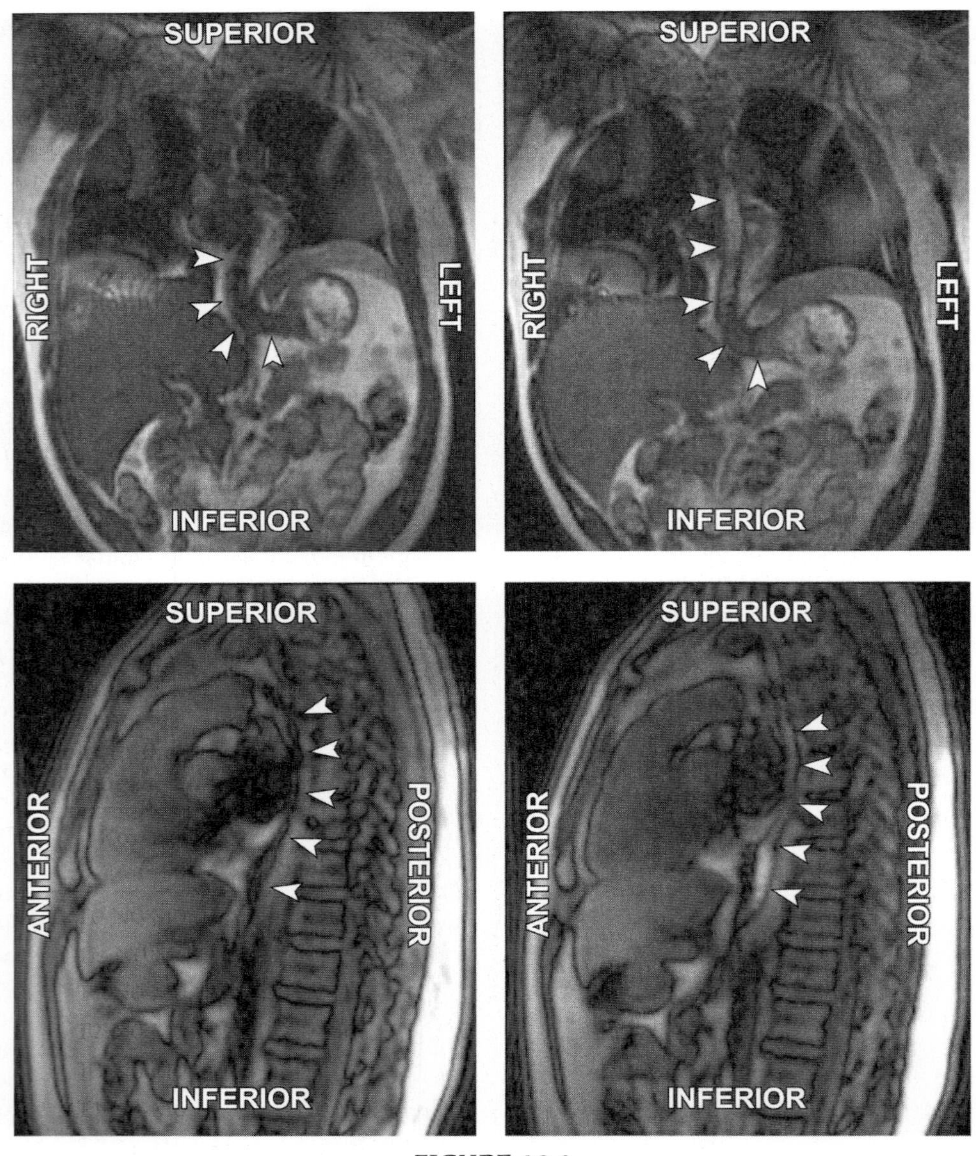

FIGURE 20.3

Use of oral contrast agents in esophageal imaging. Coronal (top) and sagittal (bottom) images of the esophagus prior to (left) and during ingestion of blueberry juice (right). Arrowheads indicate the location of the esophagus (from Chang et al. [22]).

patients and to gauge therapeutic response to chemoradiation. Given these promising results, larger-scale studies are needed to evaluate the ability of this imaging modality to determine the response to chemoradiation. Furthermore, this imaging modality may also improve prognostication, facilitate the study of new therapies for chemoradiation, and enhance the quality of clinical trials.

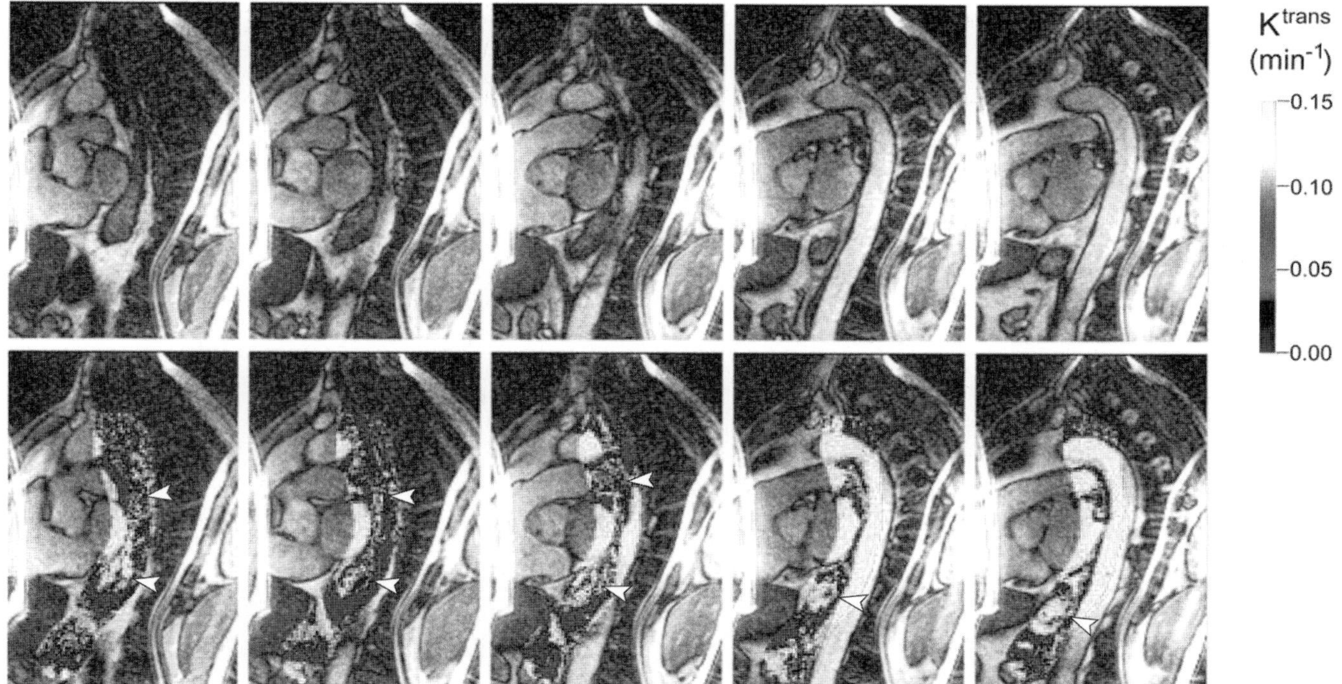

FIGURE 20.4

Parametric maps generated from K^{trans} values at each pixel, represented using color scales converted to monochromatic images. Anatomic images from a patient with esophageal adenocarcinoma are shown (top row). Parametric maps are coregistered and superimposed on anatomic images (bottom row). Each column shows a different slice position. Arrowheads indicate the location of the esophagus (from Chang et al. [22]).

References

1. Zuccaro G Jr, Rice TW, Goldblum J, et al. Endoscopic ultrasound cannot determine suitability for esophagectomy after aggressive chemoradiotherapy for esophageal cancer. *Am J Gastroenterol.* 1999;94(4):906–912.
2. Melcher L, Wong W, Sanghera B, et al. Sequential FDG-PET scanning in the assessment of response to neoadjuvant chemotherapy in perable oesophageal cancer. *J Clin Oncol.* 2004;22(14S):327s.
3. Jones DR, Parker LA Jr, Detterbeck FC, et al. Inadequacy of computed tomography in assessing patients with esophageal carcinoma after induction chemoradiotherapy. *Cancer.* 1999;85(5):1026–1032.
4. Hordijk ML, Kok TC, Wilson JH, et al. Assessment of response of esophageal carcinoma to induction chemotherapy. *Endoscopy.* 1993;25(9):592–596.
5. Laterza E, de Manzoni G, Guglielmi A, et al. Endoscopic ultrasonography in the staging of esophageal carcinoma after preoperative radiotherapy and chemotherapy. *Ann Thorac Surg.* 1999;67(5):1466–1469.
6. Knopp MV, von Tengg-Kobligk H, Choyke PL. Functional magnetic resonance imaging in oncology for diagnosis and therapy monitoring. *Mol Cancer Ther.* 2003;2(4):419–426.
7. Knopp MV, Weiss E, Sinn HP, et al. Pathophysiologic basis of contrast enhancement in breast tumors. *J Magn Reson Imaging.* 1999;10(3):260–266.
8. Tofts PS. Modeling tracer kinetics in dynamic Gd-DTPA MR imaging. *J Magn Reson Imaging.* 1997;7(1):91–101.
9. Tofts PS, Berkowitz B, Schnall MD. Quantitative analysis of dynamic Gd-DTPA enhancement in breast tumors using a permeability model. *Magn Reson Med.* 1995;33(4):564–568.
10. Couvelard A, Paraf F, Gratio V, et al. Angiogenesis in the neoplastic sequence of Barrett's oesophagus. Correlation with VEGF expression. *J Pathol.* 2000;192(1):14–18.
11. Lord RV, Park JM, Wickramasinghe K, et al. Vascular endothelial growth factor and basic fibroblast growth factor expression in esophageal adenocarcinoma and Barrett esophagus. *J Thorac Cardiovasc Surg.* 2003;125(2):246–253.
12. Torres C, Wang H, Turner J, et al. Prognostic significance and effect of chemoradiotherapy on microvessel density (angiogenesis) in esophageal Barrett's esophagus-associated adenocarcinoma and squamous cell carcinoma. *Hum Pathol.* 1999;30(7):753–758.
13. Auvinen MI, Sihvo EI, Ruohtula T, et al. Incipient angiogenesis in Barrett's epithelium and lymphangiogenesis in Barrett's adenocarcinoma. *J Clin Oncol.* 2002;20(13):2971–2979.
14. Landis CS, Li X, Telang FW, et al. Determination of the MRI contrast agent concentration time course in vivo following bolus injection: effect of equilibrium transcytolemmal water exchange. *Magn Reson Med.* 2000;44(4):563–5674.
15. Landis CS, Li X, Telang FW, et al. Equilibrium transcytolemmal water-exchange kinetics in skeletal muscle in vivo. *Magn Reson Med.* 1999;42(3):467–478.
16. Springer CS Jr. B-dependence of the CR-determined exchange regime for equilibrium transcytolemmal water transport: implications for bolus-tracking studies. *Proceedings of the International Society for Magnetic Resonance in Medicine.* 2001;3:2241.
17. Zhou R, Pickup S, Yankeelov TE, et al. Simultaneous measurement of arterial input function and tumor pharmacokinetics in mice by dynamic contrast enhanced imaging: effects of transcytolemmal water exchange. *Magn Reson Med.* 2004;52(2):248–257.
18. Yankeelov TE, Rooney WD, Li X, et al. Variation of the relaxographic "shutter-speed" for transcytolemmal water exchange affects the CR bolus-tracking curve shape. *Magn Reson Med.* 2003;50(6):1151–1169.
19. Yankeelov TE. Pharmacokinetic analysis is affected be fast-exchange-limit departure during bolus CR passage. *Proceedings of the International Society for Magnetic Resonance in Medicine.* 2002;3:2116.
20. Li X. Shutter speed analysis of CR bolus-tracking data facilitates discrimination of benign and malignant breast disease. *Proceedings of the International Society for Magnetic Resonance in Medicine.* 2004;12.
21. Wu LF, Wang BZ, Feng JL, et al. Preoperative TN staging of esophageal cancer: comparison of miniprobe ultrasonography, spiral CT and MRI. *World J Gastroenterol.* 2003;9(2):219–224.
22. Chang EY, Li X, Jerosch-Herold M, et al. The evaluation of esophageal adenocarcinoma using dynamic contrast-enhanced magnetic resonance imaging. *J Gastrointest Surg.* 2007:166–175.
23. Hiraishi K, Narabayashi I, Fujita O, et al. Blueberry juice: preliminary evaluation as an oral contrast agent in gastrointestinal MR imaging. *Radiology.* 1995;194(1):119–123.
24. Karantanas AH, Papanikolaou N, Kalef-Ezra J, et al. Blueberry juice used per os in upper abdominal MR imaging: composition and initial clinical data. *Eur Radiol.* 2000;10(6):909–913.
25. Schmid MR, Hany TF, Knesplova L, et al. 3D MR gastrography: exoscopic and endoscopic analysis of the stomach. *Eur Radiol.* 1999;9(1):73–77.

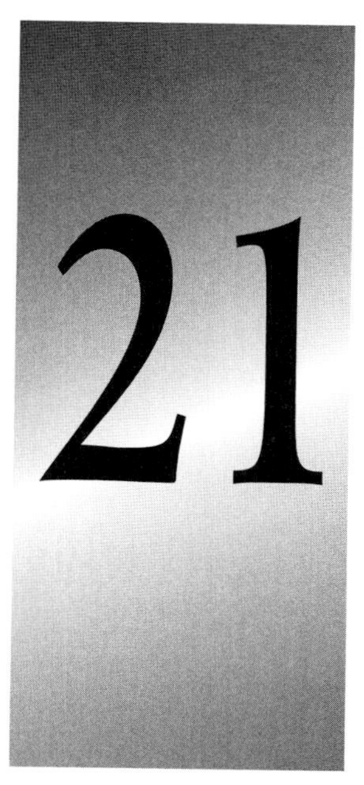

Esophageal Cancer Staging—Clinical

Yasser M. Bhat
Michael L. Kochman

Staging of any cancer is essential for both prognostication and selection of the appropriate therapeutic modality. Imprecise tools and limited treatment options have hampered esophageal cancer staging. Computed tomography (CT) scanning was the mainstay of staging and still remains an essential component for initial staging and evaluation for distant metastatic disease. Developments of complementary technologies including endoscopic ultrasound (EUS) with fine-needle aspiration (FNA) capability, positron-emission tomography (PET), and minimally invasive surgical staging (both thoracoscopic or laparoscopic) have vastly improved the accuracy of staging in this disease. This chapter focuses on clinical staging of esophageal cancer using CT scan and endoscopic ultrasound. Details concerning specifics of PET scan, magnetic resonance imaging (MRI), and molecular markers have been covered elsewhere in the text (Chapters 19–20).

The American Joint Committee on Cancer has established staging by tumor, node and metastasis classification (1). Survival outcomes are strongly related to the depth of tumor invasion with 5-year survival rates ranging from 46% (T1) to 7% (T4) (2). For node-negative disease (N0), the 5-year survival is 40% as compared to 17% for N1 disease in patients who are candidates for surgical excision. Metastatic disease to distant lymph nodes or organs significantly impacts long-term survival with 5-year survival data of 5% and 3%, respectively. In patients with complete staging information, the 5-year survival decreases as follows: stage I (60%), stage II (31%), stage III (20%), and stage IV (4%) (3).

Precise staging is extremely important in selecting patients for either definitive medical or surgical therapy and for selections of appropriate candidates for palliative therapy. This is best achieved with a combination of tests; no single technology is adequate for complete staging of all aspects of this disease. Therefore, tests for staging of newly diagnosed esophageal cancer may include combinations of cross-sectional imaging (CT scan or MRI), EUS, PET scanning, and minimally invasive surgery. Even after all efforts, metastatic disease may be seen in up to 60% of cases at attempted curative surgery, and accurate staging continues to be a challenge (4).

STAGING OF ESOPHAGEAL CANCER—COMPUTED TOMOGRAPHY SCANNING

Distant metastases are found in up to 50% of patients with esophageal cancer at presentation making them inoperable for cure. The most common sites of metastasis include the liver (35% of patients), lungs (20%), bones (9%), and adrenals or brain (2%), with the pericardium, pleura, soft tissues, stomach, pancreas, or spleen rarely infrequent at roughly 1% each (5). CT scan of the chest and abdomen includes most of these sites and is helpful to survey for these locations. Since it is inexpensive, noninvasive, and readily available, its use as an initial staging test is appropriate and effective.

Thoracic and abdominal lymph nodes >1 cm in diameter can be detected by CT scanning. Periesophageal lymph nodes are often masked by the primary tumor, and because metastatic disease may be present in normal-sized lymph nodes, this is a limitation of the test. The sensitivity of detecting mediastinal lymphadenopathy by CT scanning is 34% to 61% and for abdominal lymphadenopathy is 50% to 76% (6). Depending on the location of the primary tumor (upper third, middle third, or lower third of the esophagus), identification of celiac lymphadenopathy may be particularly important in the treatment algorithm. CT scanning is particularly poor for detection of celiac lymphadenopathy with a sensitivity of only 8% (7).

Given the increasing incidence of adenocarcinoma of the lower esophagus in the United States, evaluation for hepatic metastases is of paramount importance. CT scanning with contrast enhancement has a sensitivity of 70% to 80% for hepatic lesions >2 cm (8). Subcentimeter lesions are often missed and frequently are the cause of false-negative studies. In a study using minimally invasive surgical staging as a gold standard, the sensitivity for PET scans for the detection of distant metastases was 69% as compared to 46% for CT. In the same study, PET scans detected 23 of 33 metastatic liver lesions, and all the missed lesions were <1 cm in diameter (9).

Since CT scanning cannot delineate the individual wall layers of the esophagus, its utility for local tumor (T) staging is very limited. T4 stage disease may be excluded if the fat pad between the esophagus and the adjacent structure is preserved, although EUS is superior to CT for this assessment (10). CT criteria for aortic involvement by tumor have been studied, and a sensitivity as high as 100% and a specificity of 86% have been reported (11). Specific criteria for involvement of the tracheobronchial tree have been described. However, there is significant interobserver variability despite these defined criteria. A study of 35 patients reported good agreement for extension of the tumor to the tracheobronchial tree, pericardium, and liver, but poor agreement among 3 radiologists for detection of involvement of the aorta, pulmonary vessels, vertebrae, or stomach (12).

In summary, CT scanning is an important tool for the initial staging of esophageal carcinoma and is able to detect distant metastases with an accuracy of 60% to 90%. However, it is limited in its ability to discern locally advanced (T4) disease and disease in subcentimeter lymph nodes.

STAGING OF ESOPHAGEAL CANCER—ENDOSCOPIC ULTRASOUND

By combining endoscopy and high-frequency ultrasound, EUS allows accurate staging of local tumor by studying the wall layers of the esophagus. EUS has become an established tool in the evaluation of esophageal tumors. In addition, periesophageal, perigastric, and celiac lymph nodes can be assessed adequately, and with the advent of curvilinear echoendoscopes, FNA biopsy of both these nodes and accessible liver lesions is possible.

EUS imaging of the 5-layer esophageal wall is generally performed at frequencies of 7.5 and 12 MHz. The earliest stage is Tis (in situ), where the cancer is present in the epithelium without invading the lamina propria. This is detected by mucosal biopsies and cannot be imaged by EUS. If the cancer traverses the lamina propria, the staging is T1 and is further subclassified into T1m (confined to mucosa) and T1sm (submucosal invasion). T1m lesions rarely metastasize to regional lymph nodes, while T1sm lesions have a 15% to 30% rate of regional metastasis, and as such, EUS helps in the selection of appropriate therapy (endoscopic mucosal resection for T1m and surgery for T1sm cancers) for these lesions. The tumor is T2 if there is invasion of the muscularis propria and T3 if it progresses further to the adventitia. Involvement of regional structures (aorta, pleura, azygous vein, or other surrounding structures) is staged as T4 disease (13). The accuracy of EUS for preoperative T-staging ranges from 75% to 85% and is both operator and stage dependent. Accuracy for T3 and T4 disease is the highest at 89%, but 6% of T3 tumors and 11% of T4 tumors as pathologically proven are overstaged by EUS. Accuracy for T1 disease is 86% with 16% of tumors overstaged, and for T2 tumors it is 73% with 10% being understaged and 17% overstaged (14,15).

EUS is also useful for N staging of esophageal cancer. Periesophageal, perigastric, mediastinal, and celiac lymph nodes can be examined for features of malignancy that include size >1 cm, round, sharp and distinct borders, and diffuse hypoechogenicity (Figure 21.1). The sensitivity, specificity, positive predictive value (PPV), and negative predictive value (NPV) of EUS for N status in one review were 89%, 75%, 86%, and 79%, respectively, with an accuracy of 84%. If all 4 of the malignant features were present, the accuracy was reported to approach 100% (16). Malignant celiac lymphadenopathy (CLN) is an important predictor of survival in esophageal cancer, especially in patients without advanced T-stage or locoregional lymphadenopathy (17). The sensitivity of EUS for detection of malignant CLN was 77% with a specificity of 85%, PPV of 89%, and NPV 71% with an overall accuracy of 81% in a large study. All celiac nodes >1 cm were malignant in this study.

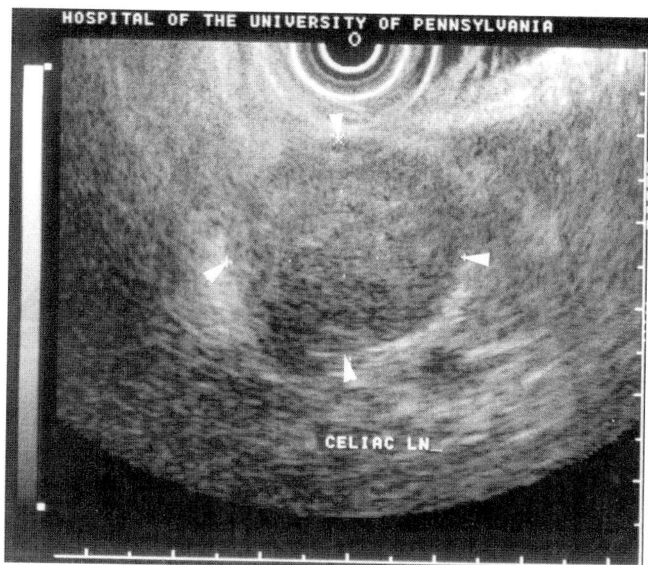

FIGURE 21.1

Endoscopic ultrasound demonstration of a typical malignant celiac axis lymph node, biopsy proven by endoscopic ultrasound fine-needle aspiration.

FNA of lymph nodes increases the accuracy (both sensitivity and specificity) even further. In the patients who underwent EUS-guided FNA biopsy of the malignant-appearing celiac lymph nodes, the sensitivity, specificity, PPV, and NPV improved to 98%, 100%, 100%, and 83%, respectively (18). EUS-FNA also allows examination and sampling of celiac nodes after neoadjuvant therapy, and patients with persistent disease in the nodes have a worse prognosis than those with eradicated disease (19).

EUS prediction of survival is helpful in the determination of therapeutic options for patients. The presence of metastatic disease to the locoregional lymph nodes is a major driver of early death, regardless of histology and T stage of the primary lesion. In a large retrospective study of 203 patients over 66 months, T stage, N stage, and presence of malignant celiac lymphadenopathy were significant predictors of survival in univariate analysis (17). When multivariate analysis was applied, only the N stage was statistically significant in predicting survival. In addition, comparison of different T stages among patients with either N stage of 0 found no statistical difference in survival, and the same results were noted in patients with N stage of 1.

In the United States, most patients present at an advanced stage once symptoms of dysphagia have developed. In up to a third of the patients, luminal stenosis is severe enough to prevent the passage of a 13 mm echoendoscope without dilation (19). Staging with EUS from positions proximal to the stricture has demonstrated decreased accuracy and an inability to access the celiac axis. Therefore, dilation of the malignant stricture may be required for complete examination of the tumor for staging purposes. While esophageal perforation was a concern with this technique initially, with perforation rates of up to 24% (20), several studies have since reported esophageal dilation to be safe and increased the rate of detection of celiac axis involvement in selected patients in whom therapy would be altered (21,22). Dilation to 14 or 15 mm is usually needed to pass the echoendoscopes, and if this is not possible, smaller-caliber, wire-guided echoendoscopes can be passed through the stenosis to complete the endosonographic examination. Even with these "miniprobes," the celiac axis is not detected in up to 10% of the cases because of retained gastric air or high-grade stenosis from the tumor. A major limitation of these probes, however, is the inability to perform FNA of lymph nodes (23,24).

EUS has consistently been shown to be more accurate than CT or MRI for staging of esophageal cancer (11,25,26). The main advantage of EUS in staging is demonstrating locoregional disease, and it is uniquely suited to determine the T stage (27). CT and PET are able to identify the primary tumor in the majority of the cases, but are not able to examine the wall layers of the esophagus, as does EUS (28). This is especially useful in early T-stage disease, where EUS can help determine the feasibility of endoscopic therapy and presence of T3 disease. In addition, EUS examination can predict long-term survival of patients with esophageal cancer well when stratified by T stage, N stage, and presence of celiac axis lymphadenopathy (17). A major limitation of EUS is the inability to detect distant metastatic disease (liver and lung), and as such, it cannot generally suffice as a single test in the evaluation of this disease.

STAGING OF ESOPHAGEAL CANCER—POSITRON-EMISSION TOMOGRAPHY

PET scanning utilizes imaging to identify areas with increased metabolism as demonstrated by ^{18}F-fluorodeoxyglucose (FDG) uptake by metabolically active lesions including active tumor foci. FDG accumulates in the majority of esophageal tumors. FDG-PET has no effective role in T staging, as it does not image the different wall layers of the esophagus. For locoregional disease, its performance is moderate, with sensitivity, specificity, and accuracy of 45%, 100%, and 48%, respectively, in one pilot study (29). In a recent study of 56 patients, PET identified locoregional lymph nodes separate from the primary tumor in 37.5% of the cases only, while EUS and CT scan identified 58.9% and 26.8% of lymph nodes, respectively (28). EUS is also superior to PET for detection of celiac axis nodes (30). PET was more sensitive than CT

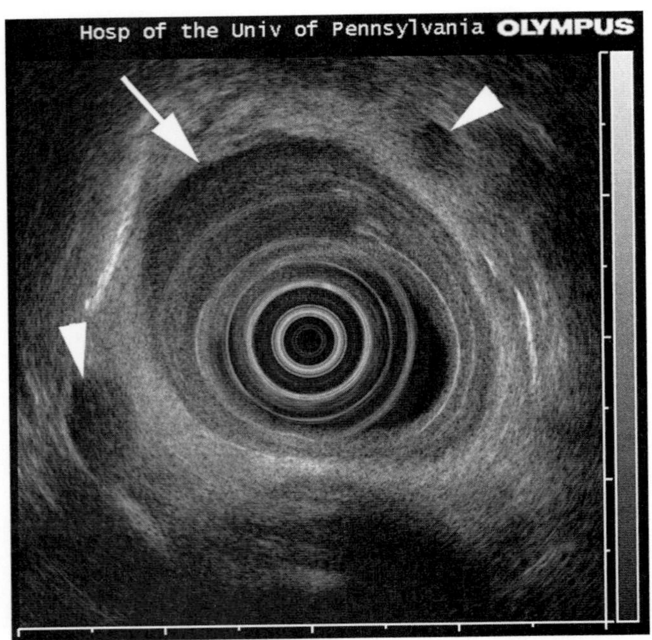

FIGURE 21.2

Endoscopic ultrasound demonstration of a typical T3N1 esophageal carcinoma.

in another study comparing them for nodal metastatic disease. The sensitivity, specificity, and accuracy for PET were 51.9%, 94.2%, and 84% as compared to 14.8%, 96.7%, and 76.6% for CT scanning (31). The major advantage of PET over CT appears to be the ability to detect distant metastatic disease, thereby potentially influencing the decision to avoid surgery. A study of 100 patients with 70 cases of distant metastasis, as confirmed by minimally invasive surgery, compared PET with CT. PET scanning was able to detect 51 of 70 cases and had sensitivity, specificity, and accuracy of 69%, 93.4%, and 84%, respectively, while CT was only 46.1% sensitive and 73% specific with an accuracy of 63%. All lesions missed by PET scans were <1 cm in size (9). The availability and cost of PET scans remain a limiting factor.

STAGING OF ESOPHAGEAL CANCER—CONCLUSION

Most patients in the United States present at an advanced stage and the typical EUS stage and clinical stage is T3N1 (Figure 21.2). There is evidence to suggest that if locoregional lymph node involvement is identified, the T stage may not influence survival. As such, accurate staging of esophageal cancer is challenging and requires a multimodality approach. A study compared the health care costs with effectiveness of various staging options using CT, EUS/FNA, PET scans, and surgical staging (32). CT followed by EUS/FNA was the most inexpensive strategy. PET followed by EUS/FNA was slightly more effective, but also more expensive. We recommend performing a CT scan as an initial screening test to determine resectability and to document the absence of distant metastatic disease, followed by EUS/FNA for tumor and lymph node staging. If patients are subsequently considered surgical candidates, PET scanning or surgical staging may be performed, but at an overall increased cost (Figure 21.3).

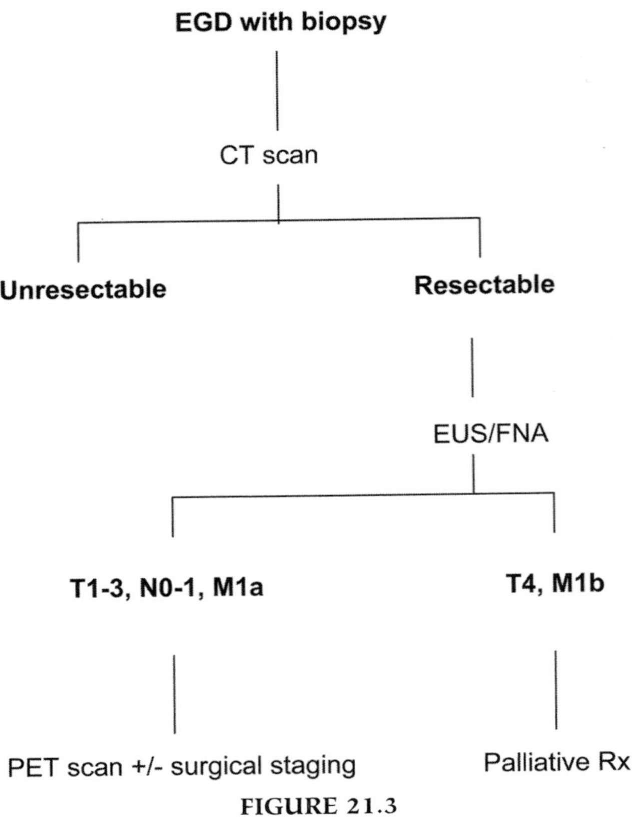

FIGURE 21.3

Proposed algorithm for clinical staging of esophageal cancer.

References

1. American Joint Committee on Cancer. Esophagus. In: AJCC, ed. *AJCC Cancer Staging Manual*. 6th ed. New York: Springer; 2002:91.
2. American Joint Committee on Cancer. Esophagus. In: Beahrs OH, Hansen DE, Hutter RVP, et al., eds. *Manual for Staging of Cancer*. 4th ed.. Philadelphia: JB Lippincott; 1992:57.
3. Ginsberg GG, Fleischer D. Esophageal tumors. In: Feldman M, Friedman L, Sleisenger M, eds. *Sleisenger and Fordtran's Gastrointestinal and Liver Disease: Pathophysiology, Diagnosis and Management*. Philadelphia: WB Saunders; 2002:647–674.
4. Ellis FH, Heatly GJ, Krasna, et al. Esophagogastrectomy for carcinoma of the esophagus and cardia: a comparison of findings and results after standard resection in three

consecutive eight-year intervals with improved staging criteria. *J Thorac Cardiovasc Surg.* 1997;113:836.
5. Quint LE, Hepburn LM, Francis IR, et al. Incidence and distribution of distant metastasis in newly diagnosed esophageal carcinoma. *Cancer.* 1995;76:1120–1125.
6. Saunders HS, Wolfman NT, Ott DJ. Esophageal cancer: radiologic staging. *Radiol Clin N Am.* 1997;35:P281–P294.
7. Reed CE, Mishra G, Sahai AV, et al. Esophageal cancer staging: improved accuracy by endoscopic ultrasound of celiac lymph nodes. *Ann Thorac Surg.* 1999;67:319–321.
8. Rice TW. Clinical staging of esophageal cancer. *Chest Surg Clin N Am.* 2000; 10:471–485.
9. Luketich JD, Friedman DM, Weigel TL, et al. Evaluation of distant metastases in esophageal cancer: 100 consecutive PET scans. *Ann Thorac Surg.* 1999;68:1133–1137.
10. Rice TW. Clinical staging of esophageal cancer. *Chest Surg Clin N Am.* 2000; 10:471–485.
11. Takashime S, Takeuchi N, Shiozake H, et al. Carcinoma of the esophagus: CT vs MRI imaging in determining resectability. *Am J Roentgenol.* 1991;156:297–302.
12. Goei R, Lamers RJ, Engelshove HA, et al. CT staging of esophageal carcinoma: a study on interobserver variation and correlation with pathologic findings. *Eur J Radiol.* 1992;15:40–44.
13. Reed CE, Eloubeidi MA. New techniques in staging esophageal cancer. *Surg Clin N Am.* 2002;82:697–710.
14. Rosch T. Endosonographic staging of esophageal cancer: a review of literature results. *Gastrointest Endosc Clin N Am.* 1995;5:537–547.
15. Mallery S, Van Dam J. EUS in the evaluation of esophageal carcinoma. *Gastrointest Endosc.* 2000;52(suppl):S6–S11.
16. Catalano MF, Sivak MVJ, Rice T, et al. Endosonographic features predictive of lymph node metastasis. *Gastrointest Endosc.* 1994;40:442–446.
17. Pfau PR, Ginsberg GG, Lew RJ, et al. EUS predictors of long term survival in esophageal carcinoma. *Gastrointest Endosc.* 2001;53:463–469.
18. Eloubeidi MA, Wallace MB, Reed CE, et al. The utility of endoscopic ultrasound and EUS-FNA in detecting celiac lymph node metastasis in patients with esophageal cancer. *Gastrointest Endosc.* 2001;54:714–719.
19. Eloubeidi MA, Wallace MB, Hoffman BJ, et al. Predictors of survival for esophageal cancer patients with and without celiac lymphadenopathy: impact of staging endosonography. *Ann Thorac Surg.* 2001;72:212–219.
20. Van Dam J, Rice TW, Catalano MF, et al. High-grade esophageal stricture is predictive of esophageal tumor stage. Risks of endosonographic evaluation. *Cancer.* 1993;71:2910–2917.
21. Pfau PR, Ginsberg GG, Lew RJ, et al. Esophageal dilation for endosonographic evaluation of malignant strictures if safe and effective. *Am J Gastroenterol.* 2000;95:2813–2815.
22. Wallace MB, Hawes RH, Sahai AV, et al. Dilation of malignant esophageal stenosis to allow EUS guided FNA: safety and effect on patient management. *Gastrointest Endosc.* 2000;51:309–313.
23. Binmoeller KF, Seifert H, Seitz U, et al. Ultrasonic esophagoprobe for TNM staging of highly stenosed esophageal carcinoma. *Gastrointest Endosc.* 1995;41:547–552.
24. Mallery S, Van Dam J. Increased rate of complete EUS staging of patients with esophageal cancer using the nonoptical, wire-guided echoendoscopes. *Gastrointest Endosc.* 1999;50:53–57.
25. Koch J, Halverson RA. Staging of esophageal cancer: CT, MRI and EUS. *Semin Roentgenol.* 1994;29:364–372.
26. Maerz LL, Deveney CW, Lopez RR, et al. Role of CT scans in the staging of esophageal and proximal gastric malignancies. *Am J Surg.* 1993;165:558–560.
27. Van Dam J. Endosonographic evaluation of the patient with esophageal cancer. *Chest.* 1997;112:184S–190S.
28. Pfau PR, Perlman SB, Stanko P, et al. The role and clinical value of EUS in a multimodality esophageal carcinoma staging program with CT and PET. *Gastrointest Endosc.* 2007;65:377–384.
29. Luketich JD, Schauer P, Landreneau R, et al. Minimally invasive surgical staging is superior to endoscopic ultrasound in detecting lymph node metastasis in esophageal cancer. *J Thorac Cardiovasc Surg.* 1997;23:393–399.
30. Akdamar M, Cerfolio R, Ohja B, et al. A prospective comparison of CT, FDG-PET and EUS in the preoperative evaluation of operable esophageal cancer (ECA) patients. *Am J Gastroenterol.* 2005;98:s5.
31. Kim K, Park SJ, Kim BT, et al. Evaluation of lymph node metastases in squamous cell carcinoma of the esophagus with positron emission tomography. *Ann Thorac Surg.* 2001;71:290–294.
32. Wallace MB, Nietert PJ, Earle C et al. An analysis of multiple staging management strategies for carcinoma of the esophagus: computed tomography, endoscopic ultrasound, positron emission tomography and thoracoscopy/laparoscopy. *Ann Thorac Surg.* 2002;74:1026–1032.

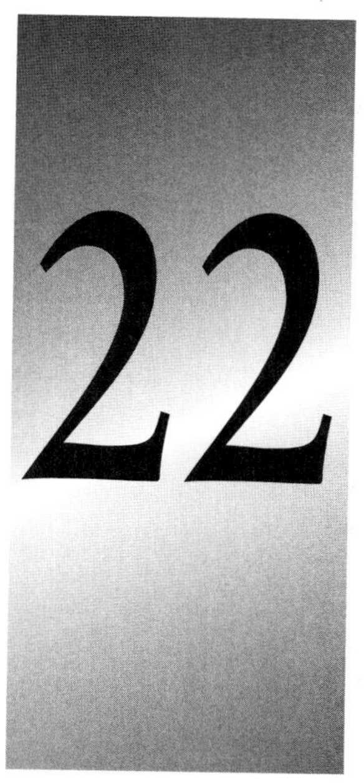

Esophageal Cancer Staging—EMR

Steven R. DeMeester

Adenocarcinoma of the esophagus has the fastest-rising incidence of any cancer in the United States and develops as a consequence of chronic gastroesophageal reflux disease (1). Barrett's esophagus is the precursor lesion from which adenocarcinoma develops, and surveillance programs have led to the detection of high-grade dysplasia and early-stage adenocarcinoma in an increasing number of patients. Both high-grade dysplasia and intramucosal adenocarcinoma, while potentially lethal, are curable lesions in most patients (2–4). However, cure is dependent on complete removal of the neoplastic tissue. Until recently, this was reliably accomplished only with esophagectomy, but new technologies have been developed that allow esophageal preservation in appropriate patients. The aim of this chapter is to explore the role of endoscopic mucosal resection (EMR) for the staging and therapy of early esophageal malignancy.

The diagnosis of Barrett's is made with endoscopy and biopsy, and the endoscopy provides critical information to guide the subsequent evaluation and treatment of the patient. The columnar mucosa in patients with Barrett's must be carefully examined for any ulcers, nodules, or abnormalities since these may represent a focus of cancer. It has been shown that despite extensive preresection biopsies, 30% to 50% of patients thought only to have high-grade dysplasia will in fact have an invasive cancer in the resected specimen (5,6). In the absence of a visible ulcer or nodule on endoscopy, these occult adenocarcinomas have always been limited to the mucosa, in our experience (5). In contrast, if a lesion of any sort is seen endoscopically within the columnar-lined portion of the esophagus, that lesion is at high risk to be a cancer. Further, any malignant, visible lesion cannot be assumed to be limited to the mucosa, regardless of the size or appearance of the lesion. Even very small cancers may penetrate into the submucosa; thus, the endoscopic appearance of the lesion cannot be used to determine the T stage.

STAGING EARLY ESOPHAGEAL CANCER

Local/regional staging of esophageal adenocarcinoma is best done with endoscopic ultrasound. Standard 7.5- and 12-MHz endoscopic ultrasound probes can accurately assess the depth of invasion once the tumor has gone through the submucosa and also provide information on the presence of abnormal or enlarged lymph nodes. However, neither the standard probes nor newer high-resolution 20-MHz probes are able to accurately distinguish intramucosal from submucosal tumor invasion (7). Currently the only method able to accurately determine the depth of invasion of a small visible lesion is endoscopic mucosal resection.

EMR excises a disc of esophageal (or stomach) wall down to the muscularis propria and provides a specimen for histologic review that includes both mucosa and submucosa. By performing an esophagectomy after EMR, we and others have demonstrated that an EMR specimen allows accurate pathologic staging of the depth of tumor invasion (8,9). Further, a recent study has suggested that EMR, by providing a larger sample, also improves diagnostic accuracy in Barrett's and reduces interobserver disagreement (10). Although several techniques have been proposed for EMR, one popular method involves the use of a cap that fits over the end of a standard endoscope. Developed by Dr. Inoue from Japan, these caps are available in various sizes and configurations (flat vs. angled) and come with a complete kit for the procedure by Olympus® (11). Using the large cap for EMR lesions up to 1.5 cm in size can be excised in 1 piece. Piecemeal excision of a lesion is acceptable but raises the potential for incomplete resection and makes pathologic evaluation of the resection margins impractical. EMR can be performed with conscious sedation, but I prefer to have the patient intubated in the operating room to minimize the chance of aspiration. The procedure is quick, and patients are typically discharged home a few hours later. In order to accurately determine margins, I have found it best to personally orient the specimen for the pathologist and have it pinned and fixed for permanent rather than frozen section. Experience at our center and elsewhere has demonstrated that patients with negative margins on the EMR specimen reliably have had complete resection of the tumor [s8,9]). However, tumor at the cauterized margin of the specimen indicates the potential for residual tumor in the esophagus, and if surgical resection is *not* planned, then repeat EMR or other ablative technique is warranted in these patients. If the EMR is done for staging and a surgical resection is planned, then the EMR resection margins are not important, and as long as an adequate portion of the tumor has been excised to allow assessment of the depth of invasion, no further efforts at excision are necessary.

INTRAMUCOSAL VERSUS SUBMUCOSAL TUMOR INVASION

The distinction between tumor invasion that is limited to the mucosa versus deeper invasion into the submucosa is critical because the likelihood of lymph node metastases changes significantly once a tumor enters the submucosa (12). While lymph node metastases are uncommon (2%–4%) in patients with an intramucosal cancer, 30% to 50% of patients with invasion into the submucosa will have at least one lymph node metastasis (9,12,13). Therefore, a therapy that does not include a lymphadenectomy is not appropriate in patients with tumors invading into the submucosa. Conversely, the low incidence of nodal disease with an intramucosal tumor obviates the need for a lymphadenectomy as part of the treatment strategy for these lesions. We recently confirmed this by comparing the survival in a group of 85 patients with intramucosal adenocarcinoma treated with a vagal-sparing esophagectomy versus either a transhiatal or en bloc resection (14). We found that cancer-specific survival was excellent in these patients (95% at 5 years) and was independent of the extent of nodal dissection. Consequently, a lymphadenectomy is not necessary in patients with tumors confined to the mucosa.

The distinction between an intramucosal and a submucosal tumor is critical if endoscopic therapy is planned for the patient or if a procedure like a vagal-sparing esophagectomy is being considered since no lymph nodes are removed with this procedure. Traditional forms of esophagectomy, including transhiatal, transthoracic, or minimally invasive thoracoscopic/laparoscopic procedures, all include a lymphadenectomy, and thus the distinction between intramucosal and submucosal lesions is less critical. While some investigators have suggested that superficial submucosal invasion may be associated with a low enough incidence of nodal metastases that endoscopic therapy could be an option for these patients, in our experience there was not a significant difference in the risk of nodal disease between superficial and deep submucosal invasion (University of Southern California data, publication pending). Therefore, in my opinion, all tumors that invade into the submucosa are best treated with esophagectomy and lymphadenectomy, provided that the patient will tolerate the procedure.

EMR AS PRIMARY THERAPY FOR ESOPHAGEAL ADENOCARCINOMA

In our initial experience with EMR, all patients had an esophagectomy after the visible lesion was excised by EMR. Further, in addition to the endoscopy at the time of the EMR, all patients had multiple endoscopies and biopsies prior to the esophagectomy, and yet on final pathology, 2 of 7 patients (29%) had an additional (undetected) cancer in the resected specimen (8). The potential for multifocal disease is concerning when considering endoscopic therapy to treat early esophageal cancer in patients with long-segment Barrett's. In addition, the potential for metachronous tumor development in the residual Barrett's is of concern. Both of these concerns were highlighted in a recent report by Ell and colleagues describing EMR as sole therapy for intramucosal adenocarcinoma (15). This report focuses on 100 highly selected and carefully screened patients that had a well-differentiated intramucosal tumor without evidence of lymphovascular invasion. The survival with EMR alone was excellent (98% at 5 years) in these patients, but despite relatively short-term follow-up, there was a high rate (11%) of metachronous tumor development. The majority of patients in this series had short-segment Barrett's, and undoubtedly the rate of metachronous tumor development will increase with longer follow-up, and it would also almost certainly be higher if more patients with long-segment Barrett's esophagus were part of the study. Thus, patients with Barrett's and one focus of adenocarcinoma are at high risk for a synchronous or metachronous tumor.

In an effort to reduce this risk, Wang and colleagues have combined EMR with photodynamic therapy to ablate the residual Barrett's. They reported that no new or recurrent cancers developed in 16 patients during a median follow-up of 13 months, although residual Barrett's was present in 47% of the patients (16). The promising combination of EMR for a visible lesion in the esophagus with ablation of residual Barrett's, along with concerns regarding the morbidity and mortality associated with esophagectomy have prompted a change in the approach to patients with early esophageal lesions at a number of centers. However, before widespread acceptance of this approach, there are several important issues to consider. First, in the report by Ell and colleagues, only intramucosal tumors with very favorable histologic features were treated endoscopically, and extension of the criteria to include less favorable tumors (moderate or poor differentiation, lymphovascular invasion) may not produce similar results (15). Second, while Ell and colleagues used the traditional 5-year cancer survival mark to evaluate the success of endoscopic therapy, they are ignoring the reality that many of these patients have a lot of years ahead of them, and cure from one or even several Barrett's cancers may not be the end of the story. Barrett's esophagus develops as a consequence of gastroesophageal reflux, and elimination of Barrett's without concomitant elimination of the reflux in these patients may be similar to pulling weeds out of a garden and expecting them never to grow again. Third, following the endoscopic resection, Ell and colleagues treated patients with pH-guided proton pump inhibitor therapy, but the efficacy of this for prevention of Barrett's recurrence is unproven. Not surprisingly, many of these patients required large doses of proton pump inhibitors to be adequately acid suppressed. This speaks to the severity of reflux disease in these patients, and, as impedance studies have demonstrated, adequate acid suppression does not equate to elimination of alkaline or weak acid reflux events (17,18). One has to suspect that lifelong maintenance of this degree of intensive medical therapy is unlikely in the majority of patients. Instead, antireflux surgery may be a more effective therapy and needs to be evaluated in this setting.

A final important issue is long-term quality of life in patients treated for high-grade dysplasia or intramucosal adenocarcinoma, since they are likely to be cured of their disease. Quality of life in patients with Barrett's is variable, but many have severe reflux disease with the accompanying problems of regurgitation, nocturnal aspiration, and dysphagia. Physicians and patients sometimes assume incorrectly that any esophageal preserving therapy is going to be better than the alternative therapy of an esophagectomy. However, I believe that this is a flawed concept, and avoidance of an esophagectomy at all cost is unfounded. The often quoted mortality of 5% to 15% for an esophagectomy is not supported by current series in patients with high-grade dysplasia or intramucosal adenocarcinoma, where mortality rates of 1% are expected (14,19,20). Esophagectomy has been the standard of care for both high-grade dysplasia and early adenocarcinoma, and the excellent results with this approach should not be quickly dismissed.

I propose that in light of the recent advances in endoscopic procedures that allow esophageal preservation and the new, less invasive, and potentially less morbid surgical techniques to remove the esophagus, it is time that we alter our approach to the evaluation of patients with high-grade dysplasia and early esophageal adenocarcinoma. In addition to determining the stage of the cancer and assessing the overall health of the patient, we should also evaluate the pathophysiologic abnormalities associated with the patient's reflux disease. In particular, an assessment should be made of the function of the stomach, lower esophageal sphincter, and esophageal body as well as the size of the hiatal hernia, length of Barrett's, and presence and severity of reflux symptoms. Esophageal preservation might be the preferred therapy in a patient with few symptoms, a small hiatal hernia, normal esophageal body function, and a short segment of Barrett's with a low-risk intramucosal carcinoma. In contrast, patients who are poor candidates for esophageal preservation are those who present with high-grade dysplasia or an intramucosal adenocarcinoma and have severe reflux symptoms or dysphagia; long-segment Barrett's with a large, fixed hiatal hernia; and poor esophageal body motility. These patients are best treated with a vagal-sparing esophagectomy since, in my opinion, esophageal preservation makes sense only if the esophagus is worth preserving, based on physiologic evaluation. Further, the long-term efficacy of EMR and Barrett's ablation in the setting of severe reflux pathophysiology is unproven, and over time recurrence of Barrett's seems likely to occur in these patients. Vagal-sparing esophagectomy is also indicated for patients with multiple lesions within long-segment Barrett's or lesions with positive lateral margins after endoscopic mucosal resection. Thus, the decision to treat high-grade dysplasia or intramucosal cancer endoscopically or with an esophagectomy takes into consideration not just the stage of the lesion, but also the pathophysiology of the esophagus and the severity of the underlying reflux disease. In this way, outcomes can be optimized for not only the dysplasia or cancer, but also the patients' reflux disease and long-term quality of life.

In conclusion, advances in both the surgical and the endoscopic therapies for Barrett's high-grade dysplasia and intramucosal adenocarcinoma offer options for these patients that were unavailable even just a few years ago. To advocate one therapy as always being the best is to take a step backward in an age of increasing individualization of therapy. Rather than a one-size-fits-all approach, our understanding of tumor biology and esophageal physiology in conjunction with patient preference, should be used to determine the best therapy for an individual patient: preserving the esophagus in those where it makes sense, and removing the esophagus when necessary to adequately address not only the cancer but also the background pathophysiology that precipitated the development of the malignancy. This approach will require a balanced and updated understanding of the advantages and disadvantages of both endoscopic and surgical therapies by the surgeons and gastroenterologist who treat these patients. Undoubtedly, future studies that assess quality of life and freedom from recurrent Barrett's and cancer will help guide the selection of therapy for an individual patient who presents with high-grade dysplasia or intramucosal adenocarcinoma of the esophagus.

References

1. Pohl H, Welch HG. The role of overdiagnosis and reclassification in the marked increase of esophageal adenocarcinoma incidence. *J Natl Cancer Inst.* 2005;97(2):142–146.
2. Oh DS, Hagen JA, Chandrasoma PT, et al. Clinical biology and surgical therapy of intramucosal adenocarcinoma of the esophagus. *J Am Coll Surg.* 2006;203(2):152–161.
3. Rice TW, Blackstone EH, Goldblum JR, et al. Superficial adenocarcinoma of the esophagus. *J Thorac Cardiovasc Surg.* 2001;122(6):1077–1090.
4. Stein HJ, Feith M, Bruecher BL, et al. Early esophageal cancer: pattern of lymphatic spread and prognostic factors for long-term survival after surgical resection. *Ann Surg.* 2005;242(4):566–573; discussion 573–575.
5. Nigro JJ, Hagen JA, DeMeester TR, et al. Occult esophageal adenocarcinoma: extent of disease and implications for effective therapy. *Ann Surg.* 1999;230(3):433–440.
6. Dar MS, Goldblum JR, Rice TW, et al. Can extent of high grade dysplasia in Barrett's oesophagus predict the presence of adenocarcinoma at oesophagectomy? *Gut.* 2003;52(4):486–489.
7. May A, Gunter E, Roth F, et al. Accuracy of staging in early esophageal cancer using high resolution endoscopy and high resolution endosonography: a comparative, prospective, and blinded trial. *Gut.* 2004;53:634–640.
8. Maish MS, DeMeester SR. Endoscopic mucosal resection as a staging technique to determine the depth of invasion of esophageal adenocarcinoma. *Ann Thorac Surg.* 2004;78:1777–1782.
9. Prasad GA, Buttar NS, Wongkeesong LM, et al. Significance of neoplastic involvement of margins obtained by endoscopic mucosal resection in Barrett's esophagus. *Am J Gastroenterol.* 2007;102(11):2380–2386.
10. Mino-Kenudson M, Hull MJ, Brown I, et al. EMR for Barrett's esophagus-related superficial neoplasms offers better diagnostic reproducibility than mucosal biopsy [see comment]. *Gastrointest Endosc.* 2007;66(4):660–666; quiz 767.
11. Tada M, Inoue H, Yabata E, et al. Colonic mucosal resection using a transparent cap-fitted endoscope [see comment]. *Gastrointest Endosc.* 1996;44(1):63–65.
12. Nigro JJ, Hagen JA, DeMeester TR, et al. Prevalence and location of nodal metastases in distal esophageal adenocarcinoma confined to the wall: implications for therapy [see comments]. *J Thorac Cardiovasc Surg.* 1999;117(1):16–23; discussion 23–25.
13. Rice TW, Zuccaro G Jr, Adelstein DJ, et al. Esophageal carcinoma: depth of tumor invasion is predictive of regional lymph node status. *Ann Thorac Surg.* 1998;65(3):787–792.
14. Peyre C, DeMeester SR, Rizzetto C, et al. Vagal-sparing esophagectomy: the ideal operation for intramucosal adenocarcinoma and Barrett's with high-grade dysplasia. *Ann Surg.* 2007;246:665–674.
15. Ell C, May A, Pech O, et al. Curative endoscopic resection of early esophageal adenocarcinomas (Barrett's cancer) [see comment]. *Gastrointest Endosc.* 2007;65(1):3–10.
16. Buttar N, Nijhawan P, Krishnadath K, et al. Combined endoscopic mucosal resection (EMR) and photodynamic therapy (PDT) for esophageal neoplasia within Barrett's esophagus. *Gastroenterology.* 2000;118:A405.
17. Tamhankar AP, Peters JH, Portale G, et al. Omeprazole does not reduce gastroesophageal reflux: new insights using multichannel intraluminal impedance technology. *J Gastrointest Surg.* 2004;8(7):890–897; discussion 897–898.
18. Katz PO. Review article: the role of non-acid reflux in gastro-oesophageal reflux disease. *Aliment Pharmacol Ther.* 2000;14(12):1539–1551.
19. Ferguson MK, Naunheim KS. Resection for Barrett's mucosa with high-grade dysplasia: implications for prophylactic photodynamic therapy. *J Thorac Cardiovasc Surg.* 1997;114(5):824–829.
20. Headrick JR, Nichols FC III, Miller DL, et al. High-grade esophageal dysplasia: long-term survival and quality of life after esophagectomy [see comment]. *Ann Thorac Surg.* 2002;73(6):1697–1702; discussion 1702–1703.

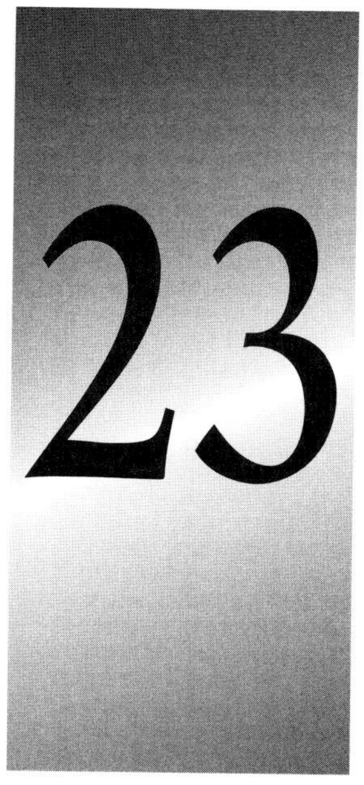

23 Esophageal Cancer Staging—Surgical

Lei Yu
Mark J. Krasna

Great progress in technology and skills in the management of esophageal cancer was not accompanied with the higher 5-year survival rate of esophageal cancer, which in patients amenable to surgery still ranges from 5% to 20%. One of the major reasons for the unsatisfactory prognosis of esophageal cancer is the lack of precise preoperative staging, which is the premise for appropriate treatment modalities. Correct staging is critical as stages I, IIA, IIB, and, depending on the surgeon, stage III are treated with surgery as well as chemotherapy and radiation therapy. Stage IV is nonsurgical. Chemotherapy and radiation treatment is generally given for palliation. If there is only local disease without nodal involvement, the prognosis increases to 40%. Unfortunately, 50% of patients are unresectable at presentation. For these patients, surgery does not increase the overall 5-year survival, and the risk of mortality from surgery may be 5% to 10%.

NONINVASIVE STAGING TECHNIQUES

Accurate tumor-node metastases (TNM) staging plays a pivotal role in cancer management and research. The purpose of cancer staging is to predict survival on the basis of anatomic extent and to direct stage-specific therapy. In 1988, a revised TNM classification was used to closely correlate stage and disease prognosis. However, the TNM staging system for esophageal cancer is frequently viewed with discontent by thoracic surgeons. The depth of wall penetration and lymph node metastases were shown to be better prognostic indicators (1), and in 2002, the American Joint Committee on Cancer (AJCC) revised the staging system to include these prognostic variables (2). Even thus, this TNM staging system still seems inadequate. Stage grouping within the constraints of AJCC definitions produces less accurate prognosis than free assignment based on survival data (3). No distinction is made in the AJCC classification between the pathologic stage (the gold standard) and the clinical stage. Attempting to stage esophageal cancer using clinical tests with an accuracy rate approaching the pathology standard has proven to be a difficult and expensive enterprise. The usual clinical tools of physical examination, blood tests, and chest X-rays remain important but are of limited value.

As imaging methods have continued to improve, clinical staging has become increasingly effective, but often falls short of pathologic perfection. Computed tomography (CT) of the chest and abdomen is the first test for staging esophageal cancer. Magnetic resonance imaging (MRI), in most cases, seems to add little if anything to the staging information can be obtained using CT. Furthermore, CT is widely available, and CT body imaging has been the best test for the detection of distant metastatic disease (M1, stage IV). If a CT scan is negative for distant metastases (M0), then endoscopic ultrasound (EUS) is often used as the next step for accurate locoregional staging. EUS uses endoscopy-guided high-frequency ultrasound transducers inside the esophageal lumen to produce detailed images of the esophageal wall and structures close to the esophagus. The great advantage of EUS for staging is that EUS is useful in the accurate assessment of the depth of mural infiltration and the detection of metastatic involvement of the regional nodes (4). Primary esophageal cancer is usually imaged as a hypoechoic disruption of the wall layers. The EUS images are highly compatible with the AJCC classification for T, depth of esophageal cancer invasion. Additionally, EUS-guided fine-needle aspiration (FNA) for cytology can be carried out with relative ease and has accuracy in the 90% range, and this procedure should also be a consideration when tissue confirmation is needed (5).

There are some drawbacks in these imaging techniques. Even the new, faster scanners and helical CT do not image the esophageal wall as a series of layers. It has become clear that staging the depth of tumor invasion on the basis of wall thickness and contour is open to frequent error. CT alone has an accuracy of 50% to 60% for staging esophageal cancer. It is best for hepatic and adrenal metastases and less sensitive for locoregional lymph nodes. Lymph nodes greater than 8 to 10 mm in diameter on CT are generally considered to be metastatic. Similar measurements have been used to assess lymph nodes on EUS, but additional EUS criteria for malignancy are nodes that are uniformly hypoechoic, sharply demarcated from surrounding fat, and rounded. Benign nodes, particularly in the mediastinum, may be greater than 10 mm but are often elongated with distinct cortical and medullary areas and are more hyperechoic with less distinct borders. These are subjective criteria and prone to greater diagnostic error than the depth of tumor invasion. Based on sizable accumulated data, the overall accuracy rate of EUS for T staging of esophageal cancer is only 84% according to collected data from 21 studies recently reported (6). Accuracy rate for T1 is 80.5%, for T2 76%, for T3 92%, and for T4 86%. The overall accuracy rate of the N staging is 77%, with 69% for N0 and 89% for N1 (7). With the aid of EUS-guided FNA, the result of N staging is significantly improved, up to 87% (8).

Like EUS, endoscopic magnetic resonance imaging offers the advantages of optical visualization combined with cross-sectional imaging and appears to be a safe technique comparable to EUS as well as with pathologic staging in esophageal cancer but with a tendency to overstage the disease (9).

Positron-emission tomography (PET) using the radiolabeled glucose analog 18-F-fluoro-deoxy-D-glucose (FDG) for esophageal cancer staging is a noninvasive method that improves detection of distant metastases and regional nodal metastases. Flamen et al. (10) presented convincing data that PET significantly improves the detection of distant lymph node and organ metastases (stage IV). PET is superior to CT and EUS combined in diagnosing stage IV disease. In the study by Flamen, PET was more accurate: 82% versus 64%n for CT and EUS combined in staging esophageal cancer. Eighteen out of 74 patients had discordant findings between PET versus CT and EUS. PET was correct in 16 out of 18 patients based on surgical findings. It upstaged 11 patients and downstaged 5 patients. In 3 other studies, PET demonstrated distant metastasis not seen on conventional imaging in (21/105 points). However, current PET scans can produce false-negative and positive results, and biopsy, cytology, or at least radiologic confirmation of positive areas on PET scans should be obtained, if possible.

The problem for all imaging modalities is detecting very small foci of cancer in lymph nodes or other distant sites and in differentiating enlarged lymph nodes that are reactive or inflammatory from those replaced by metastatic disease. In addition, CT, MRI, PET, and EUS are still inaccurate in evaluating local surgical resectability.

At the present time, there is no biochemical test or molecular marker that has proven equal to the tumor-node-metastasis description of the anatomical extent of disease for esophageal cancer staging.

THORACOSCOPIC AND LAPAROSCOPIC STAGING

In order to improve accuracy of pretherapeutic tumor staging, thoracoscopy and laparoscopy have been used in esophageal cancer staging at some surgical centers (11–13). These studies proved that minimally invasive surgical staging is a promising adjunct to esophageal cancer staging. The thoracoscopic (Ts) and laparoscopic staging (Ls) provide more accurate information for evaluating local invasion, lymph node, and distant metastasis. Thoracoscopy can allocate patients with stage IV for neoadjuvant therapy and help avoid an unnecessary thoracotomy in patients found to have gross spread of locoregional disease.

From the histologic and pathologic standpoint, freely anastomosing networks of esophageal lymphatic drainage facilitate lengthwise tumor dissemination. It has been thought that the upper third drains into cervical nodes, the middle third to paraesophageal and paratracheal mediastinal nodes, and the lower third to nodes around aorta and celiac axis. Recently, the submucosal drainage territory has shown to extend in lymphatic drainage vessels of the esophagus with and without nodal delay to the thoracic duct in the human esophagus, identified macroscopically and histologically (14,15). This explains why aggressive malignancy commonly presents as locally advanced disease with a poor prognosis. Lymph node metastasis of esophageal cancer is the major factor that influences the prognosis after surgery. Even with an invasion depth limited to the mucosa or submucosa, the prognosis is remarkably poor compared with the same invasion depth in gastric or colorectal cancer. Superficial cancer of the esophagus may metastasize into lymph nodes far distant from the primary tumor, not only into the mediastinum but also into the neck and abdomen. Therefore, some surgical investigators have suggested that thoracoscopy and laparoscopy should be routinely used for maximum accuracy in esophageal cancer staging because definitive staging of esophageal cancer facilitates allocation of patients to appropriate treatment regimens according to each patient's stage (16).

HISTORY OF SURGICAL STAGING

Mediastinoscopy remains the classic surgical approach to mediastinal lymph node sampling. Limitations of this technique include difficulty in sampling the aorticopulmonary window and the left para-aortic lymph nodes. Biopsy of subcarinal lymph nodes may also be problematic, especially if nodes are inferior and posterior. The Chamberlain mediastinotomy provides an excellent approach to biopsy of the anterior mediastinal lymph nodes. In 1977, Murray et al. (17) described the use of mediastinoscopy and minilaparotomy for preresection staging of esophageal cancer. Five of 30 patients (17%) had positive lymph nodes at mediastinoscopy, and 16 (53%) had positive lymph nodes at minilaparotomy. Operative staging could thus identify lymph node metastases before resection in esophageal cancer. Dagnini et al. (18) performed routine laparoscopy just prior to planned esophagectomy for esophageal cancer. In 369 patients, unsuspected intraabdominal visceral metastases and celiac lymph node metastases were noted in 14% and 9.7% of patients, respectively. Since describing a thoracoscopic Chamberlain procedure for staging esophageal cancer in patients with enlarged aorticopulmonary window lymph nodes, Krasna has used this technique routinely in staging esophageal cancer (19). According to another study by Krasna (20), thoracic lymph nodes were correctly staged in all of an early series of 14 patients. A multi-institutional pilot study from the Cancer and Leukemia Group B described 90% accuracy for thoracoscopic laparoscopic lymph node staging. Knowing the precise preoperative stage would then facilitate grouping patients into those likely to have residual local or lymphatic disease and those likely to have complete resections. This would allow the rational allocation of adjuvant chemotherapy and/or radiation therapy to those patient populations that would most benefit and thus limit the morbidity associated with these treatments.

SURGICAL STAGING TECHNIQUES

The patient is placed in the lateral decubitus position with 2 television monitors, one over the patient's head and the other over the patient's legs. This allows the surgeon and the first assistant to visualize the same field equally, without "mirror imaging" (21).

The patient is intubated with a double-lumen endotracheal tube for one-lung ventilation to achieve the necessary exposure. The first incision is made along the posterior axillary line in the sixth intercostal space, and the thoracoscope is inserted and the chest explored. Two additional incisions are made at the fifth intercostal space, anterior axillary line, and at the seventh or eighth intercostal space, anterior axillary line. [C0.sub.2] insufflation to compress the underlying lung has been used routinely. At surgical exploration, assessment of the entire chest for evidence of lymph node involvement, pleural metastases, pulmonary metastases, or direct spread is performed (21).

A right-sided thoracoscopy is currently used routinely for esophageal cancer staging. This avoids the aorta and allows access to a maximum number of lymph nodes from which biopsy specimens can be taken. The azygos vein can be divided with staplers or sutures to facilitate exposure. The mediastinal pleura overlying the proximal esophagus is elevated lateral to the posterior edge of the trachea. Using endoscopic shears with electrocautery, the pleura is incised from the level of the subclavical vessels down to the azygos arch. Biopsy specimens are taken from lymph nodes using hemoclips for hemostasis. The level 2R, 4R, 3P, and 10 lymph nodes can be sampled in this way. The lung is retracted anteriorly by grasping the superior segment of the right lower lobe, and the subcarinal space is identified (21).

The mediastinal pleura is incised from the azygos vein to the inferior pulmonary vein. Biopsy specimens of all nodes are again taken using hemoclips for hemostasis. The right lower lung lobe is grasped and retracted superiorly. The inferior pulmonary ligament is divided using endoscopic shears with electrocautery. Once the inferior pulmonary vein is visualized, the dissection is complete, and biopsy specimens are taken from levels 7, 8, and 9 lymph nodes. The chest is irrigated and examined for hemostasis or air leak from retraction. A single 24F chest tube is placed posteriorly and secured with 2 0-silk sutures. The remaining incisions are closed with a 3–0 polyglactin subcutaneous and subcuticular suture (21).

If preoperative noninvasive staging shows suspicious lymph nodes on the left side, a left thoracoscopy is performed. Inspection of the aorticopulmonary window will identify level 5 and 6 lymph nodes. The remainder of the hemithorax is examined for evidence of gross esophageal tumor extension or metastatic disease to the lung. The mediastinal pleura overlying the lymph nodes is incised using electrocautery. The incision is continued up to the apex of the triangle formed by the phrenic and vagus nerves. Inferiorly, the pleura is incised over the left main pulmonary artery. Lymph nodes in this region are mobilized, and the vascular pedicle is ligated with an endoscopic clip applier (21).

Laparoscopic lymph node staging is now performed routinely. The patient is placed in the supine position with both television monitors placed at the head of the table. The abdomen is prepared and draped for a standard laparotomy. The procedure is begun with 3 12-mm ports, although a fourth port may be necessary in the left upper quadrant for retraction of the stomach and placement of tension on the gastrohepatic ligament. A 30-degree laparoscope is helpful for exposure of the operative field. An operating scope was generally used to allow 4 instruments to be used with 3 trocars (21).

After thorough surgical exploration of the peritoneal cavity, the surface of the liver is inspected, and biopsy specimens are taken from gross abnormalities and sent for frozen section. The liver is retracted with an expandable fan retractor, and the lesser sac is entered using sharp dissection through the lesser omentum, just to the right of the esophagus. The dissection is carried craniad toward the right crus of the diaphragm. Most of this dissection may be performed with electrocautery, but occasional use of clips may be necessary. When very large vessels are seen in this area, we have used an endoscopic vascular stapler. Biopsy specimens are taken from lymph nodes identified along the lesser curve. Pulsations from the right gastric artery are visible caudally, and division of the omentum may stop at this point. Exposure of the celiac axis is obtained by elevation of the lesser curve of the stomach near the gastroesophageal junction. The left gastric artery is identified by its pulsation as it projects straight up from the celiac axis and enters the posterior wall of the stomach, and small lymph nodes can usually be found (21).

RECENT STUDIES AND COMPARISONS

According to a study in 1999 (22), thoracoscopic staging was done in 82 patients and found N_1 in 11 patients. Fifty-four patients had laparoscopy, which detected N_1 in 21 patients. Thirty-four cases had chemoradiation followed by surgery. Esophagectomy was performed in 47 patients after thoracoscopic staging and 33 with laparoscopic staging. Of these 47 resected patients, thoracoscopic staging showed N_0 in 42 patients and N_1 in 5 patients with an accuracy of 93.6%. Laparoscopic staging detected normal celiac lymph nodes in 20 patients and diseased lymph nodes in 11 patients with an accuracy of 93.9%. Comparing with final resection pathology, the sensitivity, specificity, and positive predictive value of staging for N_1 disease in the chest was 62.5%, 100.0%, and 100.0% by TS; 75.0%, 75.6%, and 23.1% by CT; and 0.0%, 51.4%, and 5.5% by EUS, respectively. For N_1 disease in the abdomen, it was 84.6%, 100.0%, and 100.0% by Ls.

Subsequently, a comparison of Ts/Ls staging with conventional noninvasive clinical staging in patients with esophageal cancer was done in 2002 (23). The result showed that the correlation between Ts/Ls staging and conventional noninvasive clinical staging in the diagnosis of T4 disease, mediastinal lymph node metastasis, celiac lymph node metastasis, and M1 disease was 18.8%, 14.5%, 25.5%, and 20.0%, respectively. Ts/Ls provided more accurate information for evaluating local invasion, lymph node metastasis, and distant metastasis. The poor correlation of staging diagnosis between Ts/Ls and conventional noninvasive clinical examinations suggests that the accuracy of current noninvasive clinical staging is questionable and needs to be improved.

Although surgical staging seems to make esophageal cancer treatment complicated, the greater accuracy afforded by minimally invasive staging is essential for patients who should undergo radical surgical or multimodal treatment. According to recent data, combining nonoperative staging procedures as CT/MRI and EUS with minimally invasive staging techniques may be more conducive to pretreatment staging, which will be even more important in the future for adjusting treatment to individual patient (24,25).

References

1. Rice TW, Zuccaro G, Adelstein DJ, et al. Esophageal carcinoma: depth of tumor invasion is predictive of regional lymph node status. *Ann Thorac Surg.* 1998;65:787–792.
2. Greene FL. American Joint Committee on Cancer, American Cancer Society. *AJCC Cancer Staging Manual.* 6th ed. New York: Springer; 2002:91–98.
3. Rice TW, Blackstone EH, Rybicki LA, et al. General thoracic surgery: refining esophageal cancer staging. *J Thorac Cardiovasc Surg.* 2003;125(5):1103–1113.
4. Boyce HW Jr. Endosonographic staging of esophageal cancer. *Cancer Control.* 1999;6:28–35.
5. Chang KJ, Katz KD, Durbin TE, et al. Endoscopic ultrasound-guided fine-needle aspiration. *Gastrointest Endosc.* 1994;40:694–699.
6. Ziegler K, Sanft C, Zeitz M, et al. Evaluation of endosonography in TN staging of oesophageal cancer. *Gut.* 1991;32(1):16–20.
7. Tio TL, Coene PP, den Hartog Jager FC, et al. Preoperative TNM classification of esophageal, carcinoma by endosonography. *Hepato-gastroenterology.* 1990;37(4):376–381.
8. Chang KJ, Katz KD, Durbin TE, et al. Endoscopic ultrasound-guided fine-needle aspiration. *Gastrointest Endosc.* 1994;40:694–699.

9. Dave UR, Williams, AD, et al. Esophageal cancer staging with endoscopic MR imaging: pilot study. *Radiology.* 2004;230:281–286.
10. Flamen P, Lerut A, Van Cutsem E, et al. Utility of positron emission tomography for the staging of patients with potentially operable esophageal carcinoma. *J Clin Oncol.* 2000;18(18):3202–3210.
11. Bonavina L, Incarbone R, Lattuada E, et al. Preoperative laparoscopy in management of patients with carcinoma of the esophagus and of the esophagogastric junction. *J Surg Oncol.* 1997;65(3):171–174.
12. Sugarbaker DJ, Jaklitsch MT, Liptay MJ. Thoracoscopic staging and surgical therapy for esophageal cancer. *Chest.* 1995;107(suppl 6):218S–223S.
13. Luketich JD, Schauer P, Landreneau R, et al. Minimally invasive surgical staging is superior to endoscopic ultrasound in detecting lymph node metastases in esophageal cancer. *J Thorac Cardiovasc Surg.* 1997;114(5):817–823.
14. Murakami G, Sato I, Shimada K, et al. Direct lymphatic drainage from the esophagus into the thoracic duct. *Surg Radiol Anat.* 1994;16(4):399–407.
15. Kuge K, Murakami G, et al. Submucosal territory of the direct lymphatic drainage system to the thoracic duct in the human esophagus. *J Thorac Cardiovasc Surg.* 2003;125:1343–1349.
16. Liebermann-Meffert D. Anatomical basis for the approach and extent of surgical treatment of esophageal cancer. *Dis Esophagus.* 2001;14(2):81–84.
17. Murray GF, Wilcox BR, Starek PJ. The assessment of operability of esophageal carcinoma. *Ann Thorac Surg.* 1977;23:393–399.
18. Dagnini G, Caldironi MW, Marin G, et al. Laparoscopy in abdominal staging of esophageal carcinoma: report of 369 cases. *Gastrointest Endosc.* 1986;32(6):400–402.
19. Krasna MJ, McLaughlin JS. Thoracoscopic lymph node staging for esophageal cancer. *Ann Thorac Surg.* 1993;56:671–674.
20. Krasna MJ, Reed C, Sugarbaker D. Thoracoscopic staging for esophageal cancer. *Ann Thorac Surg.* 1995;60:1337–1340.
21. Krasna MJ, Flowers JL, Attar S, et al. Combined thoracoscopic/laparoscopic staging of esophageal cancer. *J Thorac Cardiovasc Surg.* 1996;111:800–807.
22. Krasna MJ, Mao YS, Sonett J, et al. The role of thoracoscopic staging of esophageal cancer patients. *Eur J Cardiothorac Surg.* 1999;16:S31–S33.
23. Wallace MB, Nietert PJ, Earle C, et al. An analysis of multiple staging management strategies for carcinoma of the esophagus: computed tomography, endoscopic ultrasound, positron emission tomography, and thoracoscopy/laparoscopy. *Ann Thorac Surg.* 2002;74(4):1026–1032.
24. Gamliel Z, Krasna MJ. Multimodality treatment of esophageal cancer. *Surg Clin North Am.* 2005;85(3):621–630.
25. Refaely Y, Krasna MJ. Multimodality therapy for esophageal cancer. *Surg Clin North Am.* 2002;82(4):729–746.

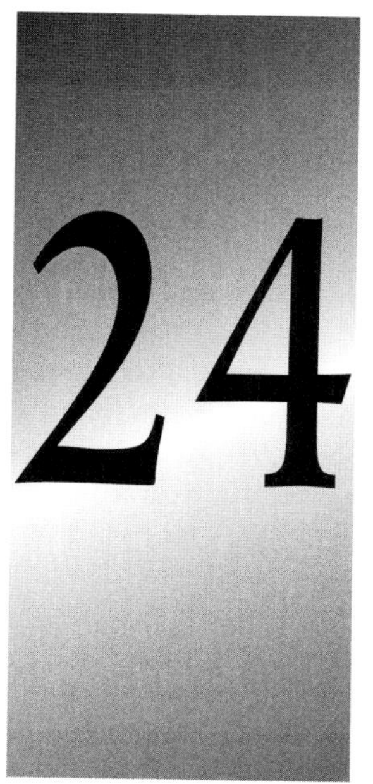

24 Restaging after Neoadjuvant Therapy

Robert J. Cerfolio
Ayesha Bryant

The long-term survival of patients with locoregionally advanced esophageal cancer (stages II–IVA) treated with surgery alone is only 6% to 40% with a median survival of 9 to 24 months (1,2). Because of these poor outcomes, multimodality approaches with chemotherapy and/or the use of concurrent chemoradiotherapy have been liberally employed and evaluated (3,4). Because of the increasing frequency of this strategy, surgeons are now often asked to evaluate patients for resection after neoadjuvant chemoradiotherapy and to determine their candidacy for resection. This decision is 2-fold. One aspect is the patient's oncologic response to the therapy, and the other is the patient's cardiopulmonary risk. Surgical resection is generally reserved for those who have responded to the neoadjuvant therapy, or at least have no evidence of disease progression. In order to ensure that surgical resection is offered to the patients who will benefit the most from the risks of surgery, the accuracy of the initial staging and the repeat staging is therefore critical. Restaging is accomplished through multimodality imaging techniques that include endoscopic ultrasound (EUS), endoscopic ultrasound with fine-needle aspiration (EUS-FNA), computed tomography (CT), and integrated computed tomography with positron-emission tomography (PET/CT). The accuracy and limitations of each of these modalities are discussed here.

COMPUTED TOMOGRAPHY

The CT scan is generally considered the standard imaging study for the monitoring and staging of solid organ tumors. However, several series have shown that its accuracy in restaging patients with esophageal cancer is poor and substantially worse than the accuracy of PET and EUS (5–8). This is related to the inability of CT to distinguish between viable tumor and reactive changes, including edema and scar tissue. Jones showed that CT had an accuracy of only 42% for T-stage assessment after induction chemoradiotherapy (8). CT's strength is in its detection of regional nodal disease and metastatic disease.

Many older series evaluated the efficacy of CT scanners that used 8 to 10 mm cuts. With the introduction of scanners that use thinner sections (usually 5 mm columinated cuts with intravenous and oral contrast), these results may improve. Thinner sections allow for improved delineation of the tumor, improved 3-dimensional measurements, and therefore more accurate and reproducible measurements of tumor volume. However, in a prospective study we performed on patients with non–small cell lung cancer, we found that even with 5 mm columinated cuts and intravenous contrast, patients were often understaged by CT scan (9). While thinner cuts may improve the accuracy of restaging somewhat, CT still remains an inferior imaging modality both for the initial staging and for restaging compared to EUS-FNA and integrated PET/CT scan. In conclusion, CT scan is a relatively poor clinical diagnostic tool for the determination of the pathologic tumor response after chemoradiotherapy of patients with esophageal cancer. Although CT is able to assess the change in size in the T, N, and M disease and detect the new development of N or M disease, it is predictive only when the tumor decreases in size. If the tumor size has increased, it does not necessarily indicate a poor response, since cancers can increase in size while undergoing cell necrosis or death (and yet have a good response to induction therapy).

ENDOSCOPIC ULTRASOUND

EUS has revolutionized the initial staging of patients with esophageal cancer during the past decade. It is a minimally invasive procedure that not only provides the best estimate of T stage but also allows pathologic confirmation of metastatic disease in various sites. Its unique visualization of the esophageal wall allows one to see 5 distinct, clearly identifiable zones (Figure 24.1). The depth of penetration is assessed as well as invasion of surrounding structures. EUS-FNA can also provide biopsy confirmation of celiac lymph node involvement (which is currently considered M1a disease for patients with distal esophageal junction tumors). In addition, it allows biopsy of distant metastases in the left and right adrenal glands and in the left side of the liver and even some lesions in the lower lobes of the lung (10). However, its value for restaging after neoadjuvant therapy is limited by its difficulty in distinguishing residual cancer from inflammation and fibrosis (11,12).

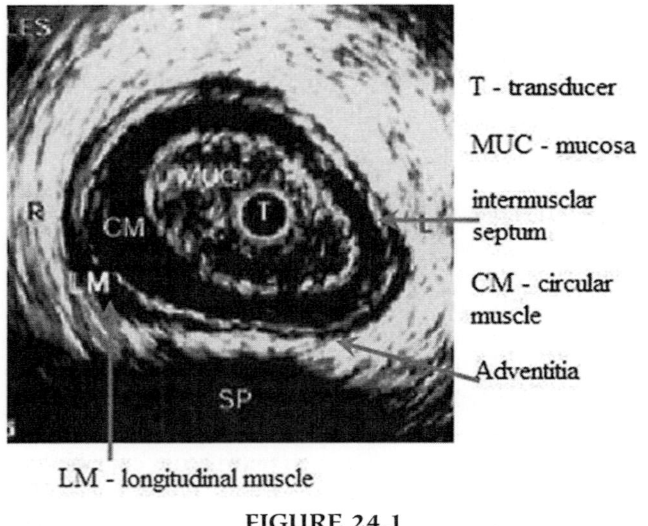

FIGURE 24.1

Five layers of the esophagus as seen by EUS.

In 2005, we reported the results of a prospective study that examined the accuracy of the restaging tests of 48 patients with esophageal cancer, all of whom underwent neoadjuvant chemoradiotherapy and then complete resection. All patients had CT scans of the chest, abdomen, and pelvis before and after induction therapy. In addition, all patients underwent an initial and repeat EUS with FNA and an initial and repeat integrated PET/CT scans. For this study we mandated that all patients underwent resection via an Ivor Lewis esophagogastrectomy, so that all lymph nodes in the abdomen and in the chest were removed and pathologically assessed (13). We found that repeat EUS-FNA was 80% accurate for predicting the overall T status. However, it should be noted that we considered a test to be correct if it predicted the T as T1, T2, or T3 and it was pathologically determined to be T1, T2, or T3. We implemented this definition since surgical resection is usually offered for a T1–T3 lesion but may not be for a T4. Since complete responders represent a different group of patients with biologically favorable disease, they were evaluated separately in our study. In this study, we found that 15 of the 48 patients were pathologic complete responders (CRs), yet repeat EUS-FNA identified only 3 of them correctly. Similarly, Beseth in 2000 found that EUS overestimated the depth of tumor penetration in 18 patients (69%) and underestimated the depth of penetration in 1 patient (4%) (14), and Kalha in 2004 showed that 19 of 22 patients who were CRs were also overstaged by EUS (10 with T2, 8 with T3, and 1 with T4) (15). Similar results were noted in a series of 137 patients treated at Memorial Sloan Kettering Cancer Center, who underwent preoperative chemoradiotherapy, followed by repeat EUS and endoscopic biopsy (16). In a preliminary report, 65% of the 104 patients who had no tumor in the endoscopic biopsies had residual tumor in the surgical specimen. Similarly, in our study, repeat EUS was noted to overestimate 12 of the 15 as having residual disease and predicted T2 in 2 patients, T3 in 7, and T4 in 3 (Table 24.1). Thus, repeat EUS-FNA is often not able to differentiate between a residual fibrotic mass and viable tumor and may overestimate the T status. Factors that have been shown to limit the accuracy of EUS are postradiation esophagitis, luminal stenosis, compression of the tumor caused by the endoscope, and experience of the endosonographer. These data suggest that different techniques besides repeat EUS-FNA are needed to predict response of locoregional disease to preoperative therapy. Measuring the change in maximal cross-sectional area pre- and postchemoradiotherapy by repeat CT scan or repeat EUS may be a more useful measure to assess the response of esophageal cancer to preoperative chemoradiotherapy, but this is not yet a standard approach (17–19).

TABLE 24.1
Restaging for T Stage Using the 3 Different Staging Modalities for Patients with Esophageal Cancer after Neoadjuvant Chemoradiotherapy and Resection via an Ivor Lewis Esophagogastrectomy [a]

Author and year	N	Accuracy of predicting pT stage		
		EUS/FNA	PET/CT	CT
Cerfolio 2005	48	80%	80%	76%
Swisher[b] 2004	103	68%	76%	62%
Kalha 2004	83	29%	ND	ND
Zuccaro 1999	59	37%	ND	ND
Laterza 1999	87	47%	ND	ND
Bowrey 1999	17	59%	ND	ND
Isenberg 1998	31	43%	ND	ND

Abbreviations: [a] p = pathologic stage; ND = not done.
[b] Accuracy in predicting pathologic nonresponse (>10% viable cancer in primary tumor).

POSITRON-EMISSION TOMOGRAPHY SCAN

During the past 10 years, whole-body PET scan using the glucose analog fluorodeoxyglucose F-18, fluoro-2-deoxy-D-glucose (FDG), has become a commonly used noninvasive method for the clinical staging of many cancers. More recently, integrated PET-CT scanners have been developed to blend the physiologic data from the FDG uptake of cells with the spatial anatomic detail of CT scan. Integrated PET-CT characterizes the maximum standardized uptake value (maxSUV) of the primary tumor as well as identifying potential nodal (N) metastases and metastatic (M1a and M1b) disease. Much confusion exists because of the multiple systems that are available and because of the often convoluted and confusing terminology. The most common types of PET systems are summarized in Table 24.2.

INTEGRATED PET-CT SUPERIOR TO DEDICATED PET

Integrated PET-CT has been shown, in 2 prospective randomized trials, to be superior to PET alone (despite the addition of the most recent CT scan for visual comparison with the PET) for staging patients with non–small cell lung cancer. PET offers superior metabolic information, but it has only limited spatial resolution and anatomic landmarks (20,21) when compared to CT. Additionally, FDG-18 is taken up by muscles, and its inflammatory processes can be mistaken for a malignant process (22,23). Additionally, some institutions utilize software that fuses CT and PET images. The problem with this technique is that patients will move or the scans may have to be performed on separate days. The improved localization with PET-CT allows the radiologists to clearly distinguish areas of normal physiologic tracer uptake from regions of increased metabolic activity. As important, sometimes there is increased metabolic activity but no anatomic abnormality that corresponds with it. By performing PET and CT studies simultaneously on an integrated system, the scanner overcomes limitations inherent in retrospective comparison of separate images and eliminates the need for postacquisition image alignment as well as the imprecision it brings.

Multiple series have examined the efficacy of PET-CT versus PET and CT alone. In 2 recently published prospective studies, PET-CT provided additional information in 41% (20/49) of patients as compared with visual correlation of PET and CT individually (24,25). Another study showed a reduction in number of false positive (3 to 0) and false negatives (16 to 2) as compared to PET alone (26). Similarly, in our prospective study we found PET-CT to be superior to PET alone for the accuracy of the T, N, and of the M staging in patients with non–small cell lung cancer. Unlike other studies, all patients in this study underwent definitive biopsies (27). Although similar data have not been generated specifically for esophageal cancer, PET-CT has been accepted as a standard in imaging solid tumors.

REPEAT PET/CT FOR RESTAGING

The greatest benefit of PET in the restaging of patients with esophageal cancer is through the measurement of maxSUV before and after induction therapy (28–31). We have shown that the best time to repeat the PET is about 1 month after the last dose of radiation for non–small cell lung cancer (32). This held true even when high-dose (60 Gy or higher) neoadjuvant radiotherapy was used. We believe the same timing holds for patients with esophageal cancer. The repeat PET allows one to calculate the change in the maxSUV. In 2004 we showed that the change in maxSUV on PET scan after neoadjuvant therapy holds a near linear relationship with pathologic response ($r^2 = 0.75$). Additionally, when the maxSUV of the primary tumor decreased by 80% or more, it was likely that the patient was a complete responder regardless of cell type, type of neoadjuvant therapy, or the final absolute maxSUV (33,34). A similar pattern was seen for SUV changes in mediastinal nodes following neoadjuvant therapy. In 2006, we showed that when the maxSUV of a mediastinal node initially involved with

TABLE 24.2
PET and PET-CT Definitions

	Definition	Advantages and disadvantages
Dedicated PET		
Full thick ring PET	Scintillation detectors cover a full 360 degrees around the volume to be imaged.	Higher sensitivity Reduction of artifacts No moving parts
Partial thick ring	Two opposed curved matrices rotate and capture image.	Decreased sensitivity compared to full thick ring Images can only be represented in 3D with this system
Coincidental gamma camera	Dual-head gamma cameras use a 15-ns window to capture images.	Lower sensitivity, longer dead time
PET-CT		
Integrated (hybrid)	The combined PET/CT scanner creates 2 images: one relies on CT, the other on PET. A computer then merges the 2 scans into a single image that helps doctors diagnose the nature and location of a disease.	Most accurate and specific system to date for the staging of patients with non–small cell lung cancer More expensive than PET or CT alone or fusion software Exam done at one time
Fusion	Software used to create a 3D model of the CT study and a 3D model of the PET transmission study and then utilizes an algorithm to compare and provide an overlay of images	Less costly than integrated PET-CT Not as accurate as integrated PET-CT CT and PET may be obtained on different dates Increased artifacts due to movement
Visually correlated	Radiologist visually compares/contrasts CT and PET scan.	Requires radiologist to manually compare a PET and CT scan side by side; decreased consistency Exam different dates

metastatic cancer decreased by >50%, it was highly likely (+LR 7.9) that the node had been rendered benign by neoadjuvant therapy. Furthermore, when the maxSUV decreased by 75% or more, there was a good likelihood (+LR 6.1) that the patient was a complete responder (35). We have shown that repeat PET had 100% accuracy when assessing this response for paratracheal lymph nodes (36). Thus, repeat PET and, even better, repeat PET-CT after neoadjuvant therapy is now a standard tool to assess the response a patient has to a certain neoadjuvant therapy to help select appropriate patients for surgical resection or to direct different, continued, or varied chemotherapeutic regimens or for the addition of radiotherapy. Moreover, the maxSUV can direct the best place to biopsy or the presence of new or suspicious N2 or N3 disease. Although much of these data are for patients with non–small cell lung cancer, it formed the basis for similar studies on patients with esophageal cancer.

In our prospective study of 48 patients with esophageal cancer described previously, we found that repeat integrated PET/CT was a superior restaging tool for predicting the nodal status and the CR rate for patients with esophageal cancer compared to repeat EUS-FNA or repeat CT scan. Rice and colleagues have shown that residual nodal disease confers a poor prognosis with a 5-year survival of 12% (37). Thus, recalcitrant or persistent nodal disease is important, and some argue that esophageal resection should be delayed and a second line of chemotherapy offered. Resection in these centers is often reserved only for those who have their nodal disease downstaged. Thus, the ability of a restaging test to predict recalcitrant nodal disease is clinically important.

In our study of 48 patients, 8 patients had regional lymph nodes that were pathologically involved with cancer despite the use of neoadjuvant chemoradiotherapy. Repeat PET/CT predicted 5 of the 8, whereas repeat EUS-FNA predicted it in only 1 patient. In addition, of the 40 patients whose lymph nodes were pathologically negative, FDG-PET predicted 33 of these 40 patients correctly, whereas repeat EUS-FNA predicted only 31. Thus, the overall accuracy for PET/CT for the nodal prediction was 93% compared to 78% for EUS-FNA ($P = 0.04$). Several other series supporting the strength of PET/CT in restaging of esophageal cancer have been summarized in Tables 24.2 and 24.3 (38–42).

PET/CT may also be more accurate for detection of M1 disease following neoadjuvant therapy. Fiore in 2006, in a study of 56 patients, showed that CT-PET was superior in identifying small mediastinal metastatic lymph nodes (N1), extrathoracic lymph nodes (M1), and hepatic metastases (#1 cm) that escaped multislice CT and EUS following neoadjuvant therapy (42). We showed in 2005 that FDG-PET/CT correctly identified M1b disease in 4 patients, falsely suggested it in 4 patients, and missed it in 2 patients, whereas for CT, it was 3, 3, and 3 patients (13).

TABLE 24.3

Restaging for N Stage Using the 3 Different Staging Modalities for Patients with Esophageal Cancer after Neoadjuvant Chemoradiotherapy and Resection via an Ivor Lewis Esophagogastrectomy [a]

		Accuracy of predicting the pN stage		
Author and year	**N**	**EUS/ FNA**	**PET/ CT**	**CT**
Cerfolio 2005	48	78%	93%	78%
Kalha 2004	83	49%	ND	ND
Zuccaro 1999	59	38%	ND	ND
Laterza 1999	87	71%	ND	ND
Bowrey 1999	17	59%	ND	ND

Abbreviation: [a] ND = not done.

PREDICTING WHO IS A COMPLETE RESPONDER

CRs represent an important subset of patients with esophageal cancer. Recently, many physicians have begun to question whether esophagogastrectomy offers any benefit in this group of patients. The only way to fully answer this provocative question would be to perform a prospective study and to randomize 2 groups of patients (both known to be CRs) to observation versus surgical resection. Since there has been no way to accurately determine who is a CR without surgical resection, this study has not been performed. In our prospective study of 48 patients, 15 patients were complete responders. Integrated PET/CT has been shown to be better than EUS-FNA and CT for the detection of CRs. We showed in this study in 2005 that the accuracy for detection of CR was 71% for CT and 70% for EUS-FNA but was 88% for integrated PET/CT. Swisher in 2004 similarly observed accuracy rates of 62%, 68%, and 76% for CT, EUS-FNA, and PET/CT, respectively. In addition to greater accuracy, the decrease in maxSUV of PET/CT scan between pre- and posttherapy scans may be an indicator of the degree of response to therapy. In our 2005 series, we found that the maxSUV fell by a median of 47% for those who were CRs and 42% for those who were downstaged. Recently, others, such as Port and colleagues, have also shown that when the maxSUV falls in patients who are pathologically CRs (43).

CONCLUSIONS/RECOMMENDATIONS

In conclusion, CT scan for the assessment of response to treatment in esophageal cancer is relatively inaccurate and useful only for M1a and M1b disease. Repeat EUS and repeat integrated PET/CT are more accurate than CT scan. EUS, unlike the other modalities, is able to provide pathologic tissue via the rebiopsy of regional lymph nodes as well as targets in selected M1a and M1b locations. However, it is not able to accurately assess the T status after neoadjuvant chemoradiotherapy. Repeat PET, which is able to measure the change in maxSUV for T, N, and M stage, is a promising restaging tool. It is most accurate when the initial PET and repeat PET are performed on the same machine at the same center using similar techniques and there has been at least 4 weeks between the end of the radiotherapy and the repeat PET. It may be the most accurate modality for the assessment of the biologic response of esophageal cancer to induction therapy. Our current treatment algorithm is depicted in Figure 24.2. Multicenter studies with large patient populations, which focus on the prediction of tumor response early in the course of neoadjuvant therapy, are needed.

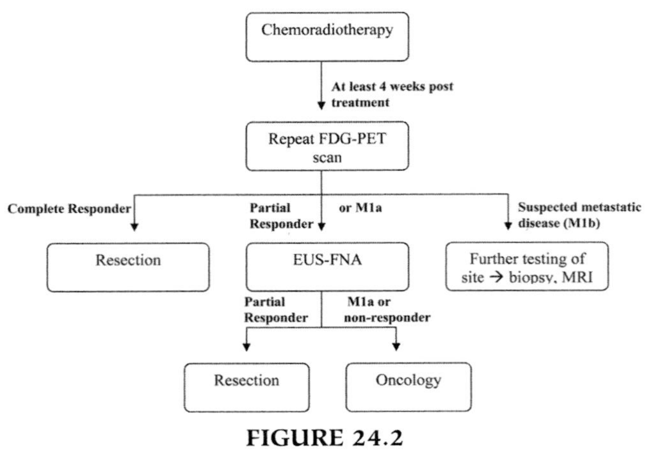

FIGURE 24.2

Recommended restaging algorithm.

References

1. Swisher SG, Hunt KK, Holmes EC, et al. Changes in the surgical management of esophageal cancer from 1970 to 1993. *Am J Surg.* 1995;69:609–614.
2. Muller JM, Erasmi H, Stelzner M, et al. Surgical therapy of oesophageal carcinoma. *Br J Surg.* 1990;77:845–857.
3. Walsh TN, Noonan N, Hollywood D, et al. A comparison of multimodal therapy and surgery for esophageal adenocarcinoma. *N Engl J Med.* 1996;335:462–467.
4. Urba SG, Orringer MB, Turrisi A, et al. Randomized trial of preoperative chemoradiation versus surgery alone in patients with locoregional esophageal carcinoma. *J Clin Oncol.* 2001;19:305–313.
5. Walker SJ, Allen SM, Steel A, et al. Assessment of the response to chemotherapy in esophageal cancer. *Eur J Cardiothorac Surg.* 1991;5:519–522.
6. Griffith JF, Chan AC, Chow LT, et al. Assessing chemotherapy response of squamous cell oesophageal carcinoma with spiral CT. *Br J Radiol.* 1999;72:678–684.
7. Kroep JR, Van Groeningen CJ, Cuesta MA, et al. Positron emission tomography using 2-deoxy-2-[18F]-flouro-D-glucose for response monitoring in locally advanced gastroesophageal cancer: a comparison of different analytical methods. *Mol Imaging Biol.* 2003;5:337–346.
8. Jones DR, Parker LA Jr, Detterbeck FC, et al. Inadequacy of computed tomography in assessing patients with esophageal carcinoma after induction cehmradiotherapy. *Cancer.* 1999;85:1026–1032.
9. Cerfolio RJ, Bryant AS. Is palpation of the lung necessary for patients with non-small cell lung cancer? *J Thorac Cardvasc Surg.* 2008;135:261–268.
10. Jhala NC, Eltoum IA, Eloubeidi MA, et al. Providing on-site diagnosis of malignancy on endoscopic-ultrasound-guided fine-needle aspirates: should it be done? *Ann Diagn Pathol.* 2007;11:176–181.
11. Hordikj ML, Kok TC, Wilson JH, et al. Assessment of response of esophageal carcinoma to induction chemotherapy. *Endoscopy.* 1993;25:592–596.
12. Zuccari G Jr, Rice TW, Golddblum J, et al. Endoscopic ultrasound cannot determine suitability for esophagectomy after aggressive chemoradiotherapy for esophageal cancer. *Am J Gastroenterol.* 1999;94:906–912.
13. Cerfolio RJ, Bryant AS, Ohja B, et al. The accuracy of endoscopic ultrasonography with fine-needle aspiration, integrated positron emission tomography with computed tomography, and computed tomography in restaging patients with esophageal cancer after neoadjuvant chemoradiotherapy. *J Thorac Cardiovasc Surg.* 2005;129:1232–1241.
14. Beseth BD, Bedford R, Isacoff WH, et al. Endoscopic ultrasound does not accurate assess pathologic stage of esophageal cancer after neoadjuvant chemoradiotherapy. *Am Surg.* 2000;66:827–831.
15. Kalha I, Kaw M, Fukami N, et al. The accuracy of endoscopic ultrasound for restaging esophageal carcinoma after chemoradiation therapy. *Cancer.* 2004;101:940.
16. Sarkaria JS, Rizk N, Bains M, et al. Does endoscopy accurately predict response to chemoradiation in patients undergoing esophagectomy? [abstract]. *J Clin Oncol.* 2006;24:184s.
17. Isenberg G, Chak A, Canto MI, et al. Endoscopic ultrasound in restaging of esophageal cancer after neoadjuvant chemoradiation. *Gastrointest Endosc.* 1998;48:158.
18. Chak A, Canto MI, Cooper GS, et al. Endosonographic assessment of multimodality therapy predicts survival of esophageal carcinoma patients. *Cancer.* 2000;88:1788.
19. Willis J, Cooper GS, Isenberg G, et al. Correlation of EUS measurement with pathologic assessment of neoadjuvant therapy response in esophageal carcinoma. *Gastrointest Endosc.* 2002;55:655.
20. Klaff V, Hicks RG, MacManus MP, et al. Clinical impact of (18) FDG positron emission tomography in patients with non-small-cell lung cancer: a prospective study. *J Clin Oncol.* 2001;19:111–118.
21. Pitterman RM, Van Putten JWG, Meuzelarr JJ, et al. Preoperative staging of non-small cell lung cancer with positron-emission-tomography. *N Engl J Med.* 2000;343:254–261.
22. Cook GJR, Maisey MN, Fogelman I. Normal variants, artifacts and interpretative pitfalls in PET imaging with 18-flouro-deoxyglycose and carbon-11 methionine. *Eur J Nucl Med.* 1999;26:1363–1378.
2. Engel H, Steinhart H, Buck A, et al. Whole body PET: physiological and artifactual flourodeoxyglucose accumulations. *J Nucl Med.* 1996;37:441–446.
24. Steinert HC, von Schulthess GK. Initial experience using a new integrated in-line PET/CT system. *Br J Radiol.* 2002;75:S36–S38.
25. Lardinois D, Weder W, Hany TF, et al. Staging of non-small-cell lung cancer with integrated positron-emission tomography-computed tomography. *N Engl J Med.* 2003;348:2500–2507.
26. Dizendorf E. PET/CT fusion worth the cost. *Diagnostic Imaging.* November 2001.
27. Cerfolio RJ, Ojha B, Bryant AS, et al. The accuracy of integrated PET-CT compared with dedicated PET alone for the staging of patients with non-small cell lung cancer. *Ann Thorac Surg.* 2004;78:1017–1023.
28. Eschmann SM, Friedel G, Paulsen F, et al. 18 F-FDG PET for assessment of therapy response and preoperative re-evaluation after neoadjuvant radio-chemotherapy in stage III non-small cell lung cancer. *Eur J Nucl Med Mol Imaging.* 2007;34:463–471.
29. Weber WA, Petersen V, Schmidt B, et al. Positron emission tomography in non-small-cell lung cancer: prediction of response to chemotherapy by quantitative assessment of glucose use. *J Clin Oncol.* 2003;21:2651–2657.
30. Dimitrakopoulou-Strauss A, Strauss LG, Rudi J. PET-FDG as predictor of therapy response in patients with colorectal carcinoma. *Q J Nucl Med.* 2003;47:8–13.
31. Weber WA, Petersen V, Schmidt B, et al. Positron emission tomography in non-small-cell lung cancer: prediction of response to chemotherapy by quantitative assessment of glucose use. *J Clin Oncol.* 2003;21:2651–2657.
32. Cerfolio RJ, Bryant AS. When is it best to repeat an FDG-PET/CT scan on patients with non-small cell lung cancer who have received neoadjuvant chemoradiotherapy? *Ann Thorac Surg.* 2007;84:1092–1097.
33. Cerfolio RJ, Bryant AS, Winokur TS, et al. Repeat FDG-PET after neoadjuvant therapy is a predictor of pathologic response in patients with non-small cell lung cancer. *Ann Thorac Surg.* 2004;78:1903–1909.
34. Eschmann SM, Friedel G, Paulsen F, et al. (18)F-FDG PET for assessment of therapy response and preoperative re-evaluation after neoadjuvant radio-chemotherapy in stage III non-small cell lung cancer. *Eur J Nucl Med Mol Imaging.* 2007;34:463–471.
35. Cerfolio RJ, Bryant AS, Ojha B. Restaging patients with N2 (stage IIIa) non-small cell lung cancer after neoadjuvant chemoradiotherapy: a prospective study. *J Thorac Cardiovasc Surg.* 2006;131:1229–1235.
36. Cerfolio RJ, Ojha B, Mukerhee S, et al. Positron emission tomography scanning with 2-fluoro-2-deoxy-d-glucose as a predictor of response of neoadjuvant treatment for non-small cell carcinoma. *Thorac Cardiovasc Surg.* 2003;125:938–944.
37. Rice TW, Blackstone EH, Adelstein DJ, et al. N1 esophageal carcinoma: the importance of staging and downstaging. *J Thorac Cardiovasc Surg.* 2001;121:454–464.

38. Flamen P, Van Cutsem E, Lerut A, et al. Positron emission tomography for assessment of the response to induction radiochemotherapy in locally advanced oesophageal cancer. *Ann Oncol.* 2002;13:361.
39. Kato H, Kuwano H, Nakajima M, et al. Usefulness of positron emission tomography for assessing the response of neoadjuvant chemoradiotherapy in patients with esophageal cancer. *Am J Surg.* 2002;184:279.
40. Song SY, Kim JH, Ryu JS, et al. FDG-PET in the prediction of pathologic response after neoadjuvant chemoradiotherapy in locally advanced, resectable esophageal cancer. *Int J Radiat Oncol Biol Phys.* 2005;63:1053.
41. Levine EA, Farmer MR, Clark P, et al. Predictive value of 18-fluoro-deoxy-glucose-positron emission tomography (18F-FDG-PET) in the identification of responders to chemoradiation therapy for the treatment of locally advanced esophageal cancer. *Ann Surg.* 2006;243:472.
42. Fiore D, Baggio V, Ruol A, et al. Multimodal imaging of esophagus and cardia cancer before and after treatment. *Radiol Torino.* 2006;111:804–817.
43. Port JL, Lee PC, Korst RJ, et al. Positron emission tomographic scanning predicts survival after induction chemotherapy for esophageal carcinoma. *Ann Thorac Surg.* 2007;84:393–400.

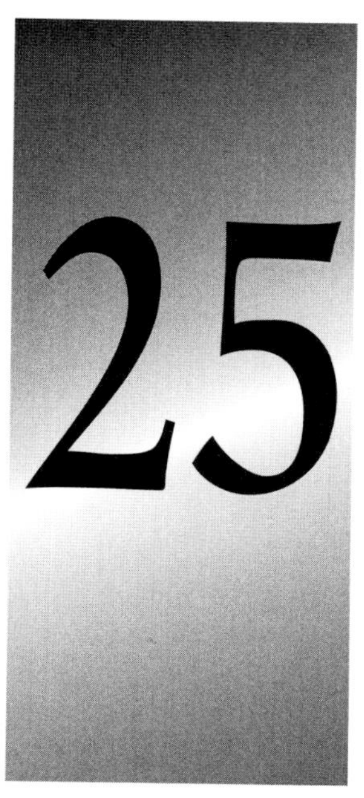

Revisions in the Staging System for Esophageal Cancer

Jeffrey A. Hagen

Esophageal cancer is staged using the tumor, nodal, and metastasis (TNM) system of classification defined by the American Joint Committee on Cancer (AJCC) in cooperation with the International Union Against Cancer (1). The goal of this staging system is to allow physicians to stratify patients according to the extent of disease present that will allow accurate determination of prognosis and selection of the most appropriate therapy. Accurate and consistent staging also allows for comparison of results reported for a variety of treatment modalities using a common language by institutions around the world. It also facilitates exchange of information among different treatment centers.

To be useful for clinical and research purposes, this staging system must include all the attributes that define the behavior of a tumor. As such, it must respond to new information that emerges in our understanding of the factors that influence prognosis. The staging system must also be viewed as a process that is responsive over time to new technologies and treatment strategies as they are developed. It must be recognized, however, that any changes made in the staging system will make it difficult to compare current and future results of therapy with those of the past. As a result, change must be undertaken cautiously and only in response to factors identified as being important in multiple large studies. In this chapter, a number of recent developments in our understanding of the management of esophageal cancer and the factors that determine outcome are reviewed. These observations emphasize several important shortcomings in the current accepted staging system, which is presently under review for revision.

CURRENT CLASSIFICATION AND STAGING OF ESOPHAGEAL CANCER USING THE TNM SYSTEM

The TNM system is designed to emphasize the important attributes of cancer that determine clinical behavior. It is based on the premise that all cancer occurring at a given site and of the same histology will have the same patterns of growth with a similar outcome. Tumors are classified on the basis of the characteristics of the primary tumor (T status), the status of the locoregional lymph nodes (N status), and the presence of systemic metastases (M status). These characteristics are used to define stage groupings that are based on the natural history of a given type of cancer and the outcomes observed. Patients can be staged on the basis of clinical examination and radiographic studies (clinical staging) and on the basis of histologic examination of tissues removed when appropriate (pathologic staging, pTNM). Cancers can also be restaged when they recur following treatment.

In the current accepted staging system, the esophagus is divided into 4 regions. The cervical esophagus is defined as extending from the cricopharyngeus to the level of the thoracic inlet, which corresponds to a distance of approximately 18 cm from the incisors. The upper third of the thoracic esophagus is defined as extending from the thoracic inlet to the carina, which is located at approximately 24 cm. Middle third tumors are defined as those located between the carina and a point half the distance between the carina and the gastroesophageal junction (GEJ). The lower third of the esophagus extends from this point to the GEJ, located between 32 and 40 cm from the incisors.

The characteristics of the primary tumor (T status) are defined on the basis of the depth of invasion into the wall of the esophagus. T_1 tumors include those that invade into but not through the submucosa. A tumor that invades into but not through the muscularis propria is designated a T_2 lesion. Tumors that invade beyond the muscularis propria into the adjacent adventitia are classified as T_3 tumors, whereas tumors that invade adjacent structures are classified as T_4.

Lymph node status is classified as a dichotomous variable in the current staging system, based on the presence or absence of regional node involvement. Regional nodes are defined differently for tumors in different locations in the esophagus (Table 25.1). For tumors located in the cervical esophagus, the cervical, supraclavicular, and upper periesophageal lymph nodes are considered regional nodes. For tumors located near the GEJ, the periesophageal nodes below the azygos vein and the diaphragmatic, pericardial, left gastric, and celiac nodes are all considered to be regional nodes. Lymph node metastases to other nonregional node stations are considered M1a disease, which, according to the current staging system, is considered stage IVA disease. Accordingly, patients with distal esophageal cancer and celiac node involvement and patients with cancers arising in the region of the GEJ and subcarinal node involvement are defined as having unresectable disease.

In addition to patients with metastases to nonregional lymph nodes, the M status of esophageal cancer includes patients with systemic metastatic disease. These later patients are classified as M1b, which is considered stage IVB disease. For tumors arising in the middle third of the thoracic esophagus, the M1b designation is also used in the presence of metastases involving nonregional lymph nodes. The AJCC staging system combines these TNM classifications into stage groupings, as defined in Table 25.2.

TABLE 25.1
Definitions of Regional and Nonregional Lymph Node Involvement by Tumor Location

Regional lymph nodes	Nonregional lymph nodes (M1a)
Tumors of the lower thoracic esophagus	
Upper periesophageal nodes (above azygos vein)	Celiac nodes
Subcarinal nodes	
Lower periesophageal nodes (below azygos vein)	
Tumors of the midthoracic esophagus	
Upper periesophageal nodes (above azygos vein)	Not applicable
Subcarinal nodes	
Lower periesophageal nodes (below azygos vein)	
Tumors of the upper thoracic esophagus	
Upper periesophageal nodes (above azygos vein)	Cervical nodes
Subcarinal nodes	
Lower periesophageal nodes (below azygos vein)	

TABLE 25.2
Stage Groupings

Stage 0	Tis	N0	M0
Stage I	T1	N0	M0
Stage IIA	T2	N0	M0
	T3	N0	M0
Stage IIB	T1	N1	M0
	T2	N1	M0
Stage III	T3	N1	M0
	T4	Any N	M0
Stage IVA	Any T	Any N	M1a
Stage IVB	Any T	Any N	M1b

INADEQUACIES IN THE CURRENT STAGING SYSTEM FOR ESOPHAGEAL CANCER

The adequacy of the current staging system for esophageal cancer has been called into question for a number of reasons. First, it does not include Barrett's-associated adenocarcinomas that arise at the GEJ. Using current definitions, a tumor arising in the region of the GEJ that involves less than 2 cm of the distal esophagus is classified as a gastric cancer in the AJCC *Staging Manual.* Second, the staging system does not consider the extent of lymph node involvement, a factor identified in several recent studies as being of prognostic importance. Third, the current version of the staging system classifies nonregional lymph node involvement in quite general terms that vary in definition depending on the location of the primary tumor. These patients are classified as having M1a (stage IVA) disease, which is considered unresectable. Fourth, when the performance of the current staging system in patients undergoing resection has been analyzed, it has been shown that survival estimates do not differ significantly between several stage groupings (i.e., the survival probabilities are not distinctive) and that some of the TNM combinations included in the same stage grouping are dissimilar (i.e., the survival probabilities are not homogeneous) (2). Finally, the adequacy of the current AJCC system has recently been questioned in the staging of patients who have received preoperative therapy.

Adenocarcinoma Arising at the GEJ

There is increasing evidence to suggest that cancers arising at the GEJ, so-called gastric cardia cancers, should be classified as esophageal in origin rather than as a gastric cancer. Similarities between these cardia cancers and esophageal adenocarcinomas and major differences from cancers arising in the more distal stomach have been observed in terms of their epidemiology, patient demographic characteristics, risk factors for occurrence, and the molecular profiles of the tumors.

The rising incidence of esophageal cancer in Western countries over the past 2 decades has been well documented (3). At the same time, population-based epidemiologic studies have shown that gastric cardia cancer has been rising in incidence in parallel with esophageal adenocarcinoma (4) at a rate of 4% to 5% per year. At the same time, the incidence of distal gastric cancer has been on the decline (5). Epidemiologic studies have also documented similarities in patient demographic characteristics between esophageal adenocarcinoma and tumors arising in the gastric cardia that contrast sharply with cancers occurring in the distal stomach. Distal gastric cancer occurs with similar frequency in men and women, while gastric cardia cancer is more than 5 times as common in men: a demographic characteristic similar to esophageal adenocarcinoma (6). Symptomatic gastroesophageal reflux disease is also common in patients with both gastric cardia cancer and esophageal adenocarcinoma (7), and an association has been documented between both types of cancer and an increased body mass index (8). On the other hand, low socioeconomic status, a well-defined demographic risk factor for distal gastric cancer, has not been associated with an increased risk of either esophageal adenocarcinoma or gastric cardia cancer (9). These similarities in epidemiology and patient demographics suggest that the etiologic factors resulting in the development of adenocarcinoma in the esophagus and cancer arising at the GEJ are similar.

Risk factors that have been identified for the development of esophageal adenocarcinoma and cancer occurring in the gastric cardia have also been shown to be similar, with important differences noted from distal gastric cancer. Chronic infection with *Helicobacter pylori* is a well-documented risk factor for distal gastric cancer, with no such relationship noted for adenocarcinoma of the gastric cardia or of the esophagus (10). In fact, it has been suggested that seropositivity for *H. pylori* may be associated with a decreased risk of cancer of the esophagus and gastric cardia (11). Dietary factors associated with the risk of gastric cardia cancer and esophageal adenocarcinoma are also similar, and they differ from those associated with distal gastric cancer. A diet high in meat (especially red meat) has been associated with an increased risk of distal gastric cancer in a dose-dependent fashion, with no such relationship found for gastric cardia cancer or for adenocarcinoma of the esophagus (12). It has also been shown that a diet high in fiber appears to be protective against the development of both gastric cardia cancer and adenocarcinoma of the esophagus (13). This effect may be mediated by the nitrate-scavenging properties of dietary fiber, especially wheat fiber (14).

There are also similarities in the molecular characteristics of cancers arising at the GEJ and esophageal adenocarcinoma that in many cases differ from the molecular profiles of distal gastric cancer. Using immunohistochemical (IHC) staining techniques, P53 alterations and expression of sucrose isomaltase (an intestinal enzyme expressed in Barrett's esophagus but not in gastric epithelium) have been shown to be common in both esophageal adenocarcinoma and gastric cardia cancer (15). Assessment of loss of heterozygosity (LOH) patterns for genes coded on the distal q arm of chromosome 17 (16) and assessment of LOH and microsatellite instability for loci of the 14q region and for p53, adenomatous polyposis coli (APC), and deleted in colorectal cancer (DCC) have also shown striking similarities between gastric cardia cancer and adenocarcinoma of the esophagus (17). On the basis of these observations, it appears that the sequence of molecular carcinogenesis may be the same for these 2 tumors. Finally, Mattioli and colleagues (18) have shown that the pattern of CK staining in tumors of the gastric cardia is similar to that of Barrett's-associated adenocarcinoma, a pattern quite dissimilar to that seen in distal gastric cancer.

Perhaps most important, a number of similarities have been identified in the clinical behavior and prognosis following therapy between esophageal adenocarcinoma and gastric cardia cancer. The frequency and patterns of lymph node involvement have been shown to be similar (19, 20), and survival following therapy appears to be the same (21). In addition, the type of operation performed for a cancer arising in the lower third of the esophagus and for a cancer of the GEJ is the same in most centers. For all these reasons, it appears that tumors that arise in the gastric cardia region should be considered together with adenocarcinoma of the esophagus rather than as a form of gastric cancer.

The Importance of the Extent of Lymph Node Involvement

The current AJCC staging system considers lymph node involvement as a dichotomous variable (present or absent), in spite of reports from centers around the world that document the importance of the extent of lymph node involvement on prognosis. It was Skinner et al. (22) who first suggested that the number of involved lymph nodes was of prognostic importance, suggesting a revised staging system in which N status was classified into 3 groups with limited node involvement defined as the presence of 2 or fewer node metastases. This proposal was later revised to a threshold of 4 or fewer node metastases on the basis of an analysis of additional patients undergoing en bloc resection (23). Since then, a number of investigators have confirmed these findings (24–26). Reports from several other investigators have also emphasized the importance of the number of lymph node metastases, although a variety of cutoff points for the number of nodes involved have been proposed (Table 25.3). On the basis of these reports, it is clear that the extent of lymph node involvement is of prognostic importance. What remains to be determined, based on studies involving many more patients than have been reported to date, is the optimal threshold for the number of involved nodes that best predicts outcome.

The extent of lymph node involvement has also been classified using the lymph node ratio (LNR) defined as the number of nodes with metastases divided by the number of nodes removed. Roder and colleagues initially reported a LNR of 20% as a threshold for defining limited versus advanced lymph node involvement (27). Since then, a number of other investigators have confirmed the value of the LNR in determining prognosis, using a variety of different thresholds (Table 25.4). When the LNR has been compared to classification schemes on the basis of the number of involved lymph nodes, the LNR has been consistently shown to be superior (26–32). It is likely that the LNR better stratifies patients with regard to prognosis because it accounts for both the number of involved lymph nodes and the extent of lymphadenectomy performed. Similar findings have been reported in patients with cancer of the breast (33), colon (34), pancreas (35), uterus (36), and stomach (37).

TABLE 25.3
Impact of the Number of Involved Lymph Nodes on Prognosis

Author	Cell type[a]	Suggested thresholds
Skinner et al. (22)	43 EAC, 43 SCCA, 5 other	0, 1–2, ≥3
Skinner et al. (23)	39 EAC, 36 SCCA, 5 other	0, 1–4, ≥5
Ellis et al. (24)	265 patients, cell types not stated	0, 1–4, ≥5
Ellis et al. (25)	303 EAC, 139 SCCA, 12 other	0, 1–4, ≥5
Hagen et al. (26)	100 EAC	0, 1–4, ≥5
Tachibana et al. (29)	76 SCCA	0, 1–4, ≥5
Rizk et al. (43)	271 EAC, 65 SCCA	0, 1–4, ≥5
Korst et al. (40)	127 EAC, 89 SCCA	0, 1–3, ≥4
Zafirellis et al. (28)	125 EAC, 31 SCCA	0, 1–3, ≥4
Kunisaki et al. (30)	113 SCCA	0, 1–3, ≥4
Hofstetter et al. (41)	766 EAC, 261 SCCA	0, 1–3, ≥4
Rice et al. (2)	401 EAC, 67 SCCA, 12 other	0, 1–2, ≥3
Wijnhoven et al. (42)	250 EAC, 42 SCCA	0, 1–2, ≥3

Abbreviations: [a]EAC = esophageal adenocarcinoma; SCCA = squamous cell carcinoma.

More recently, we have used IHC-detected micrometastases in an attempt to better classify patients with regard to survival (38). We examined 1,970 nodes removed from 37 patients who had en bloc resections for esophageal adenocarcinoma, to determine the frequency and prognostic importance of IHC-detected micrometastases. Twenty of these patients had limited lymph node involvement defined by an LNR of <10%. Five-year survival in this group of patients was 55%. Additional node metastases were identified by IHC in 14 patients (70%). When the number of IHC-detected node metastases was added to the number detected by H&E, the LNR remained <10% in 13 patients, and survival was 77% at 5 years. In contrast, in the 7 patients with an LNR >10% when the additional metastases detected by IHC were added to the H&E detected metastases, survival at 5 years was only 14%, similar to the 13% survival observed in patients with an LNR >10% based on H&E examination alone. These observations suggest that the optimal staging strategy to assess lymph node involvement may be the use of the LNR calculated on the basis of the combined findings of H&E staining and IHC examination.

TABLE 25.4
Impact of the Lymph Node Ratio on Prognosis [a]

Author	Cell type	Suggested thresholds
Roder et al. (27)	434 SCCA	0, 0.01–0.20, ≥0.20
Zafirellis et al. (28)	125 EAC, 31 SCCA	0, 0.01–0.20, ≥0.20
Lagarde et al. (44)	251 EAC	0, 0.01–0.20, ≥0.20
Wijnhoven et al. (42)	250 EAC, 42 SCCA	0, 0.01–0.20, ≥0.20
Holscher et al. (31)	137 EAC	0, 0.01–0.30, ≥0.30
van Sandick et al. (32)	86 EAC, 29 SCCA	0, 0.01–0.30, ≥0.30
Kunisaki et al. (30)	113 SCCA	0, 0.01–0.15, ≥0.15
Hagen et al. (26)	100 EAC	0, 0.01–0.10, ≥0.10
Tachibana et al. (29)	76 SCCA	0, 0.01–0.10, ≥0.10

Abbreviations: [a]EAC = esophageal adenocarcinoma; SCCA = squamous cell carcinoma.

Nonregional Lymph Node Involvement

The current classification system defines involvement of nonregional lymph nodes as metastatic disease (M1a), which results in the designation as stage IVA disease, for which surgical resection for cure is not generally recommended. A number of investigators have called this classification scheme into question, particularly in patients with lower esophageal adenocarcinoma and celiac lymph node involvement. This classification has its origin in data from Japan in patients with squamous cell carcinoma, where involvement of abdominal nodes may, in fact, portend a poor prognosis. With the dramatic rise in the frequency of adenocarcinoma of the esophagus in many parts of the world, this issue of proper classification of nonregional nodes has attracted considerable attention beginning with the report by Steup et al. in 1996 (39). In this report, they found that patients with nonregional lymph node involvement had a significantly better survival than patients with visceral M1 disease. Their findings were supported 2 years later in a report by Korst et al. (40) in which involvement of nonregional nodes was classified as N2 disease in a proposed revision to the staging system in use at the time. Since then, a number of other investigators have reported similar findings. In our experience with en bloc resections performed for distal esophageal adenocarcinoma (26), we reported 26 patients with distant lymph node involvement, including 16 with involvement of celiac nodes. Survival at 5 years in these patients with stage IVA disease was 28%, which was not statistically different from the outcome observed in patients with only regional lymph nodes involved when the number of involved nodes was greater than 4 (22% 5-year survival). Hofstetter et al. (41) have reported similar findings in a review of more than 1,000 resections for esophageal cancer of all cell types. In their series, 3-year survival in patients classified as having M1a disease was 24%, which was nearly identical to the survival they reported (23%) for patients with regional lymph node involvement alone. These findings are in disagreement with those of Rice et al. (2) and Wijnhoven et al. (42), who recommended revisions to the staging system that included elimination of the M1a group, classifying patients with involvement of nonregional nodes and those with visceral metastases as M1 disease. It is worth emphasizing, however, that these 2 reports did not compare survival in patients with celiac node metastases to patients with multiple nodes involved elsewhere in the resected specimen. This is an important distinction since the presence of celiac node metastases is significantly more common in patients with multiple lymph node metastases (31,43), with nearly two-thirds of the patients with celiac node metastases having more than 4 lymph nodes involved. Celiac node metastases are also more common in patients with extracapsular lymph node involvement (44)—an additional histopathologic factor that has been associated with a poor outcome (45). On the basis of these observations, it appears likely that the apparent prognostic importance of celiac lymph node involvement in some series may be explained by the failure of the current classification system to account for the extent of lymph node involvement and other poor prognostic indicators with which celiac node involvement is highly linked. What is clear is that survival reported after resection in patients with celiac node involvement appears to be considerably better than the 4- to 6-month median survival typically reported in patients with visceral metastases.

Performance of the Current Stage Grouping in Predicting Prognosis

For optimal performance, staging systems should result in groupings that are distinctive (defined as significant separation between classifications or stage groups based on survival), homogeneous (defined as the absence of distinct subgroups within a single classification or grouping), and with a monotonic ordering with decreasing survival with increasing stage grouping. The poor performance of the current staging system as it relates to these issues has been emphasized, beginning with the report by Skinner et al. (22) that proposed modifications based largely on the number of involved lymph nodes. Since then, others have proposed additional revisions that are summarized in Table 25.5.

More recently, Rice and colleagues (2) have clearly described several important shortcomings in the current staging system in their report of 480 patients who underwent resection alone for esophageal cancer. They noted that the T and N classifications and the defined stage groupings were monotonic, but they found a lack of homogeneity in the T1 classification, noting significant survival differences for tumors limited to the lamina propria (T1a) compared to tumors that involved the submucosa (T1b). For reasons noted previously, they also noted a lack of homogeneity in patients classified as having N1 disease, with a significant decrease in survival as the number of regional node metastases increased. They also demonstrated a lack of distinctiveness between several of the stage groupings as currently defined, with significant differences in survival between stages I, IIA, and III but no difference between stage IIB, III, and IV disease. On the basis of these observations, they recommended a number of revisions to the stage groupings, as summarized in Table 25.5.

TABLE 25.5
Proposed Revisions to the Staging System for Esophageal Cancer

Stage	Ellis et al. (25)	Korst et al. (40)	Rice et al. (2)
0	Tis N0 M0	T0 N0 M0,	Not applicable
	T1 N0 M0	Tis N0 M0	
I	T1 N1 M0,	T1 N0 M0,	Tis (HGD),
	T2 N0 M0	T2 N0 M0	T1 N0 M0
IIA		T3 N0 M0	
	T2 N1 M0, T3 N0 M0	T1 N1 M0	T1b N0 M0, T1a N1 M0, T2 N0 M0
IIB		T2 N1 M0 T3 N1 M0	
III	T3 N1 M0, any T N2 M0	T1-3 N2 M0	T3 N0 M0, T1b/ T2 N1 M0, T3 N1 M0, T4 N0 M0
IV	Any T, any N M1	T4, any N M0, any T, any N M1	T4 N1 M0, any T N2 M0, any T, any N M1

Staging after Neoadjuvant Therapy

With the recent increase in popularity of combined modality therapy in esophageal cancer, questions have arisen regarding the adequacy of the current staging system in predicting outcome after neoadjuvant therapy. It has been shown that although pTNM status following neoadjuvant therapy is an independent predictor of outcome after resection, the current staging system results in several stage groupings that are not distinctive (46). To address this shortcoming, these authors proposed an assessment of the extent of response to neoadjuvant therapy for inclusion into the staging system (47). The problem with this proposal is that it results in a classification scheme with 18 separate stage groupings, which is both cumbersome to use and difficult to translate into the context of existing AJCC staging systems. Using recursive partitioning analysis, Rizk et al. (48) developed 2 different classification schemes that are easier to use in the neoadjuvant setting since they define only 6 separate stage groupings. The problem with these proposed revisions is that they result in at least 2 stage groupings for which the predicted survival is not distinctive. Further work involving larger numbers of patients from multiple institutions may resolve these issues.

SUMMARY

The current staging system for esophageal cancer as defined by the AJCC has several inadequacies that need to be addressed on the basis of the available literature regarding outcome after current therapy. Future revisions to the staging system should consider inclusion of GEJ cancers as esophageal in origin, and they must take into account the number of lymph nodes involved (or the LNR). Multi-institutional data from high-volume centers around the world should be analyzed to best define the thresholds for the extent of lymph node involvement and the ideal system for stage groupings for patients undergoing primary surgical resection and a neoadjuvant therapy approach to treatment.

References

1. American Joint Committee on Cancer. *AJCC Cancer Staging Manual.* 6th ed. New York: Springer-Verlag; 2002.
2. Rice TW, Blackstone EH, Rybicki LA, et al. Refining esophageal cancer staging [see comment]. *J Thorac Cardiovasc Surg.* 2003;125(5):1103–1113.
3. Blot WJ, Devesa SS, Fraumeni JF Jr. Continuing climb in rates of esophageal adenocarcinoma: an update. *JAMA.* 1993;270(11):1320.
4. Blot WJ, Devesa SS, Kneller RW, et al. Rising incidence of adenocarcinoma of the esophagus and gastric cardia [see comment]. *JAMA.* 1991;265(10):1287–1289.

5. Powell J, McConkey CC. The rising trend in oesophageal adenocarcinoma and gastric cardia. *Eur J Cancer Prev.* 1992;1(3):265–269.
6. Driessen A, Van Raemdonck D, De Leyn P, et al. Are carcinomas of the cardia oesophageal or gastric adenocarcinomas? *Eur J Cancer.* 2003;39(17):2487–2494.
7. Lagergren J, Bergstrom R, Lindgren A, et al. Symptomatic gastroesophageal reflux as a risk factor for esophageal adenocarcinoma [see comment]. *N Engl J Med.* 1999;340(11):825–831.
8. Chow WH, Blot WJ, Vaughan TL, et al. Body mass index and risk of adenocarcinomas of the esophagus and gastric cardia. *J Natl Cancer Inst.* 1998;90(2):150–155.
9. Brewster DH, Fraser LA, McKinney PA, et al. Socioeconomic status and risk of adenocarcinoma of the oesophagus and cancer of the gastric cardia in Scotland. *Br J Cancer.* 2000;83(3):387–390.
10. Wu AH, Crabtree JE, Bernstein L, et al. Role of *Helicobacter pylori* CagA+ strains and risk of adenocarcinoma of the stomach and esophagus. *Int J Cancer.* 2003;103(6):815–821.
11. Kamangar F, Dawsey SM, Blaser MJ, et al. Opposing risks of gastric cardia and noncardia gastric adenocarcinomas associated with *Helicobacter pylori* seropositivity [see comment]. *J Natl Cancer Inst.* 2006;98(20):1445–1452.
12. Gonzalez CA, Jakszyn P, Pera G, et al. Meat intake and risk of stomach and esophageal adenocarcinoma within the European Prospective Investigation into Cancer and Nutrition (EPIC). *J Natl Cancer Inst.* 2006;98(5):345–354.
13. Terry P, Lagergren J, Ye W, et al. Inverse association between intake of cereal fiber and risk of gastric cardia cancer [see comment]. *Gastroenterology.* 2001;120(2):387–391.
14. Moller M, Dahl R, Bockman O. A possible role of the dietary fibre product, wheat bran, as a nitrite scavenger. *Food Chem Toxicol.* 1988;26:841–845.
15. Iannettoni MD, Lee SS, Bonnell MR, et al. Detection of Barrett's adenocarcinoma of the gastric cardia with sucrase isomaltase and p53. *Ann Thorac Surg.* 1996;62(5):1460–1465; discussion 5–6.
16. Petty EM, Kalikin LM, Orringer MB, et al. Distal chromosome 17q loss in Barrett's esophageal and gastric cardia adenocarcinomas: implications for tumorigenesis. *Mol Carcinog.* 1998;22(4):222–228.
17. Yanagi M, Keller G, Mueller J, et al. Comparison of loss of heterozygosity and microsatellite instability in adenocarcinomas of the distal esophagus and proximal stomach. *Virchows Arch.* 2000;437(6):605–610.
18. Mattioli S, Ruffato A, Di Simone MP, et al. Immunopathological patterns of the stomach in adenocarcinoma of the esophagus, cardia, and gastric antrum: gastric profiles in Siewert type I and II tumors. *Ann Thorac Surg.* 2007;83(5):1814–1819.
19. Dolan K, Sutton R, Walker SJ, et al. New classification of oesophageal and gastric carcinomas derived from changing patterns in epidemiology. *Br J Cancer.* 1999;80(5–6):834–842.
20. Nigro JJ, DeMeester SR, Hagen JA, et al. Node status in transmural esophageal adenocarcinoma and outcome after en bloc esophagectomy. *J Thorac Cardiovasc Surg.* 1999;117(5):960–968.
21. Wijnhoven BP, Siersema PD, Hop WC, et al. Adenocarcinomas of the distal oesophagus and gastric cardia are one clinical entity. Rotterdam Oesophageal Tumour Study Group [see comment]. *Br J Surg.* 1999;86(4):529–535.
22. Skinner DB, Dowlatshahi KD, DeMeester TR. Potentially curable cancer of the esophagus. *Cancer.* 1982;50(suppl 11):2571–2575.
23. Skinner DB. En bloc resection for neoplasms of the esophagus and cardia. *J Thorac Cardiovasc Surg.* 1983;85(1):59–71.
24. Ellis FH Jr, Watkins E Jr, Krasna MJ, et al. Staging of carcinoma of the esophagus and cardia: a comparison of different staging criteria. *J Surg Oncol.* 1993;52(4):231–235.
25. Ellis FH Jr, Heatley GJ, Balogh K. Proposal for improved staging criteria for carcinoma of the esophagus and cardia. *Eur J Cardiothorac Surg.* 1997;12(3):361–364; discussion 4–5.
26. Hagen JA, DeMeester SR, Peters JH, et al. Curative resection for esophageal adenocarcinoma: analysis of 100 en bloc esophagectomies. *Ann Surg.* 2001;234(4):520–530; discussion 30–31.
27. Roder JD, Busch R, Stein HJ, et al. Ratio of invaded to removed lymph nodes as a predictor of survival in squamous cell carcinoma of the oesophagus. *Br J Surg.* 1994;81(3):410–413.
28. Zafirellis K, Dolan K, Fountoulakis A, et al. Multivariate analysis of clinical, operative and pathologic features of esophageal cancer: who needs adjuvant therapy? [erratum appears in *Dis Esophagus.* 2002;15(4):345. Note: Fountolakis A (corrected to Fountoulakis A)]. *Dis Esophagus.* 2002;15(2):155–159.
29. Tachibana M, Dhar DK, Kinugasa S, et al. Esophageal cancer patients surviving 6 years after esophagectomy. *Langenbecks Arch Surg.* 2002;387(2):77–83.
30. Kunisaki C, Akiyama H, Nomura M, et al. Developing an appropriate staging system for esophageal carcinoma [see comment]. *J Am Coll Surg.* 2005;201(6):884–890.
31. Holscher AH, Bollschweiler E, Bumm R, et al. Prognostic factors of resected adenocarcinoma of the esophagus. *Surgery.* 1995;118(5):845–855.
32. van Sandick JW, van Lanschot JJB, ten Kate FJW, et al. Indicators of prognosis after transhiatal esophageal resection without thoracotomy for cancer. *J Am Coll Surg.* 2002;194(1):28–36.
33. Yildirim E, Berberoglu U. Lymph node ratio is more valuable than level III involvement for prediction of outcome in node-positive breast carcinoma patients. *World J Surg.* 2007;31(2):276–289.
34. Schumacher P, Dineen S, Barnett C Jr, et al. The metastatic lymph node ratio predicts survival in colon cancer. *Am J Surg.* 2007;194(6):827–831; discussion 31–32.
35. Pawlik TM, Gleisner AL, Cameron JL, et al. Prognostic relevance of lymph node ratio following pancreaticoduodenectomy for pancreatic cancer. *Surgery.* 2007;141(5):610–618.
36. Chan JK, Kapp DS, Cheung MK, et al. The impact of the absolute number and ratio of positive lymph nodes on survival of endometrioid uterine cancer patients. *Br J Cancer.* 2007;97(5):605–611.
37. Celen O, Yildirim E, Berberoglu U. Prognostic impact of positive lymph node ratio in gastric carcinoma. *J Surg Oncol.* 2007;96(2):95–101.
38. Waterman TA, Hagen JA, Peters JH, et al. The prognostic importance of immunohistochemically detected node metastases in resected esophageal adenocarcinoma. *Ann Thorac Surg.* 2004;78(4):1161–1169; discussion 1169.
39. Steup WH, De Leyn P, Deneffe G, et al. Tumors of the esophagogastric junction: long-term survival in relation to the pattern of lymph node metastasis and a critical analysis of the accuracy or inaccuracy of pTNM classification. *J Thorac Cardiovasc Surg.* 1996;111(1):85–94; discussion 94–95.
40. Korst RJ, Rusch VW, Venkatraman E, et al. Proposed revision of the staging classification for esophageal cancer. *J Thorac Cardiovasc Surg.* 1998;115(3):660–669; discussion 9–70.
41. Hofstetter W, Correa AM, Bekele N, et al. Proposed modification of nodal status in AJCC esophageal cancer staging system. *Ann Thorac Surg.* 2007;84(2):365–373; discussion 74–75.
42. Wijnhoven BPL, Tran KTC, Esterman A, et al. An evaluation of prognostic factors and tumor staging of resected carcinoma of the esophagus. *Ann Surg.* 2007;245(5):717–725.
43. Rizk N, Venkatraman E, Park B, et al. The prognostic importance of the number of involved lymph nodes in esophageal cancer: implications for revisions of the American Joint Committee on Cancer staging system. *J Thorac Cardiovasc Surg.* 2006;132(6):1374–1381.
44. Lagarde SM, ten Kate FJW, de Boer DJ, et al. Extracapsular lymph node involvement in node-positive patients with adenocarcinoma of the distal esophagus or gastroesophageal junction. *Am J Surg Pathol.* 2006;30(2):171–176.
45. Lerut T, Coosemans W, Decker G, et al. Extracapsular lymph node involvement is a negative prognostic factor in T3 adenocarcinoma of the distal esophagus and gastroesophageal junction [see comment]. *J Thorac Cardiovasc Surg.* 2003;126(4):1121–1128.
46. Chirieac LR, Swisher SG, Ajani JA, et al. Posttherapy pathologic stage predicts survival in patients with esophageal carcinoma receiving preoperative chemoradiation. *Cancer.* 2005;103(7):1347–1355.
47. Swisher SG, Hofstetter W, Wu TT, et al. Proposed revision of the esophageal cancer staging system to accommodate pathologic response (pP) following preoperative chemoradiation (CRT). *Ann Surg.* 2005;241(5):810–817; discussion 7–20.
48. Rizk NP, Venkatraman E, Bains MS, et al. American Joint Committee on Cancer staging system does not accurately predict survival in patients receiving multimodality therapy for esophageal adenocarcinoma [see comment]. *J Clin Oncol.* 2007;25(5):507–512.

III

PRINCIPLES OF THERAPY

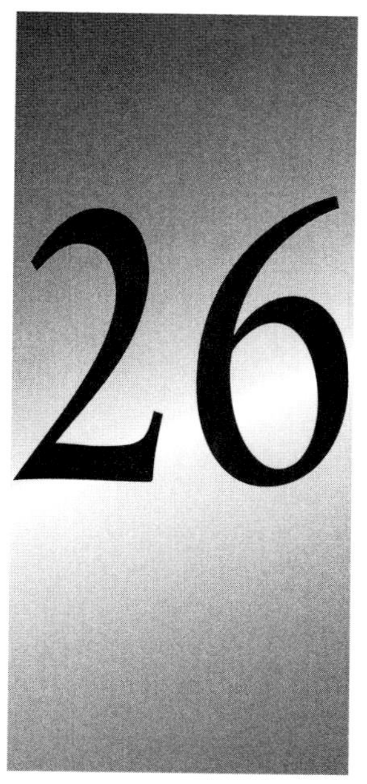

26 Rationale for Tailored Treatment

Georg Lurje
Heinz-Josef Lenz

Cancers arising from the esophagus are relatively uncommon in the United States. In 2007, an estimate of 13,900 new cases will be diagnosed, and more than 90% will die of their disease (1). Esophageal cancer is currently the most rapidly increasing cancer in the Western world and is coinciding with a shift in histologic type and primary tumor location (2–5). Despite recent improvements in the detection, surgical resection, and (radio-)chemotherapy, the overall survival (OS) of esophageal cancer remains poor. It is becoming increasingly apparent that neoadjuvant chemoradiation followed by surgery may be beneficial in terms of increasing resectability and overall survival compared to surgery alone. However, selection of the most beneficial treatment strategy in esophageal cancer remains a challenge and is hindered by the lack of predictive and prognostic markers. The introduction of "targeted therapies" that aim to inhibit specific molecular signal transduction pathways will increase our treatment options in esophageal cancer. Even though the development of biologic agents for esophageal carcinoma is still in its infancy, encouraging results have been reported with antibodies directed at the epidermal growth factor receptor (EGFR) and vascular endothelial growth factor (VEGF) ligand. A multimodal approach, including surgery, chemoradiotherapy, and "targeted agents" alone or in combination, will be necessary to improve the outlook for patients with this disease. The development of molecular markers as an adjunct to traditional staging systems will be critical in selecting more efficient treatment strategies with the means of tailoring a targeted and effective therapy to the molecular profile of both the patient and the tumor while minimizing and avoiding life-threatening toxicities.

Esophageal adenocarcinoma (EA) is now more prevalent than squamous cell carcinoma (SCC), and most tumors are located in the distal esophagus (2–5). While risk factors for SCC of the esophagus have been identified (e.g., tobacco, alcohol, diet), the risk factors associated with EA are less clear. The presence of Barrett's esophagus (BE) is associated with an increased risk of developing EA, and gastroesophageal reflux disease (GERD) is considered the predominant cause of Barrett's metaplasia (6–9).

Despite recent improvements in the detection (10–12), surgical resection (13–15), and neo-adjuvant radiochemotherapy (16,17), OS of esophageal cancer remains lower than other solid tumors. Further, esophageal cancer is regarded as a treatable but rarely curable disease with an estimated 5-year OS of 5% to 30% (1,18). At the time of diagnosis, 2 of 3 patients will have tumors that are considered inoperable because of comorbidities or tumor extension. Traditionally, surgical resection has offered the best hope for prolonged survival, even though surgical resection will only cure 15% to 20% of patients with seemingly localized esophageal cancer (18). Until recently, there was concern that the morbidity and mortality associated with primary resection of an esophageal carcinoma could outweigh the likelihood of a long-term benefit. This concern has been addressed through the development of improved surgical techniques and better postoperative care (13–15).

Despite these recent advancements, selection of the most beneficial treatment strategy in esophageal cancer remains a challenge and is hindered by the lack of predictive and prognostic markers. A multidisciplinary approach, including surgery, radiotherapy, and chemotherapy, alone or in combination, will be necessary to improve the outlook for patients with this disease. In addition, the high incidence of tumor drug resistance remains a major stumbling block for effective cancer treatment. In recent years, research efforts on a global scale have attempted to identify subsets of molecular markers that can predict both response to neoadjuvant treatment and prognostic markers to assess the aggressiveness of the disease and the likelihood of recurrence after surgery. The science of pharmacogenomics is emerging as a useful molecular tool to investigate the disparity in drug efficacy by simultaneous analysis of variables in the patient and the disease, such as genetic polymorphisms in drug targets, metabolizing enzymes, transporters, and influential receptors (19). Accordingly, the development of validated predictive and prognostic markers not only may be helpful in identifying patients who are at high risk but also will be critical in selecting more efficient treatment strategies with the means of a targeted and effective therapy to the molecular profile of both the patient and the disease while minimizing and avoiding life-threatening toxicities.

BIOLOGY OF ESOPHAGEAL CANCER

More than 90% of esophageal cancers occur in 2 major histologic forms: SCC and EA. SCC occurs in more than 80% of cases in chronic tobacco smokers and is further potentiated by heavy alcohol consumption (20). Other known risk factors for SCC include Plummer-Vinson syndrome, scleroderma, achalasia, and nutritional factors, such as the presence of nitrosamines in the food or vitamin deficiency (21,22). In contrast to SCC, the most important risk factor for the development of EA is the presence of columnar-lined esophagus, also known as BE. It is estimated that up to 90% of all EA arise from BE, and the presence of BE is associated with an increased risk of EA by a factor of 30 to 125. Although the development of BE represents an acquired pathologic response to duodenogastroesophageal reflux, hereditary and genetic changes may contribute to the carcinogenesis because the majority of patients with GERD do not develop BE (23). Approximately 70% of all EA are found in the distal esophagus, whereas SCC are more commonly located within the middle and upper third (24,25).

Despite ongoing efforts to characterize the molecular and morphologic changes of esophageal carcinoma, its pathogenesis remains poorly understood. SCC and EA may share some biologic features; however, it is being increasingly recognized that SCC and EA are separate and distinct disease groups in terms of molecular biology, comorbidities, and treatment and therefore need to be considered individually (26,27). EA development is regarded as a multistep process that starts with the mucosal injury of the squamous epithelium of the distal esophagus by GERD and progresses through intestinal metaplasia and dysplasia to invasive adenocarcinoma (28). Numerous molecular events associated with this metaplasia-dysplasia-adenocarcinoma sequence have recently been identified (7,8). In vivo studies suggest that oxidative damage from factors such as smoking or GERD, which cause inflammation and consecutive esophagitis with increased cell turnover, may initiate a carcinogenic process that ultimately leads to EA. In this regard, Lagergren et al. reported that symptomatic GERD is a major risk factor for EA and that the frequency, severity, and duration of reflux symptoms are strongly associated with malignant transformation of the esophageal mucosa (9). Prior to macroscopic or even microscopic evidence of inflammatory damage, there are molecular changes occurring within the mucosal cells. These molecular changes result in alterations in the expression of genes that affect cellular integrity, proliferation, and migration. Recently, acid reflux disease has been shown to alter gene expression of inflammatory and carcinogenic genes in the esophageal mucosa (8,29). In fact, overexpression of interleukin-8 (IL-8) and cyclooxygenase-2 (COX-2) was recently reported to represent one of the earliest changes associated with GERD and esophageal cancer development (8,29–31). In vivo studies about severe reflux in rodents reported that inhibition of COX-2 with selective inhibitors resulted in a reduced rate of intestinal metaplasia and cancer development (32,33). Chemoprevention strategies might therefore be applied earlier in the neoplastic process, since the use of selective COX-2 inhibitors may prevent progression of disease at an early stage (34–36). In addition to their potential as chemoprevention, several phase II trials have recently been reported with combinations of COX-2 inhibitors and concurrent chemoradiotherapy for locally advanced esophageal cancer. Even though preliminary, reports from these studies revealed encouraging complete pathologic response rates of 44% with no increased risk for thrombembolic events (37).

The potential influence of histology and molecular biology has been largely ignored in clinical trials of treatment for esophageal cancer, mainly because histology influences neither the surgical technique nor the prognosis after radical surgery alone. With the use of nonsurgical approaches, histology and molecular biology could have a more important influence on outcome. The molecular biology of a SCC induced by alcohol and tobacco is likely to be very different from that of an adenocarcinoma arising from BE. Furthermore, differences in molecular biology may have implications for response rates after chemotherapy, radiotherapy, or chemoradiation. A better selection of patients, based on the unique molecular profile of both the patient and the tumor, will be critical in selecting more efficient treatment strategies with the means of tailoring a targeted and individualized treatment approach.

MANAGEMENT OF ADVANCED ESOPHAGEAL CANCER

More than 50% of patients present with metastatic or unresectable esophageal cancer. Even though chemotherapy is considered palliative, both SCC and EA of the esophagus are responsive to chemotherapy. However, clinical and radiographic responses typically last no longer than 4 months, and survival is short, rarely exceeding 1 year (18,38).

Although a survival benefit has yet to be proven with chemotherapy in advanced esophageal cancer, chemotherapy is considered to improve quality of life and dysphagia in 60% to 80% of patients (39–42). Shrinkage of the tumor typically occurs in 15% to 30% of patients who are treated with single-agent 5-FU, taxanes (Paclitaxel or Docetaxel), or irinotecan. Thus, combination regimens, containing cisplatin, tend to produce higher response rates (30%–57%) (39–41,43–46), and the median survival time remains less than 10 months. Therefore, the therapeutic benefit of more intense combination therapies should be balanced against its greater potential for toxic side effects.

Recently, advances in molecular pharmacology have refined the understanding of the mechanisms of action of drugs and resistance to chemotherapy. Several mechanisms of resistance have been identified among the most commonly used agents in the treatment of patients with esophageal cancer (5-FU, cisplatin). Numerous studies have shown that an increased gene expression of thymidylate synthase (TS) and excision cross-complementing gene 1 (ERCC1) is associated with a decrease in survival and increase of chemoresistance to neoadjuvant chemoradiotherapy (47–49). However, further validation in biomarker-embedded and prospective clinical trials is needed.

The development of molecular markers of prognosis and novel targeted therapies will enable oncologists to tailor patient specific chemotherapy regimens by maximizing drug efficacy and minimizing adverse and possibly severe side effects.

MANAGEMENT OF LOCALLY ADVANCED ESOPHAGEAL CANCER

Surgery

Surgical resection is the standard treatment option for esophageal cancer, usually undertaken either by a right transthoracic or a transhiatal approach. Transthoracic resection involves a laparotomy and right-sided thoracotomy, leading to an esophagogastric anastomosis either in the upper chest (Lewis-Santy) or in the neck. Although this approach allows en bloc resection of the tumor and lymph nodes under sight, this approach increases the risk of cardiopulmonary complications (18,50). The transhiatal approach uses a laparotomy with blunt dissection of the thoracic esophagus and cervical anastomosis, a procedure that carries a higher risk for fistula formation and vocal cord paralysis (50).

Because locoregional recurrence after esophagectomy typically results in rapid death from cancer, local control remains one of the primary goals of therapy for this disease. Although the optimum procedure for esophageal cancer is still a subject of ongoing debate, transthoracic en bloc esophagectomy with gastroplasty and 2-field lymphadenectomy is currently considered the procedure of choice worldwide for patients with resectable middle to lower third esophageal carcinoma (16,50). Poor survival with surgery alone in patients with large tumors and advanced localized disease (stages IIB–III) prompted investigation into the use of neoadjuvant chemotherapy or chemoradiotherapy in addition to surgical resection. Neoadjuvant and adjuvant chemotherapy and radiation are intended to eliminate residual micrometastatic disease, decrease cancer-cell dissemination during surgical intervention, and finally improve OS.

Neoadjuvant Chemotherapy Followed by Surgical Resection

The rationale for neoadjuvant treatment of esophageal cancer is similar to that for many other tumors. Even though only 20% to 30% of tumors will show complete pathologic response, resection of responsive tumors may be accomplished with less morbidity and sacrifice of adjacent organs. Some tumors that are deemed unresectable may become resectable. In addition, manipulation of smaller, treated tumors may result in less intraoperative dislodgement of viable tumor cells, and early treatment of distant micrometastatic disease may improve oncologic outcome. Furthermore, progression, particularly distant progression, of patients on neoadjuvant treatment may indicate the futility of surgery in these patients.

Neoadjuvant chemotherapy, based on 5-fluorouracil (5-FU) and cisplatin, was compared with surgery alone in esophageal cancer in multiple randomized clinical trials (51–54). Only 1 trial, the UK Medical Research Council (MRC-OE02) trial from England (51), showed better OS in the chemotherapy group compared with the surgery-alone group. However, several details of the MRC-OE02 trial are worth reviewing. Preoperative computed tomography assessment to detect tumor extension and specific surgical techniques along with quality control of the surgery were not imposed, as an outstanding 17% of patients left the operating room with no surgical resection of the tumor. Furthermore, a most recent meta-analysis by Malthaner et al. showed that preoperative chemotherapy plus surgery did not offer a survival advantage over surgery alone for resectable thoracic esophageal cancer (55). However, the Medical Research Council Adjuvant Gastric Infusional Chemotherapy trial has recently shown that perioperative chemotherapy—chemotherapy given both before and after surgery—can also provide a significant survival benefit. The investigators suggested that a perioperative chemotherapy regimen would have advantages over postoperative chemotherapy alone, including increasing the likelihood of curative resection by downstaging the tumor, eliminating micrometastases, rapidly improving tumor-related symptoms, and determining whether the tumor is sensitive to chemotherapy (56). Another recent intergroup trial (RTOG trial 8911), conducted by Kelson and colleagues led to similar conclusions (54). The authors demonstrated that disease-free survival and OS strongly depend on performance of a complete resection, including negative microscopic margins, and that the presence of residual disease is a strong predictor of poor outcome. While preoperative chemotherapy decreased the incidence of R1 resections, the authors report that OS was not improved in the preoperative chemotherapy arm compared to the surgery alone (54). However, patients with complete pathologic response to neoadjuvant chemotherapy were reported to have a significant survival benefit, which is in accordance to previous reports (57).

Since only patients with a complete pathologic response to neoadjuvant therapy will have a significant survival benefit, the identification of validated predictive markers is critical in successfully selecting patients who will benefit from this therapy.

Neoadjuvant Radiotherapy Followed by Surgical Resection

Five randomized clinical trials investigating neoadjuvant radiotherapy followed by surgery compared to surgery alone have been reported (58–62). Only 1 study reported a 3-year survival advantage in patients receiving neoadjuvant radiotherapy (62). However, a recent meta-analysis of 5 randomized clinical trials analyzing data from 1,147 patients did not show any significant survival benefit for patients receiving neoadjuvant radiotherapy (63). Therefore, preoperative radiotherapy does not have a role in the treatment of resectable esophageal cancer.

Neoadjuvant Chemoradiotherapy Followed by Surgical Resection

There are 3 major advantages of neoadjuvant chemoradiation. First, chemotherapy could reach (micro-)metastases outside the radiation field; second, preoperative chemoradiation could decrease the rate of locoregional recurrences; and, third, local efficacy of radiotherapy could be enhanced by a radiosensitization effect, as described for the 3 most commonly used chemotherapeutic drugs: cisplatin, 5-FU, and mitomycin (50,64).

To date, 8 randomized phase III clinical trials (62,65–71) have been reported, and out of these, only 1 single institution clinical trial, conducted by Walsh et al., showed a significant survival benefit from neoadjuvant chemoradiation therapy compared to surgery alone (67). Because only 2 trials included a large enough number of patients to achieve adequate statistical power, the Cancer and Leukemia Group B (CALGB) attempted to complete a large definitive trial (CALGB 9781) of cisplatin, 5-FU, and radiation followed by surgery versus surgery alone. However, only a total of 56 patients were entered on the study when the trial was closed because of poor patient accrual (72). Preliminary data presented at the 42nd annual meeting of the American Society of Clinical Oncology reported a long-term survival benefit with the use of neoadjuvant chemoradiation followed by surgery in the treatment of esophageal cancer (72). However, publication of these results is awaited because only 56 of the expected 500 patients have been included and information on tumor stage is not available. Two recent meta-analyses of the previously mentioned clinical trials have been published, and both concluded that preoperative chemoradiation followed by surgery is superior compared to surgery alone (73,74). The most recent meta-analysis by Gebski et al. analyzed 8 randomized clinical trials consisting of 1,724 patients and compared neoadjuvant chemotherapy followed by surgery with surgery alone (74). The authors concluded that trimodality treatment with neoadjuvant chemoradiation followed by surgery is beneficial for patients with early and locally advanced esophageal carcinoma (74).

A review of the trials allows several comparisons to be made and a few conclusions to be reached. First, it has been well established that only patients with a complete pathologic response to neoadjuvant therapy will have a significant survival benefit (57,75). Further, neoadjuvant chemoradiation is suitable for local disease control, since preoperative chemoradiation was reported to increase complete surgical resection as a result of treatment-dependent downstaging. In addition, a review of the literature does not show a significant postoperative increase in morbidity and mortality associated with neoadjuvant chemoradiotherapy. Moreover, the results of the previously mentioned clinical trials highlight the imminent need for predictive markers of response to neoadjuvant chemotherapy. Recently, molecular markers like ERCC1 and TS have been identified as highly specific to predict minor response to neoadjuvant chemotherapy regimens (49,76). However, these reports are preliminary, and further validation in biomarker-embedded and prospective clinical trials is warranted.

To conclude, there is strong evidence that neoadjuvant chemoradiation followed by surgery may be beneficial in terms of increasing respectability and OS compared to surgery alone. However, the results are not yet conclusive, and since only patients with a complete pathologic response were shown to have a clear survival benefit of neoadjuvant chemoradiotherapy, the development of validated predictive markers as an adjunct to traditional staging systems will be critical in selecting more efficient treatment strategies with the means of tailoring a targeted and effective therapy to the molecular profile of both the patient and the tumor while minimizing and avoiding life-threatening toxicities.

Positron-Emission Tomography–Guided Induction Chemotherapy

Recently, neoadjuvant treatment followed by surgery has become an accepted choice for locally advanced esophageal carcinomas (51,66,73,74). However, there is an ongoing debate as to which subgroup of patients should be offered neoadjuvant treatment (77–79). It is becoming increasingly apparent that only patients with a complete pathologic response to neoadjuvant therapy will have a significant survival benefit (80). From the surgical point of view, chemotherapy should therefore not be administered to nonresponding patients since it may cause fatal delay of a potentially curative surgery (17,77). In addition, the safety of surgery of neoadjuvant chemoradiotherapy has been repeatedly called into question, even though most trials did not show a significant postoperative increase in morbidity and mortality associated with neoadjuvant chemoradiotherapy (74). Although histopathologic response remains the most important prognosticator, identifying patients with chemosensitive disease before completion of neoadjuvant treatment has not been possible yet. Therefore, there is an urgent need for prospectively validated and reliable predictive markers to allow tailored (radio-) chemotherapy to increase the number of complete pathologic responses following neoadjuvant approaches.

18-Fluorodeoxyglucose-positron emission tomography ([^{18}F] FDG-PET) has been become generally available within the past decade. The assessment of FDG-PET-guided glucolytic activity of the tumor has provided further high-resolution imaging by evaluating the locoregional and distant extent of the disease. More recently, glucose uptake by use of FDG-PET has yielded reproducible results that are useful not only for predicting early clinical and histopathologic response to induction chemotherapy but also and more importantly for predicting improvements in survival after esophagectomy (11,12,17,81–83). Most recently, Lordick et al. presented the first clinical trial that prospectively incorporated response measured by PET ("metabolic response") into a treatment algorithm for the management of distal EA (Siewert I) and carcinomas of the gastric cardia (Siewert II) (12). The investigators could show that PET-guided induction chemotherapy and assessment of early "metabolic response" is feasible and might unmask tumors with an unfavorable biology and poor clinical prognosis. In addition, early discontinuation of induction chemotherapy for patients who were "nonmetabolic responders" did not show adverse effect in terms of overall clinical outcome (12). However, randomized and multicenter phase III clinical trials are warranted before implementing FDG-PET-guided induction chemotherapy into routine clinical practice.

MOLECULAR MARKERS AND BIOLOGIC AGENTS: DEFINING THEIR ROLE

Improvements in surgical resection, postoperative care, and chemoradiotherapy have had a modest impact on the morbidity and mortality associated with esophageal cancer. The introduction of novel biologic agents that target receptor-mediated tumor processes have shown promise to provide meaningful clinical benefit in patients with colorectal and lung cancer (84–90). However, our knowledge of the precise mechanisms of action, resistance, and optimal scheduling and administration of these agents is still in its infancy. A greater understanding of these issues will assist in identifying the population of patients who will benefit from these agents. This will not only ensure efficacy and increase histopathologic response rates but also justify the additional financial burden incurred in a therapeutic strategy that incorporates a biologic agent and will represent a major advancement in individualized esophageal cancer treatment.

Over the past decade, a number of novel targets have been identified as potential predictive and prognostic markers. These include growth-factor receptors (91–95), enzymes of angiogenesis (96–101), tumor suppressor genes (102–107), cell cycle regulators (105,107–109), and enzymes involved in the DNA repair system (47,49,110) and in the degradation of extracellular matrix (111–113). The results of these mainly retrospective studies are promising, but prospective and biomarker-embedded clinical trials are needed to confirm and validate their predictive and prognostic value. Clinical trials are in various stages of development incorporating these new agents (monoclonal antibodies, tyrosine kinase inhibitors, COX-2 inhibitors), but to date the available clinical data have been limited.

Targeting the Epidermal Growth Factor Receptor

One of the most promising targets is the Epidermal Growth Factor Receptor (EGFR), a member of the type I receptor tyrosine kinase family. EGFR is overex pressed in a variety of malignancies, including up to 92% of esophageal cancers, and is associated with tumor progression and poor prognosis (48,92,94,114,115). Activation of the epidermal growth factor (EGF)/EGFR axis triggers multiple signaling pathways that result in endothelial cell proliferation, apoptosis, angiogenesis, and metastasis (116). Conversely, inhibition of the EGFR pathways with anti-EGFR monoclonal antibodies was reported to block cell cycle progression and induce apoptosis in numerous in vitro and xenograft models (20,117,118). Multiple phase II/III clinical trials demonstrated that cetuximab has promising efficacy in patients with metastatic colon cancer (mCRC) and locally advanced head and neck cancers (85,87,119).

Given these encouraging results from the colorectal and head and neck cancer trials, research on a global scale is evaluating the efficacy of monoclonal antibody inhibition of EGFR in esophageal cancer patients. In a recent retrospective analysis, Wilkinson et al. demonstrated that poorly differentiated adenocarcinomas of the esophagus demonstrated higher EGFR expression compared to low-grade tumors based on immunohistochemical (IHC) analysis (120). In addition, Kitagawa and colleagues showed that the cumulative survival rate for patients with EGFR gene amplification in the primary tumors was significantly lower than that for patients without amplification ($P < 0.001$). A significant correlation was observed between extensive lymph node involvement at the time of surgery and EGFR gene amplification ($P < 0.05$) (121).

Cetuximab (Erbitux®™, C255, Bristol-Myers Squib, Princeton, NJ) is a chimeric IgG1 anti-EGFR monoclonal antibody that binds to the extracellular domain of the EGFR and prevents ligand binding and activation of downstream events, such as endothelial cell proliferation, apoptosis, angiogenesis, and metastasis (116). Several phase I/II clinical trials are ongoing, and the results of these are awaited. SWOG 0414 (Southwestern Oncology Group) is an ongoing prospective phase II clinical trial that has already completed patient accrual and is seeking to evaluate clinical outcome in patients with surgically or medically unresectable locally advanced esophageal cancer (T4M0) (122). All patients received chemoradiotherapy (cisplatin, CPT-11) with the addition of cetuximab. Other trials include SWOG 0415, which is evaluating the efficacy of cetuximab as a second-line therapy in patients with metastatic esophageal adenocarcinoma (123). The Memorial-Sloan Kettering Cancer Center is exploring cetuximab in irinotecan/cisplatin-refractory patients with metastatic disease (124). Recently, the Dana-Farber Cancer Institute reported preliminary data at the 42nd annual meeting of the American Society of Clinical Oncology for the combination of cetuximab with irinotecan/cisplatin and radiation as preoperative therapy in esophageal cancer (125). Even though preliminary, the authors report a lower pathologic complete response rate and higher overall toxicity than anticipated. At the same meeting, Suntharalingam et al. presented preliminary but promising results of a phase II study of cetuximab with chemoradiation for patients with esophagogastric carcinomas (126). Thus far, 30 patients have completed treatment and were evaluable for clinical and pathologic complete response. Eighteen of 27 patients (67%) have had clinical complete response. Seven patients out of 16 (43%) who have gone to surgery have had a pathologic complete response. The authors concluded that cetuximab can be safely administered with chemoradiation for patients with esophageal cancer. However, patient accrual is ongoing, and final results are awaited.

Until now, there have been only a few clinical and potential molecular markers that can identify patients who will most likely benefit from this therapy. Multiple groups in Europe and the United States are investigating why some patients show response to EGFR-targeted treatment and others show progressive disease. Recently, our group tested mRNA gene expression levels and germ-line polymorphisms within the EGF/EGFR signaling pathway in patients with mCRC treated with single agent cetuximab (ImClone 0144) (86). Intratumoral overexpression of VEGF was associated with resistance to cetuximab, whereas low expression levels of COX-2, EGFR, and IL-8 were significantly associated with improved OS (127). In addition, numerous studies reported that k-ras mutations were shown to have a major predictive impact on efficacy of EGFR targeted treatment regimens. In fact, mCRC patients with wild-type k-ras showed a higher disease control rate (48%) on cetuximab treatment than patients with k-ras mutations (10%) (128,129). However, the value of k-ras mutational analysis in esophageal carcinoma has yet to be determined.

Even though preclinical and early phase I/II studies are promising, further randomized and biomarker-embedded clinical trials are warranted before introducing k-ras mutational analysis and other predictive markers into routine clinical practice.

Targeting the HER-2/neu Receptor

The HER-2/neu gene (cERBB2) is part of a 4-member family of ErbB receptors and belongs to the type 1 receptor tyrosine kinase family (130). The ErbB receptors consist of 4 transmembrane glycoproteins (ErbB1-ErbB4), and ErbB2 is the preferred dimerization partner of Trastuzumab (Herceptin®™; Genentech, Inc., San Francisco, CA), a fully humanized anti-185 HER2 monoclonal antibody. Amplification of the HER-2/neu antigen has been identified in up to 30% of invasive breast cancer patients and increases the aggressiveness of the tumor (131). Cobleigh et al. reported a response rate of 15% in patients with metastatic and HER-2/neu-overexpressing breast cancer treated with trastuzumab (132). Consequently, trastuzumab was approved by the Food and Drug Administration for the treatment of HER-2/neu-overexpressing and metastatic breast cancer (133).

Small series have suggested that HER-2/neu amplification as determined by IHC or fluorescence in situ hybridization is similar in esophageal carcinomas to that of breast cancer (134,135). In addition, Ross et al. reported that HER-2/neu overexpression is associated with tumor progression and poor response to neoadjuvant chemotherapy (136). HER-2/neu is therefore a potential target in esophageal cancers, particularly as part of a multimodality treatment regimen. In a recent phase I/II trial of weekly trastuzumab, paclitaxel, cisplatin, and radiation in patients with locally advanced adenocarcinoma of the esophagus, Safran et al. could show that HER-2/neu was overexpressed in 12 out of 36 (33%) patients with locally advanced EA. Further, the investigators concluded that trastuzumab can be safely incorporated into concurrent chemoradiotherapy regimens without increasing side effects such as cardiotoxicity and esophagitis (135). Nevertheless, further investigation of trastuzumab in HER-2-overexpressing esophageal cancer is warranted.

Targeting VEGF

VEGF is one of the most important activators of tumor associated angiogenesis (137). Activation of the VEGF/VEGF-receptor axis triggers multiple signaling pathways that result in endothelial cell survival, mitogenesis, migration, differentiation, vascular permeability, and mobilization of endothelial progenitor cells (138). Overexpression of VEGF mRNA and protein has been associated with tumor progression and poor prognosis in a variety of malignancies, including esophageal carcinoma (98,139–144).

Bevacizumab (Avastin©™, Genentech, Inc.) is a humanized monoclonal antibody to VEGF that binds to all isoforms with high affinity and prevents the binding of VEGF to its receptor. Numerous clinical trials with bevacizumab in solid tumors are ongoing or completed, and activity has so far been shown against colon, renal cell, non–small cell lung, ovarian, and breast cancer (145–148). For esophageal cancer, bevacizumab is in the early stages of development. Nevertheless, early reports from a multicenter phase II clinical trial are encouraging. In fact, Shah et al. reported preliminary results showing that the addition of bevacizumab to CPT-11 and cisplatin appears to be active (87% partial response or stable disease) in metastatic adenocarcinoma of the esophagus (149). However, the trial was stopped because of increased incidences of thrombembolic events and associated bowel perforations.

CONCLUSION

It is becoming increasingly apparent that neoadjuvant chemoradiation followed by surgery may be beneficial in terms of increasing resectability and OS compared to surgery alone. Selection of the most beneficial treatment strategy in esophageal cancer remains a challenge and is hindered by the lack of predictive and prognostic markers. The goal is to identify predictive markers to increase complete pathologic response rates in patients treated with neoadjuvant chemoradiotherapy and to identify prognostic markers to possibly select patients for adjuvant chemotherapy who are at high risk for tumor recurrence. In fact, several biomarkers (ERCC1, TS, p53) have been evaluated over the past decades, and it is becoming increasingly apparent that disease progression is driven largely by complex pathways and that analysis of 1 single marker is unlikely to precisely predict progression of disease with sufficient resolution and reproducibility. The introduction of "targeted therapies" that aim to inhibit specific molecular signal transduction pathways will increase our treatment options in esophageal cancer. Even though the development of biologic agents for esophageal carcinoma is still in its infancy, encouraging results have been reported with antibodies directed at the EGFR and VEGF ligand. A multimodal approach, including surgery, chemoradiotherapy, and "targeted agents" alone or in combination, will be necessary to improve the outlook for patients with this disease. The development of validated molecular markers will be critical in selecting more efficient treatment strategies with the means of tailoring a targeted and effective therapy to the molecular profile of both the patient and the tumor while minimizing and avoiding life-threatening toxicities.

References

1. Jemal A, Siegel R, Ward E, et al. Cancer statistics, 2007. *CA Cancer J Clin.* 2007;57:43–66.
2. Bollschweiler E, Wolfgarten E, Gutschow C, et al. Demographic variations in the rising incidence of esophageal adenocarcinoma in white males. *Cancer.* 2001;92:549–555.
3. Pohl H, Welch HG. The role of overdiagnosis and reclassification in the marked increase of esophageal adenocarcinoma incidence. *J Natl Cancer Inst.* 2005;97:142–146.
4. Blot WJ, McLaughlin JK. The changing epidemiology of esophageal cancer. *Semin Oncol.* 1999;26:2–8.
5. Devesa SS, Blot WJ, Fraumeni JF Jr. Changing patterns in the incidence of esophageal and gastric carcinoma in the United States. *Cancer.* 1998;83:2049–2053.
6. Altorki NK, Skinner DB. Adenocarcinoma in Barrett's esophagus. *Semin Surg Oncol.* 1990;6:274–278.
7. Wijnhoven BP, Tilanus HW, Dinjens WN. Molecular biology of Barrett's adenocarcinoma. *Ann Surg.* 2001;233:322–337.
8. Lurje G, Vallbohmer D, Collet PH, et al. COX-2 mRNA expression is significantly increased in acid-exposed compared to nonexposed squamous epithelium in gastroesophageal reflux disease. *J Gastrointest Surg.* 2007;11:1105–1111.
9. Lagergren J, Bergstrom R, Lindgren A, et al. Symptomatic gastroesophageal reflux as a risk factor for esophageal adenocarcinoma. *N Engl J Med.* 1999;340:825–831.
10. Flamen P, Lerut A, Van Cutsem E, et al. Utility of positron emission tomography for the staging of patients with potentially operable esophageal carcinoma. *J Clin Oncol.* 2000;18:3202–3210.
11. Weber WA, Ott K, Becker K, et al. Prediction of response to preoperative chemotherapy in adenocarcinomas of the esophagogastric junction by metabolic imaging. *J Clin Oncol.* 2001;19:3058–3065.
12. Lordick F, Ott K, Krause BJ, et al. PET to assess early metabolic response and to guide treatment of adenocarcinoma of the oesophagogastric junction: the MUNICON phase II trial. *Lancet Oncol.* 2007;8:797–805.
13. Holscher AH, Schneider PM, Gutschow C, et al. Laparoscopic ischemic conditioning of the stomach for esophageal replacement. *Ann Surg.* 2007;245:241–246.
14. Hagen JA, DeMeester SR, Peters JH, et al. Curative resection for esophageal adenocarcinoma: analysis of 100 en bloc esophagectomies. *Ann Surg.* 2001;234:520–530; discussion 530–531.
15. Peyre CG, Demeester SR, Rizzetto C, et al. Vagal-sparing esophagectomy: the ideal operation for intramucosal adenocarcinoma and Barrett with high-grade dysplasia. *Ann Surg.* 2007;246:665–674.
16. Mariette C, Piessen G, Triboulet JP. Therapeutic strategies in oesophageal carcinoma: role of surgery and other modalities. *Lancet Oncol.* 2007;8:545–553.
17. Siewert JR, Lordick F, Ott K, et al. Induction chemotherapy in Barrett cancer: influence on surgical risk and outcome. *Ann Surg.* 2007;246:624–631.
18. Enzinger PC, Mayer RJ. Esophageal cancer. *N Engl J Med.* 2003;349:2241–2252.
19. McLeod HL, Yu J. Cancer pharmacogenomics: SNPs, chips, and the individual patient. *Cancer Invest.* 2003;21:630–640.
20. De Stefani E, Barrios E, Fierro L. Black (air-cured) and blond (flue-cured) tobacco and cancer risk. III: oesophageal cancer. *Eur J Cancer.* 1993;29A:763–766.
21. Wolfgarten E, Rosendahl U, Nowroth T, et al. Coincidence of nutritional habits and esophageal cancer in Germany. *Onkologie.* 2001;24:546–551.
22. Daly JM, Fry WA, Little AG, et al. Esophageal cancer: results of an American College of Surgeons Patient Care Evaluation Study. *J Am Coll Surg.* 2000;190:562–572; discussion 572–573.
23. Clark GW, Smyrk TC, Mirvish SS, et al. Effect of gastroduodenal juice and dietary fat on the development of Barrett's esophagus and esophageal neoplasia: an experimental rat model. *Ann Surg Oncol.* 1994;1:252–261.
24. Pisani P, Parkin DM, Bray F, et al. Estimates of the worldwide mortality from 25 cancers in 1990. *Int J Cancer.* 1999;83:18–29.
25. Siewert JR, Stein HJ, Feith M, et al. Histologic tumor type is an independent prognostic parameter in esophageal cancer: lessons from more than 1,000 consecutive resections at a single center in the Western world. *Ann Surg.* 2001;234:360–367; discussion 368–369.
26. Metzger R, Schneider PM, Warnecke-Eberz U, et al. Molecular biology of esophageal cancer. *Onkologie.* 2004;27:200–206.
27. Montesano R, Hollstein M, Hainaut P. Genetic alterations in esophageal cancer and their relevance to etiology and pathogenesis: a review. *Int J Cancer.* 1996;69:225–235.
28. Peters JH, Hagen JA, DeMeester SR. Barrett's esophagus. *J Gastrointest Surg.* 2004;8:1–17.
29. Oh DS, DeMeester SR, Vallbohmer D, et al. Reduction of interleukin 8 gene expression in reflux esophagitis and Barrett's esophagus with antireflux surgery. *Arch Surg.* 2007;142:554–559; discussion 559–560.
30. Ling FC, Baldus SE, Khochfar J, et al. Association of COX-2 expression with corresponding active and chronic inflammatory reactions in Barrett's metaplasia and progression to cancer. *Histopathology.* 2007;50:203–209.
31. Vallbohmer D, DeMeester SR, Oh DS, et al. Antireflux surgery normalizes cyclooxygenase-2 expression in squamous epithelium of the distal esophagus. *Am J Gastroenterol.* 2006;101:1458–1466.
32. Buttar NS, Wang KK, Leontovich O, et al. Chemoprevention of esophageal adenocarcinoma by COX-2 inhibitors in an animal model of Barrett's esophagus. *Gastroenterology.* 2002;122:1101–1112.
33. Oyama K, Fujimura T, Ninomiya I, et al. A COX-2 inhibitor prevents the esophageal inflammation-metaplasia-adenocarcinoma sequence in rats. *Carcinogenesis.* 2005;26:565–570.
34. Altorki N. COX-2: a target for prevention and treatment of esophageal cancer. *J Surg Res.* 2004;117:114–120.
35. Dannenberg AJ, Altorki NK, Boyle JO, et al. Cyclo-oxygenase 2: a pharmacological target for the prevention of cancer. *Lancet Oncol.* 2001;2:544–551.
36. Taketo MM. Cyclooxygenase-2 inhibitors in tumorigenesis (part I). *J Natl Cancer Inst.* 1998;90:1529–1536.
37. Enzinger P, Mamon H, Choi N, et al. Phase II cisplatin, irinotecan, celecoxib and concurrent radiation therapy followed by surgery for locally advanced esophageal cancer. In: *2004 Gastrointestinal Cancers Symposium.* San Francisco: 2004.
38. Ng T, Dipetrillo T, Purviance J, et al. Multimodality treatment of esophageal cancer: a review of the current status and future directions. *Curr Oncol Rep.* 2006;8:174–182.
39. Ilson DH, Forastiere A, Arquette M, et al. A phase II trial of paclitaxel and cisplatin in patients with advanced carcinoma of the esophagus. *Cancer J.* 2000;6:316–323.
40. Ilson DH, Saltz L, Enzinger P, et al. Phase II trial of weekly irinotecan plus cisplatin in advanced esophageal cancer. *J Clin Oncol.* 1999;17:3270–3275.
41. Petrasch S, Welt A, Reinacher A, et al. Chemotherapy with cisplatin and paclitaxel in patients with locally advanced, recurrent or metastatic oesophageal cancer. *Br J Cancer.* 1998;78:511–514.
42. Homs MY, Van der Gaast A, Siersema PD, et al. Chemotherapy for metastatic carcinoma of the esophagus and gastro-esophageal junction. *Cochrane Database Syst Rev.* 2006:CD004063.
43. Bleiberg H, Conroy T, Paillot B, et al. Randomised phase II study of cisplatin and 5-fluorouracil (5-FU) versus cisplatin alone in advanced squamous cell oesophageal cancer. *Eur J Cancer.* 1997;33:1216–1220.
44. Conroy T, Etienne PL, Adenis A, et al. Vinorelbine and cisplatin in metastatic squamous cell carcinoma of the oesophagus: response, toxicity, quality of life and survival. *Ann Oncol.* 2002;13:721–729.
45. Ilson DH, Ajani J, Bhalla K, et al. Phase II trial of paclitaxel, fluorouracil, and cisplatin in patients with advanced carcinoma of the esophagus. *J Clin Oncol.* 1998;16:1826–1834.
46. Kok TC, Van der Gaast A, Dees J, et al. Cisplatin and etoposide in oesophageal cancer: a phase II study. Rotterdam Oesophageal Tumour Study Group. *Br J Cancer.* 1996;74:980–984.
47. Joshi MB, Shirota Y, Danenberg KD, et al. High gene expression of TS1, GSTP1, and ERCC1 are risk factors for survival in patients treated with trimodality therapy for esophageal cancer. *Clin Cancer Res.* 2005;11:2215–2221.
48. Schneider S, Uchida K, Brabender J, et al. Downregulation of TS, DPD, ERCC1, GST-Pi, EGFR, and HER2 gene expression after neoadjuvant three-modality treatment in patients with esophageal cancer. *J Am Coll Surg.* 2005;200:336–344.
49. Warnecke-Eberz U, Metzger R, Miyazono F, et al. High specificity of quantitative excision repair cross-complementing 1 messenger RNA expression for prediction of minor

histopathological response to neoadjuvant radiochemotherapy in esophageal cancer. *Clin Cancer Res.* 2004;10:3794–3799.

50. DeMeester SR. Adenocarcinoma of the esophagus and cardia: a review of the disease and its treatment. *Ann Surg Oncol.* 2006;13:12–30.
51. Medical Research Council Oesophageal Cancer Working Group. Surgical resection with or without preoperative chemotherapy in oesophageal cancer: a randomised controlled trial. *Lancet.* 2002;359:1727–1733.
52. Baba M, Natsugoe S, Shimada M, et al. Prospective evaluation of preoperative chemotherapy in resectable squamous cell carcinoma of the thoracic esophagus. *Dis Esophagus.* 2000;13:136–141.
53. Kelson DP, Ginsberg R, Pajak TF, et al. Chemotherapy followed by surgery compared with surgery alone for localized esophageal cancer. *N Engl J Med.* 1998;339:1979–1984.
54. Kelson DP, Winter KA, Gunderson LL, et al. Long-term results of RTOG trial 8911 (USA Intergroup 113): a random assignment trial comparison of chemotherapy followed by surgery compared with surgery alone for esophageal cancer. *J Clin Oncol.* 2007;25:3719–3725.
55. Malthaner RA, Collin S, Fenlon D. Preoperative chemotherapy for resectable thoracic esophageal cancer. *Cochrane Database Syst Rev.* 2006;3:CD001556.
56. Cunningham D, Allum WH, Stenning SP, et al. Perioperative chemotherapy versus surgery alone for resectable gastroesophageal cancer. *N Engl J Med.* 2006;355:11–20.
57. Brucher BL, Stein HJ, Zimmermann F, et al. Responders benefit from neoadjuvant radiochemotherapy in esophageal squamous cell carcinoma: results of a prospective phase-II trial. *Eur J Surg Oncol.* 2004;30:963–971.
58. Arnott SJ, Duncan W, Kerr GR, et al. Low dose preoperative radiotherapy for carcinoma of the oesophagus: results of a randomized clinical trial. *Radiother Oncol.* 1992;24:108–113.
59. Gignoux M, Roussel A, Paillot B, et al. The value of preoperative radiotherapy in esophageal cancer: results of a study of the E.O.R.T.C. *World J Surg.* 1987;11:426–432.
60. Launois B, Delarue D, Campion JP, et al. Preoperative radiotherapy for carcinoma of the esophagus. *Surg Gynecol Obstet.* 1981;153:690–692.
61. Wang M, Gu XZ, Yin WB, et al. Randomized clinical trial on the combination of preoperative irradiation and surgery in the treatment of esophageal carcinoma: report on 206 patients. *Int J Radiat Oncol Biol Phys.* 1989;16:325–327.
62. Nygaard K, Hagen S, Hansen HS, et al. Pre-operative radiotherapy prolongs survival in operable esophageal carcinoma: a randomized, multicenter study of pre-operative radiotherapy and chemotherapy. The second Scandinavian trial in esophageal cancer. *World J Surg.* 1992;16:1104–1109; discussion 1110.
63. Arnott SJ, Duncan W, Gignoux M, et al. Preoperative radiotherapy for esophageal carcinoma. *Cochrane Database Syst Rev.* 2005:CD001799.
64. Mariette C, Triboulet JP. Is preoperative chemoradiation effective in treatment of oesophageal carcinoma? *Lancet Oncol.* 2005;6:635–637.
65. Bosset JF, Gignoux M, Triboulet JP, et al. Chemoradiotherapy followed by surgery compared with surgery alone in squamous-cell cancer of the esophagus. *N Engl J Med.* 1997;337:161–167.
66. Burmeister BH, Smithers BM, Gebski V, et al. Surgery alone versus chemoradiotherapy followed by surgery for resectable cancer of the oesophagus: a randomised controlled phase III trial. *Lancet Oncol.* 2005;6:659–668.
67. Walsh TN, Noonan N, Hollywood D, et al. A comparison of multimodal therapy and surgery for esophageal adenocarcinoma. *N Engl J Med.* 1996;335:462–467.
68. Urba SG, Orringer MB, Turrisi A, et al. Randomized trial of preoperative chemoradiation versus surgery alone in patients with locoregional esophageal carcinoma. *J Clin Oncol.* 2001;19:305–313.
69. Apinop C, Puttisak P, Preecha N. A prospective study of combined therapy in esophageal cancer. *Hepatogastroenterology.* 1994;41:391–393.
70. Le Prise E, Etienne PL, Meunier B, et al. A randomized study of chemotherapy, radiation therapy, and surgery versus surgery for localized squamous cell carcinoma of the esophagus. *Cancer.* 1994;73:1779–1784.
71. Lee JL, Park SI, Kim SB, et al. A single institutional phase III trial of preoperative chemotherapy with hyperfractionation radiotherapy plus surgery versus surgery alone for resectable esophageal squamous cell carcinoma. *Ann Oncol.* 2004;15:947–954.
72. Tepper J, Krasna M, Niedzwiecki D, et al. Superiority of trimodality therapy to surgery alone in esophageal cancer: results of CALGB 9781. *J Clin Oncol.* 2006;24(suppl 18S, pt 1):4012.
73. Fiorica F, Di Bona D, Schepis F, et al. Preoperative chemoradiotherapy for oesophageal cancer: a systematic review and meta-analysis. *Gut.* 2004;53:925–930.
74. Gebski V, Burmeister B, Smithers BM, et al. Survival benefits from neoadjuvant chemoradiotherapy or chemotherapy in oesophageal carcinoma: a meta-analysis. *Lancet Oncol.* 2007;8:226–234.
75. Zacherl J, Sendler A, Stein HJ, et al. Current status of neoadjuvant therapy for adenocarcinoma of the distal esophagus. *World J Surg.* 2003;27:1067–1074.
76. Ott K, Vogelsang H, Marton N, et al. The thymidylate synthase tandem repeat promoter polymorphism: a predictor for tumor-related survival in neoadjuvant treated locally advanced gastric cancer. *Int J Cancer.* 2006;119:2885–2894.
77. Demeester SR. Reoperative chemoradiotherapy for oesophageal cancer: a systematic review and meta-analysis. *Gut.* 2005;54:440–441.
78. Ilson DH. Cancer of the gastroesophageal junction: combined modality therapy. *Surg Oncol Clin N Am.* 2006;15:803–824.
79. Lordick F, Stein HJ, Peschel C, et al. Neoadjuvant therapy for oesophagogastric cancer. *Br J Surg.* 2004;91:540–551.
80. Greer SE, Goodney PP, Sutton JE, et al. Neoadjuvant chemoradiotherapy for esophageal carcinoma: a meta-analysis. *Surgery.* 2005;137:172–177.
81. Ott K, Weber WA, Lordick F, et al. Metabolic imaging predicts response, survival, and recurrence in adenocarcinomas of the esophagogastric junction. *J Clin Oncol.* 2006;24:4692–4698.
82. Downey RJ, Akhurst T, Ilson D, et al. Whole body 18FDG-PET and the response of esophageal cancer to induction therapy: results of a prospective trial. *J Clin Oncol.* 2003;21:428–432.
83. Rizk N, Downey RJ, Akhurst T, et al. Preoperative 18[F]-fluorodeoxyglucose positron emission tomography standardized uptake values predict survival after esophageal adenocarcinoma resection. *Ann Thorac Surg.* 2006;81:1076–1081.
84. Tyagi P. Bevacizumab, when added to paclitaxel/carboplatin, prolongs survival in previously untreated patients with advanced non-small-cell lung cancer: preliminary results from the ECOG 4599 trial. *Clin Lung Cancer.* 2005;6:276–278.
85. Cunningham D, Humblet Y, Siena S, et al. Cetuximab monotherapy and cetuximab plus irinotecan in irinotecan-refractory metastatic colorectal cancer. *N Engl J Med.* 2004;351:337–345.
86. Lenz HJ, Van Cutsem E, Khambata-Ford S, et al. Multicenter phase II and translational study of cetuximab in metastatic colorectal carcinoma refractory to irinotecan, oxaliplatin, and fluoropyrimidines. *J Clin Oncol.* 2006;24:4914–4921.
87. Saltz LB, Meropol NJ, Loehrer PJ Sr., et al. Phase II trial of cetuximab in patients with refractory colorectal cancer that expresses the epidermal growth factor receptor. *J Clin Oncol.* 2004;22:1201–1208.
88. Adams GP, Weiner LM. Monoclonal antibody therapy of cancer. *Nat Biotechnol.* 2005;23:1147–1157.
89. Altorki N, Port JL, Korst RJ, et al. A phase II trial of preoperative paclitaxel/ carboplatin with celecoxib followed by adjuvant celecoxib for esophageal cancer: preliminary report. *J Clin Oncol.* 2005;23(suppl 16S, pt 1):4205.
90. Hurwitz H, Fehrenbacher L, Novotny W, et al. Bevacizumab plus irinotecan, fluorouracil, and leucovorin for metastatic colorectal cancer. *N Engl J Med.* 2004;350:2335–2342.
91. Akamatsu M, Matsumoto T, Oka K, et al. c-erbB-2 oncoprotein expression related to chemoradioresistance in esophageal squamous cell carcinoma. *Int J Radiat Oncol Biol Phys.* 2003;57:1323–1327.
92. Gibault L, Metges JP, Conan-Charlet V, et al. Diffuse EGFR staining is associated with reduced overall survival in locally advanced oesophageal squamous cell cancer. *Br J Cancer.* 2005;93:107–115.
93. Gibson MK, Abraham SC, Wu TT, et al. Epidermal growth factor receptor, p53 mutation, and pathological response predict survival in patients with locally advanced esophageal cancer treated with preoperative chemoradiotherapy. *Clin Cancer Res.* 2003;9:6461–6468.
94. Inada S, Koto T, Futami K, et al. Evaluation of malignancy and the prognosis of esophageal cancer based on an immunohistochemical study (p53, E-cadherin, epidermal growth factor receptor). *Surg Today.* 1999;29:493–503.
95. Miyazono F, Metzger R, Warnecke-Eberz U, et al. Quantitative c-erbB-2 but not c-erbB-1 mRNA expression is a promising marker to predict minor histopathologic response to neoadjuvant radiochemotherapy in oesophageal cancer. *Br J Cancer.* 2004;91:666–672.
96. Han B, Liu J, Ma MJ, et al. Clinicopathological significance of heparanase and basic fibroblast growth factor expression in human esophageal cancer. *World J Gastroenterol.* 2005;11:2188–2192.
97. Imdahl A, Bognar G, Schulte-Monting J, et al. Predictive factors for response to neoadjuvant therapy in patients with oesophageal cancer. *Eur J Cardiothorac Surg.* 2002;21:657–663.
98. Kulke MH, Odze RD, Mueller JD, et al. Prognostic significance of vascular endothelial growth factor and cyclooxygenase 2 expression in patients receiving preoperative chemoradiation for esophageal cancer. *J Thorac Cardiovasc Surg.* 2004;127:1579–1586.
99. Kuo KT, Chow KC, Wu YC, et al. Clinicopathologic significance of cyclooxygenase-2 overexpression in esophageal squamous cell carcinoma. *Ann Thorac Surg.* 2003;76:909–914.
100. Shimada H, Hoshino T, Okazumi S, et al. Expression of angiogenic factors predicts response to chemoradiotherapy and prognosis of oesophageal squamous cell carcinoma. *Br J Cancer.* 2002;86:552–557.
101. Xi H, Baldus SE, Warnecke-Eberz U, et al. High cyclooxygenase-2 expression following neoadjuvant radiochemotherapy is associated with minor histopathologic response and poor prognosis in esophageal cancer. *Clin Cancer Res.* 2005;11:8341–8347.
102. Ikeda G, Isaji S, Chandra B, et al. Prognostic significance of biologic factors in squamous cell carcinoma of the esophagus. *Cancer.* 1999;86:1396–1405.
103. Ikeguchi M, Oka S, Gomyo Y, et al. Combined analysis of p53 and retinoblastoma protein expressions in esophageal cancer. *Ann Thorac Surg.* 2000;70:913–917.
104. Kitamura K, Saeki H, Kawaguchi H, et al. Immunohistochemical status of the p53 protein and Ki-67 antigen using biopsied specimens can predict a sensitivity to neoadjuvant therapy in patients with esophageal cancer. *Hepatogastroenterology.* 2000;47:419–423.
105. Nakashima S, Natsugoe S, Matsumoto M, et al. Expression of p53 and p21 is useful for the prediction of preoperative chemotherapeutic effects in esophageal carcinoma. *Anticancer Res.* 2000;20:1933–1937.
106. Shimada Y, Watanabe G, Yamasaki S, et al. Histological response of cisplatin predicts patients' survival in oesophageal cancer and p53 protein accumulation in pretreatment biopsy is associated with cisplatin sensitivity. *Eur J Cancer.* 2000;36:987–993.
107. Sohda M, Ishikawa H, Masuda N, et al. Pretreatment evaluation of combined HIF-1alpha, p53 and p21 expression is a useful and sensitive indicator of response to radiation and chemotherapy in esophageal cancer. *Int J Cancer.* 2004;110:838–844.

108. Itami A, Shimada Y, Watanabe G, et al. Prognostic value of p27(Kip1) and CyclinD1 expression in esophageal cancer. *Oncology.* 1999;57:311–317.
109. Kuwahara M, Hirai T, Yoshida K, et al. p53, p21(Waf1/Cip1) and cyclin D1 protein expression and prognosis in esophageal cancer. *Dis Esophagus.* 1999;12:116–119.
110. Terashita Y, Ishiguro H, Haruki N, et al. Excision repair cross complementing 3 expression is involved in patient prognosis and tumor progression in esophageal cancer. *Oncol Rep.* 2004;12:827–831.
111. Ishibashi Y, Matsumoto T, Niwa M, et al. CD147 and matrix metalloproteinase-2 protein expression as significant prognostic factors in esophageal squamous cell carcinoma. *Cancer.* 2004;101:1994–2000.
112. Sharma R, Chattopadhyay TK, Mathur M, et al. Prognostic significance of stromelysin-3 and tissue inhibitor of matrix metalloproteinase-2 in esophageal cancer. *Oncology.* 2004;67:300–309.
113. Tanioka Y, Yoshida T, Yagawa T, et al. Matrix metalloproteinase-7 and matrix metalloproteinase-9 are associated with unfavourable prognosis in superficial oesophageal cancer. *Br J Cancer.* 2003;89:2116–2121.
114. Salomon DS, Brandt R, Ciardiello F, et al. Epidermal growth factor-related peptides and their receptors in human malignancies. *Crit Rev Oncol Hematol.* 1995;19:183–232.
115. Hickey K, Grehan D, Reid IM, et al. Expression of epidermal growth factor receptor and proliferating cell nuclear antigen predicts response of esophageal squamous cell carcinoma to chemoradiotherapy. *Cancer.* 1994;74:1693–1698.
116. Herbst RS, Shin DM. Monoclonal antibodies to target epidermal growth factor receptor-positive tumors: a new paradigm for cancer therapy. *Cancer.* 2002;94:1593–1611.
117. Karnes WE Jr, Weller SG, Adjei PN, et al. Inhibition of epidermal growth factor receptor kinase induces protease-dependent apoptosis in human colon cancer cells. *Gastroenterology.* 1998;114:930–939.
118. Wu X, Fan Z, Masui H, et al. Apoptosis induced by an anti-epidermal growth factor receptor monoclonal antibody in a human colorectal carcinoma cell line and its delay by insulin. *J Clin Invest.* 1995;95:1897–1905.
119. Bonner JA, Harari PM, Giralt J, et al. Radiotherapy plus cetuximab for squamous-cell carcinoma of the head and neck. *N Engl J Med.* 2006;354:567–578.
120. Wilkinson NW, Black JD, Roukhadze E, et al. Epidermal growth factor receptor expression correlates with histologic grade in resected esophageal adenocarcinoma. *J Gastrointest Surg.* 2004;8:448–453.
121. Kitagawa Y, Ueda M, Ando N, et al. Further evidence for prognostic significance of epidermal growth factor receptor gene amplification in patients with esophageal squamous cell carcinoma. *Clin Cancer Res.* 1996;2:909–914.
122. Cetuximab, combination chemotherapy, and radiation therapy in treating patients with locally advanced esophageal cancer that cannot be removed by surgery. Available at: http://clinicaltrials.gov/ct/show/NCT00109850. Accessed October 9, 2007.
123. Cetuximab in treating patients with metastatic esophageal cancer or gastroesophageal junction cancer. Available at: http://clinicaltrials.gov/ct/show/NCT00096031. Accessed October 9, 2007.
124. Cetuximab, cisplatin, and irinotecan in treating patients with metastatic esophageal cancer, gastroesophageal junction cancer, or gastric cancer that did not respond to previous irinotecan and cisplatin. Available at: http://clinicaltrials.gov/ct/show/NCT00397904. Accessed October 9, 2007.
125. Enzinger P, Yock T, Suh W, et al. Phase II cisplatin, irinotecan, cetuximab and concurrent radiation therapy followed by surgery for locally advanced esophageal cancer. *J Clin Oncol.* 2006;24(suppl 18S, pt 1):4064.
126. Suntharalingam M, Dipetrillo T, Akerman P, et al. Cetuximab, paclitaxel, carboplatin and radiation for esophageal and gastric cancer. *J Clin Oncol.* 2006;24(suppl 18S, pt 1):4029.
127. Vallbohmer D, Zhang W, Gordon M, et al. Molecular determinants of cetuximab efficacy. *J Clin Oncol.* 2005;23:3536–3544.
128. Di Fiore F, Blanchard F, Charbonnier F, et al. Clinical relevance of KRAS mutation detection in metastatic colorectal cancer treated by Cetuximab plus chemotherapy. *Br J Cancer.* 2007;96:1166–1169.
129. Khambata-Ford S, Garrett CR, Meropol NJ, et al. Expression of epiregulin and amphiregulin and K-ras mutation status predict disease control in metastatic colorectal cancer patients treated with cetuximab. *J Clin Oncol.* 2007;25:3230–3237.
130. Yarden Y, Sliwkowski MX. Untangling the ErbB signalling network. *Nat Rev Mol Cell Biol.* 2001;2:127–137.
131. Slamon DJ, Godolphin W, Jones LA, et al. Studies of the HER-2/neu proto-oncogene in human breast and ovarian cancer. *Science.* 1989;244:707–712.
132. Cobleigh MA, Vogel CL, Tripathy D, et al. Multinational study of the efficacy and safety of humanized anti-HER2 monoclonal antibody in women who have HER2-overexpressing metastatic breast cancer that has progressed after chemotherapy for metastatic disease. *J Clin Oncol.* 1999;17:2639–2648.
133. Baselga J, Tripathy D, Mendelsohn J, et al. Phase II study of weekly intravenous recombinant humanized anti-p185HER2 monoclonal antibody in patients with HER2/neu-overexpressing metastatic breast cancer. *J Clin Oncol.* 1996;14:737–744.
134. Brien TP, Odze RD, Sheehan CE, et al. HER-2/neu gene amplification by FISH predicts poor survival in Barrett's esophagus-associated adenocarcinoma. *Hum Pathol.* 2000;31:35–39.
135. Safran H, DiPetrillo T, Nadeem A, et al. Trastuzumab, paclitaxel, cisplatin, and radiation for adenocarcinoma of the esophagus: a phase I study. *Cancer Invest.* 2004;22:670–677.
136. Ross JS, McKenna BJ. The HER-2/neu oncogene in tumors of the gastrointestinal tract. *Cancer Invest.* 2001;19:554–568.
137. Hicklin DJ, Ellis LM. Role of the vascular endothelial growth factor pathway in tumor growth and angiogenesis. *J Clin Oncol.* 2005;23:1011–1027.
138. Dvorak HF. Vascular permeability factor/vascular endothelial growth factor: a critical cytokine in tumor angiogenesis and a potential target for diagnosis and therapy. *J Clin Oncol.* 2002;20:4368–4380.
139. Decaussin M, Sartelet H, Robert C, et al. Expression of vascular endothelial growth factor (VEGF) and its two receptors (VEGF-R1-Flt1 and VEGF-R2-Flk1/KDR) in non-small cell lung carcinomas (NSCLCs): correlation with angiogenesis and survival. *J Pathol.* 1999;188:369–377.
140. Ferrer FA, Miller LJ, Lindquist R, et al. Expression of vascular endothelial growth factor receptors in human prostate cancer. *Urology.* 1999;54:567–572.
141. Masood R, Cai J, Zheng T, et al. Vascular endothelial growth factor (VEGF) is an autocrine growth factor for VEGF receptor-positive human tumors. *Blood.* 2001;98:1904–1913.
142. Takahashi Y, Tucker SL, Kitadai Y, et al. Vessel counts and expression of vascular endothelial growth factor as prognostic factors in node-negative colon cancer. *Arch Surg.* 1997;132:541–546.
143. Shih CH, Ozawa S, Ando N, et al. Vascular endothelial growth factor expression predicts outcome and lymph node metastasis in squamous cell carcinoma of the esophagus. *Clin Cancer Res.* 2000;6:1161–1168.
144. Lord RV, Park JM, Wickramasinghe K, et al. Vascular endothelial growth factor and basic fibroblast growth factor expression in esophageal adenocarcinoma and Barrett esophagus. *J Thorac Cardiovasc Surg.* 2003;125:246–253.
145. Chen HX. Expanding the clinical development of bevacizumab. *Oncologist.* 2004;9(suppl 1):27–35.
146. Hurwitz HI, Fehrenbacher L, Hainsworth JD, et al. Bevacizumab in combination with fluorouracil and leucovorin: an active regimen for first-line metastatic colorectal cancer. *J Clin Oncol.* 2005;23:3502–3508.
147. Johnson DH, Fehrenbacher L, Novotny WF, et al. Randomized phase II trial comparing bevacizumab plus carboplatin and paclitaxel with carboplatin and paclitaxel alone in previously untreated locally advanced or metastatic non-small-cell lung cancer. *J Clin Oncol.* 2004;22:2184–2191.
148. Yang JC, Haworth L, Sherry RM, et al. A randomized trial of bevacizumab, an anti-vascular endothelial growth factor antibody, for metastatic renal cancer. *N Engl J Med.* 2003;349:427–434.
149. Shah M, Ilson D, Ramanathan RK, et al. A multicenter phase II study of irinotecan (CPT), cisplatin (CIS), and bevacizumab (BEV) in patients with unresectable or metastatic gastric or gastroesophageal junction (GEJ) adenocarcinoma. *J Clin Oncol.* 2005;23(suppl 16S, pt 1):4025.

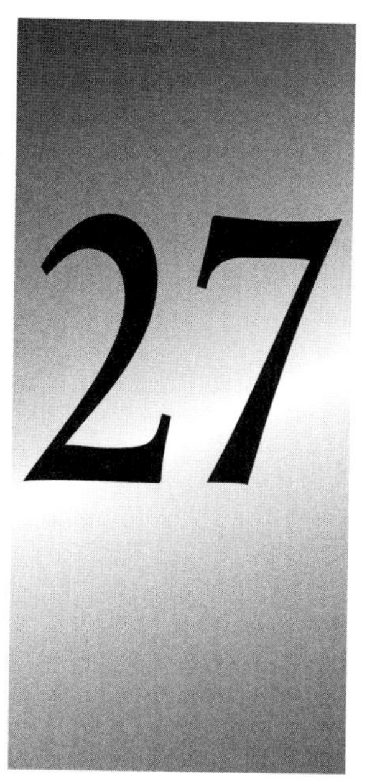

Principles of Multimodality Therapy

Daniel V. T. Catenacci
Ezra Cohen
Victoria M. Villaflor

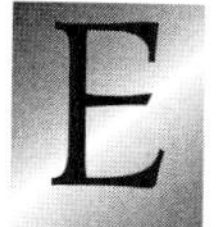

Esophageal cancer is the ninth most frequent cancer in the world and the fifth most frequent cancer in developed countries (1). In the United States, the incidence of esophageal cancer was 14,550 and accounted for 13,770 cancer deaths in 2006 (2). The incidence of esophageal cancer has increased in recent years, outstripping all other solid tumors (3–5), largely because of a dramatic increase in the incidence of adenocarcinoma (AC) of the distal esophagus and gastroesophageal junction (GEJ) (6).

AC and squamous cell carcinoma (SCC) are the 2 main histologic types of esophageal cancer. Historically, the 2 subtypes have been managed as a single disease entity because prognosis was similar. Two decades ago, AC accounted for only 5% and SCC for approximately 90% of all esophageal tumors (1). Although the incidence of SCC has increased over the past several decades in the United States, there has been a profound epidemiological shift in esophageal cancers as a result of a 350% increase in AC between 1974 and 1994, now accounting for 60% of all esophageal cancers (7). This epidemiological shift reflects a change in etiology of the disease, with SCC being associated mainly with the chronic irritation of the esophageal mucosa secondary to smoking and alcohol consumption. Other risk factors include achalasia, diverticulae, and caustic strictures. On the other hand, the increase in AC mirrors an increase in Barrett's metaplasia, a preneoplastic condition induced by chronic gastroesophageal reflux (8,9). Barrett's metaplasia is a prerequisite for the development of AC of the GEJ and distal esophagus (10). The relationship of Barrett's metaplasia to AC explains the increased incidence of AC relative to SCC and explains the shift of the site of primary tumors to the distal esophagus and GEJ (10,11). Debate regarding the differences or similarities of AC of the distal esophagus (type I GEJ) versus GEJ (type II GEJ) and gastric cardia (type III GEJ) has occurred (12,13) in relation to the optimal treatment approach (12) and is discussed in detail in a later section of this chapter.

Despite substantial improvements in screening, diagnosis, and treatment of esophageal cancer, the prognosis is bleak. Surgery has been the cornerstone of treatment for esophageal cancer, and adequate negative margins are the key to curative resection (14). Unfortunately, approximately 2 of 3 patients have unresectable or inoperable disease at the time of diagnosis, secondary to either tumor extension or comorbid disease (15). Moreover, it is estimated that only 15% to 20% of all esophageal patients are actual surgical candidates when considering all factors, including surgical exploration for staging. Survival at 5 years for all esophageal cancer patients taken together, with or without surgery, is less than 10% (15).

For those patients that are surgical candidates, resection alone is at best associated with a 20% to 25%

5-year survival (15,16). While operative mortality has almost halved as a result of improved surgical techniques (14,17–20) that are being performed at more experienced centers (21), the long-term prognosis with surgery alone remains grossly unchanged (22–24). Therefore, a multidisciplinary approach has evolved to include surgery, radiation, and chemotherapy, alone or in combination, in attempt to improve the survival of this aggressive disease.

PRINCIPLES OF MULTIMODALITY THERAPY

The poor outcome of patients undergoing surgery alone has led to a number of studies using various regimens of chemotherapy and various doses and schedules of radiation, alone or combined, administered before or after surgery. The basis of surgery, as discussed previously, is to remove the primary tumor with adequate negative margins with curative intent. However, even in cases achieving negative surgical margins by pathology, there is a significant risk of local recurrence. In addition, proportional to an increasing disease stage, the risk of distant recurrence after surgery as a result of micrometastases at the time of surgery is of concern.

Therefore, to address local recurrence, radiation therapy is used to exert its effects within the irradiated field by inducing tumor cell apoptosis and necrosis. Chemotherapy is administered primarily with the intent to treat microscopic systemic disease (25,26). The general clinical goal of administering chemotherapy and radiation simultaneously is to improve both locoregional and systemic tumor control. Spatial interaction recognizes that radiation will work within the irradiated field, while chemotherapy exerts its effect systemically, principles not requisite on simultaneous administration (27). An additional goal of concomitant chemoradiotherapy is to increase the efficacy of radiation; chemotherapy in this respect augments the effect of radiation therapy, a principle referred to as radiation sensitization (28,29). Sensitization addresses the fact the clonogenic radioresistance will ultimately cause treatment failure within the irradiated field after single-modality radiotherapy (29). Similarly, targeted agents have been shown to result in radiation sensitization, including epidermal growth factor receptor signaling pathway inhibition, antiangiogenic agents, histone deacetylation inhibition, and genetically engineered viruses that express tumor necrosis factor when exposed to radiation by using a radiation inducible promoter to allow gene transcription (30–33).

Possible sensitizing mechanisms have included synergistic DNA damage, inhibition of repair of radiation damage, hypoxic cell sensitization, cell cycle synchronization, inhibition of rapid repopulation of tumor cells, and suppression of radiation resistance pathways (29,34).

Initially, most clinical trials focused on adjuvant treatment strategies. Such postoperative treatment strategies did not result in significant clinical improvement. Adjuvant chemotherapy is not easy to administer, and only a minority of patients are actually able to tolerate it; this is exemplified by the MAGIC trial that is discussed later. Accordingly, preoperative approaches have since entailed the majority of attention; neoadjuvant therapy has a number of advantages over adjuvant therapy. First, patients have an optimum performance status prior to surgery, whereas postoperative treatment is frequently delayed 8 to 10 weeks to allow for sufficient patient recovery. Second, preoperative therapy may enable a proportion of tumors to be "downstaged," making potentially inoperable tumors (e.g., T4 lesions) (35) amenable to resection. Along these lines, tumor shrinkage after neoadjuvant therapy may also result in a less complicated surgery for those tumors initially deemed operable. Third, response to treatment can be accurately assessed pathologically after resection, and response to therapy is the best available surrogate marker of the likely outcome of treatment (36–38). Fourth, exposure of micrometastases to the so-called tumor growth–promoting postoperative milieu is best curtailed by treating with neoadjuvant chemotherapy.

The main disadvantages of preoperative therapy are the inability to predict who will respond to treatment, the inability to determine who has had a complete pathological response (R0) and therefore undergo unnecessary surgery, and treatment toxicity. Addressing treatment response, novel metabolic imaging with positron-emission tomography (PET) as early as 14 days after initiating neoadjuvant therapy may prevent a delay to surgery in those tumors not responding to treatment or may allow for an adjustment of the neoadjuvant regimen in order to better treat the tumor (39–41). Endoscopic ultrasound postchemotherapy has also been evaluated as a tool to predict therapy response and downstaging (42).

Various drug combinations have been studied in a pre- and postoperative setting, and patterns of response are emerging. However, the majority of trials are not randomized trials, and those that are randomized are poorly designed with insufficient numbers or use outdated ineffective chemotherapy regimens and/or radiation doses. Additionally, most trials fail to study the question of therapy outcome differences between the histologic subtypes of esophageal cancer: AC and SCC. The randomized clinical trials that attempt to address the multiple permutations of therapy in the neoadjuvant and adjuvant setting have been reviewed (12,43–52) and are discussed next.

TREATMENT WITH SURGERY

Surgery Alone

Surgery alone cures a minority of patients with localized esophageal cancer. Contemporary outcome data for treatment with surgery alone demonstrate the limits of surgery to control disease. Median survival is 16 months with 1-, 2-, and 3-year survival rates of 60%, 37%, and 26%, respectively, for patients in the surgery-alone group of randomized trials (53,54). Rate of failure to control local disease was high—40% of patients did not have complete resection of all gross disease, and 18% of completely resected patients recurred locally, for a total of 58% local recurrence with surgery alone (53). Median survival is approximately 13 to 16 months, and 2-year survival is 34% (25) and modest long-term survival 10% to 25% (52), depending the stage of disease included in the cited trials. As mentioned, the surgical approach and 2-field versus 3-field lymphadenectomy is a subject of ongoing debate, neither showing clear benefit over the other. It is clear, however, that postoperative morbidity, mortality, and survival are significantly better in expert centers that perform a higher number of this surgery (21). Surgery alone is probably adequate for T1 localized tumors without lymph node involvement (T1, N0). Whether T2 lesions are adequately treated with surgery alone is controversial; National Comprehensive Cancer Network guidelines suggest that only noncervical T1 disease be treated with single-modality surgery (55). As such, in more advanced local disease, poor survival after single-modality surgery has led to the consideration of therapeutic combinations with radiation, chemotherapy, and/or surgery.

Radiation versus Surgery Alone

Adjuvant Radiation versus Surgery Alone

Four phase III trials (Table 27.1) comparing surgery alone with adjuvant radiation (45–56 Gy) failed to show an overall survival advantage (53,56–58). There was, however, improved local control of disease in the radiation arm. Adjuvant radiotherapy increased complications at the gastroplasty level, including adhesions, scarring, and fistulas. A subgroup of patients who had palliative resection did show a significant decrease in locoregional recurrence, and therefore it is reasonable to consider postoperative radiotherapy for those patients who have palliative resections to enhance local disease control. One phase III trial reports improved survival with postoperative radiotherapy (59). Xiao et al. randomized 495 patients to receive surgery alone or surgery and then adjuvant radiotherapy (50–60 Gy) in 25 to 30 fractions, starting 3 to 4 weeks postoperatively. Overall, 5-year survival was 31.7% versus 41.3%, respectively, the difference of which was not statistically significant ($P= 0.45$). However, subgroup analysis did show that patients with stage III disease had 5-year overall survival of 13.1% versus 31.5%, respectively ($P < 0.002$).

TABLE 27.1
Randomized Controlled Trials of Adjuvant Radiation versus Surgery Alone for Esophageal Cancer[a]

Study/year published	Histology	TA/CA	MS TA/CA	5-Year OS (%) TA/CA	*P* value	XRT (Gy) (total dose)
Fok 1993	SCC	42/39	11/22	10/16	NS	43–53
Kunath 1984	SCC	23/21	9/6		NS	50–55
Teniere 1991	SCC	102/119	18/18	19/19	NS	45–55
Zieren 1995	SCC	33/35			NS	56
Xiao 2003[b]	SCC/AC	220/275		All patients 41.3/31.4 Stage III 35.1/13.1	$P = 0.45$ (NS) $P < 0.002$	50–60

Abbreviations: [a]TA = treatment arm; CA = control arm; MS = median survival (months); OS = overall survival; XRT = radiotherapy; SCC = squamous cell carcinoma; NS = not significant; AC = adenocarcinoma.
[b]Trial with statistically significant benefit over control.

Neoadjuvant Radiation versus Surgery Alone

Again, 5 phase III trials (Table 27.2) comparing surgery alone with neoadjuvant radiation failed to reveal significant increases in resectability or overall survival in esophageal cancer (60–64). Arnott et al. and Gignoux et al. used what is considered suboptimal radiation doses currently, 20 and 33Gy, respectively. Only Nygaard et al., who used 35 Gy, showed a 3-year survival advantage that was significant, but they pooled patients receiving preoperative chemotherapy and radiotherapy with those who had radiotherapy only. Five-year survival in these trials collectively was between 5% and 35% in the group receiving neoadjuvant radiotherapy versus 9% to 30% in the surgery alone group. Three trials using preoperative radiation (40 Gy) in a total of 690 patients found similar 5-year survival rates between patients receiving neoadjuvant radiotherapy and surgery-alone controls (60,62). A meta-analysis of the trials with a median follow-up of 9 years and data from 1,147 patients showed no significant survival benefit at 5 years (odds ratio [OR] 0.89; 95% CI 0.78–1.01; $P = 0.062$) (65). As such, radiotherapy alone in the neoadjuvant setting does not have a role in the curative treatment strategy for esophageal cancer.

Chemotherapy versus Surgery Alone

Adjuvant Chemotherapy versus Surgery Alone

Three phase III trials (Table 27.3) compared adjuvant chemotherapy with surgery alone and did not show any benefit in overall survival (66–68). Ando et al. reported a 5-year disease-free survival advantage with chemotherapy (55% vs. 45%, $P = 0.037$) but not significant overall survival difference (61% vs. 52%, $P = 0.13$) (67). Patients with pN1 disease did have significant survival advantage (52% vs. 38%, $P = 0.041$). However, a meta-analysis of randomized and nonrandomized trials using cisplatin-based chemotherapy did not show any benefit in the adjuvant setting (69), and it is, therefore, not considered a standard therapeutic option.

Neoadjuvant Chemotherapy versus Surgery Alone

Eleven randomized trials comparing neoadjuvant chemotherapy (based on cisplatin) versus surgery alone have been conducted, 8 (Table 27.4) with data that may be analyzed (25,54,64,70–77). The drugs and doses were different between studies, and no study allowed an optimum regimen to be defined. Collectively, these studies showed a complete response of 19% to 58% and a histological complete response of 2.5% to 13%, and 2 studies reported a significant overall survival benefit (25,76). The UK Medical Research Council trial of 802 patients showed a better overall survival in the chemotherapy group (median survival 16.8 vs. 13.3 months and 2-year survival 43% vs. 34%) (25). However, when criteria including tomodensitometry assessment to detect tumor extension and specific surgical techniques along with quality control of the surgery were imposed, Kelsen et al., in another large study, did not show an overall survival benefit (54). An update by Kelsen et al. of this trial reported that in patients with localized esophageal cancer, whether or not preoperative chemotherapy is administered, only an R0 resection results in substantial long-term survival (78). Even microscopically positive margins are an ominous prognostic factor. After an R1 resection, postoperative chemoradiotherapy therapy offers the possibility of long-term disease-free survival to a small percentage of patients (78). Two recent meta-analyses have been conducted addressing the question of neoadjuvant chemotherapy versus surgery

TABLE 27.2
Randomized Controlled Trials of Neoadjuvant Radiation versus Surgery Alone for Esophageal Cancer [a]

Study/year published	Histology	TA/CA	MS TA/CA	5-Year OS (%) TA/CA	*P* value	XRT (Gy) (total dose)
Lanouis 1981	SCC	47/33	12/10	12/10	NS	40
Gignoux 1987	SCC	106/102	11/11	9/10	NS	30
Wang 2001	SCC	104/102		30/35	NS	40
Arnott 1992	SCC/AC	90/86	8/8	17/9	NS	20
Nygaard 1992[b]	SCC	Group III, 48/41			Pooled group III/IV	35

Abbreviations: [a]TA = treatment arm; CA = control arm; MS = median survival (months); OS = overall survival; XRT = radiotherapy; SCC = squamous cell carcinoma; NS = not significant; AC = adenocarcinoma.
[b]Trial with statistically significant benefit over control.

TABLE 27.3
Randomized Controlled Trials of Adjuvant Chemotherapy versus Surgery Alone for Esophageal Cancer [a]

Study/year published	Histology	TA/CA	Five-Year OS (%) TA/CA	*P* value	Chemotherapy (mg/m2)
Ando 1997	SCC	100/105		NS	Cisplatin (70/vindesine (3)
Ando 2003[b]	SCC	120/122	61/52	$P = 0.13$	Cisplatin (80)/5-FU (800)
			DFS 55.45	$P < 0.037$	
Pouliquen 1996	SCC	52/68		NS	Cisplatin (100)/5-FU (500)

Abbreviations: [a]TA = treatment arm; CA = control arm; OS = overall survival; SCC = squamous cell carcinoma; NS = not significant; DFS = 5-year disease-free survival.
[b]Trial with statistically significant benefit over control (better 5-year DFS, especially those with lymph node metastases).

TABLE 27.4
Randomized Controlled Trials of Neoadjuvant Chemotherapy versus Surgery Alone for Esophageal Cancer [a]

Study/year published	Histology	TA/CA	MS	*P* value	Chemotherapy
Roth 1988	SCC/AC	19/20	9/9	NS	Cisplatin/vindesine/bloeomycin
Schlag 1992	SCC	22/24	10/10	NS	Cisplatin/5-FU
Maipang 1994	SCC	24/22	10/10	NS	Cisplatin/vindesine/bleomycin
Kok 1996[b]	SCC	74/74	19/11	$P = 0.002$	5-FU/etoposide
Law 1997	SCC	74/73	16.8/13	NS	Cisplatin/5-FU
Kelsen 1998	SCC/AC	220/221	15/16	NS	Cisplatin/5-FU
Ancona 2001	SCC	47/47		NS	Cisplatin/5-FU
MRCOCWP 2002[b]	Any	400/402	16.8/13.3	$P = 0.004$	Cisplatin (80)/5-FU (1000)

Abbreviations: [a]TA = treatment arm; CA = control arm; MS = median survival (months); SCC = squamous cell carcinoma; AC = adenocarcinoma; NS = not significant.
[b]Trial with statistically significant improved overall survival and median survival.

alone (79,80). The first concluded that compared with surgery alone, neoadjuvant chemotherapy and surgery is associated with a lower rate of esophageal resection but a higher rate of complete resection. It does not increase treatment-related mortality. This meta-analysis did not demonstrate a survival benefit for the combination of neoadjuvant chemotherapy and surgery (79). The second meta-analysis also concluded that preoperative chemotherapy did not offer a survival advantage over surgery alone (OR 0.88; 95% CI 0.75–10.4; $P = 0.15$) (80). Neoadjuvant chemotherapy alone, therefore, does not have sufficient evidence to support it as a standard therapeutic option.

Neoadjuvant and Adjuvant Chemotherapy versus Surgery Alone

Three randomized trials have looked at pre- and postoperative chemotherapy (cisplatin based) versus surgery alone (54,73,81) (Table 27.5). None of these trials showed survival benefit over surgery alone. In the case of distal esophageal/GEJ, the MAGIC trial reported that neoadjuvant chemotherapy and adjuvant chemotherapy with epirubicin, cisplatin, and 5-FU (ECF) does have significant benefit and is an acceptable approach to treating this subgroup of esophageal cancers (82). This is discussed in further detail in the section addressing GEJ cancer.

TABLE 27.5
Randomized Controlled Trials of Neoadjuvant and Adjuvant Chemotherapy versus Surgery Alone for Esophageal Cancer [a]

Study/year published	Histology	TA/CA	MS TA/CA	*P* value	Chemotherapy (mg/m2)
Roth 1988	SCC/AC	19/20			Cisplatin/vindesine/bleomycin
Saltz 1992					Cisplatin/vindesine/bleomycin
Kelsen 1998			14.9/16.1	$P = 0.53$	Cisplatin/5-FU
			HR for death/95% CI TA compared to CA		
Cunningham 2005[b]	AC GE jxn/distal esophagus	65/66	0.75/0.59–0.93	$P < 0.008$	Epirubicin/cisplatin/5-FU

Abbreviations: [a]TA = treatment arm; CA = control arm; MS = median survival (months); SCC = squamous cell carcinoma; AC = adenocarcinoma; HR = hazard ratio; CI = confidence interval; GE jxn = gastroesophageal junction.
[b]Trial with statistically significant benefit over control (none).

Adjuvant Chemoradiotherapy versus Surgery Alone

The trial evaluating efficacy of adjuvant chemoradiotherapy was in the U.S. Intergroup 0116 study that looked specifically at patients with gastroesophageal tumors (83). This trial is discussed in detail in the section on GEJ adjuvant therapy later in this chapter.

Neoadjuvant Chemoradiotherapy versus Surgery Alone

The goal of multimodality or trimodal therapy, as discussed previously, is to benefit from radiotherapy by optimizing local control alongside chemotherapy that is used to address distant metastases, to affect the primary tumor, and to allow for radiosensitization (84,85). This concept has been studied extensively in 9 phase III randomized trials (64,86–92) . One is published only in abstract (93). The 8 completed trials are displayed in Table 27.6. All the trials reported a complete pathologic response of approximately 25%. Neither of the 2 trials that actually achieved adequate statistical power (86,91) showed a survival benefit in the chemoradiotherapy arm over surgery alone. The randomized single-center trial with 113 patients showed an overall survival advantage for neoadjuvant chemoradiotherapy (40 Gy) compared to surgery alone (89). This trial included only AC histological subtype. However, the small sample size, abnormally low survival in the group who had surgery alone (6% at 3 years), and absence of preoperative tomodensitometry make interpretation of the results difficult. They did report a maintained survival advantage at 5 years (94). An ongoing trial (93) has pointed again toward a survival benefit for neoadjuvant chemoradiotherapy compared with surgery alone, and publication of these results is eagerly awaited. The CALGB 9781 trial looking at early stage esophageal cancer (stages I to III) (cisplatin/5-FU/50.4Gy) was closed early secondary to lack of accrual. Only 56 of a planned 500 patients were enrolled. Those patients receiving the neoadjuvant therapy had a better 5-year overall survival over the surgery-alone arm (39 vs. 16 months; $P = 0.0005$), again suggesting benefit from neoadjuvant chemoradiotherapy. Urba et al. conducted a study of 100 patients with potentially resectable esophageal carcinoma to receive an intensive regimen of preoperative chemoradiation with cisplatin, fluorouracil, and vinblastine and 45 Gy of radiation before surgery or surgery alone (90). At a median follow-up of 8.2 years, there was no significant difference in survival between the treatment arms. Median survival was 17.6 months in the surgery alone arm and 16.9 months in the group receiving chemoradiotherapy preoperatively. Survival at 3 years was 16% in the surgery-alone arm and 30% in those receiving neoadjuvant chemoradiotherapy ($P = 0.15$). This study was statistically powered to detect a relatively large increase in median survival from 1 year to 2.2 years, with at least 80% power. Urba et al. concluded that this randomized trial of preoperative chemoradiation versus surgery alone for patients with potentially resectable esophageal carcinoma did not demonstrate a statistically significant survival difference but did show a trend toward improved survival in the chemoradiotherapy group. Additionally, their data suggested that patients with complete pathological response had the most benefit in survival.

TABLE 27.6
Randomized Controlled Trials of Neoadjuvant Chemoradiotherapy versus Surgery Alone for Esophageal Cancer [a]

Study/year published	Histology	TA/CA	MS TA/CA *P* value	3-Year OS (%) TA/CA *P* value	Chemotherapy	XRT (Gy) (total dose)
Nygaard 1992	SCC	47/41			Cisplatin/bleomycin	35
Apinop 1994	SCC	35/34			Cisplatin/5-FU	40
Le Prise 1994	SCC	41/45			Cisplatin/5-FU	20
Walsh 1996[b]	AC	58/55	16/11 $P = 0.01$	32/6 $P = 0.01$	Cisplatin/5-FU	40
Bosset 1997	SCC	143/139	18.6/18.6 NS		Cisplatin	37
Urba 2001	AC/SCC	50/50	16.9/17.6 NS	30/15 NS	Cisplatin/5-FU/ vinblastine	45
Lee 2004	SCC	51/50	28.2/27.3 NS		Cisplatin/5-FU	45.6
Burmeister 2005	Any	128/128			Cisplatin/5-FU	35

Abbreviations: [a]TA = treatment arm; CA = control arm; MS = median survival (months); OS = overall survival; XRT = radiotherapy; SCC = squamous cell carcinoma; AC = adenocarcinoma; NS = not significant.
[b]Trial with statistically significant improved overall survival and median survival.

Several meta-analyses have been published regarding neoadjuvant chemoradiotherapy (95–99), the most recent (98) concluding that neoadjuvant chemoradiotherapy provided a survival benefit of 19% (OR 0.81; 95% CI 0.7–0.93; P = 0.002) over surgery alone. Survival advantage results for different histological subtypes were as follows: SCC 16% (OR 0.84; CI 0.71–0.99; P = 0.04) and AC 25% (OR 0.75; CI 0.59–0.95; P = 0.02). Preoperative chemotherapy that was followed sequentially by radiotherapy did not show a statistically significant survival benefit, whereas synchronous delivery of chemoradiotherapy showed a survival benefit (OR 0.76; CI 0.59–0.98; P = 0.02) (98,100).

Features common in trials evaluating neoadjuvant chemoradiotherapy were: (1) increases in complete surgical resection as a result of tumor downstaging by chemoradiotherapy, (2) patients who responded had better survival, (3) no tumor residue present in surgical samples in a quarter of patients after neoadjuvant chemoradiotherapy, and (4) no significant increase in postoperative morbidity and mortality after neoadjuvant chemoradiotherapy. In a trial considering only locally advanced tumors (T3), a large case control study showed a significant survival benefit for neoadjuvant chemoradiotherapy (100).

Given the heterogeneity of chemotherapy regimens and radiation dosing, as well as the lack of statistical significance of the various underpowered trials, the meta-analyses should be viewed as the authority in decision making until results from more definitive and statistically significant trials are available.

TREATMENT WITHOUT SURGERY

The high incidence of postoperative complications, the differences in interpatient resectability, and few long-term survivors have led to several trials evaluating the necessity of undergoing esophagectomy at all.

Radiotherapy Alone versus Surgery Alone

Preliminary results of a randomized trial comparing surgery alone with hyperfractionated accelerated radiotherapy for SCC showed similar 5-year survival of 35% versus 37%, respectively (P = 0.58). Final results are awaited since precise information on staging and surgical quality are yet to be provided. (101). Other trials comparing primary radiotherapy alone with surgery alone have been conducted (102–104). Earlam et al. abandoned the trial because of poor patient recruitment (102). Fok et al. randomized 84 patients to receive surgery alone or radiotherapy alone (45–53Gy) (104). Median survival was 9 months versus 22 months, respectively. Badwe et al., after randomizing 99 patients to surgery or radiotherapy (50 Gy), reported that outcome in terms of dysphagia relief and survival was inferior to surgery alone (103).

Definitive Chemoradiotherapy

Chemotherapy in conjunction with radiation without planned esophagectomy is referred to as definitive chemoradiotherapy. In phase II trials investigating chemoradiotherapy alone, local control varied from 40% to 75%, median overall survival from 9 to 24 months, and 5-year survival from 18% to 40% (105–110).

Chemoradiotherapy Alone versus Radiotherapy Alone

Roussel et al. reported no survival advantage in 144 patients randomized to either radiotherapy alone or single-agent methotrexate chemotherapy and radiotherapy (56 Gy) (111). Similarly, Slabber et al. showed no significant difference in 70 patients with stage III esophageal cancer randomized to chemoradiotherapy (cisplatin/5-FU) versus radiotherapy alone (112). A definitive trial using radiation (50 Gy in 5 weeks) combined with 4 cycles of chemotherapy (5-FU/cisplatin) was compared with radiotherapy alone (64 Gy) in 121 patients in the RTOG-8501 trial (113). Median survival was 12.5 versus 8.9 months, and 2-year survival was 38% versus 10%, respectively ($P = 0.005$). There was no difference seen in SCC versus AC subtypes. Grade 3 to 4 toxic effects were higher in the chemoradiotherapy arm compared to the radiotherapy-alone arm (66% vs. 28%, respectively). A similar study compared radiotherapy alone (50 Gy) with radiotherapy plus 1 cycle of 5-FU-bleomycin-mitomycin that produced similar results to those reported by Hersckovic et al. (114). A 5-year follow-up to the RTOG-8501 trial reported that 26% of those treated by chemoradiotherapy were alive, while none of those treated by radiotherapy alone survived (115). A recent meta-analysis of 13 randomized trials comparing radiotherapy alone versus chemoradiotherapy alone confirmed that chemoradiotherapy is better (116). Chemoradiotherapy provided a significant overall reduction in mortality at 1 to 2 years, an absolute reduction in mortality by 7%, and a reduction in either the presence of tumor cells in the esophageal lumen after completion of chemoradiotherapy or in recurrence by 12%. There was, however, an absolute increase in grade 3 to 4 toxic effects by 17%.

On the basis of available, albeit heterogeneous, studies, chemoradiotherapy alone provides better results than radiotherapy alone, with acceptable tolerability. Clearly, radiotherapy alone is inferior to surgery alone, as already seen in the previously reported randomized trials. Definitive chemoradiotherapy alone (with cisplatin-based and adequate radiation dose) is suitable as the standard treatment for nonoperable patients without distant metastases. However, as reported by Herskovic et al., residual tumor was seen in 40% of patients in the chemoradiotherapy arm, the majority of which had early-stage disease (92% with T1–T2 tumors and 82% with N0), suggesting that additional surgery could have improved overall survival in those patients who were able to undergo surgery (113).

Chemoradiotherapy Alone versus Neoadjuvant Chemoradiotherapy

Two phase III multicenter trials (Table 27.7) compared definitive chemoradiotherapy versus neoadjuvant chemoradiotherapy for locally advanced esophageal tumors (T3–T4, N0–N1) (117,118). The first included 177 patients with SCC tumors (117). All patients received induction chemotherapy with bolus 5-FU/leucovorin/etoposide/cisplatin every 3 weeks for 3 cycles. The patients in the surgery group underwent subsequent chemoradiotherapy (cisplatin/etoposide/45 Gy) followed by surgery. The definitive chemoradiotherapy arm received chemoradiotherapy (cisplatin/etoposide/65 Gy) after induction chemotherapy and then more chemoradiotherapy (cisplatin/etoposide/40 Gy). Although there was a trend in the group undergoing surgery toward better results than definitive chemoradiotherapy, this was not significant (median overall survival 16 vs. 15 months; 3-year survival 28% vs. 20%, respectively; $P = 0.22$). Hospital mortality was 10% in the surgery group versus 4% in the definitive chemoradiotherapy arm. Patients who responded to chemoradiotherapy had a >50% life expectancy at 3 years. However, those patients who did not

TABLE 27.7
Randomized Controlled Trials of Definitive Chemoradiotherapy versus Neoadjuvant Chemoradiotherapy for Esophageal Cancer [a]

Study/year published	Histology	TA/CA	MS TA/CA	Chemotherapy	XRT (Gy) (total dose)
Stahl 2005	SCC	86/86	16.4/14.9 NS	Cisplatin/5-FU/ etoposide	40 control 65 definitive
Bedenne 2007	SCC	129/130	19.3/17.7 NS	Cisplatin/5-FU	Induction: 46 or 15 split course Definitive: 20 or 15 split course

Abbreviations: [a]TA = treatment arm; CA = control arm; MS = median survival (months); XRT = radiotherapy; SCC = squamous cell carcinoma.

respond to induction chemotherapy had a better 3-year survival if they then went on to surgery versus those who did not (32% vs. 11%, respectively). Local progression free survival was better in the surgery group (64.3% vs. 40.7%, *P* = 0.003), but again, median overall survival and 3-year survival differences were not significant.

Bedenne et al. randomized 259 patients, mostly with SCC. All patients received 2 cycles of induction therapy with 5-FU/cisplatin/and radiotherapy (46 Gy). If there was less than a partial response to this induction, patients went on to surgery. If there was a partial response or better to induction, then patients were randomized to either surgery or 3 more cycles of the same chemotherapy with radiotherapy (20 Gy). There was no difference in median overall survival (17.7 vs. 19.3 months, respectively) or 2-year overall survival (34% vs. 40%, *P* = 0.56) between the groups. There was a significant difference between hospital mortality in the surgery versus no-surgery arms (9.3% vs. 0.8%, *P*= 0.002, respectively) and cumulative lengths of hospitalization (68 days vs. 52 days, *P* = 0.02, respectively). Progression-free survival at 2 years was better in the surgery group (64.3% vs. 40.7%, *P* = 0.003). The need for palliative procedures for dysphagia was higher in the nonsurgical group (46% vs, 24%, *P* > 0.0001). Quality of life was similar between the groups (119).

These recent studies raise the question of the necessity of surgery or, rather, who will benefit most from it. Response to neoadjuvant treatment identifies a group of patients that will do well with or without surgery. It has been suggested that patients with SCC who respond to induction chemoradiotherapy are the best candidates for definitive chemoradiotherapy (50). However, further studies using updated techniques to ascertain pathological complete response, the best marker of long-term survival, by using PET and/or biological markers need to be conducted.

OPTIMAL RADIATION DOSING

The question of the optimal radiation dose ranging from 20 to 64.8 Gy has been evaluated over time in the settings of radiation alone, neoadjuvant or adjuvant radiation, and combined neoadjuvant or definitive chemoradiotherapy. Higher doses have the advantage of improved tumor downstaging and eradication of the primary tumor and regional lymph node involvement at the expense of increased toxicity. Using modern radiation techniques, namely, intensity modulated radiotherapy and fractionated stereotactic radiotherapy, it is possible to use higher doses of radiation with acceptable toxicity profiles (120). The RTOG 85-01 trial discussed previously (107,109, 115) compared cisplatin/5-FU in combination with radiation (50 Gy in 5 weeks) versus radiation alone (64 Gy in 6.5 weeks). Median survival was 12.5 versus 8.9 months, and 2-year survival was 38% versus 10%, respectively. There was no difference seen in SCC versus AC subtypes. Minsky et al., in the phase III INT 0123 trial, reported similar findings comparing 50.4 Gy in 5 weeks versus 64.8 Gy in 6.5 weeks, confirming that higher doses of radiation used with chemotherapy does not improve local control rates or survival but does increase toxicity and mortality (121,122). Split course of radiotherapy (2 courses of 20 Gy in 5 fractions) had a significantly lower local control, 2-year survival, and disease-free survival than standard dosing schedules (Jacob Proc Am Assoc Cancer Res, abstr 1999[**B2**]). Thus, 50.4 Gy is considered the standard radiation dose in combined neoadjuvant chemoradiotherapy. It should be noted, therefore, that the majority of trials evaluating neoadjuvant chemoradiotherapy as discussed previously have used lower inadequate radiation doses, and the survival data should be viewed with this in mind.

GEJ TUMORS

As mentioned, the incidence of distal esophageal cancer and esophagastric cancer has increased significantly in recent decades. The classification and treatment approaches of GEJ AC over the years have been confusing. One factor contributing to this uncertainty is the debate concerning the definition of the GEJ, where it is located, and where the gastric cardia and subcardia begin (12,13). The GEJ is defined differently by anatomists, physiologists, endoscopists, and pathologists—accounting for the difficulty in classifying and treating cancers arising from this region. A common criterion observed by endoscopists indicated that the GEJ arises at the point where the tubular esophagus flares to become the sac-like stomach at the proximal margin of the gastric folds (13). However, peristaltic activity and movement with respiration render this task a difficult one for the endoscopist. Histologically, the gastric cardia has a distinct pattern that can be easily distinguished from the fundic-type epithelium in addition to the proximal squamous epithelium of the distal esophagus. It has been suggested that the definition of the GEJ be the squamocolumnar junction (SCJ). However, as the SCJ can shift proximally in the setting of Barrett's metaplasia, others argue that this is an incorrect reference point (13).

Stemming from the debate as to the exact definition of the GEJ is the controversy regarding the classification and treatment of AC arising in this general location (12). It is generally accepted that the tumors of debate are those arising from within 5 cm proximally and distally of the GEJ. The most widely adopted classification system for AC arising in the proximity of the esophagogastric junction is as follows: type I—the distal esophagus arising from an area with specialized intestinal metaplasia of the esophagus between 2 and 5 cm and can infiltrate the GEJ from above; type II—true carcinoma of the cardia arising from the cardia epithelium; and type III—subcardial gastric carcinoma that can infiltrate the GEJ from below (12).

Type I tumors are believed to be a distinct entity that should be treated as a distal esophageal cancer. These are the subtypes that arise in the setting of Barrett's metaplasia secondary to chronic gastric reflux. Studies have shown that these patients benefit from a transthoracic surgical approach, as the lymph node drainage is usually toward lower mediastinal and upper gastric lymph nodes. On the other hand, type III GEJ tumors are defined as 2 to 5 cm distal to the GEJ and behave more like proximal gastric cancer; the surgical approach, therefore, is usually as such, with a total gastrectomy. Type II tumors, defined as within 1 cm proximally and 2 cm distally from the GEJ, also tend to behave more like gastric carcinoma, and only approximately 10% of these tumors are associated with Barrett's metaplasia. There is support for classifying and treating type II tumors more like gastric cancer in the lymphatic drainage pathways. Types II and III tend to drain preferentially to the celiac axis nodes and have a much higher incidence of intra-abdominal metastases during laparoscopic staging (26% in type II/III vs. 6% in type I). Differences in genetic profiles of the various subtypes have been examined in an attempt to find definitive evidence that these tumors are indeed distinct from one another. However, to date, no obvious gene expression changes have been consistently identified, other than COX-2, which is overexpressed in distal esophageal AC (type I GEJ) only, and level of expression is an independent prognostic factor for survival (12).

Multimodality Therapy of the GEJ

Neoadjuvant Chemotherapy of the GEJ

Many phase II trials have looked at a variety of chemotherapy combinations for GEJ AC, and they generally suggest that neoadjuvant chemotherapy is beneficial (123–127). Cisplatin-based regimens have been shown to significantly improve survival compared to those patients who do not receive chemotherapy neoadjuvantly (128). Another regimen includes FAMTX (5-FU, doxorubicin, and methotrexate), which has been used as the reference treatment to which newer regimens are compared. A recent trial looked at ECF compared to FAMTX with improved response rates and 2-year survival (13.5% vs. 5.4%, respectively) (129) (Table 27.8). More recently, the MAGIC trial gave perioperative ECF (3 cycles before and 3 cycles after surgery) compared with surgery alone (82). The perioperative chemotherapy group had a higher overall survival and progression-free survival; the 5-year survival was 36% in the chemotherapy group versus 23% in the group undergoing surgery alone (82). Irinotecan has also shown benefit in the neoadjuvant setting, as seen in a phase II trial (130).

Neoadjuvant Chemoradiotherapy of the GEJ

Many of the trials and meta-analyses discussed in the previous sections included patients with GEJ AC. However, the majority of patients in these trials had SCC rather than AC in the proximal esophagus. Therefore, it is difficult to extrapolate the findings of these

TABLE 27.8
Neoadjuvant Chemotherapy of Gastroesophageal Junction Tumors [a]

Study/year published	Patients	Chemotherapy Arm A Arm B	RR	*P* value	Median survival	*P* value
Webb 1997[b]	274	ECF	45%	$P < 0.0002$	8.9	$P < 0.0009$
		FAMTX	21%		5.7	
		Chemotherapy versus surgery		**HR for PD**	**HR for OS**	
Cunningham 2006b	250 253	ECF surgery alone	0.66	$P < 0.001$	0.75	$P < 0.0009$

Abbreviations: [a]RR = response rates; ECF = epirubicin, cisplatin, 5-FU; FAMTX = 5-FU, doxorubicin, methotrexate; HR = hazard ratio; PD = progressive disease; OS = overall survival.
[b]Trial with statistically significant improved overall survival and progression-free survival.

studies specifically to the group of patients with GEJ tumors. One study of note, however, is that conducted by Walsh et al., in which they looked at 113 patients with predominantly lower esophageal and cardia AC (89). As discussed earlier, multimodality therapy was found to be superior to surgery alone for resectable AC of the esophagus. In fact, this is one of the few randomized trials evaluating neoadjuvant chemoradiotherapy that did show a statistically significant benefit in end points, leading some to the conclusion that AC histology may be the group of esophageal cancer patients that obtains the most benefit from multimodality therapy in the neoadjuvant setting. Clearly, more studies are needed to obtain a more definitive answer to the question of combined chemoradiotherapy in the neoadjuvant setting. As mentioned earlier, the combinations of chemoradiotherapy with novel targeted agents such as antiangiogenesis drugs and growth factor receptor inhibitors are being evaluated in clinical trials, and the results are eagerly awaited.

Adjuvant Therapy of the GEJ

After gastric resection with curative intent, there remains a 40% to 60% chance of local or regional recurrence in the gastric remnant or tumor bed, anastomosis, or regional lymph nodes (12,131). As such, locally directed adjuvant therapy has been an important aspect of therapy for GEJ tumors (132,133). Adjuvant chemotherapy compared with surgery alone did not show significant benefit (134,135). On the other hand, survival was improved with adjuvant radiation alone or radiation in combination with chemotherapy (5-FU) (136). Macdonald et al., in the U.S. Intergroup 0116 study, looked at 556 patients with gastric cancer, of whom approximately 20% had GEJ tumors (83). The survival benefit for patients with adjuvant therapy was identical for both gastric and GEJ carcinomas. Three-year overall survival and disease-free survival were 52% and 49% in the chemoradiotherapy group, respectively, while in the surgery-alone group the rates were lower at 41% and 32%, respectively (83). More studies are required to help determine which patients are more likely to benefit from this approach to therapy of GEJ tumors.

In summary, GEJ tumors appear to be a distinct pathophysiologic entity, separate from esophageal and gastric carcinomas yet with similar features of each (12). Patients can be divided into 2 groups: resectable and unresectable. The goal, as discussed earlier, is R0 resection and adequate lymphadenectomy. It has been recommended that 25 lymph nodes be evaluated to adequately stage the tumor. Those with bulky tumors (T3, T4) and locally advanced tumors should receive multimodality therapy to assist the surgeon in obtaining the R0 resection. The controversial question raised by the 2 relevant trials (MAGIC and INT 0116) as to which patient should receive sole neoadjuvant therapy and adjuvant therapy with ECF versus adjuvant chemoradiotherapy is a matter of debate (82,83). Future trials should be aimed at determining the answer to this fundamental question for those patients with GEJ tumors.

CONCLUSION

Evaluation of available randomized trials allows several conclusions. The majority of patients with esophageal cancer have systemic disease at presentation, requiring systemic treatment. For those patients who are locally advanced at diagnosis, the available trials are heterogeneous and must be interpreted in light of the various chemotherapy drug regimens and dosages, radiation scheduling and dosages, and the particular stage of disease at diagnosis. Although immediate surgery still remains a standard treatment option, neoadjuvant chemoradiotherapy is a commonly used therapeutic approach in the United States because it appears to improve outcome based on the results of numerous phase II and underpowered phase III trials. Survival, as evidenced by several meta-analyses of the various trials, has not been improved by intensifying chemotherapy, increasing radiation dose above 50.4 Gy, or giving adjuvant chemotherapy or radiotherapy (which is generally poorly tolerated and thus lacks feasibility). Further improvements in outcome will depend on identifying novel targeted agents with limited additional toxicity, an improved understanding about optimal therapy for the different histologic subtypes (AC vs. SCC), more individualized selection of therapy, and early identification of responders with the use of PET and other modalities.

Marriette et al. propose the following strategies: surgery alone for stages I and IIa or in combination with neoadjuvant chemotherapy or chemoradiotherapy for stage IIb. For locally advanced tumors (stage III T3–T4, N1), AC should be treated with neoadjuvant chemotherapy or chemoradiotherapy followed by surgery, whereas SCCs that have shown response to induction therapy could be considered for chemoradiotherapy alone, with diligent surveillance posttreatment, to be considered for salvage esophagectomy in the case of recurrence. In addition, those patients with SCC without response to induction therapy or those with residual tumor after completed definitive chemoradiotherapy should undergo salvage esophagectomy. Swisher et al., however, have reported increased morbidity and mortality in those patients undergoing salvage esophagectomy (137).

Further research in upcoming years addressing where novel targeted biologic agents fit into the scheme of therapy for esophageal carcinoma is anticipated.

Identifying patients who will best benefit from neoadjuvant treatment, both chemotherapy and chemoradiotherapy, is an ultimate goal. Moreover, better predictors and assessment of complete pathological response after neoadjuvant/definitive therapy to avoid unnecessary surgery are anticipated.

References

1. Holmes RS, Vaughan TL. Epidemiology and pathogenesis of esophageal cancer. *Semin Radiat Oncol.* 2007;17:2–9.
2. Ozols RF, Herbst RS, Colson YL, et al. Clinical cancer advances 2006: major research advances in cancer treatment, prevention, and screening—a report from the American Society of Clinical Oncology. *J Clin Oncol.* 2007;25:146–162.
3. Powell J, McConkey CC. The rising trend in oesophageal adenocarcinoma and gastric cardia. *Eur J Cancer Prev.* 1992;1:265–269.
4. Devesa SS, Blot WJ, Fraumeni JF Jr. Changing patterns in the incidence of esophageal and gastric carcinoma in the United States. *Cancer.* 1998;83:2049–2053.
5. Blot WJ, Devesa SS, Kneller RW, et al. Rising incidence of adenocarcinoma of the esophagus and gastric cardia. *JAMA.* 1991;265:1287–1289.
6. Pera M, Cameron AJ, Trastek VF, et al. Increasing incidence of adenocarcinoma of the esophagus and esophagogastric junction. *Gastroenterology.* 1993;104:510–513.
7. Pye JK, Crumplin MK, Charles J, et al. One-year survey of carcinoma of the oesophagus and stomach in Wales. *Br J Surg.* 2001;88:278–285.
8. Maley CC. Open questions in oesophageal adenocarcinogenesis. *Gut.* 2007; 56:897–898.
9. Pace F, Pallotta S, Vakil N. Gastroesophageal reflux disease is a progressive disease. *Dig Liver Dis.* 2007;39:409–414.
10. Morales TG, Bhattacharyya A, Johnson C, et al. Is Barrett's esophagus associated with intestinal metaplasia of the gastric cardia? *Am J Gastroenterol.* 1997;92:1818–1822.
11. Schuchert MJ, Luketich JD. Barrett's esophagus-emerging concepts and controversies. *J Surg Oncol.* 2007;95:185–189.
12. Gee DW, Rattner DW. Management of gastroesophageal tumors. *Oncologist.* 2007; 12:175–185.
13. Marsman WA, Tytgat GN, ten Kate FJ, et al. Differences and similarities of adenocarcinomas of the esophagus and esophagogastric junction. *J Surg Oncol.* 2005;92:160–168.
14. von Rahden BH, Stein HJ, Siewert JR. Surgical management of esophagogastric junction tumors. *World J Gastroenterol.* 2006;12:6608–6613.
15. van Meerten E, van der Gaast A. Systemic treatment for oesophageal cancer. *Eur J Cancer.* 2005;41:664–672.
16. Lerut T. Oesophageal carcinoma—past and present studies. *Eur J Surg Oncol.* 1996;22:317–323.
17. Muller JM, Erasmi H, Stelzner M, et al. Surgical therapy of oesophageal carcinoma. *Br J Surg.* 1990;77:845–857.
18. Nishihira T, Hirayama K, Mori S. A prospective randomized trial of extended cervical and superior mediastinal lymphadenectomy for carcinoma of the thoracic esophagus. *Am J Surg.* 1998;175:47–51.
19. Altorki N, Skinner D. Should en bloc esophagectomy be the standard of care for esophageal carcinoma? *Ann Surg.* 2001;234:581–587.
20. Hulscher JB, van Sandick JW, de Boer AG, et al. Extended transthoracic resection compared with limited transhiatal resection for adenocarcinoma of the esophagus. *N Engl J Med.* 2002;347:1662–1669.
21. Mariette C, Taillier G, Van Seuningen I, et al. Factors affecting postoperative course and survival after en bloc resection for esophageal carcinoma. *Ann Thorac Surg.* 2004;78:1177–1183.
22. Cheng KK, Day NE, Davies TW. Oesophageal cancer mortality in Europe: paradoxical time trend in relation to smoking and drinking. *Br J Cancer.* 1992;65:613–617.
23. Luketich JD, Alvelo-Rivera M, Buenaventura PO, et al. Minimally invasive esophagectomy: outcomes in 222 patients. *Ann Surg.* 2003;238:486–494; discussion 94–95.
24. Mariette C, Piessen G, Balon JM, et al. Surgery alone in the curative treatment of localised oesophageal carcinoma. *Eur J Surg Oncol.* 2004;30:869–876.
25. Medical Research Council Esophageal Cancer Working Party. Surgical resection with or without preoperative chemotherapy in oesophageal cancer: a randomized controlled trial. *Lancet* 2002;359:1727–1733.
26. Albertsson M. Chemoradiotherapy of esophageal cancer. *Acta Oncol.* 2002;41:118–123.
27. Kleinberg L, Gibson MK, Forastiere AA. Chemoradiotherapy for localized esophageal cancer: regimen selection and molecular mechanisms of radiosensitization. *Nat Clin Pract Oncol.* 2007;4:282–294.
28. Shewach DS, Lawrence TS. Antimetabolite radiosensitizers. *J Clin Oncol.* 2007;25:4043–4050.
29. Vokes EE, Brizel DM, Lawrence TS. Concomitant chemoradiotherapy. *J Clin Oncol.* 2007;25:4031–4032.
30. Harari PM, Allen GW, Bonner JA. Biology of interactions: antiepidermal growth factor receptor agents. *J Clin Oncol.* 2007;25:4057–4065.
31. Duda DG, Jain RK, Willett CG. Antiangiogenics: the potential role of integrating this novel treatment modality with chemoradiation for solid cancers. *J Clin Oncol.* 2007;25:4033–4042.
32. Camphausen K, Tofilon PJ. Inhibition of histone deacetylation: a strategy for tumor radiosensitization. *J Clin Oncol.* 2007;25:4051–4056.
33. Advani SJ, Weichselbaum RR, Chmura SJ. Enhancing radiotherapy with genetically engineered viruses. *J Clin Oncol.* 2007;25:4090–4095.
34. Overgaard J. Hypoxic radiosensitization: adored and ignored. *J Clin Oncol.* 2007;25:4066–4074.
35. Seto Y, Chin K, Gomi K, et al. Treatment of thoracic esophageal carcinoma invading adjacent structures. *Cancer Sci.* 2007;98:937–942.
36. Forastiere AA, Heitmiller RF, Lee DJ, et al. Intensive chemoradiation followed by esophagectomy for squamous cell and adenocarcinoma of the esophagus. *Cancer J Sci Am.* 1997;3:144–152.
37. Brucher BL, Becker K, Lordick F, et al. The clinical impact of histopathologic response assessment by residual tumor cell quantification in esophageal squamous cell carcinomas. *Cancer.* 2006;106:2119–2127.
38. Swisher SG, Hofstetter W, Wu TT, et al. Proposed revision of the esophageal cancer staging system to accommodate pathologic response (pP) following preoperative chemoradiation (CRT). *Ann Surg.* 2005;241:810–817; discussion 7–20.
39. Ott K, Weber WA, Lordick F, et al. Metabolic imaging predicts response, survival, and recurrence in adenocarcinomas of the esophagogastric junction. *J Clin Oncol.* 2006;24:4692–4698.
40. Song SY, Kim JH, Ryu JS, et al. FDG-PET in the prediction of pathologic response after neoadjuvant chemoradiotherapy in locally advanced, resectable esophageal cancer. *Int J Radiat Oncol Biol Phys.* 2005;63:1053–1059.
41. Wieder HA, Brucher BL, Zimmermann F, et al. Time course of tumor metabolic activity during chemoradiotherapy of esophageal squamous cell carcinoma and response to treatment. *J Clin Oncol.* 2004;22:900–908.
42. Ribeiro A, Franceschi D, Parra J, et al. Endoscopic ultrasound restaging after neoadjuvant chemotherapy in esophageal cancer. *Am J Gastroenterol.* 2006;101: 1216–1221.
43. McKian KP, Miller RC, Cassivi SD, et al. Curing patients with locally advanced esophageal cancer: an update on multimodality therapy. *Dis Esophagus.* 2006;19:448–453.
44. Naughton P, Walsh TN. Multimodality therapy for cancers of the esophagus and gastric cardia. *Expert Rev Anticancer Ther.* 2004;4:141–150.
45. Visser BC, Venook AP, Patti MG. Adjuvant and neoadjuvant therapy for esophageal cancer: a critical reappraisal. *Surg Oncol.* 2003;12:1–7.
46. Mooney MM. Neoadjuvant and adjuvant chemotherapy for esophageal adenocarcinoma. *J Surg Oncol.* 2005;92:230–238.
47. Varadhachary G, Ajani JA. Preoperative and adjuvant therapies for upper gastrointestinal cancers. *Expert Rev Anticancer Ther.* 2005;5:719–725.
48. Lordick F, Stein HJ, Peschel C, et al. Neoadjuvant therapy for oesophagogastric cancer. *Br J Surg.* 2004;91:540–551.
49. Shinoda M, Hatooka S, Mori S, et al. Clinical aspects of multimodality therapy for resectable locoregional esophageal cancer. *Ann Thorac Cardiovasc Surg.* 2006;12:234–241.
50. Mariette C, Piessen G, Triboulet JP. Therapeutic strategies in oesophageal carcinoma: role of surgery and other modalities. *Lancet Oncol.* 2007;8:545–553.
51. Graham AJ, Shrive FM, Ghali WA, et al. Defining the optimal treatment of locally advanced esophageal cancer: a systematic review and decision analysis. *Ann Thorac Surg.* 2007;83:1257–1264.
52. Kleinberg L, Forastiere AA. Chemoradiation in the management of esophageal cancer. *J Clin Oncol.* 2007;25:4110–4117.
53. Fok M, Sham JS, Choy D, Cheng SW, et al. Postoperative radiotherapy for carcinoma of the esophagus: a prospective, randomized controlled study. *Surgery.* 1993;113:138–147.
54. Kelsen DP, Ginsberg R, Pajak TF, et al. Chemotherapy followed by surgery compared with surgery alone for localized esophageal cancer. *N Engl J Med.* 1998;339:1979–1984.
55. Ajani J, Bekaii-Saab T, D'Amico TA, et al. Esophageal cancer clinical practice guidelines. *J Natl Compr Cancer Netw.* 2006;4:328–347.
56. Kunath U, Fischer P. [Radical nature and life expectancy in the surgical treatment of esophageal and cardial carcinoma]. *Dtsch Med Wochenschr.* 1984;109:450–453.
57. Teniere P, Hay JM, Fingerhut A, et al. Postoperative radiation therapy does not increase survival after curative resection for squamous cell carcinoma of the middle and lower esophagus as shown by a multicenter controlled trial. French University Association for Surgical Research. *Surg Gynecol Obstet.* 1991;173:123–130.
58. Zieren HU, Muller JM, Jacobi CA, et al. Adjuvant postoperative radiation therapy after curative resection of squamous cell carcinoma of the thoracic esophagus: a prospective randomized study. *World J Surg.* 1995;19:444–449.
59. Xiao ZF, Yang ZY, Liang J, et al. Value of radiotherapy after radical surgery for esophageal carcinoma: a report of 495 patients. *Ann Thorac Surg.* 2003;75:331–336.
60. Launois B, Delarue D, Campion JP, et al. Preoperative radiotherapy for carcinoma of the esophagus. *Surg Gynecol Obstet.* 1981;153:690–692.
61. Gignoux M, Roussel A, Paillot B, et al. The value of preoperative radiotherapy in esophageal cancer: results of a study of the E.O.R.T.C. *World J Surg.* 1987;11:426–432.

62. Wang M, Gu XZ, Yin WB, et al. Randomized clinical trial on the combination of preoperative irradiation and surgery in the treatment of esophageal carcinoma: report on 206 patients. *Int J Radiat Oncol Biol Phys.* 1989;16:325–327.
63. Arnott SJ, Duncan W, Kerr GR, et al. Low dose preoperative radiotherapy for carcinoma of the oesophagus: results of a randomized clinical trial. *Radiother Oncol.* 1992;24:108–113.
64. Nygaard K, Hagen S, Hansen HS, et al. Pre-operative radiotherapy prolongs survival in operable esophageal carcinoma: a randomized, multicenter study of pre-operative radiotherapy and chemotherapy. The second Scandinavian trial in esophageal cancer. *World J Surg.* 1992;16:1104–1109; discussion 10.
65. Arnott SJ, Duncan W, Gignoux M, et al. Preoperative radiotherapy for esophageal carcinoma. *Cochrane Database Syst Rev.* 2005:CD001799.
66. Ando N, Iizuka T, Kakegawa T, et al. A randomized trial of surgery with and without chemotherapy for localized squamous carcinoma of the thoracic esophagus: the Japan Clinical Oncology Group Study. *J Thorac Cardiovasc Surg.* 1997;114:205–209.
67. Ando N, Iizuka T, Ide H, et al. Surgery plus chemotherapy compared with surgery alone for localized squamous cell carcinoma of the thoracic esophagus: a Japan Clinical Oncology Group Study—JCOG9204. *J Clin Oncol.* 2003;21:4592–4596.
68. Pouliquen X, Levard H, Hay JM, et al. 5-Fluorouracil and cisplatin therapy after palliative surgical resection of squamous cell carcinoma of the esophagus: a multicenter randomized trial. French Associations for Surgical Research. *Ann Surg.* 1996;223:127–133.
69. Bhansali MS, Vaidya JS, Bhatt RG, et al. Chemotherapy for carcinoma of the esophagus: a comparison of evidence from meta-analyses of randomized trials and of historical control studies. *Ann Oncol.* 1996;7:355–359.
70. Ancona E, Ruol A, Santi S, et al. Only pathologic complete response to neoadjuvant chemotherapy improves significantly the long term survival of patients with resectable esophageal squamous cell carcinoma: final report of a randomized, controlled trial of preoperative chemotherapy versus surgery alone. *Cancer.* 2001;91:2165–2174.
71. Baba M, Natsugoe S, Shimada M, et al. Prospective evaluation of preoperative chemotherapy in resectable squamous cell carcinoma of the thoracic esophagus. *Dis Esophagus.* 2000;13:136–141.
72. Wang C, Ding T, Chang L. [A randomized clinical study of preoperative chemotherapy for esophageal carcinoma]. *Zhonghua Zhong Liu Za Zhi.* 2001;23:254–255.
73. Roth JA, Pass HI, Flanagan MM, et al. Randomized clinical trial of preoperative and postoperative adjuvant chemotherapy with cisplatin, vindesine, and bleomycin for carcinoma of the esophagus. *J Thorac Cardiovasc Surg.* 1988;96:242–248.
74. Schlag PM. Randomized trial of preoperative chemotherapy for squamous cell cancer of the esophagus. The Chirurgische Arbeitsgemeinschaft Fuer Onkologie der Deutschen Gesellschaft Fuer Chirurgie Study Group. *Arch Surg.* 1992;127:1446–1450.
75. Maipang T, Vasinanukorn P, Petpichetchian C, et al. Induction chemotherapy in the treatment of patients with carcinoma of the esophagus. *J Surg Oncol.* 1994;56:191–197.
76. Kok TC, Van der Gaast A, Dees J, et al. Cisplatin and etoposide in oesophageal cancer: a phase II study. Rotterdam Oesophageal Tumour Study Group. *Br J Cancer.* 1996;74:980–984.
77. Law S, Fok M, Chow S, et al. Preoperative chemotherapy versus surgical therapy alone for squamous cell carcinoma of the esophagus: a prospective randomized trial. *J Thorac Cardiovasc Surg.* 1997;114:210–217.
78. Kelsen DP, Winter KA, Gunderson LL, et al. Long-term results of RTOG trial 8911 (USA Intergroup 113): a random assignment trial comparison of chemotherapy followed by surgery compared with surgery alone for esophageal cancer. *J Clin Oncol.* 2007;25:3719–3725.
79. Urschel JD, Vasan H, Blewett CJ. A meta-analysis of randomized controlled trials that compared neoadjuvant chemotherapy and surgery to surgery alone for resectable esophageal cancer. *Am J Surg.* 2002;183:274–279.
80. Malthaner RA, Collin S, Fenlon D. Preoperative chemotherapy for resectable thoracic esophageal cancer. *Cochrane Database Syst Rev.* 2006;3:CD001556.
81. Saltz L, Kelsen D. Combined-modality therapy in the treatment of local-regional esophageal cancer. *Ann Oncol.* 1992;3:793–799.
82. Cunningham D, Allum WH, Stenning SP, et al. Perioperative chemotherapy versus surgery alone for resectable gastroesophageal cancer. *N Engl J Med.* 2006;355:11–20.
83. Macdonald JS, Smalley SR, Benedetti J, et al. Chemoradiotherapy after surgery compared with surgery alone for adenocarcinoma of the stomach or gastroesophageal junction. *N Engl J Med.* 2001;345:725–730.
84. Tordiglione M, Kalli M, Vavassori V, et al. Combined modality treatment for esophageal cancer. *Tumori.* 1998;84:252–258.
85. Fagerberg J, Stockeld D, Lewensohn R. Combined treatment modalities in esophageal cancer: should chemotherapy be included? *Acta Oncol.* 1994;33:439–450.
86. Bosset JF, Gignoux M, Triboulet JP, et al. Chemoradiotherapy followed by surgery compared with surgery alone in squamous-cell cancer of the esophagus. *N Engl J Med.* 1997;337:161–167.
87. Apinop C, Puttisak P, Preecha N. A prospective study of combined therapy in esophageal cancer. *Hepatogastroenterology.* 1994;41:391–393.
88. Le Prise E, Etienne PL, Meunier B, et al. A randomized study of chemotherapy, radiation therapy, and surgery versus surgery for localized squamous cell carcinoma of the esophagus. *Cancer.* 1994;73:1779–1784.
89. Walsh TN, Noonan N, Hollywood D, et al. A comparison of multimodal therapy and surgery for esophageal adenocarcinoma. *N Engl J Med.* 1996;335:462–467.
90. Urba SG, Orringer MB, Turrisi A, et al. Randomized trial of preoperative chemoradiation versus surgery alone in patients with locoregional esophageal carcinoma. *J Clin Oncol.* 2001;19:305–313.
91. Burmeister BH, Smithers BM, Gebski V, et al. Surgery alone versus chemoradiotherapy followed by surgery for resectable cancer of the oesophagus: a randomised controlled phase III trial. *Lancet Oncol.* 2005;6:659–668.
92. Lee JL, Park SI, Kim SB, et al. A single institutional phase III trial of preoperative chemotherapy with hyperfractionation radiotherapy plus surgery versus surgery alone for resectable esophageal squamous cell carcinoma. *Ann Oncol.* 2004;15:947–954.
93. Tepper JE, Krasna M, Niedzwiecki D, et al. Superiority of trimodality therapy to surgery alone in esophageal cancer: Results of CALGB 9781 [abstract]. *J Clin Oncol* 2006;24:181s.
94. Walsh TN, Grennell M, Mansoor S, et al. Neoadjuvant treatment of advanced stage esophageal adenocarcinoma increases survival. *Dis Esophagus.* 2002;15:121–124.
95. Urschel JD, Vasan H. A meta-analysis of randomized controlled trials that compared neoadjuvant chemoradiation and surgery to surgery alone for resectable esophageal cancer. *Am J Surg.* 2003;185:538–543.
96. Fiorica F, Di Bona D, Schepis F, et al. Preoperative chemoradiotherapy for oesophageal cancer: a systematic review and meta-analysis. *Gut.* 2004;53:925–930.
97. Kaklamanos IG, Walker GR, Ferry K, et al. Neoadjuvant treatment for resectable cancer of the esophagus and the gastroesophageal junction: a meta-analysis of randomized clinical trials. *Ann Surg Oncol.* 2003;10:754–761.
98. Gebski V, Burmeister B, Smithers BM, et al. Survival benefits from neoadjuvant chemoradiotherapy or chemotherapy in oesophageal carcinoma: a meta-analysis. *Lancet Oncol.* 2007;8:226–234.
99. Malthaner RA, Wong RK, Rumble RB, et al. Neoadjuvant or adjuvant therapy for resectable esophageal cancer: a systematic review and meta-analysis. *BMC Med.* 2004;2:35.
100. Mariette C, Piessen G, Lamblin A, et al. Impact of preoperative radiochemotherapy on postoperative course and survival in patients with locally advanced squamous cell oesophageal carcinoma. *Br J Surg.* 2006;93:1077–1083.
101. Yu J, Ren R, Sun X, et al. A randomized clinical study of surgery versus radiotherapy in the treatment of resectable esophageal cancer [Abstract 4013]. *Proc Am Soc Clin Oncol.* 2006;24:181s.
102. Earlam R. An MRC prospective randomised trial of radiotherapy versus surgery for operable squamous cell carcinoma of the oesophagus. *Ann R Coll Surg Engl.* 1991;73:8–12.
103. Badwe RA, Sharma V, Bhansali MS, et al. The quality of swallowing for patients with operable esophageal carcinoma: a randomized trial comparing surgery with radiotherapy. *Cancer.* 1999;85:763–768.
104. Fok M, Law SY, Wong J. Operable esophageal carcinoma: current results from Hong Kong. *World J Surg.* 1994;18:355–360.
105. Coia LR, Engstrom PF, Paul AR, et al. Long-term results of infusional 5-FU, mitomycin-C and radiation as primary management of esophageal carcinoma. *Int J Radiat Oncol Biol Phys.* 1991;20:29–36.
106. Leichman L, Herskovic A, Leichman CG, et al. Nonoperative therapy for squamous-cell cancer of the esophagus. *J Clin Oncol.* 1987;5:365–370.
107. al-Sarraf M, Martz K, Herskovic A, et al. Progress report of combined chemoradiotherapy versus radiotherapy alone in patients with esophageal cancer: an intergroup study. *J Clin Oncol.* 1997;15:277–284.
108. Seitz JF, Giovannini M, Padaut-Cesana J, et al. Inoperable nonmetastatic squamous cell carcinoma of the esophagus managed by concomitant chemotherapy (5-fluorouracil and cisplatin) and radiation therapy. *Cancer.* 1990;66:214–219.
109. Algan O, Coia LR, Keller SM, et al. Management of adenocarcinoma of the esophagus with chemoradiation alone or chemoradiation followed by esophagectomy: results of sequential nonrandomized phase II studies. *Int J Radiat Oncol Biol Phys.* 1995;32:753–761.
110. Denham JW, Burmeister BH, Lamb DS, et al. Factors influencing outcome following radio-chemotherapy for oesophageal cancer. The Trans Tasman Radiation Oncology Group (TROG). *Radiother Oncol.* 1996;40:31–43.
111. Roussel A, Jacob JH, Haegele P, et al. Controlled clinical trial for the treatment of patients with inoperable esophageal carcinoma: a study of the EORTC Gastrointestinal Tract Cancer Cooperative Group. *Recent Results Cancer Res.* 1988;110:21–29.
112. Slabber CF, Nel JS, Schoeman L, et al. A randomized study of radiotherapy alone versus radiotherapy plus 5-fluorouracil and platinum in patients with inoperable, locally advanced squamous cancer of the esophagus. *Am J Clin Oncol.* 1998;21:462–465.
113. Herskovic A, Martz K, al-Sarraf M, et al. Combined chemotherapy and radiotherapy compared with radiotherapy alone in patients with cancer of the esophagus. *N Engl J Med.* 1992;326:1593–1598.
114. Araujo CM, Souhami L, Gil RA, et al. A randomized trial comparing radiation therapy versus concomitant radiation therapy and chemotherapy in carcinoma of the thoracic esophagus. *Cancer.* 1991;67:2258–2261.
115. Cooper JS, Guo MD, Herskovic A, et al. Chemoradiotherapy of locally advanced esophageal cancer: long-term follow-up of a prospective randomized trial (RTOG 85-01). Radiation Therapy Oncology Group. *JAMA.* 1999;281:1623–1627.
116. Wong R, Malthaner R. Combined chemotherapy and radiotherapy (without surgery) compared with radiotherapy alone in localized carcinoma of the esophagus. *Cochrane Database Syst Rev.* 2006:CD002092.
117. Stahl M, Stuschke M, Lehmann N, et al. Chemoradiation with and without surgery in patients with locally advanced squamous cell carcinoma of the esophagus. *J Clin Oncol.* 2005;23:2310–2317.
118. Bedenne L, Michel P, Bouche O, et al. Chemoradiation followed by surgery compared with chemoradiation alone in squamous cancer of the esophagus: FFCD 9102. *J Clin Oncol.* 2007;25:1160–1168.

119. Bonnetain F, Bouche O, Michel P, et al. A comparative longitudinal quality of life study using the Spitzer quality of life index in a randomized multicenter phase III trial (FFCD 9102): chemoradiation followed by surgery compared with chemoradiation alone in locally advanced squamous resectable thoracic esophageal cancer. *Ann Oncol.* 2006;17:827–834.
120. Taremi M, Ringash J, Dawson LA. Upper abdominal malignancies: intensity-modulated radiation therapy. *Front Radiat Ther Oncol.* 2007;40:272–288.
121. Minsky BD, Neuberg D, Kelsen DP, et al. Final report of Intergroup Trial 0122 (ECOG PE-289, RTOG 90–12): phase II trial of neoadjuvant chemotherapy plus concurrent chemotherapy and high-dose radiation for squamous cell carcinoma of the esophagus. *Int J Radiat Oncol Biol Phys.* 1999;43:517–523.
122. Minsky BD, Pajak TF, Ginsberg RJ, et al. INT 0123 (Radiation Therapy Oncology Group 94–05) phase III trial of combined-modality therapy for esophageal cancer: high-dose versus standard-dose radiation therapy. *J Clin Oncol.* 2002;20:1167–1174.
123. Plukker JT, Mulder NH, Sleijfer DT, et al. Chemotherapy and surgery for locally advanced cancer of the cardia and fundus: phase II study with methotrexate and 5-fluorouracil. *Br J Surg.* 1991;78:955–958.
124. Plukker JT, Sleijfer DT, Verschueren RC, et al. Neo-adjuvant chemotherapy with carboplatin, 4-epiadriamycin and teniposide (CET) in locally advanced cancer of the cardia and the lower oesophagus: a phase II study. *Anticancer Res.* 1995;15:2357–2361.
125. Rougier P, Mahjoubi M, Lasser P, et al. Neoadjuvant chemotherapy in locally advanced gastric carcinoma—a phase II trial with combined continuous intravenous 5-fluorouracil and bolus cisplatinum. *Eur J Cancer.* 1994;30A:1269–1275.
126. Melcher AA, Mort D, Maughan TS. Epirubicin, cisplatin and continuous infusion 5-fluorouracil (ECF) as neoadjuvant chemotherapy in gastro-oesophageal cancer. *Br J Cancer.* 1996;74:1651–1654.
127. Waters JS, Norman A, Cunningham D, et al. Long-term survival after epirubicin, cisplatin and fluorouracil for gastric cancer: results of a randomized trial. *Br J Cancer.* 1999;80:269–272.
128. Siewert JR, Stein HJ, Sendler A, et al. Surgical resection for cancer of the cardia. *Semin Surg Oncol.* 1999;17:125–131.
129. Webb A, Cunningham D, Scarffe JH, et al. Randomized trial comparing epirubicin, cisplatin, and fluorouracil versus fluorouracil, doxorubicin, and methotrexate in advanced esophagogastric cancer. *J Clin Oncol.* 1997;15:261–267.
130. Pozzo C, Barone C, Szanto J, et al. Irinotecan in combination with 5-fluorouracil and folinic acid or with cisplatin in patients with advanced gastric or esophageal-gastric junction adenocarcinoma: results of a randomized phase II study. *Ann Oncol.* 2004;15:1773–1781.
131. Landry J, Tepper JE, Wood WC, et al. Patterns of failure following curative resection of gastric carcinoma. *Int J Radiat Oncol Biol Phys.* 1990;19:1357–1362.
132. Ku GY, Ilson DH. Esophageal cancer: adjuvant therapy. *Cancer J.* 2007;13:162–167.
133. Hundahl SA, Phillips JL, Menck HR. The National Cancer Data Base Report on poor survival of U.S. gastric carcinoma patients treated with gastrectomy: Fifth Edition American Joint Committee on Cancer staging, proximal disease, and the "different disease" hypothesis. *Cancer.* 2000;88:921–932.
134. Hermans J, Bonenkamp JJ, Boon MC, et al. Adjuvant therapy after curative resection for gastric cancer: meta-analysis of randomized trials. *J Clin Oncol.* 1993;11:1441–1447.
135. Earle CC, Maroun JA. Adjuvant chemotherapy after curative resection for gastric cancer in non-Asian patients: revisiting a meta-analysis of randomised trials. *Eur J Cancer.* 1999;35:1059–1064.
136. Moertel CG, Childs DS, O'Fallon JR, et al. Combined 5-fluorouracil and radiation therapy as a surgical adjuvant for poor prognosis gastric carcinoma. *J Clin Oncol.* 1984;2:1249–1254.
137. Swisher SG, Wynn P, Putnam JB, et al. Salvage esophagectomy for recurrent tumors after definitive chemotherapy and radiotherapy. *J Thorac Cardiovasc Surg.* 2002;123:175–183.

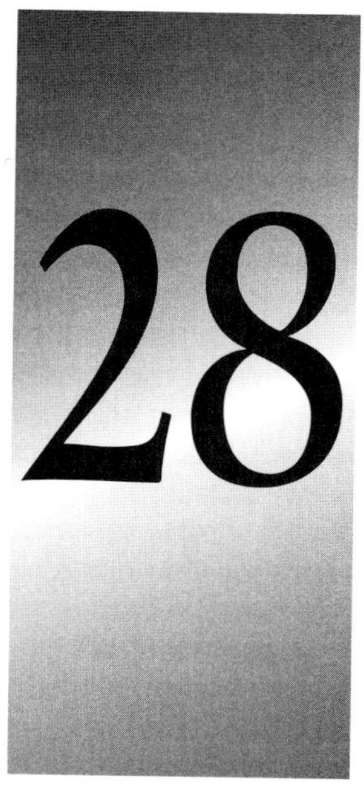

28 Principles of Chemotherapy

Syma Iqbal
Lawrence Leichman

Effective systemic treatment of cancer has roots in the wartime observation that humans exposed to mustard gas developed bone marrow lymphoid hypoplasia. This led to the first clinical tests and publications of results using alkylating agents against Hodgkin's disease and lymphomas in the 1940s (1,2). At about the same time, Sidney Farber noted that targeting folic acid with 4-amethopteroylglutamic acid (aminopterin) was an effective strategy for the treatment of acute lymphoblastic leukemia in children (3). A clear understanding of aminopterin's action and its potential to treat cancer ushered in the first class of "targeted" chemotherapeutic agents known as antimetabolites. With the exception of spindle inhibitors such as vinca alkaloids and taxanes, the newer classes of compounds (i.e., anthracylcines, topoisomerase I and topoisomerase inhibitors, alkylating agents, and the platinum compounds) act similarly to alkylating agents by interrupting the structural integrity of DNA.

The newer and ever-growing number of modern "targeted agents" are directed against specific driving forces of tumor growth, such as epidermal growth factor receptors (EGFR) and vascular endothelial growth factor receptors (VEGFR) and those molecules within the tumor cell affected by these receptors. Overall, the efficacy of any particular targeted agent depends on whether the agent can be delivered to its target and whether that target is the major driving force behind that particular tumor's growth and reproduction. To achieve the goal of individualizing cancer therapy, it will be necessary to match the systemic agent to the molecular target(s) that drive the patient's cancer cells to immortality.

THEORY

Tumor Cell Growth Kinetics

The experimental murine L1210 leukemia model has served to establish the concept that systemic chemotherapeutic agents kill cells in a logarithmic pattern. Chemotherapy kills a constant percentage of cells, not a constant number. In a sensitive, rapidly growing experimental cell line, the ability to achieve cure is directly related to the tumor burden. In animals with rapidly growing, experimental tumors, the ability to retreat before viable but sensitive tumor cells regrow is essential. Of course, initial and subsequent doses of chemotherapy must that allow for the maintenance of the animal's non-tumor cells (4).

Human tumors do not grow exponentially. Instead, human tumors grow by what is known as the Gompertzian kinetics. In the Gompertzian model, the growth fraction of the tumor is not a constant but a function the number of cells in the tumor system. The growth fraction of human tumors is highest when tumor burden is low; the growth fraction exponentially decreases at the highest tumor burdens. By the Gompertzian model, for drug-sensitive tumors, depth of response to a particular systemic agent will depend on whether tumor cells are in a rapid or slow portion of the growth curve (5). Clinically undetectable tumors will be growing more rapidly than grossly visible tumors.

Using the Gompertzian model, Norton noted that relapse-free and overall survival for patients treated for breast cancer will not differ if microscopic residual disease is 1 cell or 1 million cells (6). Thus, efforts to reduce host toxicity by planning a priori dose reductions in chemotherapy treatments in the adjuvant or neoadjuvant settings could result in decreasing overall cure rates.

Tumor Mutation

Tumors mutate as they grow. Current concepts in scheduling chemotherapy and for using drug non–cross resistant drug combination are based largely on observations of spontaneous mutations noted in the unchecked growth of *Escherichia coli* colonies (7). Goldie and Coldman developed a mathematic model designed to explain drug sensitivity of a tumor using the tumor's spontaneous mutation rate. They postulated that over time (1) untreated tumors will increase not only in absolute numbers but also in the number of resistant cells, (2) the number of resistant cells of tumors with same number of cells is a function of the mutational rate intrinsic to that tumor system, and (3) tumors develop mutational resistance to chemotherapy early in their biologic lives within a host (8). The Goldie-Coldman theory laid the groundwork for dose-intense, dose-dense combination chemotherapy in the adjuvant therapy of solid tumors.

Building on the Goldie-Coldman theory, Norton developed a mathematical model for tumor growth, suggesting that tumors from the same primary source will not mutate in a "symmetrical" fashion. Norton's theory stated that the most effective combination of agents avoid significant reductions of each drug in the combination. Moreover, combinations therapy will be most effective if delivered in a dose-intense and dose-dense schedule. Perhaps, less intuitively, Norton's model postulated that effective combinations should *not* be alternated after only 1 cycle but delivered for a number of cycles before initiating another effective combination (9). Norton's theory appears to have been validated in the postoperative adjuvant treatment combination therapy for patients with node-positive breast cancer (10).

MOLECULAR MECHANISMS UNDERLYING SENSITIVITY AND RESISTANCE TO CHEMOTHERAPY

Understanding the molecular mechanisms that make tumor cells unique from normal cells has provided insight into the failure of current chemotherapeutic agents to act in ways predicted by tumor cell kinetic theory. The process of programmed cell death known as apoptosis involves a cascade of an intricate signal transduction network that is stimulated by a death-inducing signal. The key to cancer cell immortality and resistance to cytotoxic therapy is the cell's ability to shut down or modify the process of apoptosis. Thus, a chemotherapeutic agent may interact successfully with its target, but then the cascade of events leading to an apoptotic death may be blocked by mutations within the tumor. On the other hand, sensitive cancer cells can be killed by chemotherapy and radiation because they lack the normal cell's ability to repair damage from cytotoxic or physical stress. The normal cell's ability to maintain normal cell cycle checkpoints, transcription factors, and normal mechanisms for apoptosis is the molecular basis for patient survival during chemotherapy. Unfortunately, for most classic cytotoxic agents in current use, there is a narrow therapeutic window permitting the survival advantage of normal cells over drug-sensitive tumor cells.

p53

It has been estimated that over 50% of human tumors harbor mutations of the *p53* gene, located on chromosome 17p (11). The gene's protein product mediates cell cycle arrest between the G_1 and G_2 (12). This type of arrest allows a cell to escape significant damage from a DNA damaging agent. Thus, *p53* has a key role in programmed cell death (apoptosis) (13). The signal that p53 transmits to the cell to begin the process of apoptosis remains uncertain. For the most part, studies have confirmed that mutations of p53 that lead to increased genetic instability within the tumor cell increase the likelihood of chemotherapy resistance (14).

Among its multifunctional tasks, p53 provides transcriptional activation of *p21,* a gene producing a protein that directly inhibits cyclin-dependent kinases. This inhibition is abetted because of wild-type *p53* participates in the inactivation of the retinoblastoma (*RB*) gene, another potent tumor suppressor gene. A normally functioning *RB* releases the E2F family of transcription factors that bind to and inhibit ribonucleotide reductase, dihydrofolate reductase, DNA-dependent RNA polymerase, thymidylate synthase, and the gene products of *c-myc, c-fos,* and *cmyb.* All these participate in the synthesis of DNA and move cells from the G_1 into the

S phase of the cell cycle. Thus, wild-type *p53* prevents cellular reproduction in the face of a cytotoxic agent(s); this may be critical to the host by allowing normal tissues with damaged DNA to repair and by preventing genetically unstable cancer cells from reproducing. In summary, mutations of *p53* can lead to loss of critical checkpoint functions allowing cancer cells to continue to move through the S phase despite cytotoxic treatment.

Wild-type p53 also acts to suppress *mdr-1*, a gene that affects resistance to many natural product chemotherapeutic agents. Mutant *p53* does not effectively suppress the *mdr-1* gene. The E2F family of transcription factors, released by normally functioning *RB*, appears to have an effect on the sensitivity/resistance of antimetabolites. Thus, the status of the *p53* and *RB* influence sensitivity and/or resistance to a wide variety of chemotherapeutic agents.

Bcl-2 and Caspases

Bcl-2 is a protooncogene whose protein product has been labeled bcl-2. Overexpression of bcl-2 and bcl-x_1, a functional and structural homologue of bcl-2, shelters tumors from the apoptotic effects of radiation and chemotherapy found most frequently in non-Hodgkin's lymphomas, chronic lymphocytic leukemia, prostate cancer, non–small cell lung cancer, breast cancer, and melanoma. Both chemotherapy and radiation therapy have been shown to induce overexpression of Bcl-2, while in vitro and in vivo suppression of Bcl-2 has overcome resistance to chemotherapy (15,16) The ratio of Bcl-2 to other molecules in this family, such as its heterodimer, bax, and other apoptotic-inducing family members, bcl-x_1 and bak, most likely determines the magnitude of the Bcl-2 effect on apoptosis (17).

Caspases (cysteine aspartate–specific proteases) are a highly conserved family of proteins that appear to mediate the final stages of apoptosis. The caspases cleave protein kinases and affect signal transduction proteins, cytoskeletal proteins, chromatin-modifying proteins, and DNA repair proteins. Eventually, caspases activate cellular nucleases that cause the characteristic DNA fragmentation that is a hallmark of apoptosis. Either "intrinsic" or "extrinsic" pathways to apoptosis may activate caspases. The intrinsic pathway works through the cell's mitochondria and is influenced by the Bcl-2 family of proteins. The proteins bax and bak permeate the outer mitochondrial membrane allowing release of cytochrome-c. By the action of cytochrome-c binding with Apaf-1, caspase 9 is activated, committing the cell to apoptosis. The extrinsic pathway of apoptosis is mediated by tumor necrosis factor (TNF) and its family of receptors, including TNF receptor-1, Fas, DR3, DR4 or TNF-related apoptosis-inducing ligand-R1 (TRAIL), DR5, or TRAIL-R2. The extrinsic pathway of apoptosis works primarily through caspase 8, which serves to activate other effector caspases, eventually leading to the activation of caspase 3. Genetic mouse models that engineered to survive without caspase 9 (intrinsic pathway) or caspase 3 (extrinsic pathway) are very resistant to the effects of chemotherapy (18,19).

Nuclear Transcription Factor Kappa B and Cell Survival

Cellular injury, whether induced by chemotherapy or radiation, induces transcription factor kappa B (NFκB), a potent suppressor of apoptosis. In a recent study of esophageal cancer, Izzo et al. noted that esophageal cancers with activated NFκB have both an aggressive biology and a poor outcome to therapy (20). IκB inactivates NFκB by degradation in the 26S proteosome, a cellular organelle that selectively degrades polyubiquinated proteins. The proteosome is also the principal pathway for degradation of cellular regulatory proteins, including p53, cyclins, and the cyclin-dependent kinase inhibitors p21 and p27 (21). Thus targeting NFκB by inhibiting its activation within the proteosome, a rationale approach to cancer therapy, has been successful in the treatment of multiple myeloma (22).

Tyrosine Kinase Inhibitors

Tyrosine kinases (TKs) transfer phosphate from ATP to tyrosine residues in polypeptides. The activation of a TK by its ligand is generally short lived, as activation is generally reversed by protein tyrosine phosphatases. In cancer cells, overexpression of TKs lead to unregulated cell growth, reproduction, and inhibition of apoptosis. There are close to 150 TK or TK-like genes that regulate cellular proliferation, survival, differentiation, and motility. Unregulated TKs become oncogenic by retroviral transduction, genomic rearrangements that may lead to fusion proteins, gain of function, or deletions in the TK and overexpression from gene amplification (23).

TKs may be divided into 2 general classes: receptor TKs (RTKs) and cytoplasmic TKs. Unfortunately, the complex interactions between RTKs and cytoplasmic TKs lead to overlapping descriptions and some confusion in classification. Approximately 30 RTKs and 15 cytoplasmic TKs with oncogenic potential have been identified. Agents such as imatinib mesylate and trastuzimab down-regulate or inhibit abnormal TKs.

RTKs

The RTKs are transmembrane glycoproteins possessing an N-terminal extracellular ligand-binding domain, a single anchoring transmembrane alpha helix, and a cytosolic C-terminal domain that contains the catalytic domain (24). The receptor TKs are activated on binding ligand to the extracellular domain, resulting in the formation of "receptor oligomers" and autophosphorylation of regulatory tyrosine molecule. Autophosphorylation allows for binding sites on signaling proteins within the cell. These are transported to the cell membrane, activating multiple signaling pathways. When activated, RTKs activate at least 3 signal transduction pathways: Ras, the phosphatidylinositol-3-kinase (PI3K), and phosphlipase-C-γ (PLC). Ras, a proto-oncogene, activated by the guanine nucleotide exchange factor Grb2/mSOS, induces Raf and downstream kinases MEK and ERK1/2. Activated PIK3 generates a membrane lipid, PIP3 that, in turn acts as a membrane-docking site for serine/threonine kinases, PDK1 and Akt. PDK1 serves to activate Akt and the mammalian target of rapamycin (mTOR). Akt is a potent inhibitor of apoptosis; mTOR up-regulates protein synthesis. Activation of PLC-γ is necessary for the formation of diacylglycerol, which in turn leads to an increased production of intracellular calcium and protein kinase-c (PKC) (25). The introduction of monoclonal antibodies (trastuzimab, imatinib, cetuximab, panitumimab, bevacizumab) and small molecules (erlotinib, gefitinib) aimed at receptor TKs that are overexpressed in malignant disease has been rapid and exciting. These agents and those directed against cytoplasmic TKs have broadened concepts of "targeted therapy" from hormones and antimetabolites to consideration of targeting any TK associated with cancer growth.

Cytoplasmic TKs

The cytoplasmic TKs do not contain a transmembrane domain; they are found within the cell, including the cytosol, nucleus, and inner surface of the cell membrane (26). Cytoplasmic TKs are maintained in an inactive state by cellular inhibitory proteins, lipids, and molecular autoinhibitors. Intracellular signaling appears to dissociate inhibitors, allowing recruitment to transmembrane receptors (27). The cytoplasmic oncogenic TKs include c-Src, c-Abl, JAKS and STATs, Ras/Raf, PI3K, mTOR, PDK-1, and Akt.

The first cellular homologue of a viral oncoprotein to be discovered, c-Src has a role in several human cancers, including colon cancers (28). Its oncogenic potential occurs when constraints on its kinase activity are relaxed by activation of the signal transducer and activator of transcription (STAT), a family of protein products of the Janus PTKs (JAKs). JAKs mediate signaling after instigation by cytokine receptors (29); c-Abl is the PTK on chromosome 9 that is involved in the reciprocal (9;22) translocation that defines the dominant molecular abnormality found in chronic myelocytic leukemia. Under normal circumstances, the structurally complex c-Abl is a nuclear protein functioning to induce cell growth arrest. The abnormal fusion protein, Bcr-Abl is found in the cytoplasm. The Bcr-Abl protein is a strong inhibitor of apoptosis. Several PTK pathways, including the Ras/Raf-Erk, JAK-STAT, and PI3 pathways, mediate the transformation of c-Abl, setting the stage for the formation of the abnormal fusion protein (30).

Epigenetic Changes

An epigenetic change is defined as an alteration of cellular gene expression that persists across more than 1 cell division but is not directly caused by changes in the cell's DNA code. These changes may result in aberrations of the cellular chromatin structure caused by methylation of cytosine residues in CpG dinucleotides, modification of histones by acetylation or methylation, or changes in the higher-order chromatin structure (31). Drugs that target methylation have activity in the treatment of myelodysplastic syndromes (32). Although solid tumors that exhibit marked hypermethylation tend to be aggressive, the question of whether altering the tumor's methylation status will lead to chemotherapy sensitivity is unknown.

COMBINATION CHEMOTHERAPY

While the rare tumors choriocarcinoma and African Burkitt's lymphoma may be cured with single-agent methotrexate and single-agent cytoxan, respectively, the modern era of chemotherapy began when it was recognized that by combining active drugs from different classifications and with different mechanisms of action, tumor cell kill was markedly enhanced even if lower doses of individual drugs were utilized. By combining agents with different mechanisms of actions, the risk of allowing a large number of insensitive cells to survive can be minimized by killing cells within a tumor type with different growth kinetics and different driving forces of cellular reproduction (33). In selecting drugs to use in combination therapy, it is highly relevant to consider whether each drug in the combination is active against the tumor, that toxicity overlap be kept to a minimum, and that the dose of each individual drug in the combination must provide tumor cell lethality.

Dose Intensity

Because the drug–tumor dose–response curve is sigmoidal, with an initial lag phase, a linear phase, and a plateau, tumor kill is always best if drugs can be given when tumor cells are in the linear phase. Since in vivo human tumors do not "announce" which phase they are in, adjuvant trials should be designed to administer the highest possible dose at the most frequent intervals. A useful working definition of dose intensity has been provided by Hryniuk et al. as the amount of drug delivered per unit time (usually the time period is 1 week) (34). In solid tumors, the importance of dose intensity has been documented in the treatment programs for ovarian, breast, lung, and colon cancers (35,36). Adhering to dose intensity is even more relevant in attempting curative combination chemotherapy for patient with lymphomas and acute leukemia (37).

Although dose intensity may be achieved by maximizing dose, it has now been shown that dose intensity can be improved by increasing "dose density," essentially decreasing the interval between cycles. The report of Intergroup trial C9741 clinically validated this principle. Using a 2 × 2 design, these investigators tested a 3-week cycle of sequential single-agent doxorubicin, cytoxan, and paclitaxel × 4 against a 2-week cycle of the same sequential single agents versus a conventional 3-week cycle combination doxorubicin and cytoxan × 4 followed by paclitaxel × 4 versus a 2-week cycle of dose-dense doxorubicin and cytoxan × 4 followed by paclitaxel × 4 for adjuvant therapy for patients with node-positive breast cancer. All patients in the dose-dense 2-week regimens received filgastrim. Dose-dense therapy improved the primary end point of disease free survival (risk ratio = 0.74; P = 010) and overall survival (risk ratio = 0.69; P = .013) (38).

Applying the principles of dose intensity and dose density may not be applicable in situations where the clinical goal is palliation, not cure. Combination chemotherapy is almost always more toxic than single-agent chemotherapy. In an Eastern Cooperative Oncology Group trial reported by Sledge et al., patients with disseminated breast cancer were randomized to receive sequential single-agent doxorubicin and paclitaxel versus a combination of the 2 agents. Combination therapy provided a superior response rate to sequential therapy, but this did not translate into improved overall survival or a better quality of life (39).

ACTIVE AGENTS AGAINST ESOPHAGEAL CANCER

Although 2 distinct histologic types of esophageal cancer are recognized, the panel of active chemotherapeutic agents against esophageal cancer appears to be the same whether the tumor is derived from glands (adenocarcinoma) or squamous mucosa (squamous cell carcinoma). Active compounds against esophageal cancers are found across the entire spectrum chemotherapeutic agents. These include antimetabolites such as 5-fluorouracil (5-FU); platinum compounds such as cisplatin, carboplatin, and oxaliplatin; vinca alkaloids such as vindesine; taxanes such as paclitaxel; topoisomerase poisons such as irinotecan and etoposide; and antibiotics such as mitomycin-c. Currently, there are scant data regarding response rates of EGFR- and/or VEGFR-targeted agents against primary or metastatic esophageal cancer.

Fluoropyrimidines

Antimetabolites such as 5-FU can be considered "indirect effectors" of DNA function. 5-FU was rationally designed to inhibit the incorporation of uracil into DNA by targeting the enzyme thymidylate synthase (TS) (40). TS gene expression has been shown to be a factor in resistance and/or sensitivity to 5-FU. The TS gene promoter regulates tandemly (TR) repeated sequences that are polymorphic in humans (41). Of the 3 most common TS polymorphisms (TR 2/2, TR 3/3, and TR 2/3), tumors homozygous for double TR (TR 2/2) and heterozygous (TR 2/3) appear to be more sensitive to 5-FU than those tumors homozygous for triple TR (TR 3/3) (42). In vitro studies have indicated tumors with the TS polymorphism that is homozygous for the triple TR produce an excess of TS. Since 5-FU is most effective when it can overwhelm the tumor's TS, the expression of TS and the polymorphic state of TS within the tumor are the major determinants for 5-FU sensitivity/resistance. As a single agent, response rates to 5-FU (and all the chemotherapeutic agents discussed in this chapter) will vary depending on whether investigators are measuring the primary tumor or metastatic disease (43,44). Currently, when used to treat esophageal cancer, 5-FU is most often employed as an infusion over 4 to 5 days or as a protracted infusion over 21 days in combination with a platinum analogue. Although swallowing pills can be a problem for patients with primary esophageal cancer, the oral fluoropyrimidine capecitabine has been studied in combination with oxaliplatin (45). The most common toxicities caused by protracted infusion schedules of 5-FU and capecitabine include mucositis (especially in combination with radiation), diarrhea, and palmar–plantar erythrodysesthia (hand–foot syndrome). Unless patients are deficient in the key catabolic enzyme dihydropyrimidine dehydrogenase, infusion schedules of 5-FU and the orally administered capecitabine rarely cause grade III/IV clinical or bone marrow toxicities (46).

Platinum Analogues

Platinum-containing compounds, including cisplatin, carboplatin, and oxaliplatin, form the chemotherapy backbone of almost all recent esophageal cancer neoadjuvant interventions. In general, the cytotoxic action of platinum analogues is associated with the induction of DNA intrastrand, interstrand, and DNA-protein cross-links (47). The major DNA adducts induced by cisplatin are interstrand cross-links (60%) and intrastrand bidentate N7 adducts with the bases guanine (60%) and adenine (30%) (48,49). High tumor levels of DNA repair genes in esophageal cancers have been shown to confer resistance to cisplatin and its analogues (50,51). This leads to cross-linkage of DNA strands or breaks within DNA that can be modified by families of DNA repair genes. Cisplatin, with single activity of between 17% and 70%, depending on measurement of response within the primary or metastatic lesions, is the only platinum analogue that has been tested has had substantial single-agent phase II testing in esophageal cancer (44,52,53). As doses of cisplatin less than 400 mg/m^2 rarely cause bone marrow toxicity, it is a good drug to use in combination with radiation and other agents that may cause marrow toxicity. However, cisplatin has significant emetogenic potential, requires significant pretreatment hydration to avoid renal toxicity, causes ototoxicity, and affects the peripheral vasculature (possibly through neuropathy). Thus, efforts to replace cisplatin with oxaliplatin in the treatment of esophageal cancer have been investigated and published (54,55).

Irinotecan

Irinotecan, a semisynthetic camptothecin derivative, inhibits DNA topoisomerase I. In general, topoisomerases are nuclear enzymes that catalyze the formation of single- and/or double-strand DNA breaks and promote the rejoining of DNA strands. Thus, topoisomerases are critical for DNA replication, transcription, and recombination. Topoisomerase I catalyzes the formation of single-stranded DNA breaks; topoisomerase II catalyzes both single- and double-strand breaks (56). Inhibition of topoisomerase I sends a strong cellular apoptotic signal (57). Irinotecan, essentially a prodrug, must be metabolized in the liver and other tissues to SN-38 (7-ethyl-10-hydroxy camptothecin) for activity. However, irinotecan itself is a weak acetycholinesterase inhibitor that can cause acute cholinergic side effects. Irinotecan dose–limiting toxicities include diarrhea, nausea, vomiting, granulocytopenia, thrombocytopenia, and anemia (58). The expression level of topoisomerase I within a tumor has not been associated with irinotecan sensitivity or resistance. However, hypermethylation of the topoisomerase gene and mutant *K-ras* have been associated with resistance (59,60). In phase II testing, irinotecan at 125 mg/m^2 weekly had a modest response rate of 14%. Nevertheless, with dose reductions to 65 mg/m^2 weekly in combination with cisplatin, excellent responses and acceptable toxicity have been reported in the neoadjuvant setting (61).

Taxanes

Taxanes, including paclitaxel and docetaxel, are mitotic spindle inhibitors with activity against esophageal cancers. The taxane rings of paclitaxel and docetaxel stabilize microtubules against depolymerization. The stabilization promotes the nucleation and elongation phases of microtubule polymerization, reducing the tubulin subunit concentration necessary for tubulin assembly (62). The area of taxane-microtubule lumen binding is distinct from vinca alkaloids (63). Taxane toxicities include hypersensitivity reactions; broad effects against bone marrow, including white blood cells, platelets, and hemoglobin; peripheral neuropathy; fluid retention; and occasional nausea and vomiting. In one phase II study, paclitaxel at 250 mg/m^2 was administered every 3 weeks in conjunction with 5 µ/kg granulocyte colony-stimulating factor (G-CSF). Although toxicity was substantial, the investigators reported that 11 of 50 patients (22%) had either a complete or partial response (64). To reduce toxicity, a weekly program of paclitaxel at 80 mg/m^2 q week × 4 weeks was explored. Toxicity was reduced, but the response rate was 13% (confidence interval [CI] 6%–20%) (65). Phase II trials of single-agent docetaxel at 75 and 70 mg/m^2 yielded response rates of 18% and 20%, respectively (66,67).

Vinca Alkaloids, Topoisomerase II Inhibitors, and Antibiotics

The spindle-inhibiting vinca alkaloids, vindesine and vinorelbine, have demonstrated single-agent response rates of 26% and 23%, respectively (68,69). Because vinca alkaloids have significant peripheral neurologic and bone marrow toxicities, their use in combined modality treatment programs against esophageal cancer has been largely abandoned. The topoisomerase II inhibitor etoposide has been found to have modest activity against squamous cell esophageal cancers (70). Most trials using etoposide in combined modality therapy against esophageal cancer have emanated from Europe. In combination with cisplatin and 5-FU plus radiation, the addition of etoposide appears to increase response rates, including pCR rates. However, many investigators designing combined modality programs for patients with primary esophageal cancer have eschewed etoposide because it is associated with high rates of grade III and IV neutropenic fever requiring hospitalization (71). Mitomycin-c, a Japanese antibiotic and trifunctional alkylator, is of historic interest because of early publications suggesting excellent activity when the administered with 5-FU and radiation for patients with primary, potentially curable squamous cell esophageal cancers (72,73). Unfortunately, mitomycin-c has predictable bone marrow toxicity and unpredictable but potentially life-threatening pulmonary toxicity. Pulmonary toxicity from mitomycin-c appears most often and is most severe in patients who undergo surgical excision of their esophageal cancer after chemotherapy and radiation.

APPLICATION OF CHEMOTHERAPY AGAINST ESOPHAGEAL CANCERS

Chemotherapy has an important role in the treatment of all stages of esophageal cancer. Details of specific trials in these stages are presented elsewhere in this text. For patients with incurable esophagus cancers, phase II trials have identified active agents. The need for continuing phase II trials is evident from the median overall survival of less than 8 months for patients with disseminated esophageal or gastroesophageal junction tumors. Chemotherapy for esophageal patients has also been tested after surgery, prior to surgery, with radiation therapy prior to surgery, and with radiation therapy without surgery. There is now little doubt that chemotherapy with radiation adds to survival prior to surgery and that chemotherapy and radiation enhance survival over radiation alone. Thus, chemotherapy for esophageal tumors plays a curative role.

Incurable Esophageal Cancers

The principles of chemotherapy administration for esophageal cancer are no different than those applied to patients with most solid tumors. Chemotherapy is frequently the only modality of value for patients presenting with incurable malignancies. Incurable patients with esophageal cancer may have widely disseminated cancer or tumors so locally advanced that cure is precluded. The goals for administering chemotherapy to patients with incurable esophageal cancers should include relief or palliation of symptoms, an overall improvement of quality of life, and prolongation of life. To make progress against esophageal cancer, it essential to enter patients with incurable cancer into clinical trials aimed at testing drug doses and schedules (phase I) and determining response rate or a surrogate for response rate (phase II). Eventually, efficacy of a new agent or combination of agents must be measured by improving disease-free survival (DFS), progression-free survival (PFS), or overall survival over a standard of care (phase III). The median overall survival for patients with incurable, disseminated cancer of the esophagus is less than 9 months. Standard agents, such as those briefly discussed here, rarely extend DFS or PFS beyond 6 months. Thus, new drugs that extend median DFS or median PFS beyond 6 months will be of great interest. Because the 5-year survival for patients with potentially curable esophageal cancer is dismal, new active agents identified in patients with incurable are quickly tested in neoadjuvant, combined modality setting.

Postoperative Adjuvant Therapy

A treatment program designed to improve survival for patients with solid tumors after they have received potentially curative surgery is called "postoperative adjuvant treatment." Postoperative adjuvant chemotherapy prolongs survival for patients with breast cancer and colorectal cancer (74,75). A 5-year overall survival following esophageal cancer surgery of 12% demonstrates the need for effective postoperative therapy (76). However, even with modern techniques, the surgical procedures for esophageal usually leave patients far more debilitated than surgery for breast and colorectal cancers. Although Japanese investigators have published studies demonstrating a trend for improved postoperative survival with adjuvant cisplatin and 5-FU, Western investigators have yet to undertake a large randomized postoperative trial for esophageal cancer patients (77).

Neoadjuvant Chemotherapy

Neoadjuvant cancer therapy is defined as an additional treatment administered prior to so-called established or standard therapy with the primary goals of increasing overall survival and improving the cure rate. Other objectives for neoadjuvant therapy include improved local tumor control; increased time to recurrence; less radical surgery, including organ sparing procedures; and, by using degree of response as guide, designing optimal future treatment for an individual patient (78).

At diagnosis, regardless of histology, most locally advanced solid tumors (stage III) have clinically occult distant metastases, and a lesser number of early-stage tumors (stages I and II) will also have occult distant metastases. Thus, systemic treatment of microscopic distant metastases without the delay of postoperative healing and rehabilitation the earliest is a scientifically sound strategy. Employing a local treatment such as radiation prior to surgery makes it possible to eradicate tumor cells sterilizing the periphery of the surgical margins. This will decrease both local and distant metastases and, in anal cancers, rectal cancers, and laryngeal cancers, maintains cure rates while sparing organ function and integrity (79). Whether a preoperative treatment plan utilizes systemic chemotherapy or radiation therapy or both, patients are generally treated early in their clinical course, before the necessity of recovery and rehabilitation following surgery but without the benefit of surgical staging.

Patients obtaining a complete pathologic response (pCR) after neoadjuvant therapy (or a near pCR) have the greatest chance for prolonged survival and the greatest opportunity to be cured (80–82). Therefore, pCR has become the most important early end point for clinicians and their patients. In current phase II and phase III neoadjuvant trials, pCR is frequently used as surrogate end point for overall survival. Moreover, Swisher et al. reported that after chemotherapy and radiation, the stage per stage survival was statistically the same after neoadjuvant therapy as it was for those with the same stage taken to surgery without preoperative neoadjuvant treatment. Thus, any downstaging from neoadjuvant treatment improved patient survival (83).

Chemotherapy Alone as Neoadjuvant Therapy for Esophageal Cancer

Esophageal cancer tends toward early distant dissemination. Thus, investigators have concentrated on strategies to wipe out occult distant cancer prior to surgery. Nevertheless, the value of preoperative chemotherapy without radiation for patients with esophageal and gastroesophageal junction tumors remains controversial. For most oncologists in North America, the question of administering chemotherapy prior to surgery appeared to be settled with the publication of the North American Intergroup trial 0013. The final report, in 1998, indicated no improvement in survival for the patients who received neoadjuvant chemotherapy (84). However, in 2002, the British Medical Research Council reported a far larger phase III randomized trial in which 802 patients with esophageal cancer (adenocarcinomas or squamous cell cancers) were randomized to receive either chemotherapy prior to surgery or surgery alone. Overall survival was statistically significantly better for the patients who received preoperative chemotherapy (hazard ratio 0.79; 95% CI 67–93; $P = 0.004$) (85).

Neoadjuvant Chemotherapy and Radiation Prior to Surgery

The historic basis for combining external beam radiation therapy (EBRT) with chemotherapy for esophageal cancer lay in the work of Nigro et al. at Wayne State University (WSU) in their treatment of anal cancers (86). Thus, Franklin et al., at WSU, tested infusion 5-FU with bolus mitomycin-c and radiation in essentially the same schedule and fractionation their colleagues used for anal cancer (87). Cisplatin, a radiation sensitizer, soon replaced mitomycin-c because it was less likely to cause bone marrow toxicity and pulmonary toxicity (88). Despite numerous reports noting the efficacy of infusion 5-FU with cisplatin and EBRT prior to surgery, a large randomized trial testing this combined modality program prior to surgery against surgery alone has never been completed (89). Recently, however, results of the aborted Cancer and Leukemia Group B randomized trial strongly suggested statistical significance for combined modality therapy with surgery versus surgery (90). Furthermore, metanalyses, reviewing the 6 published randomized trials, have concluded that combined chemotherapy and radiation prior to surgery results in significant benefit in disease-free survival and overall survival (91,92).

Chemotherapy and Radiation without Surgery

Chemotherapy in combination with EBRT without surgery improves overall survival for patients with esophageal cancer. With the publication of the Radiation Therapy Oncology Group trial noting a statistically significant survival for patients who received 5-FU and cisplatin with concomitant radiation versus radiation alone, chemotherapy and radiation have been defined as acceptable definitive, potentially curative therapy for patients with either squamous cell carcinoma or adenocarcinoma of the esophagus (93,94). At 5 years, 27% of the 61 patients who treated with chemotherapy and radiation group were alive; of the 62 patients randomized to receive radiation alone, none were alive beyond 3 years ($P < 0.001$) (95). At 10 years, the overall survival for the combined modality group was 21% (96). The Eastern Cancer Oncology Group reported the results of a prospectively randomized trial in which 119 patients were randomized to receive 5-FU and mitomycin-c with radiation versus radiation alone. The investigators found that chemotherapy and radiation improved median survival from 9 months to 15 months ($P = 0.04$) (97). A meta-analysis evaluated 11 randomized prospective trials comparing chemotherapy and radiation against radiation alone; the hazard ratio for overall survival was 0.73 (95% CI 0.64–0.84) in favor of the combined modality therapy (98).

Future of Chemotherapy

Although molecular-targeted agents for systemic cancer therapy are multiplying almost as fast as targets are found, not all targets drive tumor-cell turnover. Learning to fit a treatment to the patient's tumor is the most important next step in using systemic chemotherapy. This dictum will hold for patients with esophageal cancers who are treated with a combination of agents and modalities (99). Actually, the future is upon us, as investigators have demonstrated that expression levels of TS, EGFR, and the DNA repair genes *MDR* and *GSTπ1*, harbored within a primary esophageal tumor, could be used to determine success and/or failure of fluoropyrimidine/platinum-based therapy (100–104).

Targeting genes associated with carcinogenesis may prove to be useful strategy for therapy of esophageal cancers. The *COX-2* gene has been shown to be associated with carcinogenesis through increase in angiogenesis and suppression of apoptosis in response to a number of tumor-promoting factors. Overexpression of the COX-2 protein is associated with a poor prognosis for patients with esophageal cancer. Indeed, high levels of *COX-2* in esophageal cancer specimens postchemotherapy correlated with had a negative outcome (105,106). Recently, it has been demonstrated that administration of celecoxib over a 4-week period will effectively downregulate COX-2 expression within adenocarcinoma of the esophagus (107). Trials to judge whether such downregulation increases response to multiagent chemotherapy for patients with esophageal cancer are now underway.

Overexpression of HER-2 is found in approximately 20% of distal esophageal adenocarcinomas. The gene *c-erbB-2* (*HER2/neu*) is amplified in approximately 6% to 8% of these tumors. Testing of drugs such as trastuzumab and lapatinib against these patients will yield information as to whether this gene is as important in driving esophageal carcinomas as it is in breast cancers. Similarly, the role of the EGFR inhibitor cetuximab must be tested in patients with adenocarcinomas of the esophagus who are receiving radiation to find if it is as relevant to esophagus cancer patients as it is to patients with head and neck tumors receiving radiation (108).

SUMMARY

The application of chemotherapy for patients with esophageal cancer follows the same principles that apply to all solid tumor treatment. The role for chemotherapy in prolonging survival for potentially curative patients has been well documented over the past 15 years. To advance beyond the current state, investigators will have to apply their knowledge of tumor growth kinetics, the natural history of esophageal cancer, the mechanisms of drug actions, dose-intense and dose-dense therapy, as well as the mechanisms driving tumorigenesis, tumor cell growth and motility, tumor cell turnover, and tumor cell death. All these contribute to usefulness of current and future systemic therapy against esophageal cancers.

References

1. Rhoads CP. Nitrogen mustards in the treatment of neoplastic disease. *JAMA.* 1946;131:656–658.
2. Goodman LS, Wintrobe MM, Dameshek W, et al. Nitrogen mustard therapy. Use of methyl-bis(beta-chloroethyl)amine hydrochloride and tris(beta-chloroethyl)amine hydrochloride for Hodgkin's disease, lymphosarcoma, leukemia, and certain allied and miscellaneous disorders. *JAMA.* 1946;105:475–476.
3. Farber S, Diamond LK, Mercer RD, et al. Temporary remissions in acute leukemia in children produced by the folic antagonist, 4-amethopteroylglutamic acid (aminopterin). *N Engl J Med.* 1948;238:787–793.
4. Skipper HE, Schabel FM Jr, Mellet LB, et al. Implications of biochemical, cytokinetic, pharmacologic and toxicologic relationships in the design of optimal therapeutic schedules. *Cancer Chemother Rep.* 1970;54:431–450.
5. Skipper HE. Kinetics of mammary tumor cell growth and implications for therapy. *Cancer.* 1971;28:1479–1499.
6. Norton L. A Gompertzian model of human breast cancer growth. *Cancer Res.* 1988;48:7067–7071.
7. Luria SE, Delbruck M. Mutations of bacteria from virus sensitivity to virus resistance. *Genetics.* 1943;28:491–511.
8. Goldie JH, Coldman AJ. A mathematic model for relating the drug sensitivity of tumors to their spontaneous mutation rate. *Cancer Treat Rep.* 1979;63:1727–1733.
9. Norton L. Implications of kinetic heterogeneity in clinical oncology. *Semin Oncol.* 1985;12:231–245.
10. Picard MJ. Mathematics and oncology: a match for life? [editorial]. *J Clin Oncol.* 2003;21:1425–1428.
11. Hollstein M, Sidransky D, Vogelstein B, et al. p53 mutations in human cancers. *Science.* 1991;253:49–53.
12. El Deiry WS. The role of p53 in chemosensitivity and radiosensitivity. *Oncogene.* 2003;22:7486–7495.
13. Green DR. Apoptotic pathways; the roads to ruin. *Cell.* 1998;94:695–698.
14. Wu GS, El Deiry WS. p53 and chemosensitivity. *Nat Med.* 1996;2:255–256.
15. Cotter FE, Corbo M, Raynaud F, et al. Bcl-2 antisense therapy in lymphoma: *in vitro* and *in vivo* mechanisms, efficacy, pharmacokinetic and toxicity studies. *Ann Oncol.* 1996;7:32.
16. O'brien S, Moore JO, Boyd TE, et al. Randomized phase III trial of fludarabine plus cyclophosphamide with or without oblimerson sodium (Bcl-2 antisense) in patients with relapsed or refractory chronic lymphocytic leukemia. *J Clin Oncol.* 2007;25:1114–1120.
17. Korsmeyer SJ. Regulators of cell death. *Trends Genet.* 1995;11:101–105.
18. Thornberry NA, Lazebnik Y. Caspases: enemies within. *Science.* 1998;281:1312–1316.
19. Fernandez-Luna JL. Apoptosis regulators as targets for cancer therapy. *Clin Transl Oncol.* 2007;9:555–562.
20. Izzo JG, Malhotra U, Wu TT, et al. Association of activated transcription factor nuclear factor κB with chemoradiation resistance and poor outcome in esophageal carcinoma. *J Clin Oncol.* 2006;24:748–754.
21. Hamilton AL, Eder JP, Pavlick AC, et al. Proteasome inhibition with bortezomib (PS-341): a phase I study with pharmacodynamic end points using a day 1 and day 4 schedule in a 14-day cycle. *J Clin Oncol.* 2005;23:6107–6116.
22. Richardson PG, Barlogie B, Berenson J, et al. A phase II study of bortezomib in relapsed, refractory myeloma. *N Engl J Med.* 2003;348:2609–2617.
23. Blume-Jensen P, Hunter T. Oncogenic kinase signaling. *Nature.* 2001;411:355–365.
24. Krause DS, Van Etten RA. Tyrosine kinases as targets for cancer therapy. *N Engl J Med.* 2005;353:172–187.
25. Sausville EA, Elsayed Y, Monga M, et al. Signal transduction-directed cancer treatments. *Annu Rev Pharmacol Toxicol.* 2003;43:199–231.
26. Schlessinger, J. Cell signaling by tyrosine kinases. *Cell.* 2000;103:211–225.
27. Smith KM, Yacobi, R, Van Etten RA. Autoinhibition of Bcr-Abl through its SH3 domain. *Mol Cell.* 2003;12:27–37.
28. Irby RB, Mao W, Coppola D, et al. Activating SRC mutation in a subset of advanced human colon cancers. *Nat Genet.* 1999;21:187–190.
29. Ihle JN, Nosaka T, Thierfelder W, et al. Jaks and Stats in cytokine signaling. *Stem Cells.* 1997;15(suppl):105–111.
30. Deininger MW, Goldman JM, Melo JV. The molecular biology of chronic myeloid leukemia. *Blood.* 2000;96:3343–3356.
31. ggerG, Liang GN, Aparicio A, et al. Epigenetics in human disease and prospects for epigenetic therapy. *Nature.* 2004;429:457–463.
32. Silverman LR, McKenzie DR, Peterson BL, et al. Further analysis of trials with azacitidine in patients with myelodysplastic syndrome: studies 8421, 8921 and 9221 by the Cancer and Leukemia Group B. *J Clin Oncol.* 2006;24:3895–3903.
33. Schnipper LE. Clinical implications of tumor-cell heterogeneity. *New Engl J Med.* 1986;314:1423–1431.

34. Hryniuk W. Average dose intensity and the impact on design of clinical trials. *Semin Oncol.* 1987;14:65–74.
35. Wood WC, Budman DR, Korzun AH, et al. Dose and dose intensity of adjuvant chemotherapy for stage II, node positive breast cancer. *N Engl J Med.* 1994;330:1253–1259.
36. Levin L, Hryniuk W. Dose intensity analysis of chemotherapy regimens in ovarian cancinoma. *J Clin Oncol.* 1987;5:756–767.
37. Frei E III, Elias A, Wheeler C, et al. The relationship between high-dose treatment and combination chemotherapy: the concept of summation dose intensity. *Clin Cancer Res.* 1998;4(9):2027–2037.
38. Citron ML, Berry DA, Cirrincione C, et al. Randomized trial of dose-dense versus conventionally scheduled and sequential versus concurrent combination chemotherapy as postoperative adjuvant treatment of node-positive primary breast cancer: first report of Intergroup trial C9741/Cancer and Leukemia Group B Trial 9741. *J Clin Oncol.* 2003;21:1431–1439.
39. Sledge GW, Neuberg D, Bernardo P, et al. Phase III trial of doxorubicin, paclitaxel and the combination of doxorubicin and paclitaxel as front-line chemotherapy for metastatic breast cancer; an Intergroup trial (E 1193). *J Clin Oncol.* 2003;21:588–592.
40. Johnson PG, Lenz HJ, Leichman CG, et al. Thymidylate synthase gene and protein expression correlate and are associated with response to 5-fluorouracil in human colorectal and gastric tumors. *Cancer Res.* 1995;55:1407–1412.
41. Kawakami K, Omura K, Kanhehira E, et al. Polymorphic tandem repeats in the thymidylate synthase gene is associated with its protein expression in human gastrointestinal cancers. *Anticancer Res.* 1999;19:3249–3252.
42. Villafranca E, Okruzhnov Y, Dominguez M, et al. Polymorphisms of the repeated sequences in the enhancer region of the thymidylate synthase gene promoter may predict downstaging after preoperative chemoradiation in rectal cancer. *J Clin Oncol.* 2001;19:1779–1786.
43. Lokich J, Shea M, Chaffey J. Sequential infusional 5-fluorouracil followed by concomitant radiation for tumors of the esophagus and gastroesophageal junction. *Cancer.* 1987;60:275–279.
44. Miller JI, McIntyre B, Hatcher CR. Combined treatment approach in surgical management of carcinoma of the esophagus: a preliminary report. *Ann Thorac Surg.* 1985;40:289–293.
45. Jatoi A, Murphy BR, Foster NR, et al. Oxaliplatin and capecitabine in patients with metastatic adenocarcinoma of the esophagus, gastroesophageal junction and gastric cardia: a phase II study from the North Central Cancer Treatment Group. *Ann Oncol.* 2006;17:29–34.
46. Harris BE, Carpenter JT, Diasio RB. Severe 5-fluorouracil toxicity secondary to dihydropyrimidine dehydrogenase deficiency: a potentially more common pharmacologic syndrome. *Cancer.* 1993;68:499–501.
47. Roberts JJ, Thomson AJ. The mechanism of action antitumor platinum compounds. *Prog Nucleic Acid Res Mol Biol.* 1979;22:71–133.
48. Strandberg MC, Bresnick E, Eastman A. DNA crosslinking induced by 1,2-diaminoc yclohexanedichloroplatinum(II) in murine leukemia L1210 cells and comparison with other platinum analogues. *Biochim Biophys Acta.* 1982;698:128–133.
49. Erickson LC, Zwelling LA, Ducore JM, et al. Differential cytotoxicity and DNA crosslinking in normal and transformed human fibroblasts treated with cis-diaminedichloroplatinum (II). *Cancer Res.* 1981;41:2791–2794.
50. Wu X, Gu J, Wu TT, et al. Genetic variations in radiation and chemotherapy drug action pathways predict clinical outcomes in esophageal cancer. *J Clin Oncol.* 2006;24:3789–3798.
51. Leichman L, Lawrence D, Leichman CG, et al. Expression of genes related to activity of oxaliplatin and 5-fluorouracil in endoscopic biopsies of primary esophageal cancers in patients receiving oxaliplatin, 5-fluorouracil and radiation: characterization and exploratory analysis with survival. *J Chemother.* 2006;18:514–524.
52. Ezdinli EZ, Gelber R, Desai DV, et al. Chemotherapy of advanced esophageal carcinoma: Eastern Cooperative Oncology Group. *Cancer.* 1980;46:2149–2153.
53. Panettiere FJ, Leichman LP, Tilchen EJ, et al. Chemotherapy for advanced epidermoid carcinoma of the esophagus with single agent cisplatin: a final report on Southwest Oncology Group study. *Cancer Treat Rep.* 1984;68:1023–1024.
54. Kushalani NI, Leichman CG, Proulx G, et al. Oxaliplatin in combination with protracted- infusion fluorouracil and radiation: report of a clinical trial for patient with esophageal cancer. *J Clin Oncol.* 2002;20:2844–2850.
55. O'Connor BM, Chadha MK, Pande A, et al. Concurrent oxaliplatin, 5-fluorouracil and radiotherapy in the treatment of locally advanced esophageal carcinoma. *Cancer J.* 2007;13:119–124.
56. Zhang H, D'Arpa P, Liu LF. A model for tumor cell killing by topoisomerase poisons. *Cancer Cells.* 1990:2:23–27.
57. Wang JC. Cellular roles of DNA topoisomerases: a molecular perspective. *Nat Rev Mol Cell Biol.* 2002;3:430–440.
58. Pizzolato JF, Saltz LB. The camptothecins. *Lancet.* 2003;361:2235–2242.
59. Takimoto CH, Arbuck SG. Topoisomerase I targeting agents: the camptothecins. In: Chabner BA, Longo DL, eds. *Cancer Chemotherapy and Biotherapy: Principles and Practice.* 3rd ed. Philadelphia: Lippincott Williams and Wilkins; 2001:579.
60. Nemunaitis J, Cox J, Meyer W, et al. Irinotecan hydrochloride (CPT-11) resistance identified by K-ras mutation in patients with progressive colon cancer after treatment with 5-fluorouracil (5-FU). *Am J Clin Oncol.* 1997;20:527–529.
61. Ilson DH. Phase II trial of weekly irinotecan/cisplatin in advanced esophageal cancer. *Oncology (Huntingt).* 2004;18(suppl 14):22–25.
62. Jordan MA. Mechanism of action of antitumor drugs that interact with microtubules and tubulin. *Curr Med Chem Anti-Cancer Agents.* 2002;2:1–17.
63. Schiff PB, Fant J, Horwitz SB. Promotion of microtubule assembly in vitro by taxol. *Nature.* 1979;22:665–667.
64. Ajani JA, Ilson DH, Daugherty K, et al. Activity of taxol in patients with squamous cell carcinoma and adenocarcinoma of the esophagus. *J Natl Cancer Inst.* 1994;86:1086–1091.
65. Ilson DH, Wadleigh RG, Leichman LP, et al. Paclitaxel given by weekly 1-h infusion in advanced esophageal cancer. *Ann Oncol.* 2007;18:898–902.
66. Muro K, Hamaguchi T, Ohtsu A, et al. A phase II study of single-agent docetaxel in patients with metastatic esophageal cancer. *Ann Oncol.* 2004;15:955–959.
67. Heath EI, Urba S, Marshall J, et al. Phase II trial of docetaxel chemotherapy in patients with incurable adenocarcinoma of the esophagus. *Invest New Drugs.* 2002;20:95–99.
68. Kelsen DP, Bains M, Citkovic E, et al. Vindesine in the treatment of esophageal carcinoma: a phase II study. *Cancer Treat Rep.* 1979;63:2019–2021.
69. Conroy TC, Etienne PL, Adenis A, et al. Phase II trial of vinorelbine in metastatic squamous cell carcinoma of the esophagus. *J Clin Oncol.* 1996;14:164–170.
70. Harstrick A, Bokemeyer C, Preusser P, et al. Phase II study of single-agent etoposide with metastatic squamous-cell carcinoma of the esophagus. *Cancer Chemother Pharmacol.* 1992;29:321–322.
71. Stahl M, Stuschke M, Lehmann N, et al. Chemoradiation with and without surgery in patients with locally advanced squamous cell carcinoma of the esophagus. *J Clin Oncol.* 2005;23:2310–2317.
72. Franklin R, Steiger Z, Vaishampayan G, et al. Combined modality therapy for esophageal squamous cell carcinoma. *Cancer.* 1983;51:1062–1071.
73. Brierley J, Wong CS, Cummings B, et al. Squamous cell carcinoma of the oesophagus treated with radiation and 5-fluorouracil, with and without mitomycin-c. *Clin Oncol (R Coll Radiol.* 2001;13:157–163.
74. Fisher B, Redmond CK, Wolmark N, et al. Long term results from NSABP trials of adjuvant therapy for breast cancer. In: Salmon SE, ed. *Adjuvant Therapy of Cancer V.* Orlando, FL: Grune & Stratton; 1987:283–295.
75. Moertel CG, Fleming TR, Macdonald JS, et al. Levamisole and fluorouracil for adjuvant therapy of resected colon cancer. *N Engl J Med.* 1990;322:352–358.
76. King MR, Pairolero PC, Trastek VF, et al. Ivor Lewis esophagectomy for carcinoma of the esophagus: early and late functional results. *Ann Thorac Surg.* 1987;44:119–122.
77. Iizuka T. Surgical adjuvant treatment of esophageal carcinoma: a Japanese Oncology Group experience. *Semin Oncol.* 1994;21:462–466.
78. Thomas E, Holmes FA, Smith TL, et al. The use of alternate, non-cross-resistant adjuvant chemotherapy on the basis of pathologic response to a neoadjuvant doxorubicin-based regimen in women with operable breast cancer: long-term results from a prospective randomized trial. *J Clin Oncol.* 2004;22:2294–2302.
79. Chau I, Brown G, Cunningham D, et al. Neoadjuvant capecitabine and oxaliplatin followed by synchronous chemoradiation and total mesorectal excision in magnetic resonance imaging-defined poor-risk rectal cancer. *J Clin Oncol.* 2006;24:668–674.
80. O'Connell MJ. Combined modality therapy for rectal cancer [editorial]. *J Clin Oncol.* 2005;23:5450–5451.
81. Ring A, Webb A, Ashley S, et al. Is surgery necessary after complete clinical remission following neoadjuvant chemotherapy for early breast cancer. *J Clin Oncol.* 2003;21:4540–4545.
82. Chireac LR, Swisher SG, Ajani JA, et al. Posttherapy pathologic stage predicts survival in patient with esophageal carcinoma receiving preoperative chemoradiation. *Cancer.* 2005;103:1347–1355.
83. Swisher SG, Hofstetter W, Wu TT, et al. Proposed revision of the esophageal cancer staging system to accommodate pathologic response (pP) following preoperative chemoradiation (CRT). *Ann Surg.* 2005;241:810–817.
84. Kelsen DP, Ginsberg R, Pajak TF, et al. Chemotherapy followed by surgery compared with surgery alone for localized esophagus cancer. *N Engl J Med.* 1998;339:1979–1984.
85. Medical Research Council Oesophageal Cancer Working Party. Surgical resection with or without preoperative chemotherapy in oesophageal cancer: a randomised controlled trial. *Lancet.* 2002;359:1727–1733.
86. Nigro ND, Vaitkevicius VK, Considine B Jr. Combined therapy for cancer of the anal canal: a preliminary report. *Dis Colon Rectum.* 1974;17:354–356.
87. Franklin R, Steiger Z, Vaishampayan G, et al. Combined modality therapy for esophageal squamous cell carcinoma. *Cancer.* 51;1983:1062–1071.
88. Leichman L, Steiger Z, Seydel HG, et al. Pre-operative chemotherapy and radiation therapy for patients with cancer of the esophagus: a potentially curative approach. *J Clin Oncol.* 1984;2(2):75–79.
89. Suntharalingam M, Moughan J, Coia LR, et al. Outcome results of the 1996–1999 Patterns of Care Survey of the National Practice for Patients Receiving Radiation Therapy for Carcinoma of the Esophagus. *J Clin Oncol.* 2005;23:2325–2331.
90. Tepper JE, Krasna M, Niedzwiecki D, et al. Superiority of trimodality therapy to surgery alone in esophageal cancer: results of CALGB 9781. *Proc Am Soc Clin Oncol.* 2006;24:4012. Abstract.
91. Urschel JD, Vasan H. A meta-analysis of randomized controlled trials that compared neoadjuvant chemoradiation and surgery to surgery alone for respectable esophageal cancer. *Am J Surg.* 2003;185:538–543.
92. Greer SE, Goodney PP, Sutton JE, et al. Neoadjuvant chemoradiotherapy for esophageal carcinoma: a meta-analysis. *Surgery.* 2005;137:172–177.
93. Herskovic A, Martz K, Al Sarraf, et al. Combined chemotherapy and radiotherapy compared with radiotherapy alone in patients with cancer of the esophagus. *N Engl J Med.* 1992;326:1593–1598.

94. Haller DG. Treatments for esophageal cancer [editorial]. *N Engl J Med.* 1992;326:629–631.
95. Al Sarraf M, Martz A, Herskovic A, et al. Progress report of combined chemoradiotherapy versus radiotherapy alone in patients with esophageal cancer: an intergroup study. *J Clin Oncol.* 1997;15:277–284.
96. Cooper JS, Guo MD, Herskovic A, et al. Chemotherapy of locally advanced esophageal cancer: long term follow-up of a prospective randomized trial (RTOG 85–01). *JAMA.* 1999;281:1623–1627.
97. Smith TJ, Ryan LM, Douglass HO, et al. Combined chemoradiotherapy vs. radiotherapy alone for early stage esophagus squamous cell carcinoma of the esophagus: a study of the Eastern Cooperative Oncology Group. *Int J Radiat Oncol Biol Phys.* 1998;42:269–276.
98. Wong R, Malthaner R. Combine chemotherapy and radiotherapy (without surgery) compared with radiotherapy alone in localized carcinoma of the esophagus [review]. *Cochrane Database Syst Rev.* 2007:Issue 4.
99. Vallbohmer D, Peters JH, Kuramochi H, et al. Molecular determinants in targeted therapy for esophageal adenocarcinoma. *Arch Surg.* 2006;141:476–482.
100. Leichman L, Lawrence D, Leichman, CG, et al. Expression of genes related to oxaliplatin and 5-fluorouracil activities in endoscopic biopsies of primary esophageal cancer in patients receiving oxaliplatin, 5-flourouracil and radiation: characterization and exploratory analysis with survival. *J Chemother.* 2006;18:514–524.
101. Schneider S, Uchida K, Brabender J, et al. Downregulation of TS, DPD, ERCC1, GST-Pi, EGFR, and HER2 gene expression after neoadjuvant three-modality treatment in patients with esophageal cancer. *J Am Coll Surg.* 2005;200:336–344.
102. Joshi M-B M, Shirota Y, Danenberg KD, et al. High gene expression of *TS1, GSTP1,* and *ERCC1* are risk factors for survival in patients treated with trimodality therapy for esophageal cancer. *Clin Cancer Res.* 2005;11:2215–2221.
103. Harpole DH Jr, Moore MB, Herndon JE II, et al. The prognostic value of molecular marker analysis in patients treated with trimodality therapy for esophageal cancer. *Clin Cancer Res.* 2001;7:562–569.
104. Langer R, Specht K, Becker K, et al. Association of pretherapeutic expression of chemotherapy-related genes with response to neoadjuvant chemotherapy in Barrett carcinoma. *Clin Cancer Res.* 2005;11:7462–7469.
105. Sivula A, Buskens CJ, van Rees BP, et al. Prognostic role of cyclooxygenase-2 in neoadjuvant-treated patients with squamous cell carcinoma of the esophagus. *Int J Cancer.* 2005;116:903–908.
106. Xi H, Baldus SE, Warnecke-Eberz U, et al. High cyclooxygenase-2 expression following neoadjuvant radiochemotherapy is associated with minor histopathologic response and poor prognosis in esophageal cancer. *Clin Cancer Res.* 2005;11:8341–8347.
107. Tuynman JB, Buskens CJ, Kemper K, et al. Neoadjuvant selective COX-2 inhibition down-regulates important oncogenic pathways in patients with esophageal adenocarcinoma. *Ann Surg.* 2005;242:840–850.
108. Bonner JA, Harari PM, Giralt J, et al. Radiotherapy plus cetuximab for squamous-cell carcinoma of the head and neck. *N Engl J Med.* 2006;354:567–578.

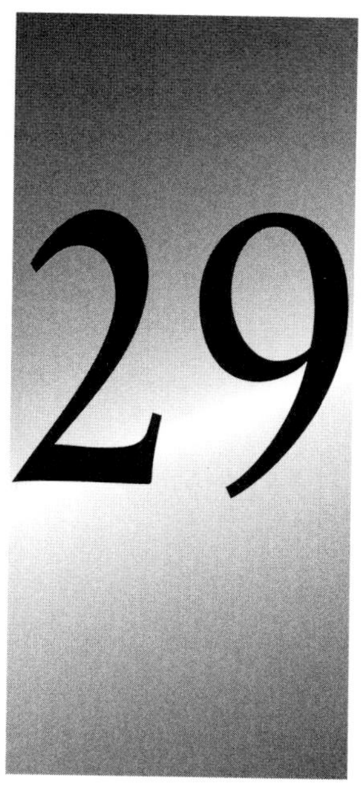

29 Principles of Systemic Therapy: Targeted Therapy

Geoffrey Y. Ku
David H. Ilson

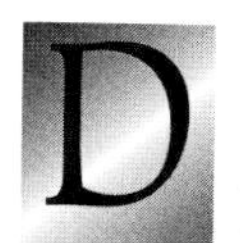

Despite ongoing research in the treatment of esophageal cancer, the prognosis for long-term survival remains poor. Surgery alone for locally advanced disease results in 5-year survival of only approximately 20% (1). The addition of preoperative strategies such as chemoradiotherapy or perioperative chemotherapy results in 5-year survival of no more than 30% to 35% (2–4). In preoperative chemoradiotherapy trials, pathologic complete responses (pCRs) are seen in approximately 10% to 40% of patients at surgery, with consistently superior 5-year survival rates of 50% to 60% seen in these patients (5,6).

Similarly, in the metastatic setting, chemotherapy is the mainstay of palliative therapy and results in response rates (RRs) of only 20% to 40% and median overall survivals (OS) of 8 to 10 months (7). Recent investigations have focused on the incorporation of a third chemotherapy agent into 2-drug regimens, resulting in modest improvements in survival but at the expense of considerable additional toxicity (8,9), potentially limiting the adaptation of these 3-drug regimens by a patient population that is often elderly and has associated medical comorbidities.

Therefore, many investigators believe that the potential for making significant progress lies in understanding and exploiting the molecular biology of these tumors. The focus of recent study has shifted toward testing newer agents that target specific molecular abnormalities known to occur in esophageal cancer.

The molecular targets of agents that are currently under active clinical evaluation include those related to growth regulation (epidermal growth factor receptor [EGFR]), angiogenesis (vascular endothelial growth factor [VEGF]), and inflammation (cyclooxygenase-2).

The results of all the trials discussed in this chapter are summarized in Table 29.1.

EPIDERMAL GROWTH FACTOR RECEPTOR

EGFR or ERBB1 is a member of the ERBB transmembrane growth factor receptor family, which initiates signal transduction by activation of a receptor-associated tyrosine kinase (TK); ERBB also includes ERBB2, ERBB3, and ERBB4 (10). These receptors possess an extracellular ligand-binding domain, a transmembrane anchoring domain, and an intracellular cytoplasmic component that carries the TK activity.

The known ligands of the EGFR are epidermal growth factor (EGF) and transforming growth factor α (TGF-α). The binding of a ligand to the EGFR causes it to dimerize, either with itself or with another member of the ERBB family. Dimerization then leads to activation of the TK, recruitment of signaling complexes, and the

TABLE 29.1
Summary of Trials of Targeted Therapies[a]

Agents	Disease stage	Histology	No. of patients	RR	pCR rate	TTP	OS	Author
Anti-epidermal growth factor receptor (EGFR) monoclonal antibodies (moAbs)								
Cetuximab +Cis/CPT/RT	Locally advanced	AdenoCA	17	N/A	13% (2/15)	NS	NS	Enzinger et al. (41)
Cetuximab + Carbo/paclitaxel/RT	Locally advanced	25 adenoCA 9 SCC 3 gastric CA	37	N/A	43% (7/16)	NS	NS	Suntharalingam et al. (45)
Cetuximab + FOLFIRI	Metastatic	4 adenoCA 34 gastric CA	38	44% (of 34)	N/A	8 mos	16 mos	Pinto et al. (46)
Cetuximab + FUFOX	Metastatic	25 adenoCA 27 gastric CA	52	65% (of 46)	N/A	7.6 mos	9.5 mos	Lordick et al. (47)
EMD72000	Metastatic (phase I)	SCC	2	1 of 2 patients with 6-month partial response				Vanhoefer et al. (48)
EMD72000 + ECX	Metastatic	11 adenoCA 6 gastric CA	17	41%	N/A	NS	NS	Rao et al. (49)
Panitumumab	Metastatic (phase I)	NS	3	1 of 3 patients with 7-month stable disease				Figlin et al. (51)
Anti-EGFR tyrosine kinase inhibitors (TKIs)								
Gefitinib	Metastatic (2nd line)	26 adenoCA 9 SCC 1 adenoSCC	36	3% (of 28)	N/A	2 mos	5.5 mos	Janmaat et al. (27)
Erlotinib	Metastatic (2nd line)	17 adenoCA 13 SCC	30	7%	N/A	NS	NS	Tew et al. (22)
Erlotinib	Metastatic (1st line)	44 adenoCA 26 gastric CA	70	9% 0%	N/A	2 mos 1.6 mos	6.7 mos 3.5 mos	Dragovich et al. (23)
Gefitinib + 5-FU/ Cis +/- RT	Locally advanced (27) Metastatic (10)	34 adenoCA 3 SCC	37	78% (of 25) 50% (of 5)	25% (1 of 4) N/A	NS	NS	Sunpaweravong et al. (61)
Anti-Her2/neu moAb								
Trastuzumab + Cis/paclitaxel/ RT	Locally Advanced	AdenoCA	19	N/A	43% (3 of 6)	NS	24 mos (median); 2-yr 50%	Safran et al. (76)
Trastuzumab + Cis	Locally advanced (1) Metastatic (16)	9 adenoCA 7 gastric CA	17	35%	N/A	NS	NS	Cortés-Funes et al. (77)
Trastuzumab + paclitaxel/IL-12	Metastatic (phase I)	NS	4	2 of 4 patients with partial response				Carson et al. (78)
Anti-vascular endothelial growth factor (VEGF) moAb								
Bevacizumab + Cis/CPT	Metastatic (1st line)	23 adenoCA 24 gastric CA	47	65%	N/A	8.3 mos	12.3 mos	Shah et al. (102)

(Continued)

TABLE 29.1
Summary of Trials of Targeted Therapies[a] (Continued)

Agents	Disease stage	Histology	No. of patients	RR	pCR rate	TTP	OS	Author
Bevacizumab + docetaxel	Metastatic (2nd line)	19 adenoCA 1 SCC 6 gastric CA	26	24% (of 17)	N/A	NS	NS	Enzinger et al. (104)
Anti-VEGF TKI								
Sunitinib	Metastatic (2nd line)	Gastric & GEJ CA	42	5%	N/A	17.1 wks	50.7 wks	Bang et al. (109)
Cyclooxygenase-2 (COX-2) inhibitors								
Celecoxib + 5-FU/Cis/RT	Locally advanced	NS	31	N/A	23% (5 of 22)	NS	NS	Govindan et al. (117)
Celecoxib + 5-FU/Cis/RT	Locally advanced	10 adenoCA 3 SCC	13	N/A	17% (1 of 6)	8.8 mos	19.6 mos	Dawson et al. (118)
Celecoxib + Cis/CPT/RT	Locally advanced	30 adenoCA 6 SCC	36	N/A	44% (11 of 25)	NS	NS	Enzinger et al. (42)
Cell-cycle inhibitors								
Flavopiridol + paclitaxel	Metastatic (paclitaxel-refractory)	NS	12	0%	N/A	NS	NS	Rathkopf et al. (121)
Bryostatin-1 + paclitaxel	Metastatic	Gastric & GEJ CA	35	29% (of 35)	N/A	4.25 mos	8 mos	Ajani et al. (123)
Bryostatin-1 + paclitaxel	Metastatic	22 adenoCA 2 SCC	24	27% (of 22)	N/A	3.7 mos	8.3 mos	Ilson et al. (124) (updated from abstract)

Abbreviations: [a]5-FU = 5-fluorouracil; AdenoCA = adenocarcinoma; AdenoSCC = adenosquamous; CA = cancer; Carbo = carboplatin; Cis = cisplatin; CPT = irinotecan; ECX = epirubicin/cisplatin/capecitabine; FOLFIRI = biweekly bolus 5-FU/leucovorin = irinotecan, infusional 5-FU; FUFOX = weekly oxaliplatin/leucovorin/infusional 5-FU; GEJ = gastroesophageal junction; N/A = not applicable; NS = not stated; OS = overall survival; pCR = pathologic complete response; RR = response rate; RT = radiation therapy; SCC = squamous cell carcinoma; TTP = time to progression.

downstream phosphorylation and activation of other effector signals (11). These downstream cascades are potent regulators of intracellular and intercellular processes, such as cell cycle progression, apoptosis and cell survival, proliferation, angiogenesis, and metastasis.

EGFR is constitutively expressed in a number of tissues, including the skin, gut, and kidney. This normal pattern of EGFR expression may explain the toxicities associated with anti-EGFR therapy, which includes an acneform skin rash (12), diarrhea, and a magnesium-wasting syndrome (13). In fact, in patients with colorectal and non–small cell lung cancer (NSCLC), the severity of the rash observed with anti-EGFR therapies may correlate with clinical response (14).

Overexpression of EGFR via immunohistochemistry (IHC) has been noted in many tumor types, including head and neck, colorectal, pancreatic, renal cell, and NSCLC. EGFR expression correlates with poor prognosis and advanced stage (15). In esophageal cancers, EGFR overexpression by IHC or gene amplification by fluorescent in situ hybridization (FISH) analysis also occur in 30% to 90% of tumors and correlate with increased invasion, a more poorly differentiated histology and a poorer prognosis (16–19). In general, EGFR overexpression is more common with the squamous cell carcinoma than adenocarcinoma histology. In addition to overexpression of EGFR, activating mutations have also been detected, most notably in NSCLC (20). Corresponding mutations in the EGFR have not been detected in esophageal cancer (21–23).

There is also an increasing body of evidence that correlates the mutational status of K-ras, an oncogene involved in an intricate array of signal transduction pathways, and responsiveness to anti-EGFR therapies. This correlation was first noted in NSCLC, where patients with mutated K-ras were found to be unresponsive to anti-EGFR tyrosine kinase inhibitor (TKI) therapy (24). Subsequently, this correlation has also been observed in patients with metastatic colorectal cancer treated with cetuximab, an anti-EGFR monoclonal antibody (moAb), where responses and survival were positively correlated with wild-type K-ras status (25,26).

In the study by Khambata-Ford et al., gene expression profiling also identified elevated expression of epiregulin and amphiregulin as being correlated with progression-free survival (PFS). Epiregulin is known to bind more weakly to EGFR and ERBB4 than EGF but is much more potent than EGF and leads to a prolonged state of receptor activation. Elevated expression of epiregulin and/or amphiregulin may produce an autocrine signaling loop through EGFR and may characterize a tumor that is EGFR dependent and, therefore, particularly sensitive to strategies to block ligand-receptor interactions.

In esophageal cancer, relatively little is known about the incidence of mutated K-ras status and its predictive value for anti-EGFR therapy. In one recent study, 2 of 23 patients (8.7%) were found to have mutated K-ras (27). In older studies, K-ras point mutations were noted in between 5% (1 of 21) to 30% (7 of 23) of adenocarcinoma samples and 0 of 27 squamous cell carcinoma samples (28,29).

Current anti-EGFR therapies that have been evaluated in upper gastrointestinal malignancies include moAbs (cetuximab, panitumimab, and EMD72000 or matuzumab) and oral TKIs (erlotinib, gefitinib).

Anti-EGFR moAbs

Cetuximab (C225, Erbitux®, Imclone Systems, Inc.) is a partially humanized murine IgG_1 moAb that binds to EGFR. It blocks binding of the ligands EGF and TGF-α to the EGFR and subsequent activation of the EGFR TK (30). Cetuximab also stimulates EGFR internalization by endocytosis, preventing interaction of the EGFR with ligand (31). Finally, binding of cetuximab to the EGFR may result in immune-mediated mechanisms, such as antibody-dependent cytotoxicity, complement-dependent cytotoxicity, and complement-dependent cell-mediated cytotoxicity (32,33).

Cetuximab has been approved by the U.S. Food and Drug Administration (FDA) for the treatment of irinotecan-refractory colorectal cancer, based on a phase III trial of cetuximab/irinotecan versus irinotecan in patients with irinotecan-refractory colorectal cancer (34). This trial demonstrated a superior RR (23% vs. 11%, $P = 0.007$) and time to progression (TTP; 4.1 vs. 1.5 months, $P < 0.001$) for the combination over irinotecan alone. Recent data presented in abstract form of a randomized phase III trial also demonstrated that the addition of cetuximab to first-line FOLFIRI chemotherapy (biweekly 5-fluorouracil or 5-FU/leucovorin/irinotecan and infusional 5-FU) in patients with metastatic colorectal cancer resulted in a modest improvement in PFS (8.9 vs. 8.0 months, $P = 0.047$) and RR (47% vs. 39%, $P = 0.005$) (35).

In addition, cetuximab has also been approved by the FDA for use with concurrent radiotherapy for the treatment of locally advanced head and neck squamous cell cancers (HNSCC), as well as for the treatment of cisplatin-refractory metastatic or recurrent HNSCC. A pivotal phase III trial that compared cetuximab and radiotherapy versus radiotherapy alone in stage III and IV HNSCC demonstrated a significant improvement in locoregional control (24.4 vs. 14.9 months, $P = 0.005$), PFS (17.1 vs. 12.4 months, $P = 0.006$), and OS (49.0 vs. 29.3 months, $P = 0.03$) with combination therapy compared to radiation alone (36). A phase II evaluation of cetuximab monotherapy in cisplatin-refractory head and neck cancers produced an RR of 13% (37), which was not clearly improved with the addition of cisplatin in 2 other phase II evaluations (38,39). More recently, data from a randomized phase III trial of patients with recurrent or metastatic HNSCC treated with first-line platinum-based chemotherapy with or without cetuximab demonstrated a survival benefit for the addition of cetuximab (median OS 10.1 vs. 7.4 months, $P = 0.036$) (40).

In esophageal cancer, cetuximab is currently being actively evaluated. In the locally advanced setting, data have been mixed. Preliminary data have been presented for a phase II study of cetuximab, irinotecan/cisplatin, and concurrent radiotherapy followed by surgery for 17 patients with locally advanced disease. The addition of cetuximab resulted in a lower-than-expected pCR rate of 13% as well as grade 3/4 toxicity in 100% of patients (41). In comparison, other phase I/II evaluations of preoperative cisplatin/irinotecan and concurrent radiation followed by surgery have reported pCR rates of 17% to 32% (42–44).

Another pilot study of 37 patients yielded more promising results. In this phase II evaluation, cetuximab was combined with carboplatin/paclitaxel and concurrent radiation for locally advanced esophageal (34 patients; 25 with adenocarcinoma, 9 with squamous cell histology) and gastric cancers (3 patients) (45). Data presented in abstract form revealed a pCR rate of 43%. Toxicities were generally manageable, with no grade 4 nonhematologic toxicities and grade 4 neutropenia seen in only 1 patient (3%). Grade 3 toxicities included esophagitis in 6 patients (20%), rash in 9 patients (30%), and a hypersensitivity reaction to cetuximab/paclitaxel in 2 patients (6%).

In the metastatic setting, 2 phase II evaluations of cetuximab with cytotoxic chemotherapy have reported promising results. In one study, cetuximab was combined with the FOLFIRI regimen as first-line therapy for patients with advanced gastric or gastroesophageal junction (GEJ) adenocarcinoma, with EGFR-positive tumors by IHC (46). In this study, 91% of patients who were screened were found to have EGFR-positive tumors, and 38 patients were enrolled (4 with primary GEJ tumors and 34 with gastric tumors). Of 34 assessable patients, the RR was 44% (including a CR rate of 12%), while 47% of patients had stable disease (SD). The median TTP was an impressive 8 months. Although the median OS for all 38 patients was not reached, it was estimated to be 16 months. Major toxicities included grade 3/4 neutropenia in 42% of patients (including 1 patient death due to febrile neutropenia, which occurred in 5% of patients). Skin rash occurred in 82% of patients but were grade 3 and 4 in only 16% and 5% of patients, respectively.

In the second evaluation in the metastatic setting, cetuximab was combined with the FUFOX regimen (weekly oxaliplatin/leucovorin/infusional 5-FU) as first-line therapy in patients with metastatic/recurrent gastric and GEJ tumors regardless of EGFR staining (47). This study enrolled 52 patients (25 with GEJ tumors and 27 with gastric tumors). Of 42 patients whose tumors were available for EGFR staining, 60% were found to be positive.

The RR was 65% (including a 9% CR rate), with SD in another 17% of patients. Median TTP was 7.6 months, with median OS of 9.5 months. Response appeared to be independent of EGFR status, and there even appeared to be a nonsignificant trend toward benefit for EGFR-negative tumors over EGFR-positive tumors in terms of RR (77% vs. 54%), TTP (9.4 vs. 7.0 months), and OS (9.1 vs. 8.1 months). These survival data may be impacted by the fact that only 33% of patients discontinued therapy because of disease progression; other reasons for treatment discontinuation included toxicity (15%), patient withdrawal (11%), and discontinuation at the recommendation of an investigator because of a good response (25%).

Toxicities seen on this trial included grade 3/4 diarrhea in 33% of patients (6% grade 4), rash in 24% (all grade 3), and neutropenia in 6% of patients (all grade 3). Two patients died on study, including 1 patient who developed febrile neutropenia and diarrhea and another who aspirated following a presumed allergic reaction to cetuximab.

EMD72000 or matuzumab is another humanized IgG_1 moAb against EGFR. In a phase I evaluation, it was found to be safe, with toxicities consisting primarily of grade 1/2 skin toxicity (48). One of 2 patients with esophageal squamous cell carcinoma had a durable 6-month partial response (PR).

Another phase I evaluation combined EMD72000 with the ECX regimen (epirubicin/cisplatin/capecitabine) as first-line therapy for patients with EGFR-positive advanced gastric and GEJ tumors (49). Seventeen patients (including 7 with GEJ and 4 with lower esophageal tumors) were subsequently enrolled. Seven patients (41%) had PRs. Major grade 3/4 toxicities included neutropenia in 59% of patients, including febrile neutropenia in 1 patient (6%).

Finally, panitumumab (ABX-EGF, Vectibix®, Amgen, Inc.) is a fully humanized IgG_2 moAb against EGFR that has been approved by the FDA for the treatment of chemorefractory EGFR-positive colorectal cancer based on a phase III trial that demonstrated improvement in RR (10% vs. 0%, $P < 0.0001$) and mean PFS (13.8 vs. 8.5 weeks, $P < 0.0001$) over best supportive care (50).

A phase I evaluation of panitumumab in refractory solid tumors demonstrated SD for 7 months in 1 of 3 patients with esophageal cancer (51).

In addition, there are also many ongoing or planned cooperative group and single-institution studies. For example, the phase III Radiation Therapy Oncology Group 04036 trial will soon open, comparing weekly cisplatin/paclitaxel and radiation with or without cetuximab as definitive therapy in locally advanced esophageal cancer.

In the metastatic setting, the Cancer and Leukemia Group B (CALGB) is conducting a randomized trial in patients with metastatic disease of cetuximab with 1 of 3 randomly assigned regimens: the ECF (epirubicin/cisplatin/infusional 5-FU) regimen, cisplatin/irinotecan, or the FOLFOX regimen. At Memorial Sloan-Kettering Cancer Center (MSKCC), there is an ongoing trial of cetuximab, cisplatin/irinotecan for patients with esophageal and GEJ cancer refractory to prior cisplatin/irinotecan. The SWOG (Southwest Oncology Group) has also completed an evaluation of cetuximab as second-line therapy for advanced esophageal adenocarcinoma, with results pending.

The REAL3 trial in the United Kingdom will also randomize patients with advanced esophagogastric cancer to the ECX regimen with or without panitumimab.

Anti-EGFR TKIs

TKIs are a class of oral, small molecules that inhibit ATP binding within the TK domain, leading to complete inhibition of EGFR autophosphorylation and signal transduction (52).

Erlotinib and gefitinib are oral TKIs against EGFR. Erlotinib (OSI-774, Tarceva®, Genentech, Inc.) has been approved by the FDA for the treatment of advanced NSCLC based on a phase III trial that demonstrated an improvement in RR (9% vs. <1%, $P < 0.001$) and OS (6.7 vs. 4.7 months, $P < 0.001$) for erlotinib over placebo (53). Gefitinib (ZD1839, Iressa®, AstraZeneca Pharmaceuticals) was initially approved by the FDA for the treatment of platinum- and docetaxel-refractory NSCLC based on a randomized phase II study of 2 different doses of gefitinib (54). However, a subsequent phase III trial comparing gefitinib with placebo did not reveal a survival benefit (55), limiting its use in clinical practice to patients already receiving gefitinib with ongoing clinical benefit. Neither erlotinib nor gefitinib has been shown to increase responses when combined with cytotoxic chemotherapy (56–59).

Erlotinib has also been approved for use with gemcitabine in the first-line treatment of pancreatic cancer based on a phase III trial that demonstrated a small improvement in OS for the combination over gemcitabine alone (median OS 6.2 vs. 5.9 months, 1-year survival 23% vs. 17%, $P = 0.038$), without any improvement in the RR (60).

Both TKIs have been evaluated in advanced esophageal cancer, with modest results. In a phase II evaluation of gefitinib as second-line therapy in 28 assessable patients with advanced disease, it produced a 3-month partial response in 1 patient (3%) and SD in 10 others (28%) (27). The median TTP was 2 months, with median OS 5.5 months. Controlled disease (objective responses plus SD) was associated with female sex and squamous cell carcinoma histology. There was also a nonsignificant trend toward improved median TTP (5.1 vs. 1.8 months) and OS (7.8 vs. 2.8 months) for high versus low tumor EGFR expression. Of note, 2 patients found to have mutated K-ras status had early progression on gefitinib therapy.

A phase II study of second-line erlotinib performed at MSKCC has been presented in abstract form (updated from presentation) (22). In this study of 30 patients with advanced esophageal and GEJ tumors, 2 (7%) had PRs, while 10 (33%) had SD. Both patients with a PR had squamous cell histology (2 of 13 patients, compared to 0 of 17 patients with adenocarcinoma histology), EGFR overexpression, and nodal-limited disease. Retrospective sequencing of EGFR mutations (in exons 18, 19, and 21) was performed from 5 patients on this trial, including 1 responder, and no EGFR mutations were detected.

A similar phase II evaluation of first-line erlotinib in advanced gastric and GEJ adenocarcinoma was performed by the SWOG, in which patients were stratified into a GEJ (44 patients) and gastric stratum (26 patients) (23). There were no responses in the patients with gastric primaries. In the GEJ stratum, the RR was 9% (1 CR and 3 PRs). The median time to failure was 1.6 and 2 months, respectively, for the gastric and GEJ strata, while the median OS was 3.5 and 6.7 months, respectively. Again, no EGFR mutations were detected out of 54 samples, and there was also no evidence of EGFR gene overamplification by FISH. There were no differences in plasma EGF levels or serum proteomic profiles between responders and nonresponders.

Toxicities on all these trials were similar. In general, therapy was well tolerated, with diarrhea and skin rash being the major toxicities. These occurred in 30% to 58% and 47% to 86% of patients, respectively, but were mostly grade 1/2.

Gefitinib has also been combined with 5-FU/cisplatin in a phase II evaluation of patients with stage II-IVb esophageal cancer, with preliminary data recently presented (61). Of 37 patients enrolled (33 with squamous cell, 4 with adenocarcinoma histology), 27 had stage II–IVa disease, while 10 had stage IVb disease. Patients with stage II-IVa disease were treated with gefitinib, 5-FU/cisplatin, and concurrent radiation, while patients with stage IVb disease received gefitinib, 5-FU/cisplatin alone.

Of the 25 evaluable patients with stage II-IVa disease, the clinical RR was 78% (including a 15% CR rate). Four of these patients underwent subsequent esophagectomy, and 1 (4% of patients enrolled or 25% of those who went to surgery) was found to have a pCR. Of 5 evaluable patients with stage IVb disease, the RR was 50%. Major grade 3/4 toxicities included neutropenia (19%), leukopenia (19%), and anemia (16%).

Although these results are encouraging, evaluation of the contribution of gefitinib to this regimen is difficult given the inclusion of both patients with locally advanced and metastatic disease and the lack of survival data. While the pCR rate is the most validated end point in assessing the efficacy of preoperative chemoradiotherapy, only 4 of 25 evaluable patients with locally advanced disease underwent esophagectomy.

At present, there are other ongoing evaluations of erlotinib or gefitinib with chemotherapy and radiation for locally advanced disease as well as evaluations of these drugs with chemotherapy in the metastatic setting.

ANTI-HER-2/NEU THERAPY

Her-2/neu (ERBB2) is another member of the ERBB TK receptor family. Peptide ligand binding to the extracellular domains of these receptors leads to homo- and heterodimerization of the receptors and subsequent tyrosine autophosphorylation. At least 9 different homo- and heterodimers of the ERBB proteins exist, with their formation displaying a distinct hierarchy. In this network, Her-2/neu plays a major coordinating role since each receptor with a specific ligand appears to prefer Her-2/neu as its heterodimeric partner. This preference is further biased by overexpression of Her-2/neu, as seen in many types of human cancer cells (62). For example, overexpression and amplification of Her-2/Neu by IHC and/or FISH has been noted in up to 20% of breast cancers and carries a poor prognosis (63,64).

Trastuzumab (Herceptin®, Genentech, Inc.) is a humanized IgG_1 moAb against Her-2/neu. Based on a number of seminal studies, it has been approved by the FDA for use in combination with chemotherapy as adjuvant therapy for Her-2/neu- and node-positive breast cancer (65–67). It is also approved for use in the metastatic setting either as monotherapy (68,69) or in combination with chemotherapy (70).

Trastuzumab is generally very well tolerated, with the exception of rare cardiac dysfunction, which is postulated to occur because Her-2 signaling is important for cardiac development (71). As a single agent, trastuzumab causes cardiac dysfunction in 3% to 7% of patients, with the risk appearing to be greatest when it is combined with anthracycline-containing regimens (27% vs. 8% compared to an anthracycline/cyclophosphamide alone) (72). As such, concurrent use of an anthracycline and trastuzumab is contraindicated.

In esophageal cancer, HER-2/neu overexpression has been variably demonstrated in esophageal squamous cell carcinoma (mean 23%, range 0%–52%) and GEJ adenocarcinoma (mean 22%, range 0%–43%) (73,74). The wide range of expression reflects the differences in receptor testing based on IHC or FISH as well as the varied cancer stages of patients. In esophageal squamous cell cancer, Her-2/neu overexpression has been correlated with extramural invasion and poor response to neoadjuvant chemotherapy (74). In GEJ adenocarcinoma, some studies have demonstrated a correlation with increasing depth of invasion, lymph node and distant organ metastasis, and overall poor survival (75).

Trastuzumab has undergone initial evaluation in esophageal cancer with encouraging results. In a phase I/II trial, increasing doses of trastuzumab were combined with cisplatin/paclitaxel and concurrent radiation for patients with locally advanced disease who were found to have 2+ (weakly positive) or 3+ (strongly positive) Her-2/neu overexpression by IHC (76). Out of 19 patients enrolled, 13 patients were treated at the full trastuzumab dose of 4 mg/kg during week 1 and then 2 mg/kg weekly for 5 weeks. The trial was closed prior to full accrual to 25 patients at the full trastuzumab dose because of slow accrual due to the fact that only approximately one-third of patients screened had tumors with Her-2/neu overexpression.

Of the 19 patients, 14 (74%) patients had either 3+ overexpression by IHC or an increase in Her-2/neu gene copy number by FISH. Of these 14 patients, 8 (57%) achieved a clinical CR. Six subsequently underwent surgery, and 3 were found to have achieved a pCR. One of 5 patients with 2+ Her-2/neu positivity by IHC but negative FISH achieved a clinical CR. At surgery, the patient was found to have residual microscopic disease. Therefore, the pCR rate was 16% for all patients enrolled and was 43% for patients who went to surgery. With a median follow-up of 54 months, the median OS was 24 months, with 2-year survival of 50%.

Toxicities were generally manageable, with only 1 incidence each (5%) of grade 3 and grade 4 esophagitis. Other grade 3/4 toxicities included neutropenia (21%) and nausea (16%). There was no cardiac toxicity.

In the metastatic setting, 2 trials combining trastuzumab with chemotherapy have been reported in abstract form. Preliminary results for an ongoing phase II evaluation of trastuzumab and cisplatin as first-line therapy for patients with locally advanced or metastatic gastric and GEJ adenocarcinoma with Her-2/neu overexpression by IHC and/or FISH were recently reported (77). Of 17 evaluable patients, 44% had involvement of the GEJ, and 16 of 17 had metastatic disease. Responses were seen in 6 patients (35%, including 1 CR), while 3 (18%) had SD. Treatment appeared tolerable, with no grade 4 toxicities.

A phase I trial has evaluated the combination of trastuzumab with paclitaxel (and increasing doses of interleukin-12) for patients with advanced Her-2/neu overexpressing tumors (78). Of 21 patients enrolled, 4 had esophageal cancer. Although the extent of prior therapy was not indicated, 2 of 4 esophageal cancer patients had a PR.

Vascular Endothelial Growth Factor

Therapies directed against vascular endothelial growth factor (VEGF) are the focus of major ongoing research in solid tumor malignancies. Folkman and others have provided compelling evidence linking tumor growth and metastases with angiogenesis (79).

Of the identified angiogenic factors, VEGF is the most potent and specific and has been identified as a crucial regulator of both normal and pathologic angiogenesis. VEGF produces a number of biologic effects, including endothelial cell mitogenesis and migration and induction of proteinases, leading to remodeling of the extracellular matrix, increased vascular permeability, and maintenance of survival for newly formed blood vessels (80).

Increased expression of VEGF has been measured in most human tumors examined to date, including tumors of the lung, breast, thyroid, gastrointestinal tract, kidney, bladder, ovary, and cervix, as well as angiosarcomas and glioblastomas (80). Nevertheless, a lack of correlation between baseline serum VEGF levels and response to anti-VEGF therapies has been noted in many tumor types, including colorectal cancer, breast cancer, and renal cell cancer. This lack of correlation may be due to complexities in the angiogenic pathway or limitations in the sensitivity of current assays for VEGF (81).

In esophageal cancer, VEGF is overexpressed in 30% to 60% of patients, with several studies demonstrating a correlation between high levels of VEGF expression, advanced stage, and poor survival in patients undergoing a potentially curative esophagectomy (82–86). Studies in squamous cancers have indicated that expression of VEGF in tumors correlates with more advanced tumor stage, the presence of nodal and distant metastases, and a poorer survival outcome (84,87).

In esophageal adenocarcinoma, increasing expression of VEGF correlates with the transition from Barrett's esophagus to high-grade dysplasia and with the transition from microinvasive to locally advanced cancer (88,89). While some investigators have not detected a relationship between VEGF expression and outcome in the adenocarcinoma histology (90), one series of 75 tumor samples obtained at esophagectomy did show that VEGF expression was correlated with the presence of angiolymphatic invasion, nodal metastases, and survival (91).

The lack of a clear correlation between baseline VEGF expression and outcome in patients with esophageal adenocarcinoma may be explained in part by the finding that tumor expression of VEGF actually increases after preoperative chemoradiation (92). Elevated serum levels of VEGF are also noted to persist following preoperative chemoradiation (even for those patients who are subsequently found to have a pCR at surgery), which suggests that nontumor cells, possibly tumor-infiltrating macrophages, may be responsible for VEGF production (93,94).

Anti-VEGF therapies that have been evaluated in esophageal cancer include the moAb, bevacizumab, and the multitarget TKI sunitinib.

Anti-VEGF moAb

Bevacizumab (Avastin®, Genentech, Inc.), a humanized IgG_1 monoclonal antibody against VEGF, has been extensively investigated in many solid tumor malignancies. The addition of bevacizumab to cytotoxic chemotherapy has been shown in several phase III clinical trials to improve the RR, TTP, and OS in patients with colorectal cancer (95), NSCLC (96), and breast cancer (97). On the basis of these studies, bevacizumab has been approved by the FDA for the treatment of metastatic colorectal cancer and NSCLC.

In addition to direct antiangiogenic effects, it has been postulated that bevacizumab may exert its antitumor effect in part by normalizing the "leaky" and disorganized vasculature within tumors. This leads to decreases in interstitial fluid pressures and increases chemotherapy drug delivery (98,99).

Bevacizumab is associated with unique side effects. In the phase III evaluation in advanced colorectal cancer, bevacizumab was noted to increase the incidence of grade 3 hypertension (11.0 vs. 2.3%, $P < 0.01$) compared to chemotherapy alone. Colonic perforation was also noted in 1.5% of patients (vs. 0% in the chemotherapy-only arm) (95). In the phase III evaluation in NSCLC, treatment with bevacizumab plus chemotherapy also led to an increased incidence of grade 3/4 proteinuria (3.1% vs. 0%, $P < 0.001$) and bleeding (4.4% vs. 0.7%, $P < 0.001$) compared to chemotherapy alone (96). Although bevacizumab is not generally thought to increase myelosuppression from chemotherapy, this trial also noted increased neutropenia (25.5% vs. 16.8%, $P = 0.002$) and thrombocytopenia (1.6% vs. 0.2%, $P = 0.04$) in the bevacizumab group. A previous randomized phase II trial in NSCLC had indicated that squamous cell histology was a risk factor for potentially fatal pulmonary hemorrhage, which led to the exclusion of such patients in the phase III trial (100). Finally, a recent meta-analysis also confirmed that bevacizumab and chemotherapy are associated with an increased incidence of arterial thromboembolism over chemotherapy alone (hazard ratio 2.0, 95% confidence interval [CI] 1.05–3.75; $P = 0.031$) (101). The increased risk was associated with more advanced age (over 65) and in patients with preexisting cardiovascular risk factors. The incidence of venous thromboembolism did not appear to be increased.

In upper gastrointestinal malignancies, bevacizumab has been evaluated in the metastatic setting. In a multicenter phase II evaluation led by MSKCC, bevacizumab and cisplatin/irinotecan were studied as first-line therapy in 47 patients with advanced gastric and GEJ adenocarcinoma (102). The addition of bevacizumab to cytotoxic chemotherapy significantly improved the TTP (8.3 months; 95% CI, 5.5–9.9 months) and OS (12.3 months; 95% CI, 11.3–17.2 months), compared to a historical TTP of 5 months. Therapy was well tolerated, although a 6% incidence of gastric perforation or near perforation and a 2% incidence of myocardial infarction were noted, possibly consistent with known toxicities of bevacizumab. Although the primary tumor was intact in 40 patients, significant upper gastrointestinal bleeding occurred in only 1 patient (2%). Grade 3/4 thromboembolic events were observed in 25.5% of patients, although this was noted to be similar to the 30% incidence previously observed in patients with locally advanced gastric cancer receiving preoperative cisplatin/irinotecan therapy (103).

Another evaluation of bevacizumab and docetaxel as second-line therapy for patients with advanced esophageal and gastric cancer has also been reported in abstract form (104). In this study, 26 patients were enrolled. Patients were allowed to have up to 1 prior therapy for metastatic disease. Of 17 patients evaluable for response, 4 PRs (24%) were noted, with an additional 4 SDs (24%). All responses occurred in patients with prior cisplatin/irinotecan therapy. In comparison, 2 prior phase II evaluations of docetaxel in chemotherapy-naive patients with gastric or esophageal adenocarcinoma reported a RR of 17% (105,106). Grade 3/4 toxicities on this trial included gastrointestinal bleeding (12%) and arterial thromboses (8%).

At present, there are ongoing trials evaluating bevacizumab in the locally advanced setting. At MSKCC, a trial is evaluating the combination of bevacizumab, cisplatin/irinotecan as induction chemotherapy followed by concurrent chemoradiotherapy with the same regimen and surgery for locally advanced esophageal adenocarcinoma. The Sarah Cannon Research Institute is also performing a phase II evaluation of carboplatin/paclitaxel/5-FU, bevacizumab, erlotinib, and radiation for locally advanced disease. In the United Kingdom, the ongoing MAGIC 2 trial randomizes patients with resectable gastric and GEJ cancer to receive perioperative ECX chemotherapy with or without bevacizumab.

In the metastatic setting, bevacizumab is being combined with a number of chemotherapy combinations and, in one trial, with erlotinib.

Anti-VEGF TKIs

Sunitinib (SU11248, Sutent®, Pfizer, Inc.) is an oral multitarget tyrosine kinase inhibitor that has activity against VEGF receptor (VEGFR). It is approved as first-line therapy for advanced renal cell cancer based on a phase III trial of sunitinib versus interferon-α that demonstrated improved PFS (11 vs. 5 months, $P < 0.001$), RR (31% vs. 6%, $P < 0.001$) and quality of life ($P < 0.001$) for sunitinib (107). In addition, it is also approved as therapy for advanced imatinib-resistant gastrointestinal stromal tumors (GISTs), based on its inhibitory activity against the c-kit TK and based on a phase III evaluation of sunitinib versus placebo for patients with imatinib-resistant GISTs (108).

Sunitinib has undergone promising initial evaluation in advanced gastric and GEJ cancer (109). In a multicenter phase II trial, 42 patients received sunitinib as second-line therapy. Of these, 2 patients (5%) had a PR, while another 15 (36%) had SD. Median TTP was 17.1 weeks, while median OS was 50.7 weeks. Toxicities were comparable to those seen on other trials with sunitinib. Significant grade 3/4 toxicities included hand–foot syndrome (10%), fatigue (10%), and anorexia (10%). Grade 3/4 hematologic toxicities included neutropenia (31%), thrombocytopenia (29%), and anemia (14%).

An evaluation of sorafenib (BAY 43-9006, Nexavar®, Bayer, Inc.), another multitarget TKI with anti-VEGFR activity that is also approved for advanced renal cell cancer, is planned at MSKCC for patients with advanced esophageal and GEJ tumors.

CYCLOOXYGENASE-2 INHIBITION

There has been growing preclinical evidence to link the expression of cyclooxygenase-2 (COX-2), an inducible enzyme that catalyzes prostaglandin synthesis, and carcinogenesis in Barrett's esophagus. COX-2 affects several pathways, including those of apoptosis, angiogenesis, inflammation, and immune surveillance (110,111). The use of aspirin and other nonsteroidal anti-inflammatory drugs (NSAIDs) to inhibit COX-2 has been associated with a lower esophageal cancer rate (112). A meta-analysis of 9 epidemiologic studies pooling 1,813 cancer cases showed a 43% risk reduction for esophageal cancer in patients who used NSAIDs (50% risk reduction for aspirin), with a trend toward a dose response (113).

Based on these preclinical and observational data, the Chemoprevention for Barrett's Esophagus Trial was implemented (114). This was a multicenter phase IIb randomized trial from April 2000 until June 2003 in which patients with Barrett's esophagus and low- or high-grade dysplasia were randomized to receive either a COX-2-specific inhibitor, celecoxib (Celebrex®, Pfizer, Inc.), 200 mg, twice daily or placebo. There was no difference in the primary outcome, which was the change from baseline to 48 weeks of therapy in the proportion of biopsy specimens with dysplasia in the celecoxib and placebo arms. Similarly, there were no differences in total surface area of the Barrett's esophagus or other biomarkers that were measured, including COX-1/2 mRNA levels, between both groups. Coupled with the cardiovascular risk that is now known to be associated with these drugs (115,116), the use of COX-2 inhibitors as chemoprevention cannot be considered routine.

In the United Kingdom, the ongoing Aspirin Esomperazole Chemoprevention trial hopes to randomize 5,000 patients with Barrett's esophagus to either 20 or 80 mg of esomeprazole (Nexium®, AstraZeneca, Inc.) daily. Half these patients will also be randomized to receive aspirin 300 mg daily. The primary end point will be the mortality or conversion rate from Barrett's esophagus to adenocarcinoma or high-grade dysplasia with aspirin or high-dose esomeprazole therapy. Trial accrual is estimated to be completed in December 2008, with the first interim analysis in 2010.

In the context of locally advanced disease, 3 trials have evaluated combinations of COX-2 inhibitors and preoperative chemoradiotherapy. In one phase II trial of 31 patients, celecoxib was combined with cisplatin/5-FU and radiation followed by surgery and adjuvant celecoxib (117). 22 patients (71%) underwent surgery, and 5 were found to have a pCR (16% of those enrolled and 23% of those who underwent surgery). Survival data were not available.

In a second, similar phase I/II trial, escalating doses of celecoxib were administered with cisplatin/5-FU and radiation to 13 patients prior to trial closure because of concerns about the safety of celecoxib (118). Seven of the 13 patients (54%) had a clinical CR, and 6 subsequently underwent surgery, with 1 pCR (8% of those enrolled and 17% of those who went to surgery). The median PFS was 8.8 months, and the median OS was 19.6 months.

The third phase II trial combined celecoxib with cisplatin/irinotecan and radiation, followed by surgery and maintenance celecoxib (42). On preliminary analysis, 25 of 36 patients had completed chemoradiotherapy and surgery, with 11 pCRs (31% of those enrolled and 44% of those who went to surgery).

Toxicities on all these trials were manageable and did not appear to be worsened by the addition of celecoxib. With the exception of the third trial, for which additional follow-up is required, however, there does not appear to be significant benefit for the addition of celecoxib when compared to historical controls.

OTHER TARGETS

In addition to the more established therapies discussed here, other tumor targets are also being actively evaluated. These include elements that control the cell cycle as well as apoptosis. Derangements in these processes have been linked to the malignant phenotype (119).

Flavopiridol is an inhibitor of cyclin-dependent kinases, which are required for cell cycling. Based on in vitro data that flavopiridol enhances paclitaxel-induced apoptosis, as well as promising data from a phase I trial (120), a phase II evaluation of sequential paclitaxel and flavopiridol was performed in patients with metastatic, paclitaxel-refractory esophageal cancer (121). Of 12 evaluable patients, 2 had SD, while the other 10 had PD; no responses were seen.

Bryostatin-1 is an inhibitor of protein kinase C, which is thought to mediate antiapoptotic signals (122). Two phase II evaluations have evaluated the combination of sequential paclitaxel and bryostatin-1 in esophagogastric cancer (123,124). While both studies suggest that this may be a potentially active combination, unexpected grade 3/4 myalgias were noted in approximately half of all patients in both studies.

Finally, other novel targets have recently been identified, including the tyrosine kinase receptor C-met, which has established oncogenic properties in several human cancers, including esophageal adenocarcinoma (125); the telomerase enzyme, which is responsible for the maintenance of telomere length in chromosomes and is thought to be important for cell immortalization as well as the early oncogenesis of esophageal squamous cell carcinoma (126, 127); and insulin-like growth factor (IGF) receptor and its ligand IGF-1, which have been implicated in the development, maintenance, and progression of human cancers, including esophageal cancer (128–131). Specific inhibitors to some of these targets have been identified and are currently undergoing preclinical and clinical evaluation in several human malignancies.

CONCLUSION

Drug development in cancer therapeutics has been transformed by our increasing understanding of the cellular mechanisms of carcinogenesis and our ability to design rational therapies to specifically target these aberrancies. In esophageal cancer, targeted therapies remain in early development, although encouraging results have been reported for anti-EGFR and anti-VEGF therapies, specifically cetuximab and bevacizumab.

In the next several years, ongoing clinical trials are expected to elucidate the role of these targeted therapies as single agents or in combination with chemotherapy or chemoradiotherapy. At the same time, researchers will continue to incorporate new targeted therapies, including novel multitarget TKIs currently undergoing phase I/II clinical evaluation, into future trials.

References

1. Orringer MB, Marshall B, Iannettoni MD. Transhiatal esophagectomy: clinical experience and refinements. *Ann Surg.* 1999;230(3):392–400; discussion 400–403.
2. Gebski V, Burmeister B, Smithers BM, et al. Survival benefits from neoadjuvant chemoradiotherapy or chemotherapy in oesophageal carcinoma: a meta-analysis. *Lancet Oncol.* 2007;8(3):226–234.
3. Walsh TN, Noonan N, Hollywood D, et al. A comparison of multimodal therapy and surgery for esophageal adenocarcinoma. *N Engl J Med.* 1996;335(7):462–467.
4. Cunningham D, Allum WH, Stenning SP, et al. Perioperative chemotherapy versus surgery alone for resectable gastroesophageal cancer. *N Engl J Med.* 2006;355(1):11–20.
5. Berger AC, Farma J, Scott WJ, et al. Complete response to neoadjuvant chemoradiotherapy in esophageal carcinoma is associated with significantly improved survival. *J Clin Oncol.* 2005;23(19):4330–4337.
6. Stahl M, Stuschke M, Lehmann N, et al. Chemoradiation with and without surgery in patients with locally advanced squamous cell carcinoma of the esophagus. *J Clin Oncol.* 2005;23(10):2310–2317.
7. Enzinger PC, Mayer RJ. Esophageal cancer. *N Engl J Med.* 2003;349(23):2241–2252.
8. Van Cutsem E, Moiseyenko VM, Tjulandin S, et al. Phase III study of docetaxel and cisplatin plus fluorouracil compared with cisplatin and fluorouracil as first-line therapy for advanced gastric cancer: a report of the V325 Study Group. *J Clin Oncol.* 2006;24(31):4991–4997.
9. Ross P, Nicolson M, Cunningham D, et al. Prospective randomized trial comparing mitomycin, cisplatin, and protracted venous-infusion fluorouracil (PVI 5-FU) with epirubicin, cisplatin, and PVI 5-FU in advanced esophagogastric cancer. *J Clin Oncol.* 2002;20(8):1996–2004.

10. Karamouzis MV, Grandis JR, Argiris A. Therapies directed against epidermal growth factor receptor in aerodigestive carcinomas. *JAMA*. 2007;298(1):70–82.
11. Yarden Y, Ullrich A. Growth factor receptor tyrosine kinases. *Annu Rev Biochem*. 1988;57:443–478.
12. Lynch TJ Jr, Kim ES, Eaby B, et al. Epidermal growth factor receptor inhibitor-associated cutaneous toxicities: an evolving paradigm in clinical management. *Oncologist*. 2007;12(5):610–621.
13. Schrag D, Chung KY, Flombaum C, Saltz L. Cetuximab therapy and symptomatic hypomagnesemia. *J Natl Cancer Inst*. 2005;97(16):1221–1224.
14. Perez-Soler R, Saltz L. Cutaneous adverse effects with HER1/EGFR-targeted agents: is there a silver lining? *J Clin Oncol*. 2005;23(22):5235–5246.
15. Salomon DS, Brandt R, Ciardiello F, et al. Epidermal growth factor-related peptides and their receptors in human malignancies. *Crit Rev Oncol Hematol*. 1995;19(3):183–232.
16. Itakura Y, Sasano H, Shiga C, et al. Epidermal growth factor receptor overexpression in esophageal carcinoma: an immunohistochemical study correlated with clinicopathologic findings and DNA amplification. *Cancer*. 1994;74(3):795–804.
17. Kitagawa Y, Ueda M, Ando N, et al. Further evidence for prognostic significance of epidermal growth factor receptor gene amplification in patients with esophageal squamous cell carcinoma. *Clin Cancer Res*. 1996;2(5):909–914.
18. Gibault L, Metges JP, Conan-Charlet V, et al. Diffuse EGFR staining is associated with reduced overall survival in locally advanced oesophageal squamous cell cancer. *Br J Cancer*. 2005;93(1):107–115.
19. Wilkinson NW, Black JD, Roukhadze E, et al. Epidermal growth factor receptor expression correlates with histologic grade in resected esophageal adenocarcinoma. *J Gastrointest Surg*. 2004;8(4):448–453.
20. Riely GJ, Politi KA, Miller VA, et al. Update on epidermal growth factor receptor mutations in non-small cell lung cancer. *Clin Cancer Res*. 2006;12(24):7232–7241.
21. Puhringer-Oppermann FA, Stein HJ, Sarbia M. Lack of EGFR gene mutations in exons 19 and 21 in esophageal (Barrett's) adenocarcinomas. *Dis Esophagus*. 2007;20(1):9–11.
22. Tew W, Shah M, Schwartz G, et al. Phase II trial of erlotonib for second-line treatment in advanced esophageal cancer. *Proc GI ASCO*. 2005:5. Abstract.
23. Dragovich T, McCoy S, Fenoglio-Preiser CM, et al. Phase II trial of erlotinib in gastroesophageal junction and gastric adenocarcinomas: SWOG 0127. *J Clin Oncol*. 2006;24(30):4922–4927.
24. Pao W, Wang TY, Riely GJ, et al. KRAS mutations and primary resistance of lung adenocarcinomas to gefitinib or erlotinib. *PLoS Med*. 2005;2(1):e17.
25. Khambata-Ford S, Garrett CR, Meropol NJ, et al. Expression of epiregulin and amphiregulin and K-ras mutation status predict disease control in metastatic colorectal cancer patients treated with cetuximab. *J Clin Oncol*. 2007;25(22):3230–3237.
26. Lievre A, Bachet JB, Le Corre D, et al. KRAS mutation status is predictive of response to cetuximab therapy in colorectal cancer. *Cancer Res*. 2006;66(8):3992–3995.
27. Janmaat ML, Gallegos-Ruiz MI, Rodriguez JA, et al. Predictive factors for outcome in a phase II study of gefitinib in second-line treatment of advanced esophageal cancer patients. *J Clin Oncol*. 2006;24(10):1612–1619.
28. Lord RV, O'Grady R, Sheehan C, et al. K-ras codon 12 mutations in Barrett's oesophagus and adenocarcinomas of the oesophagus and oesophagogastric junction. *J Gastroenterol Hepatol*. 2000;15(7):730–736.
29. Arber N, Shapira I, Ratan J, et al. Activation of c-K-ras mutations in human gastrointestinal tumors. *Gastroenterology*. 2000;118(6):1045–1050.
30. Goldstein NI, Prewett M, Zuklys K, et al.. Biological efficacy of a chimeric antibody to the epidermal growth factor receptor in a human tumor xenograft model. *Clin Cancer Res*. 1995;1(11):1311–1318.
31. Baselga J, Norton L, Masui H, et al. Antitumor effects of doxorubicin in combination with anti-epidermal growth factor receptor monoclonal antibodies. *J Natl Cancer Inst*. 1993;85(16):1327–1333.
32. Kawaguchi Y, Kono K, Mimura K, et al. Cetuximab induce antibody-dependent cellular cytotoxicity against EGFR-expressing esophageal squamous cell carcinoma. *Int J Cancer*. 2007;120(4):781–787.
33. Imai K, Takaoka A. Comparing antibody and small-molecule therapies for cancer. *Nat Rev Cancer*. 2006;6(9):714–727.
34. Cunningham D, Humblet Y, Siena S, et al. Cetuximab monotherapy and cetuximab plus irinotecan in irinotecan-refractory metastatic colorectal cancer. *N Engl J Med*. 2004;351(4):337–345.
35. Van Cutsem E, Nowacki M, Lang I, et al. Randomized phase III study of irinotecan and 5-FU/FA with or without cetuximab in the first-line treatment of patients with metastatic colorectal cancer (mCRC): the CRYSTAL trial. *J Clin Oncol*. 2007;25(18S):4000. Abstract.
36. Bonner JA, Harari PM, Giralt J, et al. Radiotherapy plus cetuximab for squamous-cell carcinoma of the head and neck. *N Engl J Med*. 2006;354(6):567–578.
37. Vermorken JB, Trigo J, Hitt R, et al. Open-label, uncontrolled, multicenter phase II study to evaluate the efficacy and toxicity of cetuximab as a single agent in patients with recurrent and/or metastatic squamous cell carcinoma of the head and neck who failed to respond to platinum-based therapy. *J Clin Oncol*. 2007;25(16):2171–2177.
38. Baselga J, Trigo JM, Bourhis J, et al. Phase II multicenter study of the antiepidermal growth factor receptor monoclonal antibody cetuximab in combination with platinum-based chemotherapy in patients with platinum-refractory metastatic and/or recurrent squamous cell carcinoma of the head and neck. *J Clin Oncol*. 2005;23(24):5568–5577.
39. Herbst RS, Arquette M, Shin DM, et al. Phase II multicenter study of the epidermal growth factor receptor antibody cetuximab and cisplatin for recurrent and refractory squamous cell carcinoma of the head and neck. *J Clin Oncol*. 2005;23(24):5578–5587.
40. Vermorken J, Mesia R, Vega V, et al. Cetuximab extends survival of patients with recurrent or metastatic SCCHN when added to first line platinum based therapy—results of a randomized phase III (extreme) study. *J Clin Oncol*. 2007;25(18S):6091. Abstract.
41. Enzinger P, Yock T, Suh W, et al. Phase II cisplatin, irinotecan, cetuximab and concurrent radiation therapy followed by surgery for locally advanced esophageal cancer. *J Clin Oncol*. 2006;24(18S):4064. Abstract.
42. Enzinger P, Mamon H, Choi N, et al. Phase II cisplatin, irinotecan, celecoxib and concurrent radiation therapy followed by surgery for locally advanced esophageal cancer. *Proc GI ASCO*. 2004;35. Abstract.
43. Ilson DH, Bains M, Kelsen DP, et al. Phase I trial of escalating-dose irinotecan given weekly with cisplatin and concurrent radiotherapy in locally advanced esophageal cancer. *J Clin Oncol*. 2003;21(15):2926–2932.
44. Ku G, Bains M, Rizk N, et al. Phase II trial of pre-operative cisplatin/irinotecan and radiotherapy for locally advanced esophageal cancer: PET scan after induction therapy may identify early treatment failure. *Proc GI ASCO*. 2007;9. Abstract.
45. Suntharalingam M, Dipetrillo T, Akerman P, et al. Cetuximab, paclitaxel, carboplatin and radiation for esophageal and gastric cancer. *J Clin Oncol*. 2006;24(18S):4029. Abstract.
46. Pinto C, Di Fabio F, Siena S, et al. Phase II study of cetuximab in combination with FOLFIRI in patients with untreated advanced gastric or gastroesophageal junction adenocarcinoma (FOLCETUX study). *Ann Oncol*. 2007;18(3):510–517.
47. Lordick F, Lorenzen S, Hegewisch-Becker S, et al. Cetuximab plus weekly oxaliplatin/5FU/FA (FUFOX) in 1st line metastatic gastric cancer. Final results from a multicenter phase II study of the AIO upper GI study group. *J Clin Oncol*. 2007;25(18S):4526. Abstract.
48. Vanhoefer U, Tewes M, Rojo F, et al. Phase I study of the humanized antiepidermal growth factor receptor monoclonal antibody EMD72000 in patients with advanced solid tumors that express the epidermal growth factor receptor. *J Clin Oncol*. 2004;22(1):175–184.
49. Rao S, Starling N, Benson M, et al. Phase I study of the humanized epidermal growth factor receptor (EGFR) antibody EMD 72000 (matuzumab) in combination with ECX (epirubicin, cisplatin and capecitabine) as first line treatment for advanced oesophagogastric (OG) adenocarcinoma. *J Clin Oncol*. 2005;23(16S):4028. Abstract.
50. Van Cutsem E, Peeters M, Siena S, et al. Open-label phase III trial of panitumumab plus best supportive care compared with best supportive care alone in patients with chemotherapy-refractory metastatic colorectal cancer. *J Clin Oncol*. 2007;25(13):1658–1664.
51. Figlin R, Belldegrun A, Crawford J, et al. ABX-EGF, a fully human anti-epidermal growth factor receptor (EGFR) monoclonal antibody (mAb) in patients with advanced cancer: phase 1 clinical results. *Proc Am Soc Clin Oncol*. 2002;21:35. Abstract.
52. Herbst RS, Fukuoka M, Baselga J. Gefitinib—a novel targeted approach to treating cancer. *Nat Rev*. 2004;4(12):956–965.
53. Shepherd FA, Rodrigues Pereira J, Ciuleanu T, et al. Erlotinib in previously treated non-small-cell lung cancer. *N Engl J Med*. 2005;353(2):123–132.
54. Fukuoka M, Yano S, Giaccone G, et al. Multi-institutional randomized phase II trial of gefitinib for previously treated patients with advanced non-small-cell lung cancer (the IDEAL 1 trial) [corrected]. *J Clin Oncol*. 2003;21(12):2237–2246.
55. Kris MG, Natale RB, Herbst RS, et al. Efficacy of gefitinib, an inhibitor of the epidermal growth factor receptor tyrosine kinase, in symptomatic patients with non-small cell lung cancer: a randomized trial. *JAMA*. 2003;290(16):2149–2158.
56. Gatzemeier U, Pluzanska A, Szczesna A, et al. Phase III study of erlotinib in combination with cisplatin and gemcitabine in advanced non-small-cell lung cancer: the Tarceva Lung Cancer Investigation Trial. *J Clin Oncol*, 2007;25(12):1545–1552.
57. Giaccone G, Herbst RS, Manegold C, et al. Gefitinib in combination with gemcitabine and cisplatin in advanced non-small-cell lung cancer: a phase III trial—INTACT 1. *J Clin Oncol*. 2004;22(5):777–784.
58. Herbst RS, Giaccone G, Schiller JH, et al. Gefitinib in combination with paclitaxel and carboplatin in advanced non-small-cell lung cancer: a phase III trial—INTACT 2. *J Clin Oncol*. 2004;22(5):785–794.
59. Herbst RS, Prager D, Hermann R, et al. TRIBUTE: a phase III trial of erlotinib hydrochloride (OSI-774) combined with carboplatin and paclitaxel chemotherapy in advanced non-small-cell lung cancer. *J Clin Oncol*. 2005;23(25):5892–5899.
60. Moore MJ, Goldstein D, Hamm J, et al. Erlotinib plus gemcitabine compared with gemcitabine alone in patients with advanced pancreatic cancer: a phase III trial of the National Cancer Institute of Canada Clinical Trials Group. *J Clin Oncol*. 2007;25(15):1960–1966.
61. Sunpaweravong P, Sunpaweravong S, Sangthawan D, et al. Combination of gefitinib, cisplatin and 5-FU chemotherapy, and radiation therapy (RT) in newly-diagnosed patients with esophageal carcinoma. *J Clin Oncol*. 2007;25(18S):4605. Abstract.
62. Casalini P, Iorio MV, Galmozzi E, et al. Role of HER receptors family in development and differentiation. *J Cell Physiol*. 2004;200(3):343–350.
63. Goldhirsch A, Glick JH, Gelber RD, et al. Meeting highlights: international expert consensus on the primary therapy of early breast cancer 2005. *Ann Oncol*. 2005;16(10):1569–1583.
64. Owens MA, Horten BC, Da Silva MM. HER2 amplification ratios by fluorescence in situ hybridization and correlation with immunohistochemistry in a cohort of 6556 breast cancer tissues. *Clin Breast Cancer*. 2004;5(1):63–69.
65. Piccart-Gebhart MJ, Procter M, Leyland-Jones B, et al. Trastuzumab after adjuvant chemotherapy in HER2-positive breast cancer. *N Engl J Med*. 2005;353(16):1659–1672.
66. Romond EH, Perez EA, Bryant J, et al. Trastuzumab plus adjuvant chemotherapy for operable HER2-positive breast cancer. *N Engl J Med*. 2005;353(16):1673–1684.

67. Smith I, Procter M, Gelber RD, et al. 2-year follow-up of trastuzumab after adjuvant chemotherapy in HER2-positive breast cancer: a randomised controlled trial. *Lancet.* 2007;369(9555):29–36.
68. Cobleigh MA, Vogel CL, Tripathy D, et al. Multinational study of the efficacy and safety of humanized anti-HER2 monoclonal antibody in women who have HER2-overexpressing metastatic breast cancer that has progressed after chemotherapy for metastatic disease. *J Clin Oncol.* 1999;17(9):2639–2648.
69. Vogel CL, Cobleigh MA, Tripathy D, et al. Efficacy and safety of trastuzumab as a single agent in first-line treatment of HER2-overexpressing metastatic breast cancer. *J Clin Oncol.* 2002;20(3):719–726.
70. Slamon DJ, Leyland-Jones B, Shak S, et al. Use of chemotherapy plus a monoclonal antibody against HER2 for metastatic breast cancer that overexpresses HER2. *N Engl J Med.* 2001;344(11):783–792.
71. Crone SA, Zhao YY, Fan L, et al. ErbB2 is essential in the prevention of dilated cardiomyopathy. *Nat Med.* 2002;8(5):459–465.
72. Seidman A, Hudis C, Pierri MK, et al. Cardiac dysfunction in the trastuzumab clinical trials experience. *J Clin Oncol.* 2002;20(5):1215–1221.
73. al-Kasspooles M, Moore JH, Orringer MB, et al. Amplification and over-expression of the EGFR and erbB-2 genes in human esophageal adenocarcinomas. *Int J Cancer.* 1993;54(2):213–219.
74. Ross JS, McKenna BJ. The HER-2/neu oncogene in tumors of the gastrointestinal tract. *Cancer Invest.* 2001;19(5):554–568.
75. Brien TP, Odze RD, Sheehan CE, et al. HER-2/neu gene amplification by FISH predicts poor survival in Barrett's esophagus-associated adenocarcinoma. *Hum Pathol.* 2000;31(1):35–39.
76. Safran H, Dipetrillo T, Akerman P, et al. Phase I/II study of trastuzumab, paclitaxel, cisplatin and radiation for locally advanced, HER2 overexpressing, esophageal adenocarcinoma. *Int J Radiat Oncol Biol Phys.* 2007;67(2):405–409.
77. Cortés-Funes H, Rivera F, Alés I, et al. Phase II of trastuzumab and cisplatin in patients (pts) with advanced gastric cancer (AGC) with HER2/neu overexpression/amplification. *J Clin Oncol.* 2007;25(18S):4613. Abstract.
78. Carson W, Roda J, Parihar R, et al. Phase I trial of interleukin-12 with trastuzumab and paclitaxel in HER2-overexpressing malignancies. *J Clin Oncol.* 2005;23(16S):2531. Abstract.
79. Folkman J. Angiogenesis and angiogenesis inhibition: an overview. *EXS.* 1997;79:1–8.
80. Ferrara N, Davis-Smyth T. The biology of vascular endothelial growth factor. *Endocr Rev.* 1997;18(1):4–25.
81. Longo R, Gasparini G. Challenges for patient selection with VEGF inhibitors. *Cancer Chemother Pharmacol.* 2007;60(2):151–170.
82. Inoue K, Ozeki Y, Suganuma T, et al. Vascular endothelial growth factor expression in primary esophageal squamous cell carcinoma. Association with angiogenesis and tumor progression. *Cancer.* 1997;79(2):206–213.
83. Kitadai Y, Haruma K, Tokutomi T, et al. Significance of vessel count and vascular endothelial growth factor in human esophageal carcinomas. *Clin Cancer Res.* 1998;4(9):2195–2200.
84. Kleespies A, Guba M, Jauch KW, et al. Vascular endothelial growth factor in esophageal cancer. *J Surg Oncol.* 2004;87(2):95–104.
85. Shih CH, Ozawa S, Ando N, et al. Vascular endothelial growth factor expression predicts outcome and lymph node metastasis in squamous cell carcinoma of the esophagus. *Clin Cancer Res.* 2000;6(3):1161–1168.
86. Imdahl A, Bognar G, Schulte-Monting J, et al. Predictive factors for response to neoadjuvant therapy in patients with oesophageal cancer. *Eur J Cardiothorac Surg.* 2002;21(4):657–663.
87. Shimada H, Hoshino T, Okazumi S, et al. Expression of angiogenic factors predicts response to chemoradiotherapy and prognosis of oesophageal squamous cell carcinoma. *Br J Cancer.* 2002;86(4):552–557.
88. Mobius C, Stein HJ, Becker I, et al. The "angiogenic switch" in the progression from Barrett's metaplasia to esophageal adenocarcinoma. *Eur J Surg Oncol.* 2003;29(10):890–894.
89. Vallbohmer D, Peters JH, Kuramochi H, et al. Molecular determinants in targeted therapy for esophageal adenocarcinoma. *Arch Surg.* 2006;141(5):476–481; discussion 81–82.
90. Kleespies A, Bruns CJ, Jauch KW. Clinical significance of VEGF-A, -C and -D expression in esophageal malignancies. *Onkologie.* 2005;28(5):281–288.
91. Saad RS, El-Gohary Y, Memari E, et al. Endoglin (CD105) and vascular endothelial growth factor as prognostic markers in esophageal adenocarcinoma. *Hum Pathol.* 2005;36(9):955–961.
92. Kulke MH, Odze RD, Mueller JD, et al. Prognostic significance of vascular endothelial growth factor and cyclooxygenase 2 expression in patients receiving preoperative chemoradiation for esophageal cancer. *J Thorac Cardiovasc Surg.* 2004;127(6):1579–1586.
93. McDonnell CO, Bouchier-Hayes DJ, Toomey D, et al. Effect of neoadjuvant chemoradiotherapy on angiogenesis in oesophageal cancer. *Br J Surg.* 2003;90(11):1373–1378.
94. McDonnell CO, Harmey JH, Bouchier-Hayes DJ, et al. Effect of multimodality therapy on circulating vascular endothelial growth factor levels in patients with oesophageal cancer. *Br J Surg.* 2001;88(8):1105–1109.
95. Hurwitz H, Fehrenbacher L, Novotny W, et al. Bevacizumab plus irinotecan, fluorouracil, and leucovorin for metastatic colorectal cancer. *N Engl J Med.* 2004;350(23):2335–2342.
96. Sandler A, Gray R, Perry MC, et al. Paclitaxel-carboplatin alone or with bevacizumab for non-small-cell lung cancer. *N Engl J Med.* 2006;355(24):2542–2550.
97. Miller K. E2100: a randomized phase III trial of paclitaxel versus paclitaxel plus bevacizumab as first-line therapy for locally recurrent or metastatic breast cancer. *Proc Am Soc Clin Oncol.* 2005. Abstract.
98. Jain RK. Normalizing tumor vasculature with anti-angiogenic therapy: a new paradigm for combination therapy. *Nat Med.* 2001;7(9):987–989.
99. Willett CG, Boucher Y, di Tomaso E, et al. Direct evidence that the VEGF-specific antibody bevacizumab has antivascular effects in human rectal cancer. *Nat Med.* 2004;10(2):145–147.
100. Johnson DH, Fehrenbacher L, Novotny WF, et al. Randomized phase II trial comparing bevacizumab plus carboplatin and paclitaxel with carboplatin and paclitaxel alone in previously untreated locally advanced or metastatic non-small-cell lung cancer. *J Clin Oncol.* 2004;22(11):2184–2191.
101. Scappaticci FA, Skillings JR, Holden SN, et al. Arterial thromboembolic events in patients with metastatic carcinoma treated with chemotherapy and bevacizumab. *J Natl Cancer Inst.* 2007;99(16):1232–1239.
102. Shah MA, Ramanathan RK, Ilson DH, et al. Multicenter phase II study of irinotecan, cisplatin, and bevacizumab in patients with metastatic gastric or gastroesophageal junction adenocarcinoma. *J Clin Oncol.* 2006;24(33):5201–5206.
103. Shah MA, Ilson D, Kelsen DP. Thromboembolic events in gastric cancer: high incidence in patients receiving irinotecan- and bevacizumab-based therapy. *J Clin Oncol.* 2005; 23(11):2574–2576.
104. Enzinger P, Fidias P, Meyerhardt J, et al. Phase II study of bevacizumab and docetaxel in metastatic esophageal and gastric cancer. *Proc GI ASCO.* 2006;68. Abstract.
105. Einzig AI, Neuberg D, Remick SC, et al. Phase II trial of docetaxel (Taxotere) in patients with adenocarcinoma of the upper gastrointestinal tract previously untreated with cytotoxic chemotherapy: the Eastern Cooperative Oncology Group (ECOG) results of protocol E1293. *Med Oncol.* 1996;13(2):87–93.
106. Heath EI, Urba S, Marshall J, et al. Phase II trial of docetaxel chemotherapy in patients with incurable adenocarcinoma of the esophagus. *Invest New Drugs.* 2002;20(1):95–99.
107. Motzer RJ, Hutson TE, Tomczak P, et al. Sunitinib versus interferon alfa in metastatic renal-cell carcinoma. *N Engl J Med.* 2007;356(2):115–124.
108. Demetri GD, van Oosterom AT, Garrett CR, et al. Efficacy and safety of sunitinib in patients with advanced gastrointestinal stromal tumour after failure of imatinib: a randomised controlled trial. *Lancet.* 2006;368(9544):1329–1338.
109. Bang Y, Kang Y, Kang W, et al. Sunitinib as second-line treatment for advanced gastric cancer: preliminary results from a phase II study. *J Clin Oncol.* 2007;25(18S):4603. Abstract.
110. Altorki NK, Subbaramaiah K, Dannenberg AJ. COX-2 inhibition in upper aerodigestive tract tumors. *Semin Oncol.* 2004;31(2 suppl 7):30–36.
111. Dannenberg AJ, Lippman SM, Mann JR, et al. Cyclooxygenase-2 and epidermal growth factor receptor: pharmacologic targets for chemoprevention. *J Clin Oncol.* 2005;23(2):254–266.
112. Morris CD, Armstrong GR, Bigley G, et al. Cyclooxygenase-2 expression in the Barrett's metaplasia-dysplasia-adenocarcinoma sequence. *Am J Gastroenterol.* 2001;96(4):990–996.
113. Corley DA, Kerlikowske K, Verma R, et al. Protective association of aspirin/NSAIDs and esophageal cancer: a systematic review and meta-analysis. *Gastroenterology.* 2003;124(1):47–56.
114. Heath EI, Canto MI, Piantadosi S, et al. Secondary chemoprevention of Barrett's esophagus with celecoxib: results of a randomized trial. *J Natl Cancer Inst.* 2007;99(7):545–557.
115. Bresalier RS, Sandler RS, Quan H, et al. Cardiovascular events associated with rofecoxib in a colorectal adenoma chemoprevention trial. *N Engl J Med.* 2005;352(11):1092–1102.
116. Bertagnolli MM, Eagle CJ, Zauber AG, et al. Celecoxib for the prevention of sporadic colorectal adenomas. *N Engl J Med.* 2006;355(9):873–884.
117. Govindan R, McLeod H, Mantravadi P, et al. Cisplatin, fluorouracil, celecoxib, and RT in resectable esophageal cancer: preliminary results. *Oncology (Huntingt).* 2004;18(suppl 14):18–21.
118. Dawson SJ, Michael M, Biagi J, et al. A phase I/II trial of celecoxib with chemotherapy and radiotherapy in the treatment of patients with locally advanced oesophageal cancer. *Invest New Drugs.* 2007;25(2):123–129.
119. Schwartz GK, Shah MA. Targeting the cell cycle: a new approach to cancer therapy. *J Clin Oncol.* 2005;23(36):9408–9421.
120. Schwartz GK, O'Reilly E, Ilson D, et al. Phase I study of the cyclin-dependent kinase inhibitor flavopiridol in combination with paclitaxel in patients with advanced solid tumors. *J Clin Oncol.* 2002;20(8):2157–2170.
121. Rathkopf D, Ilson D, Yi S, et al. A phase II trial of sequential paclitaxel and flavopiridol in patients with metastatic paclitaxel-refractory esophageal cancer. *Proc GI ASCO.* 2004;67. Abstract.
122. Philip PA, Harris AL. Potential for protein kinase C inhibitors in cancer therapy. *Cancer Treat Res.* 1995;78:3–27.
123. Ajani JA, Jiang Y, Faust J, et al. A multi-center phase II study of sequential paclitaxel and bryostatin-1 (NSC 339555) in patients with untreated, advanced gastric or gastroesophageal junction adenocarcinoma. *Invest New Drugs.* 2006;24(4):353–357.
124. Ilson D, Shah M, O'Reilly E, et al. A phase II trial of weekly one hour paclitaxel followed by bryostatin-1 in patients with advanced esophageal cancer: an active new drug combination. *Proc Am Soc Clin Oncol.* 2001;20:633. Abstract.
125. Watson GA, Zhang X, Stang MT, et al. Inhibition of c-Met as a therapeutic strategy for esophageal adenocarcinoma. *Neoplasia.* 2006;8(11):949–955.

126. Tang WK, Chui CH, Fatima S, et al. Inhibitory effects of *Gleditsia sinensis* fruit extract on telomerase activity and oncogenic expression in human esophageal squamous cell carcinoma. *Int J Mol Med.* 2007;19(6):953–960.
127. Yu HP, Xu SQ, Lu WH, et al. Telomerase activity and expression of telomerase genes in squamous dysplasia and squamous cell carcinoma of the esophagus. *J Surg Oncol.* 2004;86(2):99–104.
128. Sohda M, Kato H, Miyazaki T, et al. The role of insulin-like growth factor 1 and insulin-like growth factor binding protein 3 in human esophageal cancer. *Anticancer Res.* 2004;24(5A):3029–3034.
129. Liu YC, Leu CM, Wong FH, et al. Autocrine stimulation by insulin-like growth factor I is involved in the growth, tumorigenicity and chemoresistance of human esophageal carcinoma cells. *J Biomed Sci.* 2002;9(6 pt 2):665–674.
130. Chen SC, Chou CK, Wong FH, et al. Overexpression of epidermal growth factor and insulin-like growth factor-I receptors and autocrine stimulation in human esophageal carcinoma cells. *Cancer Res.* 1991;51(7):1898–1903.
131. Moschos SJ, Mantzoros CS. The role of the IGF system in cancer: from basic to clinical studies and clinical applications. *Oncology.* 2002;63(4):317–332.

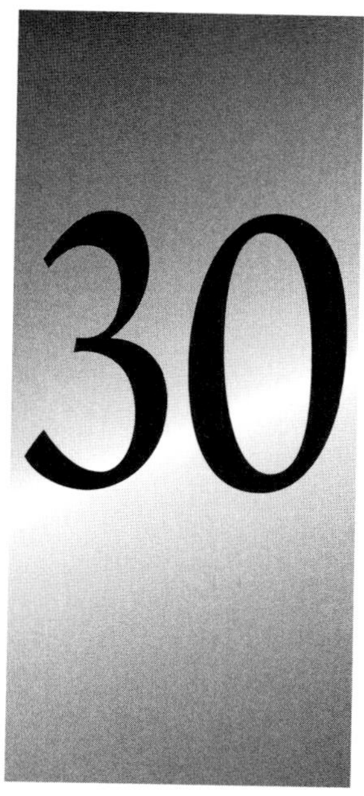

30 Principles of Radiation Therapy

Melenda Jeter

Radiation therapy has been used as a cancer treatment for more than 100 years. X-rays were first described by Roentgen. The field of radiation therapy began to grow in the early 1900s, largely due to the groundbreaking work of Nobel Prize–winning scientist Marie Curie, who discovered the radioactive element radium. In the 1930s, clinical therapy using protracted, fractionated radiation therapy was developed by Henry Coutard. The more recent treatment era began with the use of Cobalt-60 as a radiation source, which has been largely replaced by the linear accelerator. Two-dimensional therapy has been largely replaced by 3-D–conformal radiation therapy (3DCRT). Currently, it is not uncommon to treat patients with intensity modulated therapy or even have a discussion about proton therapy. Alongside the technical advances has been increasing knowledge of radiation biology. This has allowed a better understanding of the molecular biology of radiation effects and has enhanced the possibility of significant improvement in using radiation therapy for treating cancer. To understand the principles of radiation therapy, one must study 3 fundamental perspectives: physical, biologic, and clinical. This chapter will address these 3 areas.

RADIATION PHYSICS

Ionizing radiation used in radiation therapy includes both electromagnetic waves and particulate radiation. Electromagnetic waves are part of a broad spectrum that includes radio waves, visible light, X-rays, and gamma rays. In radiation therapy, X-rays and gamma rays are used. These types of radiation possess the same general properties but differ in only their source and energy. X-rays for cancer treatment are produced from a linear accelerator when energetic charged particles (usually electrons) impinge on a target and react with either atomic nuclei or orbital electrons. The maximum energy of the X-rays is in the megavoltage range, typically between 4 and 20 megavolts (MV). The penetrating megavoltage beams deliver a relatively low dose to superficial tissues. This is a property called "skin sparing" and reduces skin reactions. Gamma rays are also produced in the megavoltage range during the decay of an unstable nucleus in a radioactive element such as Cobalt-60. However, due to limited penetration and sharpness, Cobalt-60 is less frequently used and typically restricted to head and neck cancers where targets are more superficial. X-rays and gamma rays are called photons.

Particulate radiation includes electrons and protons. Electrons from a linear accelerator can be used to deliver radiation to superficial tissues. Because electrons have both mass and charge, they interact over a shorter distance in tissues compared to photons and therefore lose energy more rapidly, limiting their penetration. With few exceptions, most radiation therapy is given with megavoltage linear accelerator machines using photons. Proton treatment is not readily available for daily radiation therapy for the vast majority of cancer patients and is also considered by many to be experimental.

Radiation can be delivered by an external source over a distance (teletherapy), or from a short range by interstitial, intracavitary, or surface applicators (brachytherapy). The depth of penetration from any source depends on the energy of the photon. For example, for a 4 MV photon beam, 60% of the maximum dose is delivered to a depth of 10 cm, whereas for a 20 MV photon beam 80% of the maximum dose is delivered to this same depth (Figure 30.1) (1). For implants, the dose falls off rapidly, over a few centimeters, and follows the inverse square law (i.e., as the distance from the source is doubled, the dose falls to one-fourth its value).

Radiation may be directly or indirectly ionizing. Charged particles are directly ionizing. With sufficient energy, they can directly disrupt the molecular structure of material through which they pass producing chemical and biological changes. Electromagnetic radiation is indirectly ionizing. When absorbed in tissue, they give up their energy to produce fast-moving charged particles, which then inflict the damage. In tissue, photons may interact in several ways. These include coherent scattering, photoelectric effect, Compton effect, pair production, and photodisintegration. The dominant reaction depends on the energy of the radiation used. At the energies used in radiation therapy, the Compton effect is the dominant reaction. Here the photon interacts with a loosely bound orbital electron. Part of the energy of the incident photon is transferred to the electron. This Compton electron may then interact with other electrons in the surrounding tissue. The remaining energy is carried away by another photon (Figure 30.2). The probability of Compton interactions is essentially independent of the atomic number of the target tissue. Thus, the amount of radiation absorbed is roughly the same whether the target is bone or soft tissue. In contrast, the photoelectric effect that is seen at lower energies is highly dependent on atomic number. Therefore bone and soft tissue appear different on a diagnostic X-rays that use lower energy photons.

Protons and other heavy particles interact with the nucleus of an atom and not with the orbital electrons. They dislodge various lower-energy showers of densely ionizing protons, neutrons, and others and deposit a large amount of energy over a short distance. This redistribution of energy is called linear energy transfer (LET). The amount of energy transferred depends on the type of radiation used. Photons and electrons have a low rate of energy transfer (low LET), while heavy particles tend to deposit their energy in a track over a relatively short distance and are classified as high-LET radiations.

Radiation dose is quantified using the amount of energy absorbed per unit mass. The standard unit for reporting dose is the Gray (Gy), which is defined as 1 joule per kilogram. Older publications may refer to the dose in terms of the rad, which is equal to 0.01 Gy or 1 centigray (cGy).

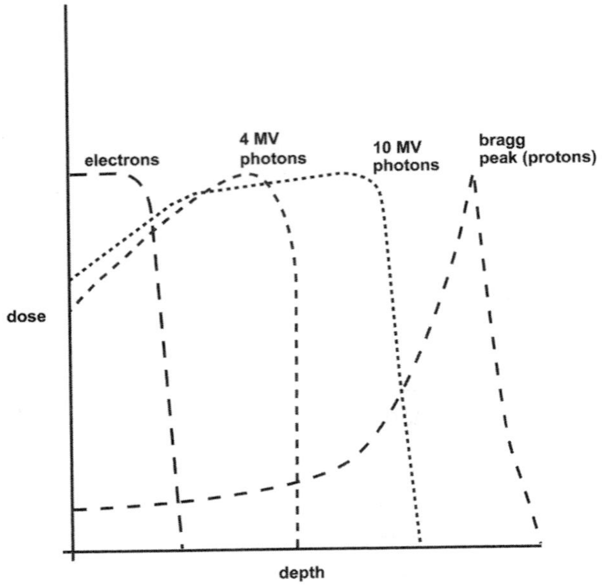

FIGURE 30.1

Depth-dose curves.

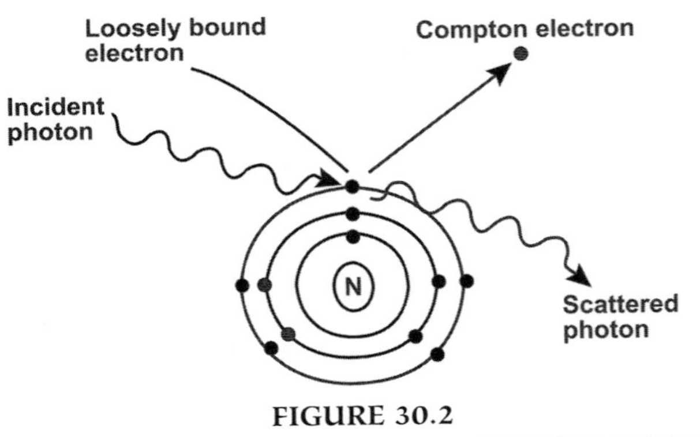

FIGURE 30.2

The Compton effect.

RADIOBIOLOGY

DNA is the ultimate target for lethal injury from radiation therapy with ionization of the atoms that make up the DNA chain (2). Radiation may directly interact with a critical intracellular structure of DNA and cause biological damage. This direct damage is the dominant process in high-LET radiation. In contrast with photon therapy, the dominant process is an indirect action. Approximately one-third of the damage may be due to the direct interaction of a recoil electron with a target molecule. The remaining two-thirds of the damage will be due to indirect action in which the recoil electron reacts with water to produce hydroxyl radicals, which may then interact with a target molecule. Various substances alter the effectiveness of hydroxyl radicals resulting in radiosensitization or radioprotection. The radiosensitivity of normal tissues in the thorax, especially normal lung and esophagus, has led investigators to seek ways of enhancing the biological antitumor effects of radiation while reducing its acute and late effects on normal tissues (3).

A cell survival curve expresses the relationship between radiation dose and the proportion of cells that survive. They are obtained by exposing a population of cells to incremental doses of radiation and counting the number of surviving cells. The data are then plotted using a logarithmic scale for surviving fraction on the ordinate and a linear scale for dose in the abscissa. The overall shape of such curves is nearly the same for all mammalian cells. With low-LET radiation, the curve usually begins with a shoulder in the low-dose region before beginning a logarithmic decline. The presence of a shoulder suggests that cells may accumulate some injury without dying or sublethal damage. This damage could then be repaired. In contrast, high-LET radiations yield a survival that is a straight line from the origin. Survival is essentially an exponential function of dose. Because cancer cells generally are undifferentiated, they reproduce more and have a diminished ability to repair sublethal damage compared to most healthy differentiated cells. The DNA damage is inherited through cell division, accumulating damage to the cancer cells causing them to die or reproduce more slowly.

One method of describing survival curves is the linear-quadratic model. This model assumes 2 components to cell killing. The linear (α) component is responsible for the initial shoulder on the cell survival curve and is caused by repairable damage to the target. The quadratic (β) component represents non-repairable damage. The linear component is proportional to the dose, while the quadratic component is proportional to the dose squared. The dose at which the 2 components of cell killing are equal is the α/β ratio. In general, cells from radiosensitive and acutely reacting tissues have a higher α/β ratio than do cells from radioresistant tumors. In contrast, tumors with a lower α/β ratio tend to be late reacting and have a higher dependence on dose per fraction and dose rate than radiosensitive tumors. Although the general shape of the curve is essentially the same for all mammalian cells, there is some variation in the inherent radiosensitivity of different cell lines and tumors. These variations are expressed mainly in the shoulder and in the slope of the curve (Figure 30.3).

Different conditions may also affect cell survival. Collectively, these factors are referred to as the 4 *R*'s of radiation biology—reoxygenation, repair, reassortment, and repopulation. Fractionating radiation therapy takes advantages of these factors: *reassortment* of cells throughout the cell cycle into more sensitive phases of the cycle and *reoxygenation* of hypoxic cells after one or more cycles of radiation increasing tumor damage, as well as *repair* of sublethal damage sparing normal tissue and *repopulation* of normal tissue cells between fractions. Radiation therapy attacks cancer cells that are dividing and also affects dividing cells in normal tissue. It is the damage to normal tissues that causes side effects. Each time radiation is given, it involves a balance between destroying the cancer cells and sparing the normal cells.

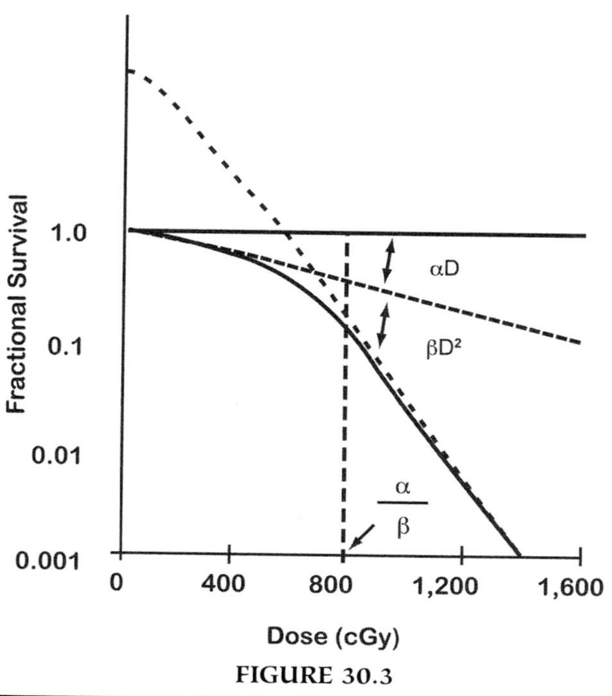

FIGURE 30.3

Typical cell survival curve with logarithmic fractional survival versus dose. With low-LET radiation, the curve usually starts with a shoulder in the low-dose area before beginning a logarithmic decline.

Reoxygenation

The effect of oxygen on cells subjected to radiation has been well documented (4). In general, the presence of oxygen enhances the effect of ionizing radiation. For sparsely ionizing radiation such as photons, the ratio of doses needed to produce the same biological effect in the absence of oxygen can by as high as 2.5 or 3.0. This is the oxygen enhancement ratio (OER). For more densely ionizing radiation, the OER approaches 1.0 where there is no oxygen effect. The exact nature of the oxygen effect is not known, but it is generally believed that oxygen aids in the production of cell damage by radiation-induced free radicals.

Repair

If sufficient damage occurs at a critical site of DNA, the cell will die during one of its subsequent divisions. This results in lethal damage. Other cells may experience sublethal damage that may be repaired if given sufficient time, energy, and nutrients. This repair of sublethal damage is the reason cells can tolerate higher total doses of radiation when the radiation is administered in multiple small fractions. Slowly responding tissues, such as the spinal cord, tend to repair damage slowly (over 6 to 8 hrs), but the repair is essentially complete. In contrast, rapidly responding tissues, such as skin and mucosa, often have incomplete repair. The implication is that slowly responding tissues are spared more by using multiple small fractions of radiation given at least 6 hours apart than acutely responding tissues.

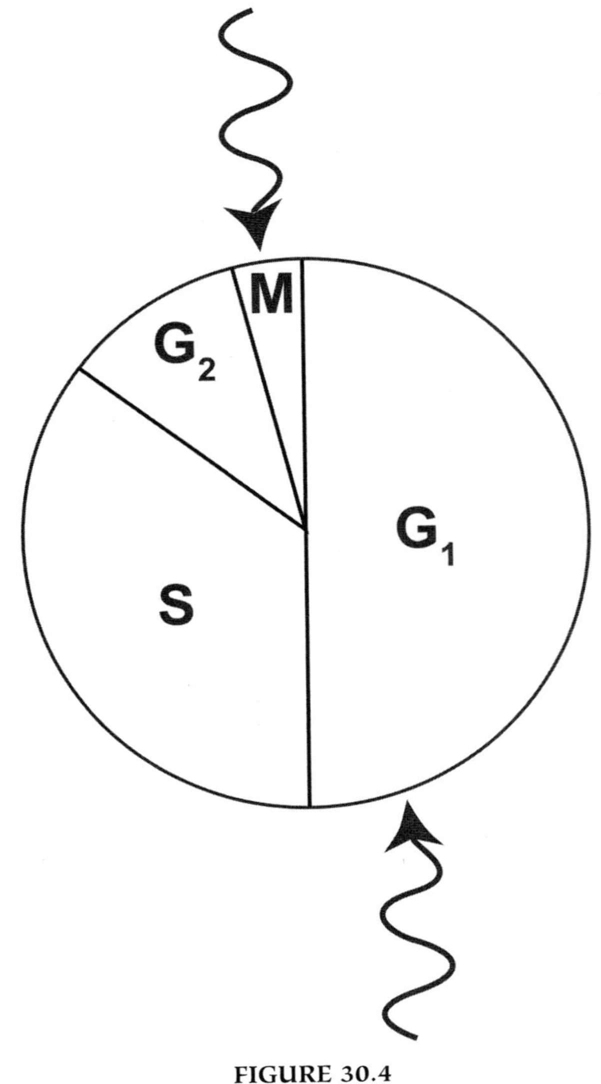

FIGURE 30.4

Cell growth cycle. Arrows demonstrate areas of the cycle which are more sensitive to radiation.

Reassortment

Individual cells will vary in their radiosensitivity throughout the cell cycle. The most sensitive stage is in mitosis (M), and the least sensitive is during the late phase of nucleic acid synthesis (S). If the first gap phase (G_1) has an appreciable length, there will be a resistant period in early G_1 followed by a sensitive phase in late G_1. Finally, the second gap phase (G_2) is also a sensitive phase (Figure 30.4). Fractionating radiation therapy may have an advantage of catching cells in different, more sensitive phases over time.

Repopulation

Both tumors and normal tissues may undergo cell division during a course of fractionated radiation therapy. Repopulation is beneficial because it can reduce the overall injury to normal tissue, which may respond by shortening the duration of the cell cycle during a fractionated course of treatment (5). In tumors, cells may divide faster than before radiation treatment. This is known as accelerated repopulation. The possibility of accelerated repopulation is a reason for completing radiation therapy as soon as feasible and avoiding delays during treatment.

CLINICAL IMPLEMENTATION

The ultimate aim of radiation therapy is to deliver radiation to a defined tumor volume with minimal damage to surrounding healthy tissue. It may be used for curative or adjuvant treatment. It is also used for palliative treatment (where cure is not possible and the aim is for local disease control or symptomatic relief). Radiation is commonly combined with surgery, chemotherapy, or a mixture of the three.

Multidisciplinary Approach

Radiation therapy is an important component of the multidisciplinary management of esophageal cancer. As re-treatment with radiation therapy within the same area is rarely possible, it is important to define the goal and course of treatment at the outset of intervention. This plan should include all disciplines involved, including a medical oncologist and thoracic surgeon. These 3 disciplines should be intimately involved in the care of esophageal cancer patients. They must closely assess the conditions relative to the patient and tumor, review the need for diagnostic and staging procedures, and determine the best treatment strategy. Once radiation therapy has been elected, treatment should be carefully planned and executed.

In curative radiation therapy, the treatment course is usually more prolonged and can be more physically taxing. Increased side effects must be accepted as the inevitable price from the possibility of cure. Patients who are physically unfit for radical curative surgery may be able to better tolerate definite radiation therapy. Definitive radiation therapy also has the advantage of organ sparing, e.g., controlling the cancer while avoiding the removal of the esophagus with preservation of normal bodily function. The aims of palliative therapy are to alleviate symptoms and to provide comfort and, if justified, prolongation of meaningful survival.

Approximately 50% of esophageal cancer patients present with locoregional disease for which chemoradiation is a critical part of the management, either as a neoadjuvant or definitive measure. It is well established that chemoradiation is the treatment of choice for nonsurgical patients, with survival rates similar to those after surgery or radiation alone (6–8). The combining of radiation therapy with chemotherapy has the advantage of potentially addressing microscopic distant subclinical disease. Also, certain chemotherapeutic agents are able to sensitize cells to irradiation. This may be additive or supra-additive; the interaction within the radiation field leads to increased cytotoxic activity either to the same degree as (additive) or more than (supra-additive) using both modalities sequentially.

Neoadjuvant chemoradiation has been shown to downstage tumors and thereby facilitating resection with an increase in the complete resection rate (9). However, this treatment approach remains investigational because there is no survival benefit realized with such an aggressive treatment. Neoadjuvant chemoradiation may help sterilize the tumor field, enhancing local/regional control and potentially reducing tumoral seeding at resection. Also, after completion of chemoradiation, patients with rapidly progressive disease who are found to have metastatic disease are spared the morbidity of a major surgical procedure. Finally, treatment with an intact vasculature, versus in the postoperative setting, may facility drug delivery and oxygenation, thereby enhancing tumoral radiosensitivity. A potential disadvantage of neoadjuvant chemoradiation is that it may interfere with normal healing of the tissues affected by radiation.

While postoperative radiation therapy is not used as frequently with esophageal cancer, it can potentially eliminate residual tumor in the operative field (10). As the postoperative field tends to be smaller, there is a possibility of delivering a higher dose directed to the volume of high risk or known residual disease than with preoperative irradiation. A potential disadvantage is that there may be a delay in the initiation of radiation until wound healing is completed. There are also vascular changes within the tumor bed by surgery that may impair the radiation effect.

Treatment Planning

After a complete staging work-up and a discussion with the multidisciplinary team, an esophageal cancer patient may be deemed a good radiation therapy candidate. Patients must first undergo a simulation where they are strictly immobilized and marked for treatment purposes, and a CT scan is obtained within the treatment position. Unlike diagnostic CT scans, this CT scan is used for treatment planning purposes. This allows both tumor volumes as well as sensitive normal tissues structures to be accurately identified and contoured.

The International Commission on Radiation Units and Measurements Report No. 50 defined treatment planning volumes (11). The gross tumor volume (GTV) includes all known gross disease including the primary tumor, regionally involved lymphadenopathy, and known metastatic disease. The clinical target volume (CTV) encompasses the GTV and also includes a margin for subclinical or microscopic disease. Both the GTV and CTV are clinical-anatomic concepts. The planning target volume (PTV) includes the CTV plus a margin for variations in treatment setup (setup margin) and other anatomic motion during treatment (internal margin), such as respirations (Figure 30.5). The PTV is a geometric concept introduced for treatment planning. It is the PTV that is used to select the appropriate beam sizes and beam arrangements to ensure that the prescribed dose is actually delivered to all parts of the CTV. The treated volume is the tissue volume that (according to the final approved treatment plan) receives at least the absorbed

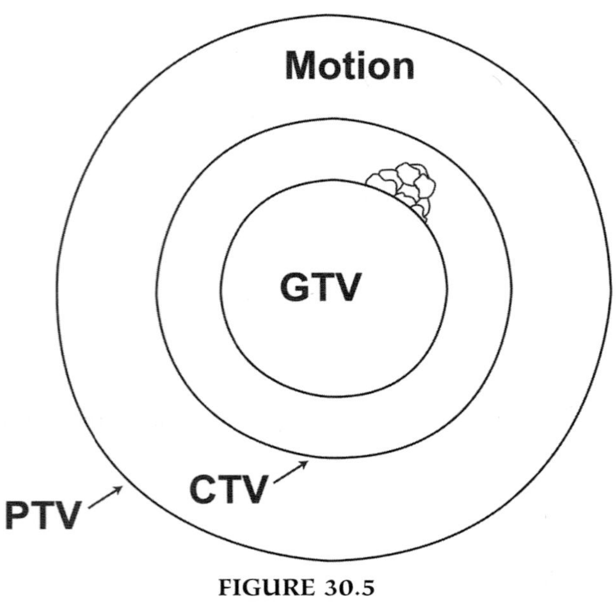

FIGURE 30.5

Treatment planning volumes. Clinical treatment volume (CTV) includes the gross treatment volume (GTV) plus microscopic disease. Planning treatment volume (PTV) includes the CTV in addition to additional margin for setup error and motion.

dose selected as the minimal dose to the PTV as specified by the radiation oncology team.

Treatment planning aims to deliver adequate dose to the target volume while minimizing dose to neighboring normal structures. The tools to do this have been revolutionized by the ability to delineate tumors and normal tissues in 3 dimensions using CT scanners and planning software. Not only are structures clearly defined, but CT planning allows recording of heterogenous tissue radiation attenuation and measurement of accumulated dose from each beam. Radiation treatment planning systems have the ability to simulate all treatment machine motions, including collimator and couch angles. Multileaf collimators (MLCs) or blocks are used to shape the beam. Plans are typically optimized by iteratively changing the beam directions and apertures and recalculating the dose distribution until an optimal plan is obtained. Plans are evaluated qualitatively using dose-display tools such as dose-volume histograms (DVHs) and 2-D isodose sections. The DVH shows the amount of target volume or critical structure receiving more or less than the specified dose. Compared to 2-D treatment planning, where volumetric and dose data could only be approximated, 3-D treatment planning optimizes dose distribution and allows radiographic verification of the volume treated. The treatment volume conforms to the shape of the tumor, and relative toxicity of radiation to the surrounding normal tissues is reduced.

While 3-D treatment is used most commonly in esophageal cancer patients, intensity modulated radiation therapy (IMRT) is growing in popularity. IMRT is the next generation of 3-D conformal treatment (12). In IMRT, the beam intensity varies across the treatment field. Rather than being treated with a single, large, uniform beam, the tumor is treated with many very small beams with different intensities. It optimizes the delivery of radiation to irregularly shaped volumes through complex inverse treatment planning and changing the shape and intensity within each beam to deliver the optimal dose. Inverse planning starts with an ideal dose distribution, finds the beam characteristics through trial and error or multiple iterations, and then produces the best approximation to the ideal dose. The radiation dose is intensified near the GTV while decreased among the neighboring tissues. Because of this, IMRT allows for higher dose to be delivered to the tumor while sparing healthy tissue as compared with conventional 2-D and 3-D conformal radiation treatment techniques (see Chapter 52, "Pre-Treatment Planning in Radiation Therapy of the Esophagus").

Side Effects

As most patients present with locoregionally advanced disease and with the larger margins necessary to encompass gross as well as microscopic disease, radiation fields for esophageal cancer tend to be large. These fields may include significant volumes of surrounding critical normal tissues including the healthy esophagus, lungs, and heart. The severity of side effects depends on the volume of critical structures irradiated, radiation dose and fractionation, and the use of chemotherapy. Acute toxicity results from the biological effects on rapidly dividing cells (e.g., esophagogastic mucosa, heart, and lung) within the irradiated field. Late-responding tissues with slowly dividing cells (e.g., connective tissue) may not express effects until months or years after radiation treatment.

Accurate assessment of the incidence and severity of esophagitis in esophageal cancer patients is difficult, as the symptoms (dysphagia, odynophagia) are non-specific and may be obscured by the effects of the tumor itself. In 1991, the National Cancer Institute created a task force that carried out an extensive literature search noting tolerance of normal tissues (13). For the esophagus, tolerance doses for a 5% chance of clinical stricture/perforation for uniform irradiation of one-third of the esophagus was 60 Gy, two-thirds was 58 Gy, and the entire esophagus was 53 Gy.

Lung Toxicity

Radiation pneumonitis is an interstitial pulmonary inflammation that can develop in patients treated with thoracic irradiation. Acute radiation pneumonitis occurs within 1 to 6 months following treatment. Symptoms can include low-grade fever and cough while radiographic findings are consistent with a diffuse infiltrate corresponding to a previously irradiated field. The clinical spectrum includes a bothersome cough to more severe effects on quality of life and, in rare cases, even death. It is treated with steroid therapy.

Emami et al. found tolerance doses for a 5% chance of pneumonitis occurring within 5 years from uniform irradiation of one-third of the lung was 45 Gy, two-thirds was 30 Gy, and whole lung was 17.5 Gy (13).

Different dosimetric parameters and dose volume histograms (DVHs) can be extracted from the 3D dose distribution to better guide a clinician for safe treatment and predict side effects. Martel reviewed the DVHs of patients with Hodgkin's disease and lung cancer for the development of radiation pneumonitis (14). A prediction was derived for low versus high risk of pneumonitis when examining risk groups stratified according to the effective volume parameter for lung (V_{eff}). Differences were also seen in mean lung dose (MLD) between patients with complications (MLD 24–26.1 Gy) versus without complications (18–21 Gy). Similar results were seen by Oetzel et al. (15) (23.8 Gy versus 20.1 Gy) as well as Kwa et al. (16).

Specific points on a DVH can also be helpful. The volume of lung receiving 20 Gy or more (V_{20}) has been shown to be predictive for increased risk of pneumonitis while most recommend keeping the $V_{20} < 40\%$ (17). Using DVH parameters does become complicated when considering the heterogeneity of patients being evaluated. Patients have varying baseline lung function, which can be further altered by receipt of chemotherapy. Also, structure volumes may be defined differently across institutions (e.g., total lung including or minus PTV, etc). This makes it more difficult to identify DVH parameters that correlate with pneumonitis risk (18).

Postoperative pulmonary complications are the most serious morbidity after esophagectomy and the leading cause of postoperative mortality among patients treated with surgery for esophageal cancer with an associated in-hospital mortality rate of 55% (19). A recent meta-analysis showed that the postoperative mortality is higher in patients treated with chemoradiation plus surgery than in those treated with surgery alone (20). Pulmonary complications including pneumonia and adult respiratory distress syndrome that develop postoperatively within 30 days after surgery are associated with a $V_{10} < 40\%$ (21). The volume of lung receiving lower doses (e.g., V_5) has also been predictive of pulmonary complications (22). This suggests that ensuring an adequate volume of lung unexposed to radiation might reduce the incidence of postoperative pulmonary complications.

Cardiac Toxicity

According to Emami et al., tolerance doses for one-third of the heart are 60 Gy, 45 for two-thirds, and 40 Gy for the entire heart with the endpoint of pericarditis (13). Previously, data regarding cardiac toxicity had been borrowed from treatment of non-esophageal cancer patients. Excess deaths have been seen in breast cancer patients receiving radiation therapy to high doses to a small portion of the left ventricle (23). More recently, a retrospective analysis of esophageal patients treated with definitive chemoradiation showed an increase in pericardial effusions at 27.7% (24). The pericardial effusion developed within 15 months after radiation therapy, with median onset of 5.3 months with risk associated with mean pericardial dose. In addition, myocardium perfusion defects including ischemia and/or scarring were identified from SPECT images in 42.3% of patients treated with chemoradiation, in contrast to only 4% of patients treated with surgery alone.

In summary, with the growing knowledge of radiation biology and physics as well as advances in technology, we are better able to achieve the ultimate goal in radiation therapy; that is, killing tumor cells while sparing normal surrounding tissues.

References

1. Howes A, Coleman C. Overall principles of cancer management: radiation therapy. In: Osteen R, ed. *Cancer Manual*. 9th ed. Boston: American Cancer Society; 1996:83–97.
2. Elkind MM, GF Whitmore. *The Radiobiology of Cultured Mammalian Cells*. 1st ed. Amsterdam: Gordon and Breach Science Pub; 1967.
3. Jeter M, Komaki R, Cox J. Radiation time, dose, and fractionation in the treatment of lung cancer. In: Jeremic B, ed. *Advances in Radiation Oncology in Lung Cancer*. New York: Springer; 2005.
4. Elkind MM, Alescio T, Swain RW, et al. Recovery of hypoxic mammalian cells from sub-lethal X-Ray damage. *Nature*. 1964;202:1190–1193.
5. Ang KK, Landuyt W, Rijnders A, et al. Differences in repopulation kinetics in mouse skin during split course multiple fractions per day (MFD) or daily fractionated irradiations. *Int J Radiat Oncol Biol Phys*. 1984;10(1):95–99.
6. Herskovic A, Martz K, al-Sarraf M, et al. Combined chemotherapy and radiotherapy compared with radiotherapy alone in patients with cancer of the esophagus. *N Engl J Med*. 1992;326(24):1593–1598.
7. al-Sarraf M, Martz K, Herskovic A, et al. Progress report of combined chemoradiotherapy versus radiotherapy alone in patients with esophageal cancer: an intergroup study. *J Clin Oncol*. 1997;15(1):277–284.
8. Cooper JS, Guo MD, Herskovic A, et al. Chemoradiotherapy of locally advanced esophageal cancer: long-term follow-up of a prospective randomized trial (RTOG 85-01). Radiation Therapy Oncology Group. *JAMA*. 1999;281(17):1623–1627.
9. Hofstetter W, Swisher SG, Correa AM, et al. Treatment outcomes of resected esophageal cancer. *Ann Surg*. 2002;236(3):376–384.

10. Rice TW, Adelstein DJ, Chidel MA, et al. Benefit of postoperative adjuvant chemoradiotherapy in locoregionally advanced esophageal carcinoma. *J Thorac Cardiovasc Surg*. 2003;126(5):1590–1596.
11. ICRU Report No. 50. Prescribing, recording and reporting photon beam therapy. Washington, DC: ICRU; 1993.
12. Galvin JM, Ezzell G, Eisbrauch A, et al. Implementing IMRT in clinical practice: a joint document of the American Society for Therapeutic Radiology and Oncology and the American Association of Physicists in Medicine. *Int J Radiat Oncol Biol Phys*. 2004;58(5):1616–1634.
13. Emami B, Lyman J, Brown A, et al. Tolerance of normal tissue to therapeutic irradiation. *Int J Radiat Oncol Biol Phys*. 1991;21(1):109–122.
14. Martel MK, Ten Haken RK, Hazuka MB, et al. Dose-volume histogram and 3-D treatment planning evaluation of patients with pneumonitis. *Int J Radiat Oncol Biol Phys*. 1994;28(3):575–581.
15. Oetzel D, Schraube P, Hensley F, et al. Estimation of pneumonitis risk in three-dimensional treatment planning using dose-volume histogram analysis. *Int J Radiat Oncol Biol Phys*. 1995;33(2):455–460.
16. Kwa SL, Theuws JC, Wagenaar A, et al. Evaluation of two dose-volume histogram reduction models for the prediction of radiation pneumonitis. *Radiother Oncol*. 1998;48(1):61–69.
17. Graham MV, Purdy JA, Emami B, et al. Clinical dose-volume histogram analysis for pneumonitis after 3D treatment for non-small cell lung cancer (NSCLC). *Int J Radiat Oncol Biol Phys*. 1999;45(2):323–329.
18. Hong TS, Crowley EM, Killoran J, et al. Considerations in treatment planning for esophageal cancer. *Semin Radiat Oncol*. 2007;17(1):53–61.
19. Fang W, Kato H, Tachimori Y, et al. Analysis of pulmonary complications after three-field lymph node dissection for esophageal cancer. *Ann Thorac Surg*. 2003;76(3):903–908.
20. Fiorica F, Di Bona D, Schepis F, et al. Preoperative chemoradiotherapy for oesophageal cancer: a systematic review and meta-analysis. *Gut*. 2004;53(7):925–930.
21. Lee HK, Vaporciyan AA, Cox JD, et al. Postoperative pulmonary complications after preoperative chemoradiation for esophageal carcinoma: correlation with pulmonary dose-volume histogram parameters. *Int J Radiat Oncol Biol Phys*. 2003;57(5):1317–1322.
22. Wang SL, Liao Z, Vaporciyan AA, et al. Investigation of clinical and dosimetric factors associated with postoperative pulmonary complications in esophageal cancer patients treated with concurrent chemoradiotherapy followed by surgery. *Int J Radiat Oncol Biol Phys*. 2006;64(3):692–699.
23. Favourable and unfavourable effects on long-term survival of radiotherapy for early breast cancer: an overview of the randomised trials. Early Breast Cancer Trialists' Collaborative Group. *Lancet*. 2000;355(9217):1757–1770.
24. Gayed IW, Liu HH, Yusuf SW, et al. The prevalence of myocardial ischemia after concurrent chemoradiation therapy as detected by gated myocardial perfusion imaging in patients with esophageal cancer. *J Nucl Med*. 2006;47(11):1756–1762.

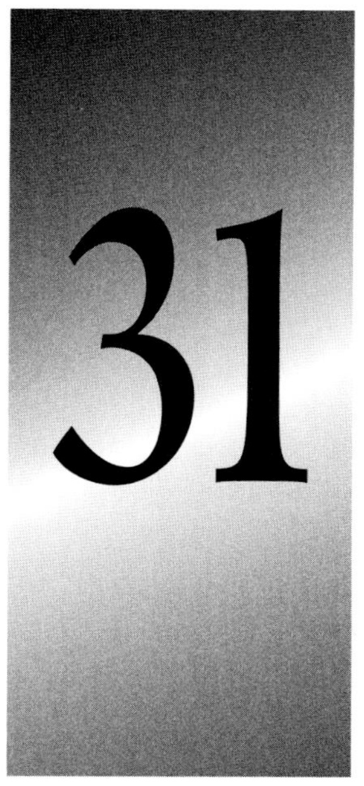

31 Principles of Surgical Therapy

Wayne L. Hofstetter

HISTORY OF ESOPHAGEAL SURGERY

According to the National Cancer Institute database, there will be an estimated 16,470 new cases of esophageal cancer diagnosed in the United States annually. Due to a number of issues, it is expected that only approximately 20% to 25% of these cases will be eligible for surgical therapy. Despite this discouraging rate of resectability, surgical therapy has been considered the gold standard for patients diagnosed with potentially curable esophageal cancer.

Yet, surgical resection of the esophagus had not been considered plausible until recent history. The recognition of esophageal cancer was described as early as the second century A.D. by Galen (1). But it would be another 1,600 years before the technology necessary for the diagnosis of neoplasms existed, including histology, endoscopy, biopsy techniques, and Roentgenology. The development of esophageal surgical techniques has evolved in parallel with medical technology.

Billroth, in 1871, described an autopsy series on patients with esophageal cancer (2). He subsequently carried out live animal studies, successfully resecting the cervical esophageal segment in dogs. However, translation to his first clinical case was a failure and his first and only patient died on the first postoperative day. In May 1877, Czerny, then a professor at Heidelberg and former assistant to Billroth in Vienna, performed the first successful resection of the cervical esophagus for carcinoma (3). His patient was a 51-year-old female who would never undergo reconstruction and survived only 1 year after the operation; her death attributed to recurrence. Czerny's effort elaborated on early collaborative work he performed with Billroth.

It would, however, be many more years before the successful resection of a thoracic esophageal lesion. Limitations in the understanding of anesthesia and pneumothorax rendered early attempts at transthoracic resection uniformly fatal. The thorax was felt to be an impenetrable cavity, and surgeons were trained to avoid traversing the pleura. Numerous surgeons and physiologists contributed to the first successful thoracic esophageal resection, including Biondi, who in 1894 described gastric mobilization into the chest with primary anastomosis. Mickulicz first attempted this in the clinical setting in 1896, avoiding pneumothorax by isolating the posterior mediastinum and suturing the diaphragm to the parietal pleura. Unfortunately, his patient died of peritonitis. In 1898, Garré resected 3 patients, but without long-term success (1).

Surgeons would remain frustrated by attempts to resect the thoracic esophagus until safe methods of managing pneumothorax were devised. It was Vesalius who first described the possibility of endotracheal intubation in the 16th century, but it would take until the 19th century for Trendelenburg to describe a modern technique for tracheotomy and positive pressure ventilation. Unfortunately, these early advances were not recognized for their significance, and modern general endotracheal anesthesia did not evolve until the early 20th century.

Sauerbruch was first to conquer the pleura, avoiding pneumothorax by method of operating in a negative pressure chamber. In 1904, he reported to the Berlin Surgical Congress on 78 experimental procedures (4). His negative pressure chamber, which was constructed based on earlier designs from other physiologists, became successful and sought after; one was constructed and used in the United States at the Rockefeller Institute in 1909. However, rapid advances in general endotracheal anesthesia by Meltzer and Auer, also at the Rockefeller Institute, quickly deposed the chamber into obsolescence (5).

Doctors Torek and Eggers, both thoracic surgeons at the German Hospital in New York City, are credited with the first total thoracic esophagectomy with general endotracheal anesthesia in 1913 (6). Dr. Torek administered anesthesia and Dr. Eggers carried out a left transthoracic resection without reconstruction. Also in 1913 Denk described transhiatal esophagectomy, again without reconstruction. In 1936, Turner performed a transhiatal esophagectomy with antethoracic skin tube reconstruction. It would be another 40 years before transhiatal esophagectomy was rediscovered by a young Dr. Orringer, whose presentation at a thoracic conference was met with dubious criticism (7).

The first reported successful transthoracic resection with reconstruction was performed as a thoracoabdominal approach by Adams and Phemister in 1938 (8). Ivor Lewis in 1946 published his lecture on the history and progress of esophageal resection (9). His contribution of 7 cases consisted of 3 from the left transthoracic approach and 4 from the right, all as thoracoabdominal approaches.

The modern era of esophageal surgery has led to several important advances in the understanding of esophageal cancer pathogenesis and treatment. Billroth erroneously concluded in 1871 that esophageal neoplasms do not spread by lymphatics and that surgical resection should result in cure. In contrast, detailed studies by Nakayama in 1962, and later by Akiyama and Skinner et al. (10–13), have led to important understanding regarding the unique anatomy of the esophageal lymphatics that facilitates the metastasis of esophageal cancer prior to any evident symptoms the patient may present with. Work by early pioneers led to our current understanding of lymphatic involvement, which occurs early on in the disease process, and it sheds light on the limitations of local-regional therapy for a disease that very often presents with occult or obvious systemic metastasis.

There are now multiple options for the surgical treatment of esophageal cancer. Various approaches to resection via transabdominal, transthoracic, three-field, or minimally invasive are utilized by today's esophageal surgeons (14). Although the stomach remains the most commonly used organ for the replacement of the thoracic esophagus, methods of reconstruction have also evolved and there are many surgeons who advocate the use of colon as an alternative. Recent work indicates that small bowel is also an excellent and facile replacement for any length of resected esophagus (15,16).

PRINCIPLES OF ESOPHAGEAL SURGERY

Historic discoveries in the development of esophageal surgery have led to the modern principles of surgical therapy for esophageal cancer. The failures of those intrepid clinicians resulted in investigations that have shaped our current practice in patient care. Among the most important principles, we will discuss the need for patient selection, preoperative assessment, individualizing treatment, minimizing mortality and morbidity, intraoperative and postoperative management, and attaining a complete surgical resection (Table 31.1).

Patient Selection and Preoperative Assessment

Esophageal cancer surgery is a challenging endeavor. Esophageal resection still carries a relatively high morbidity and mortality rate, and this is largely influenced by a surgeon's experience and volume and that of the hospital in which the resection is performed (17). Many publications have placed the minimum bar at 6 resections per year (data based on national databases), but to achieve the best results, the optimal number would be much higher. To further minimize surgically related

TABLE 31.1
The 10 Most Important Principles of Esophageal Surgery

- Patient selection
- Adequate hospital/surgeon volume
- Preoperative assessment
- Individualized therapy
- Multidisciplinary care
- Ancillary services
- Minimize morbidity and mortality
- Gentle manipulation of the conduit
- Perform a complete resection
- Systematic lymph node resection (stage appropriate)

events, patient selection is extremely important (18). Many investigators would argue that an observed increase in overall survival during the recent era is at least partially due to patient selection. One reason for this is that the definition of a *resectable patient* is constantly in flux and surgical outcomes directly correlate to patient selection. The indications for surgical resection have changed over time; what was considered potentially resectable in the past is no longer thought of as surgical disease. Objective evaluation of historic data has taught us this important lesson: operating on advanced disease with adjacent organ involvement or distant metastasis conveys a poor prognosis. These patients are more effectively treated with alternative methods of palliation. The concept of the palliative esophageal resection for any reason other than symptomatic perforation or acute hemorrhage has been surpassed by advancements in chemotherapy and radiotherapy as well as by mechanic devices proven to reliably relieve symptoms in a majority of patients (19). Recognizing when a patient is potentially curable or, alternatively, is in need of purely palliative efforts, is difficult and dependent on collected data, available therapies, and technology. Changes in the indications for surgical resection are expected to continue. As an example, most centers no longer treat cervical esophageal cancer with surgery primarily but reserve resection for patients who have failed locally after definitive chemoradiotherapy. Similar trends are being seen in patients with locally advanced squamous cell carcinoma of the thoracic esophagus. Some centers perform resection only in the subset of patients who are nonresponders after definitive chemoradiation or in those with local-regional recurrence (20). These changes in surgical indications can effectively "weed out" poor performers and will also bias overall survival results when compared to historic data.

Multidisciplinary Team

For patients who are being considered for resection, patient selection is a systematic process that involves a multidisciplinary approach. This begins with a careful history and physical examination focusing on the risk factors for the disease that do not coincidentally parallel risk factors for postoperative complications. Patients with squamous cell carcinoma of the esophagus are apt to carry neurologic, cardiac, hepatic, and pulmonary comorbidities that can significantly increase perioperative risk. Ongoing tobacco abuse in patients with either squamous cell or adenocarcinoma is associated with cardiac and pulmonary disease with the potential for a higher incidence of perioperative cardiac events or pneumonia. We strongly encourage complete abstinence for as long as possible prior to resection. Consideration is always given for testing cardiac and pulmonary physiologic reserve prior to therapy. Patients may be physiologically depleted from their comorbid risk factors or by the disease itself. Often patients presenting with dysphagia have had significant weight loss. This was more apparent in the thinner squamous population than in today's adeno-predominant esophageal cancer. However, even if a patient is overweight, significant protein malnutrition can lead to poor performance throughout therapy. Typically, a nutritionist meets with our patients at initial consultation and then remains a critical member of the care team well after resection.

A careful gastrointestinal and nutritional review to include reflux history, meal, and bowel habits can provide clues for postoperative management as well. The lifestyle changes necessitated by esophageal resection and reconstruction can be difficult for similar reasons that the patient has risk factors for the primary disease. Poor nutritional choices, obesity, over-eating and late-night dining, inflammatory bowel disease, or constipation may all signal specific behavior modifications necessary to a successful surgical outcome.

Emphasis is placed on treating these complicated patients in a multimodality setting. Presentation of findings on integrated PET/CT by the radiologists at multidisciplinary conference allows our interventional gastroenterologists to perform necessary staging studies that will affect decisions about resectability. It is common for an ambiguous finding on imaging to be confirmed by endoscopic ultrasound-guided fine needle aspiration at the time of upper endoscopy. This critical information often changes management, and this issue is discussed in more detail in other chapters (see Chapter 49, "Multidisciplinary Care Team: Structure and Format").

Individualize Treatment

Individualizing therapy is strongly recommended. There are many treatment options for patients with esophageal cancer. Some are more invasive than others and may inherently have higher risk of morbidity while others are very minimally invasive but may have higher risk of recurrence or incomplete resection.

Technical details of esophagectomy and choice of procedure will be covered in detail in other chapters, but a few general details are worth noting. Mitigating risk–benefit ratio is an astute, morbidity-reducing exercise. Existing data indicate that high-grade dysplasia and intramucosal disease carry an extremely low risk of regional lymph node involvement (21). Therefore, a less invasive option such as vagal-sparing esophagectomy that does not portend the same risk of a transthoracic en bloc resection may be appropriate so long as a complete resection can be accomplished. In other words, consideration should be given to match stage to treatment. Furthermore, patients with marginal physiologic reserves need attention to approach, such as the patient with poor pulmonary function who may be better treated by transhiatal resection, or an octogenarian who could be considered for a least-invasive, viable alternative. Choice of conduit should also be individualized. For example, a gastroesophageal junction tumor extending into the gastric cardia may require a significant proximal gastrectomy to obtain an adequate negative margin, rendering a cervical esophagogastrostomy unfeasible. Or a younger patient whose vocation requires stooping or bending at the waist may be better served with an alternate conduit such as jejunal or colon interposition rather than a gastric pull-up, to avoid significant problems with postoperative reflux, regurgitation, and aspiration.

Intra- and Postoperative Therapy

Careful attention must be paid to anatomy with focus on preservation of the arterial and venous blood supply to the reconstructive organ. Gentle handling of the interposed organ, whether it will be stomach, small bowel, or colon, is vital for avoiding postoperative events such as leak or necrosis. We use multiple techniques to advance the conduit through or around the mediastinum for reconstruction. It is important to minimize manipulation to the conduit during that process such that a healthy gastric or bowel end is delivered for anastomosis. Regarding technique of anastomosis, many units still perform a hand-sewn technique; however, there are multiple papers describing the benefits of a stapled anastomosis (22), and this is covered completely in other areas of the book (see Chapter 64, "Anastomatic Technique and Selection of Location"). Since I have converted to stapled anastomoses, I have seen a significant decrease in the need to perform anastomotic dilation. A caveat, however, is that many centers are employing neoadjuvant chemoradiotherapy for locally advanced disease. Encountering the post-irradiated edematous, boggy stomach may cause one to rethink the stapled anastomosis due to the thickness of the tissue. For that matter, one may also reconsider the use of that conduit altogether.

Minimize Surgically Related Events

Do the most to avoid iatrogenic, technical events that can lead to further difficulty. Attention to the smallest details will meaningfully contribute to an uncomplicated postoperative recovery. Among the most important is avoiding injury to the recurrent laryngeal nerves. A detailed knowledge of where one would encounter the nerves throughout the course of any approach to the esophagus and paying the utmost respect to them; avoiding traction, metal retractors, or mono-polar cautery anywhere near the nerves will help to maintain function of the cords. Traction injury to the right or left recurrent nerve is a potential pitfall, even when dissecting well away from the nerves, and care must be taken during "blunt" dissection to avoid this.

Further insults to swallowing function can be encountered during dissection for a cervical anastomosis. Strap muscles in the neck should routinely be preserved, with the exception that the omohyoid may need to be sacrificed. If possible, maintain the integrity of the ansa cervicalis to avoid denervating muscles that have secondary function in swallowing.

Postoperative hernias can be common. The incidence of hernia in midline incisions is upwards of 30%. To decrease the need for these secondary reparative procedures, our group performs either a chevron incision or minimally invasive resection in morbidly obese patients. Internal hernias are also described and can be a source of some serious side effects. Mesenteric defects during colon interposition should be properly dispositioned, and conduit to diaphragm tacking sutures may avoid subsequent intrathoracic conduit redundancy or abdominal content herniation into the chest, an event described as a potential need for redo operation to avoid significant deleterious side effects from strangulation.

During the postoperative period, the excellent care of your ancillary team is important to the overall outcome. Our nursing care unit is monitored, and the nurses are experienced in the care of esophagectomy patients. Routine in-services help to initiate the newer recruits of the care team. Respiratory, physical therapy, nutrition, speech pathology, radiology, and anesthesia pain teams also administer vital care to these patients.

Perform a Complete Resection

The most critical principle of cancer surgery is complete resection. There are differing opinions regarding techniques of resection, and in fairness to all camps, there have been only a limited number of comparative trials with none showing clear superiority of one approach over another (23). The ability to achieve adequate control of local-regional disease is the most debated issue. The more conservative, transhiatal approach has the tendency toward higher local-regional recurrence but perhaps lower morbidity, while radical resections provide excellent local control but are inherently associated with increased morbidity. The inability to demonstrate a significant survival advantage between the various approaches has as much to do with patient selection and individualizing therapy as with the fact that most of our patients are recurring systemically, thus rendering any local control issue irrelevant (24,25). What has been suggested is that the tumor location and number of nodes involved may be pertinent to the efficacy of the approach (23). There is general agreement, however, that an operation that fails locally is difficult to salvage, and a complete resection of all tumor and involved nodes (R0 resection) is superior to an incomplete resection. Retrospective review of a high volume of patients has shown that the ability to achieve an R0 resection is an independent predictor of long-term survival (26–28) (Figure 31.1). Complete resection should also take into account an appropriate lymph node resection. Goals of the operation include negative margins and the removal of all involved lymph nodes. There is some evidence that the minimum appropriate number of dissected lymph nodes that constitutes a complete resection is between 12 and 18 nodes (29,30).

Margins must be carefully considered, including proximal, distal, and radial margins. We routinely examine margins interoperatively for the presence of metaplasia or cancer. Gastric margins, particularly during Lewis-type resections, need to be carefully considered. Pretreatment endoscopy should be performed to examine for any extension of disease into the stomach, and we routinely perform biopsies into the cardia and lesser curve for tumors that extend through the gastroesophageal junction. These procedures enable us to map out the area of the tumor and plan for later resection. After anesthetic induction, the surgeon should perform an upper gastrointestinal endoscopy to aid in planning the distal resection line.

Finally, margins are checked by frozen histologic analysis with the forewarning that once the conduit is resected with a stapler, redoing this margin is more difficult. Therefore, intraoperative examination for margins can help avoid this potential pitfall. The actual optimal distance of the clear margin from tumor is not fully understood. Historically, recommendations were for 10 cm proximal and distal. This has been challenged to 5 cm, 3.8 cm, or even a microscopic negative margin (29). Our current practice is to aim for 4–5 cm margins above and below with clear radial margins microscopically.

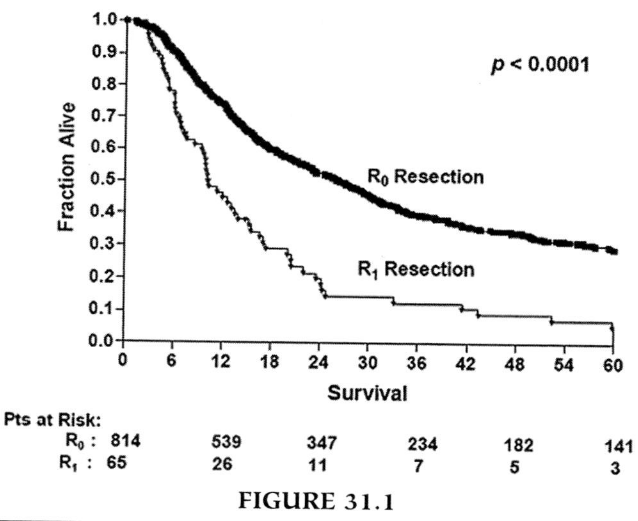

FIGURE 31.1

Comparison of overall survival in completely versus incompletely resected esophageal cancer patients.

SUMMARY

Esophageal cancer surgery is a challenging field that requires commitment and experience. There are multiple barriers to achieving perfect outcomes, due to the complexity of the disease and the patients. Most often, the unique lymphatic structure of the esophagus conspires against the patient rendering cure an elusive goal for the caregivers. However, for the patients who are potentially curable, there are several principles of surgery that can alter the outcome. There are many studies suggesting a direct relationship of volume and outcome where higher-volume centers attain comparatively excellent results. An expert esophageal multidisciplinary group will positively influence patient selection and outcomes. Appropriate intraoperative management and decision making correlates to fewer postoperative events and smooth recovery. Finally, a complete resection is the most important goal of esophageal cancer surgery. These general principles are ultimately applicable to any esophageal cancer patient being considered for any type of resection.

References

1. Pompili MF, Mark JB. The history of surgery for carcinoma of the esophagus. *Chest Surg Clin of North Am.* 2000;10(1):145–151.
2. Billroth T. Über die Resection des Oesophagus. *Arch Klin Chir.* 1871;13:65.
3. Czerny. Neue Operationen. *Zentralbl Chir.* 1877;4:433.
4. Sauerbruch F. Über die Ausschaltung der schädlichen Wirkung des Pneumothorax bei intrathorakalen Operationen. *Zentralbl Chir.* 1904;31:146.
5. Meltzer SJ, Auer J. Continuous respiration without respiratory movements. *J Exp Med.* 1909;11:622.
6. Torek F. The first successful case of resection of the thoracic portion of the oesophagus for carcinoma. *Surg Gynecol Obstet.* 1913;16:614.
7. Orringer MB, Sloan HJ. Esophagectomy without thoracotomy. *J Thorac Cardiovasc Surg.* 1978;76(5):643–654.
8. Adams WE, Phemister DB. Carcinoma of the lower thoracic esophagus. Report of a successful resection and esophagogastrostomy. *J Thorac Surg.* 1938;7:621.
9. Lewis I. The surgical treatment of carcinoma of the oesophagus with special reference to a new operation for growths of the middle third. *Br J Surg.* 1946;34:18.

10. Nakayama K, Hirota K. Experiences of about 3,000 cases with cancer of the oesophagus and the cardia. *Aust N Z J Surg*. 1962;31:222–230.
11. Akiyama H, Tsurumaru M, Kawamura T, et al. Principles of surgical treatment for carcinoma of the esophagus: analysis of lymph node involvement. *Ann Surg*. 1981;194;(4):438–446.
12. Skinner DB. En bloc resection for neoplasms of the esophagus and cardia. *J Thorac Cardiovasc Surg*. 1983;85(1):59–71.
13. Akiyama H, Tsurumaru M, Udagawa H, et al. Radical lymph node dissection for cancer of the thoracic esophagus. *Ann Surg*. 1994;220(3):364–373.
14. Seely AJ, Sundaresan RS, Finley RJ. Principles of laparoscopic surgery of the gastroesophageal junction. *J Am Coll Surg*. 200;(1):77–87.
15. Akiyama H, Miyazono H, Tsurumaru M, et al. Use of the stomach as an esophageal substitute. *Ann Surg*. 1978;188(5):606–610.
16. Ascioti A, Hofstetter W, Miller M, et al. Long-segment, supercharged, pedicled jejunal flap for total esophageal reconstruction. *J Thorac Cardiovasc Surg*. 2005;130(5):1391–1398.
17. Begg CB, Cramer LD, Hoskins WJ, et al. Impact of hospital volume on operative mortality for major cancer surgery. *JAMA*. 1998;280(20):1747–1751.
18. Dionigi G, Rovera F, Boni L, et al. Cancer of the esophagus: the value of preoperative patient assessment. *Expert Rev Anticancer Ther*. 2006;6(4):581–593.
19. Harvey JA, Bessell JR, Beller E, et al. Chemoradiation therapy is effective for the palliative treatment of malignant dysphagia. *Dis Esophagus*. 2004;17(3):260–265.
20. Bedenne L, Michel P, Bouché O, et al. Chemoradiation followed by surgery compared with chemoradiation alone in squamous cancer of the esophagus: FFCD 9102. *J Clin Oncol*. 2007;25(10):1160–1168.
21. Nigro JJ, Hagen JA, DeMeester TR, et al. Occult esophageal adenocarcinoma: extent of disease and implications for effective therapy. *Ann Surg*. 1999;230(3):433–438.
22. Orringer M, Marshall B, Chang A, et al. Two thousand transhiatal esophagectomies: changing trends, lessons learned. *Ann Surg*. 2007;246(3):363–374.
23. Omloo J, Lagarde S, Hulscher J, et al. Extended transthoracic resection compared with limited transhiatal resection for adenocarcinoma of the mid/distal esophagus: five-year survival of a randomized clinical trial. *Ann Surg*. 2007;246(6):992–1001.
24. Kelsen DP, Winter KA, Gunderson LL, et al. Long-term results of RTOG trial 8911 (USA Intergroup 113): a random assignment trial comparison of chemotherapy followed by surgery compared with surgery alone for esophageal cancer. *J Clin Oncol*. 2007;20;25(24):3719–3725.
25. Burmeister BH, Smithers BM, Gebski V, et al. Surgery alone versus chemoradiotherapy followed by surgery for resectable cancer of the oesophagus: a randomised controlled phase III trial. *Lancet Oncol*. 2005;6(9):659–668.
26. Hofstetter W, Swisher SG, Correa AM, et al. Treatment outcomes of resected esophageal cancer. *Ann Surg*. 2002;236(3):376–385.
27. Law S, Kwong DL, Kwok KF, et al. Improvement in treatment results and long-term survival of patients with esophageal cancer: impact of chemoradiation and change in treatment strategy. *Ann Surg*. 2003;238(3):339–347.
28. Lerut T, Coosemans W, De Leyn P, et al. Treatment of esophageal carcinoma. *Chest*. 1999;116(6 Suppl):463S–465S.
29. Barbour A, Rizk N, Gonen M, et al. Adenocarcinoma of the gastroesophageal junction: influence of esophageal resection margin and operative approach on outcome. *Ann Surg*. 2007;246(1):1–8.
30. Lerut T, Nafteux P, Moons J, et al. Quality in the surgical treatment of cancer of the esophagus and gastroesophageal junction. *Eur J Surg Oncol*. 2005;31(6):587–594.

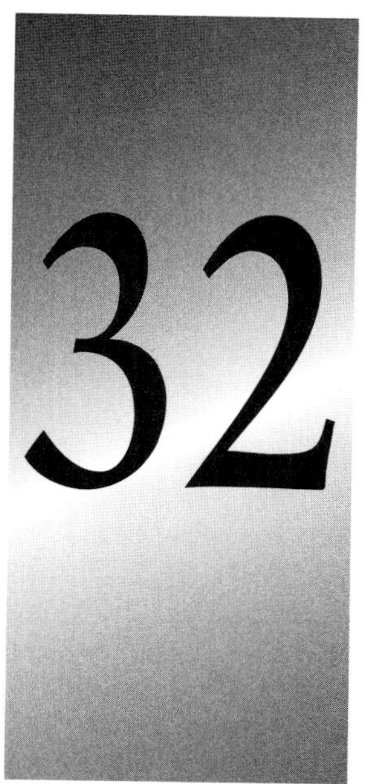

32 The Relationship Between Volume and Outcome in the Treatment of Esophageal Cancer

Ioannis Rouvelas
Jesper Lagergren

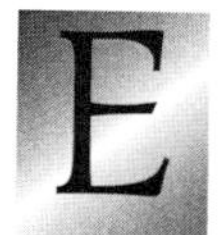

Esophageal cancer is an aggressive disease with a poor prognosis. The overall long-term survival rates remain below 15% in most Western countries (1). The long-term prognosis and treatment options are highly dependent on the tumor stage. The tumor stage also determines whether the therapeutic intention is for cure or palliation. Radical surgical resection is an established potentially curative treatment option for patients with resectable esophageal cancer (2,3). As the tumor stage is often already advanced when the diagnosis is first confirmed, only a minority of patients are eligible for curatively intended treatment. Moreover, even after an R0 surgical resection, fewer than 40% of the patients are cured (2). The anatomic location of the esophagus explains why esophagectomy for esophageal cancer is one of the most demanding surgical procedures undertaken in general surgery. The surgical trauma imposed by esophageal cancer surgery is immense, often involving surgery of the abdomen, chest, and neck (3,4). Moreover, esophagectomy is performed in patients who are typically older, have concurrent diseases, and/or are malnourished (5). Therefore, esophagectomy may be associated with a considerable risk of major postoperative complications and mortality (6,7). However, it is encouraging that the population-based survival after esophagectomy, both short- and long-term, has improved considerably in recent years (8). This improvement is probably multifactorial, including advances in noninvasive imaging, preoperative staging, anesthesia, and postoperative pain control, combined with improvements in preoperative risk evaluation, surgical technique, and postoperative care.

The outcome after such complex surgery should be influenced by the skill, knowledge, and experience not only of the surgical team but of the whole hospital staff, including anesthesiologists, intensivists, nursing staff, and dietitians. Centralization is appropriate for complex procedures with high baseline mortality risks and high costs because it provides an opportunity for the team to gain expertise through experience at patient selection, case management, and performing the appropriate operation, in order to yield the best outcome. Several studies have documented a significant relation between surgery volume of certain surgical procedures and outcome. Together with coronary artery bypass grafting, abdominal aortic aneurysm repair, heart transplantation, and pancreatic resection, esophagectomy has been found to be entailed by a decreased in-hospital mortality when performed at high-volume centers (9,10). Furthermore, several studies have demonstrated that hospital volume and experience are associated with improved clinical and economic outcomes with complex gastrointestinal procedures (11,12). Based on this evidence, there has been an increasing demand by governments and insurance companies to have complex surgical procedures referred to high-volume centers whenever possible. Although short-term mortality is an important and easily evaluated outcome, there is also a need to consider other outcome variables, including postoperative complications, long-term prognosis, and health-related quality of life. Here, we present a review of the available literature regarding the impact of hospital and surgeon volume in relation to various outcomes after surgical treatment of esophageal cancer.

IMPACT OF ESOPHAGECTOMY VOLUME ON EARLY POSTOPERATIVE MORBIDITY

The risk of serious postoperative complications after esophagectomy is high, ranging between 26% and 41% in most reports (2). Early morbidity after esophageal cancer surgery is often related to pulmonary complications and/or anastomotic leaks. These serious complications are valid indicators of the quality of the care and are associated with high risk of postoperative mortality (13,14).

An overview of published studies that have addressed the influence of surgery volume on postoperative morbidity is presented in Table 32.1.

Dimick et al. investigated the risk of developing major postoperative complications after esophageal resection at high-volume hospitals (HVHs), defined as hospitals performing more than 8 esophagectomies annually, compared to low-volume hospitals (LVHs), defined as hospitals that performed fewer than 8 esophagectomies per year (13,15). They showed that patients undergoing esophagetomy at LVH had a profound increased risk of aspiration, pulmonary failure, reintubation, renal failure, septicemia, and surgical complications, compared to those operated on at HVHs. Moreover, the risk of postoperative mortality for patients with at least 1 complication was 16.9% compared to 2.5% for those without any complications ($p < 0.001$). Thus, the authors concluded that esophagectomy should be performed at high-volume centers. Accordingly, in a population-based study from Sweden, a nearly 8-fold increased risk of anastomotic leakage was demonstrated if the operations were conducted by a low-volume surgeon (LVS), defined as < 5 operations per year, compared to those conducted by surgeons of higher annual volume (7).

Sutton et al. evaluated the performance of a single well-trained surgeon in 150 consecutive esophagectomies over a 7-year period in England, and found a reduction in single-lung operating time, intraoperative blood loss, transfusion requirement, stay at the intensive care unit, and an increased number of resected lymph nodes over this time interval (16). Similarly, Traverso et al. reviewed the surgical outcomes of 174 consecutive patients who underwent esophagectomy performed by a single surgeon over the time period 1996–2002 at the Virginia Mason medical center in Seattle, United States, and found lower intraoperative blood loss, less need for transfusion, and lower rate of reoperations, compared to other published series of esophagectomies (17). Furthermore, the mortality and length of stay was significantly lower in a high-volume surgical practice.

In a study performed by Patti et al., the incidence of infections or hemorrhage after esophageal resection was analyzed, comparing 5 volume categories, without finding any differences between them (LVH defined ≤ 5 resections per year, HVH defined > 30 resections annually) (18). The postoperative mortality rate in HVHs was, however, significantly decreased compared to LVHs despite the similar rate of infection and hemorrhage. This observation led to the conclusion that such complications can be managed considerably better in a hospital with higher surgical workload, since the hospital staff, particularly in the operating room and the intensive care units, is better trained to recognize these complications earlier and treat them more effectively.

In summary, these studies taken together indicate that as far as postoperative complications are concerned, high surgery volume is to be recommended.

IMPACT OF ESOPHAGECTOMY VOLUME ON EARLY POSTOPERATIVE MORTALITY

Historically, esophageal cancer surgery was associated with high early postoperative mortality. In a critical review of outcomes following esophagectomy for cancer based on 122 reports published between 1960 and 1979, Earlam and Cunha-Melo documented postoperative mortality as high as 29% and a dismal 5-year survival of 4% after surgical treatment (19). A subsequent review covering the period 1980–1988 reported a substantial decrease of postoperative mortality after esophagectomy to 13% and an increase of 5-year survival to 20% (20). Finally, in the latest corresponding review documenting postoperative mortality rates over the period 1990–2000, a continuing improvement in survival was reported with an overall postoperative mortality dropping to 6.7% (30-day mortality rate 4.9% and in-hospital mortality rate 8.8%) and a 5-year survival of 27.9% (6). Since all these studies used data from other published series, it was not possible to identify a clear explanation for the improvements in survival. Nevertheless, these encouraging results are most likely due to a combination of better patient selection, improved surgery techniques, and improved perioperative management. Surgery volume has been used as a surrogate of quality for complex surgical procedures. Regarding esophageal surgery, studies have repeatedly demonstrated an inverse correlation between hospital volume and postoperative mortality after

TABLE 32.1
Overview of Studies Investigating the Relation between Hospital Volume and Clinical and Economical Outcomes

Author (year)	*Country (region)*	*Years*	*Patient number*	*Main findings*	*Major conclusions*
Patti (1998) (18)	U.S. (California)	1990–1994	1,561	No difference in length of hospital stay, higher rate of home discharges and hospital charges with increasing volume	Esophagectomy for cancer should be restricted to experienced centers
Sutton (1998) (16)	U.K. (Newcastle)	1990–1996	150	Reduced single-lung operating time, transfusion, ICU-stay, hospital stay, higher number of resected lymph nodes	Continuing improvement in a surgeon's performance over a 7-year period
Swisher (2000) (24)	U.S. (national)	1994–1996	340	Decreased complication, reduced length of stay, and decreased hospital charges with increasing volume	Support for selective referral to high-volume centers
Dimick (2001) (40)	U.S. (Maryland)	1984–1999	1,136	Reduced length of stay and decrease in hospital charges with increasing volume	HVHs have superior clinical and economical outcomes
Kuo (2001) (39)	U.S. (Massachusetts)	1992–2000	1,193	Reduced hospital and ICU stay increased home discharges with increasing volume. No difference in hospital charges	HVHs have better results with early clinical outcomes
Dimick (2003) (13)	U.S. (national)	1996–1997	1,226	Decreased rate of pulmonary, renal, infectious, and surgical complications with increasing volume	HVHs have a decreased rate of postoperative complications
Dimick (2003) (15)	U.S. (Maryland)	1994–1998	366	Decreased rate of pulmonary, renal, infectious, and surgical complications with increasing volume	Increased risk for postoperative complications and death for patients undergoing surgery at LVHs
Goodney (2003) (38)	U.S. (national)	1994–1999	—	No significant differences in length of stay and readmission rate	No relationship between volume and length of hospital stay or readmission rate
Traverso (2004) (17)	U.S. (Seattle)	1996–2002	174	Lower mortality, reduced length of stay, reduced intraoperative blood loss, less need for transfusion, and reduced reoperation rate	Improved results with increasing experience
Viklund (2006) (7)	Sweden	2001–2003	275	8-fold increased risk of anastomotic leakage for LVSs	LVSs seem to increase the risk for anastomotic leakage

esophagectomy for cancer, either expressed as 30-day mortality or in-hospital mortality.

In Table 32.2, a selection of published series evaluating the impact of hospital or surgeon volume on postoperative mortality is presented. In 1986, Mathews et al. revealed 39.4% in-hospital mortality for surgeons performing less than 6 esophagectomies per year, compared to 21.6% for surgeons performing more than 6 procedures per year ($p < 0.01$) (21). Likewise, Miller et al. demonstrated a significantly lower operative mortality among patients operated on by high-volume surgeons (HVSs) (> 5 cases per year), compared to those operated on by LVSs (22). Furthermore, in a series of 1,561 patients who underwent esophagectomy for cancer at hospitals in California from 1990 to 1994, Patti et al. demonstrated a striking correlation between hospital volume and the outcome of this operation with an in-hospital mortality below 5% for hospital performing more than 30 esophagectomies per year compared to 18% at hospitals with less than 5 cases annually (18). The conclusion was that this form of surgery should be restricted to hospitals that can exceed a yearly minimum experience.

In 2 well-designed studies using the Medicare database, Begg et al. (23) and Swisher et al. (24) also reported a significant impact of hospital volume on mortality with levels as low as 3.4% and 3.0% respectively at HVHs. Moreover, Swisher and colleagues demonstrated at their series that volume of esophagectomies was the independent risk factor for operative mortality, not the number of non-esophageal operations, hospital size, or cancer specialization. In one of the most renowned studies addressing the relation between hospital volume and operative mortality for different cardiovascular and cancer operations, including esophageal cancer surgery, Birkmeyer et al. reported a significantly decreased risk of mortality by selecting HVH (20.3% at hospitals with less than 2 cases per year compared to 8.4% for hospitals with more than 19 cases per year) (9). This study was followed by another focusing on the relation between surgeon volume and postoperative mortality using the same database (25). For esophageal cancer, there was significantly higher postoperative mortality among patients operated on by LVSs (< 2 resections/year): 18.8% compared to those operated on by HVSs (> 6 resection/year): 9.2%. The authors could also demonstrate that surgeon volume accounted for a large proportion of the apparent effect of the hospital volume (46% for esophagectomy).

Similar results have been found in studies from the Netherlands, Canada, and Sweden. Van Lanschot and colleagues analyzed hospital mortality after esophagectomy for cancer in the Netherlands between 1993 and 1998 and found a linear relation between hospital volume and mortality (26). Hospitals with < 10 procedures per year had 12.1% in-hospital mortality, while hospitals with > 20 resections per year had a corresponding 4.9% mortality. This volume-outcome trend was also supported in a study of hospitals in Ontario, Canada, by Urbach et al., in which it was estimated that 4 lives potentially would be saved annually if esophageal resection was performed only at high-volume centers in the province (27). Correspondingly, Rouvelas et al. showed in a Swedish population-based study that the 30-day mortality rate was twice as high at LVHs (9%), defined < 10 cases per year, compared to HVHs conducting at least 10 such operations annually (4%) (28). In another Swedish nationwide study based on a different database, patients operated on by HVSs (> 6 esophagectomies annually) had a 58% lower 30-day mortality risk compared to those operated on by LVSs (29).

The conclusion based on a substantial literature is that esophageal cancer surgery should be conducted at HVHs and by HVSs to reduce the risk of early postoperative mortality.

IMPACT OF ESOPHAGECTOMY VOLUME ON LONG-TERM PROGNOSIS

Although the postoperative mortality in relation to surgery volume after esophageal cancer surgery has been investigated extensively, resulting in an established inverse association, the effect of surgical workload on long-term survival remains uncertain. Only a limited number of studies have been conducted addressing this question and the results have been conflicting. A difference between early postoperative mortality and long-term survival is that tumor stage must be considered in the latter, since it is the dominating prognostic factor with regard to long-term prognosis.

In Table 32.3, publications reporting on the relation between surgery volume and long-term survival are presented. Three population-based studies, with inherent less risk of selection bias, have assessed the relation between hospital volume and long-term survival after esophageal resection for cancer with similar findings. In a retrospective case-note study in the West Midlands region of England, performed by Gillison et al., no relation between increasing hospital volume and improved long-term surgical outcome was found. The 5-year survival was approximately 18% for the 3 hospital volume categories (30). Equivalent results were demonstrated by Rouvelas et al. in a national, retrospective Swedish study performed during 1987–2000, in which patients operated on at hospitals performing > 10 esophagectomies per year had 27.4% 5-year survival compared to 23.8% at LVHs, but the difference was statistically non-significant, and when tumor stage was adjusted for, no difference in risk was found (HR = 0.99, 95% CI 0.84-1.18) (28). Similarly, a recently published study by Thompson and colleagues in Edinburgh, Scotland, found

TABLE 32.2
Selected Publications Reporting Relation between Hospital Volume and Postoperative Mortality

Author (year)	Country (region)	Years	Patient number	Operative volume (cases/year) Mortality rate (%)[a]					Hospital/ surgeon
Matthews (1986) (21)	U.K. (W. Midlands)	1957–1976	1,119	1–3	>6				Surgeon
				39.4	21.6				
Miller (1997) (22)	Canada (S. W. Ontario)	1989–1993	231	1–5	>5				Surgeon
				22	0				
Patti (1997) (18)	U.S. (California)	1990–1994	1,561	1–5	6–10	11–20	21–30	>30	Hospital
				18	19	11	15	5	
Begg (1998) (23)	U.S. (national)	1984–1993	503	<5	5–10	>11			Hospital
				17.3	3.9	3.4			
Swisher (2000) (24)	U.S. (national)	1994–1996	340	<5	>5				Hospital
				12.2	3.0				
van Lanschot (2000) (26)	Netherlands (national)	1993–1998	1,900	1–10	11–20	>20			Hospital
				12.1	7.5	4.9			
Birkmeyer (2001) (41)	U.S. (national)	1999	2,055	1–7	>7				Hospital
				15.8	5.9				
Dimick (2001) (40)	U.S. (Maryland)	1984–1999	1,136	3	4–15	>15			Hospital
				16	12.7	2.7			
Kuo (2001) (39)	U.S. (Massachusetts)	1992–1999	1,193	<6	>6				Hospital
				9.2	2.5				
Gillison (2002) (30)	U.K. (W. Midlands)	1992–1996	1,125	<4	4–11	>12			Surgeon
				15.1	6.6	11.8			
					<20	>20			Hospital
					9.8	10.2			
Birkmeyer (2002) (9)	U.S. (national)	1994–1999	6,337	<2	2–4	5–7	8–19	>19	Hospital
				20.3	17.8	16.2	11.4	8.4	
Birkmeyer (2003) (25)	U.S. (national)	1998–1999	—	<2	2–6	>6			Surgeon
				18.8	13.1	9.2			
Dimick (2003) (15)	U.S. (Maryland)	1994–1998	366	<8	>8				Hospital
				15.4	2.5				
Urbach (2003) (27)	Canada (Ontario)	1994–1999	613	2.8	8.8	16.6	19		Hospital
				18.6	12.6	12	10.2		
Metzger (2004) (35)	Worldwide	1984–1999	18,032	<5	5–10	11–20	>20		Hospital
				18.0	13.8	11.0	4.9		
Rouvelas (2006) (29)	Sweden (national)	2001–2005	607	<2	2–6	>6			Surgeon
				7.1	2.1	2.6			
Rouvelas (2007) (28)	Sweden (national)	1987–2000	1,199	<10	>10				Hospital
				9.3	4.5				

[a] Postoperative mortality is generally reported at 30 days.

TABLE 32.3
Publications Reporting Relation between Hospital Volume and Long-Term Survival

				Operative volume (cases/year)				
Author (year)	**Country (region)**	**Years**	**Patient number**	**Survival (%)[a]**				**Hospital/surgeon**
Gillison (2002) (30)[b]	U.K. (W. Midlands)	1992–1996	1,125	<4	4–11	>12		Hospital
					Approximately 18			
Wenner (2005) (33)	Sweden (national)	1987–1996	1,425	<5	5–15	>15		Hospital
				17	19	22		
Rouvelas (2007) (28)[b]	Sweden (national)	1987–2000	1,199	<10	>10			Hospital
				23.8	27.4			
Birkmeyer (2007) (32)	U.S. (national)	1992–2002	822	0.3–3.8	14.4–107			Hospital
				17.4	33.7			
Thompson (2007) (31)	Scotland (national)	1997–1999	1,302	13	13–19	20–34	>35	Hospital
				43.4	38.5	37.6	36.8	

[a]Survival refers to overall survival at 5 years.
[b]Tumor stage was included in the analysis

no relationship between hospital volume and long-term survival after surgery for esophageal cancer (31). All these studies included tumor stage in their analyses, but one of the studies had missing data on a high frequency of cases and did not include stage in its analyses (31). In conflict with these results, Birkmeyer et al., in a study using the Medicare database, demonstrated that HVHs have better late survival rates than LVHs (33.7% vs. 17.4% respectively) (32), a finding supported by a study by Wenner and colleagues (33). However, the results of both these studies must be interpreted very cautiously since tumor stage was not available.

In summary, more research is needed before the role of surgery volume with regard to tumor stage specific survival is established, but based on the few valid studies that included tumor stage, it seems that tumor biology has a greater impact on the long-term survival than does surgery volume.

DEFINITION OF VOLUME

The recommendations of the minimum number of esophagectomies needed to be performed annually to allow such surgery to be as safe as possible deserve attention. First, an important issue is whether hospital or surgeon volume is a better measure of comparison. Hospital volume may be a better parameter, since it represents a multidisciplinary and complex system of independent contributing process and structure variables that relate to patient care. This system includes preoperative patient selection, experience of the surgical, anaesthesiologic, medical, and nursing staff with major surgery, intraoperative technical skills, and postoperative prevention, early diagnosis and management of complications. It is not only the single surgeon that makes the difference, but all the contributors to the multidisciplinary treatment that influence patient outcome after such a complex surgery such as esophagectomy for cancer. Since it has been well established that the early postoperative morbidity and mortality is higher at LVHs, the vast majority of the experts in treatment of esophageal cancer agree that these patients should be discussed and treated in a multidisciplinary setting, and esophageal cancer surgery should be performed in high-volume centers by skilled and experienced esophageal surgeons.

Given the heterogeneity of the definition of hospital and surgeon volume in the literature, it has been difficult to identify minimum volume thresholds at which satisfactory performance is achieved. The Leapfrog Group, a consortium of health care purchasers and providers in the United States and perhaps the best-known promoter of volume-based selective referral, in one of its initial (2000) guidelines for selective referral to HVHs suggested an annual volume threshold of 7 esophagectomies a year, but after a revision in 2003, this threshold was increased to 13 cases a year. Christian et al. tested whether this latter threshold represented the optimal cutoff to discriminate between high- and low-mortality hospitals (34). They concluded that there was a lack of correlation between volume and mortality when based on the Leapfrog Group threshold and suggested an empirical cutoff of 22 esophagectomies per year. A meta-analysis by Metzger et al. tried to identify the lower limit of esophageal cancer operations performed per year required to achieve the best results concerning early postoperative mortality (35). They reviewed 13 studies between the years 1990 and 2003 and the hospital volume was categorized in 4 groups with the very low-volume hospitals (VLVHs) defined as < 5 esophagectomies per year and HVHs defined as > 20 resections performed annually. The postoperative mortality was significantly higher in VLVHs (18%) compared to HVHs (4.9%). The conclusion drawn based on these results was that esophageal cancer surgery should be performed only by specialists who operate in HVHs with at least 20 or more cases per year, and furthermore, that only by referring to experienced specialized teams the patients have a chance of decreased postoperative mortality. Finally, in the United Kingdom, the National Health Service Executive guidance in 2001 recommended that the hospitals that managed esophageal cancer patients should evaluate at least 100 patients yearly, approximately corresponding to an annual resection frequency of 40 esophagectomies (36).

VOLUME AND OTHER RELEVANT OUTCOMES

Although mortality is usually considered as the major endpoint in studies examining the effect of hospital volume in the clinical outcomes after surgery, health-related quality of life should be another very important endpoint, particularly in oncologic surgery. To our knowledge, besides a study conducted in Sweden finding a non-significantly improved quality of life among patients operated at HVHs compared to those operated at LVHs (37), no other study has specifically addressed this question. However, it is documented that postoperative complications, especially surgery-related, have a negative impact on the global quality of life 6 months after esophageal cancer surgery (37). Speculatively, decreasing the risk for postoperative morbidity after esophageal resection by centralization should also increase the chances for improved quality of life after such a procedure. Nevertheless, more prospective studies investigating patient-related outcomes (PRO) are warranted. This is of obvious importance, since the majority of esophageal cancer patients are not cured even after successful esophageal resection, making quality of life measurements the decisive parameters of the clinical outcome. Current cooperative group, multi-institutional clinical trials incorporate PRO survey instruments prospectively.

Other potential informative indicators on the effect of hospital volume to the clinical outcome after esophageal resection for cancer may be related to the health economics that pertain to length of hospital stay, need for intensive care unit (ICU) stay, and readmission rates (Table 32.1). These measures are likely mainly mirroring the occurrence of postoperative complications. Patti et al. found no difference in length of hospital stay depending on the hospital volume, but a substantially increased rate of home discharges and a linear increase in hospital charges was demonstrated with increasing surgical volume (18). No significant differences in length of hospital stay or readmission rates in relation to surgical workload were either found by Goodney and colleagues (38). Opposite to these findings, Kuo et al. showed that compared to LVH surgery, patients undergoing surgery at HVH (> 6 cases/year) had a 2-day shorter median length of stay ($p < 0.001$), a 3-day reduction in ICU stay ($p < 0.001$), and a non-significant increase in the median hospital costs (39). Similar results with reduced length of stay and decreased hospital charges by increasing hospital volume were also demonstrated both by Dimick and colleagues (40) and Swisher and colleagues (24). In summary, the health economics may be superior in high-volume surgery centers, likely due to less postoperative complications.

CONCLUSION

Esophagectomy is a complex surgical procedure where the risk for severe postoperative complications is considerably high and the chance for cure remains low. This review of the available literature has shown, however, that this surgery can be performed safely with low rate of postoperative morbidity and postoperative mortality in experienced, specialized centers with high annual surgical workload and in a multidisciplinary setting. Furthermore, higher surgical volume seems also to be related with better health economic outcomes most likely due to decreased risk and better management of complications. Nevertheless, there is no striking evidence regarding improved long-term outcome with increasing volume where the tumor biology seems to have a greater impact.

Centralization to dedicated centers, performing at least 20 esophageal resection per year, is advocated for the vast majority of experts in treatment of esophageal cancer. In this way, a further improvement in the prognosis of esophageal cancer patients can be achieved. However, further investigation, focusing on parameters like disease-free interval and health-related quality of life, is warranted.

References

1. Jemal A, Murray T, Samuels A, et al. Cancer statistics, 2003. *CA Cancer J Clin.* 2003;53(1):5–26.
2. Enzinger PC, Mayer RJ. Esophageal cancer. *N Engl J Med.* 2003;349(23):2241–2252.
3. Wu PC, Posner MC. The role of surgery in the management of oesophageal cancer. *Lancet Oncol.* 2003;4(8):481–488.
4. Lerut T, Coosemans W, Decker G, et al. Surgical techniques. *J Surg Oncol.* 2005;92(3):218–229.
5. Law S, Wong KH, Kwok KF, et al. Predictive factors for postoperative pulmonary complications and mortality after esophagectomy for cancer. *Ann Surg.* 2004;240(5):791–800.
6. Jamieson GG, Mathew G, Ludemann R, et al. Postoperative mortality following oesophagectomy and problems in reporting its rate. *Br J Surg.* 2004;91(8):943–947.
7. Viklund P, Lindblad M, Lu M, et al. Risk factors for complications after esophageal cancer resection: a prospective population-based study in Sweden. *Ann Surg.* 2006;243(2):204–211.
8. Rouvelas I, Zeng W, Lindblad M, et al. Survival after surgery for oesophageal cancer: a population-based study. *Lancet Oncol.* 2005;6(11):864–870.
9. Birkmeyer JD, Siewers AE, Finlayson EV, et al. Hospital volume and surgical mortality in the United States. *N Engl J Med.* 2002;346(15):1128–1137.
10. Dudley RA, Johansen KL, Brand R, et al. Selective referral to high-volume hospitals: estimating potentially avoidable deaths. *JAMA.* 2000;283(9):1159–1166.
11. Sosa JA, Bowman HM, Gordon TA, et al. Importance of hospital volume in the overall management of pancreatic cancer. *Ann Surg.* 1998;228(3):429–438.
12. Gordon TA, Bowman HM, Bass EB, et al. Complex gastrointestinal surgery: impact of provider experience on clinical and economic outcomes. *J Am Coll Surg.* 1999;189(1):46–56.
13. Dimick JB, Pronovost PJ, Cowan JA Jr, et al. Variation in postoperative complication rates after high-risk surgery in the United States. *Surgery.* 2003;134(4):534–541.
14. Junemann-Ramirez M, Awan MY, Khan ZM, et al. Anastomotic leakage post-esophagogastrectomy for esophageal carcinoma: retrospective analysis of predictive factors, management and influence on longterm survival in a high volume centre. *Eur J Cardiothorac Surg.* 2005;27(1):3–7.
15. Dimick JB, Pronovost PJ, Cowan JA, et al. Surgical volume and quality of care for esophageal resection: do high-volume hospitals have fewer complications? *Ann Thorac Surg.* 2003;75(2):337–341.
16. Sutton DN, Wayman J, Griffin SM. Learning curve for oesophageal cancer surgery. *Br J Surg.* 1998;85(10):1399–1402.
17. Traverso LW, Shinchi H, Low DE. Useful benchmarks to evaluate outcomes after esophagectomy and pancreaticoduodenectomy. *Am J Surg.* 2004;187(5):604–608.
18. Patti MG, Corvera CU, Glasgow RE, et al. A hospital's annual rate of esophagectomy influences the operative mortality rate. *J Gastrointest Surg.* 1998;2(2):186–192.
19. Earlam R, Cunha-Melo JR. Oesophogeal squamous cell carcinoms: II. A critical view of radiotherapy. *Br J Surg.* 1980;67(7):457–461.
20. Muller JM, Erasmi H, Stelzner M, et al. Surgical therapy of oesophageal carcinoma. *Br J Surg.* 1990;77(8):845–857.
21. Matthews HR, Powell DJ, McConkey CC. Effect of surgical experience on the results of resection for oesophageal carcinoma. *Br J Surg.* 1986;73(8):621–623.
22. Miller JD, Jain MK, de Gara CJ, et al. Effect of surgical experience on results of esophagectomy for esophageal carcinoma. *J Surg Oncol.* 1997;65(1):20–21.
23. Begg CB, Cramer LD, Hoskins WJ, et al. Impact of hospital volume on operative mortality for major cancer surgery. *JAMA.* 1998;280(20):1747–1751.
24. Swisher SG, Deford L, Merriman KW, et al. Effect of operative volume on morbidity, mortality, and hospital use after esophagectomy for cancer. *J Thorac Cardiovasc Surg.* 2000;119(6):1126–1132.
25. Birkmeyer JD, Stukel TA, Siewers AE, et al. Surgeon volume and operative mortality in the United States. *N Engl J Med.* 2003;349(22):2117–2127.
26. van Lanschot JJ, Hulscher JB, Buskens CJ, et al. Hospital volume and hospital mortality for esophagectomy. *Cancer.* 2001;91(8):1574–1578.
27. Urbach DR, Bell CM, Austin PC. Differences in operative mortality between high- and low-volume hospitals in Ontario for 5 major surgical procedures: estimating the number of lives potentially saved through regionalization. *CMAJ.* 2003;168(11):1409–1414.
28. Rouvelas I, Lindblad M, Zeng W, et al. Impact of hospital volume on long-term survival after esophageal cancer surgery. *Arch Surg.* 2007;142(2):113–118.
29. Rouvelas I, Jia C, Viklund P, et al. Surgeon volume and postoperative mortality after oesophagectomy for cancer. *Eur J Surg Oncol.* 2007;33(2):162–168.
30. Gillison EW, Powell J, McConkey CC, et al. Surgical workload and outcome after resection for carcinoma of the oesophagus and cardia. *Br J Surg.* 2002;89(3):344–348.
31. Thompson AM, Rapson T, Gilbert FJ, et al. Hospital volume does not influence long-term survival of patients undergoing surgery for oesophageal or gastric cancer. *Br J Surg.* 2007;94(5):578–584.
32. Birkmeyer JD, Sun Y, Wong SL, et al. Hospital volume and late survival after cancer surgery. *Ann Surg.* 2007;245(5):777–783.
33. Wenner J, Zilling T, Bladstrom A, et al. The influence of surgical volume on hospital mortality and 5-year survival for carcinoma of the oesophagus and gastric cardia. *Anticancer Res.* 2005;25(1B):419–424.
34. Christian CK, Gustafson ML, Betensky RA, et al. The Leapfrog volume criteria may fall short in identifying high-quality surgical centers. *Ann Surg.* 2003;238(4):447–457.
35. Metzger R, Bollschweiler E, Vallbohmer D, et al. High volume centers for esophagectomy: what is the number needed to achieve low postoperative mortality? *Dis Esophagus.* 2004;17(4):310–314.
36. NHS Executive. *Guidance on Commissioning Cancer Services. Improving Outcomes in Upper Gastro-intestinal Cancers, the Manual Department of Health.* London: Department of Health; June 2001.
37. Viklund P, Lindblad M, Lagergren J. Influence of surgery-related factors on quality of life after esophageal or cardia cancer resection. *World J Surg.* 2005;29(7):841–848.
38. Goodney PP, Stukel TA, Lucas FL, et al. Hospital volume, length of stay, and readmission rates in high-risk surgery. *Ann Surg.* 2003;238(2):161–167.
39. Kuo EY, Chang Y, Wright CD. Impact of hospital volume on clinical and economic outcomes for esophagectomy. *Ann Thorac Surg.* 2001;72(4):1118–1124.
40. Dimick JB, Cattaneo SM, Lipsett PA, et al. Hospital volume is related to clinical and economic outcomes of esophageal resection in Maryland. *Ann Thorac Surg.* 2001;72(2):334–341.
41. Birkmeyer JD, Finlayson EV, Birkmeyer CM. Volume standards for high-risk surgical procedures: potential benefits of the Leapfrog initiative. *Surgery.* 2001;130(3):415–422.

IV

TUMOR TYPES

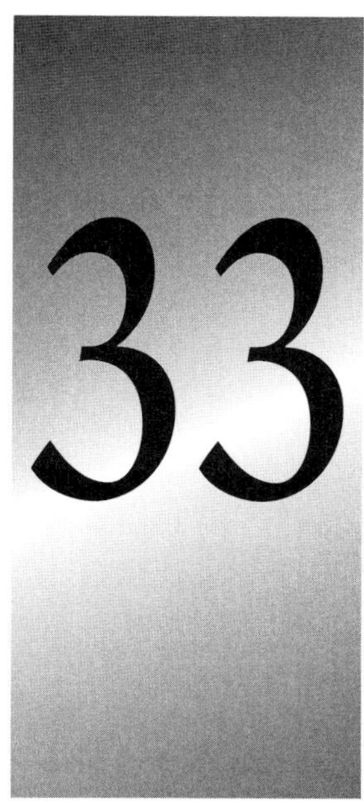

33 Benign: Lipoma

Shigeru Tsunoda
Glyn Jamieson

A lipoma of the alimentary tract is a relatively rare disease, with the incidence being 4.1% in 4,000 cases of benign gastrointestinal tumors (1). The majority (64%) of them occur in the small intestine. Lipoma of the esophagus is extremely rare, with an incidence of only 2% of lipomas of the gastrointestinal tract, and they constitute only 2% of benign esophageal tumors (2). On the other hand, a lipoma is the third most common polypoid tumor (17%) in the hypopharynx and the esophagus (3).

The majority of lipomas of the esophagus are pedunculated and found in the cervical esophagus, while intramural lipomas tend to arise in the thoracic esophagus (4,5). As pedunculated polyps of the esophagus have been variously reported as a hamartoma, fibroma, lipoma, and fibrolipoma (6,7), pedunculated lipomas might be better classified as fibrovascular polyps, a term recommended by the World Health Organization's international histological classification (8).

CLINICAL PRESENTATION

As with other esophageal tumors, lipomas of the esophagus commonly present with dysphagia (9). Odynophagia, recurrent melena (10), and mechanical compression of the upper respiratory tract (11,12) have also been described. The pedunculated lesions in the cervical esophagus can cause polyp aspiration and fatal asphyxiation (13–15).

DIAGNOSTIC EVALUATION

An initial evaluation should include a thorough history and physical examination, followed by a barium swallow and upper endoscopy. Endoscopic clues to a diagnosis of lipoma include the "tenting" sign (easy retractability of normal mucosa overlying a lesion) and the "cushion" sign (a sponge-like impression made by biopsy forceps as they are advanced into the lesion) (16,17). Most lipomas are covered by normal mucosa, but they sometimes present with ulceration over the distal part of the tumor due to the reflux of acid (18). However, in one report it was found that 22% of initial contrast studies and 33% of initial endoscopic examinations failed to identify the presence of polyps (3). Proximal dilation of the esophagus was mentioned in 24% of the contrast studies, and the free passage of barium into the stomach was universally noted (3). Therefore, one has to be careful before dismissing those patients who present with symptoms of dysphagia and yet have a nondiagnostic initial work-up. Repeat studies should be considered, and if the problem is severe enough, consideration should be given to obtaining a computed tomographic (CT) scan, magnetic resonance imaging (MRI), or endoscopic ultrasonography (EUS) (19). Lipomas are demonstrated on CT scan as homogeneous low density tumors (20), whereas liposarcomas are usually heterogeneous with septa and areas of non-fatty tissue (20) that show enhancement with contrast by CT or by MRI (21). As most lipomas of the esophagus are pedunculated, the most likely observation is of a low density mass surrounded by a single ring of normal esophageal wall (22). Rarely, a lipoma presents as an intramural mass rather than a pedunculated one (23,24). With regard to MRI, fatty elements are identified easily as areas of T1-weighted hyperintensity that follow the signal of subcutaneous fat on all pulse sequences and appear hypointense on the fat-suppressed images (25,26). With EUS, a lipoma may present as a hyperechoic submucosal tumor with a distinct margin (27,28). However, it can be difficult to exclude the possibility of liposarcoma especially if the lesion is well differentiated, unless of course there is clear evidence of invasion or metastatic lesions (26,29). However, if lipomas are rare, then liposarcomas are much rarer again in the esophagus. As a lipoma of the esophagus is a submucosal tumor, endoscopic biopsy rarely provides a definite preoperative diagnosis (29).

TREATMENT

Because of the potential for disastrous complications, surgical or endoscopic removal of proximal pedunculated tumors is strongly recommended (3). When managed conservatively, it has been reported that the tumors can increase in size (16). Treatment strategies need to be individualized with such factors as the tumor location and the size of the tumor being important. Pedunculated polyps can be removed by means of endoscopic ligation or stapling. If it is difficult or impossible to resect endoscopically, surgical intervention should be considered. The approach can be transcervical, transthoracic, or thoracoscopic (4,30). There is a report of a transgastric laparoscopic resection of a giant pedunculated lipoma of the thoracic esophagus with a 5 cm stalk, which was resected using an endoscopic linear stapler (31). If a lipoma is intramural, the enucleation of the tumor is the preferred approach. However, occasionally esophagectomy can be indicated (32).

PROGNOSIS

As a lipoma is a benign disease, recurrences do not usually occur. There is a report of a series of cases where intentional "subtotal"endoscopic resections of lipomas of the colon were undertaken without recurrence in a 1- to 8-year follow-up period (33). However, there is also a report of a laryngoscopic ligation of a pedunculated hypopharyngeal lipoma from a patient who had a history of laryngoscopic removal of similar hypopharyngeal polyp 6 years earlier (34). As stalks of pedunculated polyps of the esophagus are often elongated by the repetitive forces of esophageal peristalsis (35), when managed via an open approach any redundant esophageal mucosa around the stalk of the polyp should be resected to prevent further recurrence (3).

References

1. Mayo CW, Pagtalunan RJ, Brown DJ. Lipoma of the alimentary tract. *Surgery*. 1963;53:598–603.
2. Nabeya K, Nakata Y. Benign tumours of the oesophagus in Japan along with personal experience. *Dis Esophagus*. 1991;4(1):21–30.
3. Caceres M, Steeb G, Wilks SM, et al. Large pedunculated polyps originating in the esophagus and hypopharynx. *Ann Thorac Surg*. 2006;81(1):393–396.
4. Salo JA, Kiviluoto T, Heikkila L, et al. Enucleation of an intramural lipoma of the oesophagus by videothoracoscopy. *Ann Chir Gynaecol*. 1993;82(1):66–69.
5. Wang CY, Hsu HS, Wu YC, et al. Intramural lipoma of the esophagus. *J Chin Med Assoc*. 2005;68(5):240–243.
6. Patel J, Kieffer RW, Martin M, et al. Giant fibrovascular polyp of the esophagus. *Gastroenterology*. 1984;87(4):953–956.
7. Levine MS. Benign tumors of the esophagus: radiologic evaluation. *Semin Thorac Cardiovasc Surg*. 2003;15(1):9–19.
8. Watanabe H, Jass J, Sobin LH. World Health Organization. *International Histological Classification of Tumours: Histological Typing of Oesophageal and Gastric Tumours*. 2nd ed. Tokyo: Springer-Verlag; 1990.
9. Sossai P, De Bernardin M, Bissoli E, et al. Lipomas of the esophagus: a new case. *Digestion*. 1996;57(3):210–212.
10. Zschiedrich M, Neuhaus P. Pedunculated giant lipoma of the esophagus. *Am J Gastroenterol*. 1990;85(12):1614–1616.
11. Samad L, Ali M, Ramzi H, et al. Respiratory distress in a child caused by lipoma of the esophagus. *J Pediatr Surg*. 1999;34(10):1537–1538.
12. Hasan N, Mandhan P. Respiratory obstruction caused by lipoma of the esophagus. *J Pediatr Surg*. 1994;29(12):1565–1566.
13. Penfold JB. Lipoma of the hypopharynx. *Br Med J*. 1952;1(4771):1286.
14. Allen MS, Jr., Talbot WH. Sudden death due to regurgitation of a pedunculated esophageal lipoma. *J Thorac Cardiovasc Surg*. 1967;54(5):756–758.
15. Cochet B, Hohl P, Sans M, et al. Asphyxia caused by laryngeal impaction of an esophageal polyp. *Arch Otolaryngol*. 1980;106(3):176–178.
16. Kang JY, Chan-Wilde C, Wee A, et al. Role of computed tomography and endoscopy in the management of alimentary tract lipomas. *Gut*. 1990;31(5):550–553.
17. De Beer RA, Shinya H. Colonic lipomas. An endoscopic analysis. *Gastrointest Endosc*. 1975;22(2):90–91.
18. Akiyama S, Kataoka M, Horisawa M, et al. Lipoma of the esophagus—report of a case and review of the literature. *Jpn J Surg*. 1990;20(4):458–462.
19. Berenstein E, Ghigliani M, Caro L, et al. Endoscopic ultrasonography in the diagnosis of submucosal tumors of the upper digestive tract [in Spanish]. *Acta gastroenterologica Latinoamericana*. 1998;28(1):5–8.
20. Heiken JP, Forde KA, Gold RP. Computed tomography as a definitive method for diagnosing gastrointestinal lipomas. *Radiology*. 1982;142(2):409–414.
21. Ruppert-Kohlmayr AJ, Raith J, Friedrich G, et al. Giant liposarcoma of the esophagus: radiological findings. *J Thorac Imaging*. 1999;14(4):316–319.
22. Marom EM, Goodman PC. Double-ring esophageal sign: pathognomonic for esophageal lipomatosis. *J Comput Assist Tomogr*. 2002;26(4):584–586.
23. Nora PF. Lipoma of the Esophagus. *Am J Surg*. 1964;108:353–356.
24. Tolis GA, Shields TW. Intramural lipoma of the esophagus. *Ann Thorac Surg*. 1967;3(1):60–62.
25. Borges A, Bikhazi H, Wensel JP. Giant fibrovascular polyp of the oropharynx. *Ajnr*. 1999;20(10):1979–1982.

26. Maruyama K, Motoyama S, Okuyama M, et al. Cervical approach for resection of a pedunculated giant atypical lipomatous tumor of the esophagus. *Surg Today*. 2007;37(2):173–175.
27. Okanobu H, Hata J, Haruma K, et al. A classification system of echogenicity for gastrointestinal neoplasms. *Digestion*. 2005;72(1):8–12.
28. Murata Y, Yoshida M, Akimoto S, et al. Evaluation of endoscopic ultrasonography for the diagnosis of submucosal tumors of the esophagus. *Surg Endosc*. 1988;2(2):51–58.
29. Liakakos TD, Troupis TG, Tzathas C, et al. Primary liposarcoma of esophagus: a case report. *World J Gastroenterol*. 2006;12(7):1149–1152.
30. von Rahden BH, Stein HJ, Feussner H, et al. Enucleation of submucosal tumors of the esophagus: minimally invasive versus open approach. *Surg Endosc*. 2004;18(6):924–930.
31. Weigel TL, Schwartz DC, Gould JC, et al. Transgastric laparoscopic resection of a giant esophageal lipoma. *Surg Laparosc Endosc Percutan Tech*. 2005;15(3):160–162.
32. Algin C, Hacioglu A, Aydin T, et al. Esophagectomy in esophageal lipoma: Report of a case. *Turk J Gastroenterol*. 2006;17(2):110–112.
33. Yu HG, Ding YM, Tan S, et al. A safe and efficient strategy for endoscopic resection of large, gastrointestinal lipoma. *Surg Endosc*. 2007;21(2):265–269.
34. Som ML, Wolff L. Lipoma of the hypopharynx producing menacing symptoms. *AMA*. 1952;56(5):524–531.
35. Bernatz PE, Smith JL, Ellis FH Jr, et al. Benign, pedunculated, intraluminal tumors of the esophagus. *J Thorac Surg*. 1958;35(4):503–512.

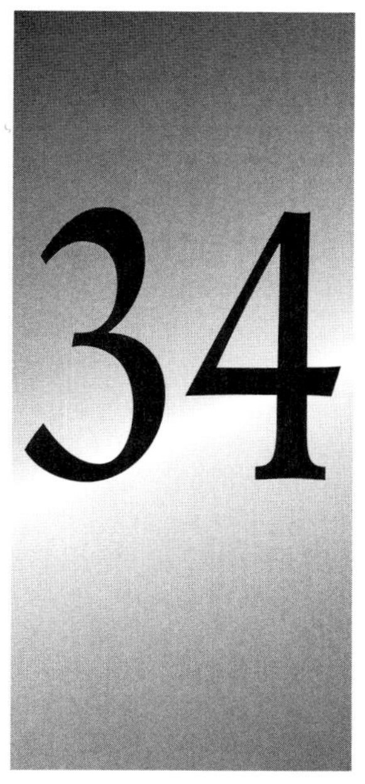

Benign: Fibrovascular Polyp

Shigeru Tsunoda
Glyn Jamieson

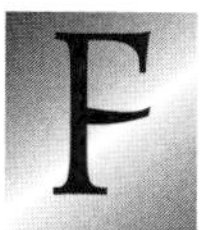

Fibrovascular polyps are a rare benign disease comprising 1% to 2% of all benign esophageal tumors (1–3). However, they are the most common histological type of hypopharyngeal and esophageal polyps with an incidence of 34% (4).

Fibrovascular polyps consist of a varying mixture of fibrous and lipomatous tissue, associated with abundant vascularization. They are covered by normal squamous epithelium (5). Depending on the predominant histologic components, theses tumors have variously been called hamartomas, fibromas, myomas, fibrolipomas, pedunculated lipomas, and fibroepithelial polyps (5,6). This peculiar composition of a mixture of normal or near-normal stromal tissues suggests that a fibrovascular polyp is not a neoplasm (7). They may be acquired malformations or hamartomas of lamina propria, or they may be some unusual form of inflammatory polyp or post-injury phenomenon, although neither preceding inflammation nor injuries have been described (7). Indeed, all of these lesions have been classified together as fibrovascular polyps, a term recommended by the World Health Organization's international histologic classification (8).

Fibrovascular polyps almost always originate from Laimer's triangle, just inferior to the cricopharyngeus muscle, although a more proximal origin in the oropharnx has been described (9). It is thought that a nodular submucosal thickening evolves into a fibrovascular polyp. The lack of muscular support in this region associated with the pressure differences between a contracted cricopharyngeus and peristaltic waves of the pharyngeal and esophageal musculature might contribute to polyp formation (10). The polyps sometimes grow to a very large size, and they can reach the distal third of the esophagus and even prolapse into the stomach (5).

CLINICAL PRESENTATION

Fibrovascular polyps of the esophagus commonly present with progressive dysphagia are often associated with weight loss, retrosternal discomfort, pharyngeal pain, or feeling of a lump in the throat (1). Regurgitation of the polyp (4) is a quite common and distinctive feature and has been observed in almost half the patients (1). A polyp can cause asphyxiation resulting from impaction of the polyp in the glottis, and this is the most likely complication to be fatal (2,11–14). Respiratory symptoms vary from coughing to respiratory distress due to the polyp causing mechanical obstruction (15). Odynophagia and melena have also been described as presenting symptoms (16).

DIAGNOSTIC EVALUATION

An initial evaluation should include a thorough history and physical examination, followed by a barium swallow and upper endoscopy (Figure 34.1). However, the presence of a fibrovascular polyp can be difficult to diagnose (17), and up to 30% of patients may die before a correct diagnosis is made (17). Even though endoscopy is recognized as the best modality for accurate diagnosis (18), a polyp may be missed at endoscopy as it is covered by normal mucosa and can be easily displaced (19). A barium esophagogram is useful for the detection of fibrovascular polyp as well. This usually demonstrates an intraluminal smooth, sausage-shaped or crescent-shaped filling defect (1,20). However, a polyp can be obscured if too much radiocontrast is used and the impression then may be a dilated esophagus suggestive of achalasia (1). An endoscopic ultrasound may demonstrate a tumor originating from submucosa (21), and it also provides information on the vascularity of the polyp and the stalk location (22,23). At computed tomography (CT), fibrovascular polyps can show different attenuation values in accordance with the proportions of fibrous and adipose tissues present (24). Therefore, polyps that contain different amounts of fibrovascular and adipose tissues show heterogeneous attenuation (20). CT with multiplanar reformatting may provide the location of the tumor as well as the proximal attachment (25). Feeding vessels of the tumor within the stalk are well visualized by contrast-enhanced helical CT (24). This may be crucial information in deciding whether to remove the polyp by endoscopic snare polypectomy or by transcervical esophagotomy (24). Magnetic resonance imaging can also be employed for optimal characterization of the tumor. Sagittal and coronal sections are ideal for showing the extent of the lesion. Different pulse sequences, including T1-weighted, T2-weighted, fat-saturated, and contrast-enhanced T1-weighted imaging, may provide valuable information regarding the composition of the mass (9). Fatty elements are identified easily as areas of T1-weighted hyperintensity that follow the signal of subcutaneous fat on all pulse sequences and appear hypointense on the fat-suppressed images (9). Similarly, areas of T1 and T2 hypointensity may reflect the presence of fibrovascular elements.

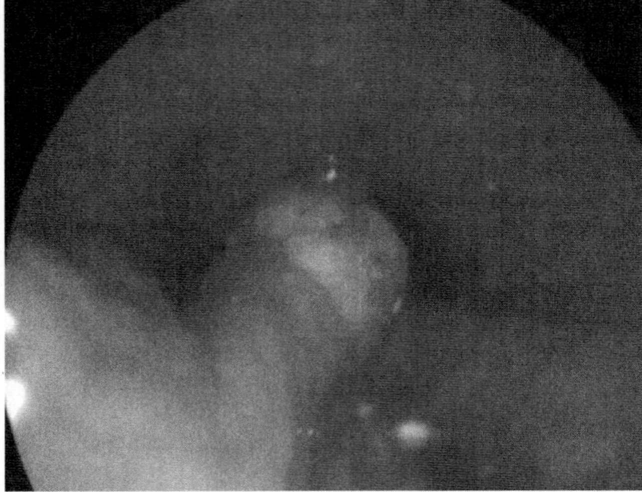

FIGURE 34.1

An endoscopic image showing a large pedunculated tumor of the esophagus.

TREATMENT

Because of the potential for disastrous complications, surgical or endoscopic removal of the tumor is strongly recommended (4). The treatment strategies are individualized based on the tumor location and/or the size of the tumor. Pedunculated polyps may be able to be removed by means of endoscopic ligation unless there is a large feeding artery within a stalk of the polyp (24), when stapling may be more appropriate, or open operation. In masses composed predominantly of adipose tissue, the risk of bleeding is low (26). In such cases, endoscopic treatment may be preferred, especially in old or frail patients. If it is difficult to resect a polyp endoscopically, surgical intervention needs to be considered because of the potential for hemorrhage from endoscopic removal (5,27). Left cervical esophagotomy is the preferred approach (28). However, occasionally it may even be necessary to undertake an esophagectomy due to difficulty with an accurate preoperative diagnosis (29).

PROGNOSIS

As the nature of the lesion is benign, the prognosis of the patients with fibrovascular polyps is good, although the potential for fatal asphyxiation exists. However, occasionally a recurrent polyp develops, although it has been reported only in patients that underwent either endoscopic removal or cervical esophagotomy (1), and there has been no report of recurrence after thoracotomy.

The literature also contains several reports of the development of squamous cell carcinoma associated with fibrovascular polyps (30,31) and also the development of liposarcoma (32). Whether this represented true malignant degeneration of a polyp is a moot point, however.

References

1. Drenth J, Wobbes T, Bonenkamp JJ, et al. Recurrent esophageal fibrovascular polyps: case history and review of the literature. *Dig Dis Sci.* 2002;47(11):2598–2604.
2. Carrick C, Collins KA, Lee CJ, et al. Sudden death due to asphyxia by esophageal polyp: two case reports and review of asphyxial deaths. *Am J Forensic Med Pathol.* 2005;26(3):275–281.
3. Wu MH, Chuang CM, Tseng YL. Giant intraluminal fibrovascular polyp of the esophagus. *Hepatogastroenterology.* 1998;45(24):2115–2116.
4. Caceres M, Steeb G, Wilks SM, et al. Large pedunculated polyps originating in the esophagus and hypopharynx. *Ann Thorac Surg.* 2006;81(1):393–396.
5. Patel J, Kieffer RW, Martin M, et al. Giant fibrovascular polyp of the esophagus. *Gastroenterology.* 1984;87(4):953–956.
6. Levine MS. Benign tumors of the esophagus: radiologic evaluation. *Semin Thorac Cardiovasc Surg.* 2003;15(1):9–19.
7. Lewin KJ, Appleman HD. Tumors of the esophagus and stomach. In: *Atlas of Tumor Pathology, 3rd Series, Vol. 18.* American Registry of Pathology; 1996:154–158.
8. Watanabe H, Jass J, Sobin LH. World Health Organization. *International Histological Classification of Tumours: Histological Typing of Oesophageal and Gastric Tumours.* 2nd ed. Tokyo: Springer-Verlag; 1990.
9. Borges A, Bikhazi H, Wensel JP. Giant fibrovascular polyp of the oropharynx. *Am J Neuroradiol.* 1999;20(10):1979–1982.
10. Zonderland HM, Ginai AZ. Lipoma of the esophagus. *Diagn Imaging Clin Med.* 1984;53(5):265–268.
11. Cochet B, Hohl P, Sans M, et al. Asphyxia caused by laryngeal impaction of an esophageal polyp. *Arch Otolaryngol.* 1980;106(3):176–178.
12. Allen MS, Jr., Talbot WH. Sudden death due to regurgitation of a pedunculated esophageal lipoma. *J Thorac Cardiovasc Surg.* 1967;54(5):756–758.
13. Penfold JB. Lipoma of the hypopharynx. *Br Med J.* 1952;1(4771):1286.
14. Sargent RL, Hood IC. Asphyxiation caused by giant fibrovascular polyp of the esophagus. *Arch Pathol Lab Med.* 2006;130(5):725–727.
15. Hasan N, Mandhan P. Respiratory obstruction caused by lipoma of the esophagus. *J Pediatr Surg.* 1994;29(12):1565–1566.
16. Zschiedrich M, Neuhaus P. Pedunculated giant lipoma of the esophagus. *Am J Gastroenterol.* 1990;85(12):1614–1616.
17. Timmons B, Sedwitz JL, Oller DW. Benign fibrovascular polyp of the esophagus. *South Med J.* 1991;84(11):1370–1372.
18. Eberlein TJ, Hannan R, Josa M, et al. Benign schwannoma of the esophagus presenting as a giant fibrovascular polyp. *Ann Thorac Surg.* 1992;53(2):343–345.
19. Reed CE. Benign tumors of the esophagus. *Chest Surg Clin N Am.* 1994;4(4):769–783.
20. Levine MS, Buck JL, Pantongrag-Brown L, et al. Fibrovascular polyps of the esophagus: clinical, radiographic, and pathologic findings in 16 patients. *Am J Roentgenol.* 1996;166(4):781–787.
21. Devereaux BM, LeBlanc JK, Kesler K, et al. Giant fibrovascular polyp of the esophagus. *Endoscopy.* 2003;35(11):970–972.
22. Lawrence SP, Larsen BR, Stacy CC, et al. Echoendosonographic and histologic correlation of a fibrovascular polyp of the esophagus. *Gastrointest Endosc.* 1994;40(1): 81–84.
23. Avezzano EA, Fleischer DE, Merida MA, et al. Giant fibrovascular polyps of the esophagus. *Am J Gastroenterol.* 1990;85(3):299–302.
24. Kim TS, Song SY, Han J, et al. Giant fibrovascular polyp of the esophagus: CT findings. *Abdom Imaging.* 2005;30(6):653–655.
25. Ridge C, Geoghegan T, Govender P, et al. Giant oesophageal fibrovascular polyp [abstract taken from 2005:12b]. *Eur Radiol.* 2006;16(3):764–766.
26. Ascenti G, Racchiusa S, Mazziotti S, et al. Giant fibrovascular polyp of the esophagus: CT and MR findings. *Abdom Imaging.* 1999;24(2):109–110.
27. Carter MM, Kulkarni MV. Giant fibrovascular polyp of the esophagus. *Gastrointest Radiol.* 1984;9(4):301–303.
28. Solerio D, Gasparri G, Ruffini E, et al. Giant fibrovascular polyp of the esophagus. *Dis Esophagus.* 2005;18(6):410–412.
29. Schuhmacher C, Becker K, Dittler HJ, et al. Fibrovascular esophageal polyp as a diagnostic challenge. *Dis Esophagus.* 2000;13(4):324–327.
30. Cokelaere K, Geboes K. Squamous cell carcinoma in a giant oesophageal fibrovascular polyp. *Histopathology.* 2001;38(6):586–587.
31. Petry JJ, Shapshay S. Squamous cell carcinoma in an esophageal polyp. *Arch Otolaryngol.* 1981;107(3):192–193.
32. Ginai AZ, Halfhide BC, Dees J, et al. Giant esophageal polyp: a clinical and radiological entity with variable histology. *Eur Radiol.* 1998;8(2):264–269.

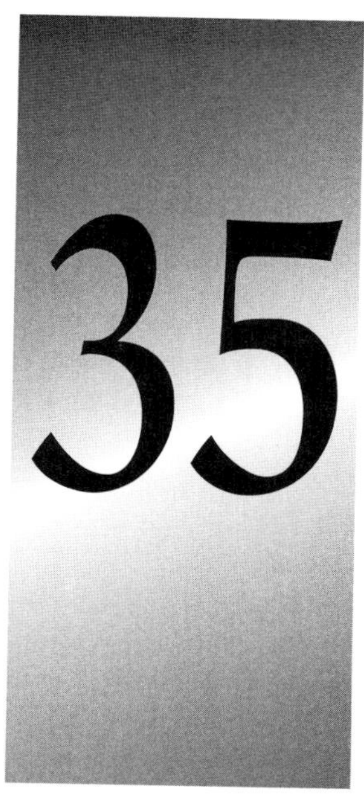

35 Benign: Fibrolipoma

Shigeru Tsunoda
Glyn Jamieson

Fibrolipoma is a pathologic variant of a lipoma originating from mesodermal tissue and is composed of fibrous and lipomatous elements (1). It has been suggested that fibrolipomas arise from the maturation of lipoblastomatosis. Further maturation of both adipose and fibrous tissue results in mature strands of collagen separating fat cells into lobules, characteristic of a fibrolipoma (2,3).

It is a very rare tumor and there were only 2 cases of fibrolipoma of the esophagus in 4,000 cases of benign neoplasms of the digestive tract in a 27-year study reported from the Mayo Clinic (4). Another review of 110 cases of pedunculated esophageal and hypopharyngeal polyps gave the incidence of fibrolipoma as 11% (5). However, pedunculated fibrolipomas might have been confused with fibrovascular polyp due to the fact that fibrovascular polyps have been variously called hamartomas, fibroma, and fibrolipomas (6,7). In fact, these lesions have all been recently classified together as fibrovascular polyps, a term recommended by the World Health Organization's international histologic classification (8).

CLINICAL PRESENTATION

The clinical features of fibrolipoma of the esophagus are not always specific and, in fact, 13% of all such patients are asymptomatic (9). Symptoms are usually related to the size of the tumor, which tends to be pedunculated and intraluminal. Pedunculated esophageal polyp can cause progressive dysphagia, weight loss, retrosternal discomfort, pharyngeal pain, or a feeling of a lump in the throat (10). Regurgitation of the mass (5) is a quite common and distinctive feature of pedunculated esophageal polyps, which may be observed in almost half the patients (10). At times it may cause asphyxiation resulting from impaction of the polyp in the glottis, which is often a fatal complication (11–16).

DIAGNOSTIC EVALUATION

Fibrolipoma is a subclass of lipoma and their clinical and histologic features are overlapped by those of fibrovascular polyps (17). (See Chapter 33 "Benign: Lipoma" and Chapter 34 "Benign: Fibrovascular Polyp.")

TREATMENT

There are not many references specific for the treatment of fibrolipomas of the esophagus due to its extreme rarity. However, they should be treated in the same way as lipomas and fibrovascular polyps of the esophagus. In other words, endoscopic or surgical removal via cervical esophagotomy or thoracotomy can be adopted in accordance with the location of the tumor, the size of the stalk, and vascularity. (See Chapter 33 "Benign: Lipoma" and Chapter 34 "Benign: Fibrovascular Polyp.")

PROGNOSIS

There are no reports of recurrence of esophageal fibrolipoma, but there is one report of recurrence of a hypopharyngeal fibrolipoma that extended into the esophagus (18). Another report documented the development of a liposarcoma that arose 9 years after excision of a fibrolipoma in the pharynx (19). In general terms, however, these are benign lesions which are treated as documented in Chapters 33 and 34.

References

1. Hsu JS, Kang WY, Liu GC, et al. Giant fibrolipoma in the mediastinum: an unusual case. *Ann Thorac Surg*. 2005;80(4):e10–12.
2. Migliore M, Jeyasingham K. Pedunculated intraluminal oesophageal fibrolipoma. A case report. *J Cardiovasc Surg*. 1998;39(4):519–521.
3. Perez B, Campos ME, Rivero J, et al. Giant esophageal fibrolipoma. *Otolaryngol Head Neck Surg*. 1999;120(3):445–446.
4. Mayo CW, Pagtalunan RJ, Brown DJ. Lipoma of the alimentary tract. *Surgery*. 1963;53:598–603.
5. Caceres M, Steeb G, Wilks SM, et al. Large pedunculated polyps originating in the esophagus and hypopharynx. *Ann Thorac Surg*. 2006;81(1):393–6.
6. Patel J, Kieffer RW, Martin M, et al. Giant fibrovascular polyp of the esophagus. *Gastroenterology*. 1984;87(4):953–956.
7. Levine MS. Benign tumors of the esophagus: radiologic evaluation. *Sem Thorac Cardiovasc Surg*. 2003;15(1):9–19.
8. Watanabe H, Jass J, Sobin LH. World Health Organization. *International Histological Classification of Tumours: Histological Typing of Oesophageal and Gastric Tumours*. 2nd ed. Tokyo: Springer-Verlag; 1990.
9. Nabeya K, Nakata Y. Benign tumours of the oesophagus in Japan along with personal experience. *Dis Esophagus*. 1991;4(1):21–30.
10. Drenth J, Wobbes T, Bonenkamp JJ, et al. Recurrent esophageal fibrovascular polyps: case history and review of the literature. *Dig Dis Sci*. 2002;47(11):2598–2604.
11. Taff ML, Schwartz IS, Boglioli LR. Sudden asphyxial death due to a prolapsed esophageal fibrolipoma. *Am J Forensic Med Pathol*. 1991;12(1):85–88.
12. Carrick C, Collins KA, Lee CJ, et al. Sudden death due to asphyxia by esophageal polyp: two case reports and review of asphyxial deaths. *Am J Forensic Med Pathol*. 2005;26(3):275–281.
13. Cochet B, Hohl P, Sans M, et al. Asphyxia caused by laryngeal impaction of an esophageal polyp. *Arch Otolaryngol*. 1980;106(3):176–178.
14. Allen MS, Jr., Talbot WH. Sudden death due to regurgitation of a pedunculated esophageal lipoma. *J Thorac Cardiovasc Surg*. 1967;54(5):756–758.
15. Penfold JB. Lipoma of the hypopharynx. *BMJ*. 1952;1(4771):1286.
16. Sargent RL, Hood IC. Asphyxiation caused by giant fibrovascular polyp of the esophagus. *Arch Pathol& Lab Med*. 2006;130(5):725–727.
17. Lewin KJ, Appleman HD. Tumors of the esophagus and stomach. In: *Atlas of Tumor Pathology, 3rd Series, Vol. 18*. American Registry of Pathology; 1996:154–158.
18. Sakamoto K, Mori K, Umeno H, et al. Surgical approach to a giant fibrolipoma of the supraglottic larynx. *J Laryngol Otol*. 2000;114(1):58–60.
19. Reibel JF, Greene WM. Liposarcoma arising in the pharynx nine years after fibrolipoma excision. *Otolaryngol Head Neck Surg*. 1995;112(4):599–602.

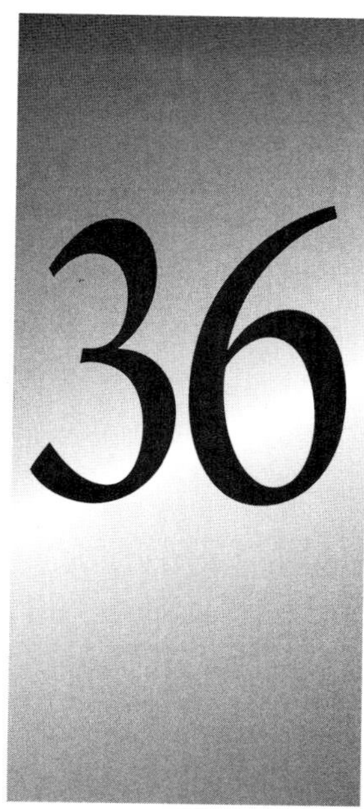

36 Benign: Hemangioma

Elizabeth Louise Wiley
Gregorio Chejfec

Hemangiomas were first described in the esophagus in 1896 (1). They are extremely infrequent and all reports in the literature consist of single cases. In a review of 99 cases of benign tumors of the esophagus published until 1960, Plachta cited only 9 hemangiomas, an incidence of 2.1% (2). The absolute majority of benign tumors were leiomyomas (51%); fibromas and lipomas were twice as frequent as hemangiomas (4.8%). Curiously, only 4 cases of neurofibromas had been reported (0.9%). The rarity of benign tumors of the esophagus was reported in a combined series of 13,460 autopsies between 2 institutions, where only 11 cases were identified, none of which were hemangiomas (3). In 1981, Hanel et al. reviewed 24 cases of hemangiomas; most of the cases were of cavernous type (4); in his report, he cited a series by Gentry et al. of 21 cases of hemangiomas among 344 cases of benign and malignant vascular tumors of the gastrointestinal tract, an incidence of 6.1% (5).

Yamashita et al. reviewed the literature in Japan; until 1993, 45 cases of hemangiomas of the esophagus had been reported in the Japanese literature (6). Also in Japan, Araki et al. found 29 cases reported in English, diagnosed from 1926 until 1997 (7). From 1997 until 2007 an additional handful of cases were reported (8–20).

CLINICAL ASPECTS

Hemangiomas of the esophagus occurred more frequently in men; in one of the series, there were 17 males and 12 females (7). The tumors are more commonly diagnosed from the fourth to the seventh decade, with a range from infancy (21) to age 72 (7). The tumors occurred throughout the length of the esophagus; 50% appeared in the upper esophagus, 28% in mid-esophagus, and 245 in the distal third (1,2,7).

Most of the reported hemangiomas were asymptomatic; their discovery occurred during routine radiologic studies or endoscopic procedures (7,8,12,19).

When symptoms motivated a consultation, dysphagia was the most common complaint (10,13,15,16,17, 20), followed by hematemesis or melena (1,11,14,15). Retrosternal pain was present in 2 cases (9,14). In the pediatric literature, 4 infants were first examined because of stridor (20).

At endoscopy, the tumors were described as bluish, polypoid masses; some were sessile (2), while others were pedunculated (1,7–9). The surface was reported as normal mucosa (7), though in several cases there was a focal ulceration (11,15). Some of the tumors were biopsied without significant bleeding (9,11).

Other diagnostic modalities included barium swallow (7,8), endoscopic ultrasonography (12–14,17), computerized tomography (CT) (18,19) and magnetic resonance (MRI) (12,19).

PATHOLOGY

Macroscopically, the tumors were extremely congested, "vascular" lesions, sometimes described as "blood clots" (1), measuring from 0.5 to 20 cm in maximum diameter (Figures 36.1 and 36.2).

Microscopically, the hemangiomas had several histologic arrangements; some were described as capillary hemangiomas, consisting of small vessels lined by normal appearing endothelial cells (8) (Figures 36.3 and 36.4). Two cases were reported as lobular capillary hemangiomas, and also referred to as "pyogenic granulomas" (8,15).

One case, initially diagnosed at biopsy as hemangioma, was reclassified as arteriovenous malformation after the lesion was resected. Microscopic examination of the case revealed thick- and thin-walled blood vessels in close proximity.

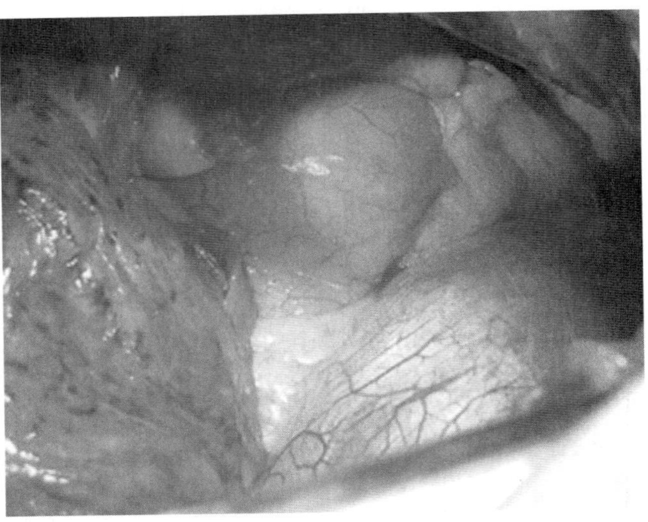

FIGURE 36.1

Intraoperative photo of a large cavernous hemangioma of the esophagus. Courtesy of Dr. Anthony Kim.

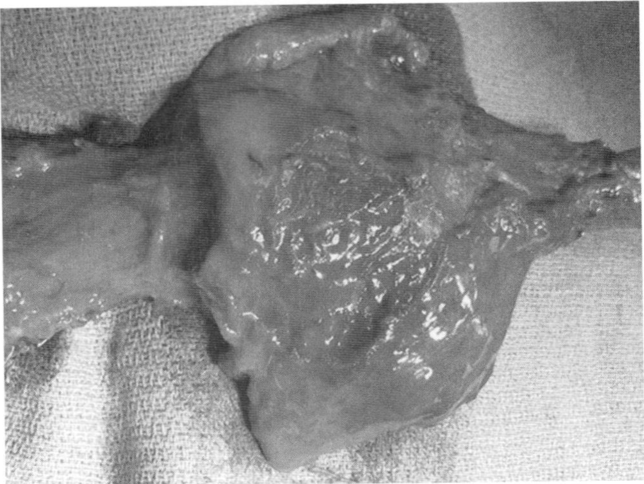

FIGURE 36.2

Surgical specimen of the large cavernous hemangioma. Courtesy of Dr. Anthony Kim.

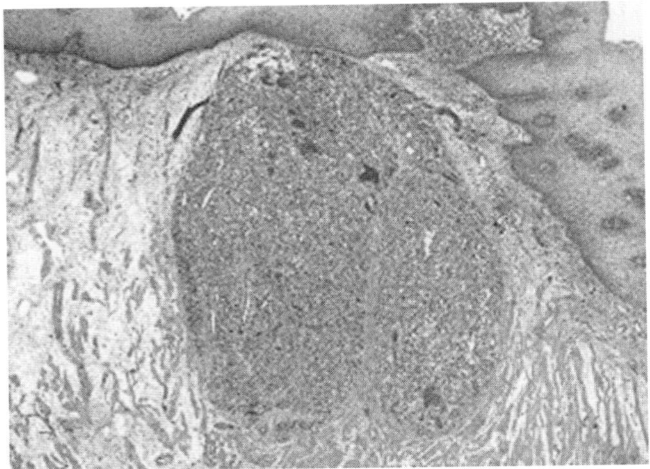

FIGURE 36.3

Low-power view of a capillary hemangioma, beneath squamous epithelium of the esophagus (H&E x 400).

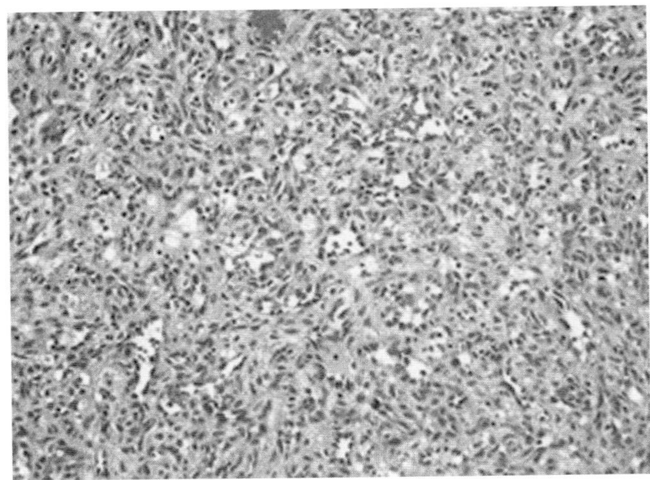

FIGURE 36.4

Higher magnification of capillary hemangioma (H&E x 200).

By far, however, the most common type of hemangioma consisted of cystically dilated, irregular vascular cavities, separated by thin septa containing thin endothelial cells. Such hemangiomas were diagnosed as cavernous. In one series, 16 of 20 hemangiomas were the cavernous type (7). One of the reports included hamartomas among the types of hemangiomas of the esophagus (17).

The microscopic diagnosis was based on examination of the classic stain, e.g., hematoxylin-eosin. Only once were immunohistochemic stains used to differentiate the hemangioma from Kaposi's sarcoma; the authors utilized antibodies to factor VIII, smooth muscle actin (SMA), and herpes virus 8 (HHV8) (15).

TREATMENT

In the early case reports, the treatment consisted of endoscopic polypectomy, enucleation, through an incision into the overlying normal mucosa (2,4,18); sclerotherapy, similar to that used for esophageal varices (1). Surgical intervention was favored in some of the reported cases, either excising the lesions (14) or performing a partial esophagectomy, which revealed an extension of the lesions into the muscular layer (17).

Other therapeutic modalities included high frequency electrocoagulation (12) fulguration using potassium titanyl/yttrium aluminum garnet (KTP/YAG), video assisted thoracic surgery (VATS) (14), and intralesional steroid injections, which successfully reduced the size of the lesion (21).

References

1. Takubo K. *Hemangioma in Pathology of the Esophagus.* Tokyo: Educa Publishing; 2000.
2. Plachta A. Benign Tumors of the esophagus. *Am J Gastroenterol.* 1962;38:639–652.
3. Harrington SW. Surgical treatment of benign and secondary malignant tumors of the esophagus. *Arch Surg.* 1949;58:646–661.
4. Hanel K, Talley NA, Hunt DR. Hemangioma of the esophagus. An unusual cause of upper gastrointestinal bleeding. *Dig Dis Sci.* 1981;26:257–263.
5. Gentry RW, Dockerty MB, Clagett OT. Vascular malformations and vascular tumors of the gastrointestinal tract. *Int Abstr Surg.* 1949;88:281–323.
6. Yamashita Y, Hirai T, Iwata T, et al. A case report of esophageal hemangioma resected by opening opposite side. *Jpn J Gastrenterol Surg.* 1993;26:1018–1022.
7. Araki K, Ohno S, Egashira A, et al. Esophageal hemangioma: A case report and review of the literature. *Hepato-Gastroenterol.* 1999;46:3148–3154.
8. Okamura T, Tanove S, Chiba K, et al. Lobular capillary hemangioma of the esophagus. *Acta Pathol Jpn.* 1983;1303–1308.
9. Cantero D, Yoshida T, Ito T, et al. Esophageal hemangioma: endoscopic diagnosis and treatment. *Endoscopy.* 1994;26:250–253.
10. Konstantakos AK, Douglas WI, Abdul-Karim FW, et al. Arteriovenous malformation of the esophagus diagnosed as a leiomyoma. *Ann Thorac Surg.* 1995;60:1798–1800.
11. Taylor FH, Fowler FC, Betsill WL, et al. Hemangioma of the esophagus. *Ann Thorac Surg.* 1996;61:726–728.
12. Tominaga K, Arakawa T, Ando K, et al. Oesophageal cavernous hemangioma diagnosed histologically, not be endoscopic procedures. *J Gastroenterol Hepatol.* 2000;15:215–219.
13. Shigemitsu K, Naomota Y, Yamatsuji T, et al. Esophageal hemangioma successfully treated by fulguration using potassium titanyl phosphate / yttrium aluminum garnet (KTP/YAG) laser: a case report. *Dis Esoph.* 2000;13:161–164.
14. Wu Y, Liu HP, Liu YH, et al. Minimal access Thoracic Surgery for esophageal hemangioma. *Ann Thorac Surg.* 2001;72:1754–1755.
15. Van Eaden S, Offerhaus GJA, Morsink FH, et al. Pyogenic granuloma: an unrecognized course of gastrointestinal bleeding. *Virchows Arch.* 2004; 444:590–593.
16. Palomino Besada AB, Garcia EG, Lopez-Calleja AR. Hemangioma cavernoso de esofago. *Rev Cub Med Militar.* 2004;33:1–6.
17. Chella B, Nosotti M, Baisi A, et al. Unusual presentation of a transparietal cavernous hemangioma of esophagus. *Dis Esoph.* 2005;18:349–354.
18. Sogabe M, Taniki T, Fukui T, et al. A patient with esophageal hemangioma treated by endoscopic mucosal resection: a case report and review of the literature. *J Med Invest.* 2006;53:177–182.
19. Kim AW, Korst RJ, Port JL, et al. Grant cavernous hemangioma of the distal esophagus treated with esophagectomy. *J Thorac Cardiovasc Surg.* 2007;133:1665–1667.
20. Folia M, Naiman N, Dubois R, et al. Management of postcricoid and upper esophageal hemangioma. *Int J Pediat Otorhinolaryng.* 2007;71:147–151.
21. Chen MT, Yeong EK, Horng SY. Intralesional corticosteroid therapy in proliferating head and neck hemangiomas: a review of 155 cases. *J Pediatr Surg.* 2000;35(3): 420–423.

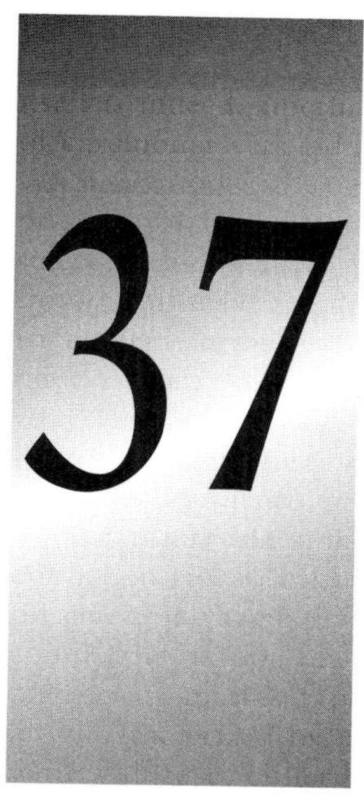

Benign: Granular Cell Tumors

Elizabeth Louise Wiley
Gregorio Chejfec

Abrikossoff first described granular cell tumors (GCTs) and, based on morphologic features, designated them as granular cell myoblastomas. His paper published in 1926 was a series of 5 cases of the tongue (1), and in 1931, he reported finding a single GCT in the esophagus (2). Fischer and Wechsler in 1962 characterized these tumors as showing Schwann cell differentiation (3).

Most commonly located in the skin and tongue, GCTs are found in every organ of the body, including the oral cavity, breast, orbit, skin skeletal muscles, and peripheral and central nervous systems (4,5). The gastrointestinal tract is an uncommon location and accounts for only 8% of all GCTs (6). Johnston and Helwig reported a large series of 74 gastrointestinal GCTs in 1981. In their series, one-third of GI GCTs were located in the esophagus, making the esophagus the most common gastrointestinal site outside the mouth (7) or 1% to 2% of GCTs overall. Some 300 GCTs of the esophagus are reported in the literature (8), with the largest series of 52 cases being published by Voskuil et al. from the national Dutch pathology register (1988–1994) in 2001 (9).

Most granular cell tumors are benign, occur as a single lesion (4,7,9) with more than half occurring in the distal esophagus. There is a female (2:1) preponderance. GCTs are more common in African Americans than Caucasians (8), and patients present most frequently in the fourth, fifth, and sixth decades of life (10,11). Almost virtually all reported cases are in adults, but rare pediatric cases are known (8). Of all esophageal tumors, 5% to 12% are multiple, being diagnosed concurrently or metachronously and independently (9,11,12). Multiple tumors may be confined to the esophagus or associated with other organ sites (8,11–16). Malignant GCT account for 1% to 2% of all GCT (16,17). The exact incidence is difficult to obtain because of the difficulty in distinguishing multiplicity from metastases in some cases and recurrences in up to 10% of resected cases (8,18).

CLINICAL PRESENTATION DIAGNOSES

Voskuil, in his report of the Dutch registry, found that 90% of patients had no symptoms or symptoms unrelated to the esophageal GCT (9), and the GCT were found incidentally in work-up for other reasons. Other case series suggest that symptomatic tumors are larger. Several published series find that symptoms are more common in tumors larger than 10 mm and also in the setting of multiple tumors (8). Ordonex and Mackay reported that more than one-half of their patients were symptomatic with dysphagia, epigastric pain, heartburn, and dyspepsia (4,11).

Endoscopically, most tumors are described as submucosal masses located in the distal esophagus, rarely associated with luminal narrowing. Differential diagnoses include fibroma, cholesterol deposit, xanthelasmata, papilloma, gastric heterotopia, leiomyoma, lipoma, Barrett's mucosa, ulceration, carcinoma (9). Both computerized tomography and esophageal ultrasound have detected GCT. Esophageal ultrasound is useful in delineating GCT, showing a hypoechoic solid pattern with smooth borders located in the submucosa and/or muscularis propria (8).

GROSS FINDINGS

Excision specimens are a nondescript nodule, which on cut section shows a white to pale yellow, firm poorly circumscribed mass with distinct margins. Most GCT are small; one-half of Voskuil's series were 5 mm or less. Only 20% were 10 to 30 mm at greatest diameter (9). The tumors usually arise in the submucosa or muscularis with little extension into the mucosa. Occasionally, GCT may lie completely within the muscularis propria (7). Like the dermatofibroma of the skin, esophageal GCT are associated with hyperplasia of the overlying epithelium. The overlying mucosa may be thickened and keratotic, sometimes being mistaken for dysplasia or tumor (Figure 37.1) (11,14). Rarely, the overlying mucosa is ulcerated.

Microscopic sections show plump, spindle, or polygonal cells with abundant finely granular amphophilic to eosinophilic cytoplasm. The cells are tightly packed into sheets, nests, and bands that infiltrate the stroma at the edges of the tumor. The typical GCT has small round nuclei with occasional small nucleoli (Figure 37.2). The cytoplasm contains numerous phagolysomes and glycolipids, which account for the characteristic cytoplasmic PAS positivity of these tumors. In keeping with electron microscopic features of Schwannian differentiation, the tumors are positive for S-100 protein by immunohistochemistry (Figure 37.3). They also are reactive to antibodies against enolase, myelin proteins, laminin, calretinin, TFE3, and nestin (19), but lack muscle and melanoma markers as well as glial fibrillary protein, CD34, and CD-117.

Similar to the dermatofibroma, about one-half of GCT show pseudoepitheliomatous hyperplasia of the overlying squamous mucosa (11,14). Mucosal biopsies

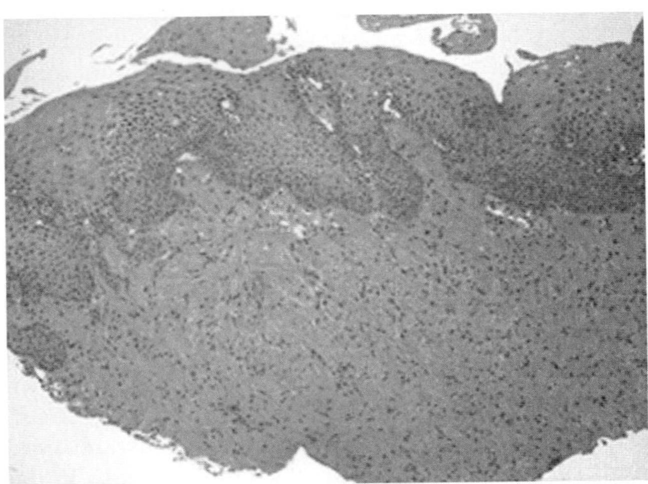

FIGURE 37.1

Low-power view of GCT showing diffuse infiltrate beneath the squamous epithelium, which is thickened (H&E x 100).

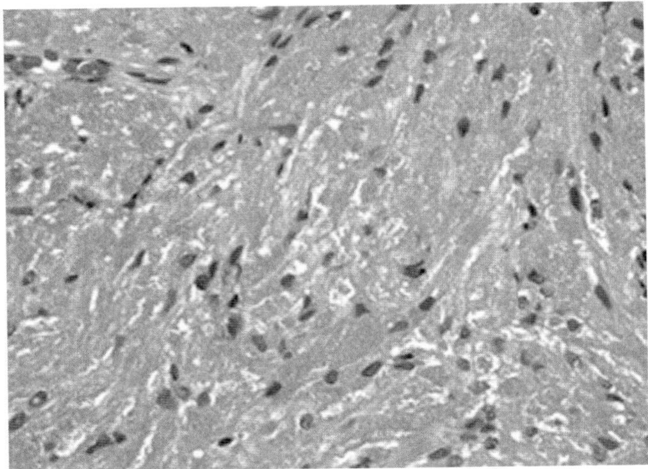

FIGURE 37.2

High-power view of GCT with the characteristic appearance (H&E x 400).

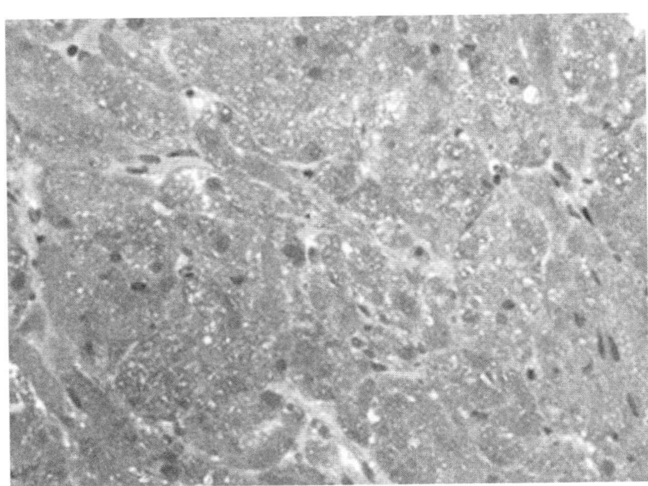

FIGURE 37.3

S100 immunostain showing diffuse and strong reactivity of the granular cells (x 400).

often are dominated by the hyperplastic squamous epithelium and little of the submucosa is present with lesional cells. Not only can the GCT be overlooked, but the squamous hyperplasia may be sufficiently atypical to lead to an incorrect diagnosis of well-differentiated squamous carcinoma (10,11).

A very small subset (~ 2%) of GCT is malignant, showing local invasion and/or metastases. Several reports have attempted to set criteria for distinguishing benign from malignant GCT (4,11,18,20,21) despite published cases of tumors with benign appearance and metastastic disease (4,22). Adverse characteristics of GCT include rapid growth, nuclear pleomorphism, high nuclear to cytoplasmic ratio, elevated mitotic index or high proliferation rate as determined by Ki-67 inex, p53 positivity in a majority of nuclei by immunohistochemistry, tumoral necrosis, and increased cellularity (12,18,20,21). David (20) and others (4,11) have suggested that an infiltrative growth pattern is important in distinguishing benign from potentially malignant tumors; of 13 cases with an infiltrative pattern, 2 metastasized (4,10,11,18). In one series of GCT, benign tumors were exclusively negative for PCNA, bcl-2, and p53 (21). Malignant GCT in the literature were diagnosed by rapid growth or rapid recurrence after excision, tracheal infiltration, lymph node metastases, abundant mitotic figures. and multiple infiltrative tumors with pleural effusion and liver metastases and infiltrative pattern (12,18,20,23).

Esophageal GCT can be found associated with malignancies; the most common is squamous carcinoma of the esophagus (10). GCT has also been found with lingual, laryngeal, lung, gastric, mammary, and Ampulla of vater carcinomas (10,23).

There are a few lesions that GCT may resemble. Differential diagnosis includes histiocytes and foreign body response. The cells of most GCT resemble histiocytes with small nondescript nuclei. However, most histiocytes nuclei have a nuclear notch and are CD68 positive and S-100 negative. The 2 tumors most closely resembling GCT are rhabdomyoma and alveolar soft part sarcoma (ASPS); both tumors are extremely rare in the esophagus. Although both GCT and ASPS have reactivity to TFE3, ASPS has rich vascularity, an alveolar pattern, nucleoli in nearly every cell, and rhomboid PAS positive crystals. Rhabdomyomas express pan-muscle and striated muscle antigens by immunohistochemistry.

As most GCT are small with low to absent cell proliferation at diagnosis, most are stable and require no therapy (11). Excision should be restricted to symptomatic lesions, lesions greater than 1 cm, and those with histologic features of malignancy (11,14). The Dutch series reported no treatment in 90% and no follow-up in one-half of patients (9). Complete excision is the only option at present for malignant GCT, as radiotherapy and chemotherapy have been shown to be of little use (24). Those cases of GCT with coexisting malignancies should have treatment indicated for the cancer (25).

References

1. Abrikossoff AI, Über Myome, ausgehend von der quergestreiften willkürlichen Muskulatur. *Virchows Arch Pathol Anat.* 1926;260:215–233.
2. Abrikossoff A. Weitere Unterschunger ueber Myoblastenmyome. *Virchows Arch Pathol Anat.* 1931; 280:723–740.
3. Fischer ER, Wechsler H. Granular cell myoblastoma—a misnomer: electron microscopy and histochemical evidence concerning it Schwann cell derivation and nature (granular cell schwannoma). *Cancer.* 1962;15:936–954.
4. Ordonez NG, Mackay B. Granular cell tumor: a review of the pathology and histogenesis. *Ultrastructurt Pathol.* 1999;23:207–222.
5. Lack EE, Worsham GF, Callihan MD, et al. Granular cell tumor: a clinicopathologic study of 110 patients. *J Surg Oncol.* 1980;13:301–316.
6. Morrison JG, Gray GF, Dao AH, et al. Granular cell tumors. *Am Surg.* 1987;53:156–160.
7. Johnston J, Helwig EB. Granular cell tumors of the gastrointestinal tract and perianal region: a study of 74 cases. *Dig Dis Sci.* 1981;26:807–816.
8. Buratti S, Savides TJ, Newbury Ro, et al. Granular cell tumor of the esophagus: report of a pediatric case and literature review. *J Pediatr Gastroenterol Nutr.* 2004;38:97–101.
9. Voskuil JH, Van Dijk MM, Wagenaar SSC, et al. Occurrence of esophageal granular cell tumors in the Netherlands between 1988 and 1994. *Dig Dis Sci.* 2001;46:1610–1614.
10. Szumilo J, Dabrowski A, Skomra D, et al. Co-existence of esophageal granular cell tumor and squamous cell carcinoma: a case report. *Dis Esophagus.* 2002;15:88–92.
11. Orlowska J, Pachlewski J, Gugulski A, et al. A conservative approach to granular cell tumors of the esophagus: four case reports and literature review. *Am J Gastroenterol.* 1993;88:311–315.
12. Maekawa H, Maekawa T, Yabuki K, et al. Multiple esophagogastric granular cell tumors. *J Gastroenterol.* 2003;38:776–780.
13. Rubesin S, Herlinger H, Sigal H. Granular cell tumors of the esophagus. *Gastrointestinal Radiol.* 1985;10:11–15.
14. Goldblum JR, Rice TW, Zuccaro G, et al. Granular cell tumors of the esophagus: a clinical and pathologic study of 13 cases. *Ann Thorac Surg.* 1996;62:860–865.
15. Kuroda N, Kohno N, Iwamura SI, et al. Granular cell tumor arising metachronously in the bronchus and esophagus. *APMIS.* 2006;144:659–62.
16. Ohmori T, Arita N, Uraga N, et al. Malignant granular cell tumor of the esophagus. A case report with light and electron microscopic, histochemical, and immunohistochemical study. *Acta Pathol Jpn.* 1987;37:775–783.
17. Strong EW, McDivitt RW, Brasfield RD. Granular cell myoblastoma. *Cancer.* 1970; 25:415–422.
18. Yoshizawa A, Ota H, Sakaguchi N, et al. Malignant granular cell tumor of the esophagus. *Virchows Arch.* 2004;444:304–306.
19. Parfitt JR, McLean CA, Joseph MG, et al. Granular cell tumours of the gastrointestinal tract: expression of nestin and clinicopathological evaluation of 11 patients. *Histopathology.* 2006;48:424–430.
20. David O, Jakate S. Multifocal granular cell tumor of the esophagus and proximal stomach with infiltrative pattern. A case report and review of the literature. *Arch Pathol Lab Med.* 1999;123:967–973.
21. Fanburg-Smith JC, Meis-Kindblom JM, Fante R, et al. Malignant granular cell tumor of the soft tissue; diagnostic criteria and clinicopathologic correlation. *Am J Surg Pathol.* 1998;22:779–794.
22. Dzubow LM, Kramer EM. Treatment of a large, ulcerating granular cell tumor by microscopically controlled excision. *J Dermatol Surg.* 1985;11:392–395.
23. Vinco A, Vettoretto N, Cervi E, et al. Association of multiple granular cell tumors and squamous carcinoma of the esophagus: case report and review of the literature. *Dis Esophagus.* 2001;14:262–264.
24. Lassaletta L, Alonso S, Granell J, et al. Synchronous glottic granular cell tumor. *Auris Nasus Larynx.* 1999;26:305–310.
25. Gabriel JB, Thomas L, Mendoza CD, et al. Granular cell tumor of the bronchus co-existing with a bronchogenic adenocarcinoma: a case report. *J Surg Oncol.* 1983;24:103–106.

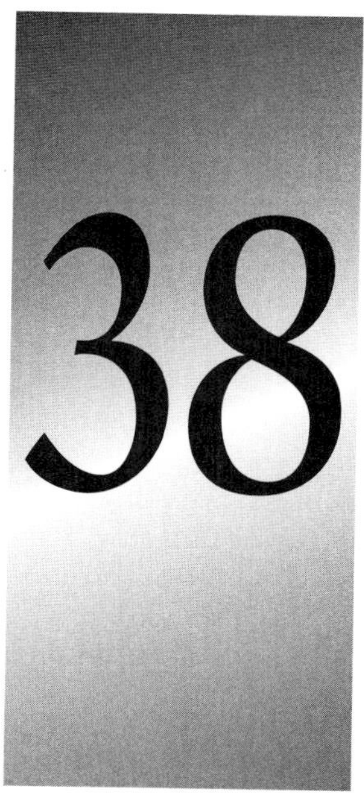

38 Benign: Neurofibroma

Elizabeth Louise Wiley
Gregorio Chejfec

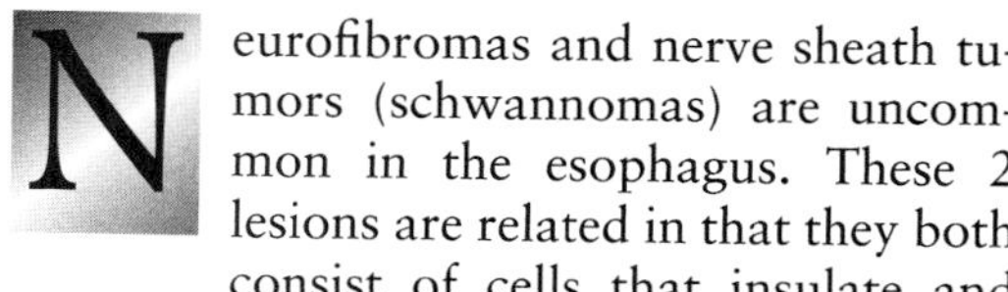

Neurofibromas and nerve sheath tumors (schwannomas) are uncommon in the esophagus. These 2 lesions are related in that they both consist of cells that insulate and protect axons and dendritic processes. These tumors differ in that the neurofibroma intimately involves a nerve with the neoplastic cells intertwining and splaying apart the axons or dendritic fibers of a nerve, whereas the schwannoma never does.

NEUROFIBROMAS

In 1950, Engelking (1) published a case of an upper esophageal neurofibroma. As Reichelt (2) reported in 1973, patients with neurofibromatosis type I (von Recklinghausen's disease) and MEN II (3) may present with esophageal manifestations, most commonly caused by plexiform neurofibromas, but also malignant peripheral nerve sheath tumors (4). By 1997, Lee had found 200 cases of benign neural tumors of the esophagus in the literature (5).

Clinical Aspects

Although solitary esophageal neurofibromas occur (5–11), most are associated with neurofibromatosis (2–4,10,12–16), an autosomal dominant inherited disorder caused by a mutation in the gene located on the long arm of chromosome 17 (17). Patients with neurofibromatosis frequently present with symptoms of obstruction but can also present with signs of esophageal dysmotility (13) and gastrointestinal hemorrhage (16). The tumors may be single (10), encasing surrounding structures (14), or multiple (12,13,15). The few reported solitary neurofibromas presented with dysphagia, stenosis, radiologic findings mimicking esophageal varix, and diaphragmatic hernia (5,10,18,19). Unlike those associated with neurofibromatosis, they commonly affect late-middle-aged women and are located in the midesophagus (5–10). Most solitary neurofibromas are treated with resection of the lesion; some of the cases of neurofibromatosis were treated with esophagectomy and colonic interposition (11,13).

Pathology

Grossly neurofibromas of the esophagus are like their counterparts in other organs, presenting as a tan to gray mass, unencapsulated, located in the submucosa. Rarely it presents as an intraluminal polypoid mass (Figure 38.1) (6). The typical neurofibroma is a fusiform mass that irregularly expands a segment of peripheral nerve. Plexiform neurofibromas, as their name implies, are complex anastamosing bundles of irregular fibers and nodules (Figures 38.2 and 38.3). Patients with neurofibromatosis may have tumors that show extensive infiltration into adjacent structures.

Microscopically, a neurofibroma consists of interlacing bundles of spindle cells with twisted "fish-like" hyperchromatic nuclei. These cells are separated by bundles of dense collagen fibers and myxoid ground substance. The plexiform neurofibroma differs from typical neurofibromas in that it consists of a torturous mass of nerve branches. It also is embedded in myxoid matrix material found in typical neurofibromas. In the setting of neurofibromatosis, the tumors are more cellular than those occurring as solitary masses.

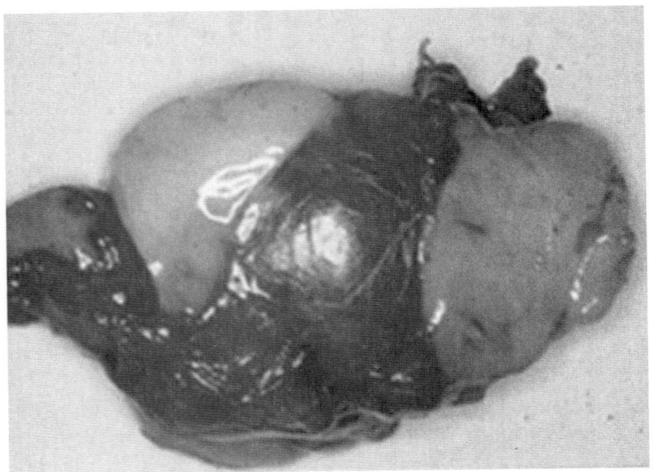

FIGURE 38.1

Gross picture of neurofibromas appearing as a polypoid mass covered by mucosa.

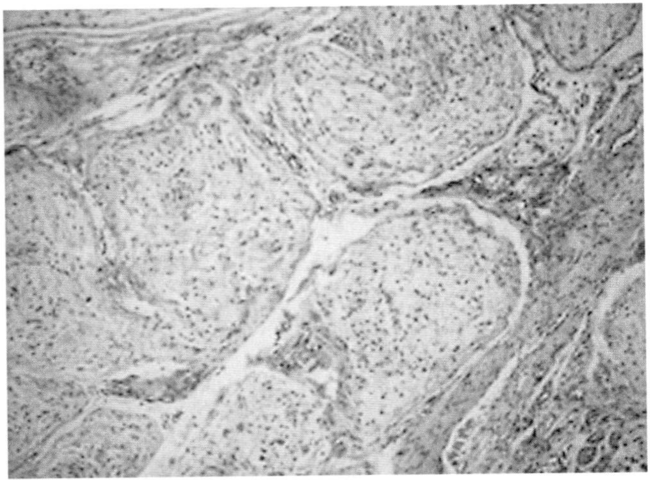

FIGURE 38.2

Medium-sized view of plexiform neurofibromas, showing discrete, irregular-sized nodules (H&E x 200).

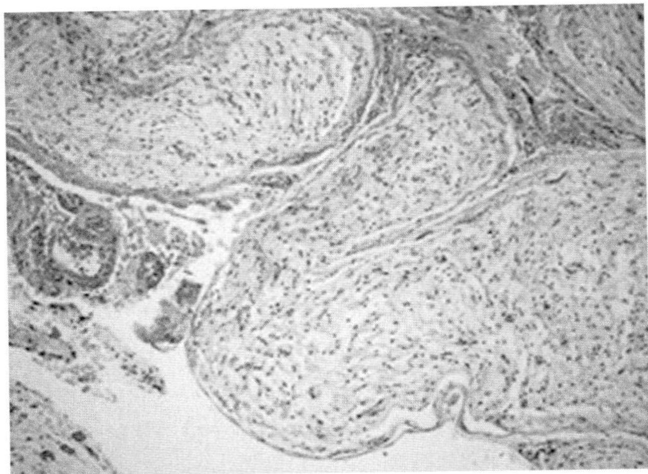

FIGURE 38.3

Medium-sized view of a different field from Figure 38.2 of plexiform neurofibroma (H&E x 200).

The neurofibromas are immunoreactive for vimentin and S-100 protein. Unlike the schwannoma, immunohistochemic staining for epithelial membrane antigen (Muc 1) is negative. Staining for neurofilament protein reveals nerve fibers embedded in the tumor mass.

SCHWANNOMAS

Clinical Aspects

Schwannomas are rarely found in the esophagus; they occur more commonly in the stomach (20,21). They are not associated with neurofibromatosis (22,23). Murase reviewed 18 cases, found mainly in women (F:M = 13:5) (24), with a peak occurrence in the sixth decade of life (25,26). A majority of patients presented with dysphagia. One tumor presented as a polyp (26). Tumor size ranged from < 0.5 to 14 cm (average 6.4 cm). Ten of the tumors were located in the upper esophagus. Eleven patients were treated with enucleation and the remainder with local resection of their tumors.

Pathology

In the esophagus, schwannomas are circumscribed but lack a true capsule that is present in most soft tissue schwannomas. Schwannomas most commonly involve the muscularis propria and the submucosa. There may be ulceration of the overlying mucosa or formation of an intraluminal polyp. As in other sites, esophageal

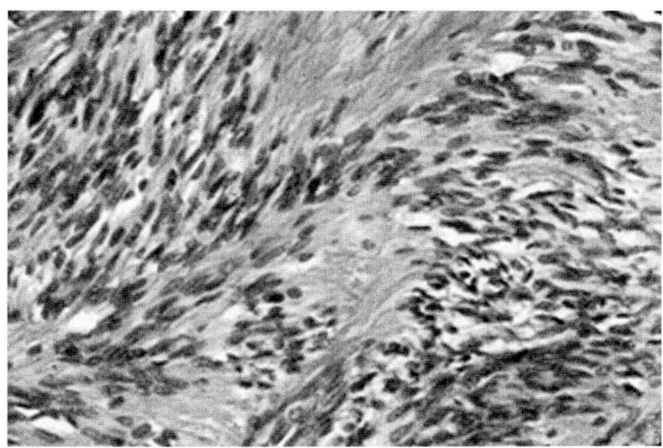

FIGURE 38.4

High power view of Verocay bodies, characteristic of schwannomas (H&E x 200).

schwannomas are composed of spindle cells with buckled or wavy nuclei. Within a tumor, cellularity often varies; areas may be paucicellular with prominent myxoid or fibrous components while others may be highly cellular with pallisaded nuclei, fasciles whorls and pigmentation (27). Verocay bodies, although present, may be inconspicuous (Figure 38.4). Mitotic activity is low but scattered cells with atypical nuclei may be present. These are more prominent in tumors showing hyalinization, vessel hyalinization, and xanthomatous changes or so-called ancient schwannoma. Electron microscopic examination shows well-developed external lamina, separating these tumors from gastrointestinal stromal tumors (25). Immunohistochemically, schwannomas are S-100 protein positive and variably CD34 positive. Most of the cases are benign.

Murase reported 1 case of malignant schwannoma with lymph node metastasis (24). Microscopic examination of the case revealed palisaded spindled cells with marked atypia and mitotic figures (1 per high power field). Immunohistochemic stains for S-100 and neuron-specific enolase were positive, and stains for actin, CD34, and CD-117 were negative. Iwata reported a schwannoma with mitoses and infiltration of the muscular wall (22). Morita reported a patient with a schwannoma that invaded surrounding tissue and had nuclear atypia (23). All 3 patients were treated with local resection of the tumors with repair of the esophagus.

References

1. Engelking CF, Knight MD, Brauns WH, et al. Benign tumors of the esophagus; report of a case of neurofibroma. *Arch Otolaryngol.* 1950;52(2):150–156.
2. Reichelt H. Unusual case of von Recklinghausen's neurofibromatosis with X-ray evidence of manifestations of the disease in the thorax, mediastinum, skull, esophagus, stomach and colon [in German]. *Rontgenblätter.* 1973;26(8):361–366.
3. Peterson JM, Ferguson DR: Gastrointestinal manifestations of type I neurofibromatosis (von Recklinghausen's disease). *Histopathology.* 1991;19:1–11.
4. Fuller CE, Williams GT: Gastrointestinal neurofibromatosis. *J Clin Gastroenterol.* 6:529–534.
5. Lee R, Williamson WA. Neurofibroma of the esophagus. *Ann Thorac Surg.* 1997;64(4):1173–1174.
6. Madrid G, Pardo J, Perez C, et al. The neurofibroma of the oesophagus. Case report. *Eur J Radiol.* 1986;6(1):67–69.
7. Ramírez Rodríguez JM, Deus Fombellida J, Lozano Mantecón R, et al. Solitary neurofibroma of the esophagus [in Spanish]. *Rev Esp Enferm Dig.* 1992;82(1):47–49.
8. Saitoh K, Nasu M, Kamiyama R, et al. Solitary neurofibroma of the esophagus. *Acta Pathol Jpn.* 1985;35(2):527–531.
9. Hishikawa Y, Miura T, Kakudo K, et al. Neurofibroma of the esophagus. *Radiat Med.* 1984;2(4):224–225.
10. Hutton L. Unusual presentations of benign intrathoracic neurogenic tumors. *J Can Assoc Radiol.* 1983;34(1):26–28.
11. Chou SH, Cheng YJ, Kao EL, et al. Histopathologic studies of gastric mucosa following gastric substitution in benign and malignant esophageal disease. *Eur Surg Res.* 1995;27(1):27–30.
12. Maunoury V, Fabre S, Wacrenier A, et al. Extensive ganglioneuromatosis of the esophagus: uncommon location of Von Recklinghausen's disease [in French]. *Gastroenterol Clin Biol.* 2005;29(11):1181–1182.
13. Sica GS, Sujendran V, Warren B, et al. Neurofibromatosis of the esophagus. *Ann Thorac Surg.* 2006;81(3):1138–1140.
14. Ganeshan A, Hon LQ, Soonawalla Z, 'et al. Plexiform neurofibroma of the oesophagus: a mimicker of malignancy. *Br J Radiol.* 2005;78(936):1095–1097.
15. Ishii T, Nitta M, Masaki T, et al. A case of multiple neurofibroma of the larynx and cervical esophagus. *Acta Otolaryngol Suppl.* 2002;(547):54–56.
16. DeVault KR, Miller LS, Yaghsezian H, et al. Acute esophageal hemorrhage from a vagal neurilemoma. *Gastroenterology.* 1992;102(3):1059–1061.
17. Fountain JW, Wallace MR, Bruce MA, et al. Physical mapping of a translocation breakpoint in neurofibromatosis. *Science.* 1989;244:1085–1087.
18. Ballabio D, Tisi E, Benenti C, et al. Unusual cause of esophageal stenosis. *Minerva Med.* 1985;76(8):341–344.
19. Tricarico C. On a case of neurofibroma of the esophagus clinically manifested by diaphragmatic hernia [in Italian]. *Riv Patol Clin.* 1964;19:163–173.
20. Dainaru Y, Kido H, Hashimoto H, et al. Benign schwannoma of the gastrointestinal tract. A clinicopathologic and immunohistochemical study. *Hum Pathol.* 1981;19:257–264.
21. Prevot S, Bienvenu L, Vaillant JC, et al. Benign schwannoma of the digestive tract; a clinicopathologic and immunhistochemical study of five cases, including a case of esophageal tumor. *Am J Surg Pathol.* 1999;23:431–436.
22. Iwata H, Kataoka M, Kureyama Y, et al. Two cases of esophageal schwannoma. *Jpn J Gastroenterol Surg.* 1992;25:401.
23. Morita I, Mushiaki H, Shinozaki Y, et al. A case of the esophageal submucosal schwannoma with pathological malignant findings [in Japanese]. *Geka.* 1996;58:506–510.
24. Murase K, Hino A, Ozeki Y, et al. Malignant schwannoma of the esophagus with lymph node metastasis: literature review of schwannoma of the esophagus. *J Castroenterol.* 2001;36:772–777.
25. Arai T, Sugrimura H, Suzuki M, et al. Benign schwannoma of the esophagus; report of two cases with immunohistochemical and ultrastructural studies. *Pathol Int.* 1994;44:460–465.
26. Eberlein TJ, Hanan R, Josa M, et al. Benign schwannoma of the esophagus present as a giant fibrovascular polyp. *Ann Thorac Surg.* 1992;53:343–345.
27. Weiss SW, Goldblum JR. Schwannoma (Neurilemoma). In *Enzinger and Weiss's soft tissue tumors.* Fourth ed. St. Louis, MO: Mosby; 2001:1146–1167.

39 Benign: Leiomyoma

Kemp H. Kernstine
Lawrence M. Weiss

Leiomyomas of the esophagus are benign tumors that histologically appear to be of smooth muscle origin. They are uncommon, accounting for between 0.5% and 0.8% of all esophageal neoplasms, with esophageal cancer being 50 times more common. It is the most common benign tumor of the esophagus, accounting for nearly 60% to 70% of all benign esophageal tumors, the remaining being cysts in 20% and polyps in 5%. At autopsy, the true prevalence is dependent upon the precision of the prosector, reported to be as high as 5% (1,2). In one autopsy series, 60% of the lesions found were less than 2 mm in diameter (3). In 95% of clinical cases, a single leiomyoma is present. In adults, the male to female ratio is 2.5:1. When leiomyomas present in childhood, females are more common than males. In over 95%, the tumors originate from the inner circular muscle of the muscularis propria, and the remainder occurs in the muscularis mucosa. In 80%, the growth pattern is intramural (4). In 13%, the leiomyoma will partially or very nearly completely encircle the esophagus. In less than 10%, the mass will have either an intraluminal or extraluminal growth pattern. In the symptomatic or incidentally discovered cases, 90% are found in the distal two-thirds of the esophagus, where the esophageal muscle is composed of smooth muscle rather than skeletal muscle found in the proximal third of the esophagus. A very rare form of familial-associated esophageal leiomyoma is leiomyomatosis (5), in which there are a number of leiomyomata along the entire length of the esophagus and stomach. The syndrome occurs in females, along with hypertrophy of the vulva and clitoris and leiomyomata of the uterus and air passages. Affected patients also have congenital nephritis and hematuria and, in some cases, there are associated cataracts and deafness.

Leiomyomas are of mesenchymal origin. At one time leiomyomata were felt to be a subset of gastrointestinal stromal tumors (GISTs) of the gastrointestinal tract, but more recently they have been found to be distinct from GISTs by electron microscopy, immunohistochemistry, and genetic expression (6). In the esophagus, leiomyomas are far more common than GISTs, but in the stomach and small intestine, GISTs are far more common than leiomyomas. Clinically, leiomyomas are from 2 to 6 cm in diameter and of those resected the mean diameter is between 4 to 5 cm. They can be as large as 1 kg (7,8). They rarely calcify, although there is one case presentation of an esophageal leiomyoma presenting as mediastinal calcification on chest radiograph (9) and in one series, calcification was found as high as 6% on pathological examination (10). They are firm, round to oval to lobulated, gray to yellowish-appearing, encapsulated masses that are relatively avascular and surrounded by stretched and somewhat attenuated normal esophageal smooth muscle. Histologically, they appear to be spindle-shaped interlacing bundles of smooth muscle cells with elongated nuclei, lacking pleomorphism (Figure 39.1). Previously, potential malignant degeneration was felt to be an indication for resection of esophageal leiomyomas, but we now know that malignant degeneration is an exceedingly rare event, only in case reports; a malignant degeneration rate of 0.2% of all leiomyomas has been reported (11,12). Features suggestive of malignancy include intratumoral hemorrhage or cystic degeneration, histologic pleomorphism and a mitotic rate of more than 5/50 high power fields (13). For treatment planning, leiomyoma must be differentiated from GIST. Immunohistochemic studies are usually necessary to differentiate leiomyoma from GIST tumors. Leiomyomas, being of smooth muscle origin, express the desmin and/or smooth-muscle actin (Figure 39.2), but do not express CD34 or CD 117 (c-kit). In contrast, GISTs do not express desmin and/or actin but do express CD34 or CD117.

Clinically, over 90% of patients present between 20 and 60 years of age. However, there have been cases reported in patients as young as 12. Most patients are found incidentally on barium swallow or endoscopy for indications other than a symptomatic esophageal mass. Nearly 50% have symptoms that include dysphagia in 50%, retrosternal pain, heartburn, cough, food sticking, odynophagia, weight loss, and bleeding period (14). In most patients, symptoms have been present for nearly 1 year by the time a diagnosis is made and in nearly 25%, the symptoms have been present for more than 5 years (4). In most reports, symptoms are completely resolved after resection, but the retrosternal pain may persist for a significant period of time (15). Unlike leiomyomas of the stomach or intestine, bleeding in esophageal leiomyomas is very

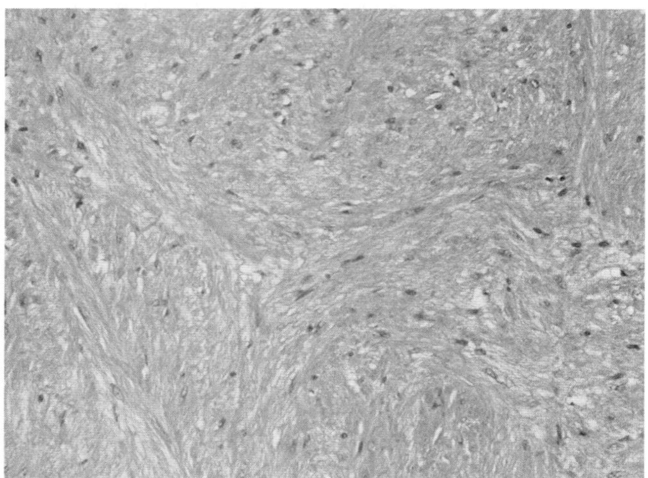

FIGURE 39.1

Hematoxylin and eosin stain of an esophageal leiomyoma.

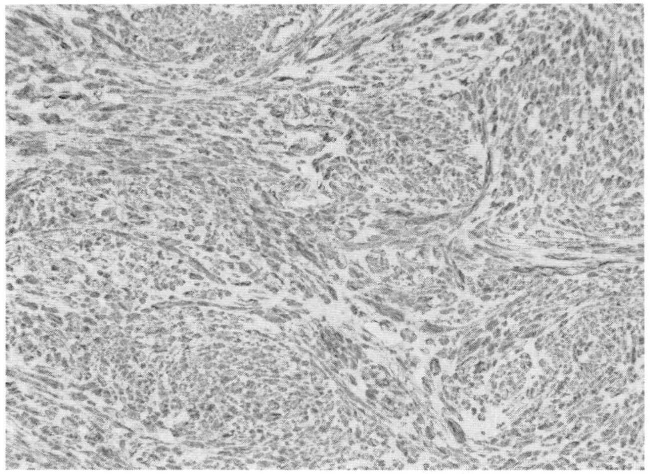

FIGURE 39.2

Smooth muscle actin immunostain of an esophageal leiomyoma.

rare. When it occurs, other causes of bleeding should be pursued. The most common concomitant defect is a hiatal hernia occurring in 4.5% to 23% (16,17) and as a result, the patients may have reflux esophagitis, which can be the source of bleeding. Symptoms can occur in tumors that are smaller than 5 cm. Lesions as small as 0.8 cm were found to be symptomatic in a large series reported from the Massachusetts General Hospital with a mean tumor diameter of 5.3 cm. They concluded that there is no correlation between symptoms and size or location of the leiomyoma. There is a case report of pulmonary osteoarthropathy of 6 months' duration being associated with an esophageal leiomyoma that completely resolved after resection (18). Even relatively small leiomyomas in a specific location along the course of the esophagus may cause debilitating dysphagia or pain.

The diagnostic evaluation should not only provide information about the esophageal leiomyoma, but also coexistent abnormalities, the physiology, possible confirmation of the diagnosis and a means to develop an operative plan. A barium swallow will demonstrate the smooth, crescent-shaped, concave defect into the lumen of the esophagus that moves with swallowing. It allows for the assessment of coexistent hiatal hernia, diverticula, and reflux (Figure 39.3). In most cases, endoscopy demonstrates a smooth, round, raised/protruding firm mass with movable mucosa. Ulceration is rare. Chest computed tomography provides the size of the lesion, location along the length of the esophagus, relationship to other mediastinal structures, right-sidedness or left-sidedness, additional associated defects, and operative planning information (Figure 39.4). Endoscopic

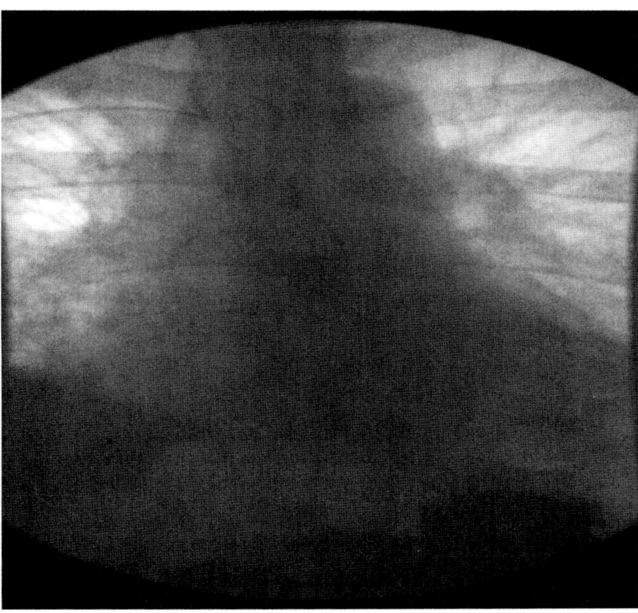

FIGURE 39.3

Air-Contrast Barium Contrast Swallowing Study demonstrates the location of the esophageal mass and assesses motility and anatomy. Up to 25% of leiomyoma patients will have a coexistent hiatal hernia.

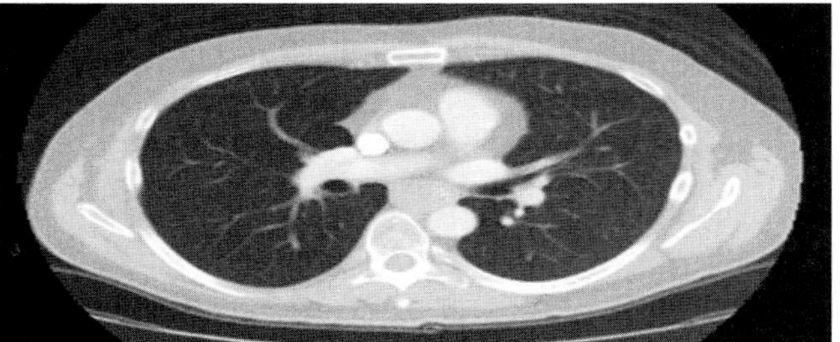

FIGURE 39.4

A contrast-enhanced computed tomogram provides further information necessary for mass evaluation and operative planning.

ultrasound (EUS) classically demonstrates that the mass arises from the fourth wall layer or the muscularis propria and is homogeneous, hypoechoic with sharp margins (19). Rarely, it can arise from the second wall layer or the muscularis mucosa. Although it is not specific for the diagnosis of malignancy rather than leiomyoma, the EUS findings in malignant esophageal wall mass include nodular shape, heterogeneity, ulceration depth greater than 0.5 mm, lesion size larger than 3 cm and associated suspicious lymphadenopathy (20). Fine-needle aspiration (FNA) and EUS-FNA does not provide sufficient accuracy to confirm the absence of malignancy (21). The differential diagnosis of esophageal wall masses includes: esophageal cancer, GIST, leiomyosarcoma, leiomyoblastoma, angioma, fibroma, angiokeratoma, lipoma, hamartoma, neurofibroma, schwannoma, granular cell tumor lymphangioma, intramural cysts such as duplication cysts, polypoid lesions that include squamous papilloma or fibrovascular polyps, and extrinsic compression or displacement from mediastinal abnormalities such as mediastinal tumors, lymphadenopathy, cysts, or aneurysms. For lesions larger than 3 to 5 cm or when the suspicion for malignancy warrants further investigation, a fluorodeoxyglucose-positron emission tomogram may offer some advantages in determining the potential for malignancy and the presence of a coexisting malignancy or metastatic disease. In patients with a significant history or findings consistent with reflux or esophageal dysfunction, a pH study and/or esophageal manometry may be indicated. A small asymptomatic leiomyoma with a low probability for malignancy may be observed, and EUS may regularly be performed at a 1- to 2-year interval.

In 1932, Sauerbruch reported performing an esophagogastrectomy to resect a benign esophageal tumor (22). Later that year, Ohsawa reported the first enucleation for an esophageal leiomyoma (23). Today, fewer than 10% of leiomyomas require surgical resection, the indications being symptomatic, lesions larger than 3 to 5 cm, increasing size on surveillance, and high suspicion for malignancy. Historically, the mortality has been reported to be as high as nearly 2%, but today most reports claim 0% mortality and almost no morbidity. Techniques have evolved to minimize encumbrance and risk. For patients with a leiomyoma smaller than 2 cm that is intraluminally polypoid, usually arising for the muscularis mucosa, excision can be performed by endoscopic removal using a snare and suction cylinder technique (24). For high-risk surgical patients, ethanol injection and debridement can be performed with low risk to reduce the likelihood for recurrence (25).

The standard surgical technique is performed by thoracotomy for lesions that are more than 4 to 5 cm above the gastroesophageal junction and by laparotomy for those within the area of the gastroesophageal junction. Upper and middle third tumors are approached by right thoracotomy. Middle third tumors associated with a hiatal hernia or lower third tumors are approached via a left thoracotomy. Today, placing an esophageal endoscope may assist in localizing the tumor and providing a means of assessing the integrity of the remaining surgically treated esophageal mucosa after resection. Once the esophageal mass is identified, the pleura and the adjacent mediastinal tissue are incised and dissected away from the longitudinal muscle. The azygous vein may need to be divided to gain exposure and/or allow for the esophagus to be rotated to achieve direct access to the tumor. Then, the longitudinal muscle is incised over the mass. A traction suture may be placed into the tumor to allow for retraction away from the mucosa. Both sharp and blunt dissection is used to separate the tumor from the adjacent muscle fibers. Electrocautery should be avoided to reduce the likelihood for mucosal injury. If a small perforation occurs, it may be primarily repaired, reapproximating the muscular layer over it. For larger defects, a pedicled intercostal muscle, thymic or omental flap may be used in the esophageal repair. For extensive tumors such as the "horseshoe" leiomyomas, the leiomyoma may need to be divided to facilitate removal. Once the mass is removed, the mucosa is examined for any defects by insufflating esophageal lumen with air after the defect is submerged beneath surgical irrigant. Closure of the muscular defect is controversial. Some feel that it may prevent mucosal herniation and improve the post-resection esophageal muscular propulsive function. For lesions resected at the gastroesophageal junction, dysfunction of the lower esophageal sphincter should be anticipated, and it is recommended that an anti-reflux procedure be performed. For large lesions, a segment of the esophagus may need to be resected and replaced with a segment of isoperistaltic colon or small bowel. In the rare cases in which lesions are larger than 8 cm, have an annular growth pattern, have significant adherence to the adjacent muscular wall, or in cases in which there is a large mucosal defect/tear after leiomyoma excision, an esophagectomy may be necessary. A vagal-sparing esophagectomy may offer fewer postoperative symptoms (26). Large lesions up to 8 to 10 centimeters have been resected without any esophageal dysfunction (27). In routine cases, a drain is left adjacent to the resection site until a swallowing study is performed on the first or second postoperative day. Many do not routinely use nasogastric tube decompression. Most surgeons advance the diet slowly, leaving patients on a soft or liquid diet for the first several postoperative days. Mucosal tear is reported to occur in 8%, but the rate increases to 40% to 50% if prior endoscopic biopsy has been performed. Other potential complications include: diverticula, fistulas, reflux, esophagitis, ulceration, and stenosis. Recurrence is rare (4). Approximately 90% of patients are symptom-free at 5 years (28). If a GIST is found on final pathology, a chest and liver computed tomogram with a liver ultrasound should be performed. Esophageal GISTs have been resected with long-term follow-up without evidence of recurrence (29). Unless there is other disease or residual margin, the use of adjuvant chemotherapy or targeted therapy, such as imatinib, is controversial.

In the last 15 years, minimally invasive surgery has evolved as it produces less discomfort and allows for earlier return to preoperative function (17, 30–35). Operating time for thoracotomy and the minimally invasive approach appears to be similar, approximately 95 minutes to 150 minutes (34,38). However, the minimally invasive approach has less pain, less analgesic requirement and a shorter hospital stay, 7 days versus 10 days for the open thoracotomy. Most have preoperative symptom resolution in the first few days to weeks (although it may take up to 2 years to resolve) and no mortality and minimal morbidity (34). For lesions within 4 to 5 cm of the lower esophageal sphincter, the laparoscopic approach appears preferable to the thoracoscopic approach for visibility, simplicity, and recovery. There may be more discomfort with the transthoracic approach due to the torque on the instrumentation (37). Iatrogenic perforations that occur intraoperatively can be safely treated by intracorporeal suture placement. Esophagectomy may be necessary for severe perforations with minimal risk of mortality (34). Pedicled-vascular flaps of intercostal muscle-parietal pleura, thymus-pericardial fat, or omentum may be used to reinforce the repair and provide supplemental blood supply. Techniques to reduce the likelihood or mucosal damage include the placement of an illuminating endoscope or an endoscopic balloon to assist in pushing the lesion out and away from the lumen (32). The hand-assisted laparoscopic technique is thought to reduce the operative time for laparoscopic resection, but there is no prospective trial to confirm this supposition (38). The largest series of minimally invasive resected benign esophageal lesions to date describes the placement of ports and the approach used (39). No nasogastric tube was placed routinely. Five patients required subsequent reoperation for reflux. Two patients had mucosal injuries, both of them having had prior needle biopsy of the total of 5 patients that had prior biopsies. There have been 4 reported cases of leiomyoma excision from the esophagus using computer-assisted technology or robotics (40,41). The 3-dimensional view and multiple arcs of rotation may reduce the likelihood for mucosal perforation. As technologies advance, resection of esophageal leiomyomas will become simpler and safer.

In summary, the leiomyoma of the esophagus is relatively rare. It is a distinct pathologic entity, which is unlikely to degenerate into malignancy. Resection should be reserved for thoroughly evaluated patients with symptoms or those in whom malignancy cannot be ruled out—usually lesions larger than 3 cm. Typically, surgical resection can be performed by a minimally invasive approach with minimal morbidity and mortality. The long-term outlook for enucleation of esophageal leiomyoma is good to excellent.

References

1. Takubo K, Nakagawa H, Tsuchiya S, et al. Seedling leiomyoma of the esophagus and esophagogastric junction zone. *Hum Pathol.* 1981:12(11):1006–1010.
2. Seremetis MG, et al. leiomyomata of the esophagus. An analysis of 838 cases. *Cancer.* 1976;38:2166–2177.
3. Postelthwait R, Musser H. Changes in the esophagus in 1000 autopsy specimens. *J Thorac Cardiovasc Surg.* 1974;68:953.
4. Hatch GF III, Wertheimer-Hatch L, Hatch KF, et al. Tumors of the esophagus. *World J Surg.* 2000;24:401–411.
5. Guarner V, Torres R. Diffuse leiomyomatosis of the esophagus; tracheobronchial, genital and renal insufficiency. In: DeMeester TR, Skinner DB, eds. *Esophageal Disorders: Pathophysiology and Therapy.* New York: Raven Press; 1985:447.
6. Miettinen M, Sarlomo-Rikala M, Sobin LH, et al. Gastrointestinal stromal tumors: a clinicopathologic, immunohistochemical, and molecular genetic study of 17 cases and comparison with esophageal leiomyomas and leiomyosarcomas. *Am J Surg Pathol.* 2000;24:211–222.
7. Kramer MD, Gibb P., Ellis FH. Giant leiomyoma of the esophagus. *J Surg Oncol.* 1986;33:166–169.
8. Tsuzuki T., Kakegawa T, Arimori M, et al. Giant leiomyoma of the esophagus and cardia weighing more than 1,000 gms. *Chest.* 1971;60:396–399.
9. Gutman E.. Posterior mediastinal calcification to esophageal leiomyoma. *Gastroenterology.* 1972;63(4):665-666.
10. Mutrie CJ, Donahue DM, Wain JC, et al. Esophageal leiomyoma: a 40-year experience. *Ann Thorac Surg.* 2005;79:1122–1125.
11. Gray S, Skondalakis J, Shepard D. Smooth muscle tumors of the esophagus. *Int Abstr Surg.* 1961;113:205.
12. Arnorsson T, Aberg C, Aberg T. Benign tumours of the oesophagus and oesophageal cysts. *Scand J Thorac Surg.* 1984;18:145–150.
13. Sugar I, Forgacs B, Istvan G, et al. Gastrointestinal stromal tumors (GIST). *Hepatogastroenterology.* 2005;52:409–413.
14. Solomon MP, Rosenblum H., Rosato FE. Leiomyoma of the esophagus. *Ann Surg.* 1984;80:246–248.
15. Skinner DB, Belsey RHR. Benign tumors of the esophagus. In: [Skinner DB, Belsey RHR] *Management of Esophageal Disease.* Philadelphia: W.B. Saunders Co.; 1988:717–727.
16. Shaffer HA Jr. Multiple leiomyomas of the esophagus. *Radiology.* 1976;118:29–34.
17. Bonavina L, Segalin A, Rosati R, et al. Surgical therapy of esophageal leiomyoma. *J Am Coll Surg.* 1995;181:257–262.
18. Ullal S. Hypertrophic osteoarthropathy and leiomyoma of the esophagus. *Am J Surg.* 1972;123:356.
19. Massari M, De Simone M, Cioffi U, et al. Endoscopic ultrasonography in the evaluation of leiomyoma and extramucosal cysts of the esophagus. *Hepatogastroenterology.* 1998;45:938–943.
20. Yasuda K, Nakajima M, Kawai K. Endoscopic ultrasonographic imaging of submucosal lesions of the upper gastrointestinal tract. *Gastrointest Endosc Clin North Am.* 1992;2:318.
21. Rice TW. Benign esophageal tumors: esophagoscopy and endoscopic esophageal ultrasound. *Semin Thorac Cardiovasc Surg.* 2003;15:20–26.
22. Sauerbruch F. Presentations in the field of thoracic surgery. *Arch Klin Chir.* 1932;173:457.
23. Ohsawa T. Surgery of the esophagus. *Arch Jpn Chir.* 1933;10:605.
24. Kajiyama T, Sakai M, Torii A, et al. Endoscopic aspiration lumpectomy of esophageal leiomyomas derived from the muscularis mucosae. *Am J Gastroenterol.* 1995;90:417–422.
25. Eda Y, Asaki S, Yamagata L, et al. Endoscopic treatment for submucosal tumors of the esophagus: studies in 25 patients. *Gastroenterol Jpn.* 1990;25:411–416.
26. Banki F, Mason RJ, DeMeester SR, et al. Vagal-sparing esophagectomy: a more physiologic alternative. *Ann Surg.* 2002;236:324–335.
27. Aures P, Grazia M, Petrella F, et al. Giant leiomyoma of the esophagus. *Eur J Cardiothorac Surg.* 2002;22:1008–1010.
28. Preda F, Alloisio M, Lequaglie C, et al. Leiomyoma of the esophagus. *Tumori.* 1986;72:503–506.
29. Palanivelu C, Rangarajan M, Senthilkumar R, et al. Thoracoscopic management of benign tumors of the mid-esophagus: a retrospective study. *Int J Surg.* 2007;5:328–333.
30. Bardini R, Segalin A, Ruol A, et al. Videothoracoscopic enucleation of esophageal leiomyoma. *Ann Thorac Surg.* 1992;54:576–577.
31. Everitt NJ, Glinatsis M, McMahon MJ. Thoracoscopic enucleation of leiomyoma of the oesophagus. *Br J Surg.* 1992;79(7):643.
32. Izumi Y, Inoue H, Endo M. Combined endoluminal-intracavitary thoracoscopic enucleation of leiomyoma of the esophagus: a new method. *Surg Endosc.* 1996;10:457–458.
33. Roviaro GC, Maciocco M, Varoli F, et al. Videothoracoscopic treatment of oesophageal leiomyoma. *Thorax.* 1998;53:190–192.
34. Zaninotto G, Portale G, Costantini M, et al. Minimally invasive enucleation of esophageal leiomyoma. *Surg Endosc.* 2006;20:1904–1908.
35. Coral RP, Madke G, Westphalen A, et al. Thoracoscopic enucleation of a leiomyoma of the upper thoracic esophagus. *Dis Esophagus.* 2003;16:339–341.
36. Von Rahden BH, Stein HJ, Feussner H, et al. Enucleation of submucosal tumors of the esophagus: minimally invasive versus open approach. *Surg Endosc.* 2004;18:924–930.
37. Hutter J, Miller K, Moritz E. Chronic sequels after thoracoscopic procedures for benign diseases. *Eur J Cardiothorac Surg.* 2000;17:687–690.
38. Redan JA, Gardner JC, Tylutki FJ. Hand-assisted laparoscopy for the removal of esophageal leiomyoma. *JSLS.* 2001;5:167–169.
39. Kent M, d'Amato T, Nordman C, et al. Minimally invasive resection of benign esophageal tumors. *J Thorac Cardiovasc Surg.* 2007;134:176–181.
40. Galvani C, Horgan S. Robots in general surgery: present and future. *Cir Esp.* 2005;78:138–147.
41. Augustin F, Schmid T, Bodner J. The robotic approach for mediastinal lesions. *Int J Med Robot.* 2006;2:262–270.

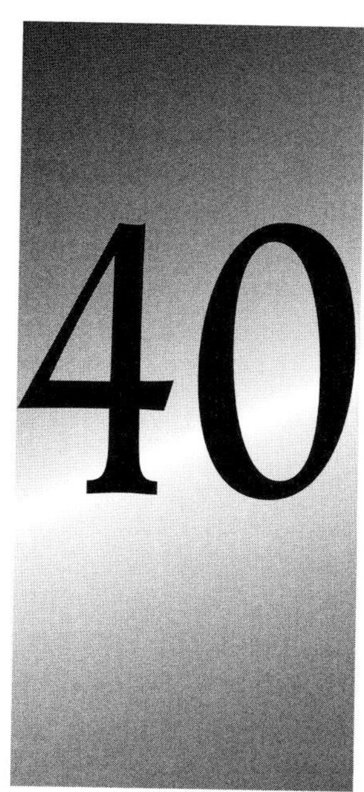

Benign: Hamartoma

Kemp H. Kernstine
Lawrence M. Weiss

Hamartoma of the esophagus accounts for 6% of all polyps, a rare entity (1,2). Most polyps occur in the upper esophagus and hypopharynx. In a Mayo Clinic series, there are 2 esophageal polyps found in 7,459 autopsies (3). Patients with polyps present with dysphagia and mass regurgitation. The masses may obtain gigantic size and can become exceedingly elongated. The male to female ratio is 2.2:1. The average age of diagnosis is 54 years, but ranges from 19 months to 88 years.

These polyps are the result of hamartomatous growth of mature normal cells and may contain elements of cartilage, bone marrow, bone, adipose tissue, fibrous tissue, skeletal muscle, or smooth muscle (4) (Figure 40.1). The mucosa over the polyp is usually intact, rarely being ulcerated. They are usually larger than 1 cm in diameter, but can be as largest 20 cm. Seventy-six percent are attached at the upper esophageal sphincter, with 3% in the middle esophagus and 6% in the distal esophagus (5). Sixteen percent originate in the hypopharynx and are more commonly found on the left lateral wall. The length of the average polyp is 13.3 cm and ranges in size from 5 cm to 28 cm and in width from 2.6 cm to 4.8 cm. Vascular compromise and resultant congestion, edema, necrosis, and ulceration may occur in 16%.

Patients may present with obstructive symptoms, rarely hematemesis. They can regurgitate the polyp into the mouth and out of the mouth in some cases, 38% of the time in subjects (Figure 40.2). Dysphagia is the most common symptom, occurring in approximately 62%. The average duration of symptoms prior to seeking medical attention is 3.7 years. Other symptoms include "lump in the throat," weight loss averaging 18 pounds, food regurgitation, non-exertional chest pain, odynophagia, vomiting, abdominal pain, melena, sore throat, and persistent cough. Aspiration into the larynx and resultant asphyxiation has also been reported.

Polyp regurgitation is pathognomonic of a polyp. Most clinicians attempt clinical confirmation and assess the polyp anatomically for treatment planning. Barium swallow and upper gastrointestinal endoscopy have a sensitivity of 78% to 67%, respectively. The sensitivity is improved by repeat contrast swallow and/or endoscopic examination. Computed tomography, endoscopic ultrasound, and magnetic resonance imaging of may provide supplemental information. In particular, the endoscopic ultrasound may be useful in identifying large feeding vessels.

Given the potential of asphyxiation, surgical resection is advised in all cases. Endoscopic excision may be performed in small lesions. Ligation and laser resection

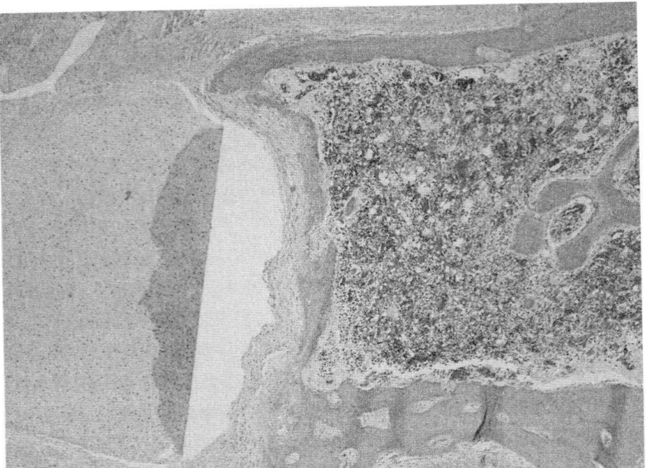

FIGURE 40.1

Hematoxylin and eosin stain of a hamartoma demonstrating elements of cartilage, bone, and bone marrow.

has been used both laryngoscopically and endoscopically. For large lesions, surgical resection is advised. For particularly large polyps, open esophagotomy by either cervical or transthoracic route with a combined laparoscopic/laparotomy to perform the transgastric resection of the bulk of the mass is advised (6).

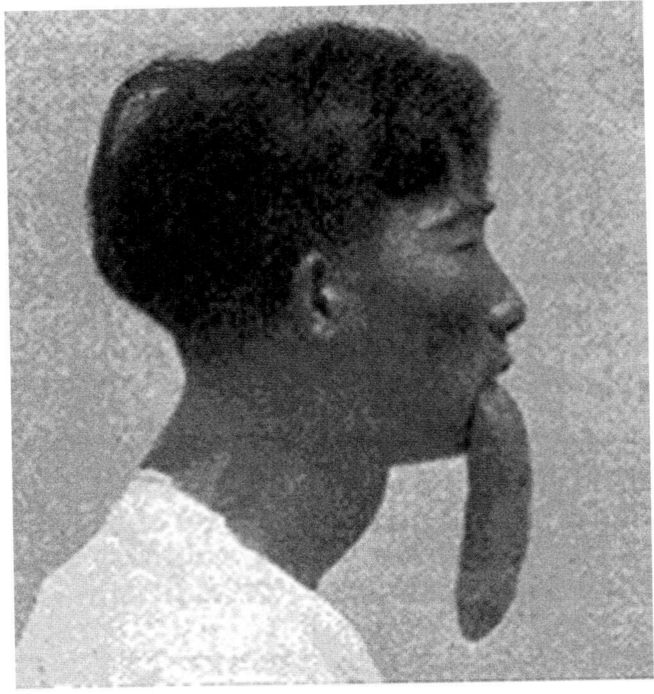

FIGURE 40.2

Fibrovascular polyp regurgitated from the mouth (7).

References

1. Beckerman RC, Taussig LM, Froede RC, at al. Fibromuscular hamartoma of the esophagus in an infant. *Am J. Dis Child.* 1980;134:153–155.
2. Caceres M, Steeb G, Wilks SM, et al. Large pedunculated polyps originating in the esophagus and hypopharynx. *Ann Thorac Surg.* 2006;81:393–396.
3. Moersch JH, Harrington SW. Benign tumor of the esophagus. *Ann Otol Rhinol Laryngol.* 1944;53:800–817.
4. Saitch U, Inomata Y, Tadaki N, et al. Pedunculated intraluminal osteochondromatous hamartoma of the esophagus. *J Otolaryngol.* 1990;19:339–342.
5. Halfhide BC, Ginai AZ, Spoejstra HAA, et al. Case report: a hamartoma presenting as a giant oesophageal polyp. *Br J Radiol.* 1995;68:85–88.
6. Hitty EC. A case of esophageal polypus accompanied by a tumor of an accessory thyroid gland. *Br J Surg.* 1938;26:195–197.

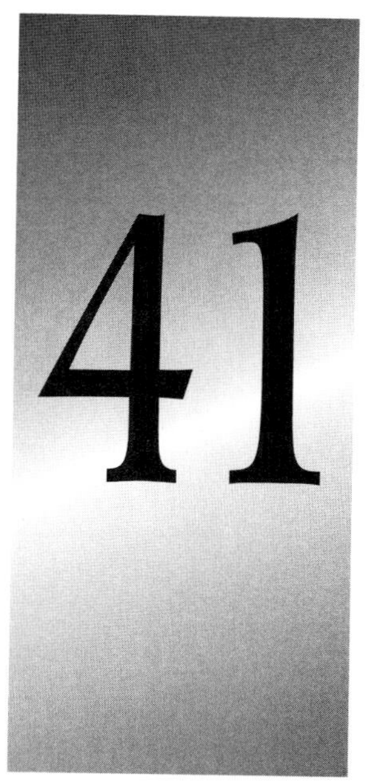

41 Benign: Congenital—Duplication Cysts

Piero Marco Fisichella
Marco G. Patti

Esophageal duplications are developmental malformations that arise from disturbances in the normal embryonic development of the alimentary tract (1). In the normal individual, the upper gastrointestinal tract embryologically develops from the posterior division of the primitive foregut. During the fourth week of gestation, the primitive foregut develops an anterior diverticulum, which becomes the respiratory bud. Meanwhile, the posterior division develops into the esophagus and upper gastrointestinal tract (1). In patients with esophageal duplications, a disturbance from this normal embryonic development of the alimentary tract occurs during organogenesis. However, the causative factor has not been identified and many theories have been proposed to clarify the etiology of these malformations. Lewis and Thyng hypothesized the persistence of embryonic diverticula during the development of the alimentary tract (2); Bremer suggested a possible abnormal luminal recanalization at 5–8 weeks' gestation (1); Mellish and Koop hypothesized the occurrence of hypoxia and trauma during the early fetal development (3); Bentley suggested that excessive traction to the endoderm from the developing notochord would result in abnormal vacuolization of the alimentary tract (4). This theory is the only one that would explain the association of the esophageal duplication with vertebral defects.

Esophageal duplications may occur as a separate tubular structure alongside the esophagus or present as a cyst in continuity to the esophagus. In rare instances, duplication cysts have been found within the wall of the esophagus. Most esophageal duplications do not communicate with the esophageal lumen (5).

The architecture of the esophageal duplications is typical as it replicates somewhat the double smooth muscle layer structure of the esophageal wall. The diagnostic features of these malformations are well recognized by the pathologist. The pathologic diagnosis requires the presence of the cyst adjacent to the esophagus, covered by 2 layers of muscularis propria, and lined by squamous columnar, cuboidal, pseudostratified, ciliated epithelium, and gastric mucosa, similar to that present in the alimentary tract (6).

Esophageal duplications are rare and the true incidence is unknown, as fewer than 100 cases of esophageal duplication cysts have been reported. They account only for 3% of the mediastinal masses (7) and are the second most common duplication of the alimentary tract, after jejuno-ileal duplications (8).

Up to 80% of esophageal duplications are diagnosed during childhood and most adults with esophageal cysts are asymptomatic (6). Symptoms are caused by compression of surrounding structures and by the size and location of the duplication. Two-thirds of the esophageal duplications are located in the distal esophagus, and dysphagia from esophageal compression by the cyst is the most common symptom (9,10). When the duplication is located higher in the esophagus, dyspnea, shortness of breath, or stridor from compression of the tracheobronchial tree can also be present (11). Cardiac arrhythmias from retrocardiac esophageal duplication cysts have been reported (5). Hematemesis can occur if heterotopic gastric mucosa is present inside the cyst. Although rare, malignant degeneration of both esophageal and gastric duplications can occur, and few cases of carcinoids, neuroendocrine tumors, and adenocarcinomas arising from the duplication or invading the stomach have been reported (12,13).

The diagnosis of esophageal duplications can be difficult. An esophagogram, CT scan, MRI, and endoscopic ultrasound usually confirm the diagnosis (14). A chest radiograph may reveal a mediastinal mass; an esophagogram will show a narrowing of the esophageal lumen; an upper endoscopy will show extrinsic compression of an intact mucosa (Figures 41.1 and 41.2). A biopsy of the lesion should not be performed, because the adhesion of the cyst wall to the esophagus caused by the biopsy can complicate the subsequent resection of the cyst (15). The CT scan identifies and localizes the cyst in contiguity to the esophagus or the stomach. The radiologic characteristics of esophageal and gastric duplications cysts found on CT scan are well documented (16). The CT density can vary from typical water density to densities characteristic of soft tissue or muscle, thus making it sometimes difficult to distinguish these lesions from solid tumors (Figures 41.1 and 41.2); MRI has been used as a more sensitive imaging tool to delineate the anatomy of the cyst in relation to surrounding structures and distinguish between a cystic lesion and a solid tumor based on its different appearance on T1- and T2-weighted images (17). Trans-esophageal endoscopic ultrasonography can clearly distinguish a cyst from a submucosal tumor such as a leiomyoma. The diagnosis of esophageal duplication cysts with endoscopic ultrasonography is based on the following features: presence of an air–fluid interface and the demonstration of echo density of fluid within the lesion (Figures 41.1 and 41.2) (18).

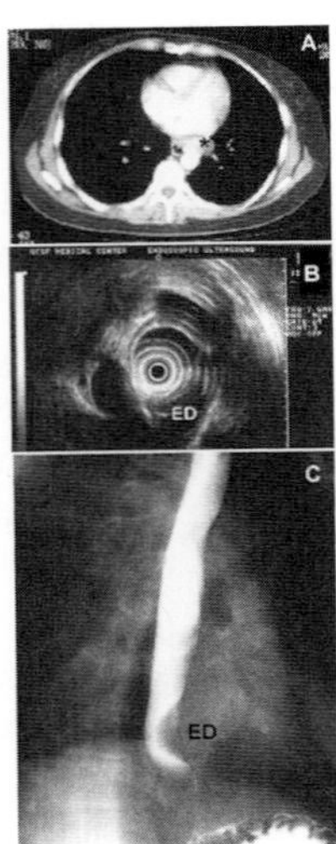

FIGURE 41.1

Abdominal computerized tomography (A), endoscopic ultrasound (B), and esophagogram (C). ED: esophageal duplication. From Herbella FA, Tedesco P, Muthusamy R, et al. Thoracoscopic resection of esophageal duplication cysts. *Dis Esophagus*. 2006;19:132–134. Reprinted with permission from Blackwell Publishing.

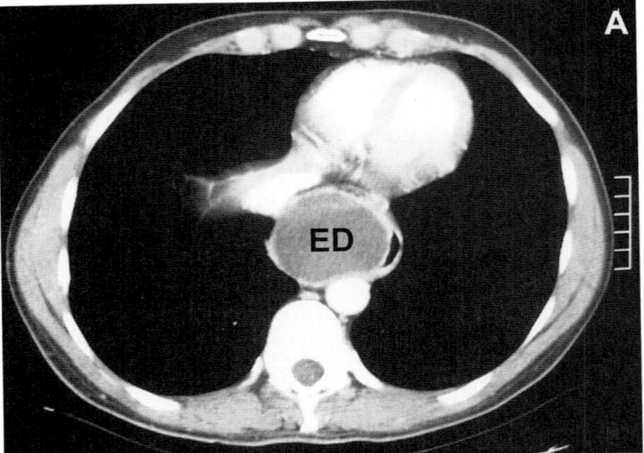

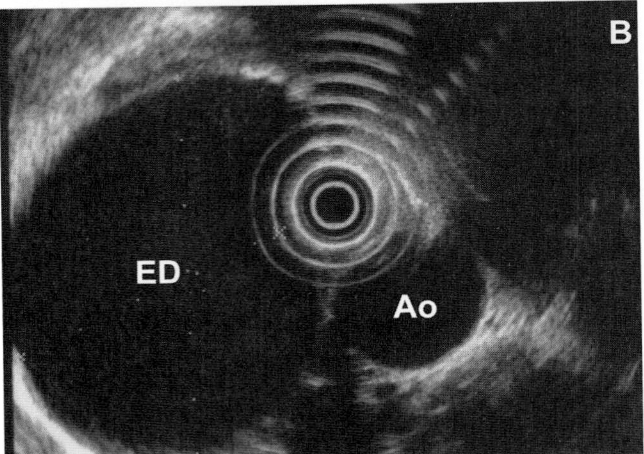

FIGURE 41.2

Abdominal computerized tomography (A) and endoscopic ultrasound (B). ED: esophageal duplication. Ao: Aorta. From Herbella FA, Tedesco P, Muthusamy R, et al. Thoracoscopic resection of esophageal duplication cysts. *Dis Esophagus*. 2006;19:132–134. Reprinted with permission from Blackwell Publishing.

The demonstration of continuity between the muscularis propria of the cyst and the muscularis propria of the esophagus is a specific sign that can lead to accurate diagnosis. This procedure is able to delineate the extent of the cyst, the layer composition of the cyst, and its relationships with the intrathoracic structures (19).

All duplications should be surgically resected. Even though duplication cysts are often asymptomatic at the time of diagnosis, surgical excision is advised because definitive diagnosis is better done on the surgical specimen and because most patients with esophageal duplication will eventually become symptomatic or develop complications such as infection and rupture and hemorrhage or perforation secondary to the presence of heterotopic gastric mucosa (15).

Traditionally, the resection of the esophageal duplications is accomplished via a posterolateral thoracotomy. Today, however, a left thoracoscopic approach is the preferred modality of treatment. It allows great visualization for resection, and it is associated with a shorter hospital stay, minimal postoperative discomfort, and fast recovery. Laparoscopic and thoracoscopic resection of esophageal duplications have been reported with excellent results and represent today the surgical approach of choice (14,15,20–23).

The surgical technique must emphasize evaluation of the integrity of the esophageal mucosa after resection of the cyst, approximation of the muscle edges over the area where the cyst was present in order to avoid a pseudodiverticulum, and identification of the vagi (15). Transillumination through an esophagoscope and decompression of the cyst are useful adjuncts that can be used during surgery to verify the integrity of the mucosa after the resection and facilitate the removal of the specimen. Partial resection can be performed in difficult cases in which the duplication firmly adheres to vital structures. Nevertheless, recurrence of foregut duplications has been reported after incomplete surgical removal (24).

References

1. Bremer JL. Diverticula and duplications of the intestinal tract. *Arch Pathol.* 1944;38:132–140.
2. Lewis FT, Thyng FW. Regular occurrence of intestinal diverticula in embryo of pig, rabbit, and man. *Am J Anat.* 1908;7:505–519.
3. Mellish RWP, Koop CE. Clinical manifestations of duplication in the bowel. *Pediatrics.* 1961;27:397–407.
4. Bentley JRR, Smith JR. Developmental posterior enteric remnants and spinal malformations: the split notochord syndrome. *Arch Dis Child.* 1960;35:76–86.
5. Holcomb GW III, Gheissari A, O'Neill JA Jr, et al. Surgical management of alimentary tract duplications. *Ann Surg.* 1989;209:167–174.
6. Cioffi U, Bonavina L, De Simone M: Presentation and surgical management of bronchogenic and esophageal duplication cysts in adults. *Chest.* 1998;113:1492–1496.
7. Lee MY, Jensen E, Kwak S, et al. Metastatic adenocarcinoma arising in a congenital foregut cyst of the esophagus: a case report with review of the literature. *Am J Clin Oncol.* 1998 Feb;21:64–6.
8. Arbona JL, Fazzi JG, Mayoral J. Congenital esophageal cysts: case report and review of literature. *Am J Gastroenterol.* 1984;79:177–182.
9. Ildstad ST, Tollerud DJ, Weiss RG, et al. Duplications of the alimentary tract. Clinical characteristics, preferred treatment, and associated malformations. *Ann Surg.* 1988;208:184–189.
10. Kim DH, Kim JS, Nam ES, et al. Foregut duplication cyst of the stomach. *Pathol Int.* 2000;50:142–145.
11. Espeso A, Verma S, Jani P, et al. Mediastinal foregut duplication cyst presenting as a rare cause of breathing difficulties in an adult. *Eur Arch Otorhinolaryngol.* 2007; 264(11)1357–1360.
12. Horne G, Ming-Lum C, Kirkpatrick AW, et al. High-grade neuroendocrine carcinoma arising in a gastric duplication cyst: a case report with literature review. *Int J Surg Pathol.* 2007;15:187–191.
13. Kuraoka K, Nakayama H, Kagawa T, et al. Adenocarcinoma arising from a gastric duplication cyst with invasion to the stomach: a case report with literature review. *J Clin Pathol.* 2004;57:428–431.
14. Hirose S, Clifton MS, Bratton B, et al. Thoracoscopic resection of foregut duplication cysts. *J Laparoendosc Adv Surg Tech A.* 2006;16:526–529.
15. Herbella FA, Tedesco P, Muthusamy R, et al. Thoracoscopic resection of esophageal duplication cysts. *Dis Esophagus.* 2006;19:132–134
16. Jeung MY, Gasser B, Gangi A, et al. Imaging of cystic masses of the mediastinum. *Radiographics.* 2002 Oct;22 Spec No:S79–S93.
17. Kanemitsu Y, Nakayama H, Asamura H, et al. Clinical features and management of bronchogenic cysts: report of 17 cases. *Surg Today.* 1999;29:1201–1205.
18. Geller A, Wang KK, DiMagno EP. Diagnosis of foregut duplication cysts by endoscopic ultrasonography. *Gastroenterology.* 1995;109:838–842.
19. Bhutani MS, Hoffman BJ, Reed C. Endosonographic diagnosis of an esophageal duplication cyst. *Endoscopy.* 1996 May;28:396–397.
20. Bratu I, Laberge JM, Flageole H, et al. Foregut duplications: is there an advantage to thoracoscopic resection? *J Pediatr Surg.* 2005;40:138–141.
21. Nelms CD, White R, Matthews BD, et al. Thoracoabdominal esophageal duplication cyst. *J Am Coll Surg.* 2002;194:674–675.
22. Kin K, Iwase K, Higaki J, et al. Laparoscopic resection of intra-abdominal esophageal duplication cyst. *Surg Laparosc Endosc Percutan Tech.* 2003;13:208–211.
23. Harvell JD, Macho JR, Klein HZ. Isolated intra-abdominal esophageal cyst. Case report and review of the literature. *Am J Surg Pathol.* 1996;20:476–479.
24. Gharagozloo F, Dausmann MJ, McReynolds SD, et al. Recurrent bronchogenic pseudocyst 24 years after incomplete excision. Report of a case. *Chest.* 1995;108: 880–883.

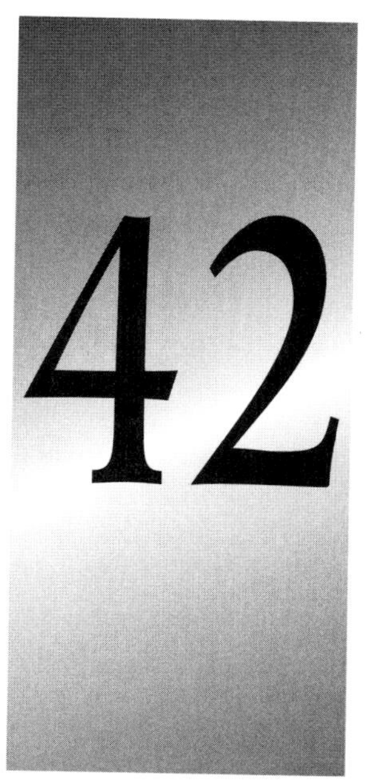

42 Benign: Congenital—Bronchogenic Cysts

Piero Marco Fisichella
Marco G. Patti

Bronchogenic cysts, like esophageal duplications, are congenital anomalies that arise from disturbances in the normal embryonic development of the foregut. Because of their common etiology, both bronchogenic cysts and esophageal duplications are often identified as foregut duplication (1).

In the normal individual, during the fourth week of gestation, the primitive foregut develops an anterior diverticulum, which becomes the respiratory bud and then the tracheobronchial tree, and a posterior or dorsal diverticulum, which grows to become the gastrointestinal tract. Bronchogenic cysts result from the abnormal budding or branching of the ventral primitive foregut while esophageal duplications arise from the dorsal primitive foregut. Therefore, esophageal duplications and bronchogenic cysts are part of the same spectrum of anomalies rather than separate entities, as they share common origin and histologic features (1). Histologically, a bronchogenic cyst is lined by ciliated mucus-secreting respiratory columnar epithelium and may contain cartilage, whereas esophageal duplications are covered by 2 layers of muscularis propria and are lined by squamous columnar, cuboidal, pseudostratified, and gastric mucosa.

Bronchogenic cysts are the most common cystic lesions of the mediastinum. They usually present as a single or, less commonly, as multiple lesions of varied size that may adhere to the bronchial wall and rarely communicate with it. Occasionally they may be located remarkably distant from the tracheobronchial tree: behind the pharynx (2), into the pericardium (3), inside the diaphragm. They can also be found outside the chest such as in the gastric fundus, or in the retroperitoneal space, where they may present as an adrenal mass (4) or a pancreatic cystic tumor (5). Because extrathoracic, subdiaphragmatic bronchogenic cysts originate from the embryonic foregut and migrate to the abdominal cavity before the fusion of the pleuroperitoneal membrane, they may be also confused with extralobar sequestrations (6). Extralobar sequestrations, however, are characterized by the presence of pulmonary parenchyma and pleural investment.

Bronchogenic cysts are rare and their true incidence is unknown. The natural history of bronchogenic cysts is also very variable. Many lesions decrease in size before birth, and some are no longer radiologically detectable after birth. In the newborn period, bronchogenic cysts can produce immediate respiratory distress or no symptom at all and may be found incidentally at any age (7).

Half of the patients are asymptomatic (8). When symptoms are present, they are mostly non-specific, as

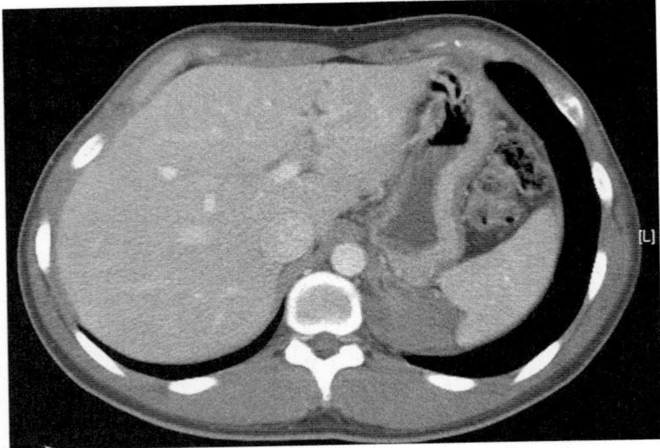

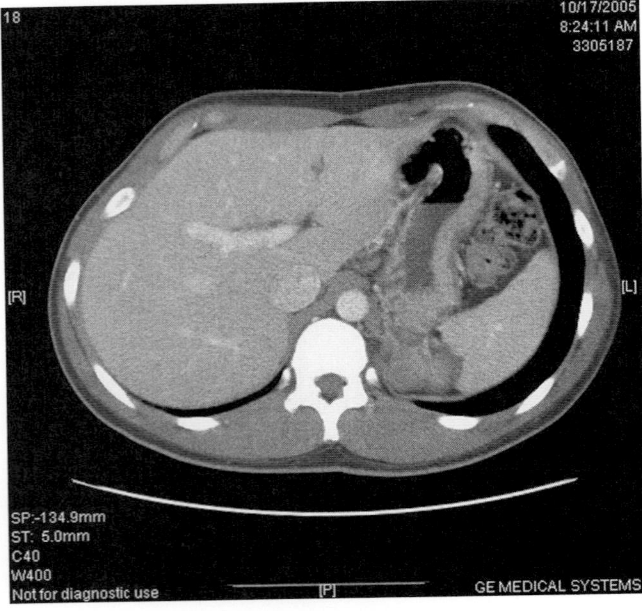

FIGURE 42.1

CT scans with and without contrast and delayed scans demonstrated a 3.5 x 2.1 cm non-enhancing lesion extending from the left adrenal gland into the left pleural space. Courtesy of Seema Pasha MD, University of Illinois at Chicago.

they are caused by compression of surrounding structures and by the size and location of the duplication along the tracheobronchial tree. The most common symptoms are dysphagia from esophageal compression, or cough, dyspnea, hemoptysis, infection, shortness of breath, and stridor from compression of the tracheobronchial tree (9).

Modern imaging techniques such as CT scan, endoscopic ultrasound, and magnetic resonance imaging (MRI) may help in providing the definitive diagnosis. In addition, they are useful for evaluating the topographic relationship of the mass and for planning the resection (10). CT scan is able to correctly diagnose bronchogenic cysts in 62% to 100% of patients (11) (Figure 42.1). MRI often improves the diagnostic accuracy as it can distinguish between a cystic lesion and a solid tumor based on the different appearance of the thick viscous content of some cysts on T1- and T2-weighted images (11).

Once diagnosed, surgical excision of symptomatic bronchogenic cysts is indicated to avoid long-term cyst related complications, such as infection, bleeding, compression, and rupture (12). Malignant degeneration is a rare event.

The management of asymptomatic cysts is controversial (13). Observation alone has been proposed for small and asymptomatic cysts. However, because preoperative differential diagnosis between congenital or acquired and benign or malignant is often difficult, the definitive diagnosis is best established on the pathologic examination of the surgical specimen. Nonetheless, surgical treatment is warranted because the majority may ultimately become symptomatic or complicated (13).

Transbronchial or percutaneous needle aspiration of bronchogenic cysts has been suggested as an alternative to surgery, especially in small asymptomatic cysts. However, needle aspiration can potentially infect the cyst, and even though cysts may regress after aspiration, they usually recur months to years later (13).

Today, thoracoscopic resection of bronchogenic cysts is the surgical approach of choice (13–16). When compared to thoracotomy, thoracoscopy reduces the length of hospitalization and it is associated to less postoperative pain and a faster recovery (13). The rate of conversion to thoracotomy ranges from to 8% to 35% and it is mainly related to the presence of dense adhesions to the adjacent organs, such as the trachea or the esophagus (14,16). In these cases, aspiration of the cyst and partial resection, leaving portions of the cyst wall behind, can be performed (17). However, recurrence of mediastinal duplications has been reported after incomplete surgical removal (18,19).

References

1. Cioffi U, Bonavina L, De Simone M. Presentation and surgical management of bronchogenic and esophageal duplication cysts in adults. *Chest*. 1998;113:1492–1496.
2. Jacob JK, George S, Roy BR, et al. Retropharyngeal bronchogenic cyst. *Otolaryngol Head Neck Surg*. 2007;136:1025–1026.
3. Kobza R, Oechslin E, Jenni R. An intrapericardial bronchogenic cyst. *Interact Cardiovasc Thorac Surg*. 2003;2(3):279–280.
4. Terry NE, Senkowski CK, Check W, et al. Retroperitoneal foregut duplication cyst presenting as an adrenal mass. *Am Surg*. 2007;73:89–92.

5. Kim EY, Lee WJ, Jang KT. Retroperitoneal bronchogenic cyst mimicking a pancreatic cystic tumour. *Clin Radiol.* 2007;62:491–494.
6. Melo N, Pitman MB, Rattner DW. Bronchogenic cyst of the gastric fundus presenting as a gastrointestinal stromal tumor. *J Laparoendosc Adv Surg Tech A.* 2005; 15:163–165.
7. Eber E. Antenatal diagnosis of congenital thoracic malformations: early surgery, late surgery, or no surgery? *Semin Respir Crit Care Med.* 2007;28:355–366.
8. Suen HC, Mathisen DJ, Grillo HC, et al. Surgical management and radiological characteristics of bronchogenic cysts. *Ann Thorac Surg.* 1993;55:476–481.
9. Espeso A, Verma S, Jani P, et al. Mediastinal foregut duplication cyst presenting as a rare cause of breathing difficulties in an adult. *Eur Arch Otorhinolaryngol.* 2007;264(11):1357–1360.
10. Jeung MY, Gasser B, Gangi A, et al. Imaging of cystic masses of the mediastinum. *Radiographics.* 2002 Oct;22 Spec No:S79–S93.
11. Kanemitsu Y, Nakayama H, Asamura H, et al. Clinical features and management of bronchogenic cysts: report of 17 cases. *Surg Today.* 1999;29:1201–1205.
12. Pages ON, Rubin S, Baehrel B. Intra-esophageal rupture of a bronchogenic cyst. *Interact Cardiovasc Thorac Surg.* 2005;4:287–288.
13. Tolg C, Abelin K, Laudenbach V, et al. Open vs. thorascopic surgical management of bronchogenic cysts. *Surg Endosc.* 2005;19:77–80.
14. Martinod E, Pons F, Azorin J, et al. Thoracoscopic excision of mediastinal bronchogenic cysts: results in 20 cases. *Ann Thorac Surg.* 2000;69:1525–1528.
15. Chang YC, Chen JS, Chang YL, et al. Video-assisted thoracoscopic excision of intradiaphragmatic bronchogenic cysts: two cases. *J Laparoendosc Adv Surg Tech A.* 2006;16:489–492.
16. Weber T, Roth TC, Beshay M, et al. Video-assisted thoracoscopic surgery of mediastinal bronchogenic cysts in adults: a single-center experience. *Ann Thorac Surg.* 2004;78:987–991.
17. Yoshida M, Kondo K, Toba H, et al. Two cases of bronchogenic cyst with severe adhesion to the trachea. *J Med Invest.* 2007;54:187–190.
18. Gharagozloo F, Dausmann MJ, McReynolds SD, et al. Recurrent bronchogenic pseudocyst 24 years after incomplete excision. Report of a case. *Chest.* 1995;108:880–883.
19. Hasegawa T, Murayama F, Endo S, et al. Recurrent bronchogenic cyst 15 years after incomplete excision. *Interact Cardiovasc Thorac Surg.* 2003;2:685–687.

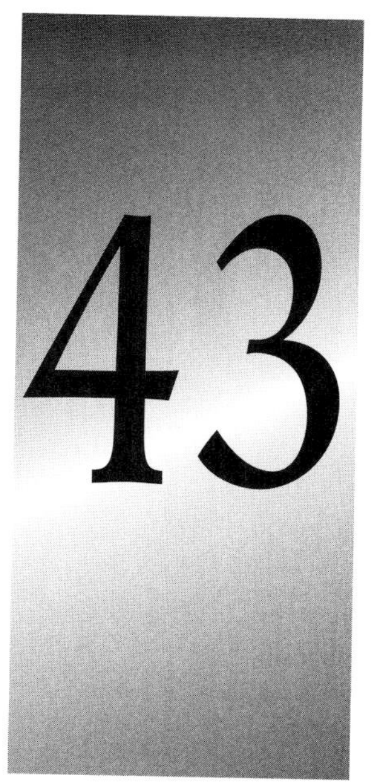

Malignant: Squamous Cell Carcinoma and Variants

Kenneth M. Gatter
Dustin V. Shackleton

Squamous cell carcinoma of the esophagus (SCC) was defined in 2000 by the World Health Organization as "a malignant epithelial tumor with squamous cell differentiation, microscopically characterized by keratinocyte-like cells with intercellular bridges and/or keratinization" (1). Its incidence shows significant geographic variability, 10 times higher in some regions compared with others. High-risk areas include portions of China, Japan, Iran, southern South America, South Africa, and northwestern France. Low-risk areas for SCC include North America, where the incidence is about 5.2 per 100,000, and where, unlike esophageal adenocarcinoma, the incidence of SCC does not appear to be increasing (1). Some Western countries have seen an increasing incidence of adenocarcinoma, and in some areas greater than 50% of primary esophageal malignancies are adenocarcinoma, not SCC. In contrast, high-risk regions for SCC see an overwhelming predominance of SCC and relatively little adenocarcinoma of the esophagus. For example, in Japan more than 90% of primary esophageal malignancies are SCC and there has been no increase in the incidence of adenocarcinoma (2).

This geographic variability, sometimes within a single country, suggests that there are several different etiologies for SCC. Risk factors include tobacco, alcohol, nutrition, and burning hot beverages, and these show a complex interaction with different etiologies more important in different regions. Human papilloma virus, or HPV, has been implicated in the pathogenesis of SCC and remains controversial (3–5).

Chapter 44 contains more detailed information about the etiology and distribution of esophageal malignancies.

INVASIVE SQUAMOUS CELL CARCINOMA

SCC arises predominantly in the middle and lower third of the esophagus. The gross appearance varies. Superficially invasive cancers often have a plaque-like appearance, but may show no significant gross mucosal abnormality. Verrucous carcinomas are typically cauliflower-like. Clearly invasive tumors may be ulcerated, fungating, or may show a relatively small mucosal defect but infiltrate deeply into the underlying tissue (6).

Invasion occurs when neoplastic squamous epithelium breaks through the basement membrane and invades into surrounding tissue (Figure 43.1). Typically, early lesions arise from carcinoma in situ (Figure 43.2) and show slender projections of atypical squamous cells extending into the lamina propria with foci of individual atypical cells or small clusters of atypical squamous cells within the lamina propria. As the tumor

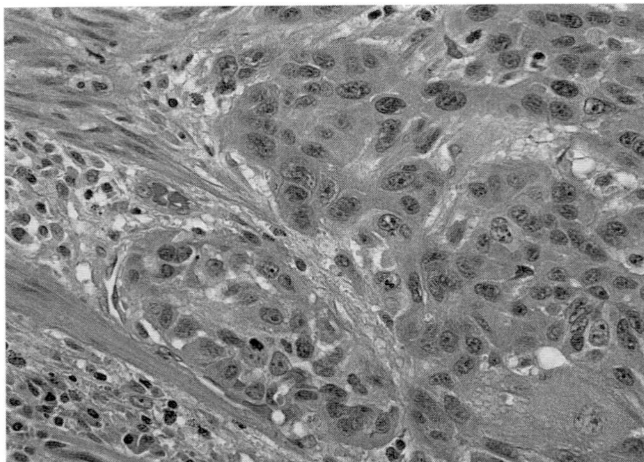

FIGURE 43.1

Invasive squamous cell carcinoma.

grows it typically extends vertically into deeper tissue and horizontally undermines the adjacent normal squamous mucosa at the tumor's periphery. Angiolymphatic invasion is more likely the deeper the tumor invades, and it may be identified some distance away from the tumor. This lymphatic spread may rarely result in intramural metastases (1). The amount of stromal reaction, defined as desmoplastic response, and the degree of inflammation vary.

Conventional SCCs are generally divided into 2 broad growth patterns: infiltrative and expansile. The infiltrative pattern is characterized by smaller tongues and nests of tumor cells infiltrating through connective tissue, often with a surrounding chronic inflammatory response. The expansile pattern consists of sheets of tumor cells advancing through the connective tissue on a broad front.

On occasion, an SCC will have small foci of glandular differentiation, forming glands or scattered mucin producing cells, which may be confirmed by special stains such as mucicarmine or Alcian blue PAS stains. Notwithstanding these foci of glandular differentiation, the diagnosis should remain SCC unless the adenomatous component represents a significant portion of the tumor (6).

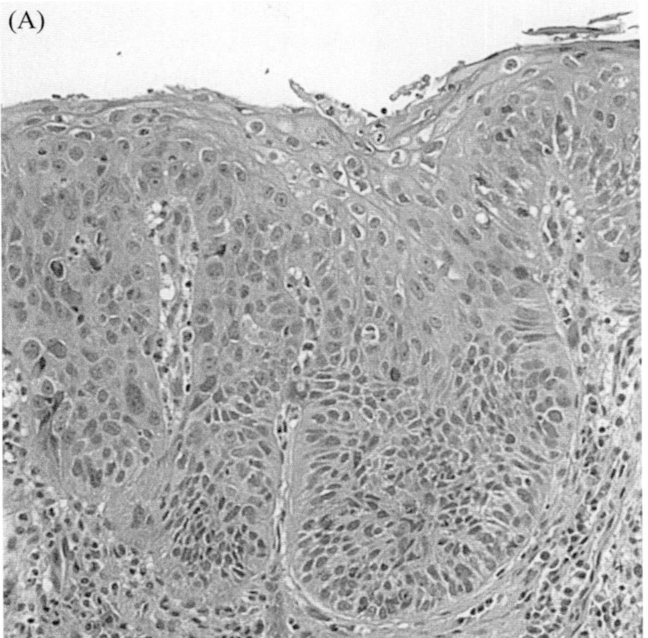

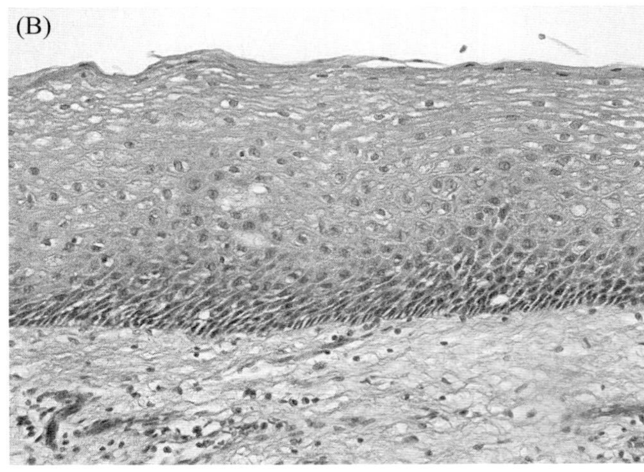

FIGURE 43.2

(A) Carcinoma in situ or high-grade dysplasia of esophageal squamous epithelium. Note that the squamous cell atypia extends from the basal layer to the surface. (B) Normal squamous epithelium and normal maturation of squamous cells.

Tumor Grade

The histologic grading of esophageal SCC is similar to the grading of SCC in other sites and is based on the degree of differentiation, mitotic activity, and nuclear pleomorphism (1). A well-differentiated tumor is easy to recognize as a SCC because the tumor resembles squamous epithelium. The cells have moderate to abundant pink cytoplasm and often show clear evidence of keratin production. Intracellular bridges are visible at high magnification. Basal cells are present, but located at the periphery of the epithelial tumor nests, and do not represent a dominant portion of the tumor.

In contrast, poorly differentiated SCCs do not resemble normal squamous epithelium. The cells typically have less cytoplasm and are predominantly basaloid. Poorly differentiated tumors have higher proliferative rates and mitotic figures are easily spotted. The most common grade of SCC is moderately differentiated (Figure 43.1), and these tumors show features between well-differentiated and poorly differentiated tumors. For example, a moderately differentiated tumor may have significant nuclear pleomorphism but clearly shows keratin production and has a moderate mitotic index.

Undifferentiated carcinomas lack definitive evidence of squamous differentiation by conventional microscopy, but some may show evidence of squamous differentiation by staining with keratins by immunohistochemistry, such as CK5, or AE1/AE3, or electron microscopy evidence of desmosomes and tonofilaments. The important differential in these cases is small cell carcinoma, which should stain with some neuroendocrine markers like neuron-specific enolase, chromogranin, or synaptophysin. Melanoma, too, is often in the differential and should stain with either S-100, HMB-45, or Melan-A, as well as lymphoma, which should be positive for CD45 or CD43 (7).

SUPERFICIAL SQUAMOUS CELL CARCINOMA OF THE ESOPHAGUS

The term *superficial squamous cell carcinoma of the esophagus* is defined by WHO as invasive SCC that has invaded into the mucosa or the submucosa, but no deeper, and the term is used regardless of lymph node metastasis. These are T1 lesions, according to the TNM classification. One team of investigators concluded after reviewing a number of articles that about 5% of superficial SCC that have invaded no deeper than the lamina propria show lymph node metastasis (6). Others have shown that the risk of modal involvement increases to 30% to 48% with invasion into the submucosa (8) and that patients with submucosal carcinoma have a disappointing 5-year survival rate of 69% (2).

The term superficial SCC differs from the term *early esophageal carcinoma*, which has been used in China and Japan and refers to SCCs that have invaded no deeper than the submucosa but have no lymph node metastasis (1). Recently, investigators in Japan demonstrated that superficial SCCs that invade the lamina propria, but do not extend into the muscularis mucosa, have no lymph node metastasis. Patients with tumors extending into the muscularis mucosa, but not the submucosa, showed a 5-year survival of greater than 95%. A recent Japanese schema proposes that early carcinoma of the esophagus is defined as mucosal carcinoma with or without lymph node metastasis, with the supporting rationale that a malignancy given the designation *early* should equate with a good prognosis (2).

SCCs that have invaded beyond the submucosa into the muscularis propria are advanced esophageal carcinomas and show a significantly higher rate of lymph node metastasis, about 35%. (9,10).

VARIANTS OF SQUAMOUS CELL CARCINOMA

Spindle cell carcinoma, also known as carcinosarcoma, pseudosarcomatous squamous cell carcinoma, and polypoid carcinoma, is a rare but diagnostically challenging variant of SCC. The typical gross characteristics reflect one of its names; it is a polypoid tumor with or without a stalk and the surrounding squamous mucosa is normal. Microscopically, it is biphasic with a spindle cell, or sarcomatous component, and a carcinomatous component. The amount of sarcomatoid spindle cells varies, and sometimes the sarcomatous cells form mature islands of bone, cartilage, or skeletal muscle. The spindle cells may show significant pleomorphism indistinguishable from a high-grade sarcoma. This is especially challenging for the pathologist when interpreting a biopsy, because one of the most important diagnostic features of a spindle cell carcinoma is that the properly sampled tumor will show some areas of squamous differentiation. Typically, the well-sampled tumor will show a gradual transition from sarcomatous histology to areas of more differentiated SCC. The biopsy, however, represents focal sampling and may only show sarcomatous histology, making a definite diagnosis difficult. Immunohistochemistry, however, may be useful in confirming the diagnosis of spindle cell SCC. For example, positive staining for p53 has good sensitivity for poorly differentiated SCCs (11).

Basaloid squamous cell carcinoma is a relatively rare variant of SCC, which in the esophagus appears indistinguishable from basaloid squamous cell carcinoma of the upper aerodigestive region. Often accompanied by intraepithelial dysplasia and areas of more common squamous cell carcinoma, these tumors are composed of basal-like cells with hyperchromatic nuclei and moderate to scant basophilic cytoplasm (Figure 43.3). The cells are typically in nests or trabeculae with a focal cribiform pattern, giving a gland-like appearance. The proliferative activity and degree of apoptosis is greater than the average squamous cell carcinoma. Originally thought to behave more aggressively than typical squamous cell carcinomas, recent opinion is that there is no significant difference in prognosis (12).

The immunohistochemical characteristics of basaloid SCC help distinguish this entity from adenoid cystic carcinoma of the esophagus, with which it may be confused. The basal cells of basaloid SCC stain with CK14 and CK19, whereas the basal cells of adenoid cystic carcinoma are positive for actin and S100 (13).

Another rare variant is verrucous carcinoma. Similar to verrucous carcinomas in other sites, the gross appearance is exophytic, often papillary and warty. These are slow-growing, low-grade, well-differentiated tumors. The microscopic features show well-differentiated keratinized squamous cells with mild atypia and a pushing margin.

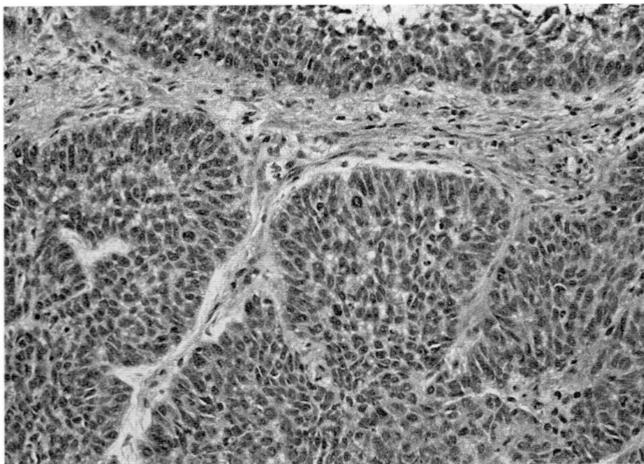

FIGURE 43.3

Basaloid squamous cell carcinoma.

This lack of a clearly invasive margin can be problematic on a biopsy because the pathologist may not see clear evidence of invasion and instead favor a squamous cell papilloma. The diagnosis of verrucous carcinoma may become clear with good communication between the clinician and pathologist.

INTRAEPITHELIAL NEOPLASIA OR SQUAMOUS CELL DYSPLASIA

Current evidence is that intraepithelial neoplasia or squamous dysplasia is a precursor lesion to invasive squamous cell carcinoma (1,15). It is often seen adjacent to invasive SCC and is more common in populations that are high risk for invasive SCC (14). Most pathologists divide these lesions into low- and high-grade lesions based on the degree and extent of cytologic atypia. Low-grade lesions or low-grade dysplasia is limited to the lower half, adjacent to the basal layer, and high-grade dysplasia shows a lack of apparent maturation and cytologic atypia extending to more than half of the epithelial thickness. Mitotic figures are often seen in the upper half of the epithelium in high-grade dysplasia. Carcinoma in situ is high-grade dysplasia in which the dysplastic cytology extends throughout the epithelium with virtually no maturation (Figure 43.2). There is epidemiologic evidence that they show increased risk for invasive cancer with increasing grade of dysplasia (15).

Although typically dysplasia leads to a thickened epithelium, atrophic or thinner epithelium may be dysplastic. Dysplasia may also involve submucosal ducts, which should not be interpreted as invasive cancer. In all cases of dysplasia, including carcinoma in situ, the basement membrane is intact.

BIOPSY

The diagnosis of SCC is typically made on biopsy. The most important differential is reactive regenerative squamous proliferation, which can show significant cytologic atypia with increased mitotic activity and long, thin prongs extending into the surrounding lamina propria. These may be at the edges or base of an ulcer. Due to sectioning artifact, there may be apparent small nests of these atypical cells within the lamina propria. Distinguishing hyperplastic regenerative squamous proliferation from superficial invasive SCC can be difficult.

The second potential pitfall when interpreting a biopsy is radiation- and chemotherapy-induced changes. The overall orientation of the epithelium is intact, but there may be marked cytologic atypia with giant bizarre nuclei and hyperchromasia. Fortunately, the nuclear to cytoplasmic ratio is typically not increased, so that although the nuclei are quite large, the cytoplasm is abundant. This is in contrast to carcinoma, in which the nuclei are typically large and the cytoplasm scant, even after radiation. The pitfall of radiation- and chemotherapy-induced atypia being overinterpreted as malignant is less likely if the pathologist is given the patient's clinical history of prior radiation or chemotherapy.

The third caveat for interpreting biopsies when SCC enters the diagnosis is to pay attention to the lamina propria, because there may be an underlying mesenchymal tumor inducing a reactive squamous proliferation. The prototypic example is the granular cell tumor causing the overlying squamous epithelium to undergo pseudoepitheliomatous hyperplasia. This squamous mucosal hyperplastic reaction may be confused with a well-differentiated superficially invasive SCC.

References

1. Gabbert HE, Shimoda T, Hainaut P, et al. *WHO Classification of Tumours: Pathology and Genetics Tumours of the Digestive System Squamous Cell Carcinoma of the Oesophagus*. Lyon, France: IARC Press, 2000.
2. Takubo K, Aida J, Sawabe M, et al. Early squamous cell carcinoma of the oesophagus: the Japanese viewpoint. *Histopathology.* 2007;51:733–742.
3. Yao P-F, Li G-C, Li J, et al. Evidence of human papilloma virus infection and its epidemiology in esophageal squamous cell carcinoma. *World J Gastroenterol.* 2006;12(9):1352–1355.
4. Matsha T, Donninger H, Erasmus, RT, et al. Expression of p53 and its homolog, p73, in HPV DNA positive oesophageal squamous cell carcinomas. *Virology.* 2007;369(1):182–190.
5. Turner JR, Shen LH, Crum CP, et al. Low prevalence of human papillomavirus infection in esophageal squamous cell carcinomas from North America: analysis by a highly sensitive and specific polymerase chain reaction-based approach. *Hum Pathol.* 1997;28(2):174–178.

6. Lewin KJ, Appelman HD. Squamous cell carcinoma. In: Juan Rosai, ed. *Tumors of the Esophagus and Stomach*. 3rd series, Fascicle 18. Washington, DC: Armed Forces Institute of Pathology, 1996:43–97.
7. Takahashi H, Shikata N, Senzaki H, et al. Immunohistochemical staining patterns of keratins in normal oesophageal epithelium and carcinoma of the oesophagus. *Histopathology*. 1995;26(1):45–50.
8. Tajima T, Nakanishi Y, Ochiai A, et al. Histopathologic findings predicting lymph node metastasis and prognosis of patients with superficial esophageal carcinoma. *Cancer*. 2000;88:1285–1293.
9. Mandard AM, Marnay J, Gignoux M, et al. Cancer of the esophagus and associated lesions: detailed pathologic study of 100 esophagectomy specimens. *Hum Path*. 1984;15:660–669.
10. Pesko P, Rakic S, Milicevic M, et al. Prevalence and clinicopathologic features of multiple squamous cell carcinoma of the esophagus. *Cancer*. 1994;73:2687–2690.
11. Kaufmann O, Fietze E, Mengs J, et al. Value of p63 and cytokeratin 5/6 as immunohistochemical markers for the differential diagnosis of poorly differentiated and undifferentiated carcinomas. *Am J Clin Pathol*. 2001;116:823–830.
12. de Sampaio G, Grizzo FC, Oliveira DT, et al. Prognoses of oral basaloid squamous cell carcinoma and squamous cell carcinoma: a comparison. *Arch Otolaryngol Head Neck Surg*. 2004;130(1):83–86.
13. Abe K, Sasano H, Itakura Y, et al., Basaloid-squamous carcinoma of the esophagus: a clinicopathologic, DNA ploidy, and immunohistochemical study of seven cases. *Am J Surg Path*. 1996;20:453–461.
14. Kuwano H, Matsuda H, Matsuka H, et al. Intra-epithelial carcinoma concomitant with esophageal squamous cell carcinoma. *Cancer*. 1987;59:783–787.
15. Dawsey SM, Lewin KJ, Wang GQ, et al. Squamous esophageal histology and subsequent risk of squamous cell carcinoma of the esophagus. A prospective follow-up study from Linxian, China. *Cancer*. 1994;74:1686.

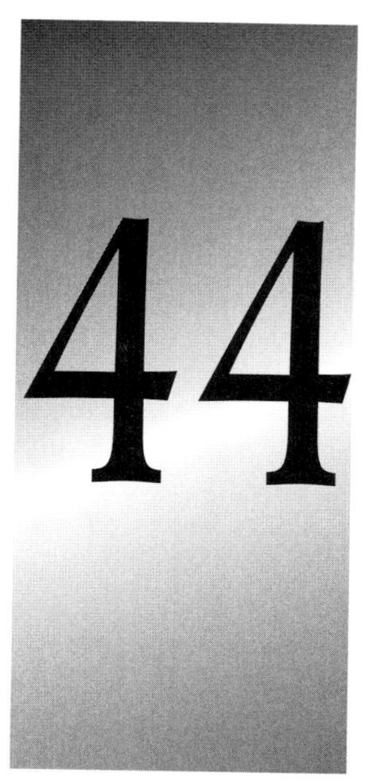

44 Malignant: Esophageal Adenocarcinoma and Variants

Laura H. Tang

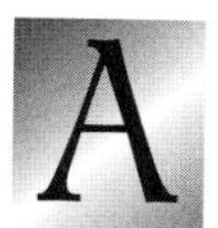

Adenocarcinoma of the esophagus is defined by a malignant epithelial tumor of the esophagus with glandular differentiation. The majority of these tumors arise from Barrett's esophagus in the lower third of the esophagus. While Barrett's esophagus, an intestinal type epithelial metaplastic process, may not always be evident as a precursor lesion, most cases of primary esophageal adenocarcinoma are likely associated with the pathology of the gastroesophageal junction (1). The degree of glandular differentiation in these tumors may vary, depending upon tumor differentiation and tumor grade. For example, adenocarcinoma may exhibit signet ring cell features, hepatoid morphology, squamous differentiation, a sarcomatous component, or characteristics of a high-grade neuroendocrine carcinoma. The presence of such features is often indicative of a more aggressive behavior of the tumor. The rare salivary type adenocarcinoma, which includes adenoid cystic carcinoma and mucoepidermoid carcinoma, arises from esophageal submucosal glands. Very infrequently, adenocarcinoma of the esophagus can originate from heterotopic gastric mucosa or pancreatic ductal epithelium, and the pathologic characteristics of these lesions closely resemble those of the site of origin of the carcinoma. This chapter discusses all the variants of primary adenocarcinoma of the esophagus.

ADENOCARCINOMA IN ASSOCIATION WITH BARRETT'S ESOPHAGUS

The detailed issues of Barrett's esophagus, including its definition, epidemiology, pathology, and molecular biology, are considered in Chapters 5 to 10. The relevant pathologic topics are discussed briefly in this chapter.

Barrett's esophagus has been documented, from both a historic perspective as well as contemporary evidence, to be associated with the development of adenocarcinoma of the gastroesophageal junction (GEJ) (2). Furthermore, this type of intestinal metaplastic change is almost invariably evident in the epithelium surrounding most GEJ adenocarcinoma. As a result of such observations, Barrett's esophagus has been considered a major risk factor for the development of adenocarcinoma at the GEJ. The similar recognition that adenocarcinoma of the GEJ has been increasing at a dramatic rate has led to the emergence of a high level of interest in the pathology, early identification, and treatment of the condition (1,3).

As with neoplasia elsewhere, the transformation from normal to a malignant mucosa in the esophagus occurs through a sequence of morphologic changes accompanied by specific molecular genetic events (4,5). While the morphologic transformation of the Barrett-type epithelium has been well recognized, the exact sequence of molecular events occurring in GEJ adenocarcinoma is not as well established as those identified in colonic adenocarcinoma. The identification and isolation of markers with potential for screening and possibly prognostic information are therefore areas of considerable clinical and scientific interest.

Macroscopic Pathology

The majority of primary adenocarcinomas of the esophagus arise in the lower third of the esophagus within the segment of Barrett's mucosa (6,7), which may be recognizable adjacent to the tumor as typical salmon-pink flat mucosa, particularly at early stage of the carcinoma (Figure 44.1). Superficial adenocarcinoma, which is usually identified in the course of surveillance of Barrett's esophagus, may exhibit subtle macroscopic alterations within Barrett's mucosa, such as mucosal bumps or plaques. However, at the time of diagnosis, most tumors have attained an advanced stage with an ulcerative or mass lesion infiltrating into the esophageal wall. In some of these advanced cases, Barrett's mucosa may be displaced by overgrowth of the tumor and is no longer recognizable in the adjacent mucosa by either gross or microscopic examination.

Histopathology

When evaluating patients in surveillance cohorts, it has been established that the presence of dysplasia indicates an increased risk of adenocarcinoma. However, the natural history of dysplasia per se, particularly low-grade dysplasia, is very difficult to predict in individual patients (8). Studies produced over the last 2 decades indicate that the detection of high-grade dysplasia in Barrett's esophagus is indicative of a synchronous adenocarcinoma. It is claimed that this neoplasia remains undetected even by the most rigorous biopsy protocols, only to be discovered in surgically resected specimens. The reported prevalence of such adenocarcinoma ranges from 0% to 75% in some series, and it has been estimated that an average 40% of occult adenocarcinoma occurs in high-grade dysplasia (9,10). A figure of such magnitude requires more rigorous evaluation and the presentation of more robust data (11,12). As a consequence of such conflicting data regarding the likelihood of occult adenocarcinoma, the reported biopsy protocols that lead to the surgical resection vary widely between centers (13–17).

Adenocarcinoma arising in Barrett's esophagus with high-grade dysplasia is defined by neoplastic cells that have penetrated through the basement membrane and infiltrated into the lamina propria or beyond (Figure 44.1). Most pathologists are unlikely to miss submucosal invasive carcinomas, particularly when provided with the clinical and endoscopic impression of a mass lesion. However, the diagnosis of a superficial adenocarcinoma may be a delicate issue in certain clinical settings. When the biopsy is superficial or the lesion

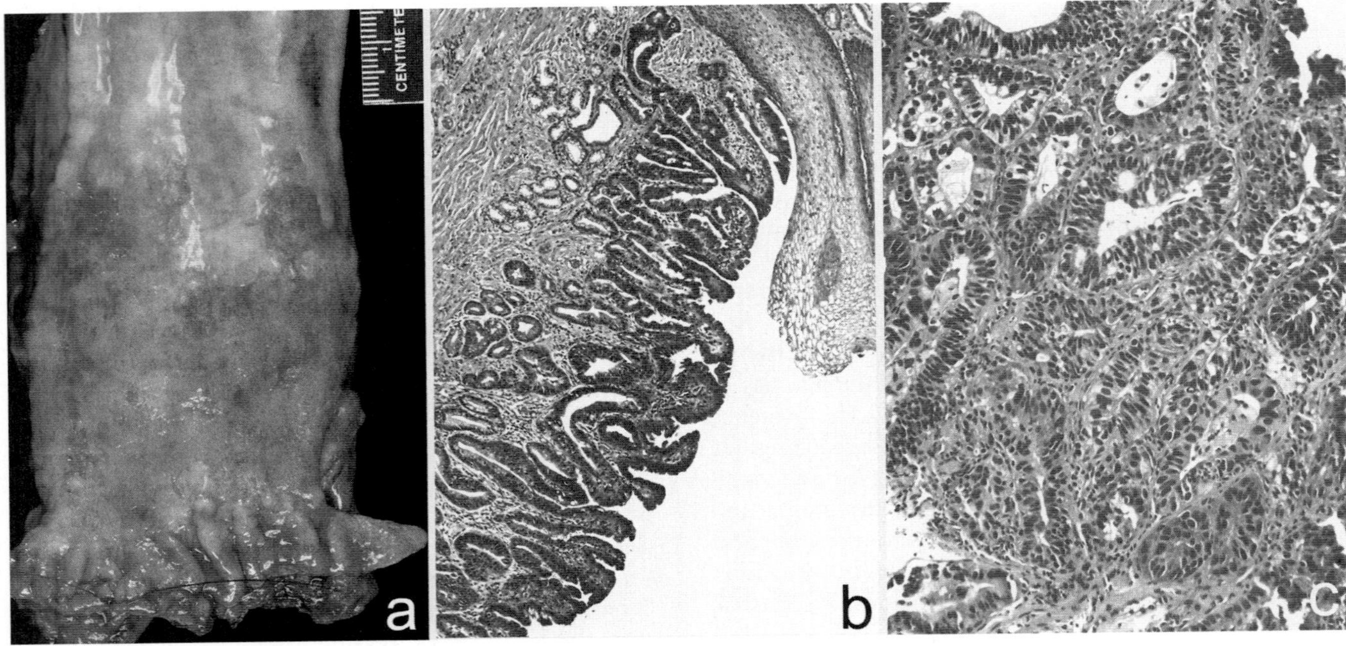

FIGURE 44.1

Gross and microscopic Barrett's esophagus with dysplasia and early adenocarcinoma. (a) Barrett's mucosa extends from the distal esophagus and up 5.0 cm into the squamous lined mucosa. (b) High-grade glandular dysplasia is evident at the squamocolumnar junction. (c) While no mass lesion is grossly identified (a), early carcinoma is detected within Barrett's mucosa.

itself is indeed superficial, the impact of the diagnosis of carcinoma versus high-grade dysplasia may require serious consideration. In view of the fact that even the presence of lamina propria invasion alone carries the risk of regional lymph node metastasis, considerable caution must be exercised (1). Thus the diagnosis of a superficially invasive carcinoma usually leads to surgical intervention.

Most cases of adenocarcinoma in association with Barrett's esophagus are well to moderately differentiated, and frequently present with architectural and cytologic transformation from the dysplastic glandular epithelium to an adenocarcinoma (Figure 44.1). The presence of variable areas of a poorly differentiated component is not uncommon. The poorly differentiated areas in this type of adenocarcinoma are usually characterized by lack of glandular differentiation with a diffuse, either signet ring cell or undifferentiated cell, infiltration. Sometimes the tumor may present with other types of epithelial differentiation, such as hepatocytic (hepatoid) or trophoblastic (choriocarcinoma) differentiation (18–20). These tumors not only bear morphologic features of exogenous epithelial differentiation, they also express their corresponding immunophenotypic markers (hepatocyte antigen and human chorionic gonadotropin, respectively). In these situations, the possibility of a metastasis should be clinically excluded. The presence of a squamous or a mesenchymal component within an adenocarcinoma may be designated as adenosquamous carcinoma and sarcomatoid carcinoma (see sections "Adenocarcinoma of Salivary Gland Type" and "Adenosquamous Carcinoma" in this chapter). When tumor cells are largely undifferentiated, particularly in a limited biopsy material, the differential diagnosis should include a poorly differentiated squamous cell carcinoma or a melanoma (Figure 44.2). The location of the lesion, the presence of an in situ carcinoma component or pre-neoplastic changes, and an immunohistochemical work-up should enable the establishment of a definitive diagnosis. The differentiation of an adenocarcinoma should be defined by the presence of >25% of its worst differentiated component; for example, a moderately differentiated carcinoma with evidence of a 25% poorly differentiated component should be classified as a poorly differentiated carcinoma.

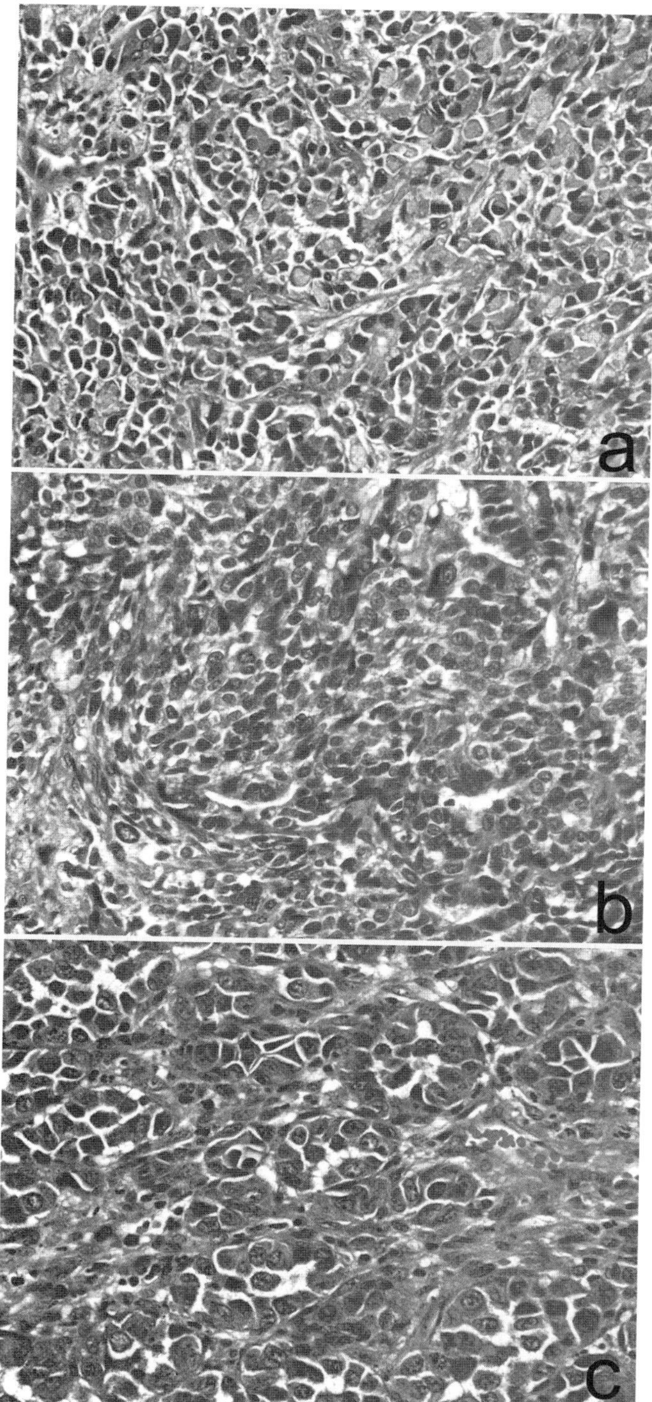

FIGURE 44.2

Examples of poorly differentiated malignant neoplasm of the esophagus. (a) An example of diffuse variant of adenocarcinoma of distal esophagus, signet ring cell type. (b) An example of an undifferentiated carcinoma with minimal recognizable features of an epithelial neoplasm. (c) A poorly differentiated malignant neoplasm, which is proven to be a primary melanoma of the esophagus by immunohistochemistry, located in the mid esophagus.

Evaluation of Barrett's Adenocarcinoma in Surgical Specimens

In order to ensure accurate tumor staging and postoperative management, the specimen should be processed with a particular focus on tumor location, depth of invasion, pathology of the surrounding mucosa, adequate lymph node dissection from the specimen, and treatment-related changes. When the tumor straddles the GEJ, the proportion of the lesion in the esophagus and in the stomach should be carefully documented. The tissue sections are best oriented and assessed after at least several hours of formalin fixation. If possible, gross photographs should be taken prior to and subsequent to fixation to assure optimal depiction of the lesion. This provides important topographic information complementary to the histologic assessment. In the absence of a large tumor mass, it is best to block the GEJ involved by tumor and submit the entire area sequentially for histologic evaluation.

An issue not yet resolved is the question of lymph node assessment. The sixth edition of American Joint Committee on Cancer (AJCC) staging includes adenocarcinoma of the GEJ in the esophageal tumor staging system but does not require extensive lymph node assessment (21). However, the clinical prognosis of GEJ adenocarcinoma is best predicted by adequate lymph node evaluation, thus, adoption of the lymph node staging for gastric carcinoma, which requires evaluation of a minimum of 15 lymph nodes, has been proposed (22).The pathologic assessment of GEJ carcinoma in response to radiation/chemotherapy involves both the gross and the microscopic examination of the resected surgical specimen (1). The gross appearance of treated tumors varies from mucosal ulceration to a fibrous scar, or a prominent mass lesion in the case of a less than obvious tumor regression. At the microscopic level, a positive treatment-related effect is observed as abolition of the malignant epithelium and replacement by reactive fibrosis or fibro-inflammation within the mucosa or the gastroesophageal wall. The ultimate pathologic response to treatment is thus determined by the amount of residual viable carcinoma in relation to areas of fibrosis or fibro-inflammation within the gross lesion, which is inversely associated with, and expressed as percentage of a favorable treatment response. Thus, a 100% treatment response indicates fibrosis or fibro-inflammation within an entire gross lesion without microscopic evidence of residual carcinoma, and a 0% response represents an entirely viable tumor in the absence of any fibrosis of fibro-inflammation. Acellular mucin is regarded as a form of positive treatment response, not as residual/viable tumor. The pathologic stage of the residual carcinoma is determined by the presence of viable malignant epithelium in the deepest layer of the gastroesophageal wall. Positive lymph nodes are defined as having at least one focus of viable tumor cells in lymph nodes (1).

Pathologists are often confronted with adenocarcinomas that straddle the GEJ; and there has been considerable debate regarding the tumor genesis and the relationship between GEJ and gastric cardia adenocarcinoma. Various criteria have been used to categorize tumors situated at the GEJ. In most classification systems, the anatomic location of the epicenter or predominant mass of the tumor is used to determine whether the neoplasm is esophageal or gastric (cardia) in origin (23–25). However, it is almost impossible to document that in a given location, such as the GEJ, tumors will grow to the same extent in a proximal and distal direction. This renders it difficult to derive any certain conclusion in regard to the epicenter of the origin. In this respect, a further problem is posed by the fact that there exists no consensus regarding the definition of cancer of the gastric cardia. The majority of the data available on cardia mucosa, cardiac mucosal dysplasia, and cardiac cancer are not comparable because of lack of diagnostic criteria. Uniformity in classification, terminology, and diagnostic criteria are still required to clarify the issue of cardia, mucosal carditis, and cardiac adenocarcinoma and its relationship with adenocarcinoma of the GEJ (23,24,26). At present, however, it would appear that the similarities between adenocarcinoma of the GEJ or cardia and Barrett's adenocarcinoma outnumber their dissimilarities.

ADENOCARCINOMA ARISING IN HETEROTOPIC EPITHELIUM

In rare cases, when an adenocarcinoma of the esophagus arises completely independent of Barrett's esophagus, the histogenesis of the tumor arising from ectopic gastric glands (gastric inlet) (27), heterotopic pancreatic tissue, or from periesophageal glands (see below "Adenocarcinoma of Salivary Type") should be considered. In contrast to Barrett's associated adenocarcinoma located in the distal esophagus of the squamocolumnar junctional mucosa, carcinomas arising from the gastric inlet are usually found in the upper and middle portion of the esophagus, whereas tumors from heterotopic pancreas can be located in both the proximal esophagus and the distal esophagus (28). Histopathologic features of these tumors at their ectopic site are similar to those of their primary carcinoma, which may display a spectrum of grades and differentiation as discussed in other variants of adenocarcinoma throughout this chapter. Careful histopathologic assessment may enable the identification of the original benign or dysplastic epithelium from which the carcinoma arises (Figure 44.3).

Given their rarity, there exist insufficient data to evaluate the clinical outcome of these tumors. It is, however, plausible to consider that they will behave in a similar fashion to any de novo adenocarcinoma of the esophagus or stomach or pancreas, in which the tumor stage is the deciding variable that dictates the prognosis.

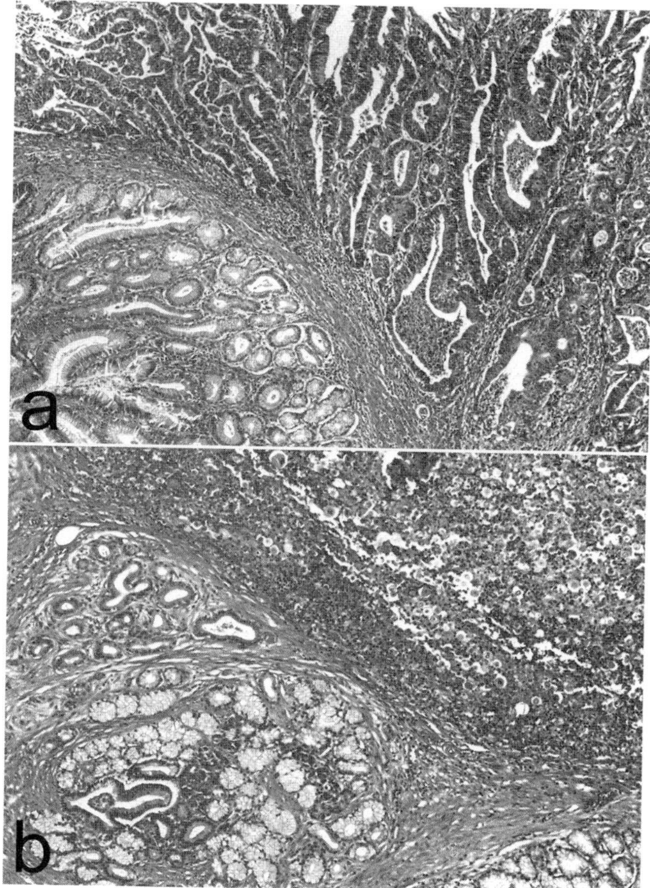

FIGURE 44.3

Adenocarcinoma of the esophagus in association with heterotopia. (a) An example of an adenocarcinoma (right upper) located in mid-esophagus and arising in heterotopic gastric mucosa (left lower). (b) A poorly differentiated adenocarcinoma (upper right) arising in distal esophagus with associated ectopic pancreatic tissue in the proximity (lower left).

ADENOCARCINOMA OF SALIVARY GLAND TYPE

The primary salivary gland type adenocarcinoma of the esophagus, which constitute <1% of all esophageal epithelial malignancies, is extremely rare, with only scattered cases reported. This type of tumor is believed to arise in the esophageal submucosal glands or the epithelium of tracheobronchial rests (29,30). Two types of this entity have been described in the esophagus: adenoid cystic carcinoma and mucoepidermoid carcinoma (30–32).

Adenoid Cystic Carcinoma

Adenoid cystic carcinoma (ACC) has been well recognized in the salivary glands, oropharynx, respiratory tract, mammary tissue, and uterine cervix. A primary ACC of the esophagus can occur in any segment of the esophagus. The morphologic features of carcinoma are similar to those of ACC of the salivary glands of the head and neck.

The most common growth pattern in ACC is cribriform, which imparts a sieve-like appearance to the tumor with islands of neoplastic epithelial cells that contain several small and round pseudocystic structures of variable diameter. The tumor is composed of 2 cell lineages. The majority of the neoplastic cells are of an abluminal type, which exhibit myoepithelial differentiation. Among the prominent basaloid myoepithelial cells, the second type of cells are scattered foci of ductal epithelial cells, which surround tiny lumens (Figure 44.4).

While most ACCs of the head and neck region are considered low-grade carcinomas, many investigators

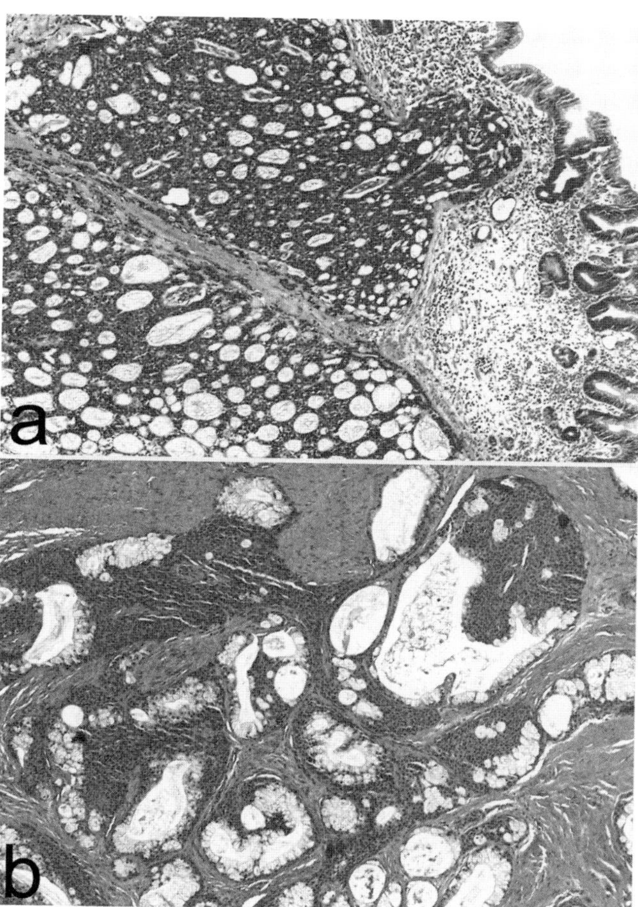

FIGURE 44.4

Adenocarcinoma of salivary gland type. (a) An example of adenoid cystic carcinoma arising in columnar mucosa of distal esophagus. (b) An example of mucoepidermoid carcinoma with mucous (goblet) cells and epideromid (squamoid) cells intimately admixed with each other.

have reported ACC of the esophagus to exhibit aggressive behavior and diffuse metastasis (30,31). This difference has been considered as due to some adverse histopathologic features including greater polymorphism, higher mitotic activity, and a more solid growth pattern. However, an alternative explanation might be that many cases of basaloid squamous cell carcinoma may have been misdiagnosed and included in the database of ACC of the esophagus. This highly regressive variant of poorly differentiated squamous cell carcinoma may exhibit a growth pattern that mimics that of an ACC and is thus liable to misclassification (33,34). The identification of a squamous cell carcinoma component, either in situ or invasive, in a carcinoma with an adenoid cystic histologic pattern, should suggest the diagnosis of a basaloid squamous cell carcinoma. A further diagnostic point important in securing the diagnosis is that basaloid squamous cell carcinoma lack the ductal epithelial component, which is required to establish the diagnosis of an ACC.

Thus a genuine ACC of the esophagus should be considered as a well-differentiated carcinoma and is anticipated to have a better prognosis than most conventional-type and moderately to poorly differentiated adenocarcinoma (35).

Mucoepidermoid Carcinoma

Mucoepidermoid carcinoma (MEC) is even rarer than ACC in the esophagus (36,37). The real incidence of MEC is difficult to estimate due not only to its rarity but also to misdiagnosis and underreporting. As a malignant mixed epithelial neoplasm, MEC is composed of varying proportions of mucous, epidermoid, intermediate, columnar, and clear cells. The characteristic histologic pattern of MEC is a prominent cystic component and small duct-like structure (Figure 44.4). The cysts are usually lined by mucous, intermediate, or epidermoid cells, which also exhibit extramural proliferation, while the lumina are typically filled with mucin. On the basis of morphologic and cytologic features, MECs are graded into low-, intermediate-, and high-grade type with a corresponding progressively worse prognosis.

Due to its mixed cell amalgamation, particularly the presence of the epidermoid (squamoid) and the mucinous (goblet) cells, MEC is often interpreted as an adenosquamous cell carcinoma (Figure 44.5). The latter entity is considered as a subtype of conventional tubular/ductal adenocarcinoma at many sites of the digestive system.

Despite its distinct histogenesis of salivary gland/duct, the prognosis of MEC, similar to that of other variants of adenocarcinoma of the esophagus, is largely dependent on clinical stage and tumor grade (36). Most cases of MEC are presented at an advanced

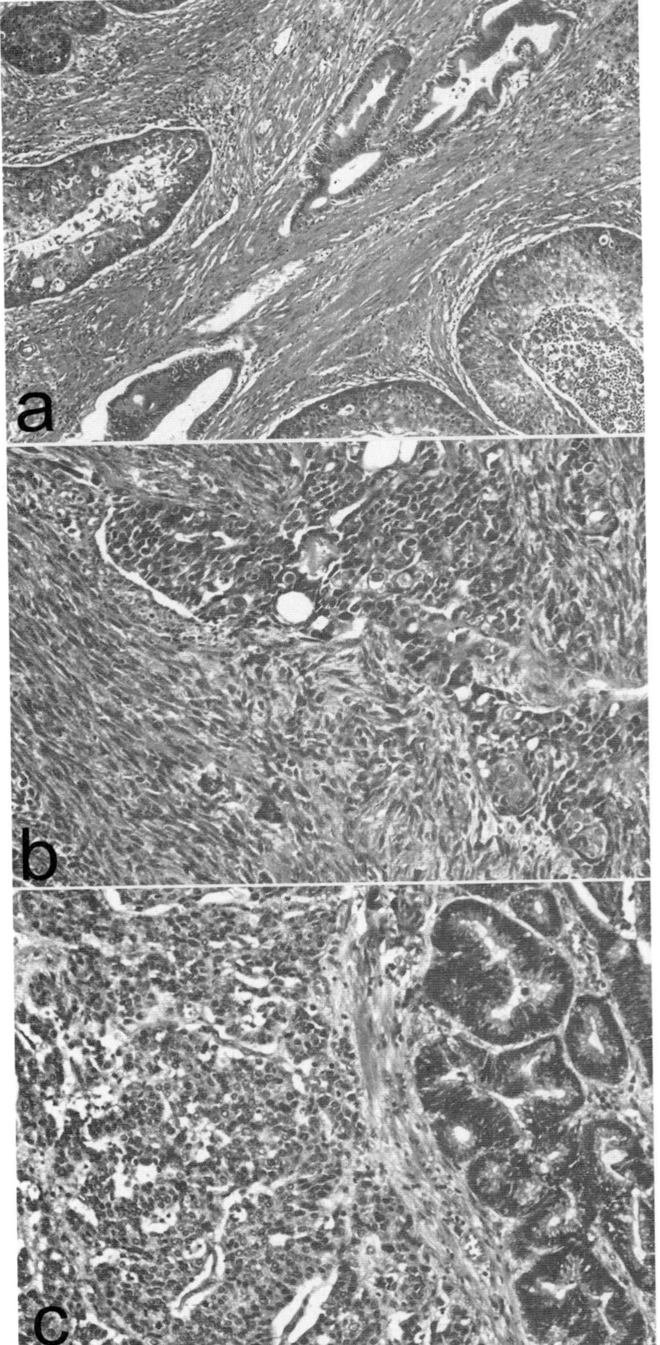

FIGURE 44.5

Other variants of adenocarcinoma of the esophagus. (a) An example of adenosquamous cell carcinoma with the malignant glandular and squamous carcinoma coexist in the same tumor, but distinct from each other. (b) An example of sarcomatoid carcinoma with a poorly differentiated epithelial component (upper right) and a malignant spindle cell element (lower left). (c) An example of high-grade neuroendocrine carcinoma (left) arising in association with Barrett's esophagus with glandular dysplasia (right).

stage, possibly due to an early underdetected submucosal lesion and a late mucosal surface involvement and associated clinical symptoms. These tumors have been reportedly more resistant to adjuvant therapy and have a poor clinical outcome (36).

ADENOSQUAMOUS CARCINOMA

Squamous differentiation is not an uncommon event in conventional type adenocarcinomas of the gastrointestinal tract and the pancreaticobiliary system. When the component represented by squamous differentiation is >25%, the carcinoma is classified as an adenosquamous carcinoma. It is uncommon to find glandular differentiation in a de novo squamous cell carcinoma; thus, regardless of the proportion of squamous component present in an adenocarcinoma, the presence of any glandular element or mucin-containing cells is adequate for a diagnosis of adenosquamous carcinoma. In this entity, the adenocarcinomatous component is usually tubular/glandular, as might be evident in a Barrett's associated adenocarcinoma. The squamous component of the tumor is usually moderately to well differentiated. Of note is the fact that the 2 components, squamous and the glandular foci, are more distinct from each other than when present in a mucoepidermoid carcinoma, in which the 2 components are intimately intermingled (see section above).

Other than the morphologic evidence of squamous differentiation, the prognosis of adenosquamous carcinomas is comparable with that of genuine adenocarcinomas of the GEJ. Thus, a high-tumor stage and the presence of poorly differentiated carcinoma predict a poor clinical outcome.

SARCOMATOID (SARCOMATOUS) CARCINOMA

This entity is defined by the morphologic presence of a sarcomatous, or malignant spindle cell component in a malignant epithelial tumor. Sarcomatoid carcinoma can occur in any carcinoma at any anatomic site, including the esophagus. While morphologically or even immunophenotypically distinct from an epithelial neoplasia, it is generally accepted that the sarcomatous elements in a sarcomatoid carcinoma represent a dedifferentiated component of the malignant epithelial origin. The term *carcinosarcoma* is not preferred in a true epithelial tumor; it is better applied to a tumor with dual histogenesis of epithelial and mesenchymal differentiation, and is most commonly found in the Mullerian system.

In the esophagus, sarcomatoid carcinoma can be present in a squamous cell carcinoma, more commonly than in an adenocarcinoma. The sarcomatous component often loses its immunoreactivity to most low molecular weight cytokeratins, but may have some degree of preserved reactivity to high molecular weight cytokeratins. Due to its poorly or dedifferentiated nature, sarcomatoid carcinoma is inevitably more aggressive and is indicative of a poor clinical outcome.

HIGH-GRADE NEUROENDOCRINE CARCINOMA

While high-grade neuroendocrine carcinoma (HGNEC) is rare in the gastrointestinal tract in general, the esophagus is a relatively common site with an estimated prevalence of 1% to 2.8% of all esophageal malignancies (38,39). Similar to the HGNEC at other locations of the gastrointestinal tract, HGNEC of the esophagus represents a heterogeneous group of clinically aggressive tumors. It remains a poorly characterized category, principally because of its rarity and the lack of consistent diagnostic criteria. HGNECs can display a spectrum of morphologic characteristics, which range from small cell to large cell neuroendocrine carcinoma of their pulmonary counterparts, and some have features intermediate between these 2 extremes. In addition, admixed components of adenocarcinoma or other non-neuroendocrine elements are commonly identified in association with >50% of any subtypes of HGNECs. At present, there are no defined criteria for classification of tumors within this spectrum. Both the WHO and AJCC recognize the small cell carcinoma variant; however, HGNECs of non-small cell type are not currently included in the classification of carcinomas of the gastrointestinal tract. As a consequence of the lack of a clear understanding of the pathobiology and molecular biology of HGNECs, there exists an inconsistency in diagnosis and clinical management.

Recent studies have classified HGNECs of the GI tract into 3 categories: (a) small cell carcinoma, (b) large cell carcinoma, and (c) mixed neuroendocrine carcinoma (40). Further analysis has demonstrated that most HGNECs arising in the squamous mucosa-lined esophagus are small cell type (83%), whereas most involving the GEJ glandular mucosa are of a large cell or mixed (67%) cell type. The presence of Barrett's metaplasia with dysplasia or an adenocarcinoma component is more frequently associated with large cell or mixed type of HGNEC; conversely, in situ squamous cell carcinoma is more commonly observed in conjunction with small cell carcinoma.

Although both well-differentiated neuroendocrine neoplasm (carcinoid) and poorly differentiated HGNEC express general neuroendocrine markers (chromogranin and synaptophysin), in most cases, they do not appear to be related in their pathogenesis. The former arises in the diffuse neuroendocrine cell system of the tubular gastrointestinal tract or the pancreaticobiliary system, and the latter most likely originates from the surface epithelium of the gastrointestinal tract. It is extremely unusual to find them in juxtaposition in individual tumors.

Gastrointestinal tract HGNECs are typically diagnosed at an advanced stage; most tumors exhibit regional lymph node involvement at the time of initial presentation, and more than half have overt distant metastasis to the liver, followed by distant lymph nodes, peritoneum, bones, and brain. The estimated 2-year disease-specific survival is <25%.

References

1. Tang LH, Klimstra DS. Barrett's esophagus and adenocarcinoma of the gastroesophageal junction: a pathologic perspective. *Surg Oncol Clin N Am.* 2006;15:715–732.
2. Morales CP, Souza RF, Spechler SJ. Hallmarks of cancer progression in Barrett's oesophagus. *Lancet.* 2002;360:1587–1589.
3. Shaheen NJ. Advances in Barrett's esophagus and esophageal adenocarcinoma. *Gastroenterology.* 2005;128:1554–1566.
4. Appelman HD. What is dysplasia in the gastrointestinal tract? *Arch Pathol Lab Med.* 2005;129:170–173.
5. Geboes K, Van Eyken P. The diagnosis of dysplasia and malignancy in Barrett's oesophagus. *Histopathology.* 2000;37:99–107.
6. Haggitt RC, Tryzelaar J, Ellis FH, et al. Adenocarcinoma complicating columnar epithelium-lined (Barrett's) esophagus. *Am J Clin Pathol.* 1978;70:1–5.
7. Paraf F, Flejou JF, Pignon JP, et al. Surgical pathology of adenocarcinoma arising in Barrett's esophagus. Analysis of 67 cases. *Am J Surg Pathol.* 1995;19:183–191.
8. Goldblum JR, Lauwers GY. Dysplasia arising in Barrett's esophagus: diagnostic pitfalls and natural history. *Semin Diagn Pathol.* 2002;19:12–19.
9. Falk GW, Rice TW, Goldblum JR, et al. Jumbo biopsy forceps protocol still misses unsuspected cancer in Barrett's esophagus with high-grade dysplasia. *Gastrointest Endosc.* 1999;49:170–176.
10. Heitmiller RF, Redmond M, Hamilton SR. Barrett's esophagus with high-grade dysplasia. An indication for prophylactic esophagectomy. *Ann Surg.* 1996;224:66–71.
11. Flejou JF. Barrett's oesophagus: from metaplasia to dysplasia and cancer. *Gut.* 2005;54 Suppl 1:i6–12.
12. Tschanz ER. Do 40% of patients resected for Barrett's esophagus with high-grade dysplasia have unsuspected adenocarcinoma? *Arch Pathol Lab Med.* 2005;129:177–180.
13. Larghi A, Lightdale CJ, Memeo L, et al. EUS followed by EMR for staging of high-grade dysplasia and early cancer in Barrett's esophagus. *Gastrointest Endosc.* 2005;62:16–23.
14. Rusch VW, Levine DS, Haggitt R, et al. The management of high grade dysplasia and early cancer in Barrett's esophagus. A multidisciplinary problem. *Cancer.* 1994;74:1225–1229.
15. Savoy AD, Wallace MB. EUS in the management of the patient with dysplasia in Barrett's esophagus. *J Clin Gastroenterol.* 2005;39:263–267.
16. Sujendran V, Sica G, Warren B, et al. Oesophagectomy remains the gold standard for treatment of high-grade dysplasia in Barrett's oesophagus. *Eur J Cardiothorac Surg.* 2005;28:763–766.
17. Tseng EE, Wu TT, Yeo CJ, et al. Barrett's esophagus with high grade dysplasia: surgical results and long-term outcome—an update. *J Gastrointest Surg.* 2003;7:164–171.
18. Motoyama T, Higuchi M, Taguchi J. Combined choriocarcinoma, hepatoid adenocarcinoma, small cell carcinoma and tubular adenocarcinoma in the oesophagus. *Virchows Arch.* 1995;427:451–454.
19. Tanigawa H, Kida Y, Kuwao S, et al. Hepatoid adenocarcinoma in Barrett's esophagus associated with achalasia: first case report. *Pathol Int.* 2002;52:141–146.
20. Wasan HS, Schofield JB, Krausz T, et al. Combined choriocarcinoma and yolk sac tumor arising in Barrett's esophagus. *Cancer.* 1994;73:514–517.
21. American Joint Committee on Cancer (AJCC). *AJCC Cancer Staging Manual.* 6th edition. Springer; New York: 2002.
22. Rizk NP, Venkatraman E, Bains MS, et al. American Joint Committee on Cancer staging system does not accurately predict survival in patients receiving multimodality therapy for esophageal adenocarcinoma. *J Clin Oncol.* 2007;25:507–512.
23. Corley DA, Buffler PA. Oesophageal and gastric cardia adenocarcinomas: analysis of regional variation using the Cancer Incidence in Five Continents database. *Int J Epidemiol.* 2001;30:1415–1425.
24. Ectors N, Driessen A, De Hertog G, et al. Is adenocarcinoma of the esophagogastric junction or cardia different from Barrett adenocarcinoma? *Arch Pathol Lab Med.* 2005;129:183–185.
25. Siewert JR, Stein HJ. Classification of adenocarcinoma of the oesophagogastric junction. *Br J Surg.* 1998;85:1457–1459.
26. De Hertogh G, Van Eyken P, Ectors N, et al. On the existence and location of cardiac mucosa: an autopsy study in embryos, fetuses, and infants. *Gut.* 2003;52:791–796.
27. von Rahden BH, Stein HJ, Becker K, et al. Heterotopic gastric mucosa of the esophagus: literature-review and proposal of a clinicopathologic classification. *Am J Gastroenterol.* 2004;99:543–551.
28. Tang P, McKinley MJ, Sporrer M, et al. Inlet patch: prevalence, histologic type, and association with esophagitis, Barrett esophagus, and antritis. *Arch Pathol Lab Med.* 2004;128:444–447.
29. Bergmann M, Charnas RM. Tracheobronchial rests in the esophagus; their relation to some benign strictures and certain types of cancer of the esophagus. *J Thorac Surg.* 1958;35:97–104.
30. Lin YK, Wang LS, Fahn HJ, et al. Primary uncommon malignant tumors of the esophagus: an analysis of 30 cases. *Zhonghua Yi Xue Za Zhi (Taipei).* 1995;55:463–471.
31. Morisaki Y, Yoshizumi Y, Hiroyasu S, et al. Adenoid cystic carcinoma of the esophagus: report of a case and review of the Japanese literature. *Surg Today.* 1996;26:1006–1009.
32. Cerar A, Jutersek A, Vidmar S. Adenoid cystic carcinoma of the esophagus. A clinicopathologic study of three cases. *Cancer.* 1991;67:2159–2164.
33. Li TJ, Zhang YX, Wen J, et al. Basaloid squamous cell carcinoma of the esophagus with or without adenoid cystic features. *Arch Pathol Lab Med.* 2004;128:1124–1130.
34. Tsubochi H, Suzuki T, Suzuki S, et al. Immunohistochemical study of basaloid squamous cell carcinoma, adenoid cystic and mucoepidermoid carcinoma in the upper aerodigestive tract. *Anticancer Res.* 2000;20:1205–1211.
35. Kabuto T, Taniguchi K, Iwanaga T, et al. Primary adenoid cystic carcinoma of the esophagus: report of a case. *Cancer.* 1979;43:2452–2456.
36. Hagiwara N, Tajiri T, Miyashita M, et al. Biological behavior of mucoepidermoid carcinoma of the esophagus. *J Nippon Med Sch.* 2003;70:401–407.
37. Kuwano H, Ueo H, Sugimachi K, et al. Glandular or mucus-secreting components in squamous cell carcinoma of the esophagus. *Cancer.* 1985;56:514–518.
38. Brenner B, Tang LH, Klimstra DS, et al. Small-cell carcinomas of the gastrointestinal tract: a review. *J Clin Oncol.* 2004;22:2730–2739.
39. Brenner B, Tang LH, Shia J, et al. Small cell carcinomas of the gastrointestinal tract: clinicopathological features and treatment approach. *Semin Oncol.* 2007;34:43–50.
40. Shia J, Tang LH, Weiser MR, et al. Is non-small cell type high grade neuroendocrine carcinoma of the tubular gastrointestinal tract a distinct disease entity? *Am J Surg Path.* 2008;32(5):719–731.

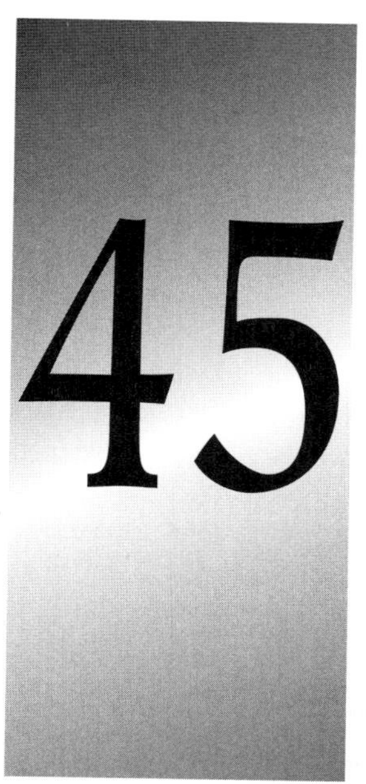

Malignant: Esophageal Adenocarcinoma of the Cardia and Proximal Stomach

John S. Macdonald
Lawrence Leichman

Gastric and gastroesophageal adenocarcinomas are important health problems. A 2005 analysis (1) of the worldwide incidence of and mortality from cancer showed that 934,000 cases of gastric cancer occurred in 2002 and that 700,000 patients die annually of this disease.

Adenocarcinoma of the body and distal stomach has been decreasing in incidence in North America and Western Europe over the last 70 years. This tumor was the number one cause of cancer death in the United States in 1900. It now is substantially less common as a cause of cancer mortality in the Western world. Although body and distal stomach cancers have declined in the developed world, this type of gastric adenocarcinoma is a continued health problem and results, as noted above, in at least 700,000 deaths annually worldwide. The reasons for the decrease in the endemic form of stomach cancer in Western societies is not known with certainty, but appears to be associated with less exposure to environmental factors known to increase the risk of stomach cancer. For example, in the West, the advent of ready access to refrigeration of food early in the 20th century led to a decrease in the ingestion of preserved and smoked foods and an increased consumption of fresh meats, fresh fruits, and vegetables. It is known that there are potential carcinogens (nitrates, nitrites, and nitrosamines) in preserved foods and that societies with high rates of the endemic form of gastric cancer have a higher consumption (2) of preserved and smoked meats.

Another factor important in gastric body and distal stomach carcinogenesis is the presence of the bacterium *Helicobacter pylori* (3). The *H. pylori* infection can result in gastritis. The development of chronic gastritis leads to dysplasia, anaplasia, and eventually carcinoma. In Western societies there is a significantly lower frequency of *H. pylori* gastric colonization and infection than there is in developing countries. With the absence of a necessary component of the gastritis to cancer sequence (*H. pylori*), there is a decreased occurrence of the endemic form of stomach cancer and, thus, body and distal gastric tumors have decreased in incidence.

While the endemic, *H. pylori*–associated stomach cancer may have decreased in Western societies, a more proximal group of cancers have increased in incidence in developed countries in the last 20 years. These cancers included adenocarcinomas of the proximal stomach, gastroesophageal junction (GEJ), and distal esophagus. Although the precise reasons for these tumors increasing is not known, it is clear that the mechanisms of carcinogenesis are certainly different from those seen in the distal endemic forms of stomach cancer. It appears that a common factor in these tumors is a relatively high frequency of gastroesophageal reflux disease (GERD). Although GERD is usually thought to cause symptoms of pain because of acid reflux causing painful proximal gastritis and/or distal esophagitis, GERD can occur without pain. One of the characteristics of neoplasia in the distal esophagus and GEJ/proximal stomach is the presence of intestinal metaplasia of the distal esophagus termed *Barrett's esophagus*. This condition is defined by the presence of areas of intestinal cell metaplasia in the distal esophagus. The precise cause of Barrett's esophagus is not known, but it clearly is associated with GERD. The GERD syndrome is more common in obese Caucasian males with a history of cigarette smoking and alcohol ingestion (4). There is a possibility that obese individuals who have relatively increased intra-abdominal pressure may have lax gastroesophageal sphincters and thus may be more prone to GERD. Chronic GERD may lead to Barrett's metaplasia in the distal esophagus. Not only is *H. pylori* gastritis not associated with proximal gastric-distal esophagus neoplasms but *H. pylori* gastritis that results in achlorhydria may actually reduce or at least ameliorate GERD and thus decrease the likelihood of Barrett's metaplasia occurring.

There is a clear sequence of carcinogenesis that may occur in patients with endoscopically documented Barrett's metaplasia, and management guidelines are based upon understanding this sequence. Patients with Barrett's metaplasia who have no evidence of dysplasia on endoscopic biopsy may be treated with acid suppression strategies and be monitored by repeat endoscopy performed on a regular basis, at least annually. If dysplasia or anaplasia is pathologically documented, then the risk of esophageal/proximal gastric cancer increases significantly and such patients require more aggressive therapy. The standard conservative approach for these cases is to perform esophagectomy. Investigational approaches for these patients include ablative techniques such as endoscopic mucosal resection and photodynamic therapy.

When cancers occur in the distal esophagus/GEJ/proximal stomach, the most pressing issue is what is the most appropriate therapy for patients with these malignancies? The management of gastroesophageal cancer, like the management of most gastrointestinal cancers, is based on surgical resection of the primary tumor. When cancers are localized and minimally invasive (5,6), surgical cure is possible in up to 90% of cases. However, the detection of early gastroesophageal cancer is unusual in Western countries. More commonly, resectable cancer is detected when it is locally advanced—that is, when the tumor extends into or through the gastric wall and there are regional lymph-node metastases (7,8). Less than 20% of such cases are cured by gastroesophagectomy. Because of the poor outcomes of surgery alone for gastroesophageal cancers, there has been much interest in adjunctive therapies that, when used in addition to surgical removal of the primary tumor, may improve survival (8–10). Adjuvant cytotoxic chemotherapy is successful in other gastrointestinal cancers (11), and many phase-3 clinical trials have explored this approach in gastroesophageal cancer (8,9). However, the survival benefit gained from the use of adjuvant chemotherapy in these tumors is not generally felt to be clinically significant (8,9), and for this reason, adjuvant chemotherapy has not become part of the standard of care in gastroesophageal cancer. There is evidence that postoperative chemoradiation (10) and perioperative chemotherapy (12) may be effective in decreasing recurrence for patients with gastroesophageal cancers. Extensive discussions of the role of various surgical techniques and approach to adjuvant and neoadjuvant therapy of gastroesophageal cancers will be presented elsewhere in this book.

In summary, proximal gastric/GEJ/distal esophageal cancers represent an important subset of upper abdominal adenocarcimomas. These tumors have different etiologies and epidemiologies than other tumors occurring in the stomach, for example, the more distal adenocarcinomas associated with *H. pylori* infection and the epidermoid carcinomas of the esophagus, which are typically seen in patients with histories of heavy alcohol and tobacco abuse. These upper gastrointestinal cancers require special consideration in regard to screening, prevention, and treatment.

References

1. Parkin DM, Bray F, Ferlay J, et al. Global cancer statistics, 2002. *CA Cancer J Clin.* 2005;55:74–108.
2. Steinmetz KA, Potter JD. Vegetables, fruit and cancer prevention: a review. *J Am Diet Assoc.* 1996:96(10):1027–1039.
3. Nomura A, Stemmermann GN, Chyou P-H, et al. Helicobacter pylori infection and gastric carcinoma among Japanese Americans in Hawaii. *N Engl J Med.* 1991;325:1132–1136.
4. Brown LM, Swanson CA, Gridley G. Adenocarcinoma of the oesophagus: role of obesity and diet. *J Nat Cancer Inst.* 1995;87:104–109.
5. Sue-Ling HM, Johnston D, Martin IG, et al. Gastric cancer: a curable disease in Britain. *BMJ.* 1993;307:591–596.
6. Sasako M, Sano T, Katai H, et al. Radical surgery. In: Sasako M, ed. *Gastric Cancer.* Oxford, England: Oxford University Press, 1997:223–248.
7. Siewert JR, Bottcher K, Roder JD, et al. Prognostic relevance of systematic lymph node dissection in gastric carcinoma. *Br J Surg.* 1993;80:1015–1018.
8. Earle CC, Maroun JA. Adjuvant chemotherapy after curative resection for gastric cancer in non-Asian patients: revisiting a meta-analysis of randomized trials. *Eur J Cancer.* 1999;35:1059–1064.
9. Hermans J, Bonenkamp JJ, Boon MC, et al. Adjuvant therapy after curative resection for gastric cancer: meta-analysis of randomized trials. *J Clin Oncol.* 1993;11: 1441–1447.
10. Macdonald JS, Smalley SR, Benedetti J, et al. Chemoradiotherapy after surgery compared with surgery alone for adenocarcinoma of the stomach or gastroesophageal junction. *N Engl J Med.* 2001;345:725–730.
11. Andre T, Boni C, Mounedji-Boudiaf L, et al. Oxaliplatin, fluorouracil, and leucovorin as adjuvant treatment for colon cancer. *N Engl J Med.* 2004;350:2343–2351.
12. Cunningham D, Allum WH, Stenning SP, et al. Perioperative chemotherapy versus surgery alone for resectable gastroesophageal cancer. *N Engl J Med.* 2006;355:11–20.

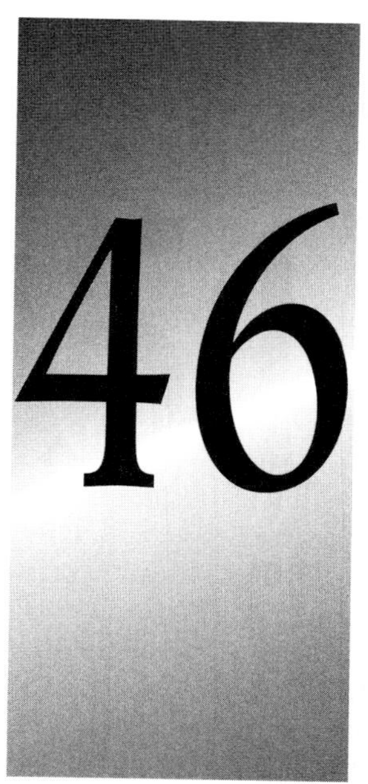

Malignant: Mesenchymal Tumors

Cameron D. Wright

Malignant mesenchymal tumors of the esophagus are very rare, representing only about 1% of all malignant tumors of the esophagus (Table 46.1). Accurate diagnosis is often difficult since they are submucosal until late in their course and are not suspected in the differential diagnosis due to their rarity. If symptomatic, patients present with the typical symptoms of esophageal obstruction. In the absence of metastatic disease, the treatment is surgical resection. The various sarcomas of the esophagus respond poorly to chemotherapy or radiation therapy. Gastrointestinal stromal tumors (GISTs) of the esophagus respond to imatinib mesylate (Gleevec, Novartis Pharmaceuticals), which can be used as an adjuvant and to treat unresectable, recurrent, or metastatic GISTs.

GASTROINTESTINAL STROMAL TUMORS

GISTs are c-kit (CD 117) positive mesenchymal spindle or epitheliod tumors of the gastrointestinal tract. The cell of origin is the interstitial cell of Cajal, or its precursor in the wall of the gastrointestinal tract, and has the expression of the tyrosine kinase receptor kit in almost all cases. They are quite rare, representing only about 3% of all gastrointestinal malignant tumors, but are the most common mesenchymal tumor of the gastrointestinal tract. They are most common in the stomach (50%–70%) and small bowel (20%–30%); they rarely occur in the esophagus (about 1% of all cases). Depending on the size and mitotic index of the tumor, GISTs are categorized into low-, intermediate-, and high-risk groups. Tumors greater than 5 cm and those with a mitotic index greater than 2/10 high power fields are at greater risk for metastases. GISTs stain for c-kit and CD 34. However, even small tumors with rare mitoses can metastasize. The largest case series of 17 cases of esophageal GISTs reported that 12 of 17 were high risk (1). Metastases are most common in the liver and are rare to the lymph nodes, although a recent case report noted nodal metastases (2). Efron and Lillemoe recently reviewed the management of GISTs (3).

About one-half of patients present with symptoms such as dysphagia, pain, odynophagia, or weight loss. GISTs occur in the older population, and most are in the distal esophagus. Most tumors present with an intraluminal polypoid mass with an intact mucosa. Mucosal biopsies are usually non-diagnostic. Contrast radiography, computed tomography (CT), and endoscopic ultrasound (EUS) are often used to assess the lesion and delineate the possibility for resection. Most patients are resected without a tissue diagnosis. Lymph node dissection is not thought to be important since nodal metastases are rare

TABLE 46.1
Malignant Mesenchymal Tumors of the Esophagus

Gastrointestinal stromal tumors (GISTs)
Leiomyosarcoma
Liposarcoma
Fibrosarcoma
Myxofibrosarcoma
Rhabdomyosarcoma
Chondrosarcoma
Carcinosarcoma
Ewing's sarcoma
Synovial cell sarcoma
Malignant schwannoma

but certainly any enlarged nodes should be removed, as nodal metastases can rarely occur (4–6).

Patients need to be followed even with low-grade GISTs, as their malignant potential is variable and capricious. The tyrosine kinase inhibitor imatinib mesylate (Gleevec, Novartis Pharmaceuticals) is very active in treating this tumor and has been used as an adjuvant treatment, and for treatment of unresectable, recurrent, or metastatic disease.

LEIOMYOSARCOMA OF THE ESOPHAGUS

Leiomyosarcoma is probably the most common sarcoma of the esophagus, with about 200 reported cases (7). They are still quite rare, as illustrated by a recent Mayo Clinic series, in which only 19 cases were reported among 6,359 patients (0.3%) with an esophageal malignancy over a 76-year period (8). Most patients are older—in the sixth or seventh decade of life—and there is a slight male predominance (1.5:1). Leiomyosarcomas are commonly found in the middle and distal third of the esophagus, but also present in the cervical esophagus. About two-thirds are polypoid and one-third are infiltrative in gross appearance. Microscopy reveals interlacing whorls of spindle cells with increased mitoses. The cells are often pleomorphic and stain for desmin and smooth muscle antigen (SMA). Lymph node metastases are rare. The most common sites of metastases are the liver and lung. There have been rare reported cases of leiomyosarcomas arising from leiomyomas of the esophagus (7,9).

Patients usually present with dysphagia, but many are asymptomatic as well. Endoscopy usually reveals intact mucosa with a polypoid mass, though ulceration may be present in larger lesions. Endoscopic biopsies are usually non-diagnostic; CT scans usually show sizable tumors that are often inhomogeneous with areas of necrosis (10–12). The diagnosis is usually made at the time of resection. Long-term survival and apparent cure have been reported with resection. One report suggested a 5-year survival rate of 32% in collected series, while the Mayo Clinic report had a 47% 5-year survival (8, 13). Polypoid tumors and well-differentiated tumors are thought to have a better prognosis.

LIPOSARCOMA OF THE ESOPHAGUS

Liposarcomas are the most common soft tissue tumors, usually arising from the lower extremities or retroperitoneum. They are rare in the gastrointestinal tract, representing only about 1% of gastrointestinal liposarcomas. Only a handful of esophageal liposarcomas have been reported (14–16). The histologic types are well-differentiated, myxoid, round cell, and pleomorphic. Esophageal liposarcomas tend to be slow-growing polypoid tumors that typically present with dysphagia. Many are pedunculated, and more have been reported in the cervical esophagus than in the chest. The mucosa is normal at endoscopy, and typically a large polypoid mass is seen, suggesting slow, indolent growth. CT and magnetic resonance (MR) scans can demonstrate the fatty nature of the tumor as well as EUS. Since the mucosa is normal, endoscopic biopsies are unrevealing. Resection can be performed by esophagectomy or, in the case of pedunculated tumors, by local resection of the base of the lesion (14). Long-term survival has been reported.

FIBROSARCOMA OF THE ESOPHAGUS

Fibrosarcomas of the esophagus are very rare with, again, only a handful of cases reported (17). Patients present with a submucosal mass, typically with normal overlying mucosa. Leiomyoma is the usual preoperative diagnosis. Malignant fibroblastic cells are seen that are arranged in sweeping fascicles and stain for vimentin and CD34. Esophagectomy is usually performed once the definitive diagnosis has been made at operation. Long-term survival has been reported. Variants of fibrosarcoma have been reported, including inflammatory fibrosarcoma and myxofibrosarcoma (18,19).

OTHER ESOPHAGEAL SARCOMAS

A variety of other sarcomas of the esophagus have been rarely reported, including rhabdomyosarcoma, chondrosarcoma, carcinosarcoma, Ewing's sarcoma, and synovial cell sarcoma (20–25). Accurate diagnosis is difficult preoperatively, as with other sarcomas of the esophagus, and the treatment is resection when possible.

Immunohistochemic staining is often very important to precisely characterize the tumor.

MALIGNANT ESOPHAGEAL SCHWANNOMA

Schwannomas of the esophagus separate from the vagus nerve have been reported, including malignant ones. Fewer than 20 cases have been reported. At least 4 of 16 cases have been noted to be malignant with features of gross invasion, nuclear atypia, and increased mitoses (26,27). Patients present with a submucosal mass with intact overlying mucosa. The diagnosis is usually made after resection. Cells are spindle shaped and thin and are arranged in fascicles. The cells satin for S-100 protein and vimentin and are negative for desmin. At least 2 cases have been documented with nodal involvement (27).

References

1. Miettinen M, Sarlomo-Rikala M, Sobin LH, et al. Esophageal stromal tumors: a clinicopathologic, immunohistochemical, and molecular genetic study of 17 cases and comparison with esophageal leiomyomas and leiomyosarcomas. *Am J Surg Path.* 2000;24:211–222.
2. Masuda T, Toh Y, Kabashima A, et al. Overt lymph node metastases from a gastrointestinal stromal tumor of the esophagus. *J Thorac Cardiovasc Surg.* 2007;134:1810–1811.
3. Efron DT, Lillemoe KD. The current management of gastrointestinal stromal tumors. *Adv Surg.* 2005;39:193–221.
4. Manu N, Richard P, Howard S. Bleeding esophageal GIST. *Dis Esoph.* 2005;18:281–282.
5. Gouveia AM, Pimenta AP, Lopes JM, et al. Esophageal GIST: therapeutic implications of an uncommon presentation of a rare tumor. *Dis Esoph.* 2005;18:70–73.
6. Basoglu A, Kaya E, Celik B, et al. Giant gastrointestinal stromal tumor of the esophagus presenting with dyspnea. *J Thorac Cardiovasc Surg.* 2006;131:1198–1199.
7. Hatch GF III, Wertheimer-Hatch L, Hatch KF, et al. Tumors of the esophagus. *World J Surg.* 2000;24:401–411.
8. Rocco G, Trastek VF, Deschamps C, et al. Leiomyosarcoma of the esophagus: results of surgical treatment. *Ann Thorac Surg.* 1998;66:894–896.
9. Rahili A, D'Amata G, Avallone S, et al. Concomitant leiomyoma and leioyosarcoma of the esophagus. *J Exp Clin Cancer Res.* 2005;24:487–491.
10. Kimura H, Konishi K, Kawamura T, et al. Smooth muscle tumors of the esophagus: clinicopathological findings in six patients. *Dis Esoph.* 1999;12:77–81.
11. Jutley RS, Gray RD, MacKenzie JM, et al. A leiomyosarcoma of the esophagus presenting incidentally without dysphagia. *Eur J Cardiothorac Surg.* 2002;21: 127–129.
12. Pramesh CS, Pantvaidya GH, Moonim MT, et al. Leiomyosarcoma of the esophagus. *Dis Esoph.* 2003;16:142–144.
13. Koga H, Iida M, Suekane H, et al. Rapidly growing esophageal leiomyosarcoma: case report and review of the literature. *Abdom Imaging.* 1995;20:15–19.
14. Temes R, Quinn P, Davis M, et al. Endoscopic resection of esophageal liposarcoma. *J Thorac Cardiovasc Surg.* 1998;116:365–367.
15. Brehant O, Pessaux P, Hennekinne-Mucci S, et al. Giant pedunculated liposarcoma of the esophagus. *J Am Coll Surg.* 2004;198:320–321.
16. Liakakos TD, Troupis TG, Tzathas C, et al. Primary liposarcoma of esophagus: a case report. *World J Gastroenterol.* 2006;12:1149–1152.
17. Caldwell CB, Bains MS, Burt M. Unusual malignant neoplasms of the esophagus: oat cell carcinoma, melanoma, and sarcoma. *J Thorac Cardiovasc Surg.* 1991;101:100–107.
18. Magovern CJ, Mack CA, Gu M, et al. Primary inflammatory fibrosarcoma of the esophagus. *Ann Thorac Surg.* 1996;62:1848–1850.
19. Song HK, Miller JI. Primary myxofibrosarcoma of the esophagus. *J Thorac Cardiovasc Surg.* 2002;124:196–197.
20. Thorek P, Neiman BM. Rhabdomyosarcoma of the esophagus. *J Thorac Surg.* 1950;20:77–89.
21. Yaghami I, Ghahremani GG. Chondrosarcoma of the esophagus. *Am J Roentgenol.* 1976;126:1175–1177.
22. Ohtaka M, Kumasaka T, Nowbukawa B, et al. Carcinosarcoma of the esophagus characterized by myoepithelial and ductal differentiation. *Pathol Int.* 2002;52:657–663.
23. Maesawa C, Iijma S, Sato N, et al. Esophageal extraskeletal Ewing's sarcoma. *Hum Pathol.* 2002;33:130–132.
24. Butori C, Hofman V, Attias R, et al. Diagnosis of primary esophageal synovial sarcoma by demonstration of t(X;18) translocation: a case report. *Virchows Arch.* 2006;449:262–267.
25. Perch SJ, Soffen EM, Whittington R, et al. Esophageal sarcomas. *Surg Oncol.* 1991;48:194–198.
26. Saito R, Kitamura M, Suzuki H, et al. Esophageal schwannoma. *Ann Thorac Surg.* 2000;69:1947–1949.
27. Sanchez A, Mariangel P, Carrasco C, et al. Malignant nerve sheath tumor of the esophagus (malignant esophageal schwannoma). *Gastroenterol Hepatol.* 2004;27:467–469.

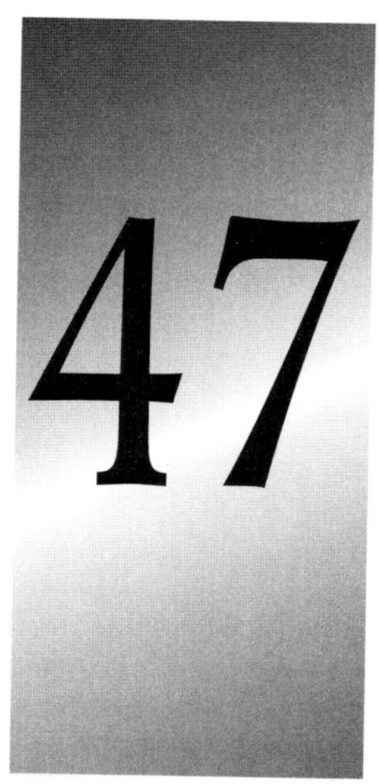

47 Malignant: Lymphoma

Abraham J. Wu
Karyn A. Goodman

Involvement of the esophagus by lymphoma is uncommon and is more likely to occur secondarily as a result of direct extension from mediastinal adenopathy. Primary esophageal lymphoma, in which the disease arises in the wall of the esophagus, is particularly rare. Little published data exist to guide management of this entity, apart from sporadic case reports and small series. However, esophageal lymphoma should not be overlooked in the differential diagnosis of dysphagia and may be particularly prevalent in patients with HIV infection or other causes of chronic immunosuppression. Reported approaches to esophageal lymphoma treatment are consistent with strategies for lymphomas in general.

EPIDEMIOLOGY

Carcinomas account for the vast majority of esophageal malignancies. Lymphomatous involvement of the esophagus is comparatively rare, accounting for less than 1% of all malignant tumors of the esophagus. Lymphomas often arise in the gastrointestinal tract, most commonly in the stomach, small and large intestines; the esophagus is involved in less than 1% of cases (1,2). In 1 series of 1,467 extranodal lymphomas, only 3 cases of primary esophageal lymphoma were recorded (3). Secondary involvement of the esophagus through contiguous spread from mediastinal or cervical lymph nodes is also more likely to be observed than primary esophageal lymphoma. In a retrospective review from the Mayo Clinic, 27 cases of lymphomatous involvement of the esophagus were identified (4). Only 3 were primary esophageal lymphomas; the remainder occurred at relapse or due to contiguous spread from mediastinal adenopathy.

Human immunodeficiency virus (HIV) infection, which is associated with an increased risk of non-Hodgkin's lymphoma, also appears to be a risk factor for the development of primary esophageal lymphoma (5,6). Fewer than 35 cases of primary esophageal lymphoma, many of which have been diagnosed in HIV-infected patients, have been reported in the modern medical literature (5,7,8). Esophageal lymphoma has also been reported in conjunction with chronic immunosuppression for hepatitis C (9). The role of Epstein-Barr virus in the development of esophageal lymphoma is unknown (10).

Sample sizes are too small to reliably assess demographic trends, although males may be more commonly affected than females. Also, esophageal lymphoma in HIV-infected patients may present at a younger age than those not associated with HIV infection, with a mean age of 40 years observed for the former group (5) and 60 years for the latter (11).

PATHOLOGY

Lymphomas are classified based on their lymphocytic origin. Hodgkin's lymphoma arises from a precursor B-cell called the *Reed-Sternberg cell*, which can be identified by its classic "binucleate" appearance and positive staining for cell surface markers CD30 and CD15 (Figure 47.1). Non-Hodgkin's lymphomas arise from a monoclonal expansion of malignant B- or T-cells. There are multiple subtypes of B- or T-cell malignancies, each with distinguishing cell surface markers and cytogenetics. The most common B-cell surface marker is CD20, while the T-cell lineage can be identified by the presence of CD2, CD3, and CD7. Several classification schemes have been developed for NHL, the most recent of which is the World Health Organization classification (Table 47.1).

Non-Hodgkin's lymphoma is the predominant histology of esophageal lymphoma, accounting for 89% of cases in the Mayo series, compared to 11% with Hodgkin's lymphoma (4) Among the reported cases of primary non-Hodgkin's lymphoma, large B-cell lymphomas appear predominant (Figure 47.2) (9,12). However, T-cell non-Hodgkin's lymphomas have also been reported (12,13).

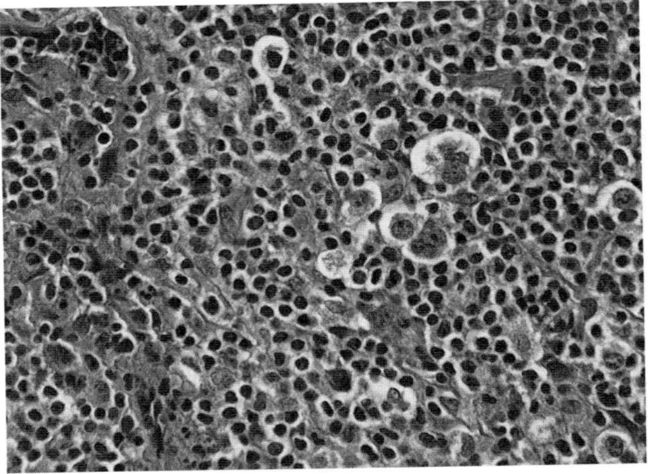

FIGURE 47.1

Hodgkin's lymphoma, nodular sclerosing type.

TABLE 47.1
World Health Organization Classification of Non-Hodgkin's Lymphoma

B-cell neoplasms
- *Precursor B-cell neoplasms*
  - B-cell lymphoblastic lymphoma/leukemia
- *Peripheral B-cell neoplasms*
  - CLL, SLL
  - Mantle cell lymphoma
  - Follicular center lymphoma (grade 1-small cell, 2-mixed, 3-large)
  - Marginal zone lymphoma
    - Extranodal (MALT) type +/– monocytoid B-cell
    - Nodal +/– monocytoid B-cell
    - Splenic
  - Hairy cell leukemia
  - Plasmacytoma/plasma cell myeloma
  - Diffuse large B-cell lymphoma
  - Burkitt's lymphoma, Burkitt's-like high-grade B-cell lymphoma

T-cell neoplasms
- *Precursor T-cell neoplasms*
  - T-cell lymphoblastic lymphoma/leukemia
- *Peripheral T-cell & NK-cell neoplasms*
  - T-cell CLL
  - Large granular lymphocyte leukemia
  - Mycosis fungoides/Sezary syndrome
  - Peripheral T-cell lymphoma
  - Angioimmunoblastic T-cell lymphoma
  - Angiocentric lymphoma
  - Intestinal T-cell lymphoma
  - Adult T-cell lymphoma/leukemia
  - Anaplastic large cell lymphoma CD30+

Extra-nodal marginal zone B-cell lymphoma of mucosa-associated lymphoid tissue (MALT type lymphoma), which is typically associated with *Helicobacter pylori* infection of the stomach, has recently been reported in the esophagus (Figure 47.3) (14). In these cases, no consistent relationship with *H. pylori* infection has been established (14,15).

CLINICAL PRESENTATION

Dysphagia is the most common presenting symptom of esophageal lymphoma, being present in 89% of patients in 1 series (4). Other symptoms may include odynophagia, chest pain, abdominal pain, weight loss, and hoarseness. The onset of such symptoms is often insidious, with progression of dysphagia over months to years (16). Serious complications such as tracheoesophageal fistula may arise from destructive involvement of lymphoma (17).

There appear to be no characteristic physical examination findings for primary esophageal lymphoma. Palpable lymphadenopathy would suggest that esophageal involvement by lymphoma is secondary. Primary lymphoma can arise in all segments of the esophagus (11). Secondary involvement of the distal esophagus, however, is particularly common from contiguous spread from the stomach (18).

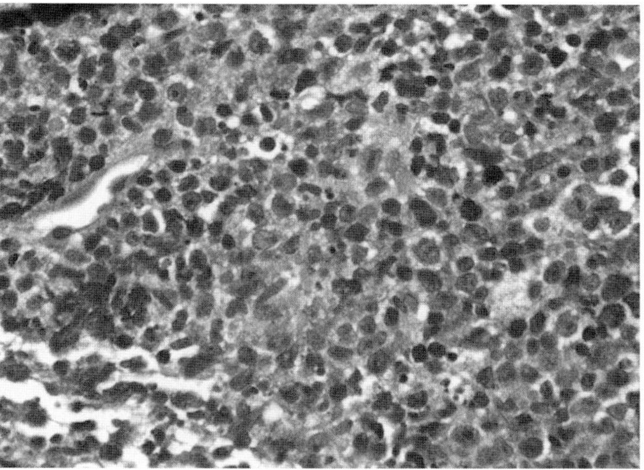

FIGURE 47.2

Diffuse large B-cell lymphoma.

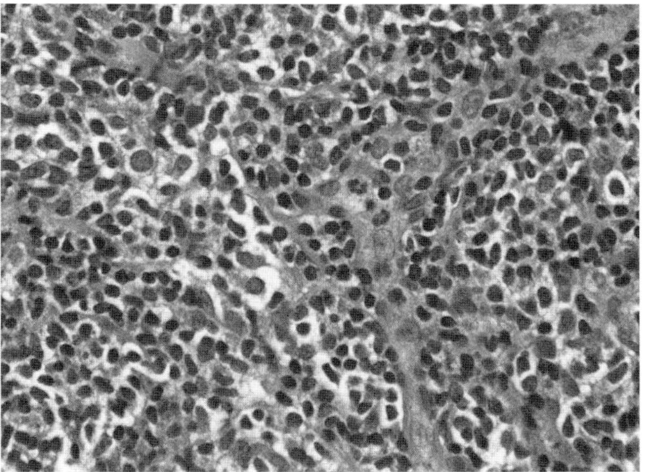

FIGURE 47.3

Marginal zone lymphoma.

DIAGNOSIS

The rarity of this disease, combined with the absence of specific signs and symptoms, makes the diagnosis of esophageal lymphoma a challenge. Investigators have typically invoked the criteria set out by Dawson to distinguish primary esophageal lymphoma from secondary involvement. These criteria include: no superficial lymphadenopathy, no apparent mediastinal adenopathy, normal white blood cell count, no liver or spleen involvement, and primary lesion in the esophagus with involvement of only the regional nodes (19).

Radiographic manifestations of esophageal lymphoma are again varied and nonspecific. Commonly, it is visualized as an irregular narrowing of the distal esophagus, particularly when caused by local extension from gastric tumor (20). Barium swallow or computed tomography of the chest may reveal stricture formation, intramural mass, or polypoid protrusion (21). Positron-emission tomography, which is now widely used in the staging of lymphoma, can also be incorporated into the work-up of suspected esophageal lymphoma.

Endoscopic ultrasound may assist in characterizing the submucosal masses and in guiding fine-needle aspiration for pathologic analysis. The ultrasound appearance of esophageal lymphoma may demonstrate a heterogeneous tumor with mixed isoechoic and hypoechoic areas (22).

Ultimately, diagnosis must be established through biopsy of malignant tissue, which is typically obtained with fiberoptic endoscopy of the upper aerodigestive tract. However, endoscopic biopsy may yield only normal or chronically inflamed tissue without evidence of malignancy, which has led to reported false-negative rates in excess of 30% (21). Sampling error is the predominant cause: primary esophageal lymphoma usually arises in submucosal lymphoid patches, which are not always reliably visualized or accessible by biopsy forceps. Consequently, histologic diagnosis may require repeat biopsy or even surgical excision.

TREATMENT

No standardized approach to the treatment of esophageal lymphoma has been established. However, surgery, chemotherapy, and radiation therapy have all been utilized, in varying combinations. Secondary involvement of the esophagus by lymphoma is typically managed with chemotherapy (11). Primary esophageal lymphoma, however, has been managed with any combination of local and systemic modalities. Surgical resection may be required to establish a firm pathologic diagnosis or to manage complications related to locally advanced disease. However, as with lymphomas in general, most reports have advocated the use of chemotherapy and/or radiotherapy as the initial therapeutic approach.

A recent review of patients with non-Hodgkin's lymphoma of the esophagus showed that 7 of 13 patients underwent radiotherapy, with or without subsequent chemotherapy (23). External beam doses in the range of 40Gy have been employed (12). The choice of chemotherapy regimens reflects standard treatment for lymphoma, with the CHOP regimen (cyclophosphamide, vincristine, prednisone, and doxorubicin) being particularly widely used (23,13). Older series have reported the successful use of MOPP chemotherapy (meclorethamine, procarbazine, vincristine, prednisone) in cases of primary Hodgkin lymphoma (24). However, this regimen has been replaced by less toxic chemotherapeutic combinations such as ABVD (doxorubicin, bleomycin, vinblastine, dacarbazine) and Stanford V (doxorubicin, vinblastine, mechlorethamine, vincristine, bleomycin, etoposide, prednisone).

PROGNOSIS

The paucity and diversity of reported cases of esophageal lymphoma makes prognostic generalizations difficult. One series of patients with lymphomatous involvement of the esophagus included 2 patients with primary non-Hodgkin's lymphoma, both of whom achieved long-term remission with radiation followed by chemotherapy (4). On the other hand, in 1 series of 6 patients, 2 of whom had HIV infection, only 1 of the patients achieved survival in excess of 14 months (23). Encouraging results of therapy for Hodgkin's lymphoma of the esophagus have been reported, with 1 review showing survival of 5 years or more in 4 of 6 patients, all of whom underwent active treatment with 1 or more modalities (24). The successful management of patients with esophageal lymphomas depends on the accurate diagnosis of the histologic subtype, as treatment recommendations vary substantially between Hodgkin's lymphoma and non-Hodgkin's lymphoma, and even within the subtypes of non-Hodgkin's lymphoma. Clinical outcomes are related to the type of lymphoma involving the esophagus, with MALT lymphomas and Hodgkin's lymphomas associated with better prognoses than diffuse large B-cell or T-cell sub-types.

References

1. Herrmann R, Panahon AM, Barcos MP, et al. Gastrointestinal involvement in non-Hodgkin's lymphoma. *Cancer*. 1980;46:215–222.
2. Rosenberg SA, Diamond HD, Jaslowitz B, et al. Lymphosarcoma: a review of 1269 cases. *Medicine (Baltimore)*. 1961;40:31–84.
3. Freeman C, Berg JW, Cutler SJ. Occurrence and prognosis of extranodal lymphomas. *Cancer*. 1972;29:252–260.
4. Orvidas LJ, McCaffrey TV, Lewis JE, et al. Lymphoma involving the esophagus. *Ann Otol Rhinol Laryngol*. 1994;103:843–848.
5. Weeratunge CN, Bolivar HH, Anstead GM, et al. Primary esophageal lymphoma: a diagnostic challenge in acquired immunodeficiency syndrome—two case reports and review. *South Med J*. 2004;97:383–387.
6. Hamed KA, Hoffman MS. Primary esophageal lymphoma in AIDS. *AIDS Patient Care STDS*. 1998;12:5–9.
7. Hosaka S, Nakamura N, Akamatsu T, et al. A case of primary low grade mucosa associated lymphoid tissue (MALT) lymphoma of the oesophagus. *Gut*. 2002;51:281–284.
8. Coppens E, El Nakadi I, Nagy N, et al. Primary Hodgkin's lymphoma of the esophagus. *Am J Roentgenol*. 2003;180:1335–1337.
9. Golioto M, McGrath K. Primary lymphoma of the esophagus in a chronically immunosuppressed patient with hepatitis C infection: case report and review of the literature. *Am J Med Sci*. 2001;321:203–205.
10. Valbuena JR, Retamal Y, Bernal C, et al. Epstein-Barr virus-associated primary lymphoepithelioma-like carcinoma of the esophagus. *Diagn Mol Pathol*. 2007;16:27–31.
11. Gupta NM, Goenka MK, Jindal A, et al. Primary lymphoma of the esophagus. *J Clin Gastroenterol*. 1996;23:203–206.
12. George MK, Ramachandran V, Ramanan SG, et al. Primary esophageal T-cell non-Hodgkin's lymphoma. *Indian J Gastroenterol*. 2005;24:119–120.
13. Kim JH, Lee JH, Lee J, et al. Primary NK-/T-cell lymphoma of the gastrointestinal tract: clinical characteristics and endoscopic findings. *Endoscopy*. 2007;39:156–160.
14. Chung JJ, Kim MJ, Kie JH, et al. Mucosa-associated lymphoid tissue lymphoma of the esophagus coexistent with bronchus-associated lymphoid tissue lymphoma of the lung. *Yonsei Med J*. 2005;46:562–566.
15. Shim CS, Lee JS, Kim JO, et al. A case of primary esophageal B-cell lymphoma of MALT type, presenting as a submucosal tumor. *J Korean Med Sci*. 2003;18:120–124.
16. Salerno CT, Kreykes NS, Rego A, et al. Primary esophageal lymphoma: a diagnostic challenge. *Ann Thorac Surg*. 1998;66:1418-1420.
17. Perry RR, Rosenberg RK, Pass HI. Tracheoesophageal fistula in the patient with lymphoma: case report and review of the literature. *Surgery*. 1989;105:770–777.
18. Carnovale RL, Goldstein HM, Zornoza J, et al. Radiologic manifestations of esophageal lymphoma. *Am J Roentgenol*. 1977;128:751–754.
19. Dawson IM, Cornes JS, Morson BC. Primary malignant lymphoid tumors of the intestinal tract. Report of 37 cases with a study of factors influencing prognosis. *Br J Surg*. 1961;49:80–89.
20. Gaskin CM, Low VH. Isolated primary non-Hodgkin's lymphoma of the esophagus. *Am J Roentgenol*. 2001;176:551–552.
21. Doki T, Hamada S, Murayama H, et al. Primary malignant lymphoma of the esophagus. A case report. *Endoscopy*. 1984;16:189–192.
22. Soon MS, Yen HH, Soon A, et al. Primary esophageal B-cell lymphoma: evaluation by EUS. *Gastrointest Endosc*. 2005;61:901–903.
23. Chadha KS, Hernandez-Ilizaliturri FJ, et al. Primary esophageal lymphoma: case series and review of the literature. *Dig Dis Sci*. 2006;51:77–83.
24. Taal BG, Van Heerde P, Somers S. Isolated primary oesophageal involvement by lymphoma: a rare cause of dysphagia: two case histories and a review of other published data. *Gut*. 1993;34:994–998.

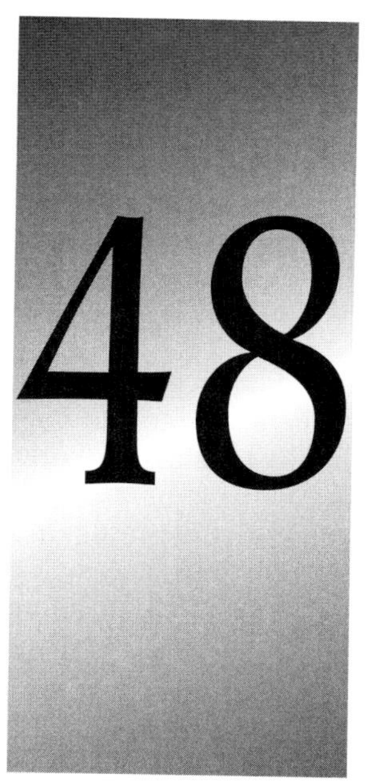

48 Malignant: Metastatic

Sai Yendamuri
Jeffrey H. Lee
David C. Rice

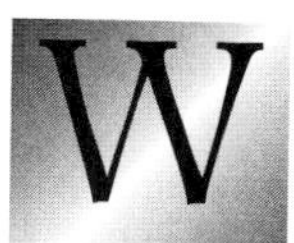

While primary esophageal cancer, in particular adenocarcinoma, is becoming increasingly common in the United States, the incidence of secondary malignancy to the esophagus remains rare. The most common mode of secondary involvement of the esophagus is by direct extension of primary cancer elsewhere in the chest or in the abdomen. The incidence of distant cancer metastasizing to the esophagus is rarer still, especially in clinical series. This chapter will review the pathology, clinical presentation, modes of diagnosis, and treatment options for patients with secondary tumors to the esophagus that have metastasized from primary tumors elsewhere.

PATHOLOGY

While the ante-mortem diagnosis of metastatic disease to the esophagus is exceedingly rare, autopsy studies suggest that the overall incidence of metastases to the esophagus in patients dying of any kind of cancer is approximately 6% (1). The most common histology in autopsy series performed in North America is breast cancer (2). For example, Holyoke et al. reported that as many as 9% of women dying of breast cancer had foci of tumor within the esophagus (3). Breast cancer is also probably the most common clinically reported metastatic disease to the esophagus, and in particular, lobular carcinoma appears to have a predisposition to metastasize to this location (4). In the most recently reported autopsy series, which was performed in Japan, 1,835 cases were reviewed for possible metastatic esophageal disease in patients dying of cancer (1). Contrary to North American series, lung cancer was most common primary histology, followed by breast cancer. In this study, 11% of patients who died from lung cancer developed metastases to the esophagus. In contrast, data from a large U.S. autopsy series including 5,000 cases revealed that only 4% of patients dying of lung cancer had metastases to the esophagus (5). In the recent Japanese study, the most common histologic subtype of lung cancer metastatic to the esophagus was adenocarcinoma, followed by small cell carcinoma. Aside from lung and breast cancer, there are numerous clinical reports of other tumors metastatic to the esophagus, including cancers of the endometrium, kidney, prostate, colon, and malignant melanoma. In fact, the first documented case of metastases to the esophagus was reported by Gross and Friedman in 1942 in a patient with prostate cancer (6). Table 48.1 lists includes case reports and cases series of malignant disease metastatic to the esophagus.

As mentioned previously, the most common mode of spread to esophagus is by contiguous extension of a primary cancer in adjacent organs. This should be

TABLE 48.1
Case Reports of Primary Tumors with Metastases to the Esophagus

Primary cancer	Reference
Lung cancer	Abrams et al. (2), Mizobuchi et al. (1), Simchuk and Low (8), Oka et al. (19)
Breast cancer	Rampado et al. (10), Varanasi et al. (14), Ayantunde et al. (23), Borst and Ingold (4), Shimada et al. (20)
Renal cancer	Trentino et al. (24), de los Monteros-Sanchez et al. (22)
Malignant melanoma	Eng et al. (25)
Endometrial carcinoma	Zarian et al. (26)
Ovarian cancer	Mizobuchi et al. (1), Haney and D'Amico (21)
Colorectal cancer	Kagaya et al. (11)
Prostate cancer	Gross and Friedman (6)

classified as direct invasion versus true metastatic disease. A review of 62 cases of secondary esophageal neoplasms estimated that 45% were the result of direct extension, 36% were due to lymphatic spread from mediastinal nodes, and 19% occurred from hematogenous seeding (7). The majority of lymphatogenous metastases develop either in the esophageal submucosa, most likely facilitated by the extensive submucosal lymphatic plexus, or in the periesophageal lymphatic tissue and secondarily invade the esophageal muscle. Differentiation between the 2 mechanisms is difficult and therefore the term *secondary* esophageal cancer may be more accurate than *metastatic* esophageal cancer. Mucosal involvement by secondary esophageal cancer is unusual (8).

CLINICAL PRESENTATION

The most common clinical presentation of disease metastatic to the esophagus is progressive dysphagia. In most clinical series, the duration of onset of dysphagia after diagnosis of the primary malignancy is impressively long. This is particularly true in cases of breast carcinoma where the mean interval from treatment of the primary tumor to the development of dysphagia has been reported to be as long as 7 to 10 years (9,10). However, in cases of patients with lung carcinoma, the interval between the presentation of the primary tumor and esophageal metastases is usually shorter, and it is not uncommon that dysphagia symptoms lead to the diagnosis of the primary lung cancer.

The usual mode of diagnosis follows the typical work-up of dysphagia. Esophagograms generally show a tight smooth stricture with normal mucosal pattern and indeed the appearance may resemble a benign esophageal stricture. Involvement of a short segment is the rule; however, secondary cancer arising from the breast may occasionally involve a long segment of the esophagus. Such strictures may taper asymmetrically and are usually located in the middle third of the esophagus (9,10). In a series of 25 cases of secondary esophageal malignancy of breast origin, Rampado et al. reported stricture location to be in the upper, middle, and lower esophagus in 20%, 52%, and 28%, respectively (10). Similarly, in a small series of secondary esophageal cancers of breast and lung origin, Simchuk and Low reported tumor location to be in the mid esophagus in 4 out of 6 patients (8). When tumor infiltration progresses and the esophagus becomes circumferentially involved, the radiographic findings may mimic primary esophageal cancer. Computed tomography (CT) scanning consistently demonstrates esophageal wall thickening but usually without an endoluminal or extrinsic mass, however, is not diagnostic. Data regarding the use of positron-emission tomography (PET) in the diagnosis of these metastases are scarce, but at least 2 case reports have demonstrated that secondary esophageal cancers show increased uptake (10,11).

Esophagoscopy typically reveals an intramural stricture with smooth, normal-appearing overlying mucosa. In fact, this is a hallmark of metastatic disease to the esophagus and this entity must be suspected in any patient with this endoscopic feature with a compatible clinical history. Occasionally erythematous mucosal will be present; however, mucosal biopsies obtained at EGD rarely yield a diagnosis. Endoscopic ultrasound (EUS) may further delineate the anatomy and may allow histologic diagnosis via transesophageal fine needle aspiration (FNA) (12). The usual appearance at EUS is esophageal wall thickening mainly involving the submucosa or muscularis propria layers with normal mucosa (Figure 48.1). Sobel et al. established diagnoses, using EUS-FNA, in all 5 cases of patients with metastatic breast cancer who had esophageal wall thickening, and in 6 of 7 patients who had hypoechoic and/or enlarged periesophageal lymph nodes. A recent case report described the use of EUS and endoscopic mucosal resection (EMR) to provide tissue diagnosis in a patient with secondary esophageal cancer (13); however, given the proficiency and apparent accuracy of EUS-FNA, it is uncertain whether the more invasive procedure of EMR would be justified for routine use, especially in cases where the major involvement is

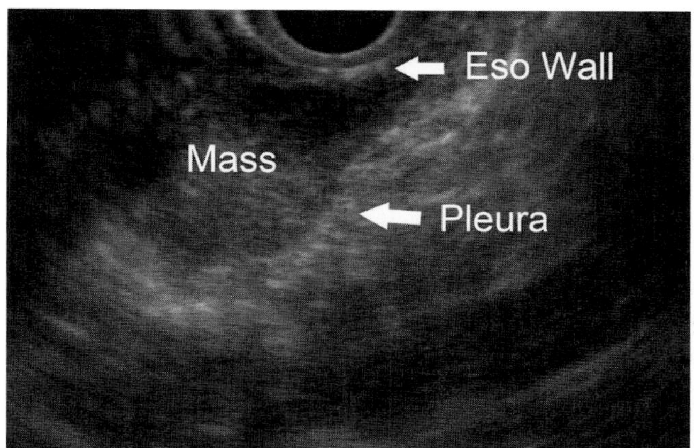

FIGURE 48.1

Patient with breast cancer metastasis to esophagus. Endoscopic ultrasound shows an intact mucosa and submucosa with thickened esophageal wall and paraesophageal mass.

in the submucosal and muscularis propria layers with normal mucosa.

Biopsy material obtained aids in determination of the site of the primary tumor, and immumohistochemic analysis for estrogen and progesterone receptors, c-erb, CA-125, as well as thyroid transcription factor-1 (TTF-1) may be useful to confirm breast, ovarian, or lung cancer as the original primary. As secondary tumors progress, invasion of adjacent organs such as the trachea and bronchus may occur resulting in hemoptysis, stridor, or tracheoesophageal fistula in addition to worsening dysphagia (Figures 48.2 and 48.3).

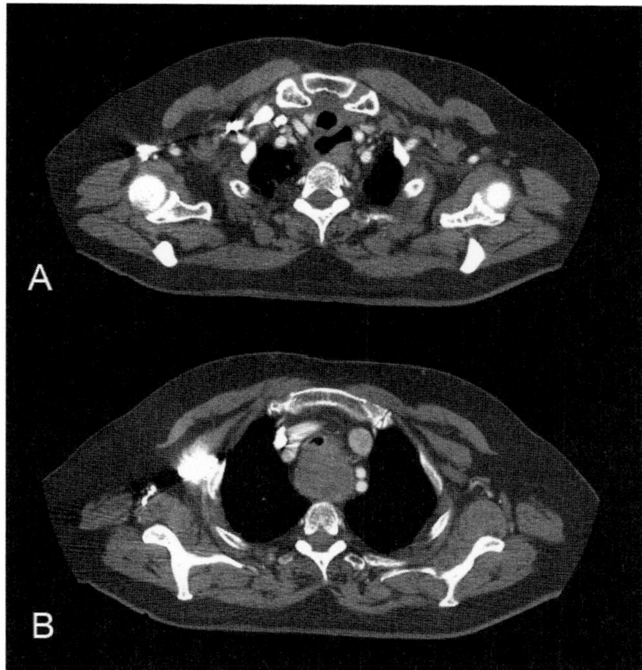

FIGURE 48.2

CT of 64-year-old male with anaplastic thyroid cancer metastatic to the esophagus who presented with stridor due to tracheal invasion. (A) Esophageal wall thickening with proximal dilatation; (B) Tumor mass invading posterior trachea with luminal compromise.

TREATMENT

Therapy for secondary cancers of the esophagus is directed toward both local treatment of symptomatic strictures and therapy for the primary tumor. The latter will depend on the histology of the primary tumor, prior therapeutic endeavors, and patient performance status, but in general will involve systemic chemotherapy or hormonal treatment. Local therapeutic options for luminal narrowing may involve any of the various treatment modalities available for the management of esophageal strictures in general and can include balloon dilation, endoluminal ablative therapy, laser fulgaration, electrocoagulation, argon plasma coagulatgion (APC), photodynamic therapy (PDT), and /or stent placement. These can be used in combination with appropriate therapy for the primary malignancy.

Endoscopic options include sequential endoscopic dilation using either hydrostatic pressure or serial mechanical dilators, and placement of self-expanding stents. Caution must be exercised in the use of endoscopic dilation as several reports have noted a high rate of perforation in the use of these treatments (10,14,15). It is best to be conservative when dilating malignant strictures, and dilation to a luminal diameter of 10 mm is usually sufficient to allow passage of food. Furthermore, placement of covered self-expanding stents will usually provide further radial expansion over time. Use of non-covered stents is to be discouraged as there have been reports of tumor in-growth and stenosis despite initially intact mucosa (11).

The use of radiation therapy for treatment of secondary esophageal malignancy has been infrequently reported. Of 25 patients with metastatic breast cancer to the esophagus reported by Rampado et al., only 2 received radiation therapy as a part of treatment (type and dose not specified) (10). Both patients had prolonged initial tumor-free intervals (14 and 21 years respectively) and had survival of 2.2 and 6.3 years, respectively, following treatment. Experience with endolunimal brachytherapy for palliative management of malignant strictures in inoperable esophageal cancer has shown efficacy in dysphagia in 50% to 80% of patients (16,17). A recent randomized trial from the Netherlands

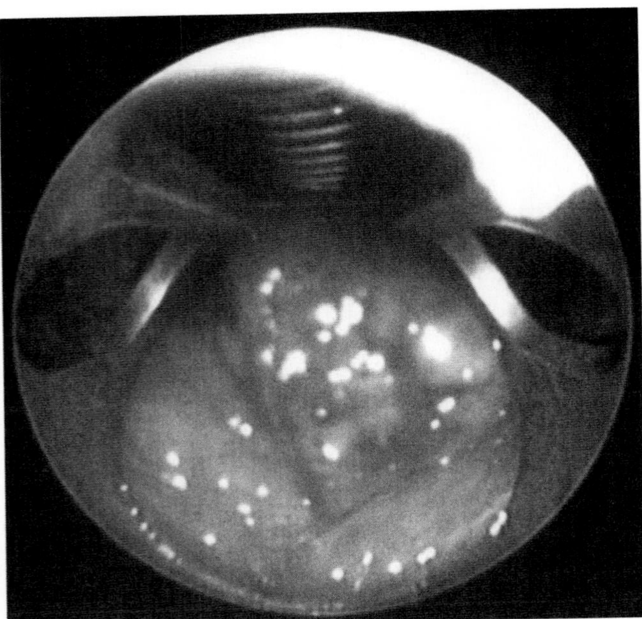

FIGURE 48.3

Rigid bronchoscopy showing secondary esophageal tumor invading posterior wall of trachea. The patient has been intubated with an armoured 6 mm endotracheal tube (arrow) to maintain the airway. Laser fulgaration and endotracheal stent placement was subsequently performed.

showed that brachytherapy was associated with longer dysphagia-free survival, better quality of life, and was less expensive compared to covered stent (Ultraflex, Boston Scientific) placement for malignant esophageal stricture (18). Persistent or recurrent stenosis can occur in as many as 40% of patients, which is similar to that seen with endoluminal stents, and perforation rates range between 5% and 10% (16,17).

For select patients with isolated secondary cancers of the esophagus, surgical resection has also been reported (1,11,19–22). However, the presence of submucosal esophageal metastatic disease from a distant primary is usually indicative of widespread metastatic disease, and the patient is unlikely to respond to local therapy alone. Nevertheless, in situations where the disease is confirmed by other imaging studies to be localized to the esophagus and the disease-free interval is long, esophageal resection may be a viable option, as it provides good palliation and may occasionally prolong survival. Mizobuchi et al. performed esophagectomy on 3 patients with metastatic disease to the esophagus. A patient with lung cancer with synchronous metastasis to the esophagus died after 6 months; however, the other 2 patients (with breast and ovarian cancer) had longer metastasis-free intervals (7 and 16 months respectively) and survived 4 and 14 years, respectively, after esophagectomy (1). Others have reported better than expected survival, particularly in patients with long disease-free intervals (Table 48.2).

CONCLUSION

Esophageal metastatic disease from distant primary cancer is exceedingly rare. The most common primaries that metastasize to the esophagus are lung and breast cancers, but numerous other histologic types have been reported. This entity must be suspected in patients with cancer with

TABLE 48.2
Case Reports of Esophageal Resection for Secondary Cancers of the Esophagus

Author	Year	Primary tumor	Tumor-free interval	Treatment	Survival	Vital status
Shimada et al. (20)	1989	Breast	9	Esophagectomy	5	Alive
Oka et al. (19)	1993	Lung	5	Esophagectomy	2	Alive
Mizobuchi et al. (1)	1997	Ovarian	16	Esophagectomy + pre-op XRT	14	Dead
Mizobuchi et al. (1)	1997	Breast	7	Esophagectomy	4	Dead
Mizobuchi et al. (1)	1997	Lung	0	Esophagectomy	0.6	Dead
Haney and D'Amico (21)	2004	Ovarian	4	Esophagectomy	NR	NR
de los Monteros-Sanchez et al. (22)	2004	Kidney	NR	Esophagectomy	1	Dead
Kagaya et al. (11)	2007	Colon	1	Esophagectomy	0.5	Alive

an esophageal stricture, normal-appearing mucosa, and a previous history of malignancy elsewhere. Along with therapy for the primary malignancy, palliative options include endoscopic dilation, stenting, and, in selected patients, surgical resection. Therapy should be individualized the overall prognosis of the patient.

References

1. Mizobuchi S, Tachimori Y, Kato H, et al. Metastatic esophageal tumors from distant primary lesions: report of three esophagectomies and study of 1835 autopsy cases. *Jap J Clin Oncol.* 1997;27:410–414.
2. Abrams HL, Spiro R, Goldstein N. Metastases in carcinoma; analysis of 1000 autopsied cases. *Cancer.* 1950;3:74–85.
3. Holyoke ED, Nemeto T, Dao TL. Esophageal metastases and dysphagia in patients with carcinoma of the breast. *J Surg Oncol.* 1969;1:97–107.
4. Borst MJ, Ingold JA. Metastatic patterns of invasive lobular versus invasive ductal carcinoma of the breast. *Surgery.* 1993;114:637–641; discussion 641–632.
5. Luomanen RKJ, Watson WL. Autopsy findings. In: Watson WL, ed. *Lung Cancer: A Study of Five Thousand Memorial Hospital Cases.* St Louis: Mosby, 1968:505–510.
6. Gross P, Friedman LJ. Obstructing secondary carcinoma of the esophagus. *Arch Pathol.* 1942;33:3.
7. Agha FP. Secondary neoplasms of the esophagus. *Gastrointest Radiol.* 1987;12:187–193.
8. Simchuk EJ, Low DE. Direct esophageal metastasis from a distant primary tumor is a submucosal process: a review of six cases. *Dis Esoph.* 2001;14:247–250.
9. Anderson MF, Harell GS. Secondary esophageal tumors. *AJR Am J Roentgenol.* 1980;135:1243–1246.
10. Rampado S, Ruol A, Guido M, et al. Mediastinal carcinosis involving the esophagus in breast cancer: the "breast-esophagus" syndrome: report on 25 cases and guidelines for diagnosis and treatment. *Ann of Surg.* 2007;246:316–322.
11. Kagaya H, Kitayama J, Hidemura A, et al. Metastatic esophageal tumor from cecal carcinoma. *Jpn J Clin Oncol.* 2007;37:628–631.
12. Sobel JM, Lai R, Mallery S, et al. The utility of EUS-guided FNA in the diagnosis of metastatic breast cancer to the esophagus and the mediastinum. *Gastrointest Endosc.* 2005;61:416–420.
13. Sunada F, Yamamoto H, Hanatsuka K et al. A case of esophageal stricture due to metastatic breast cancer diagnosed by endoscopic mucosal resection. *Jpn J Clin Oncol.* 2005;35:483–486.
14. Varanasi RV, Saltzman JR, Krims P, et al. Breast carcinoma metastatic to the esophagus: clinicopathological and management features of four cases, and literature review. *Am J Gastroenterol.* 1995;90:1495–1499.
15. Anaya DA, Mujun Y, Riyad KJ. Esophageal perforation in a patient with metastatic breast cancer to esophagus. *Ann Thorac Surg.* 2006;81:1136–1138.
16. Sharma V, Mahantshetty U, Dinshaw KA, et al. Palliation of advanced/recurrent esophageal carcinoma with high-dose-rate brachytherapy. *Int J Rad Oncol Biol Phys.* 2002;52:310–315.
17. Sur RK, Levin V, Donde B, et al. Prospective randomized trial of HDR brachytherapy as a sole modality in palliation of advanced esophageal carcinoma—an International Atomic Energy Agency study. *Int J Rad Oncol Biol Phys.* 2002;53:127–133.
18. Horns MYV, Steyerberg EW, Eijkenboom WMH, et al. Single-dose brachytherapy versus metal stent placement for palliation of dysphagia from oesophageal cancer: multicenter randomised trial. *Lancet.* 2004;364:1497–1504.
19. Oka T, Ayabe H, Kawahara K, et al. Esophagectomy for metastatic carcinoma of the esophagus from lung cancer. *Cancer.* 1993;71:2958–2961.
20. Shimada Y, Imamura M, Tobe T. Successful esophagectomy for metastatic carcinoma of the esophagus from breast cancer—a case report. *Surg Today.* 1989;19:82–85
21. Haney JC, D'Amico TA. Transhiatal esophagogastrectomy for an isolated ovarian cancer metastasis to the esophagus. *J Thorac Cardiovasc Surg.* 2004;127: 1835–1836.
22. de los Monteros-Sanchez AE, Medina-Franco H, Arista-Nasr J, et al. Resection of an esophageal metastasis from a renal cell carcinoma. *Hepatogastroenterology.* 2004;51:163–164.
23. Ayantunde AA, Agrawal A, Parsons SL, et al. Esophagogastric cancers secondary to a breast primary tumor do not require resection. *World J Surg.* 2007;31:1597–1601.
24. Trentino P, Rapacchietta S, Silvestri F, et al. Esophageal metastasis from clear cell carcinoma of the kidney. *Am J Gastroenterol.* 1997;92:1381–1382.
25. Eng J, Pradhan GN, Sabanathan S, et al. Malignant melanoma metastatic to the esophagus. *Ann Thorac Surg.* 1989;48:287–288.
26. Zarian LP, Berliner L, Redmond P. Metastatic endometrial carcinoma to the esophagus. *Am J Gastroenterol.* 1983;78:9–11.

V

THERAPY

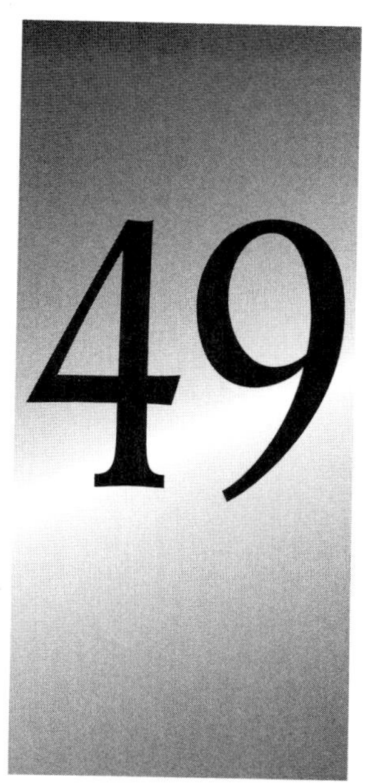

49 Multidisciplinary Care Team: Structure and Format

Kyle A. Perry
Blair A. Jobe

The multidisciplinary care team (MDCT) approach to the treatment of various malignancies has become more prevalent in recent years due to the increasing complexity of cancer therapy. Currently, most solid tumors require multimodality therapy, often with multiple possible treatment approaches. For cancers with complex treatment algorithms, a productive discussion between multiple specialists should lead to more accurate preoperative staging and appropriate triage into defined treatment pathways.

Esophageal cancer is no exception. Although surgical resection remains the only curative treatment option, several treatment approaches may be considered, especially for patients presenting with advanced disease. MDCTs play a significant role in determining both which modalities will be utilized and the sequence of treatment strategies. The rapid evolution of chemotherapeutic regimens and the development of laparoscopic and endoscopic approaches to both curative resection and palliation require interactions of experts from multiple disciplines to discuss treatment options and ensure delivery of the best possible care.

The MDCT approach has been defined as the creation of a tailored treatment plan for each esophageal cancer patient based on input from multiple disciplines (1). Table 49.1 shows a list of potential team members broken down into functional subgroups. The team consists of a coordinator and members from multiple departments, including treating physicians, diagnostic services, support services, and research staff. The roles of various team members and the interactions between them will be described in detail later in this chapter.

Many studies have addressed the role of MDCTs in cancer treatment. In the past, retrospective studies looking at extremity sarcoma and ovarian cancer found improvements in limb salvage and cancer-free survival (2,3). In 2006, two retrospective studies compared the treatment of esophageal cancer using a MDCT approach to the results achieved by individual practicing surgeons. Davies et al. demonstrated improved preoperative clinical staging and determination of appropriate therapy (4), while Stephens et al. found improved preoperative clinical staging, decreased operative mortality, and improved 5-year survival with the MDCT approach (5). Although no randomized trials have definitively confirmed these findings, these studies support the common sense conclusion that the effective flow of information between specialists leads to the best possible patient care.

This chapter describes a model for an esophageal cancer MDCT. We will outline the goals that the care team seeks to accomplish and describe a team structure and organization of patient flow designed to achieve these goals. It concludes with an evaluation of some potential pitfalls of MDCT development and potential

TABLE 49.1
Multidisciplinary Care Team Members

- Administrative staff
  - MDCT coordinator
- Oncologists
  - Esophageal surgeons
  - Medical oncologists
  - Radiation oncologists
- Diagnostic Services
  - Gastroenterologists
  - Pathologists
  - Radiologists
- Support Services
  - Nurse specialists
  - Nutritionists
  - Palliative care team
  - Physical therapy
  - Smoking cessation team
  - Social workers
- Research Staff

TABLE 49.2
Goals of the Multidisciplinary Care Team

1. Development of an institution-wide, unified vision for treatment of esophageal cancer
2. Creation of defined diagnostic and treatment pathways
3. Accurate preoperative clinical staging of disease
4. Clear communication with patients regarding disease staging, prognosis, and treatment options
5. Provision of psychosocial support for patients and their families
6. Provision of a framework for research and development
7. Provision of a forum for education and continued evolution of team function

future directions to ensure quality and ongoing evolution of team function.

GOALS OF THE MDCT APPROACH

The goals of the MDCT approach to esophageal cancer treatment are outlined in Table 49.2. They begin with steps to optimize the care rendered to individual patients and their families in both medical and psychosocial areas. The MDCT also plays an important role by providing a framework for research and education. Clinical and basic science research advance the understanding of esophageal cancer and lead to development of new diagnostic and treatment modalities, while a well-structured educational program encourages continued MDCT growth and development.

Development of a Unified Vision of Patient Care and Defined Treatment Pathways

Using ongoing dialogue between physicians in surgery, medical oncology, radiation oncology, and palliative care medicine, the MDCT develops an institution-wide unified approach to the care of esophageal cancer patients. Once this has been achieved, this vision can be translated into defined diagnostic and treatment pathways based on the patient's overall medical condition and clinical stage of disease.

Accurate Preoperative Staging

After the collection of diagnostic studies, cooperative evaluation of the results by surgeons, oncologists, gastroenterologists, radiologists, and pathologists in MDCT meetings leads to more accurate preoperative clinical staging, as suggested by the aforementioned studies. This approach results in more accurate triage of patients into the treatment pathways developed by the MDCT.

Clear Communication with Patients and Families

Conclusions reached in MDCT meetings regarding stage of disease, prognosis, and treatment options must be clearly and concisely communicated to patients and their families. This communication may occur separately in each specialist's own clinic or in a common esophageal cancer care clinic in which each group of treating physicians is represented. In the latter setting, patients have one cohesive group discussion with multiple team members involved in their case during a single office visit, rather than via several isolated discussions with different doctors at different times. Although logistically more difficult, this approach provides the most streamlined flow of information from physicians to their patients.

Patient and Family Psychosocial Support

Nursing specialists, social workers, and palliative care specialists form the psychosocial support network of the MDCT. These services are available to help patients and their families through the difficult process of cancer diagnosis and treatment. Participation in team meetings provides these professionals with detailed knowledge of a patient's clinical condition, prognosis, and treatment plan, giving them insight into the particular stresses faced by individual patients and their family members. They can then provide psychosocial support within the context of the overall care plan developed by the MDCT.

Provide a Framework for Research and Development

Treatment of patients within the context of a MDCT places them in an environment conducive to prospective data collection regarding diagnostic work-up, treatment, quality of life, and other variables. Our experience suggests that the streamlined process of diagnostic testing and effective flow of communication in this setting leads to increased patient satisfaction and enrollment in research protocols. Dedicated research specialists can organize research efforts, identify patient eligibility for trials, and facilitate patient participation as the MDCT deems appropriate.

Provide a Forum for Education and Innovation

A well-organized education program, including CME (continuing medical education) credit for the participating members, encourages ongoing education and discussion about the evolving field of esophageal cancer care. These meetings can ultimately lead to implementation of new approaches and evolution of the team's diagnostic and treatment pathways. These efforts also support the group's research interests by providing a forum for generating hypotheses for new directions in research and development.

MDCT STRUCTURE AND FUNCTION

The MDCT consists of members from several disciplines who work together to guide patients through the diagnosis, treatment, and surveillance of their disease. Several small groups within the MDCT work in conjunction with one another to carry out the team's care plans. The structure of these subgroups and their interactions with one another create the framework for patient flow within the MDCT system.

Team Members

Administrative Staff

The team coordinator leads the administrative staff, which is responsible for monitoring the administration of the entire system. The coordinator schedules meetings and clinics and ensures that all relevant patient information is available for team meetings. This group also records all decisions regarding patient diagnosis and treatment plans and coordinates efforts to track successful treatment plan implementation and follow-up.

Treating Physicians

This portion of the team consists of the treating physicians, including surgeons, medical oncologists, radiation oncologists, and in some cases, gastroenterologists and palliative care physicians. These members develop a cohesive description of the patient's clinical stage of disease and treatment options and communicate this information to the patient. They also work together with the patient to decide upon a definitive course of treatment and carry out this plan.

Diagnostic Services

This unit is composed of gastroenterologists, pathologists, and radiologists. The gastroenterologist serves as the point of entry for patients into the MDCT and coordinates the diagnostic work-up of the patients according to the team's established protocols. When the desired diagnostic testing is complete, these physicians collaborate with the treating physicians in the MDCT meeting to accurately stage the patient's cancer.

Support Services

Palliative care specialists, nurse specialists, social workers, psychologists, nutritionists, physical therapists, and the smoking cessation team comprise this diverse group. These services work to deliver day-to-day care and support to patients and their families as dictated by the individual treatment plan. The participation of each group in MDCT meetings provides a context for the MDCT to understand the challenges facing patients and their family to a degree that would not be possible if each group worked in isolation.

Research Staff

The research staff works to coordinate basic science research efforts and clinical trials within the MDCT. They also oversee patient enrollment and follow-up within the context of clinical trials. The research staff is also involved in the educational component of the MDCT and development of new research and development protocols.

Patient Flow and Interaction of Various Patient Care Groups

Although the patient care groups within the MDCT may often work in isolation, efficient communication of information between these groups is imperative for the optimal functioning of the MDCT. Figure 49.1 outlines

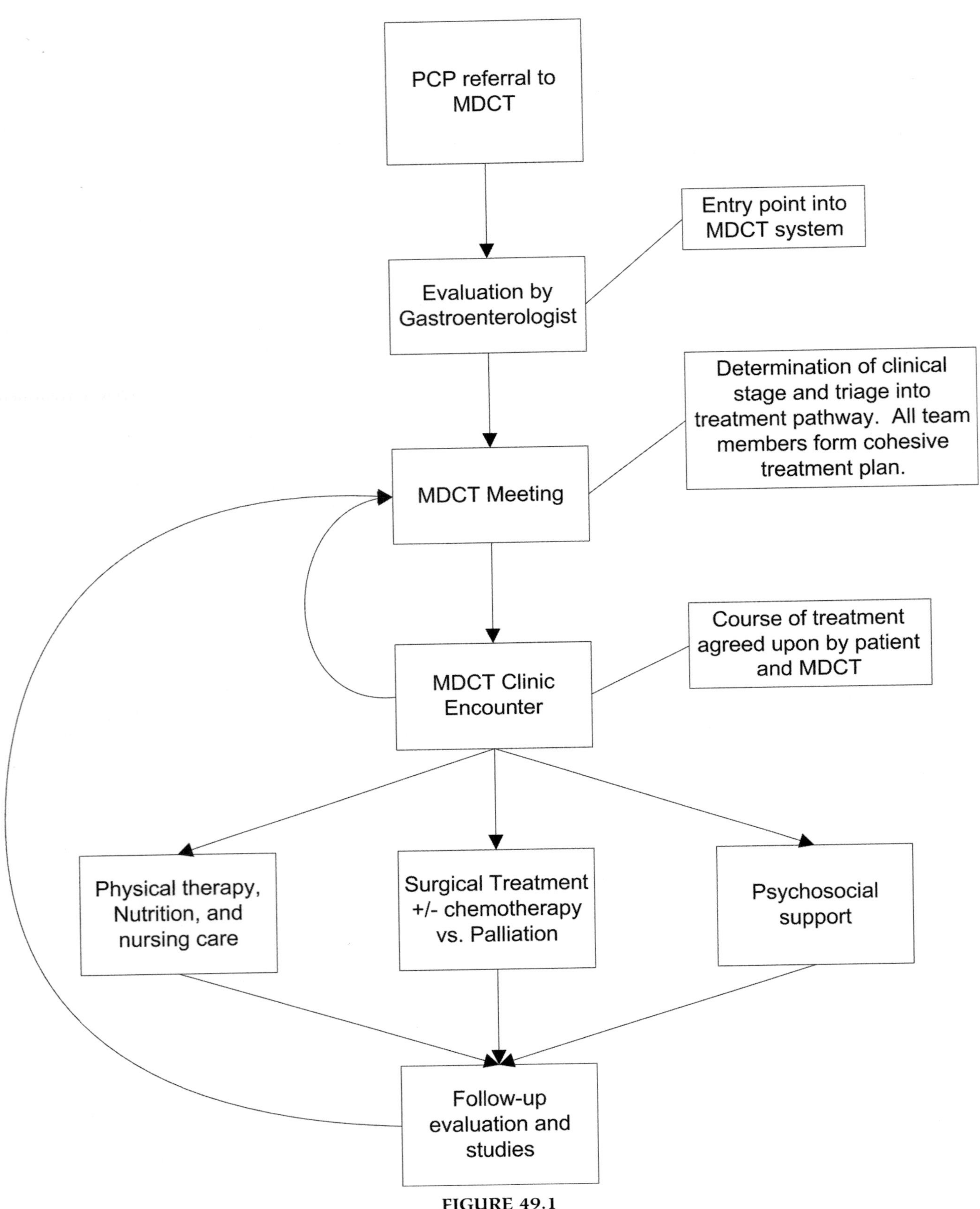

FIGURE 49.1

Patient flow in the multidisciplinary care team system.

patient flow through the MDCT system and highlights the times when the MDCT meet together to ensure effective communication. Each patient's diagnosis and treatment plan are discussed by all team members during the first MDCT meeting. At this time all members of the team develop a clear understanding of the patient's prognosis and treatment plan and can form their own action plan within this context.

After this meeting is completed, the patient is seen by members of the team in the common esophageal care clinic. Coherent discussions with patients determine a definitive course of action. The entire MDCT meets again after the initiation of treatment so that all team members have a detailed understanding of the patient's progression through the treatment plan.

The research and educational meetings occur outside of the realm of direct patient care. It is important to organize a CME program to encourage participation of all team members. These meetings serve to keep team members abreast of new developments in the field of esophageal cancer and to stimulate discussion and generate questions for research projects within the group.

CONCLUSION AND FUTURE DIRECTIONS

The development of patient MDCTs for the treatment of esophageal cancer is an important step in the treatment of this infrequent and complex disease. The cooperation of multiple disciplines and the efficient flow of information between physicians are vital to ensuring the best possible patient care.

In order to achieve this level of care, however, a couple of important situations must exist. First, the esophageal cancer MDCT requires a great deal of support from the hospital in order to succeed. This support comes in the form of physical space within cancer centers for the multispecialty cancer care clinic as well as support of the group's educational and research activities. This should include the development of a CME program for attendance of the group's academic conferences.

The second important step is the development of ways to monitor team function and evaluate outcomes. Team meetings and combined clinics will only work to the degree that the treatment plans formulated by the team are enacted properly and fully by all team members. In the United Kingdom, Blazeby et al. tracked the rate of successful implementation of MDCT treatment plans for upper gastrointestinal cancers and found a 15% failure rate (6). The most common reasons for alterations in treatment were unrecognized comorbidities and patient choice, highlighting the need for improved communication between physicians and patients. To allow critical assessment and improvement of team function, MDCTs must develop effective systems for monitoring treatment plan implementation and treatment outcomes.

The MDCT approach to the treatment of esophageal cancer is still in the early stages of its development, and much work remains to refine the process. The pursuit of highly functioning MDCTs will ultimately provide the highest possible level of oncologic and psychosocial care for esophageal cancer patients and their families.

References

1. Jobe BA, Enestvedt CK, Thomas CR Jr. Disease-specific multidisciplinary care: a natural progression in the management of esophageal cancer. *Dis Esophagus.* 2006;19:417–418.
2. Morton DL, Eilber FR, Townsend Jr. CM, et al. Limb salvage from a multidisciplinary treatment approach for skeletal and soft tissue sarcomas of the extremity. *Ann Surg.* 1976;184:268–278.
3. Junor EJ, Hole DJ, Gillis CR. Management of ovarian cancer: referral to a multidisciplinary team matters. *Br J Cancer.* 1994;70:363–370.
4. Davies AR, Deans DA, Penman I, et al. The multidisciplinary team meeting improves staging accuracy and treatment selection for gastro-esophageal cancer. *Dis Esophagus.* 2006;19:496–503.
5. Stephens MR, Lewis WG, Brewster AE, et al. Multidisciplinary team management is associated with improved outcomes after surgery for esophageal cancer. *Dis Esophagus.* 2006;19:164–171.
6. Blazeby JM, Wilson L, Metcalfe C, et al. Analysis of clinical decision-making in multidisciplinary cancer teams. *Ann Oncol.* 2006;3:457–460.

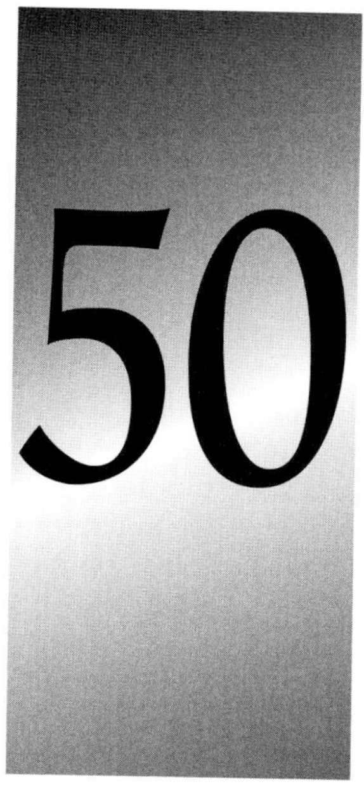

50 Informed Consent in the Esophageal Cancer Patient

Scott R. Sommers
Paul R. Helft

The foundation of traditional theories of consent to treatment lies in the law of battery. The notion of informed consent can be traced to 2 landmark cases from the early 20th century. In the most recognized decision addressing informed consent, Justice Cardozo stated: "Every human being of adult years and sound mind has a right to determine what shall be done with his own body; and a surgeon who performs an operation without his patient's consent commits an assault for which he is liable in damages" (1). Justice Cardozo's statement is the hallmark of most appellate cases about consent, informed consent, or the right to refuse treatment. Additionally, *Mohr v. Williams* affirmed "the right to the inviolability of [a patient's] person," which no surgeon, no matter how eminent or skillful, may violate without consent (2). In this case, the physician obtained Anna Mohr's consent for an operation on her right ear. In the course of her surgery, a surgically correctable problem concerning the patient's left ear was instead discovered, and the surgeon proceeded to operate on the left ear. The Minnesota Supreme Court found that the physician should have obtained the patient's consent to the surgery on the left ear. The judge decided that a physician needs to advise a patient of all the information related to a particular procedure and must review all the risks and benefits. Only after this exchange does the patient enter into a contract, a contract that authorizes the physician to operate *only* to the extent of the consent given. Regrettably, legal history has shaped our understanding of informed consent and created a culture in which informed consent represents a legalistic protection from liability.

In fundamentally important ways, informed consent should be viewed as a *process* rather than as an *event*. Informed consent in the *ethical* sense can only evolve from a meaningful discussion between patients and physicians that deepens a patient's understanding and takes account of patients' preferences, desires, and fears. This mutual or bilateral method of informed consent has been called *shared decision making* (3,4). Others have described this as patient-centered communication (5) or as the doctor-patient accommodation (6). Informed consent in the context of such a shared dialogue removes the "doctor knows best" paternalism and generates a discussion that helps properly inform patients and ultimately enhances their autonomy.

This idealized concept of shared decision making becomes complex in the patient with esophageal cancer. Although physicians and patients must find ways to accommodate the 4 main elements of informed consent for a medical decision or treatment—competence, disclosure of information, comprehension, and voluntariness—the disclosure of useful and pertinent information and assuring patients' comprehension cannot be accomplished in straightforward ways. We believe that there are 5 issues that complicate the process of informed consent in patients with esophageal cancer. First, the overall outcomes for esophageal cancer are poor, even in patients with ostensibly curable stages of disease at presentation. Second, the precise relative and absolute benefits of therapy, particularly in the adjuvant setting, remain uncertain and controversial. Third, both the therapies employed in the treatment of esophageal cancer as well as the disease itself greatly affect patients' quality of life. The actual impact of disease and therapy on quality of life is challenging to communicate successfully to patients. Fourth, helping patients to arrive at an adequate understanding of prognosis, potential risks, and benefits of therapy is dependent upon the physician's ability to communicate information and patients' ability to receive and process information in ways that achieve understanding. Fifth, patients have varying information and decision-making preferences. These preferences vary with respect to the quantity of information desired, the format in which information is presented, and change with time and with altered clinical status. Also, patients' preference for engagement in decision making varies considerably. Such preferences must be taken into account in an idealized model of shared decision making.

Thus, assuring informed consent in patients with esophageal cancer is problematic. We will discuss each of these issues in turn. Subsequently, we will make suggestions to help those caring for patients with esophageal cancer to recognize and address the complexities surrounding shared decision making in this patient group.

ISSUE 1: POOR OUTCOMES

The 5-year survival rate for esophageal cancer was 4% from 1961 to 1989 and increased to 10.5% from 1990 to 1996 (7). Some authors have suggested that these increases in survival are related to improvements in detection (attributed to the increasing frequency of endoscopy), advancements in surgical techniques, and improvement in therapies, including concomitant radiation and chemotherapy (7,8). Despite these advances, the relative 5-year survival rates in the United States for patients at diagnosis was 14.3% from 1995 to 2000 for all stages (9). Even in patients undergoing surgical resection of limited regional disease with curative intent, 5-year survival rates are 20% to 40% in clinical trials (10,11). Such statistically poor outcomes make careful assessment and communication of risks and benefits of therapy vital for patients facing difficult therapeutic decisions.

ISSUE 2: UNCERTAIN BENEFITS OF THERAPY

The most controversial clinical question in the therapy of patients with esophageal cancer concerns the benefits of adjuvant therapy. Establishing the benefits of adjuvant therapy definitively has been complicated by difficulties in accruing patients to clinical trials, imperfect trial methodologies, and by the changing epidemiology of the disease over the past 2 decades. Most important, because of the major shift in North America and, to a lesser extent, Western Europe from predominantly squamous cell histology to adenocarcinoma, further uncertainties regarding the validity and applicability of previous clinical research to current patient groups have arisen (8,12). Indeed, most of the salient studies are limited to patients with squamous cell histology. Several studies have demonstrated that squamous cell carcinomas can behave quite differently from adenocarcinoma clinically (7,8). Our purpose is not to provide a systematic review of the many studies, but rather to highlight the reasons why the evidence has not definitively answered important therapeutic questions.

Table 50.1 outlines several selected studies concerning preoperative chemotherapy. A Cochrane Review of 11 randomized clinical trials in 2006 compared preoperative chemotherapy and surgery versus surgery alone (21). Preoperative chemotherapy provided a statistically significant survival difference at 5 years (RR = 1.44, 95% CI; 1.05–1.97; *P* = 0.02). Another recent meta-analysis evaluated the patient-based data from 9 trials (2,102 patients). The overall survival favored preoperative chemotherapy (HR = 0.87, 95% CI 0.79–0.95, *P* = 0.003) (22). Conversely, in a meta-analysis by Urschel and colleagues (23), no significant difference in survival was noted at 1, 2, and 3 years. Many believe the contradictory evidence is largely due to the heterogeneity of the study protocols, but these conflicted analyses make definitive conclusions regarding the benefits of neoadjuvant chemotherapy problematic. Although all of the protocols used cisplatin-based regimens, concomitant agents, doses, and cycles completed varied among studies. Moreover, most of these studies included primarily patients with squamous cell cancers.

Preoperative chemoradiation has been the de facto standard of care for operable esophageal cancer in the United States for several years. Table 50.2 summarizes several trials of preoperative chemoradiation in patients with respectable esophageal cancer. Walsh and colleagues (27) did detect a statistically significant survival advantage in patients who received neoadjuvant chemoradiation; however, this study has been widely criticized for the poor outcome in its surgical arm, lack of preoperative CT scans, premature closure, and short follow-up (32,33). Three meta-analyses have undertaken the

TABLE 50.1
Preoperative Chemotherapy and Surgery versus Surgery Alone

Reference	Histology & number	Treatment regimen	Median survival (chemo/surg vs. surg) (in months)	Three-Year survival (chemo/surg vs. surg)
Law et al., 1997 (13)	SC, 147 patients	FUP x 2 cycles + esophagectomy vs. esophagectomy alone	16.8 vs. 13 (p=0.03)	38% vs. 14%
Schlag et al., 1992 (14)	SC, 46 patients	FUP x 3 cycles + esophagectomy vs. esophagectomy alone	7.5 vs. 5	NR
Nygaard et al., 1992 (15)	SC, 106 patients	Cisplatin/Bleomycin + esophagectomy vs. esophagectomy alone	7 vs. 7	3% vs. 9%
Miapang et al., 1994 (16)	SC, 46 patients	Cisplatin/Vinblastine/Bleomycin + esophagectomy vs. esophagectomy alone	17 vs. 17	31% vs. 36%
Kok et al., 1997 (17)	SC, 160 patients	Cisplatin/Etoposide x 2 cycles (responders received an extra 2 cycles) + esophagectomy vs. esophagectomy alone	18.5 vs. 11 (p=0.002)	NR
Kelson et al., 1998 (18)	SC + AC, 467 patients	FUP x 3 cycles + esophagectomy (responders received an extra 2 cycles postoperatively) vs. esophagectomy alone	14.9 vs. 16.8	42% vs. 45%
Ancona et al., 2001 (19)	SC, 94 patients	FUP x 2 cycles + esophagectomy vs. esophagectomy alone	25 vs. 24	44% vs. 41%
MRC 2002 (20)	SC + AC, 802 patients	FUP x 2 cycles + esophagectomy vs. esophagectomy alone	16.8 vs. 13.3 (p=0.004)	48% vs. 36%

Note: Only statistically significant *P* values shown; if not shown, results were not significant. Abbreviations: NR = not reported; SC = squamous cell; AC = adenocarcinoma; FUP = cisplatin/fluorouracil; MRC = Medical Research Council.

task of evaluating preoperative chemoradiation. Of the 3, 1 favored chemoradiation, while the remaining 2 did not find a benefit (32,34,35). As noted with preoperative chemotherapy, these studies are quite heterogeneous and include mostly patients with squamous cell histology. Many of the others were plagued with poor patient accrual and thus underpowered. Definitive randomized trials of adjuvant chemoradiation are thus lacking.

There have been 3 randomized clinical trials (36–38) evaluating postoperative chemotherapy (using cisplatin regimens) to surgery alone in patients with squamous cell carcinoma of the esophagus. These studies failed to demonstrate a significant survival advantage with postoperative chemotherapy (32,39). In evaluating patients with gastric and gastroesophageal junction tumors, MacDonald and colleagues (40) evaluated postoperative fluorouracil and radiation. Median overall survival was 36 months versus 27 months, favoring the postoperative tri-modal therapy.

In metastatic disease, treatment outcomes are quite dismal. Levard and colleagues (41) compared cisplatin and 96-hour infusional fluorouracil to the best supportive care in the palliative setting. There was no survival benefit for chemotherapy over supportive care. Indeed, there are no definitive trials in the setting of metastatic esophageal cancer that have been proven to prolong survival over the best supportive care.

Cisplatin-based regimens have been the standard for combination therapy in metastatic or locally advanced disease. The earliest platinum-based regimens with combination cisplatin included bleomycin, mitomycin, methotrexate/bleomycin, vindesine, and vinblastine and were associated with response rates of 23% to 33% (42–48). More recent regimens have produced similar survival rates and improvements in quality of life (i.e., improvement in dysphagia) with fewer side effects (42). Selected cisplatin regimens are summarized in Table 50.3. Usual response rates are around 30%. Few

TABLE 50.2
Preoperative Chemoradiation and Surgery versus Surgery Alone

Reference	Histology & number	Treatment regimen	Median survival (chemoradiation/surg vs. surg.) (in months)	Three-Year survival (chemo/surg vs. surg)
Nygaard et al., 1992 (15)	SC, 103 patients	Cisplatin/Bleomycin x 2 cycles + 35 Gy XRT + esophagectomy vs. esophagectomy alone	7 vs. 7	17% vs. 9%
Le Prise et al., 1994 (24)	SC, 86 patients	FUP x 2 cycles + 20 Gy XRT+ esophagectomy vs. esophagectomy alone	11 vs.11	19% vs. 14%
Apinop et al., 1994 (25)	SC, 69 patients	FUP x 2 cycles +40 Gy XRT + esophagectomy vs. esophagectomy alone	9.7 vs. 7.4	26% vs. 20%
Bosset et al., 1994 (26)	SC, 282 patients	Cisplatin x 2 cycles + 37 Gy XRT + esophagectomy vs. esophagectomy alone	18.6 vs. 18.6	39% vs. 37%
Walsh et al., 1996 (27)	AC, 113 patients	FUP x 2 cycles + 40 Gy XRT + esophagectomy vs. esophagectomy alone	16 vs. 11 (p=0.01)	32% vs. 6%
Urba et al., 2001 (28)	SC + AC, 100 patients	Cisplatin/Vinblastine x 2 cycles + 21 days 5-FU + 45 Gy XRT + esophagectomy vs. esophagectomy	17.6 vs. 16.9	30% vs. 14%
Burmeister et al., 2002 (29)	SC + AC, 256 patients	FUP + 35Gy + esophagectomy vs. esophagectomy	22.2 vs. 19.3	NR
Natsugoe et al., 2006, (30)	SC, 53 patients	FUP + 40 Gy XRT + esophagectomy vs. esophagectomy alone	NR	**5 year 57% vs. 14%* (p=0.58)
Tepper et al., 2007 (31)	SC + AC, 56 patients	FUP x 2 cycles + 50 Gy XRT + esophagectomy vs. esophagectomy	**Median Survival* 4.5yrs vs. 1.8yrs	**5 year 39% vs. 16%*

Note: Only statistically significant *P* values shown; if not shown, results were not significant. Abbreviations: NR = not reported; SC = squamous cell; AC = adenocarcinoma; FUP = cisplatin/fluorouracil; Gy = Gray; XRT = radiotherapy; 5-FU = fluorouracil.

patients achieve a complete response, and median survival times are less than 11 months.

Many non-cisplatin regimens have also been evaluated. These regimens also provide similar response rates and median survival times. Many have argued that some regimens provide improved toxicity profiles, but there is little consensus agreement. Table 50.4 summarizes some selected non-cisplatin regimens.

In none of the treatment settings summarized are there definitive data to answer important clinical questions, and so recommendations to patients and practice patterns must necessarily be based on inadequate evidence. This lack of definitive data makes informing patients of the benefits of adjuvant therapy challenging. Patients may equate uncertainty of data with uncertainty of their physician's recommendation. Moreover, in cases in which patients are at greater risk of toxicity from therapy, physicians may feel even greater pressure to help patients achieve a nuanced understanding of the risks and benefits of the treatments offered.

ISSUE 3: QUALITY OF LIFE

For patients with early stage disease, the morbidity and mortality of esophagectomy are considerable. Operative mortality currently ranges approximately from 6% to 10% overall (76,77). Significant morbidity occurs in

TABLE 50.3
Cisplatin-Based Regimens for Advanced Esophageal Cancer

References	Treatment regimen	Histology	Number pt (n)	Response rate (95% CI)	CR rate (%)	Median survival (mo)
Bleiberg et al., 1997 (49)	Cisplatin/FU	SC	88	34% (24%–44%)	2%	7.9
Hayashi et al., 2001 (50)	Cisplatin/FU	SC	36	33% (19%–55%)	3%	6.7
Hsu et al., 2002 (51)	Cisplatin/methotrexate/ FU +LV	SC + AC	26	28% (12%–49%)	0	5
Ilson et al., 1998 (52)	Cisplatin/FU/paclitaxel	SC + AC	60	48% (35%–61%)	12%	10.8
Polee et al., 2001 (53)	Cisplatin/FU/LV/ etoposide	SC	69	34% (22%–46%)	4%	9.5
Conroy et al., 2002 (54)	Cisplatin/Vinorelbine	SC	75	34% (23%–46%)	0	6.8
Kok et al., 1996 (55)	Cisplatin/etoposide	SC	65	48% (35%–60%)	8%	NR
Spiridonidis et al., 1996 (56)	Cisplatin/etoposide	AC	27	48% (36%–74%)	19%	9.8
Ilson et al., 2000 (57)	Cisplatin/ paclitaxel	SC + AC	32	38% (24%–54%)	NR	6.9
Petrasch et al., 1998 (58)	Cisplatin/paclitaxel	SC + AC	20	40% (NR)	15%	NR
Ajani et al., 2005 (59)	Cisplatin/docetaxel +/-FU (DC vs. DCF)	AC	DC = 76 DCF = 79	26% = DC 43% = DCF	NR	9.6 = DC 10.5 = DCF
Ilson et al., 1999 (60)	Cisplatin/ irinotecan	SC + AC	35	57% (41%–73%)	6%	14.6
Mackay et al., 2001 (61)	Cisplatin/epirubicin/ raltitrexd	AC	21	29% (11%–52%)	NR	4.5
Corporaal et al., 2006 (62)	Cisplatin/epirubicin/ capecitabine	AC	23	57%	NR	9.0
Urba et al., 2004 (63)	Cisplatin/gemcitabine	SC + AC	64	NR	NR	7.3
Millar et al., 2005 (64)	Cisplatin/gemcitabine	SC + AC	42	45%	7%	11.0

Note: Some of these studies included locally advanced cancer which cannot be evaluated by RECIST criteria. Abbreviations: NR = not reported; SC = squamous cell; AC = adenocarcinoma; CI = confidence interval; IFF = irinotecan/FU/FA; IC = irinotecan/cisplatin; FU = fluorouracil; LV = leucovorin; FA = folinic acid; DC = docetaxel/cisplatin; DCF = docetaxel/cisplatin/FU.

up to 50% of patients undergoing esophagectomy (78). When 7,500 surgical patients were evaluated for types of surgical complications, they ranged from cardiac (6%–20%), pulmonary (13%–19%), anastomotic leak (7%–14%), vocal cord paralysis (4%–10%), wound infection (4%–8%), and chylous leakage (1%–2%) (77). Several studies have shown that quality of life (QoL) significantly deteriorates in the early postoperative period with the exception of emotional QoL (79–82). Length of full recovery after surgery is generally estimated to be

TABLE 50.4
Non-Cisplatin–Based Regimens for Advanced Esophageal Cancer

References	Treatment regimen	Histology	Number pt (n)	Response rate (95% CI)	CR rate (%)	Median survival (mo)
Kelsen et al., 1992 (65)	Interferon α-2a/FU	SC + AC	37	27% (13%–41%)	3%	6.4
Airoldi et al., 2003 (66)	Docetaxel/ vinorelbine	SC	20	60%	15%	10.5
Morgan-Meadows et al., 2005 (67)	Gemcitabine/ FU/LV	SC + AC	35	31%	3%	9.8
Burge et al., 2006 (68)	Irinotecan/ capecitabine	AC	31	32% (16%–52%)	NR	10.0
Pozzo et al., 2004 (69)	Irinotecan/FU/FA (IFF) vs. Irinote-can/cisplatin (IC)	AC	59 (IFF) 56 (IC)	42% (IFF) 32% (IC)	5% (IFF) 2% (IC)	10.7 (IFF) 6.9 (IC)
Jatoi et al., 2002 (70)	Irinotecan/ docetaxel	AC	46	26% (14%–41%)	0	7.3
Lordick et al., 2003 (71)	Irinotecan/ docetaxel	SC + AC	24	12.5% (3%–32%)	0	NR
Lorenzen et al., 2005 (72)	Capecitabine/ docetaxel	SC + AC	24	46%	4%	15.8
Mauer et al., 2005 (73)	Oxaliplatin/ LV/FU	SC + AC	34	40% (24%–57%)	3%	7.1
El-Rayes et al., 2004 (74)	Carboplatin/ paclitaxel	SC + AC	35	43% (30%–58%) [a]	NR	9.0
Braybrooke et al., 1997 (75)	Mitomycin C/etoposide	AC	26	15% (4%–35%)	NR	6.0

[a]These were 90% CI.
Note: Some of these studies included locally advanced cancer which cannot be evaluated by RECIST criteria. Abbreviations: NR = not reported; SC = squamous cell; AC = adenocarcinoma; CI = confidence interval; IFF = irinotecan/FU/FA; IC = irinotecan/cisplatin; FU = fluorouracil; LV = leucovorin; FA = folinic acid; DC= docetaxel/cisplatin; DCF = docetaxel/cisplatin/FU.

around 9 to 12 months (77). Unfortunately, most recurrences occur within 18 to 24 months after surgery (83). In 1 study of patients undergoing tri-modal therapy, all patients who relapsed did so in the 18 months after esophagectomy (84). The obvious implication is that between half and two-thirds of patients' time to recurrence is occupied with surgical recovery and poor QoL. Long-term data concerning QoL in patients with esophageal cancer have been difficult to obtain because the 1-year survival rate following esophagectomy is only 65% (81). High attrition rates make the QoL data difficult to interpret. In 1 study of patients who died within 2 years of surgery, QoL continued to worsen after surgery and never recovered before death (78). With a long recovery period and early recurrence, patients who have recurrent disease may never achieve and/or sustain good QoL before death.

Although surgical therapy of esophageal cancer entails the greatest morbidity, neoadjuvant therapy, particularly chemoradiation, causes significant morbidity as well. The Cancer and Leukemia Group B trial 9781 reported grade 3 esophagitis/dysphagia in 40% of patients undergoing preoperative chemoradiation (31). Herskovic and colleagues reported that 50% of patients receiving combination chemoradiation developed at least 1 grade 3 toxicity (85). Treatment-related mortality for chemoradiation has been reported to be between 1% and 6% in selected studies (86).

Scores of QoL have been noted to deteriorate quickly during neoadjuvant chemotherapy and then fall further during concomitant radiation therapy (87). Scores generally recover prior to esophagectomy. In 1 study, patients who underwent surgery alone reported significantly worse QoL after surgery than those who received neoadjuvant therapy. In another prospective study, QoL scores in the first year after surgery did not differ between the 2 groups (79).

The evidence regarding the impact of chemotherapy on QoL in advanced disease is less clear. Epirubicin, cisplatin, and 5-fluorouracil in 74 patients with metastatic esophageal cancer showed no benefit in QoL between responders and non-responders, though pain scores were improved in the responders (88). In another study, 35 patients receiving irinotecan and cisplatin for metastatic disease, scores improved in both responders and non-responders (60). In a study of 71 patients receiving vinorelbine and cisplatin for metastatic disease, response to chemotherapy was associated with an improvement in QoL scores (54). Patients with stable or progressive disease generally had no decrease in QoL scores after 2 cycles.

Thus, the therapies available for the treatment of esophageal cancer all involve significant toxicity and have a major impact on quality of life. Helping patients to arrive at a fuller understanding of these significant risks is an important challenge in informed consent for treatment.

ISSUE 4: PATIENTS' UNDERSTANDING

Most authorities on informed consent agree that an informed consent discussion should include the following elements: (a) the nature of the decision/procedure, (b) realistic alternatives to the planned decision/intervention, (c) the relevant risks, (d) possible benefits, (e) an appraisal of patient understanding, and (f) acceptance of the intervention by the patient. In addition, a patient must possess sufficient decision-making capacity to make the decision, and the decision must be arrived at in a voluntary way. In many cases, assuring that patients understand enough about each of these elements is problematic. For example, there is a significant body of evidence that suggests that multiple features of patients' psychology, educational level, socioeconomic and cultural circumstances, and health literacy and numeracy may affect their ability to understand important information presented to them during the course of making a major medical decision (89). Thus, the clinician must find ways of accounting for all of these factors in leading patients through an informed consent process.

Unfortunately, several studies have found that many patients do not understand the status of their disease or the intentions of treatment. Survival is often greatly overestimated. One study revealed that only 44% of patients correctly recalled side effects of treatment and only 33% correctly recalled the prognosis properly (90). Such misconceptions may influence patients' decisions to undertake therapy (91). Despite reports by physicians that discussions of prognosis occurred, patients' estimates of survival remain inadequate (92,93).

Finally, we note that patients' choices are not always strictly logical. Jansen and colleagues found that 40% of breast cancer patients would choose to undergo chemotherapy, even when there was zero likelihood of benefit (94).

ISSUE 5: INFORMATION AND DECISION-MAKING PREFERENCES

To complicate matters further, patients' preferences for both information and level of engagement in decision making often vary. For example, much of the literature about prognostic communication suggests that patients desire full information about prognosis (5). In evaluating a group of heterogeneous cancer patients, Jenkins and colleagues found that 87% of patients wanted all information, whether it was good or bad (95). Patients tend to desire information regarding chances of cure, extent of disease spread, possible side effects of treatment, life expectancy, and the effects of the malignancy on their life (96,97). Patients almost universally prefer that their physicians discuss their preferences for information (98,99).

Concerning the format for communicating prognostic information, Kaplowitz and colleagues (98) found that 80% of patients preferred qualitative information such as "you will probably live a long time" or "you will/will not die from this disease," compared to only 50% of patients who wanted a quantitative prognosis, such as estimates of survival or percentages of mortality. The evidence about information preferences in patients with more advanced disease is less developed, but suggests that patients with incurable disease may desire less information (100). Cancer patients uniformly desire that difficult information be conveyed with a sense of hope and sensitivity (101,102).

Patients' preferences for engagement in decision making may also vary and are not universally correlated with information preferences. In a randomized study, Swenson and colleagues (103) found that 69% of patients appreciated the shared decision-making method. The remaining 31% reported that they would prefer more of the decision making be relegated to the physician. Winefield and colleagues (104) further delineated which patients may prefer a physician-centered approach in a general practice setting. They found great satisfaction among patients whose care was characterized by the shared decision-making model when decision/intervention outcomes are equally acceptable. However, it must be noted that patients with either highly complex or very straightforward problems favored physician-centered styles of decision making (105). Furthermore, those noted to have high levels of anxiety or carry a poor prognosis tended to prefer a physician-directed approach to decision making (98,106). In a group of patients undergoing esophagectomy for esophageal cancer, McKneally and Martin (107) stated, "The patients described themselves as relieved, encouraged, and hopeful when the surgeon recommended an operation. They felt 'in control' of the decision process based on trust, rather than information." They found that these patients considered trust and confidence in their physician as the most important factor that provided them with comfort when making decisions. Patients preferred to have an "expert" or "specialist" doctor to proceed with a physician-centered decision-making process versus shared decision making.

CONCLUSION

We have tried to suggest the many reasons why assuring informed consent for patients with esophageal cancer is complex. These include the poor outcomes; complexity and toxicity of therapy; the uncertain benefits and significant risks associated with most therapies for this disease; and the considerable variations in patients' preferences, understanding, information needs, and desires for participation in decision making. We believe that effort spent both on recognizing these complexities and taking account of them during the informed consent process will pay off in terms of patients' satisfaction with their decisions. We advocate a shared decision-making model, which might best be described as *collaborative* between patients and the care team, since medical providers are experts in disease and therapy and patients are experts in their own needs and preferences. Eliciting the patients' needs and wants for physician-patient communication and tailoring informed consent discussions to those will ultimately provide the patient with the most comfort and confidence.

We offer several suggestions for improving the process:

1. Spread the informed consent process out over more than 1 encounter. This strategy allows patients to digest more complicated information over time and for them to formulate new questions, which may lead to deeper understanding. Multiple encounters can additionally strengthen the doctor-patient trust relationship, which allows a better grasp of patient understanding (see #3).
2. Provide concurrent, multidisciplinary consultation if possible. This allows specific questions concerning each type of therapy to be answered in detail when questions arise. Such an approach works especially well if the multidisciplinary group evaluates the patient's circumstances and arrives at a mutually agreeable recommendation for treatment ahead of time.
3. Verify understanding. This last step in medical communication is frequently omitted but can be vital for identifying knowledge deficits or misunderstandings. Nurses can be invaluable in this process. Multiple encounters along with consultation with other specialists also can provide several chances to ensure comprehension.
4. Seek a careful understanding of patients' preferences and needs prior to explanations. Time spent understanding how patients think and analyze decisions will pay off in providing information and helping them to grapple with complex decisions. A good way to approach patients when seeking to understand their decision-making preferences is to ask how they have approached other big decisions in their lives: Do they ask and accept the advice of an expert? Do they gather all of the information and spend time weighing the pros and cons of each? Do they rely on input from close friends or family? These questions help to shape a recommendation which takes into account an individual's previous style of approaching difficult choices.

References

1. *Schloendorff v. New York Hospital*, 211 NY 125, 105 NE 92 (1914).
2. *Mohr v. Williams*, 95 Minn 261, 104 NW 12 (1905).
3. de Haes H. Dilemmas in patient centeredness and shared decision making: a case for vulnerability. *Patient Educ Couns*. 2006;62:291–298.
4. Braddock CH, Edwards KA, Hasenberg NM, et al. Informed decision making in outpatient practice. *JAMA*. 1999;282:2313–2320.
5. Hagerty RG, Butow PN, Ellis PM, et al. Communicating prognosis in cancer care: a systematic review of the literature. *Ann Oncol*. 2005;16:1005–1053.
6. Siegler M. The doctor-patient accommodation: a critical event in clinical medicine. *Arch Intern Med*. 1982;142:1899–1902.
7. Lieberman MD, Franseschi D, Marsan B, et al. Esophageal carcinoma: the unusual variants. *J Thorac Cardiovasc Surg*. 1994;108:1138–1146.
8. Polednak AP. Trends in survival for both histological types of esophageal cancer US surveillance, epidemiology and end results in areas. *Int J Cancer*. 2003;105: 98–100.
9. Jemal A, Clegg LX, Ward E, et al. Annual report to the nation of the status of cancer, 1975–2001, with a special feature regarding survival. *Cancer*. 2004;101:3–27.
10. Brenner B, Ilson D, Minsky BD. Treatment of localized esophageal cancer. *Semin Oncol*. 2004;31:554–565.
11. Kelson D. Preoperative chemoradiotherapy for esophageal cancer. *J Clin Oncol*. 2001;19:283–285.
12. Malthaner RA, Wong RKS, Rumble RB, et al. Neoadjuvant or adjuvant therapy for resectable esophageal cancer: a systematic review and meta-analysis. *BMC Med*. 2004;2:35–39.
13. Law S, Fok M, Chow S, et al. Preoperative chemotherapy versus surgical therapy alone for squamous cell carcinoma of the esophagus: a prospective randomized trial. *J Thorac Cardiovasc Surg*. 1997;114:210–217.
14. Schlag PM. Randomized trial of preoperative chemotherapy for squamous cell cancer of the esophagus. The Chirurgische Arbeitsgemeinschaft fuer Onkologie der Deutschen Gesellschaft fuer Chirugie Study Group. *Arch Surg*. 1992;127:1446–1450.

15. Nygaard K, Hagen S, Hansen HS, et al. Pre-operative radiotherapy prolongs survival in operable esophageal carcinoma: a randomized, multi-center study of pre-operative radiotherapy and chemotherapy. The second Scandinavian trial in esophageal cancer. *World J Surg*. 1992;16:1104–1109.
16. Miapang T, Vasinankorn P, Petpichetchian C, et al. Induction chemotherapy in the treatment of patients with carcinoma of the esophagus. *J Surg Oncol*. 1994;56:191–197.
17. Kok TC, van Lanschot J, Siersma PD, et al. Neoadjuvant chemotherapy in operable esophageal squamous cell cancer: final report of a phase III multicenter randomized controlled trial [abstract 984]. *Proc Ann Meet Soc Clin Oncol*. 1997;16:277a.
18. Kelson D, Ginsberg R, Pajak TF, et al. Chemotherapy followed by surgery compared with surgery alone for localized esophageal cancer. *N Engl J Med*. 1998;339:1979–1984.
19. Ancona E, Ruol A, Santi S, et al. Only pathologic complete response to neoadjuvant chemotherapy improves significantly the long term survival of patients with resectable esophageal squamous cell carcinoma. *Cancer*. 2001;91:2165–2174.
20. Oesophageal Medical Research Council Oesophageal Cancer Working Party. Surgical resection with or without preoperative chemotherapy in oesophageal cancer: a randomized controlled trial. *Lancet*. 2002;359:1727–1733.
21. Malthaner RA, Collin S, Fenlon D. Preoperative chemotherapy for respectable thoracic esophageal cancer. *Coch Data Sys Rev*. 2001;3:CD001556.
22. Thirion PG, Michiels S, Le Maitre A, et al. Individual patient data-based meta-analysis assessing pre-operative chemotherapy in resectable oesophageal carcinoma [Abstract]. *J Clin Oncol*. 2007;25:4512.
23. Urschel JD, Vasan H, Blewett CJ. A meta-analysis of randomized controlled trials that compared neoadjuvant chemotherapy and surgery to surgery alone for resectable esophageal cancer. *Am J Surg*. 2002;183:274–279.
24. Le Prise E, Etienne PL, Meunier B, et al. A randomized study of chemotherapy, radiation therapy, and surgery versus surgery for localized squamous cell carcinoma of the esophagus. *Cancer*. 1994;73:1779–1784.
25. Apinop C, Puttisak P, Preecha N. A prospective study of combined therapy in esophageal cancer. *Hepatol Gastroenterol*. 1994;41:391–393.
26. Bosset JF, Gignoux M, Triboulet JP, et al. Chemoradiotherapy followed by surgery compared with surgery alone in squamous-cell cancer of the esophagus. *N Engl J Med*. 1997;337:161–167.
27. Walsh TN, Noonan N, Hollywood D, et al. A comparison of multimodal therapy and surgery for esophageal adenocarcinoma. *N Engl J Med*. 1996;33:462–467.
28. Urba SG, Orringer MB, Turrisi A, et al. Randomized trial of preoperative chemoradiation versus surgery alone in patients with locoregional esophageal carcinoma. *J Clin Oncol*. 2001;19:305–313.
29. Burmeister BH, Smithers BM, Gebski V, et al. Surgery alone versus chemoradiotherapy followed by surgery for resectable cancer of the oesophagus: a randomized controlled phase III trial. *Lancet Oncol*. 2005;6:659–668.
30. Natsugoe S, Okumura H, Uchikado Y, et al. Randomized controlled study on preoperative chemoradiotherapy followed by surgery versus surgery alone for esophageal squamous cell cancer in a single institution. *Dis Esophagus*. 2006;19:468–472.
31. Tepper JE, Krasna M, Niedzwiecki D, et al. Superiority of trimodality therapy to surgery alone in esophageal cancer: Results of CALGB 9781 [Abstract]. *J Clin Oncol*. 2006;24:4012.
32. Malthaner RA, Wong RS, Rumble RB, et al. Neoadjuvant or adjuvant therapy for respectable esophageal cancer: a systematic review and meta-analysis. *BMC Med*. 2004;2:35–39.
33. Burak WE. Is adjuvant chemotherapy the answer to adenocarcinoma of the esophagus? *Am J Surg*. 2003;186:296–300.
34. Fiorica F, Camma C, Venturi A, et al. Preoperative radiotherapy and chemotherapy in patients with esophageal carcinoma: a meta-analysis [abstract]. *Int J Radiat Oncol Biol Phys*. 2002;54:220.
35. Urschel JD, Vasan H. A meta-analysis of randomized controlled trials that compared neoadjuvant chemoradiation and surgery to surgery for esophageal cancer. *Am J Surg*. 2003;185: 538–543.
36. Pouliquen X, Levard H, Hay JM, et al. Fluorouracil and cisplatin therapy after palliative surgical resection of squamous cell carcinoma of the esophagus. A multicenter randomized trial. French Association for Surgical Research. *Ann Surg*. 1996;223:127–133.
37. Ando N, Iizuka T, Kakegawa J, et al. A randomized trial of surgery with and without chemotherapy for localized squamous cell of the thoracic esophagus: the Japan Clinical Oncology Study. *J Thorac Cardiovasc Surg*. 1997;114:205–209.
38. Ando N, Iizuka T, Idle H, et al. A randomized trial of surgery alone vs. surgery plus postoperative chemotherapy with cisplatin and 5-fluorouracil for localized squamous carcinoma of the thoracic esophagus: The Japan Clinical Oncology Group Study (JCOG 9204) [abstract 1034]. *Proc Ann Meet Am Soc Clin Oncol*. 1999;18:269a.
39. Mooney MM. Neoadjuvant and adjuvant chemotherapy for esophageal adenocarcinoma. *J Surg Oncol*. 2005;92:230–238.
40. MacDonald JS, Smalley SR, Benedetti J, et al. Chemotherapy after surgery compared with surgery alone for adenocarcinoma of the stomach or gastroesophageal junction. *N Engl J Med*. 2001;345:725–730.
41. Levard H, Pouliquen X, Hay JM, et al. 5-Fluorouracil and cisplatin as palliative treatment of advanced oesophageal squamous cell carcinoma: a multicenter randomized controlled trial. *Eur J Surg*. 2003;164:849–857.
42. Shah MA, Schwartz GK. Treatment of metastatic esophagus and gastric cancer. *Semin Oncol*. 2004;31:574–587.
43. Vogl SE, Greenwald E, Kaplan BH. Effective chemotherapy for esophageal cancer with methotrexate, bleomycin, and cis-diamminedichloroplatinum II. *Cancer*. 1981;48:2555–2558.
44. Kelsen DP, Fein R, Coonley C, et al. Cisplatin, vindesine, and mitoguazone in the treatment of esophageal cancer. *Cancer*. 1986;70:255–259.
45. Coonley CJ, Bains M, Hilaris M, et al. Cisplatin and bleomycin in the treatment of esophageal carcinoma, a final report. *Cancer*. 1984. 54:2351–2355.
46. Engstrom PF, Lavin PT, Klaassen DJ. Phase II evaluation of mitomycin and cisplatin in advanced esophageal carcinoma. *Cancer Treat Rep*. 1983;67:713–715.
47. Kelsen D, Hilaris B, Coonley C, et al. Cisplatin, vindesine, and bleomycin chemotherapy of local-regional and advanced esophageal carcinoma. *Am J Med*. 1983;75:645–652.
48. Dinwoodie WR, Bartolucci AA, Lyman GH, et al. Phase II evaluation of cisplatin, bleomycin, and vindesine in advanced squamous cell carcinoma of the esophagus: a Southeastern Cancer Study Group trial. *Cancer Treat Rep*. 1986;70: 267–270.
49. Bleiberg H, Conroy T, Paillot B, et al. Randomised phase II study of cisplatin and 5-fluorouracil (5-FU) versus cisplatin alone in advanced squamous cell oesophageal cancer. *Eur J Cancer*. 1997;33:1216–1220.
50. Hayashi K, Ando N, Watanabe H, et al. Phase II evaluation of protracted infusion of cisplatin and 5-fluorouracil in advanced squamous cell carcinoma of the esophagus: a Japan Esophageal Oncology Group Trial (JCOG9407). *Jap J Clin Oncol*. 2001;31:419–423.
51. Hsu CH, Cheng AL, Hsu C, et al. A phase II study of weekly methotrexate, cisplatin, and 24-hour infusion of high-dose 5-fluorouracil and leucovorin (MP-HDFL) in patients with metastatic and recurrent esophageal cancer-improving toxicity profile by infusional schedule and double biochemical modulation of 5-fluorouracil. *Anticancer Res*. 2002;22:3621–3627.
52. Ilson DH, Ajani J, Bhalla K, et al. Phase II trial of paclitaxel, fluorouracil, and cisplatin in patients with advanced carcinoma of the esophagus. *J Clin Oncol*. 1998;16:1826–1834.
53. Polee MB, Kok TC, Siersema PD, et al. Phase II study of the combination of cisplatin, etoposide, 5-fluorouracil, and folinic acid in patients with advanced squamous cell carcinoma of the esophagus. *Anti-Cancer Drugs*. 2001;12:513–517.
54. Conroy T, Etienne PL, Adenis A, et al. Vinorelbine and cisplatin in metastatic squamous cell carcinoma of the oesophagus: response, toxicity, quality of life and survival. *Ann Oncol*. 2002;13:721–729.
55. Kok TC, Van der Gaast A, Dees J, et al. Cisplatin and etoposide in oesophageal cancer: a phase II study. *Brit J Cancer*. 1996;74:980–984.
56. Spiridonidis CH, Laufman LR, Jones JJ, et al. A phase II evaluation of high dose cisplatin and etoposide in patients with advanced esophageal adenocarcinoma. *Cancer*. 1996;78:2070–2077.
57. Ilson DH, Forastiere A, Arquette M, et al. A phase II trial of paclitaxel and cisplatin in patients with advanced carcinoma of the esophagus. *Cancer J*. 2000;6:316–323.
58. Petrasch S, Welt A, Reinacher A, et al. Chemotherapy with cisplatin and paclitaxel in patients with locally advanced, recurrent or metastatic oesophageal cancer. *Brit J Cancer*. 1998;78:511–514.
59. Ajani JA, Fodor MB, Tjulandin SA, et al. Phase II multi-institutional randomized trial of docetaxel plus cisplatin with or without fluorouracil in patients with untreated, advanced gastric or gastroesophageal adenocarcinoma. *J Clin Oncol*. 2005;23:5660–5667.
60. Ilson DH, Saltz L, Enzinger P, et al. Phase II trial of weekly irinotecan plus in advanced esophageal cancer. *J Clin Oncol*. 1999;17:3270–3275.
61. Mackay HJ, McInnes A, Paul J, et al. A phase II study of epirubicin, cisplatin, and raltitrexed combination chemotherapy in patients with advanced oesophageal and gastric adenocarcinoma. *Ann Oncol*. 2001;12:1407–1410.
62. Corporaal S, Smit WM, Russel MG, et al. Capecitabine, epirubicin and cisplatin in the treatment of oesophagogastric adenocarcinoma. *Netherlands J Med*. 2006;64:141–146.
63. Urba SG, Chansky K, VanVeldhuizen PJ, et al. Gemcitabine and cisplatin for patients with metastatic or recurrent esophageal carcinoma. *Investigational New Drugs*. 2004;22:91–97.
64. Millar J, Scullin P, Morrison A, et al. Phase II study of gemcitabine and cisplatin in locally advanced/metastatic oesophageal cancer. *Brit J Cancer*. 2005;93:1112–1116.
65. Kelsen D, Lovett D, Wong J, et al. Interferon alfa-2a and fluorouracil in the treatment of patients with advanced esophageal cancer. *J Clin Oncol*. 1992;10:269–274.
66. Airoldi M, Cortesina G, Giordando C, et al. Docetaxel and vinorelbine: an effective regimen in recurrent squamous cell esophageal cancer. *Med Oncol*. 2003;20:19–24.
67. Morgan-Meadows S, Mulkerin D, Berlin JD, et al. A phase II trial of gemcitabine, 5-fluorouracil, and leucovorin in advanced esophageal carcinoma. *Oncology*. 2005;69:130–134.
68. Burge ME, Smith D, Topham C, et al. A phase I and II study of 2-weekly irinotecan with capecitabine in advanced gastroesophageal adenocarcinoma. *Brit J Cancer*. 2006;94:1281–1286.
69. Pozzo C, Barone C, Szanto J, et al. Irinotecan in combination with 5-fluorouracil and folinic acid or with cisplatin in patients with advanced gastric or esophageal-gastric junction adenocarcinoma: results of a randomized phase II study. *Ann Oncol*. 2004;15:1773–1781.
70. Jatoi A, Tirona MT, Cha SS, et al. A phase II trial of docetaxel and CPT-11 in patients with metastatic adenocarcinoma of esophagus, gastroesophageal junction, and gastric cardia. *Int J Gastro Cancer*. 2002;32:115–123.
71. Lordick F, von Schilling C, Bernhard H, et al. Phase II trial of irinotecan plus docetaxel in cisplatin-pretreated relapsed or refractory oesophageal cancer. *Brit J Cancer*. 2003;89:630–633.
72. Lorenzen S, Duyster J, Lersch C, et al. Capecitabine plus docetaxel every 3 weeks in first- and second-line metastatic oesophageal cancer: final results of a phase II trial. *Brit J Cancer*. 2005;92:2129–2133.

73. Mauer AM, Kraut EH, Krauss SA, et al. Phase II trial of oxaliplatin, leucovorin, and fluorouracil in patients with advanced carcinoma of the esophagus. *Ann Oncol.* 2005;16:1320–1325.
74. El-Rayes BF, Shields A, Zalupski M, et al. A phase II study of carboplatin and paclitaxel in esophageal cancer. *Ann Oncol.* 2004;15:960–965.
75. Braybrooke JP, O'Bryne KJ, Saunders MP, et al. A phase II study of mitomycin C and oral etoposide for advanced adenocarcinoma of the upper gastrointestinal tract. *Ann Oncol.* 1997;8:294–296.
76. Sihvo ET, Luostarinen ME, Salo JA. Fate of patients with adenocarcinomas of the esophagus and the esophagogastric junction: a population-based analysis. *Am J Gastroenterol.* 2004;99:419–424.
77. Hulscher JF, Tijssen JP, Obertop H, et al. Transthoracic versus transhiatal resection for carcinoma of the esophagus: a meta-analysis. *Ann Thorac Surg.* 2001;72:306–313.
78. Thierry C, Marchal F, Blazeby JM. Quality of life in patients with oesophageal and gastric cancer: an overview. *Oncology.* 2006;70:391–402.
79. Brooks JA, Kesler KA, Johnson CS, et al. Prospective analysis of quality of life after surgical resection for esophageal cancer: preliminary results. *J Surg Oncol.* 2002;81:185–194.
80. de Boer AG, van Lanschot JJ, van Sandick JW, et al. Quality of life after transhiatal compared with extended transthoracic resection for adenocarcinoma of the esophagus. *J Clin Oncol.* 2004;22:4202–4208.
81. Blazeby JM, Farndon JR, Donovan J, et al. A prospective longitudinal study examining the quality of life of patients with esophageal carcinoma. *Cancer.* 2000;88:1781–1787.
82. Viklund P, Wengstrom Y, Rouvelas I, et al. Quality of life and persisting symptoms after esophageal cancer surgery. *Euro J Cancer.* 2006;42:1407–1414.
83. Mao YS, Suntharalingam M, Krasna MJ. Management of late distant metastases after trimodality therapy for esophageal cancer. *Ann Thorac Surg.* 2003;76:1742–1743.
84. Bhogaraju AK, Hanna N, Brooks JA, et al. Survival and disease recurrence for esophageal cancer patients achieving pathologic complete response (pCR) at surgery after neoadjuvant chemoradiation [abstract 582]. *Proc Am Soc Clin Oncol.* 21:2002.
85. Herskovic A, Martz K, al-Sarraf M, et al. Combined chemotherapy and radiotherapy compared with radiotherapy alone in patients with cancer of the esophagus. *N Engl J Med.* 1992;326:1593–1598.
86. Shah MA, Kelsen DP. Combined modality therapy of esophageal cancer: changes in the standard of care? *Ann Surg Oncol.* 2004;11:641–643.
87. Blazeby JM, Sanford E, Falk SJ, et al. Health-related quality of life during neoadjuvant treatment and surgery for localized esophageal carcinoma. *Cancer.* 2005;103:1791–1799.
88. Bamias A, Hill ME, Cunningham D, et al. Epirubicin, cisplatin, and protracted venous infusion of 5-fluorouracil for esophagogastric adenocarcinoma: response, toxicity, quality of life, and survival. *Cancer.* 1996;77:1978–1985.
89. Ancker JS, Kaufman D. Rethinking health numeracy: A multidisciplinary literature review. *J Am Med Inform Assoc.* 2007; 14:713–721.
90. Kim MK, Alvi A. Breaking the bad news of cancer: the patient's perspective. *Laryngoscope.* 1999;109:1064–1067.
91. Weeks JC, Cook EF, O'Day SJ, et al. Relationship between cancer patients' predictions of prognosis and their treatment preferences. *JAMA.* 1998;279:1709–1714.
92. Seale C. Communication and awareness about death: a study of a random sample of dying people. *Soc Sci Med.* 1991;32:943–952.
93. Haidet P, Harmel MB, Davis RB, et al. Outcomes, preferences for resuscitation, and physician-patient communication among patients with metastatic colorectal cancer. *Am J Med.* 1998;105:222–229.
94. Jansen ST, Kievit J, Nooij MA, et al. Patients' preferences for adjuvant chemotherapy in early-stage breast cancer: is treatment worthwhile? *Brit J Cancer.* 2001;84:1577–1585.
95. Jenkins V, Fallowfield L, Saul J. Information needs of patients with cancer: results from a large study in UK cancer centres. *Brit J Cancer.* 2001;84:48–51.
96. Butow PN, McLean M, Dunn S, et al. The dynamics of change: cancer patients' preference for information, involvement and support. *Ann Oncol.* 1997;8:857–863.
97. Butow PN, Kazemi J, Beeney LJ, et al. When the diagnosis is cancer: patient communication experiences and preferences. *Cancer.* 1996;77:2630–2637.
98. Kaplowitz SA, Campo S, Chui WT. Cancer patients' desire for communication of prognosis information. *Health Comm.* 2002;14:221–241.
99. Lobb EA, Butow PN, Kenny DT, et al. Communicating prognosis in early breast cancer; do women understand the language used? *Med J Australia.* 1999;171: 290–294.
100. Kutner JS, Steiner JF, Corbett KK, et al. Information needs in terminal illness. *Soc Sci Med.* 1999;48:1341–1352.
101. Peteet JR, Abrams HE, Ross DM, et al. Presenting a diagnosis of cancer: patients' views. *J Family Prac.* 1991;32:577–581.
102. Sardell AN, Trierweiler SJ. Disclosing the cancer diagnosis. Procedures that influence patient hopefulness. *Cancer.* 1993;72:3355–3365.
103. Swenson SL, Buell S, Zettler P, et al. Patient-centered communication: do patients really prefer it? *J Gen Inter Med.* 2004;19:1069–1079.
104. Winefield HR, Murrell TC, Clifford JV, et al. The usefulness of distinguishing different types of general practice consultation, or are needed skills always the same? *Fam Prac.* 1995;12:402–407.
105. Elwyn G, Edwards A, Kinnersley P, et al. Shared decision making and the concept of equipoise: the competences of involving patients in healthcare choices. *Brit J Gen Pract.* 2000;50:892–899.
106. Graugaard PK, Finset A. Trait anxiety and reactions to patient-centered and doctor centered styles of communication; an experimental study. *Psychosom Med.* 2000;62:33–39.
107. McKneally MF, Martin DK. An entrustment model of consent for surgical treatment of life-threatening illness: perspective of patients requiring esophagectomy. *J Thorac Cardiovasc Surg.* 2000;120:264–269.

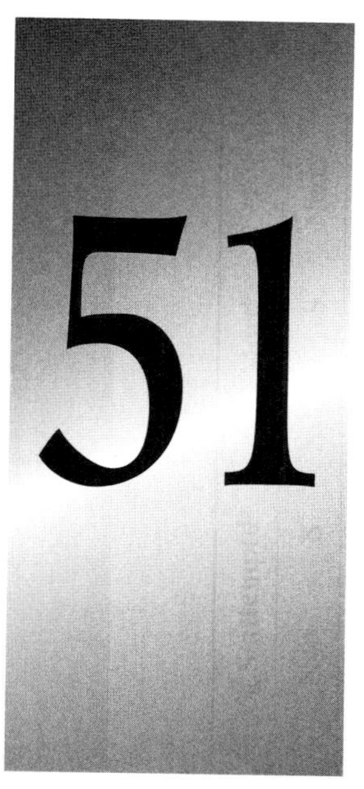

51 Review and Synthesis of Clinical Trials in Esophageal Cancer

Geoffrey Y. Ku
David H. Ilson

For locally advanced esophageal cancer, surgery remains the mainstay of treatment. Various reviews have reported 5-year overall survival (OS) rates from 10% up to 30% to 40% with surgical resection alone (1,2). Primary radiation therapy was previously used for local tumor control, though less successfully. In 1 large series, the 3-year survival after radiotherapy alone was only 6% (3). For metastatic disease, chemotherapy alone results in response rates of only 20% to 40% and median survivals of 8 to 10 months (4).

Given the activity of all 3 modalities, numerous studies have combined them in distinct neoadjuvant (preoperative) strategies for locally advanced disease. Multimodality approaches have included chemotherapy or radiation or concurrent chemoradiotherapy followed by surgery, in an effort to improve the dismal prognosis of this aggressive cancer. Relatively few studies have focused on an adjuvant (postoperative) approach.

The results of these studies have been mixed and their combined outcomes have failed to elevate any preoperative strategies to a clear standard for resectable esophageal cancer. However, trials involving preoperative chemoradiotherapy and chemotherapy have demonstrated a trend toward improved survival over surgery alone. Based on these data, many clinicians now treat locoregional disease with preoperative multimodality therapy.

PALLIATIVE CHEMOTHERAPY

Although several chemotherapeutic agents have modest antitumor activity in esophageal cancer, the duration of response to both single agents and combination regimens is only generally 4 to 6 months. In the palliative setting, this approach may be considered appropriate treatment. However, chemotherapy is rarely used alone with curative intent.

Commonly used drugs include cisplatin (5–7), 5-fluorouracil (5-FU) (8,9), and mitomycin (10–12), with single-agent response rates ranging from 10% to 25%. Newer agents include the oral 5-FU pro-drugs (capecitabine [13,14] and S-1 [15]), the taxanes (paclitaxel [16–18] and docetaxel [19–21]), irinotecan (22) and oxaliplatin (23,24), with response rates of 15% to 45%. Some of these trials have primarily enrolled patients with gastric cancer but also include patients with gastroesophageal junction (GEJ) cancer.

The majority of data for single-agent chemotherapy are derived from phase II trials, which makes comparison across different trials difficult. In addition, the confidence limits largely overlap across trials in most cases.

Given the modest activity of single agents in esophageal cancer, combination chemotherapy has been extensively studied. In metastatic disease, cisplatin-containing regimens have shown 25% to 45% activity. In locoregional disease, response rates as high as 45% to 75% have been reported. Disappointingly, these responses have been no more durable than those of single agents. As such, no clearly superior first-line regimen has been identified in the metastatic setting.

The combination of cisplatin/infusional 5-FU has been studied extensively, with toxicity consisting mainly of mucositis, diarrhea, nausea/vomiting, renal toxicity, and myelosuppression. Despite the common use of this regimen, only a single phase II trial has compared cisplatin with the combination regimen in patients with advanced squamous cell carcinoma (25). While there was a higher response rate in favor of the combination regimen, there was no statistically significant survival benefit. In addition, the combination group had a significantly higher rate of treatment-related deaths (16% versus 0%).

Randomized trials have compared numerous other drug combinations to cisplatin/5-FU. For example, the ECF regimen (epirubicin/cisplatin/infusional 5-FU) has been compared to the FAMTX regimen (bolus 5-FU/doxorubicin/methotrexate) (26). The ECF arm achieved superior median OS (8.9 versus 5.7 months), response rate (45% versus 21%), and quality of life at 24 weeks compared with FAMTX.

A subsequent study compared the ECF and MCF regimen, where mitomycin was substituted for epirubicin, in previously untreated patients with advanced esophageal cancer (27). The study reported no significant differences in response rate or median survival but found that quality of life was better maintained with ECF. The equivalent response rates and outcomes that were seen with both of these regimens have led some to question whether either regimen offers any advantage over the conventional 2-drug standard. The data from the ECF trials, however, support the use of continuous infusion 5-FU over bolus 5-FU, as well as lower doses of cisplatin (60 mg/m^2) more commonly used in the 2-drug 5-FU/cisplatin combination (75–100 mg/m^2).

In the recent REAL-2 study, Cunningham and colleagues from the United Kingdom compared the ECF regimen to the ECX regimen (which involves the substitution of 5-FU with capecitabine), the EOF regimen (substitution of oxaliplatin for cisplatin), and the EOX regimen (a double substitution of both capecitabine and oxaliplatin) in patients with locally advanced esophageal, GEJ and gastric cancer (24). In this trial, designed to demonstrate non-inferiority in OS between the 5-FU and capecitabine groups and between the cisplatin and oxaliplatin groups, all the combinations had similar response rates and comparable toxicities. The EOX regimen was associated with improved median OS compared to the ECF regimen (11.2 versus 9.9 months, $P = 0.02$), leading the investigators to propose that the EOX regimen could replace the ECF regimen in future trials.

The oral 5-FU prodrug S-1 has also been evaluated in combination regimens. In a single-arm phase II evaluation in gastric and GEJ cancer, the combination of S-1/cisplatin produced a response rate of 51%, with an encouraging median OS of 10.9 months (15). Two recent randomized phase III trials performed in Japan also compared S-1 versus S-1/cisplatin in one trial and S-1 versus infusional 5-FU versus cisplatin/irinotecan in the other (28,29). As these trials enrolled patients with gastric cancer (with the proportion of those with GEJ involvement not stated), their applicability to patients with GEJ/lower esophageal adenocarcinoma is unclear.

Taxanes have also been evaluated in combination regimens. The addition of docetaxel to cisplatin/5-FU was recently evaluated by Van Cutsem et al. in a phase III randomized trial in gastric and GEJ cancer that compared the DCF regimen (docetaxel/cisplatin/ infusional 5-FU) to cisplatin/infusional 5-FU (30). Although response rate and time-to-progression (TTP) were improved with the 3-drug regimen over the 2-drug regimen, OS was only slightly improved (median OS 9.2 versus 8.6 months, 2-year OS 18% versus 9%). In addition, the 3-drug regimen was associated with significantly more toxicity, including a grade 3/4 neutropenia rate of 82% (versus 57% for CF) and febrile neutropenia in 29% of patients (versus 12% for CF).

A slight variant of the DCF regimen used by Van Cutsem et al. (termed TCF, employing a 14- versus 5-day 5-FU infusion at a lower dose) was also recently compared to the ECF regimen in a phase II randomized trial (which included a third arm of docetaxel/cisplatin) (31). TCF was associated with a superior response rate (the primary endpoint) when compared to ECF (37% versus 25%) but the toxicity—particularly rates of neutropenia and neutropenic fever—was again substantial. This phase II trial also included a third arm with the TC (docetaxel/cisplatin) regimen. Activity and survival were comparable between the TC and TCF arms and there was a suggestion of superior toxicity profile for the 2-drug TC regimen compared to the 3-drug TCF regimen. Based on the toxicity seen with TCF, the authors commented that further evaluation of this regimen might not be warranted.

Similarly, another randomized phase II study demonstrated comparable activity for a regimen of DF (docetaxel/5-FU) versus ECF, although the study was not powered for a head-to-head comparison of both regimens (32). Response rates (38% versus 36% respectively) and median TTP (5.5 versus 5.3 months) and OS (9.5 versus 9.7 months) were very similar, with differing but manageable toxicities for both regimens. Although the DF regimen had significant grade 3/4 neutropenia, neutropenic fever occurred in only 4.4% of patients. This trial enrolled patients with gastric cancer but, as 29% of patients had involvement of the gastric cardia, these results may also be applicable to patients with GEJ/lower esophageal adenocarcinoma.

Other investigators have combined cisplatin with paclitaxel, both with and without 5-FU in phase II evaluations (33–36). Response rates ranged from 43% to 50% but toxicity included significant diarrhea, neurotoxicity, and myelosuppression.

Irinotecan is another active agent in upper gastrointestinal tumors that has been combined with mitomycin, 5-FU/leucovorin or cisplatin in phase II evaluations, with response rates ranging from 30% to 65% (37–41). In a randomized phase II trial, Pozzo and colleagues compared the FUFIRI regimen (weekly irinotecan/5-FU/leucovorin) with irinotecan/cisplatin administered every 3 weeks in patients with advanced gastric and GEJ cancer (39). FUFIRI was associated with a superior response rate, TTP, and OS, and less neutropenia than the irinotecan/cisplatin arm. This led to a subsequent phase III trial of FUFIRI versus cisplatin/5-FU. Both regimens had comparable efficacy but there was less neutropenic fever and grade 3/4 stomatitis and nausea in the FUFIRI arm (42). Only the incidence of grade 3/4 diarrhea was increased in the FUFIRI arm, although more patients withdrew from the cisplatin/5-FU arm than the FUFIRI arm (22% versus 10%, $P = 0.004$) for drug-related adverse events.

NEOADJUVANT CHEMOTHERAPY

Despite the short-lived responses using chemotherapy alone in advanced disease, neoadjuvant chemotherapy is associated with many theoretical benefits (43). This approach has the potential to assess tumor response to chemotherapy and direct the possible use of chemotherapy postoperatively or in the metastatic setting. Chemotherapy may also improve baseline dysphagia, downstage the primary tumor, increase resection rates, and treat micrometastatic disease that is undetectable at diagnosis.

Kok and colleagues reported a small randomized phase III trial, in which 148 patients with squamous cell carcinoma were randomized to surgery alone or preoperative cisplatin/etoposide followed by surgery (44). Preoperative chemotherapy was associated with a significant improvement in median OS (18.5 months versus 11 months). No final report of this study has been published.

However, the large North American Intergroup 0113 trial failed to show a survival benefit for perioperative cisplatin/5-FU plus surgery compared with surgery alone in 440 patients (45). Patients in the combined-modality arm received 3 cycles of cisplatin/5-FU preoperatively and 2 cycles postoperatively. Pathologic complete responses (pCR) were seen in only 2.5% of patients receiving preoperative chemotherapy, and there was no improvement in the curative resection rate. The median OS was not significantly different in the 2 groups and the 5-year OS with or without chemotherapy was 20%. The addition of chemotherapy did not change the rate of recurrence either locally or at distant sites.

Renewed interest in preoperative chemotherapy was generated by a trial performed by the Medical Research Council Oesophageal Cancer Working Group (46). This study randomized 802 patients (nearly double the number of patients in the Intergroup trial) to surgery alone versus 2 cycles of preoperative cisplatin/5-FU. At a relatively short median follow-up of only 2 years, the chemotherapy-treated group demonstrated improved median OS (16.8 months versus 13.3 months) and 2-year survival (43% versus 34%). The curative resection rate was improved marginally from 55% to 60% and the pCR rate was 4% in the preoperative chemotherapy group. It may be that the larger sample size compared to the Intergroup trial facilitated the detection of a small improvement with chemotherapy. In addition, a larger proportion of patients on this trial had adenocarcinoma histology compared to the Intergroup 113 trial (66% versus 54%). Two recent meta-analyses (described in detail subsequently) suggest greater benefit from preoperative chemotherapy for patients with adenocarcinoma versus squamous cell cancer (47,48).

Additional evidence to support the use of perioperative chemotherapy comes from the recent MAGIC trial performed in the United Kingdom (49). This trial randomized 503 patients with gastric or GEJ adenocarcinoma to 3 cycles each of pre- and postoperative ECF chemotherapy and surgery or surgery alone. Perioperative chemotherapy resulted in significant improvement in 5-year OS (36% versus 23%). However, there was no improvement in the curative resection rate and there were no cases of pCR. As 26% of patients on this trial had tumors in the GEJ and lower esophagus, the results may apply to esophageal cancer.

Finally, data from a French trial of 224 patients with gastric or lower esophageal adenocarcinoma were recently presented (50). Patients were randomized to 2 or 3 cycles of preoperative cisplatin/5-FU followed by surgery versus surgery alone. Preoperative chemotherapy was associated with a significant improvement in R0 resection rate (84% versus 73%), 5-year disease-free survival (34% versus 21%), and 5-year OS (38% versus 24%).

Although comparisons between different clinical trials must be made cautiously, the survival benefit seen with preoperative cisplatin/5-FU on this trial appears to be very similar to that seen with perioperative ECF in the MAGIC trial. Because of the smaller sample size of this trial, however, outcome differences in as few as 10 to 15 patients would have changed the trial outcome. Also, the trial did not consistently stage patients with endoscopic ultrasound or stratify them by pre-therapy stage. In a small-scale trial, even a slight imbalance in pre-therapy stage might impact the trial outcome. Finally, a multivariate analysis indicated a greater survival benefit for patients with gastric versus esophageal primary tumors, making the relative benefit of this therapy in patients with esophageal adenocarcinoma possibly less certain.

These data are summarized in Table 51.1. Overall, recent trials suggest a survival benefit for perioperative chemotherapy, although preoperative chemotherapy alone is associated with a low pCR rate and only borderline improvement in the resection rate. Such a survival benefit was also demonstrated in a recent large, individual patient data meta-analysis of 12 randomized trials involving preoperative chemotherapy (48). This meta-analysis revealed a 5-year survival benefit of only 4% with preoperative chemo, with a suggestion of lesser benefit for squamous (4%) compared to adenocarcinoma histology (7%).

NEOADJUVANT RADIATION THERAPY

Trials that have evaluated the use of preoperative radiation have largely reported no benefit.

Kelsen and colleagues performed a randomized trial comparing preoperative radiation to preoperative chemotherapy in 96 patients with esophageal cancer (51). Although there was no increase in operative morbidity or mortality for patients treated with preoperative therapy compared with historic controls treated with surgery alone, there was also no additional treatment benefit. Another randomized trial involving 176 patients also failed to identify a benefit for preoperative radiation (52).

TABLE 51.1

Results of Phase III Preoperative Chemotherapy Trials in Esophageal Cancer

Treatment	Histology	Pts	Survival	Reference
Surgery alone	Squamous	41	9% at 3 years	Nygaard et al. (53)
Cis/bleo + surgery		50	3% at 3 years	
RT + surgery		48	21 % at 3 years	
Cis/bleo/RT/surgery		47	17% at 3 years	
Cis/etop + surgery	Squamous	74	18.5 months	Kok et al. (44)
Surgery alone		74	11 months	
Pre-op Cis/5-FU + surgery + post-op cis/5-FU	Squamous + adenocarcinoma	213	14.9 months (median); 23% at 3 years	Kelsen et al. (45)
Surgery alone		227	16.1 months (median); 26% at 2 years	
Cis/5-FU + surgery	Squamous + adenocarcinoma	400	16.8 months (median); 2-year survival 43%	Medical Research Council (46)
Surgery alone		402	13.3 months (median); 2-year survival 34%	
Pre-op ECF + surgery + post-op ECF	Adenocarcinoma	250	24 months (median); 5-year survival 36%	Cunningham et al. (49)
Surgery alone		253	20 months (median); 5-year survival 23%	
Cis/5-FU + surgery	Adenocarcinoma	113	5-year survival 38%	Boige et al. (50)
Surgery alone		111	5-year survival 24%	

Abbreviations: bleo = bleomycin; cis = cisplatin; ECF = epirubicin, cisplatin, 5-fluoruoracil; etop = etoposide; 5-FU = 5-fluorouracil; RT = radiotherapy.

A prospective, multicenter Scandinavian trial reported by Nygaard et al. randomized 186 patients with esophageal squamous cell carcinoma to 4 treatment groups: surgery alone; preoperative chemotherapy (cisplatin/bleomycin) and surgery; preoperative radiation and surgery or; preoperative chemotherapy and radiation, followed by surgery (53). The 3-year OS was significantly higher in the pooled groups receiving radiation compared with the non-radiation groups. The results indicated an intermediate-term survival benefit for preoperative radiation but found that the chemotherapy regimen did not influence survival.

However, a subsequent meta-analysis was unable to establish a significant benefit for preoperative radiation (54). With a median follow-up of 9 years, an analysis of more than 1,100 patients from 5 randomized trials suggested a survival benefit of 3% at 2 years and 4% at 5 years that was not statistically significant ($P = 0.062$).

ADJUVANT (POSTOPERATIVE) THERAPY

Combined-modality therapy in esophageal carcinoma has long focused on preoperative strategies. The role of adjuvant therapy has not been studied extensively, and the data that are available suggest equivocal results.

Postoperative chemotherapy without preoperative therapy was studied in 2 Japanese randomized trials, where patients with squamous cell histology were randomized to receive 2 cycles of chemotherapy with cisplatin/vindesine (55) or cisplatin/5-FU (56) respectively. While the trial with cisplatin/vindesine did not show any survival benefit, the trial with cisplatin/5-FU did reveal a survival benefit, but only for patients with lymph node involvement (5-year disease-free survival 52% versus 38%).

These results are consistent with those of a randomized French trial, which also found no survival benefit for 6 to 8 months of adjuvant chemotherapy with cisplatin/5-FU (57). In fact, there were significantly more complications in the chemotherapy group.

In contrast, a recent pilot Eastern Cooperative Oncology Group (ECOG) trial recently evaluated 4 cycles of postoperative paclitaxel/cisplatin in patients with esophageal or GEJ adenocarcinoma (58). Two-year OS was 60%, which is statistically superior compared to the historic control (38%, derived from Intergroup 113 trial).

Trials involving adjuvant radiotherapy have generally reported negative results. A French study randomized 221 patients to surgery alone versus surgery followed by radiation and found no survival benefit from radiation (59).

Another randomized study of 130 patients from Hong Kong actually demonstrated increased mortality with postoperative radiation (8.7 versus 15.2 months, in favor of the no adjuvant therapy group), with the difference attributed to radiation-related deaths and early metastatic disease (60).

Finally, a large prospective Chinese study also failed to detect an OS benefit among 495 patients randomized to adjuvant radiation or no further therapy (61). However, a subgroup analysis of stage III patients did show a 5-year survival benefit, up from 13.1% in the surgery-only group to 35.1% in the group that received adjuvant radiation.

While trials of adjuvant radiotherapy alone have not suggested significant benefit, there may be benefit from adjuvant concurrent chemoradiotherapy, as suggested the results of the Intergroup trial 116 in gastric adenocarcinoma (62). This trial revealed a significant improvement in overall and disease-free survival for the delivery of postoperative therapy with 5-FU/leucovorin and radiation compared to surgery alone. As 20% of the patients treated had proximal gastric cancers (with involvement of the GEJ) and primary GEJ cancers, these data may justify the use of postoperative therapy in such patients who have not received preoperative therapy.

NEOADJUVANT (PREOPERATIVE) CHEMORADIOTHERAPY

Although recent pre- and perioperative chemotherapy trials have indicated a survival benefit, the low rate of pCR and the inconsistent improvement in operability have led researchers to investigate neoadjuvant chemoradiotherapy.

Chemoradiotherapy typically involves regimens of cisplatin or mitomycin and continuous infusion 5-FU, with radiotherapy dosages from 30 to 40 Gy and up to 60 Gy in more recent trials. This approach results in pCR rates in the range of 20% to 40%, with long-term survival of no more than 25% to 35% (63,64). Superior survival is consistently achieved, though, in patients achieving a pCR to chemoradiotherapy (up to 50%–60% at 5 years) (65–69).

These results are at the expense of significant toxicities—primarily hematologic and gastrointestinal—which have been greatest in trials employing a higher dose of or twice-daily radiation or in which radiotherapy overlapped all cycles of preoperative chemotherapy (70). The gastrointestinal toxicity associated with cisplatin/5-FU and radiation includes nausea, mucositis, and esophagitis, leading some investigators to mandate placement of enteral feeding tubes prior to treatment initiation.

The seminal phase III U.S. Radiation Therapy Oncology Group (RTOG) trial 85–01 demonstrated the superiority of chemoradiotherapy over radiation alone

(71). This nonoperative study compared standard-fractionation radiation (64 Gy) to radiation (50 Gy) plus concurrent cisplatin/5-FU. The trial was stopped when data from 121 patients showed an improved median OS in favor of chemoradiotherapy (12.5 months versus 8.9 months). Two-year survival was also improved in the chemoradiotherapy group (38% versus 10%), as was 5-year survival (21% versus 0%) (72). Long-term survival was also seen in the small number of adenocarcinoma patients on the trial, with 13% of patients alive at 5 years.

In addition to a survival benefit, disease recurrence was significantly reduced by the addition of chemotherapy to radiation. At 1 year, recurrent disease was observed in 62% of the group that received radiation versus 44% in the chemoradiotherapy arm; distant recurrence rates were 38% and 22% respectively. Based on this study, chemoradiotherapy was established as the standard of care in the nonsurgical management of locally advanced squamous cell esophageal cancer.

Building on these results, alternative treatment strategies have also been investigated. In the non-operative RTOG 90–12 chemoradiotherapy study, "induction" chemotherapy with cisplatin/5-FU followed by chemoradiotherapy with the same regimen did not appear to afford any additional benefit (73). The RTOG 94–05 study compared a total radiation dose of 64.8 Gy versus 50.4 Gy during concurrent cisplatin/5-FU and also failed to demonstrate superior results with the more intense regimen (74). This study confirmed 50.4 Gy as the standard radiation dose when given in combined therapy with cisplatin/5-FU. Finally, the phase I/II RTOG 92–07 trial, which attempted to "boost" radiation with brachytherapy following external beam radiation, revealed significant toxicity, including a 12% incidence of treatment-related fistulas (75).

PHASE III TRIALS OF CHEMORADIOTHERAPY

Subsequently, 5 randomized trials have compared preoperative chemoradiotherapy followed by surgery versus surgery alone. Four of these have been published, while the last is reported in abstract form. The results are summarized in Table 51.2. Only 2 trials indicated a survival benefit for the addition of preoperative chemoradiotherapy compared to surgery alone. However, unlike the larger preoperative chemotherapy trials (treating in excess of 200 to up to 800 patients), trials of preoperative chemoradiotherapy have generally been small (treating only 100–250 patients) and have lacked sufficient statistic power to detect modest survival differences between treatment arms. Many trials failed to meet planned accrual goals.

Urba and colleagues from the University of Michigan randomized 100 patients to preoperative cisplatin/5-FU/vinblastine and radiation or to surgery alone (76). Despite a statistically significant decrease in the rate of local recurrence favoring preoperative therapy (19%

TABLE 51.2
Results of Phase III Preoperative Chemoradiotherapy Trials in Esophageal Cancer

Treatment	Histology	No. of patients	Pathologic CR (%)	Survival		Local failure	Reference
				Median	Overall		
Preop CRT	24% SCC 76% Adeno	50	28	16.9 mos	30% 3-yr	19%	Urba et al. (76)
Surgery		50	N/A	17.6 mos	16% 3-yr	42%	
Preop CRT	100% Adeno	58	25	16 mos	32% 3-yr	NS	Walsh et al. (77)
Surgery		55	N/A	11 mos	6% 3-yr	NS	
Preop CRT	100% SCC	143	26	18.6 mos	26% 5-yr	NS	Bosset et al. (79)
Surgery		139	N/A	18.6 mos	26% 5-yr	NS	
Preop CRT	35% SCC 63% Adeno 2% other	128	16	22.2 mos	NS	15%	Burmeister et al. (80)
Surgery		128	N/A	19.3 mos	NS	26%	
Preop CRT	25% SCC 75% Adeno	30	40	4.5 yrs	39% 5-yr	NS	Tepper et al. (81)
Surgery		26	N/A	1.8 yrs	16% 5-yr	NS	

Abbreviations: Adeno = adenocarcinoma; CR = complete response; NS = not stated; Preop CRT = preoperative chemoradiotherapy; SCC = squamous cell carcinoma.

versus 42%), 3-year OS trended toward improvement but was not statistically significant (30% versus 16%, $P = 0.15$). Rates of curative resection were equivalent in both groups (90%).

Walsh and associates from Ireland randomized 113 patients with esophageal adenocarcinoma to preoperative cisplatin/5-FU/radiation or surgery alone (77). Rates of negative margin resection were not reported, although it was noted that the preoperative therapy group had a significantly lower incidence of positive lymph nodes or metastatic disease at surgery (42% versus 82%). A significant improvement in 3-year OS was noted (32% versus 6%). Interpretation of this study is confounded by the very poor survival of the surgical control arm—6% at 3 years—which is inconsistent with the minimum 20% 5-year survival rates reported for modern surgical series (78). Other shortcomings of this trial include inadequate pre-therapy staging (endoscopic ultrasound was not performed and computed tomography was performed only if chest radiographs or abdominal sonograms were abnormal) that could have led to an imbalance in prognostic factors between both groups, the variable surgical procedures used, premature termination based on an unplanned interim analysis and the relatively short follow-up period for surviving patients (18 months).

Bosset et al., on behalf of the European Organization for Research and Treatment of Cancer (EORTC), randomized 282 patients with esophageal squamous cell carcinoma to preoperative cisplatin and concurrent split-dose radiation or surgery (79). Compared to the surgery-only group, the chemoradiotherapy group had a significantly higher rate of curative resection (81% versus 69%), as well as an improvement in disease-free survival (hazard ratio [HR] 0.6, 95% CI 0.4 to 0.9) and a decreased risk of local recurrence (HR 0.6, 95% CI 0.4 to 0.9). However, OS (the primary trial endpoint) was not significantly different. It might be that the significantly higher postoperative mortality in the chemoradiotherapy arm (12% versus 4%) outweighed any potential survival benefit for the chemoradiotherapy group.

In a recent Australian trial, Burmeister and colleagues randomized 256 patients to 1 cycle of preoperative cisplatin/5-FU and radiation or to surgery alone (80). While the trial failed to show a survival advantage for patients who received chemoradiotherapy, they did have a significantly higher curative resection rate compared to the surgery-only patients (80% versus 59%). In this study, the administration of a single chemotherapy cycle may represent suboptimal delivery of chemotherapy. This is reflected by the rather low pCR rate of 9% reported for patients with adenocarcinoma histology.

Finally, results of the Cancer and Leukemia Group B (CALGB) trial 9781 have been presented in abstract form (81). This trial randomized patients to 2 cycles of preoperative cisplatin/5-FU and radiation or to surgery alone. Fifty-six patients were randomized before the trial was closed for poor accrual. Patients assigned to chemoradiotherapy had substantially improved median survival (4.5 versus 1.8 years) and 5-year OS (39% versus 16%) compared to patients undergoing surgery alone.

Overall, these randomized trials are associated with methodologic concerns, are significantly smaller than randomized preoperative chemotherapy trials, and produce conflicting results. However, they do suggest improved curative resection rates as well as decreased local recurrence. Significant rates of pCR are achieved with combined chemoradiotherapy, compared to preoperative chemotherapy alone. A survival advantage for preoperative chemoradiotherapy over surgery alone is not clearly demonstrated, although several studies suggest such a trend.

These observations are further supported by a recent meta-analysis, in which 10 randomized trials of preoperative chemoradiotherapy versus surgery alone and 8 trials of preoperative chemotherapy versus surgery alone were analyzed (47). Preoperative chemoradiotherapy was associated with a hazard ratio of all-cause mortality of 0.81 versus surgery alone (95% CI 0.70–0.93, $P = 0.002$), which translated to a 13% absolute difference in mortality at 2 years. This benefit was irrespective of histology. Preoperative chemotherapy was associated with a hazard ratio of 0.90 (95% CI 0.81–1.00, $P = 0.05$) compared to surgery alone, which related to a 2-year absolute survival benefit of 7%. There did not appear to be any benefit for patients with squamous histology (HR 0.88; 95% CI 0.75–1.03, $P = 0.12$), although there was a benefit for patients with adenocarcinoma histology (HR 0.78; 95% CI 0.64–0.95, $P = 0.014$).

The possible superiority of preoperative chemoradiotherapy over preoperative chemotherapy has also been suggested by a randomized study recently presented in abstract form (82). In this study by Stahl and colleagues for the German Esophageal Cancer Study Group, patients were randomized to preoperative chemotherapy with cisplatin/5-FU/leucovorin followed by surgery versus cisplatin/5-FU/leucovorin followed by chemoradiotherapy with cisplatin/etoposide and then surgery. One-hundred and twenty eligible patients were randomized before the trial was closed due to poor accrual. As such, the study did not meet its planned accrual and is statistically underpowered. The results did reveal a trend toward improved local progression-free survival (77% versus 59%), median OS (32.8 versus 21.1 months) and 3-year survival (43% versus 27%) for the chemoradiotherapy over chemotherapy group but these results were not statistically significant ($P = 0.14$). Both the pCR rate (16% versus 2%) and node-negative status (64% versus 37%) were significantly higher in the chemoradiotherapy group. Strengths of this trial include the careful pre-therapy staging (which included endoscopic ultrasound and laparoscopy), the enrollment only of high-risk patients with at least T3 or node-positive tumors and the careful balancing of pre-therapy stage between the 2 treatment arms.

CHEMORADIOTHERAPY WITH OR WITHOUT SURGERY

Two recent randomized trials have compared definitive chemoradiotherapy versus chemoradiotherapy followed by surgery. The first study was performed by the German Esophageal Cancer Study Group, which assigned 172 patients with squamous cell carcinoma to preoperative therapy (3 cycles of cisplatin/5-FU/leucovorin/etoposide, then cisplatin/etoposide and concurrent radiation to 40 Gy) followed by surgery or to the preoperative therapy alone with a higher radiation dose (to at least 65 Gy) in lieu of surgery (67). Although local progression-free survival was improved with the addition of surgery (64% versus 41%, $P = 0.003$), there was only a non-significant trend towards improvement in 3-year OS (31.3% versus 24.4%). Treatment-related mortality was also significantly higher in the surgery group compared to the chemoradiotherapy-only group (12.8% versus 3.5%).

The second study is the French FFCD 9102 trial, where 444 patients with mostly squamous cell histology underwent initial chemoradiotherapy with cisplatin/5-FU (83) Those who responded to initial therapy were then randomized either to undergo surgery or to receive an additional 3 cycles of cisplatin/5-FU with radiation as the authors felt that it would be inappropriate to continue chemoradiotherapy in patients not responding to therapy. Of the 444 patients, 259 responding patients were randomized. The 2-year survival rate was not significantly different between both groups (34% in surgery group versus 40% in chemoradiotherapy-only group, $P = 0.44$). However, locoregional recurrence was higher in the chemoradiotherapy-only group (43% versus 34%), and there was also a higher incidence of stent placement in this group (32% versus 5%). Three-month mortality was significantly higher in the surgery group (9.3% versus 0.8%). Based on these data, the authors concluded that patients with tumors, especially of squamous cell histology, that respond to initial chemoradiotherapy did not derive any survival benefit from subsequent surgery. Patients who underwent surgery did have improved local control of their disease, albeit at the cost of increased treatment-related mortality.

As a related issue, definitive chemoradiotherapy alone versus surgery alone has also recently been compared in a Scandinavian phase III trial of 91 patients, who were randomized to receive either cisplatin/5-FU and radiation alone or surgery (84). At a median follow-up of 51.8 months, there was no survival difference between both groups. Although this study may be underpowered to detect small survival differences, the data collectively support definitive chemoradiotherapy an acceptable approach for patients who have contraindications to surgery.

NEWER CHEMORADIOTHERAPY REGIMENS

The poor results obtained with conventional cisplatin/5-FU-based regimens have led to the search for more effective and better tolerated regimens.

Paclitaxel-based chemotherapy has undergone extensive evaluation in combined modality therapy trials with radiation. These phase II trials have combined a conventional schedule of paclitaxel/cisplatin every 3 weeks (85,86), weekly paclitaxel with cisplatin every 3 weeks (87) or weekly paclitaxel with weekly cisplatin (88,89), with weekly carboplatin (90) or with 5-FU (91). They have reported pCR rates of 19% to 46%, with toxicities generally less in trials with weekly chemotherapy regimens. Consistently, pCR rates in recent trials are higher in patients with squamous cancer compared to patients with adenocarcinoma histology (80).

Other trials have combined paclitaxel and continuous infusion 5-FU and cisplatin or carboplatin (92–95). These 3-drug trials have reported substantial toxicities, including severe myelosuppression and esophagitis, but have not consistently demonstrated superior results. Retrospective data from the Massachusetts General Hospital indicated similar pCR rates and 3-year survival for a 3-drug regimen of paclitaxel/cisplatin/5-FU and radiation compared to cisplatin/5-FU and radiation (96).

The relative efficacy and toxicity of paclitaxel-based chemotherapy will be answered in the recently completed RTOG trial 0113. In this trial, a regimen of weekly paclitaxel/cisplatin and radiation was compared to weekly paclitaxel/5-FU and radiation in locally advanced esophageal cancer, as definitive therapy without surgery.

In addition, irinotecan-based regimens have also been investigated. Based on a response rate of 57% in the metastatic setting (41), a regimen of weekly irinotecan/cisplatin and radiation has been evaluated in phase I and II studies (97–99). The regimen was found to be tolerable and is associated with pCR rates of 19% to 35%.

Based on these positive results, the CALGB 80302 trial is currently evaluating induction chemotherapy with weekly irinotecan/cisplatin followed by irinotecan/cisplatin with concurrent radiation as preoperative therapy for locally advanced esophageal cancer. The ECOG 1201 trial recently compared weekly irinotecan/cisplatin versus weekly paclitaxel/cisplatin, with concurrent radiation, followed by surgery in patients with esophageal adenocarcinoma (100). The results—presented in abstract form—revealed a disappointingly low pCR rate of 15% and 16% respectively, with a toxicity profile comparable to that historically noted with standard cisplatin/5-FU and radiation. However, these pCR rates are within the range of 9% to 22% reported as the pCR rates for adenocarcinoma histology in the phase III trials of chemoradiotherapy described earlier. Survival data are pending.

CONCLUSION

The treatment of esophageal cancer remains a great challenge to medical, surgical, and radiation oncologists. Although it is clear that patients with advanced disease can be palliated by chemotherapy, trials evaluating newer drugs may help to identify more efficacious and tolerable systemic regimens that can be combined with other treatment modalities.

Chemoradiotherapy is now the standard of care in the treatment of inoperable, localized disease. The use of preoperative chemoradiotherapy continues to be investigated but appears to lead to improved OS in patients who have had a pCR. Several recent trials have suggested that perioperative chemotherapy is also a valid strategy in adenocarcinoma. The use of preoperative chemotherapy alone in squamous cell cancer is less supported by the literature, given the equivocal phase III data and limited survival benefit seen in meta-analyses. For patients undergoing primary resection of esophageal adenocarcinoma, postoperative chemoradiotherapy also appears to improve survival compared to surgery alone.

Although surgery remains the standard curative treatment for early-stage disease, there are data that definitive chemoradiotherapy results in similar survival rates as surgery alone, at least in patients with squamous cell carcinoma. Similarly, patients who respond to initial chemoradiotherapy do not appear to derive a survival benefit from subsequent surgery in squamous cell carcinoma.

References

1. Muller JM, Erasmi H, Stelzner M, et al. Surgical therapy of oesophageal carcinoma. *Br J Surg.* 1990;77(8):845–857.
2. Hulscher JB, van Sandick JW, de Boer AG, et al. Extended transthoracic resection compared with limited transhiatal resection for adenocarcinoma of the esophagus. *N Engl J Med.* 2002;347(21):1662–1669.
3. Earlam R, Cunha-Melo JR. Oesophageal squamous cell carcinoma: I. A critical review of surgery. *Br J Surg.* 1980;67(6):381–390.
4. Enzinger PC, Mayer RJ. Esophageal cancer. *N Engl J Med.* 2003;349(23):2241–2252.
5. Davis S, Shanmugathasa M, Kessler W. cis-Dichlorodiammineplatinum(II) in the treatment of esophageal carcinoma. *Cancer Treat Rep.* 1980;64(4–5):709–11.
6. Murthy SK, Prabhakaran PS, Chandrashekar M, et al. Neoadjuvant Cis-DDP in esophageal cancers: an experience at a regional cancer centre, India. *J Surg Oncol.* 1990;45(3):173–176.
7. Kantarjian H, Ajani JA, Karlin DA. Cis-diaminodichloroplatinum (II) chemotherapy for advanced adenocarcinoma of the upper gastrointestinal tract. *Oncology.* 1985;42(2):69–71.
8. Ezdinli EZ, Gelber R, Desai DV, et al. Chemotherapy of advanced esophageal carcinoma: Eastern Cooperative Oncology Group experience. *Cancer.* 1980;46(10):2149–2153.
9. Lokich JJ, Shea M, Chaffey J. Sequential infusional 5-fluorouracil followed by concomitant radiation for tumors of the esophagus and gastroesophageal junction. *Cancer.* 1987;60(3):275–279.
10. Desai PB, Borges EJ, Vohra VG, et al. Carcinoma of the esophagus in India. *Cancer.* 1969;23(4):979–989.
11. Engstrom PF, Lavin PT, Klaassen DJ. Phase II evaluation of mitomycin and cisplatin in advanced esophageal carcinoma. *Cancer Treat Rep.* 1983;67(7–8):713–715.
12. Whittington RM, Close HP. Clinical experience with mitomycin C (NSC-26980). *Cancer Chemother Rep.* 1970;54(3):195–198.
13. Hong YS, Song SY, Lee SI, et al. A phase II trial of capecitabine in previously untreated patients with advanced and/or metastatic gastric cancer. *Ann Oncol.* 2004;15(9):1344–1347.
14. Koizumi W, Saigenji K, Ujiie S, et al. A pilot phase II study of capecitabine in advanced or recurrent gastric cancer. *Oncology.* 2003;64(3):232–236.
15. Ajani JA, Lee FC, Singh DA, et al. Multicenter phase II trial of S-1 plus cisplatin in patients with untreated advanced gastric or gastroesophageal junction adenocarcinoma. *J Clin Oncol.* 2006;24(4):663–667.
16. Ilson D, Wadleigh R, Leichman L, et al. Paclitaxel given by a weekly 1-h infusion in advanced esophageal cancer. *Ann Oncol.* 2007;18(5):898–902.
17. Ajani JA, Ilson DH, Daugherty K, et al. Activity of taxol in patients with squamous cell carcinoma and adenocarcinoma of the esophagus. *J Natl Cancer Inst.* 1994;86(14):1086–1091.
18. Anderson SE, O'Reilly EM, Kelsen DP, et al. Phase II trial of 96-hour paclitaxel in previously treated patients with advanced esophageal cancer. *Cancer Invest.* 2003;21(4):512–516.
19. Einzig AI, Neuberg D, Remick SC, et al. Phase II trial of docetaxel (Taxotere) in patients with adenocarcinoma of the upper gastrointestinal tract previously untreated with cytotoxic chemotherapy: the Eastern Cooperative Oncology Group (ECOG) results of protocol E1293. *Med Oncol.* 1996;13(2):87–93.
20. Heath EI, Urba S, Marshall J, et al. Phase II trial of docetaxel chemotherapy in patients with incurable adenocarcinoma of the esophagus. *Invest New Drugs.* 2002;20(1):95–99.
21. Muro K, Hamaguchi T, Ohtsu A, et al. A phase II study of single-agent docetaxel in patients with metastatic esophageal cancer. *Ann Oncol.* 2004;15(6):955–959.
22. Enzinger PC, Kulke MH, Clark JW, et al. A phase II trial of irinotecan in patients with previously untreated advanced esophageal and gastric adenocarcinoma. *Dig Dis Sci.* 2005;50(12):2218–2223.
23. Al-Batran S, Hartmann J, Probst S, et al. A randomized phase III trial in patients with advanced adenocarcinoma of the stomach receiving first-line chemotherapy with fluorouracil, leucovorin and oxaliplatin (FLO) versus fluorouracil, leucovorin and cisplatin (FLP). [abstract LBA4016] *J Clin Oncol.* 2006;24(18S).
24. Cunningham D, Starling N, Rao S, et al. Capecitabine and oxaliplatin for advanced esophagogastric cancer. *N Engl J Med.* 2008;358(1):36–46.
25. Bleiberg H, Conroy T, Paillot B, et al. Randomised phase II study of cisplatin and 5-fluorouracil (5-FU) versus cisplatin alone in advanced squamous cell oesophageal cancer. *Eur J Cancer.* 1997;33(8):1216–1220.
26. Webb A, Cunningham D, Scarffe JH, et al. Randomized trial comparing epirubicin, cisplatin, and fluorouracil versus fluorouracil, doxorubicin, and methotrexate in advanced esophagogastric cancer. *J Clin Oncol.* 1997;15(1):261–267.
27. Ross P, Nicolson M, Cunningham D, et al. Prospective randomized trial comparing mitomycin, cisplatin, and protracted venous-infusion fluorouracil (PVI 5-FU) with epirubicin, cisplatin, and PVI 5-FU in advanced esophagogastric cancer. *J Clin Oncol.* 2002;20(8):1996–2004.
28. Boku N, Yamamoto S, Shirao K, et al. Randomized phase III study of 5-fluorouracil (5-FU) alone versus combination of irinotecan and cisplatin (CP) versus S-1 alone in advanced gastric cancer (JCOG9912). [abstract LBA4513]. *J Clin Oncol.* 2007;25(18S).
29. Narahara H, Koizumi W, Hara T, et al. Randomized phase III study of S-1 alone versus S-1 + cisplatin in the treatment for advanced gastric cancer (The SPIRITS trial) SPIRITS: S-1 plus cisplatin vs S-1 in RCT in the treatment for stomach cancer [abstract 4514]. *J Clin Oncol.* 2007;25(18S).
30. Van Cutsem E, Moiseyenko VM, Tjulandin S, et al. Phase III study of docetaxel and cisplatin plus fluorouracil compared with cisplatin and fluorouracil as first-line therapy for advanced gastric cancer: a report of the V325 Study Group. *J Clin Oncol.* 2006;24(31):4991–4997.
31. Roth AD, Fazio N, Stupp R, et al. Docetaxel, cisplatin, and fluorouracil; docetaxel and cisplatin; and epirubicin, cisplatin, and fluorouracil as systemic treatment for advanced gastric carcinoma: a randomized phase II trial of the Swiss Group for Clinical Cancer Research. *J Clin Oncol.* 2007;25(22):3217–3223.
32. Thuss-Patience PC, Kretzschmar A, Repp M, et al. Docetaxel and continuous-infusion fluorouracil versus epirubicin, cisplatin, and fluorouracil for advanced gastric adenocarcinoma: a randomized phase II study. *J Clin Oncol.* 2005;23(3):494–501.
33. Ilson DH, Ajani J, Bhalla K, et al. Phase II trial of paclitaxel, fluorouracil, and cisplatin in patients with advanced carcinoma of the esophagus. *J Clin Oncol.* 1998;16(5):1826–1834.
34. Ilson DH, Forastiere A, Arquette M, et al. A phase II trial of paclitaxel and cisplatin in patients with advanced carcinoma of the esophagus. *Cancer J.* 2000;6(5):316–323.

35. Polee MB, Eskens FA, van der Burg ME, et al. Phase II study of bi-weekly administration of paclitaxel and cisplatin in patients with advanced oesophageal cancer. *Br J Cancer.* 2002;86(5):669–673.
36. Polee MB, Verweij J, Siersema PD, et al. Phase I study of a weekly schedule of a fixed dose of cisplatin and escalating doses of paclitaxel in patients with advanced oesophageal cancer. *Eur J Cancer.* 2002;38(11):1495–1500.
37. Gold P, Carter G, Livingston R. Phase II trial of irinotecan (CPT-11) and mitomycin c (MMC) in the treatment of metastatic esophageal and gastric cancers [abstract]. *Proc Am Soc Clin Oncol.* 2001;20:644.
38. Ajani JA, Baker J, Pisters PW, et al. CPT-11 plus cisplatin in patients with advanced, untreated gastric or gastroesophageal junction carcinoma: results of a phase II study. *Cancer.* 2002;94(3):641–646.
39. Pozzo C, Barone C, Szanto J, et al. Irinotecan in combination with 5-fluorouracil and folinic acid or with cisplatin in patients with advanced gastric or esophageal-gastric junction adenocarcinoma: results of a randomized phase II study. *Ann Oncol.* 2004;15(12):1773–1781.
40. Slater S, Shamash J, Wilson P, et al. Irinotecan, cisplatin and mitomycin in inoperable gastro-oesophageal and pancreatic cancers—a new active regimen. *Br J Cancer.* 2002;87(8):850–853.
41. Ilson DH, Saltz L, Enzinger P, et al. Phase II trial of weekly irinotecan plus cisplatin in advanced esophageal cancer. *J Clin Oncol.* 1999;17(10):3270–3275.
42. Dank M, Zaluski J, Barone C, et al. Randomized phase 3 trial of irinotecan (CPT-11) + 5FU/folinic acid (FA) vs CDDP + 5FU in 1st-line advanced gastric cancer patients [abstract 4003]. *J Clin Oncol.* 2005;23(16S)
43. Harris DT, Mastrangelo MJ. Theory and application of early systemic therapy. *Sem Oncol.* 1991;18(6):493–503.
44. Kok T, Lanschot J, Siersema P, et al. Neoadjuvant chemotherapy in operable esophageal squamous cell cancer: final report of a phase III multicenter randomized controlled trial [abstract 984]. *Proc Am Soc Clin Oncol.* 1997.
45. Kelsen DP, Ginsberg R, Pajak TF, et al. Chemotherapy followed by surgery compared with surgery alone for localized esophageal cancer. *N Engl J Med.* 1998;339(27):1979–1984.
46. Medical Research Council Oesophageal Cancer Working Group. Surgical resection with or without preoperative chemotherapy in oesophageal cancer: a randomised controlled trial. *Lancet.* 2002;359(9319):1727–1733.
47. Gebski V, Burmeister B, Smithers BM, et al. Survival benefits from neoadjuvant chemoradiotherapy or chemotherapy in oesophageal carcinoma: a meta-analysis. *Lancet Oncol.* 2007;8(3):226–234.
48. Thirion P, Michiels S, Le Maître A, et al. Individual patient data-based meta-analysis assessing pre-operative chemotherapy in resectable oesophageal carcinoma [abstract 4512]. *J Clin Oncol.* 2007;25(18S)
49. Cunningham D, Allum WH, Stenning SP, et al. Perioperative chemotherapy versus surgery alone for resectable gastroesophageal cancer. *N Engl J Med.* 2006;355(1):11–20.
50. Boige V, Pignon J, Saint-Aubert B, et al. Final results of a randomized trial comparing preoperative 5-fluorouracil (F)/cisplatin (P) to surgery alone in adenocarcinoma of stomach and lower esophagus (ASLE): FNLCC ACCORD07-FFCD 9703 trial [abstract 4510]. *J Clin Oncol.* 2007;25(18S)
51. Kelsen DP, Minsky B, Smith M, et al. Preoperative therapy for esophageal cancer: a randomized comparison of chemotherapy versus radiation therapy. *J Clin Oncol.* 1990;8(8):1352–1361.
52. Arnott SJ, Duncan W, Kerr GR, et al. Low dose preoperative radiotherapy for carcinoma of the oesophagus: results of a randomized clinical trial. *Radiother Oncol.* 1992;24(2):108–113.
53. Nygaard K, Hagen S, Hansen HS, et al. Pre-operative radiotherapy prolongs survival in operable esophageal carcinoma: a randomized, multicenter study of pre-operative radiotherapy and chemotherapy. The second Scandinavian trial in esophageal cancer. *World J Surg.* 1992;16(6):1104–1109; discussion 1110.
54. Arnott SJ, Duncan W, Gignoux M, et al. Preoperative radiotherapy for esophageal carcinoma. *Cochrane Database Syst Rev.* 2005(4):CD001799.
55. Ando N, Iizuka T, Kakegawa T, et al. A randomized trial of surgery with and without chemotherapy for localized squamous carcinoma of the thoracic esophagus: the Japan Clinical Oncology Group Study. *J Thorac Cardiovasc Surg.* 1997;114(2):205–209.
56. Ando N, Iizuka T, Ide H, et al. Surgery plus chemotherapy compared with surgery alone for localized squamous cell carcinoma of the thoracic esophagus: a Japan Clinical Oncology Group Study—JCOG9204. *J Clin Oncol.* 2003;21(24):4592–4596.
57. Pouliquen X, Levard H, Hay JM, et al. 5-Fluorouracil and cisplatin therapy after palliative surgical resection of squamous cell carcinoma of the esophagus. A multicenter randomized trial. French Associations for Surgical Research. *Ann Surg.* 1996;223(2):127–133.
58. Armanios M, Xu R, Forastiere AA, et al. Adjuvant chemotherapy for resected adenocarcinoma of the esophagus, gastro-esophageal junction, and cardia: phase II trial (E8296) of the Eastern Cooperative Oncology Group. *J Clin Oncol.* 2004;22(22):4495–4499.
59. Teniere P, Hay JM, Fingerhut A, et al. Postoperative radiation therapy does not increase survival after curative resection for squamous cell carcinoma of the middle and lower esophagus as shown by a multicenter controlled trial. French University Association for Surgical Research. *Surg Gynecol Obstet.* 1991;173(2):123–130.
60. Fok M, Sham JS, Choy D, et al. Postoperative radiotherapy for carcinoma of the esophagus: a prospective, randomized controlled study. *Surgery.* 1993;113(2):138–147.
61. Xiao ZF, Yang ZY, Liang J, et al. Value of radiotherapy after radical surgery for esophageal carcinoma: a report of 495 patients. *Ann Thorac Surg.* 2003;75(2):331–336.
62. Macdonald JS, Smalley SR, Benedetti J, et al. Chemoradiotherapy after surgery compared with surgery alone for adenocarcinoma of the stomach or gastroesophageal junction. *N Engl J Med.* 2001;345(10):725–730.
63. Coia LR, Engstrom PF, Paul AR, et al. Long-term results of infusional 5-FU, mitomycin-C and radiation as primary management of esophageal carcinoma. *Intl J Radiat Oncol Biol Phys.* 1991;20(1):29–36.
64. Valerdi JJ, Tejedor M, Illarramendi JJ, et al. Neoadjuvant chemotherapy and radiotherapy in locally advanced esophagus carcinoma: long-term results. *Int J Radiat Oncol Biol Phys.* 1993;27(4):843–847.
65. Berger AC, Farma J, Scott WJ, et al. Complete response to neoadjuvant chemoradiotherapy in esophageal carcinoma is associated with significantly improved survival. *J Clin Oncol.* 2005;23(19):4330–4337.
66. Makary MA, Kiernan PD, Sheridan MJ, et al. Multimodality treatment for esophageal cancer: the role of surgery and neoadjuvant therapy. *Am Surg.* 2003;69(8):693–700; discussion 700–702.
67. Stahl M, Stuschke M, Lehmann N, et al. Chemoradiation with and without surgery in patients with locally advanced squamous cell carcinoma of the esophagus. *J Clin Oncol.* 2005;23(10):2310–2317.
68. Heath EI, Burtness BA, Heitmiller RF, et al. Phase II evaluation of preoperative chemoradiation and postoperative adjuvant chemotherapy for squamous cell and adenocarcinoma of the esophagus. *J Clin Oncol.* 2000;18(4):868–876.
69. Forastiere AA, Orringer MB, Perez-Tamayo C, et al. Preoperative chemoradiation followed by transhiatal esophagectomy for carcinoma of the esophagus: final report. *J Clin Oncol.* 1993;11(6):1118–1123.
70. Geh JI. The use of chemoradiotherapy in oesophageal cancer. *Eur J Cancer.* 2002;38(2):300–313.
71. Herskovic A, Martz K, al-Sarraf M, et al. Combined chemotherapy and radiotherapy compared with radiotherapy alone in patients with cancer of the esophagus. *N Engl J Med.* 1992;326(24):1593–1598.
72. Cooper JS, Guo MD, Herskovic A, et al. Chemoradiotherapy of locally advanced esophageal cancer: long-term follow-up of a prospective randomized trial (RTOG 85–01). Radiation Therapy Oncology Group. *JAMA.* 1999;281(17):1623–1627.
73. Minsky BD, Neuberg D, Kelsen DP, et al. Final report of Intergroup Trial 0122 (ECOG PE-289, RTOG 90–12): phase II trial of neoadjuvant chemotherapy plus concurrent chemotherapy and high-dose radiation for squamous cell carcinoma of the esophagus. *Intl J Radiat Oncol Biol Phys.* 1999;43(3):517–523.
74. Minsky BD, Pajak TF, Ginsberg RJ, et al. INT 0123 (Radiation Therapy Oncology Group 94–05) phase III trial of combined-modality therapy for esophageal cancer: high-dose versus standard-dose radiation therapy. *J Clin Oncol.* 2002;20(5):1167–1174.
75. Gaspar LE, Winter K, Kocha WI, et al. A phase I/II study of external beam radiation, brachytherapy, and concurrent chemotherapy for patients with localized carcinoma of the esophagus (Radiation Therapy Oncology Group Study 9207): final report. *Cancer.* 2000;88(5):988–995.
76. Urba SG, Orringer MB, Turrisi A, et al. Randomized trial of preoperative chemoradiation versus surgery alone in patients with locoregional esophageal carcinoma. *J Clin Oncol.* 2001;19(2):305–313.
77. Walsh TN, Noonan N, Hollywood D, et al. A comparison of multimodal therapy and surgery for esophageal adenocarcinoma. *N Engl J Med.* 1996;335(7):462–467.
78. Orringer MB, Marshall B, Iannettoni MD. Transhiatal esophagectomy: clinical experience and refinements. *Ann Surg.* 1999;230(3):392–400; discussion 400–403.
79. Bosset JF, Gignoux M, Triboulet JP, et al. Chemoradiotherapy followed by surgery compared with surgery alone in squamous-cell cancer of the esophagus. *N Engl J Med.* 1997;337(3):161–167.
80. Burmeister BH, Smithers BM, Gebski V, et al. Surgery alone versus chemoradiotherapy followed by surgery for resectable cancer of the oesophagus: a randomised controlled phase III trial. *Lancet Oncol.* 2005;6(9):659–668.
81. Tepper J, Krasna M, Niedzwiecki D, et al. Superiority of trimodality therapy to surgery alone in esophageal cancer: results of CALGB 9781 [abstract 4012]. *J Clin Oncol.* 2006;24(18S)
82. Stahl M, Walz M, Stuschke M, et al. Preoperative chemotherapy (CTX) versus preoperative chemoradiotherapy (CRTX) in locally advanced esophagogastric adenocarcinomas: first results of a randomized phase III trial [abstract 4511]. *J Clin Oncol.* 2007;25(18S)
83. Bedenne L, Michel P, Bouche O, et al. Chemoradiation followed by surgery compared with chemoradiation alone in squamous cancer of the esophagus: FFCD 9102. *J Clin Oncol.* 2007;25(10):1160–1168.
84. Carstens H, Albertsson M, Friesland S, et al. A randomized trial of chemoradiotherapy versus surgery alone in patients with resectable esophageal cancer [abstract 4530]. *J Clin Oncol.* 2007;25(18S)
85. Adelstein DJ, Rice TW, Rybicki LA, et al. Does paclitaxel improve the chemoradiotherapy of locoregionally advanced esophageal cancer? A nonrandomized comparison with fluorouracil-based therapy. *J Clin Oncol.* 2000;18(10):2032–2039.
86. Blanke CD, Choy H, Teng M, et al. Concurrent paclitaxel and thoracic irradiation for locally advanced esophageal cancer. *Semin Radiat Oncol.* 1999;9(2 Suppl 1):43–52.
87. Urba SG, Orringer MB, Ianettonni M, et al. Concurrent cisplatin, paclitaxel, and radiotherapy as preoperative treatment for patients with locoregional esophageal carcinoma. *Cancer.* 2003;98(10):2177–2183.
88. Brenner B, Ilson DH, Minsky BD, et al. Phase I trial of combined-modality therapy for localized esophageal cancer: escalating doses of continuous-infusion paclitaxel with cisplatin and concurrent radiation therapy. *J Clin Oncol.* 2004;22(1):45–52.
89. Safran H, Gaissert H, Akerman P, et al. Paclitaxel, cisplatin, and concurrent radiation for esophageal cancer. *Cancer Invest.* 2001;19(1):1–7.

90. van Meerten E, Muller K, Tilanus HW, et al. Neoadjuvant concurrent chemoradiation with weekly paclitaxel and carboplatin for patients with oesophageal cancer: a phase II study. *Br J Cancer.* 2006;94(10):1389–1394.
91. Schnirer, II, Komaki R, Yao JC, et al. Pilot study of concurrent 5-fluorouracil/paclitaxel plus radiotherapy in patients with carcinoma of the esophagus and gastroesophageal junction. *Am J Clin Oncol.* 2001;24(1):91–95.
92. Henry LR, Goldberg M, Scott W, et al. Induction cisplatin and paclitaxel followed by combination chemoradiotherapy with 5-fluorouracil, cisplatin, and paclitaxel before resection in localized esophageal cancer: a phase II report. *Ann Surg Oncol.* 2006;13(2):214–220.
93. Meluch AA, Greco FA, Gray JR, et al. Preoperative therapy with concurrent paclitaxel/carboplatin/infusional 5-FU and radiation therapy in locoregional esophageal cancer: final results of a Minnie Pearl Cancer Research Network phase II trial. *Cancer J.* 2003;9(4):251–260.
94. Weiner LM, Colarusso P, Goldberg M, et al. Combined-modality therapy for esophageal cancer: phase I trial of escalating doses of paclitaxel in combination with cisplatin, 5-fluorouracil, and high-dose radiation before esophagectomy. *Semin Oncol.* 1997;24(6 Suppl 19):S19–93—S19–95.
95. Wright CD, Wain JC, Lynch TJ, et al. Induction therapy for esophageal cancer with paclitaxel and hyperfractionated radiotherapy: a phase I and II study. *J Thorac Cardiovasc Surg.* 1997;114(5):811–815; discussion 816.
96. Roof KS, Coen J, Lynch TJ, et al. Concurrent cisplatin, 5-FU, paclitaxel, and radiation therapy in patients with locally advanced esophageal cancer. *Int J Radiat Oncol Biol Phys.* 2006;65(4):1120–1128.
97. Enzinger P, Mamon H, Choi N, et al. Phase II cisplatin, irinotecan, celecoxib and concurrent radiation therapy followed by surgery for locally advanced esophageal cancer [abstract 35]. *Proc Gastrointest Am Soc Clin Oncol.* 2004.
98. Ilson DH, Bains M, Kelsen DP, et al. Phase I trial of escalating-dose irinotecan given weekly with cisplatin and concurrent radiotherapy in locally advanced esophageal cancer. *J Clin Oncol.* 2003;21(15):2926–2932.
99. Ku G, Bains M, Rizk N, et al. Phase II trial of pre-operative cisplatin/irinotecan and radiotherapy for locally advanced esophageal cancer: PET scan after induction therapy may identify early treatment failure [abstract 9]. *Proc Gastrointest Am Soc Clin Oncol.* 2007.
100. Kleinberg L, Powell M, Forastiere A, et al. E1201: An Eastern Cooperative Oncology Group (ECOG) randomized phase II trial of neoadjuvant preoperative paclitaxel/cisplatin/RT or irinotecan/cisplatin/RT in endoscopy with ultrasound (EUS) staged adenocarcinoma of the esophagus [abstract 4533]. *J Clin Oncol.* 2007;25(18S).

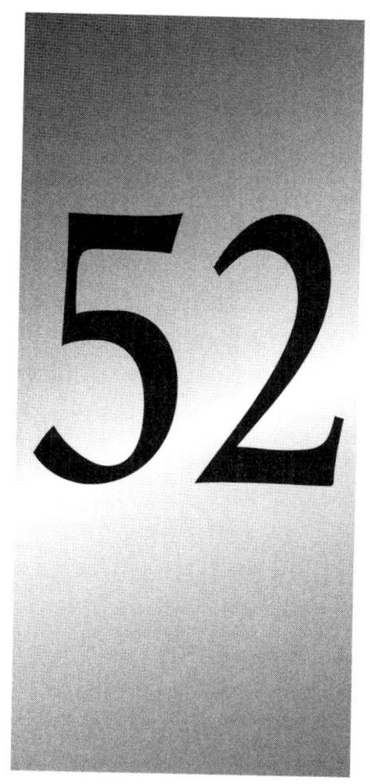

52 Pretreatment Planning in Radiation Therapy of the Esophagus

Theodore Sunki Hong
Lisa A. Kachnic

Radiation therapy is an important modality in the management of esophageal cancer, both in the preoperative setting and as definitive therapy in combination with chemotherapy. Optimal implementation of radiation therapy, however, requires thoughtful pretreatment planning not only to assure tumor and regional nodal coverage in order to optimize local efficacy, but also to treat as little normal tissue as possible in attempts to minimize toxicity and, hence, increase the therapeutic ratio.

The radiation pretreatment planning process for esophageal cancer is quite complex. Because of the advanced presentation of esophageal cancers, large radiation fields are commonly employed. The treatment volume is further increased by generous longitudinal margins to acknowledge the high risk of submucosal spread, as well as coverage of the regional nodal basins, including celiac nodes for distal tumors and supraclavicular nodes for more proximal cancers. These large fields, in turn, encompass significant volumes of critical normal organs including the heart and lungs. Inherent difficulties in target delineation and significant organ motion temper our ability to decrease the large treatment volumes. Together, these complex planning and delivery issues can impact both the local efficacy of radiation therapy, as well as treatment-related toxicity.

In this chapter, we will begin by discussing the key considerations in the radiation pretreatment planning procedures. We will then focus on the many challenges associated with accurately defining the treatment volume, including a review of normal tissue tolerances and how these impact treatment planning. Finally, we will discuss the various radiation planning techniques for esophageal cancer.

RADITION PRE-PLANNING PROCEDURES

Computed Tomography–Based Simulation

Positioning

Patients may be simulated supine or prone, with a computed tomography (CT)-slice distance of < 5mm. The advantage of prone simulation is that it theoretically increases the distance between the esophagus and spine, allowing for less shallow off-cord obliques and consequently less lung dose. The advantage of supine positioning is that this position is more comfortable for patients, especially given common medical comorbidities such as obesity, chronic obstructive pulmonary disease (COPD), and other debilitative conditions. If the patient is supine, it is recommended to use a mold or alpha cradle for immobilization. For thoracic and gastroesophageal junction tumors, arms should be raised.

For patients with cervical esophageal cancers, patients should be positioned with arms down, masked, with chin extended, as would be standard for a patient with a head and neck cancer. This allows treatment of the supraclavicular fossa and neck nodal groups without skin folds.

Contrast

Intravenous contrast should be used if available in the radiation oncology department for proper delineation of regional nodal volumes (IV contrast ISOVUE 300, 40 second delay, 100cc, 1.5 cc/s, 2.5 mm slices). Prior to administration, patients should be screened for history of contrast reaction and also have a normal serum creatinine documented.

Oral contrast is also recommended to visualize the esophageal lumen. A paste such as (Esopho-Cat 3% Barium sulfate w/w, E-Z-EM, Westbury, NY) has worked well at our institutions. Paste specifically designed for esophageal is preferable to standard barium contrast as standard contrast can pool in the lower esophageal sphincter and cause significant artifact and consequently may obscure the tumor. Typically, a teaspoon of esophageal contrast is sufficient, as giving more can cause dilation of the esophagus that will not be present during treatment.

Target Volume Definitions

Defining the Tumor

Accurate delineation of the gross tumor volume (GTV) requires integration of the clinical history with endoscopy findings, computed tomography (CT) imaging, and other imaging modalities such as positron-emission tomography (PET) scan and barium swallow. Physical examination will be helpful in denoting bulky supraclavicular and/or cervical lymphadenopathy. Prior to simulation, all relevant studies should be carefully reviewed to most accurately define the local as well as regional extent of the tumor.

Endoscopy is often the first study reviewed, as it assists in defining the superior and inferior extent of the esophageal tumor. Endoscopy also provides information regarding tumor circumferentiality as well as bleeding. If an ultrasound is performed at the time of endoscopy (endoscopic ultrasound [EUS]), further information regarding depth of penetration (T-stage) and peritumoral nodal involvement (N-stage) will be obtained. Typically, longitudinal distances are given in centimeters from the incisors. Useful general landmarks are the postcricoid space at 15 cm, thoracic inlet at 18 cm, carina at 25 cm, and gastroesophageal junction (GEJ) at 40 cm. These are general estimates and may vary with head position at the time of endoscopy, patient size, and the presence of a hiatal hernia. Close attention should also be given to tumor extension into the GEJ or gastric cardia. It is often helpful to communicate directly with the gastroenterologist to determine the location of gastric extension. With or without regional nodal fine needle aspirate findings, EUS may also guide the definition of nodal gross tumor, as well as elective nodal volumes. The diagnostic staging (non-radiation planning) CT scan is also an important data set as it most closely represents the images obtained during CT simulation. Often, the quality of the diagnostic scan is superior to that of the radiation planning CT, particularly for distal esophageal and GEJ lesions. This is due to the difference in technique that is employed by diagnostic radiology. Diagnostic CT scans are often obtained in breath-hold to minimize motion artifact. The stomach is mildly inflated to better ascertain gastric involvement. Furthermore, the intravenous contrast is pushed as opposed to dripped, which provides clearer visualization of pertinent vessels. The diagnostic CT scan should be carefully reviewed to help define the extent of the esophageal tumor, as well as regional nodal coverage.

If a barium swallow is performed, it is a useful technique to visualize the site of a malignant stricture, as well as the extent of local disease. However, with the increased use of high-resolution CT scans with 3-dimensional (3-D) reconstruction, the use of barium swallow in our institutions has markedly decreased.

[^{18}F]-fluoro-2-deoxy-D-glucose positron-emission tomography (FDG-PET)–based planning may be useful in defining local and regional tumor extent. PET scanning has also demonstrated increased sensitivity in the staging of distant metastatic disease. Several studies have demonstrated that the inclusion of PET information changes GTV definition in the majority of patients (1–5).

There are caveats, however, to PET-based radiation planning. One major concern is the lack of consensus on how best to segment tumor from normal tissue. Differences in segmentation methods can lead to significant inter-observer variability. In the most qualitative approach, the planner can simply window the PET images in the treatment planning system and the apparent tumor length can consequently change. Another approach is to use a semiquantitative approach. One such method is to use standard uptake values (SUV) as a threshold level to define tumor. Two fundamental problems exist with this approach. First, the SUV concept is limited by the need for accurate recording of time of injection and scanning, as well as accurate calculation of patient size. Second, it is unknown what lower threshold should be used. One common practice for lung cancer is to use a minimal SUV threshold of 2.5. Alternatively, acknowledging that each tumor has a unique SUV, one can define tumor enclosed by an area of 40% or 50% of maximum intensity (1,5). However, this approach can lead to drastic differences in tumor length. A final approach is to use an automated tumor segmentation method whereby a lower threshold can be calculated based on internal control (such as liver) (2,3). However, no standard approach currently exists, nor has one been validated with pathology in a large cohort of patients. Another limitation of PET scanning is that the acquisition of data occurs over a prolonged period of time. Inherently, PET scanning lacks reliable resolution beyond 5 mm. The smearing of the image due to organ motion further increases this uncertainty. This limitation may be partially overcome by the simultaneous use of 4-dimensional (4-D) CT scanning (see section below).

The 2 most commonly used methods of incorporating PET into radiation pretreatment planning are the "side-by-side" comparison, whereby the planner evaluates the PET scan on a separate screen from the planning CT, and the "fused" method in which the PET scan is actually fused to the planning CT scan, and the physician contours on either or both datasets. In our institutions, we are routinely fusing FDG-PET/CT scans done for diagnostic purposes to planning CT scans as an aid to defining the GTV, for both involved primary and nodal areas. Currently, the greatest utility in PET-based planning may be in detecting (Figure 52.1) non-continuous disease, especially nodal groups that may not be encompassable in a reasonable radiation portal (6).

Elective Target Coverage

Elective radiation field coverage beyond the gross primary esophageal and nodal tumor volume has been heterogeneously described in the published literature. Elective coverage includes both the longitudinal esophageal extension beyond the GTV, as well as potential areas of regional nodal spread. This elective coverage is contained in the clinical target volume (CTV).

Longitudinal margins have ranged from including the whole esophagus, as in the Radiation Therapy Oncology Group (RTOG) 8501 study (7), to an additional 5 cm to the local esophageal tumor edge (Figure 52.2). These margins acknowledge the risk of submucosal microscopic extension beyond the gross tumor volume. With the advent of the 3D-simulation era, new planning definitions were created to mirror the historical 2-dimensional (2D) conventions. As an example, RTOG esophageal protocol 0123 specifically defined GTV, CTV, and PTV (planning target volume) (8). The CTV was defined to include the GTV with 4 cm proximal and distal margins, and 1 cm lateral margins. The PTV represented a 1–2 cm expansion beyond the CTV to allow for variability in daily set-up, as well as intra-fraction motion of the patient and/or targets.

Elective nodal coverage has also been variable, with some studies excluding celiac and supraclavicular coverage unless it was involved (9–11). In contrast,

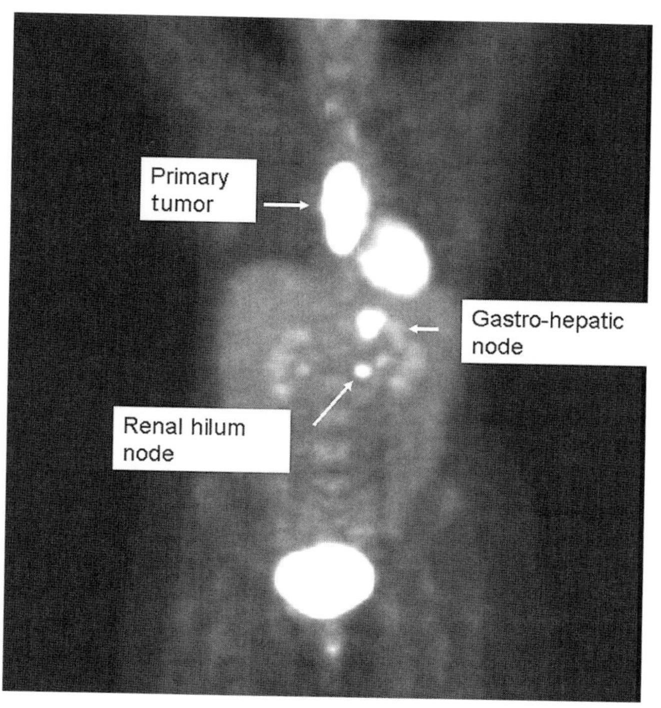

FIGURE 52.1

FDG avidity seen in a node (renal hilar) not previously identified as tumor bearing on staging CT scan.

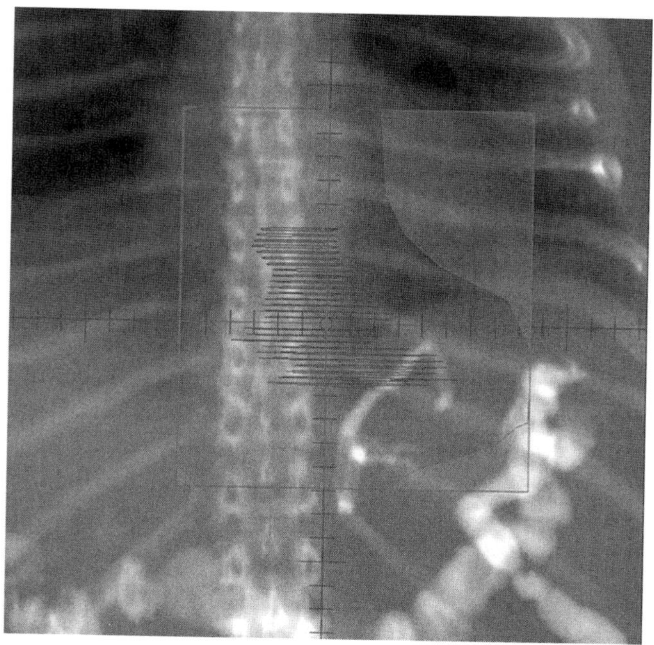

FIGURE 52.2

Conventional anterior radiation field (digital reconstruction) with 5 cm longitudinal margins beyond the gross esophageal tumor.

studies in the United States have recommended supraclavicular coverage for proximal esophageal tumors and celiac coverage for distal or gastroesophageal junction tumors (8,12).

In general, it is reasonable to define the CTV as 3.5 to 4 cm longitudinally from the GTV and 1 to 2 cm radially. The celiac axis is included for distal esophageal and gastroesophageal junction tumors and supraclavicular nodes can be included for tumors above the carina. This CTV can be treated in general to 45 Gy in 1.8 Gy Monday through Friday daily fractions.

Internal Organ Motion and Patient Setup

In considering appropriate margins for uncertainty in tumor location, one must consider both setup variations and organ motion. Typically, patients are set up on a daily base to external cutaneous tattoos marked laterally and midline, and then aligned via laser coordinates in the treatment room (3-point landing). However, even with a rigid setup, this technique can lead to daily setup variations greater than 5 mm (13). Daily electronic imaging and image-guided techniques (such as cone beam CT scanning) currently employed in our institutions may improve this but thus far have not been validated for esophageal cancer.

Internal organ motion, particularly for distal tumors, is another source of uncertainty in tumor location. Four-dimensional (4-D) CT can be used ascertain tumor motion. 4-D CT scanning employs a surface array that is tracked by a camera system and placed on the patient's abdomen. This array is used to monitor a patient's respiratory phases. CT slices are then obtained and "binned" according to the specific respiratory phase during which it was acquired. These CT data can then be formatted into a movie that re-creates tumor and respiratory motion. A recent study from the Massachusetts General Hospital (MGH) analyzing the effect of respiratory motion in 10 patients with esophageal tumors using 4-D CT, demonstrated a median superior-inferior tumor motion of 2 cm, with 1 patient having a 4.8 cm excursion (14). An example of this phenomenon is shown in Figure 52.3. This study highlights the variability in internal organ motion and the utility of individualizing PTV expansions. In general, a 1 to 2 cm margin superiorly and inferiorly, and a 1 cm margin radially, should be considered beyond the CTV.

RADIATION PLANNING CONSIDERATIONS

Owing to the advanced presentation of esophageal cancers, large radiation fields are commonly used. The treatment volume is further enlarged by the generous longitudinal margins necessary to cover submucosal spread and also the need to cover distant nodal basins (15), including celiac nodes for distal or GEJ tumors and supraclavicular nodes for more proximal cancers. These large fields encompass significant volumes of normal tissue including the heart and lungs. In this section, normal tissue considerations will be discussed as well as treatment planning techniques.

Normal Tissue Considerations

Lung Dose and Pulmonary Toxicity

As with any normal tissue, radiation can cause complications in the lung. The clinical spectrum of this toxicity is broad and can potentially be life-threatening. The 2 most commonly described pulmonary complications are radiation pneumonitis and postoperative pulmonary morbidity.

Radiation Pneumonitis

Radiation pneumonitis, a common dose-limiting complication of radiation therapy for lung cancer, is characterized by persistent cough or shortness of breath arising 6 weeks to 6 months after therapy, with radiologic abnormalities showing correlation with the photon beam path. This syndrome can have a significant impact on a patient's quality of life, and in rare instances, can be responsible for treatment-related mortality.

Numerous publications have evaluated dose-volume histogram (DVH) parameters predicting the risk of radiation pneumonitis. Many parameters of lung dose have been described to correlate with risk of clinically significant radiation pneumonitis. The largest clinical series, reported by Kwa and colleagues, studied 540 patients from 5 institutions who were pooled to determine the relationship of dose distribution in the lung and grade > 2 radiation pneumonitis (16). This analysis demonstrated that the risk of grade 2 or greater pneumonitis correlated with mean lung dose normalized to 2-Gy fraction equivalents (normalized total dose [NTD]). The authors concluded that using an NTD_{mean} of 20 Gy was associated with a normal tissue complication rate (NTCP) of 13% to 24%, which the authors deemed acceptable. Others have seen a similar relationship between the mean lung dose and the rate of clinically significant pneumonitis (17–20). Other DVH parameters that have been found to be informative include V20 < 40% (19) and V30 < 18% (20). (Note: V20 represents the percentage of the lung that receives a dose of 20 Gy.) There remains no consistent evidence that any one of these characteristics is more accurate than another. Lung DVH analysis may also be complicated by regional anatomic differences in lung sensitivity. A study by Yorke and colleagues examining DVH predictors of pneumonitis found that the dose received

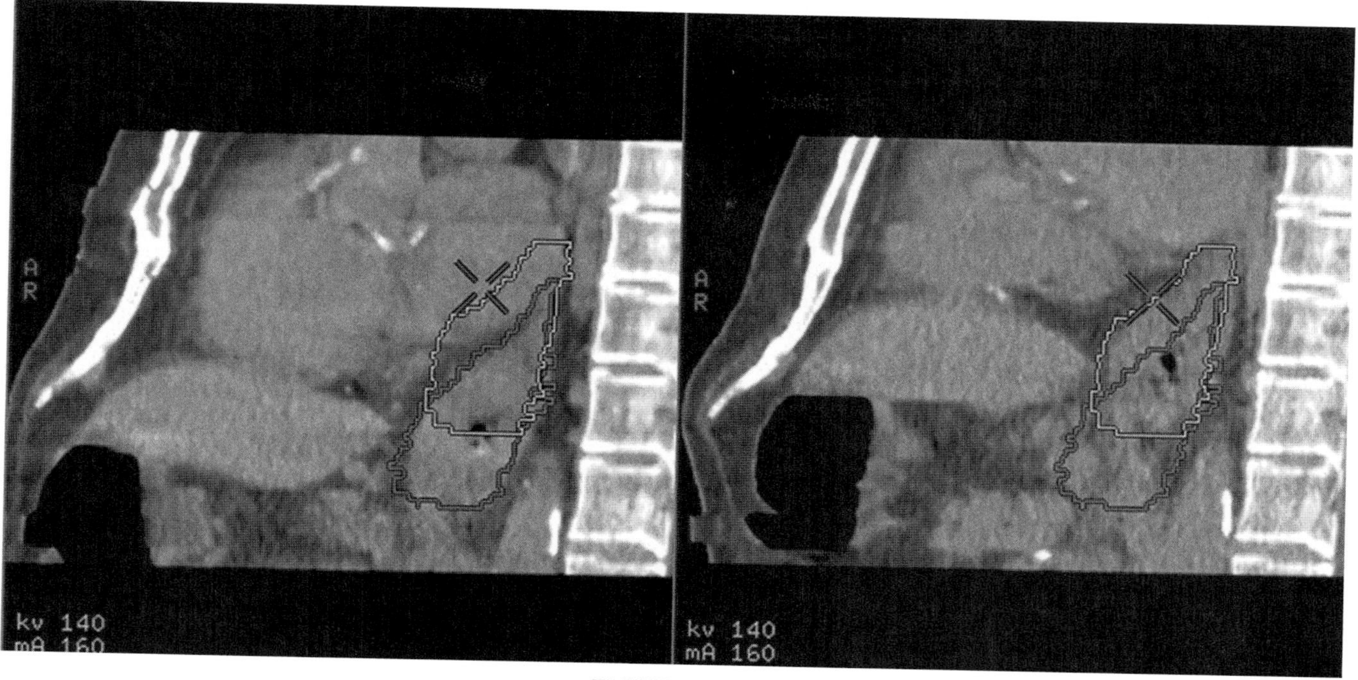

FIGURE 52.3

4-D CT display of esophageal tumor motion. Panel on left shows location of tumor (circled in black) during inspiration and panel on right shows location of tumor (circled in white) in expiration. Courtesy of Abhi Patel.

by the contralateral lung and the upper portion of the lungs were not strong predictors of complications (17).

In spite of the significant efforts to predict toxicity risk using DVH parameters, the concept of using dosimetric parameters has some flaws. Firstly, the subjects included in these studies constitute a heterogeneous population of patients with respect to lung function and performance status. Secondly, chemotherapy regimens have evolved over time and remain a confounding variable in any pneumonitis study (21). Finally, varying definitions of "lung" have been used (ipsilateral lung, combined lung, combined lung minus PTV, etc.). Hence, it is challenging to identify a definitive set of DVH parameters that correlate with a low pneumonitis risk.

Postoperative Pulmonary Complications

Postoperative pulmonary complications represent a clinically separate entity, which encompass any respiratory or pulmonary complications that occur in the postoperative period. In contrast to radiation pneumonitis, postoperative pulmonary complications are generally regarded as an acute complication. In 1 large series from Hong Kong, pulmonary complications occurred in over 15% of patients and accounted for 55% of the hospital deaths after esophagectomy (22).

The correlation between lung irradiation and postoperative lung complications was examined by Wang and colleagues from the MD Anderson Cancer Center (23). In their study, 110 patients who underwent preoperative chemoradiation followed by esophagectomy were evaluated. The trial endpoint was postoperative lung complications as defined by pneumonia or adult respiratory distress syndrome (ARDS) occurring within 30 days of surgery. Eighteen patients developed postoperative pulmonary complications. The only independent predictor associated with postoperative pulmonary complications was the absolute lung volume spared from 5 Gy (also referred to as V5). The authors hypothesized that low-dose radiation may sensitize the lung to the physiologic strain of surgery, which triggers subclinical damage that would not otherwise become clinically evident.

Cardiac Dose and Toxicity

Long-term cardiac morbidity and mortality from esophageal radiation remain largely unknown. This is likely due to the lack of long-term follow-up and small patient numbers. However, it is clear that radiation can be cardiotoxic. The Early Breast Cancer Trialists' Collaborative Group demonstrated an excess in cardiac deaths after 20 years of follow-up in the patients receiving radiotherapy (24), who generally received high doses to a small portion of the left ventricle. Modest dose to the whole heart can also place a patient at risk for cardiac toxicity. In an analysis by Ng and colleagues, survivors of Hodgkin's disease had an absolute excess risk (AER, per 10,000 patient-years) of 5 to 7 in the time interval from 0 to 15 years after radiotherapy (25). However, the risk markedly increased to 13.9 between 15 and 20 years, and to 41.1 beyond 20 years after therapy. Eriksson and colleagues similarly noted an increased risk of cardiac mortality (26). In an attempt to correlate these findings with DVH parameters, 3 risk groups were identified. The high-risk group received > 38 Gy to 35% of the whole cardiac volume. The intermediate-risk group received < 38 Gy to 35% of volume and > 35 Gy to 30% of volume. The low-risk group received < 35 Gy to no more than 30% of the volume. The excess risk of cardiovascular disease at 15 years was 7.9, 5.5, and 3.8% for the high-, intermediate-, and low-risk groups, respectively. These values had wide confidence intervals, reflecting the relatively limited numbers of patients with long follow-up.

Although these data are not specific for patients with esophageal cancer treated with radiation, it is likely that these patients (if they are long-term survivors) may see a similarly increased risk of cardiac events. The cardiac dose may become more important as cure rates improve. Thus, it is desirable, when performing radiation pre-planning, to reduce cardiac dose as much as possible. For now, it seems that limiting the volume of heart, and in particular the left ventricle, to a radiation dose of < 40 Gy, is a reasonable goal, pending further investigation. As will be described, however, this goal is often not easily achievable, particularly when treating distal and GEJ tumors.

Current Normal Tissue Dose Recommendations

In the presence of multiple recommendations for these various endpoints, it has been our practice to integrate multiple DVH parameters into treatment planning. Currently, for lung, we employ a mean combined lung dose-PTV of < 20 Gy, V5 < 50%, V13 < 40%, V20 < 30%, and a V30 < 20%. Regarding heart, we limit the V40 < 10%, with particular attention in keeping the high-dose radiation regions off of the left ventricle. Spinal cord dose is held to a maximum dose below 45 Gy.

Treatment Planning Techniques

The implementation of complete target coverage while maintaining normal tissue radiation dose constraints is dependent on quality radiation treatment planning. There has recently been the rapid development of novel radiation planning and delivery technologies in the past several years. Here, we will highlight the more commonly used technologies, and their limitations.

Three-Dimensional Conformal Radiation Therapy

Three-dimensional conformal radiation therapy (3-D CRT) specifically refers to the method of treatment planning whereby CT data are directly used for radiation treatment planning and dose calculation. Conceptually, this differs from the historic method of treatment planning with 2-D techniques. Briefly, the traditional 2-D techniques relied on isocentric plain films that mimic the geometry of treatment beams. Fields were based on bony anatomy and radio-opaque oral contrast. With 2-D, accurate assessment of radiation dose to different normal structures is not feasible.

3-D CRT treatment planning allows for target definition directly based on CT information. Furthermore, a better assessment of radiation dose to normal structures can be performed. In 3-D CRT, a patient will undergo simulation as previously. These CT data are transferred to a treatment planning system where the radiation oncologist will contour the tumor as well as normal tissues. The radiation oncologist and dosimetrist then design beam arrangements.

The specific beam arrangement used is at the discretion of the treating physician, but strives to achieve the normal tissue dose objectives previously outlined, as well as > 95% of the PTV covered by the prescription isodose line. One standard approach is to treat with parallel-opposed anterior and posterior fields (AP/PA) until spinal cord tolerance is reached. Afterwards, oblique angled beams that avoid the spinal cord are used to complete the treatment. Most commonly, parallel-opposed fields from right/anterior (RAO) and left/posterior (LPO) are used to decrease the cardiac dose. Another alternative method is to treat the tumor and nodal PTVs with AP/PA fields to approximately 30.6 to 36 Gy, and then to treat with 3 fields (an anterior [AP] field, and 2 posterior off/cord oblique fields) to 45 to 50.4 Gy (see Figure 52.4). We often employ a boost field from 45 to 50.4 Gy using lateral or oblique fields to the GTV plus 2 to 3 cm. While these are commonly used beam arrangements, the treatment planner should strive to creatively meet treatment planning goals acknowledging the highly variable anatomy from patient to patient.

Intensity Modulated Radiation Therapy

Intensity modulated radiation therapy (IMRT) affords the potential to shape high-dose radiation around normal structures while fully dosing the tumor and other at-risk areas. Conventional radiation techniques for

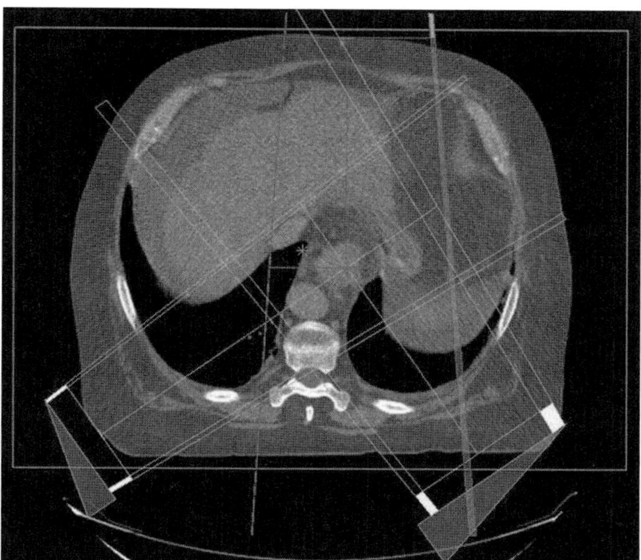

FIGURE 52.4

3-D CRT beam arrangement with an anterior field and 2 posterior off/cord oblique fields.

esophageal cancer utilize large static fields that produce somewhat homogeneous dose distributions and generous field coverage. The fundamental difference between IMRT and 3-D CRT is the concept of inverse planning. As described before, in 3-D CRT, the treatment planner chooses static beams, and the radiation dose is analyzed after computation of relative dose from each beam. This process is known as *forward planning*. In contrast, in IMRT planning, the treatment planning system is given goals for tumor coverage and normal tissue sparing. The treatment planning system then creates an optimal intensity map from the chosen beam angles to achieve these treatment goals. This *inverse planning* process allows for the creation of highly conformal radiation plans. However, in spite of its potential, data regarding the use of IMRT for esophageal cancer remain quite sparse. The integration of IMRT into clinical practice for esophageal cancer is complicated by the continuously evolving literature on dose-volume predictors of pulmonary and cardiac complications, as already discussed.

In general, IMRT has been employed to either allow for dose escalation or greater normal tissue sparing. Because of the lack of benefit with dose escalation (8), the primary goal of IMRT in esophageal cancer is to reduce radiation dose to adjacent normal structures. Organs of particular interest include the lungs, heart, spinal cord, liver, and kidneys. With a conventional planning, the doses to the spinal cord, liver, and kidneys are kept within tolerance with little difficulty. Of greater interest is the potential of IMRT to reduce lung and cardiac dose. However, as described above, the precise dose-volume parameters predicting pulmonary and cardiac toxicity continue to evolve. Furthermore, it is unlikely that any definitive data will soon become available, as late effect data, by definition, take years to mature. Hence, the benefit of IMRT in esophageal cancer may continue to be limited until better dosimetric predictors of toxicity are established.

Dosimetric Studies

Little clinical data exist on the use of IMRT in esophageal cancer. Most of the published current research to date has evaluated potential dosimetric advantages of IMRT over 3-D CRT. Wu and colleagues compared IMRT plans with forward and inverse 3-D CRT plans on 15 patients with mid-esophageal cancers (27). Plans were evaluated for target conformality as well as the dose received by the heart and lungs. A dose of 60 Gy was prescribed to isocenter with 95% of the PTV receiving 58 Gy. The IMRT plans generated the most conformal high-dose distribution around the PTV ($P = 0.008$) as well as lower mean lung and cardiac dose. The authors concluded that IMRT might afford better potential for dose escalation. Fu and co-investigators reached a similar conclusion when comparing the ability of 3-D and IMRT to deliver simultaneous integrated boost (SIB) dose-escalated plans in which the GTV received 67.2 (2.4 Gy/fraction) and 50.4 (1.8 Gy/fraction) Gy over 28 fractions (28). Upper esophageal locations were specifically evaluated in 5 patients. The IMRT appeared to produce lower V20 and V30 in lung. Cardiac dose was not specifically addressed, due to the upper esophageal location.

In contrast to the 2 studies above, a study by Chandra et al. specifically addressed the potential advantage of IMRT in distal esophageal cancers (29). Standard preoperative and definitive doses of 50.4 Gy were evaluated in 1.8 Gy/fractions. Ten patients were analyzed in this study. The IMRT plans showed significant reduction in mean lung dose, as well as lung V10 and V20. There was no significant reduction in cardiac dose over the 3-D CRT plans.

Because of the large volume treated for esophageal cancer, as well as the proximity of critical organs, IMRT has attractive potential in delivering better plans. However, much remains unknown about the routine use of IMRT for esophageal cancer. Firstly, it is unclear how one should balance dose constraints for lung and heart. The MD Anderson optimized plans to improve lung DVHs, but were then unable to significantly lower cardiac dose. Furthermore, attempts to limit cardiac dose or produce greater conformality of the high isodose lines may be associated with a "spraying" of the low dose isodose cloud into more lung tissue.

To examine this point, investigators at the MGH performed a dosimetric study with the goal of decreasing cardiac dose in distal esophageal cancers (30). The CTV was defined by the CT-based GTV with a 5 cm cranial-caudal and a 2 cm radial expansion. Expansions of PTV were individualized based on 4-D CT. To treat the CTV to 50.4 Gy in 1.8 Gy fractions, 3-D CRT and IMRT plans were created. A "combined" plan was also created that treated the CTV to 36 Gy in 20 fractions using 3-D, followed by an IMRT boost for the final 14.4 Gy. In all plans, a cone down was performed after 45 Gy, Figure 52.5. The treatment planning goals were, in order of priority: (a) spinal cord maximum dose < 45 Gy; (b) > 95% of the PTV covered by the prescription isodose line; (c) lung dose restricted to a combined V20 < 30% and a mean lung dose of 20 Gy; (d) cardiac dose restricted to V40 < 20%; and (e) global hot spot of less than 15%.

DVH results for 15 3-D CRT, IMRT, and combined distal esophageal plans are depicted in Table 52.1. The full IMRT plans were best able to reduce dose to the heart as measured by V40 and mean cardiac dose but were also associated with the highest V5 and V20 in the heart. 3-D CRT plans were least successful in achieving the cardiac planning constraints. The combined plans achieved both cardiac and pulmonary planning dose constraints, and displayed a superior lung V20. Mean lung doses were not significantly different and equivalent uniform dose (EUD) analyses on 9 of the plans suggest that EUD for the high-dose CTV does not differ between plans. In this preliminary analysis for the treatment of distal esophageal cancers, a combined 3-D/IMRT plan (in contrast to full-course IMRT) achieved adequate cardiac sparing while maintaining lower lung DVH parameters, as defined a priori.

These studies highlight the difficulty in clinical translation of IMRT in the radiotherapeutic management of esophageal cancer. Because an IMRT plan can be optimized in any number of ways, trade-offs in dose to the normal structures are left to the discretion of the treatment planners. Currently, 3-D or IMRT approaches that achieve the above-stated dosimetric goals are considered reasonable.

TABLE 52.1
Comparative Dosimetry of 3-D, IMRT, and Combined Plan for Distal Esophageal Cancer

	3-D CRT	IMRT	Combined
Heart			
V40	26.0%	10.3%	17.9%
Mean dose	33.0 Gy	23.9 Gy	29.9 Gy
Lung			
V5	56.3%	74.5%	64.9%
V20	27.2%	28.1%	22.3%
Global hot spot	56.6 Gy	58.1 Gy	56.0 Gy

While IMRT was able to meet all planning constraints, it produced the highest lung V5 and V20. Values are averaged over 5 plans.

CONCLUSION

Radiation therapy planning for esophageal cancer has multiple layers of complexity. Careful attention is warranted to the discussed issues of target definitions, normal tissue sparing, organ motion, and treatment delivery strategies. While acknowledging the commonalities in treatment planning, radiation planning and treatment should remain individualized based on patient factors.

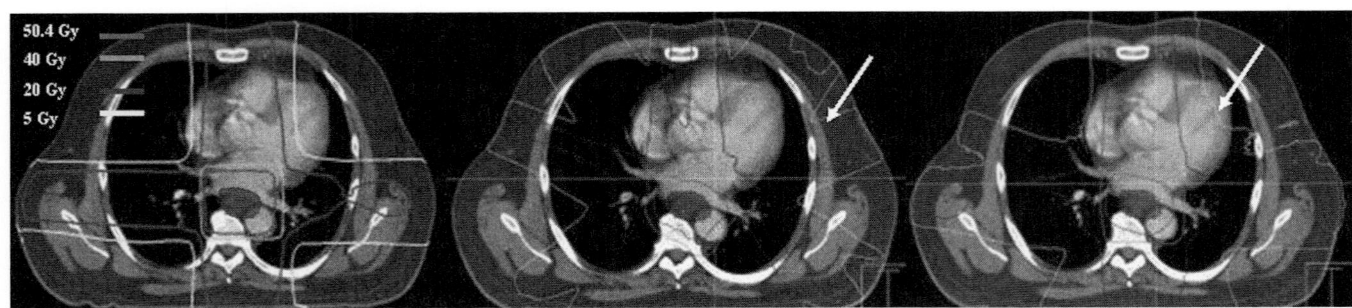

FIGURE 52.5

Comparative dosimetric trade-offs between (a) 3-D, (b) IMRT only, and (c) combined 3-D and IMRT. Note the increased lung volume receiving 5 Gy with the IMRT only plan (arrow).

References

1. Bradley J, Thorstad WL, Mutic S, et al. Impact of FDG-PET on radiation therapy volume delineation in non-small-cell lung cancer. *Int J Radiat Oncol Biol Phys.* 2004;59(1):78–86.
2. Gondi V, Bradley K, Mehta M, et al. Impact of hybrid fluorodeoxyglucose positron-emission tomography/computed tomography on radiotherapy planning in esophageal and non-small-cell lung cancer. *Int J Radiat Oncol Biol Phys.* 2007;67(1):187–195.
3. Heron DE, Andrade RS, Flickinger J, et al. Hybrid PET-CT simulation for radiation treatment planning in head-and-neck cancers: A brief technical report. *Int J Radiat Oncol Biol Phys.* 1419;60(5):1419–1424.
4. Mah K, Caldwell CB, Ung YC, et al. The impact of 18FDG-PET on target and critical organs in CT-based treatment planning of patients with poorly defined non-small-cell lung carcinoma: a prospective study. *Int J Radiat Oncol Biol Phys.* 2002;52(2):339–350.
5. Nestle U, Kremp S, Schaefer-Schuler A, et al. Comparison of different methods for delineation of F-18-FDG PET-positive tissue for target volume definition in radiotherapy of patients with non-small cell lung cancer. *J Nucl Med.* 1342;46(8):1342–1348.
6. Nestle U, Kremp S, Grosu A-L. Practical integration of [F-18]-FDG-PET and PET-CT in the planning of radiotherapy for non-small cell lung cancer (NSCLC): The technical basis, ICRU-target volumes, problems, perspectives. *Radiother Oncol.* 2006;81(2):209–225.
7. Herskovic A, Martz K, al-Sarraf M, et al. Combined chemotherapy and radiotherapy compared with radiotherapy alone in patients with cancer of the esophagus. *N Engl J Med.* 1992;326(24):1593–1598.
8. Minsky BD, Pajak TF, Ginsberg RJ, et al. INT 0123 (Radiation Therapy Oncology Group 94–05) Phase III trial of combined-modality therapy for esophageal cancer: high-dose versus standard-dose radiation therapy. *J Clin Oncol.* 2004;20(5):1167–1174.
9. Bosset J-F, Gignoux M, Triboulet J-P, et al. Chemoradiotherapy followed by surgery compared with surgery alone in squamous-cell cancer of the esophagus. *N Engl J Med.* 1997;337(3):161–167.
10. Urba SG, Orringer MB, Turrisi A, et al. Randomized trial of preoperative chemoradiation versus surgery alone in patients with locoregional esophageal carcinoma. *J Clin Oncol.* 2001;19(2):305–313.
11. Walsh TN, Noonan N, Hollywood D, et al. A comparison of multimodal therapy and surgery for esophageal adenocarcinoma. *N Engl J Med.* 1996;335(7):462–467.
12. Tepper JE, Krasna M, Niedzwiecki D, et al. Superiority of trimodality therapy to surgery alone in esophageal cancer: Results of CALGB 9781. *J Clin Oncol.* 2006;24(18S):4012.
13. Hong TS, Tome WA, Chappell RJ, et al. The impact of daily setup variations on head-and-neck intensity-modulated radiation therapy. *Int J Radiat Oncol Biol Phys.* 2005;61(3):779–788.
14. Patel AA, Wolfgang JA, Niemierko A, et al. Implications of respiratory motion as measured by 4D CT for radiation treatment planning of esophageal tumors. *Int J Radiat Oncol Biol Phys.* 2006;66(3):S607.
15. Hosch SB, Stoecklein NH, Pichlmeier U, et al. Esophageal cancer: the mode of lymphatic tumor cell spread and its prognostic significance. *J Clin Oncol.* 2001;19(7):1970–1975.
16. Kwa SL, Theuws JC, Wagenaar A, et al. Evaluation of two dose-volume histogram reduction models for the prediction of radiation pneumonitis. *Radiother Oncol.* 1998;48(1):61–69.
17. Yorke ED, Jackson A, Rosenzweig KE, et al. Dose-volume factors contributing to the incidence of radiation pneumonitis in non-small-cell lung cancer patients treated with three-dimensional conformal radiation therapy. *Int J Radiat Oncol Biol Phys.* 2002;54(2):329–339.
18. Oetzel D, Schraube P, Hensley F, et al. Estimation of pneumonitis risk in three-dimensional treatment planning using dose-volume histogram analysis. *Int J Radiat Oncol Biol Phys.* 1995;33(2):455–460.
19. Graham MV, Purdy JA, Emami B, et al. Clinical dose-volume histogram analysis for pneumonitis after 3D treatment for non-small cell lung cancer (NSCLC). *Int J Radiat Oncol Biol Phys.* 1999;45(2):323–329.
20. Hernando ML, Marks LB, Bentel GC, et al. Radiation-induced pulmonary toxicity: a dose-volume histogram analysis in 201 patients with lung cancer. *Int J Radiat Oncol Biol Phys.* 2001;51(3):650–659.
21. Lingos TI, Recht A, Vicini F, et al. Radiation pneumonitis in breast cancer patients treated with conservative surgery and radiation therapy. *Int J Radiat Oncol Biol Phys.* 1991;21(2):355–360.
22. Law S, Wong KH, Kwok KF, et al. Predictive factors for postoperative pulmonary complications and mortality after esophagectomy for cancer. *Ann Surg.* 2004;240(5):791–800.
23. Wang SL, Liao Z, Vaporciyan AA, et al. Investigation of clinical and dosimetric factors associated with postoperative pulmonary complications in esophageal cancer patients treated with concurrent chemoradiotherapy followed by surgery. *Int J Radiat Oncol Biol Phys.* 2006;64(3):692–699.
24. Early Breast Cancer Trialists' Collaborative Group. Favourable and unfavourable effects on long-term survival of radiotherapy for early breast cancer: an overview of the randomised trials. *Lancet.* 2000;355(9217):1757–1770.
25. Ng AK, Bernardo MP, Weller E, et al. Long-term survival and competing causes of death in patients with early-stage Hodgkin's disease treated at age 50 or younger. *J Clin Oncol.* 2002;20(8):2101–2108.
26. Eriksson F, Gagliardi G, Liedberg A, et al. Long-term cardiac mortality following radiation therapy for Hodgkin's disease: analysis with the relative seriality model. *Radiother Oncol.* 2000;55(2):153–162.
27. Wu Q, Mohan R, Morris M, et al. Simultaneous integrated boost intensity-modulated radiotherapy for locally advanced head-and-neck squamous cell carcinomas. I: dosimetric results. *Int J Radiat Oncol Biol Phys.* 2003;56(2):573–585.
28. Fu WH, Wang LH, Zhou ZM, et al. Comparison of conformal and intensity-modulated techniques for simultaneous integrated boost radiotherapy of upper esophageal carcinoma. *World J Gastroenterol.* 2004;10(8):1098–1102.
29. Chandra A, Guerrero TM, Liu HH, et al. Feasibility of using intensity-modulated radiotherapy to improve lung sparing in treatment planning for distal esophageal cancer. *Radiother Oncol.* 2005;77(3):247–253.
30. Crowley EM, Kachnic LA, Mamon HJ, et al. Optimizing the cardiac and pulmonary dose in treatment planning for distal esophageal cancer: does IMRT always produce the best plan? *Int J Radiat Oncol Biol Phys.* 2006;66(3):S281–S282.

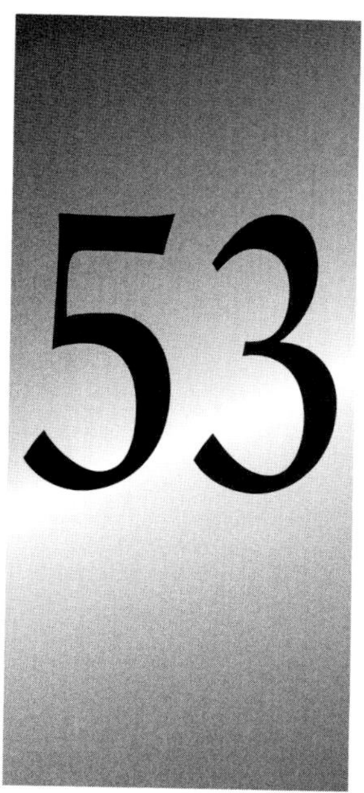

53 Adjuvant (Postoperative) Therapy

Parag Sanghvi
Mehee Choi
John Holland
Charles R. Thomas, Jr.

Despite major advances in surgical techniques, systemic therapy, and radiation treatment planning and delivery, 5-year survival rates for patients with locally advanced esophageal cancer remain dismally low, at around 10% to 15% (1). Surgical resection, when possible, remains the cornerstone of treatment; however, its utility as a monotherapy has been challenged (2,3). Since the early 1990s, there has been a developing trend to incorporate concurrent chemotherapy and radiotherapy (chemoradiotherapy [CRT]) into the treatment regimen, to both control distant micrometastatic disease and enhance local radiation effects (4–6). For locally advanced unresectable disease, definitive nonoperative treatment with CRT became the standard of care with the publication of the RTOG 85–01 trial, which demonstrated a significant survival benefit for concurrent cisplatin-based CRT compared with radiotherapy (RT) alone (median survival 14 vs. 9 months) (7–9). At present, 50 Gy RT plus 4 courses of cisplatin and 5-FU (with the first 2 courses given concurrently with RT) remains a standard approach (7,10,11). For patients with clinically resectable cancer, optimal treatment remains a very controversial topic. The most common approaches include surgery alone, neoadjuvant chemotherapy or chemoradiotherapy, and adjuvant chemoradiotherapy. In this chapter, we review the role of both neoadjuvant and adjuvant CRT in the treatment of locally advanced resectable esophageal cancer, with focus on the adjuvant approach.

The main advantage to neoadjuvant, or induction, CRT includes clinical downstaging of the tumor, thereby increasing the likelihood of achieving a complete resection and improving local control. Additionally, there appears to be general preference for neoadjuvant over adjuvant CRT in patients who will ultimately require RT. This is primarily due to the increased morbidity of radiation after surgery, as normal tissue tolerances are lower in a devascularized tumor bed, particularly following a gastric pull-up or intestinal interposition (12).

At least 9 randomized controlled trials (RCT) have compared neoadjuvant CRT versus surgery alone, with conflicting results (13–21). Of these, only 2 trials have shown an overall survival benefit with neoadjuvant CRT, both using a concurrent rather than sequential approach (14,18). In the first study, known as the Irish trial, Walsh and colleagues randomized 113 patients to concurrent CRT with cisplatin, 5-FU, and 40 Gy RT followed by surgery versus surgery alone (14). Two courses of cisplatin and 5-FU were administered during weeks 1 and 6 of RT, which was delivered to a total dose of 40 Gy in 15 fractions over 3 weeks via either an AP-PA field or a 3-field technique. Surgery was performed approximately 4 to 6 weeks after induction CRT. Approximately 25% of patients who underwent neoadjuvant therapy were noted to achieve a complete pathologic response, and when the surgical specimens were compared, regional nodal involvement was less frequent in the CRT group (42% vs. 82%). Trimodality therapy was associated with significantly longer median survival (16 months vs. 11 months) and 3-year survival (32% vs. 6%). (P = 0.001). In the second trial, CALGB 9781, Tepper and colleagues randomized patients with adenocarcinoma or squamous cell carcinoma of the esophagus to either neoadjuvant CRT with cisplatin and 5-FU followed by surgery or surgery alone. RT was delivered in standard fractions to a total dose of 50.4 Gy. The study was closed prematurely with only 56 patients enrolled due to poor accrual. Preliminary results showed that 40% of the patients undergoing neoadjuvant therapy achieved a pathologic complete response. It also showed a statistically significant improvement in both local control and overall survival in the induction arm. The 5-year survival rate was 39% in the trimodality arm versus 16% in the surgery alone arm (P = 0.008) (18). Neither the Irish trial nor the CALGB 9781 trial showed a difference in perioperative morbidity or mortality with trimodality therapy.

Other randomized trials have not shown a statistically significant survival advantage with neoadjuvant CRT (13,15–17,19–21). However, these trials have been criticized for using suboptimal chemotherapy regimens, inadequate RT dose-fractionation schedules, or sequential rather than concurrent CRT.

Two meta-analyses of the RCTs comparing neoadjuvant CRT versus surgery alone have shown a significant benefit to neoadjuvant treatment (22,23). In a meta-analysis of 6 trials, Fiorica and colleagues demonstrated a significant reduction in 3-year mortality after neoadjuvant CRT compared with surgery alone (odds ratio 0.53, P = 0.03) as well as more frequent downstaging of the tumor (odds ratio 0.43, P = 0.001) (22). The second meta-analysis by Urschel and colleagues included patients enrolled on 9 RCTs. When trials using both concurrent and sequential CRT were included, the study showed a nonsignificant trend towards improved 3-year survival with neoadjuvant CRT compared with surgery alone (odds radio 0.66, P = 0.36). The improvement became statistically significant when the analysis was restricted to the subset of trials using concurrent CRT only (odds ratio 0.45, P = 0.005) (23). A third meta-analysis of 10 RCTs comparing preoperative CRT versus surgery alone came to the same conclusion (24).

In current practice, neoadjuvant CRT followed by surgery is the most common approach for patients with locally advanced resectable esophageal cancer. Whether this approach adds benefit to surgery for potentially resectable disease remains a controversial area.

ROLE OF ADJUVANT RADIOTHERAPY

Adjuvant radiotherapy has been used to decrease the risk of locoregional recurrence and to attempt to improve survival in the settings of locally advanced (T3 or T4) tumors, gross residual disease, microscopically positive margins, multiple positive nodes, or extracapsular extension.

Adjuvant Radiotherapy versus Surgery Alone

There are 5 published phase III trials that have compared adjuvant RT versus surgery alone (25–29). No overall survival advantage for adjuvant RT was seen in these studies, though they consistently showed improved local control with adjuvant RT, especially in the subgroup of patients receiving palliative resections.

Teniere and colleagues from France performed a multi-institutional trial from 1979 to 1985 randomizing 221 patients with squamous cell carcinoma of the mid-lower esophagus postoperatively to either RT or no further treatment (26). All patients underwent R0 resection. Those randomized to radiation received postoperative standard fractionation RT to a total dose of 45–55 Gy within 3 months of surgery. Extended field RT was used, with bilateral supraclavicular fossae and mediastinum covered in all patients, and celiac fields covered only for pathologically positive celiac nodes. There was no difference in overall survival at 5 years (19% in both arms). In node-positive patients, there was a trend towards improved locoregional recurrence with adjuvant RT compared with surgery alone (local failure 30% vs. 38%). The improvement in locoregional control was significant in the subset of patients with node-negative disease, with a local failure rate of 10% in irradiated patients versus 15% in patients treated with surgery alone.

The second trial by Fok and colleagues at the University of Hong Kong randomized 130 patients with esophageal cancer of predominantly squamous histology to postoperative radiotherapy versus no further treatment (27). Of the total 130 patients enrolled on the study, 60 patients underwent curative resection and 70 patients underwent palliative resection prior to randomization. Radiation was delivered to a total dose of 49 Gy for the patients with curative resection, and 52.5 Gy for those with palliative resection. The dose per fraction was 3.5 Gy. The target volume covered a 5 cm margin at both cephalad and caudad ends of the initial tumor as shown by a preoperative barium swallow. Standard circumferential margins were used. If the resection margin was positive, the irradiation was extended to cover the esophageal anastomosis, if the anastomosis was not already within the target volume. There was a statistically significant reduction in overall survival in patients who received RT. Median survival was 8.7 months in the postoperative RT arm versus 15.2 months in the surgery alone arm (P = 0.02). In patients undergoing a curative resection, the local recurrence rate was similar between the 2 treatment arms (10% S+RT versus 13% S, P > 0.05). However, among patients undergoing a palliative resection, the local recurrence rate was significantly lower after adjuvant RT (20% vs. 46%, P = 0.04). It was also noted that patients who had residual disease after resection were less likely to die of a tracheobronchial obstruction if they received adjuvant RT (7% vs. 33%, P = 0.07). There was no difference in the rate of distant metastases between treatment arms (S+RT 42% vs. S 55%, P = 0.16). Treatment-related morbidity (gastric pull-up complications) was substantially higher with RT (S+RT 37% vs. S 6%, P < 0.0001). Six fatal bleeds were reported in the RT arm. The authors concluded that postoperative RT was associated with significantly increased morbidity and mortality with decreased overall survival. The high rate of treatment-related complications was felt to be due possibly to the large radiation fractions and total dose delivered leading to a high overall biologically equivalent dose.

Zieren and colleagues from Germany randomized 68 patients who underwent curative resection for squamous cell carcinoma of the esophagus to adjuvant RT versus observation. Patients with stage II to IV tumors who underwent a R0 resection were enrolled. Radiation was delivered in standard fractions to 55.8 Gy. For upper thoracic esophagus tumors, bilateral supraclavicular fossae were included. The celiac nodes were covered for tumors in the lower thoracic esophagus. Results showed no difference in overall or disease-free survival between the treatment arms. The overall survival at 3 years was 22% in the irradiation arm and 20% in the observation arm. Postoperative RT significantly increased the incidence of fibrotic esophagogastric or esophagocolonic strictures (28).

Xiao and colleagues from China randomized 495 patients with squamous cell carcinoma of the esophagus to adjuvant RT versus no further treatment from 1986 to 1997. Most tumors were located in the mid-thoracic esophagus (67%) and at least T3 (69%). Nearly half of the patients had node-positive disease (48%). Patients received RT to a total dose of 60 Gy, with 40 Gy delivered AP-PA and the remaining 20 Gy delivered with an off-cord technique. Extended field RT was used covering supraclavicular, mediastinal, periesophageal, and perigastric nodes. Overall, no survival benefit was seen with adjuvant RT. The 5-year overall survival rate was 41.3% in the RT arm versus 37.1% in the surgery arm (P = 0.45). A subanalysis of patients with node-negative disease did not show any improvement in 5-year survival with RT (S+RT 52.8% vs. S 51%, P = 0.95). However, in the subset of patients with positive lymph nodes, there was a trend toward improved survival at 5 years (S+RT 29.2% vs. S 14.7%, P = 0.07). When stratified by stage, the subset of patients with stage III disease who received adjuvant RT had a significantly higher 5-year survival rate compared with patients receiving surgery as monotherapy (S+RT 35.1% vs. S 13.1%, P = 0.003). Patients receiving RT also had significantly lower rates of intrathoracic failure (16.2% vs. 25%, P = 0.015), supraclavicular failure (3.1% vs. 13.8%, P < 0.05), and anastomotic recurrence (0.5% vs. 5.8%, P = 0.003). There was no significant increase in anastomotic stenosis or rate of distant failure between the 2 arms.

A 2005 update of the above study further examined the impact of RT in node-positive versus node-negative patients (30). Patients were stratified into 3 groups: no lymph node involvement, 1 to 2 lymph nodes involved, and 3 or more lymph nodes involved. In patients with node-positive disease, the 5-year overall survival rate was significantly higher with adjuvant RT versus surgery alone (34.1% vs. 17.6%, P = 0.038). In patients with node-negative disease, 5-year overall survival was similar between treatment arms (51.4% S+R vs. 53% S, P > 0.05). Overall, patients with 3 or more positive lymph nodes fared worse than patients with 1 to 2 positive lymph nodes. Among patients with 1 to 2 positive lymph nodes, the 5-year overall survival rate was 45.1% with adjuvant RT and 23.5% with surgery alone. Among patients with 3 or more positive lymph nodes, the 5-year overall survival rate was 20.6% with adjuvant RT; there were no survivors among those receiving surgery alone.

Adjuvant Radiotherapy versus Adjuvant Chemotherapy

The Japanese Esophageal Oncology Group performed a phase III trial comparing RT and chemotherapy as adjuvant treatments for esophageal cancer (31). Total 258 patients who had undergone uncomplicated curative resection were enrolled between 1985 and 1987. There was no surgery alone control arm. Histology was not specified. There were no restrictions in terms of staging. Approximately 40% patients in both arms were stage II or lower. Nearly 30% were node-negative in both arms. Patients randomized to the RT arm received 50 Gy standard fractionation adjuvant RT to an extended radiation field. Patients randomized to the chemotherapy arm received 2 cycles of cisplatin (50 mg/m^2) and vindesine (3 mg/m^2) separated by 3 weeks. Protocol-prescribed treatment was completed in 91% of patients. There was no significant difference in 5-year survival rates between the RT and chemotherapy arms (44% vs. 42%, respectively).

Local recurrence rates were similar as well (RT 22% vs. C 25%, $P > 0.05$).

Adjuvant Chemoradiotherapy versus Surgery Alone

MacDonald and colleagues evaluated the role of adjuvant CRT following surgery in 556 patients with resectable adenocarcinoma of the stomach or gastroesophageal junction (GEJ) who were treated between 1991 and 1998 (32). Approximately 20% of the patients had GEJ tumors. Patients were randomly assigned postoperatively to CRT versus observation. Patients with stage IB to stage IV were eligible for enrollment; 85% had node-positive disease. A total dose of 45 Gy RT was delivered to the tumor bed and regional lymph nodes in 25 fractions. Chemotherapy consisted of 1 cycle of 5-FU and leucovorin prior to radiation, followed by concurrent 5-FU during radiation and 2 additional cycles of 5-FU and leucovorin after radiation was completed. Three-year survival rates were significantly improved in the CRT arm compared with the surgery-only arm (50% vs. 41%, $P = 0.005$). Median duration of survival was 36 months in the CRT arm versus 27 months in the surgery-only arm (hazard ratio 1.35). Three-year relapse-free survival rates (48% vs. 31%) and the median duration of relapse-free survival was significantly greater in the CRT arm versus the surgery-only arm (30 versus 19 months, $P < 0.0001$). The local failure rate was higher in the surgery-only arm (29% vs. 19%).

Bedard and colleagues performed a retrospective review of 70 patients with resected node-positive esophageal carcinoma who either received adjuvant CRT or no further treatment between 1991 and 1997 (33). Patients with squamous cell carcinoma or adenocarcinoma histology and thoracic esophagus or GEJ location were included. Patients in the CRT arm received concurrent CRT consisting of 4 cycles of chemotherapy (cisplatin, 5-FU with or without epirubicin), the first 2 prior to radiation, then 2 concurrent with radiation. RT was delivered in standard fractions to a total dose of 50 Gy, with the first 36 Gy delivered AP-PA followed by 14 Gy using an off-cord technique with CT-based planning. No specific data on the number of positive lymph nodes or extracapsular extension were provided. The median overall survival was significantly better in the adjuvant CRT arm at 47.5 months versus 14.1 months in the surgery alone arm ($P = 0.001$). The 5-year overall survival was 48% in the adjuvant CRT arm; there were no survivors in the surgery alone arm at 5 years. There was an increased rate of locoregional recurrence in the surgery alone arm (35% vs. 13%, $P = 0.09$). Toxicities in the CRT arm were acceptable. There were no treatment-related deaths. Grade 3 GI toxicity was reported in 46% of patients; there was no grade 4 GI toxicity. Grade 3 and grade 4 hematologic toxicities were reported in 21% and 16% of the patients, respectively. The authors concluded that adjuvant concurrent CRT was safe, feasible, and improved overall survival in patients with locally advanced resectable esophageal cancers.

Rice and colleagues reported retrospective data on 31 patients with locally advanced esophageal cancer (T3+, N1 or M1a) treated with adjuvant CRT at the Cleveland Clinic (34). Results were compared against those of 52 patients with similar advanced disease who received no adjuvant therapy after surgery. Radiation consisted of 50.4 to 59.4 Gy in standard fractions. Chemotherapy consisted of two 4-day cycles of intravenous 5-FU (1000 mg/m^2/d) and cisplatin (20 mg/m^2/d). Patients who received adjuvant CRT showed an improved median survival of 28 versus 15 months in patients who underwent surgery alone ($P = 0.05$). The 4-year overall survival rates for the adjuvant CRT versus surgery alone arms were 44% versus 0%.

Adjuvant Chemoradiotherapy versus Adjuvant Radiotherapy

Liu and colleagues from Taiwan reported a nonrandomized study that prospectively enrolled 60 patients with T3–4 N0–1 squamous cell carcinoma of the esophagus from 1999 to 2002 (35). Patients were assigned to receive either adjuvant RT or adjuvant concurrent CRT (30 patients per treatment arm). RT delivery was identical between treatment arms. The postoperative tumor bed and surrounding regional lymph nodes were treated initially to 40 Gy using an AP-PA technique followed by an off-cord boost of 15 to 20 Gy using 3-D conformal treatment planning with longitudinal and radial margins of 5 cm and 3 cm, respectively. The mean dose delivered was 58.2 Gy. Patients in the CRT arm received concurrent chemotherapy that consisted of weekly cisplatin (30mg/m^2) during RT. Subsequently, adjuvant chemotherapy with cisplatin (100 mg/m^2) and bolus 5-FU (1000 mg/m^2) was delivered in 4 monthly cycles given over 5 days every month. In the CRT arm, all patients completed protocol-prescribed RT, 50% received all 6 weekly cycles of concurrent chemotherapy, 34% received 4 of 6 cycles of concurrent chemotherapy, 16% received fewer than 4 cycles of concurrent chemotherapy, and 50% received all 4 cycles of adjuvant chemotherapy. In the RT alone arm, 80% received the intended radiation dose. The CRT arm showed significantly improved

3-year overall survival of 70% compared with 33.7% in the RT alone arm (P = 0.003). Mean survival was 31.7 months in the CRT arm versus 20.7 months in the RT alone arm. Locoregional and distant failure rates were lower in the CRT arm versus the RT alone arm (40% vs. 60% and 27% vs. 57%, respectively). Toxicity rates with the CRT regimen were modest compared with adjuvant CRT regiments used in previous studies. The only grade 3 or 4 toxicities that occurred were hematologic, affecting 20% of patients in the CRT arm versus 17% in the RT arm. The authors concluded that adjuvant CRT improved overall survival in locoregionally advanced esophageal cancers with an acceptable toxicity profile.

CONCLUSION

Despite the controversial findings regarding survival benefit, improvements in postoperative morbidity and mortality, and tumor response, the authors feel that there is a therapeutic role for trimodality therapy with CRT and surgery for locally advanced resectable esophageal carcinoma. Adjuvant chemoradiation should be considered in patients with T3 or T4 lesions, node-positive disease, and/or positive margins because it can provide a meaningful benefit in terms of locoregional control. We recommend treating the tumor bed and the involved locoregional lymph nodes to a dose of 45–50.4 Gy with concurrent Cisplatin and 5-FU based chemotherapy.

References

1. Jemal A, Siegel R, Ward E, et al. Cancer Statistics, 2008. *CA Cancer J Clin.* 2008.
2. O'Reilly S, Forastiere AA. Is surgery necessary with multimodality treatment of oesophageal cancer. *Ann Oncol.* 1995;6:519–521.
3. Coia LR. Esophageal cancer: is esophagectomy necessary? *Oncology (Williston Park).* 1989;3:101–110; discussion 110–101, 114–105.
4. McGinn CJ, Kinsella TJ. The experimental and clinical rationale for the use of S-phase-specific radiosensitizers to overcome tumor cell repopulation. *Semin Oncol.* 1992;19:21–28.
5. Forastiere AA. Treatment of locoregional esophageal cancer. *Semin Oncol.* 1992;19: 57–63.
6. Herscher LL, Cook JA, Pacelli R, et al. Principles of chemoradiation: theoretical and practical considerations. *Oncology (Williston Park).* 1999;13:11–22.
7. Herskovic A, Martz K, al-Sarraf M, et al. Combined chemotherapy and radiotherapy compared with radiotherapy alone in patients with cancer of the esophagus. *N Engl J Med.* 1992;326:1593–1598.
8. al-Sarraf M, Martz K, Herskovic A, et al. Progress report of combined chemoradiotherapy versus radiotherapy alone in patients with esophageal cancer: an intergroup study. *J Clin Oncol.* 1997;15:277–284.
9. Cooper JS, Guo MD, Herskovic A, et al. Chemoradiotherapy of locally advanced esophageal cancer: long-term follow-up of a prospective randomized trial (RTOG 85-01). Radiation Therapy Oncology Group. *JAMA.* 1999;281:1623–1627.
10. Minsky BD, Pajak TF, Ginsberg RJ, et al. INT 0123 (Radiation Therapy Oncology Group 94-05) phase III trial of combined-modality therapy for esophageal cancer: high-dose versus standard-dose radiation therapy. *J Clin Oncol.* 2002; 20:1167–1174.
11. Rebecca WO, Richard MA. Combined chemotherapy and radiotherapy (without surgery) compared with radiotherapy alone in localized carcinoma of the esophagus. *Cochrane Database Syst Rev.* 2003:CD002092.
12. Czito BG, Denittis AS, Willett CG. Esophageal cancer. In: Halperin EC, Perez CA, Brady LW, et al., eds. *Perez and Brady's Principles and Practice of Radiation Oncology.* 5th ed. Philadelphia: Lippincott Williams & Wilkins; 2008:1131–1153.
13. Urba SG, Orringer MB, Turrisi A, et al. Randomized trial of preoperative chemoradiation versus surgery alone in patients with locoregional esophageal carcinoma. *J Clin Oncol.* 2001;19:305–313.
14. Walsh TN, Noonan N, Hollywood D, et al. A comparison of multimodal therapy and surgery for esophageal adenocarcinoma. *N Engl J Med.* 1996;335:462–467.
15. Bosset JF, Gignoux M, Triboulet JP, et al. Chemoradiotherapy followed by surgery compared with surgery alone in squamous-cell cancer of the esophagus. *N Engl J Med.* 1997;337:161–167.
16. Bains MS, Stojadinovic A, Minsky B, et al. A phase II trial of preoperative combined-modality therapy for localized esophageal carcinoma: initial results. *J Thorac Cardiovasc Surg.* 2002;124:270–277.
17. Burmeister BH, Smithers BM, Gebski V, et al. Surgery alone versus chemoradiotherapy followed by surgery for resectable cancer of the oesophagus: a randomised controlled phase III trial. *Lancet Oncol.* 2005;6:659–668.
18. Tepper JE, Krasna M, Niedzwiecki D, et al. Superiority of trimodality therapy to surgery alone in esophageal cancer: results of CALGB 9781. *J Clin Oncol, 2006 ASCO Annual Meeting Proceedings (Post-Meeting Edition).* 2006;24:4012.
19. Stahl M, Stuschke M, Lehmann N, et al. Chemoradiation with and without surgery in patients with locally advanced squamous cell carcinoma of the esophagus. *J Clin Oncol.* 2005;23:2310–2317.
20. Nygaard K, Hagen S, Hansen HS, et al. Pre-operative radiotherapy prolongs survival in operable esophageal carcinoma: a randomized, multicenter study of pre-operative radiotherapy and chemotherapy. The second Scandinavian trial in esophageal cancer. *World J Surg.* 1992;16:1104–1109; discussion 1110.
21. Le Prise E, Etienne PL, Meunier B, et al. A randomized study of chemotherapy, radiation therapy, and surgery versus surgery for localized squamous cell carcinoma of the esophagus. *Cancer.* 1994;73:1779–1784.
22. Fiorica F, Di Bona D, Schepis F, et al. Preoperative chemoradiotherapy for oesophageal cancer: a systematic review and meta-analysis. *Gut.* 2004;53:925–930.
23. Urschel JD, Vasan H. A meta-analysis of randomized controlled trials that compared neoadjuvant chemoradiation and surgery to surgery alone for resectable esophageal cancer. *Am J Surg.* 2003;185:538–543.
24. Gebski V, Burmeister B, Smithers BM, et al. Survival benefits from neoadjuvant chemoradiotherapy or chemotherapy in oesophageal carcinoma: a meta-analysis. *Lancet Oncol.* 2007;8:226–234.
25. Kunath U, Fischer P. Radical nature and life expectancy in the surgical treatment of esophageal and cardial carcinoma [in German]. *Dtsch Med Wochenschr.* 1984;109:450–453.
26. Teniere P, Hay JM, Fingerhut A, et al. Postoperative radiation therapy does not increase survival after curative resection for squamous cell carcinoma of the middle and lower esophagus as shown by a multicenter controlled trial. French University Association for Surgical Research. *Surg Gynecol Obstet.* 1991;173:123–130.
27. Fok M, Sham JS, Choy D, et al. Postoperative radiotherapy for carcinoma of the esophagus: a prospective, randomized controlled study. *Surgery.* 1993;113:138–147.
28. Zieren HU, Muller JM, Jacobi CA, et al. Adjuvant postoperative radiation therapy after curative resection of squamous cell carcinoma of the thoracic esophagus: a prospective randomized study. *World J Surg.* 1995;19:444–449.
29. Xiao ZF, Yang ZY, Liang J, et al. Value of radiotherapy after radical surgery for esophageal carcinoma: a report of 495 patients. *Ann Thorac Surg.* 2003;75:331–336.
30. Xiao ZF, Yang ZY, Miao YJ, et al. Influence of number of metastatic lymph nodes on survival of curative resected thoracic esophageal cancer patients and value of radiotherapy: report of 549 cases. *Int J Radiat Oncol Biol Phys.* 2005;62:82–90.
31. Japanese Esophageal Oncology Group. A comparison of chemotherapy and radiotherapy as adjuvant treatment to surgery for esophageal carcinoma. *Chest.* 1993;104:203–207.
32. Macdonald JS, Smalley SR, Benedetti J, et al. Chemoradiotherapy after surgery compared with surgery alone for adenocarcinoma of the stomach or gastroesophageal junction. *N Engl J Med.* 2001;345:725–730.
33. Bedard EL, Inculet RI, Malthaner RA, et al. The role of surgery and postoperative chemoradiation therapy in patients with lymph node positive esophageal carcinoma. *Cancer.* 2001;91:2423–2430.
34. Rice TW, Adelstein DJ, Chidel MA, et al. Benefit of postoperative adjuvant chemoradiotherapy in locoregionally advanced esophageal carcinoma. *J Thorac Cardiovasc Surg.* 2003;126:1590–1596.
35. Liu HC, Hung SK, Huang CJ, et al. Esophagectomy for locally advanced esophageal cancer, followed by chemoradiotherapy and adjuvant chemotherapy. *World J Gastroenterol.* 2005;11:5367–5372.

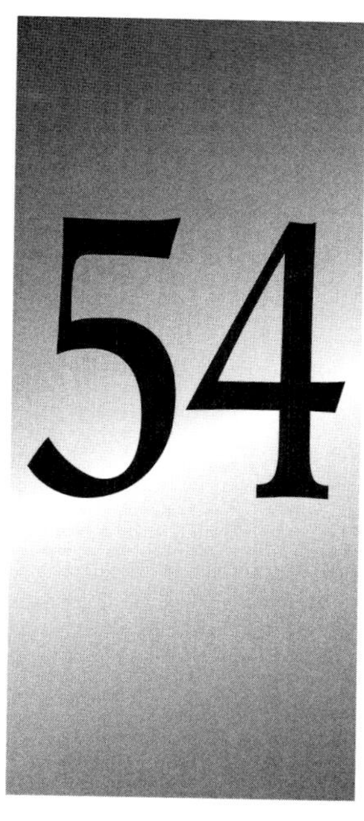

Neoadjuvant Therapy

Daniel J. Boffa
Frank C. Detterbeck

This chapter is focused on neoadjuvant therapy for esophageal cancer, sometimes also referred to as induction therapy. This is defined as preoperative therapy with intent to cure. Neoadjuvant therapy can consist of radiotherapy alone (RT), chemotherapy alone (CT), or chemoradiotherapy (CRT). Some of the more recent neoadjuvant treatment strategies also administered adjuvant (or postoperative) chemo- or radiotherapy. These are included in this chapter with part of a neoadjuvant treatment plan, but adjuvant therapy given without an induction component is discussed in Chapter 62.

This chapter focuses on randomized clinical trials that have compared a form of neoadjuvant therapy to surgery alone. We have carried out a careful literature search for randomized clinical trials in esophageal cancer that involved surgery and neoadjuvant or induction therapy. We have also used the reference lists of randomized trials and meta-analyses to search for articles. We have included all trials that have been fully published in English, omitting trials published only in abstract form. In addition, we have included meta-analyses of such randomized trials.

This review of randomized trials spans more than 3 decades (1970 to 2002) and includes publications through the end of 2007. During this time many changes have occurred in the care of esophageal cancer patients. For example, surgical technique and patient care have contributed to operative mortalities declining from 20% in the earliest trials to less than 5% in the most recent trials. In most of the studies, staging was typically limited to history, endoscopy, barium swallow, chest radiograph (CXR), and blood testing. Chemotherapy regimens and the ability to minimize toxicity have changed. There have also been major advances in the technology of radiotherapy, resulting in much more accurate targeting and less toxicity to nearby normal tissues. Therefore, attempts to make comparisons between treatment strategies as well as individual trials must be mindful of the era in which the patients were cared for.

It is quite possible that inaccurate staging allowed patients with undetected distant metastases to be included into the randomized trials; however, the process of randomization should balance any staging inaccuracies between the treatment arms.

PATIENT POPULATION OF PHASE III STUDIES

Patient Characteristics

The patients included in randomized studies of neoadjuvant therapy for esophageal cancer over the past 3 decades have been predominantly men, with a mean age of 63, and good to excellent performance status (PS). Approximately two-thirds of the patients were PS 0 several studies (1,2), while the majority of patients were PS 1 in others (3,4). This is fairly representative of patients in general with esophageal cancer (Table 54.1). In fact, a review of U.S. National Cancer Database (NCDB) of 5,044 esophageal cancer patients in 1994 disclosed a 3:1 ratio of men to women and a mean age of 67 years (5). That being said, the randomized studies do include some data from patients outside of this narrow description. For example, the oldest randomized patients ranged from 65 to 84 years of age (median 74). With respect to performance status, 3% of the patients in one of the largest neoadjuvant studies (n = 802) were a performance status of 2 or more (1).

The extent of weight loss was infrequently specified for the randomized patients. Several studies excluded patients who had lost more than 15% of their total body weight prior to being evaluated (2,6,7). At the other end of the spectrum, the neoadjuvant studies reported by Kelsen et al. and Lee et al. stand out as including particularly large fractions of patients with a substantial weight loss (23% and 17%, respectively of patients with a loss of > 10% of their total body mass prior to randomization) (8,4).

Tumor Characteristics

Squamous cell carcinoma (SCC) has been the most widely studied esophageal tumor, reflecting the predominance of this histology worldwide. Thirteen of the 20 randomized studies reviewed in this chapter contained exclusively SCC, and 1 included only adenocarcinoma (Table 54.1). Among the 6 remaining trials, SCC made up a median of 37% of the patients (range 25% to 45%). That being said, adenocarcinoma has been becoming much more common, especially in the United States and western Europe (1,5,8). More recent trials conducted in these regions have reflected the inclusion of many patients with adenocarcinoma (1,8).

All studies excluded patients with systemic metastases, which in the present era translates to more than a third of all patients with esophageal cancer (9). The trials that required CT scanning offer the best estimate of preoperative stage. In general the trials included relatively few stage I patients (range 0%–18%) (2,4,10,11), which is similar to the fraction of stage I patients in the 1994 NCDB review (14%) (5). On the other hand, the randomized studies varied substantially in the prevalence of clinically detected lymph node metastases: Burmeister, 16% (3); Ancona, 33% (10); Baba, 38% (12); Urba, 42% (13); Lee, 65% (4). The NCDB reports the prevalence of clinically detected lymph nodes at that time to be between 23% and 45% (clinical stage II and III, as stage II was not separated into IIA and IIB) (5).

Tumor Staging

The patients included in the randomized studies were relatively poorly staged by modern standards. Esophageal ultrasound (EUS) was used in only a minority of studies (Table 54.1), and PET was not used in any of them. In fact, not even a CT scan was required in 9 out of the 20 studies. This fact must be kept in mind when interpreting the data regarding resectability and survival. Indeed, it appears that there was a slightly higher 2-year survival in those trials that required CT scanning vs. those in which it was optional (38% vs. 29%), but a more detailed analysis would be required to establish this definitively.

Nevertheless, the staging performed in the randomized trials is not that different from what was routine at the time. The 1994 NCDB study reported that a CT scan was included in the work-up in 64% of the patients (5). Furthermore, the effect of modern staging tests may be less than one might intuitively guess. For example, only 5% of patients deemed resectable had unsuspected distant metastases detected by PET scan in the American College of Surgeons Oncology Group (ACOSOG) Z0060 trial (14).

TOXICITY AND TREATMENT-RELATED MORTALITY

Neoadjuvant Therapy

Mortality due to neoadjuvant therapy has generally been quite low. As seen in Table 54.2, mortality during neoadjuvant RT has been extremely rare. Mortality during neoadjuvant CT or CRT has also been low in most studies (range 0%–6%). The 2 outliers are the relatively small studies by Maipang et al. and Schlag et al., with a mortality of 17% and 9% (11,15). It is not clear why such high rates were seen in these studies. The regimens used were not markedly different, nor is there evidence that the patients were appreciably more ill on study entry.

Toxicity due to neoadjuvant therapy has also been acceptable. There is almost no toxicity from the relatively low doses of RT that have been used in neoadjuvant RT studies. The rate of grade 3 or 4 toxicity in CT or CRT studies has varied significantly but is generally around 25%. The variation in reported rates appears to be due to variation in how toxicity was reported rather than details of the treatment. In most studies, the compliance with neoadjuvant treatment has been good at around 80% to 90%. The notable exceptions are the studies by Maipang et al., Kelsen et al. and Urba et al. (11,8,13). No consistent reason is apparent why compliance was poor in these studies. The study by Kelsen et al. was one of the few that involved a third cycle of neoadjuvant CT (8).

TABLE 54.1
Patient Population Included in Phase III Studies

Study name	N elig	Accrual years	% Sq hist	Treatment			Mean age	Men (%)	Elig PS	>10% wt loss (%)	Preop stage (%)			Staging tests	
				Chemo	Sequence	RT (Gy)					T3	N1	M1a	CT	EUS
Launois (57)	124	73–76	100			RT (40)	—	—	—	—	—	—	—	No	No
Gignoux (6)	208	76–82	100			RT (33)	—	—	—	—	4	Y	0	optional	No
Wang (34)	206	77–85	—			RT (40)	53	71	—	—	—	—	—	No	No
Arnott (58)	176	79–83	32			RT (20)	63	64	—	—	—	—	—	No	No
Nygaard (16)	108	83–88	100			RT (35)	63[a]	61	0–2	—	0	Y	Y	Yes	No
Roth (59)	39	82–86	95	BVP × 2			—	—	—	39	—	—	—	Yes	No
Nygaard (16)	109	83–88	100	BP × 2			63[a]	61	0–2	—	0	Y	Y	Yes	No
Maipang (11)	46	88–90	100	BPV × 2			65	87	0–2	—			Y	Yes	No
Schlag (15)	46	?	100	PF × 3			57	91	0,1	—	Y	Y	Y	Yes	No
Law (60)	147	89–95	100	PF × 2			64	85	—	—	—	Y	0	few	few
Baba (12)	42	93–95	100	PF × 2			62	93	0,1	—	26	38	Y	Yes	Yes
Kelsen (8)	440	90–95	45	PF × 3			62[a]	79	—	23	Y	Y	0	Yes	optional
Ancona (10)	94	92–97	100	PF × 2–3			58	81	—	—	Y	35	0	Yes	optional
MRC (1)	802	92–98	31	PF × 2			63[a]	76	0–4	—	Y	Y	Y	optional	No
Nygaard (16)	103	83–88	100	BP ×2	Seq	RT (35)	63[a]	61	0–2	—	0	Y	Y	Yes	No
Le Prise (7)	86	88–91	100	PF × 2	conc	RT (20)	58[a]	93	0,1	—	Y	Y	0	optional	No
Apinop (17)	69	86–92	100	PF × 2	conc	RT (20)	60	78	0,1	—			Y	optional	No

(Continued)

TABLE 54.1

Patient Population Included in Phase III Studies (Continued)

Study name	N elig	Accrual years	% Sq hist	Treatment			Mean age	Men (%)	Elig PS	>10% wt loss (%)	Preop stage (%)			Staging tests	
				Chemo	Sequence	RT (Gy)					T3	N1	M1a	CT	EUS
Urba (13)	100	89–94	25	PFV × 2	conc	RT (45)	63	85	0–2	—	Y	42	Y	Yes	No
Walsh (42)	113	90–95	0	PF × 2	conc	RT (40)	65[a]	74	0–2	—	Y	Y	Y	Few	No
Bosset (2)	282	89–95	100	P × 2	conc	RT[b] (37)	57	93	0–2	—	27	23	0	Yes	No
Burmeister (3)	256	94–00	37	PF × 1	conc	RT (35)	61[a]	81	0,1	—	Y	16	0	Yes	Few
Lee (4)	101	99–02	100	PF	conc	RT[c] (45)	63[a]	92	0,1	17	Y	65	0	Yes	Yes

[a] median age [b] Split course RT [c] hyperfractionated RT (twice daily)

Abbreviations: B = bleomycin; chemo = chemotherapy; CT = Computed Tomography scan; conc = concurrent; elig = eligible; EUS = Esophageal Ultrasound; F = 5-fluorouracil; Gy = Gray; P = cisplatin; Preop = preoperative; PS = Performance Status (World Health Organization scale); RT = radiotherapy; seq = sequential; Sq hist = squamous histologic type; wt = weight; V = vinblastine; Y = Yes (included, percent not specified); ? = data not provided.

Chemotherapy regimens:

Roth: 2 cycles (Bleomycin 40 U/m², Vindesine 3 mg/m²d 1,8,15,22, Cisplatin 120 mg/m²)

Nygaard: 2 cycles (Cisplatin 100 mg/m² + Bleomycin 50 mg/m²)

Maipang: 2 cycles (cisplatin 100 mg/m² + bleomycin 50 mg/m² + vinblastine 12 mg/m²)

Schlag: 3 cycles (Cisplatin 20 mg/m²/day + Fluorouracil 1000 mg/m²/day × 5 days)

Law: 2 cycles (cisplatin 100 mg/m² + Fluorouracil 500 mg/m²/day × 5 days)

Baba: 2 cycles (Cisplatin 70 mg/m² + Fluorouracil 700 mg/m²/day × 5 days)

Kelsen: 3 cycles (cisplatin 100 mg/m² + Fluorouracil 1000 mg/m²/day × 5 days)

Ancona: 2 cycles (cisplatin 100 mg/m² + Fluorouracil 500 mg/m²/day × 5 days) 3rd cycle given if response to 1st two

MRC: 2 cycles (cisplatin 80 mg/m² + Fluorouracil 1000 mg/m²/day × 4 days)

Nygaard: 2 cycles (Cisplatin 100 mg/m² + Bleomycin 50 mg/m²); RT (35 Gy) sequential

La Prise: 2 cycles Cisplatin 100 mg/m² + Fluorouracil 600 mg/m²/d × 4 days; RT (20 Gy) sequential, sandwiched on alternate weeks between chemotherapy

Apinop: 2 cycles (cisplatin 100 mg/m² + Fluorouracil 1000 mg/m²/day × 4 days)

Urba: 2 cycles Cisplatin 20 mg/m²/day × 5 days—Fluorouracil 300 mg/m²/day × 21 days—2 cycles Vinblastine 1 mg/m²/d × 4 days; concurrent RT (45 Gy)

Walsh: 2 cycles (Cisplatin75 mg/m² + Fluorouracil 15 mg/kg/day × 5 days); concurrent RT (40 Gy)

Bosset: 2 cycles (Cisplatin 80 mg/m²) × RT (37Gy) concurrent, RT split by 2 week break

Burmeister: 1 cycle (Cisplatin 80 mg/m² + Fluorouracil 800 mg/m² × 4 days); concurrent RT (35 Gy)

Lee: 1 cycle (Cisplatin 120 mg/m² fluorouracil 1000 mg/m²/d × 4 days); concurrent RT (45.6 Gy)

TABLE 54.2

Safety of Neoadjuvant Therapy

Study name	N elig	Accrual years	Treatment: Chemo	Treatment: Sequence	Treatment: RT(Gy)	% Neo compli[a]	Gr 3,4 tox %[a]	% Neo mort[a]	Interval (days)	% S attemptd[a] Neo	% S attemptd[a] S	% S Mort[b] Neo	% S Mort[b] S	% S Morb[b] Neo	% S Morb[b] S
Launois (57)	124	73–76			RT (40)	100	1	0	8	93	84	23	23	—	—
Gignoux (6)	208	76–82			RT (33)	—	2	1	5	95	100	25	18	—	—
Arnott (58)	176	79–83			RT (20)	—	0	0	—	93	94	12	10	13	10
Wang (34)	206	77–85			RT (40)	100	—	0	14–28	100	100	(5)[c]	(6)[c]	(1)[d]	(6)[d]
Nygaard (16)	108	83–88			RT (35)	100	—	—	21	75	93	11	13	33	34
Average[e]	**822**					**100**	**0.5**	**0.2**		**91**	**94**	**18**	**16**	**23**	**22**
Roth (59)	39	82–86	BVP × 2			—	—	0	—	—	—	10	0	29	47
Nygaard (16)	109	83–88	BP × 2			95	—	—	21	82	93	15	13	34	34
Maipang (11)	46	88–90	BPV × 2			63	46	17	14	—	100	—	0	—	—
Schlag (15)	46	?	PF × 3			—	—	9	14–24	91	100	—	—	—	—
Law (60)	147	89–95	PF × 2			84	11	0	—	91	100	8	8	(≥30)[f]	(≥32)[f]
Baba (12)	42	93–95	PF × 2			95	24[g]	0	35	100	100	5	0	(≥43)[f]	(≥29)[f]
Kelsen (8)	440	90–95	PF × 3			73	(≥29)[f]	6	14–28	80	96	6	6	31	26
Ancona (10)	94	92–97	PF × 2–3			68	21	2	21–28	85	100	3	5	37	39
MRC (1)	802	92–98	PF × 2			88	—	3	21–35	90	96	10	10	40	42
Average[e]	**1719**					**81**	**26**	**4**		**88**	**98**	**8**	**5**	**34**	**31**
Nygaard (16)	103	83–88	BP × 2	seq	RT (35)	90	—	—	21	72	93	24	13	47	34
Le Prise (7)	86	88–91	PF × 2	seq	RT (20)	—	—	0	17	85	93	9	7	40	43
Apinop (17)	69	86–92	PF × 2	conc	RT (20)	—	—	6	28	74	100	19	15	27	15
Urba (13)	100	89–94	PFV × 2	conc	RT (45)	61	(≥78)	0	21	94	100	2	4	14	10
Walsh (42)	113	90–95	PF × 2	conc	RT (40)	—	14	—	14	88	100	9	4	28	32
Bosset (2)	282	89–95	P × 2	conc	RT[h] (37)	96	—	1	21	97	99	12	4	33	26
Burmeister (3)	256	94–00	PF × 1	conc	RT (35)	82	(≥16)	2	21–42	92	86	4	6	53	64
Lee (4)	101	99–02	PF	conc	RT[i] (45)	96	—	0	21–36	69	96	3	2	—	—
Average	**1110**					**85**	**—**	**2**		**84**	**96**	**10**	**7**	**35**	**32**

[a] % of all patients randomized per arm [b] % of attempted resections [c] % of resected patients [d] Anastomotic leak [e] Excluding values in parentheses [f] Only partial list of morbidity reported [g] Includes grade 2 and 3 hematologic toxicity [h] Split course RT [i] hyperfractionated RT (twice daily)

Abbreviations: B = bleomycin; chemo = chemotherapy; compli = compliance (% of planned dose given); conc = concurrent; elig = eligible; F = 5-fluorouracil; Gr 3,4 Tox = Grade 3 or 4 Toxicity; Gy = Gray; morb = morbidity; mort = mortality; Neo = neoadjuvant arm; P = cisplatin; RT = radiotherapy; S = Surgery only arm; seq = sequential; V = vinblastine; ? = data not provided.

Another measure of the toxicity of the neoadjuvant treatment is in how often a surgical resection is attempted. This is also shown in Table 54.2. In trials involving neoadjuvant RT, the rate of attempted resection is high, with little difference between the neoadjuvant and the primary surgical resection arm. The notable exception to this is the study by Nygaard et al. (16), which seems to show low rates of surgery no matter what type of neoadjuvant treatment was used. In studies involving either neoadjuvant CT or CRT, approximately 10% fewer patients underwent attempted resection after neoadjuvant therapy. This difference is clearly a trade-off that must be taken into account when assessing the value of neoadjuvant therapy. Studies with particularly low rates of attempted resection include the smaller studies of Apinop and Lee (4,17) but also large multicenter studies, such as by Kelsen et al. (8). There is no correlation between neoadjuvant toxicity, mortality or rate of attempted resection with patient, tumor, or treatment characteristics (i.e., poor PS, stage, or a more intense treatment regimen).

Surgical Resection

Neoadjuvant therapy does not significantly impact the risk of complication and death following esophagectomy. In Table 54.2, it can be seen that there is little difference in these rates between the neoadjuvant and the control arms, although there is a suggestion of a 2% to 3% increase in mortality with neoadjuvant therapy. In contrast to the minimal toxicity and mortality of neoadjuvant RT by itself, the surgical mortality in these studies was quite high. This is undoubtedly because these are the oldest studies. A clear trend can be seen toward progressively lower surgical mortality rates in more recent studies, and the mortality in the more recent neoadjuvant CT and CRT studies is acceptable. The observed mortality rates in the neoadjuvant studies are very similar to what has been published in other series of esophagectomy in contemporary studies.

It is also clear that surgical morbidity rates are similar between neoadjuvant and control arms. Only a few studies reported any appreciable difference between the study cohorts. A large amount of variability is seen between studies in morbidity rates, which is primarily related to differences in which complications were assessed and how the complications were defined. No differences were detected when investigators examined specific complications such as anastomotic leaks, infection, respiratory and cardiac complications (18–20).

MEASURES OF TREATMENT EFFECT

Clinical or Radiographic Response

Response to induction therapy has been shown to correlate with improved survival in several studies (10,21,22). However, radiographic assessment of response in esophageal cancer has not been standardized. Simple measurement of tumor diameter and length has not typically been used, and not all studies have even employed CT scanning routinely. Radiographic response to neoadjuvant therapy was typically assessed by barium swallow in most studies. Approximately 40% to 50% of patients have had a response to either neoadjuvant CT or CRT (Table 54.3). One of the most recent studies, by Lee et al., used EUS before and after induction CRT and found a clinical response rate of 86% (4).

The ability of restaging tests to detect the presence of viable tumor is poor. The accuracy of noninvasive restaging following induction therapy for esophageal cancer is suboptimal (EUS, 60%; CT scan, 62%; PET, 75%) (23–26). The false negative rate for each of these tests is approximately 50%, and this is true for repeat endoscopy as well (25–28). More recently, the change in maximum SUV from pretreatment to posttreatment PET scans has been suggested to offer additional value in assessing response (29).

Improvement in Dysphagia

The randomized trials did not consistently examine dysphagia during neoadjuvant therapy. However, other retrospective studies have found that the majority of patients experienced an improvement in dysphagia and were either stable or gained weight during neoadjuvant therapy (25,30,31). Therefore, routine placement of a feeding tube should not be done, and this intervention should be reserved for patients with refractory dysphagia and progressive malnutrition. However, there is controversy about where the threshold should be. For example, in one of the randomized studies, 63% of neoadjuvant patients received a feeding tube prior to attempted resection (13). It is interesting to note that this study reported one of the lowest operative mortalities (3% for all patients). This study came from one of the most experienced esophageal surgical centers in the United States, and it is unclear whether the operative mortality can be attributed to placement of a feeding tube.

Should the clinician deem a feeding tube necessary, it has been shown that initial placement of a gastrostomy tube does not complicate the subsequent use of the stomach for reconstruction after esophagectomy (32).

TABLE 54.3

Response to Neoadjuvant Therapy

Study name	N elig	Accrual years	Treatment Chemo	Treatment Sequence	Treatment RT(Gy)	Clinical resp[a] %	% pCR[b]	% pN1[c] Neo	% pN1[c] S	% pM1a[c] Neo	% pM1a[c] S	% R_0^a Neo	% R_0^a S	% Unresect[a] Neo	% Unresect[a] S
Launois (57)	124	73–76			RT (40)	—	0	—	—	—	—	76	70	—	—
Gignoux (6)	208	76–82			RT (33)	—	2	56	58	—	—	47	58	22	18
Arnott (58)	176	79–83			RT (20)	—	0	44	40	—	—	69[d]	81[d]	18	23
Wang (34)	206	77–85			RT (40)	—	23	27	35	—	—	—	—	—	—
Nygaard (16)	108	83–88			RT (35)	—	—	—	—	—	—	40	37	25	24
Average						**—**	**6**	**42**	**44**			**58**	**62**	**22**	**22**
Roth (59)	39	82–86	BVP × 2			—	6	—	—	—	—	35	21	—	—
Nygaard (16)	109	83–88	BP × 2			—	—	—	—	—	—	44	37	24	24
Maipang (11)	46	88–90	BPV × 2			25	0	—	—	—	—	—	—	—	—
Schlag (15)	46	?	PF × 3			42	5	—	—	—	—	32	42	27	21
Law (60)	147	89–95	PF × 2			42	6	70	88	—	—	67	33	1	5
Baba (12)	42	93–95	PF × 2			60	0	62	57	19	29	81	86	—	—
Kelsen (8)	440	90–95	PF × 3			19	3	—	—	—	—	62	59	24	11
Ancona (10)	94	92–97	PF × 2–3			—	15	—	—	—	—	79	74	0	13
MRC (1)	802	92–98	PF × 2			—	4	58	65	23	25	58	53	8	16
Average						**37**	**5**	**63**	**70**			**60**	**52**	**18**	**17**
Nygaard (16)	103	83–88	BP × 2	seq	RT (35)	—	—	—	—	—	—	55	37	6	24
Le Prise (7)	86	88–91	PF × 2	conc	RT (20)	29	11	28	38	0[e]	10[e]	85	84	0	10
Apinop (17)	69	86–92	PF × 2	conc	RT (20)	54[c]	—	—	—	—	—	—	—	—	—
Urba (13)	100	89–94	PFV × 2	conc	RT (45)	—	30	—	—	—	—	88	88	6	0
Walsh (42)	113	90–95	PF × 2	conc	RT (40)	—	25	41	75	—	—	—	—	—	—
Bosset (2)	282	89–95	P × 2	conc	RT[f] (37)	—	23	38	55	38[g]	41[g]	78[h]	68[h]	—	—
Burmeister (3)	256	94–00	PF × 1	conc	RT (35)	29[i]	16	43	67	—	—	80	59	5	10
Lee (4)	101	99–02	PF	conc	RT[j] (45)	86	43	37	78	6	2	69	84	0	4
Average						**50**	**25**	**37**	**63**	**15**	**18**	**76**	**70**	**3**	**10**

[a] % of the total number randomized to the respective arm; [b] % of attempted resections; [c] % of resected patients; [d] upper and lower margins clear of tumor; [e] Includes both celiac node involvement and mediastinal involvement; [f] Split course RT; [g] the number of patients with celiac lymph nodes that could be evaluated were 115 in CRS and 117 in S; [h] Free of all macroscopic disease; [i] only 73 patients were reevaluated for clinical response; [j] hyperfractionated RT (twice daily)

Abbreviations: B = bleomycin; chemo = chemotherapy; conc = concurrent; elig = eligible; F = 5-fluorouracil; Gy = Gray; Neo = neoadjuvant arm; P = cisplatin; pCR = pathologic Complete Response (No viable tumor cells present); resp = response; R_0 = complete resection (no macro or microscopic residual disease); RT = radiotherapy; S = Surgery only arm; seq = sequential; Unresect = unresectable tumors (due to local extent of disease); V = vinblastine; ? = data not provided.

Tumor Downstaging by Neoadjuvant Therapy

The ability to determine downstaging by neoadjuvant therapy requires the accurate assessment of stage before and after treatment. This is not possible in the majority of trials, especially given the limited staging tests that were employed. An indirect way of assessing downstaging is to compare the pathologic stage between induction and control arms. The lymph node status is the factor most consistently reported among the trials, and there are data suggesting that downstaging of the lymph node status with neoadjuvant therapy provides a survival advantage (21). Table 54.3 suggests that there is a lower prevalence of lymph metastases in the neoadjuvant patients (46%) compared to control patients (60%). This effect is more dramatic among the neoadjuvant CRT trials (37% vs. 63% with pN1 in the neoadjuvant vs. control arms). There appears to be little effect of RT on downstaging (42% vs. 44% pN1), and a more limited effect of neoadjuvant CT (63% vs. 70% pN1).

Rate of Pathologic Complete Response

Pathologic complete response (pCR), defined as the absence of any residual tumor within the resected specimen, provides the most definitive evidence of response to induction therapy. As one might expect, patients with a pCR have markedly increased survival compared to patients with an incomplete or no response (10,13,22,33). However, a pCR does not guarantee a cure. The rate of pCR probably also depends on the extent and diligence with which the pathologist examines the resected tissue. The median survival of patients with a pathologic complete response following neoadjuvant therapy and esophagectomy is about 50 months and the 5-year survival is approximately 40% to 50% (13,22,33).

Complete response rates have ranged from 0% to 43% in the randomized neoadjuvant therapy trials (Table 54.3). At the low end of the spectrum are the induction RT trials, but the interval between RT and resection was generally short (< 10 days) and probably insufficient to assess the impact of RT. The one neoadjuvant RT study which extended the interval between the last dose of RT and surgery to 14 to 28 days reported a pCR rate of 23% (34). Neoadjuvant CT alone also resulted in a low pCR rate (average 5%). Neoadjuvant CRT led to the highest pCR rates (average 25%).

Interestingly, one study reports the pattern of failure to be similar between patients who had a pCR and those who did not (locoregional failure in 12% and 8% respectively) (22). Therefore, pCR should be viewed as a marker of sensitivity to neoadjuvant therapy that is generally associated with better prognosis, and not as a literal indicator of whether viable tumor cells are or are not present.

Resectability

The ability to achieve a complete (R_0) resection (removal of all gross and microscopic cancer with clear margins) is a measure of the activity of neoadjuvant therapy that is related to downstaging and the pCR rate. Long-term survival is more likely following a R_0 resection than resections in which disease is left behind ($R_{1,2}$) (4,35,36). In Table 54.3, the R_0 resection rate is shown, expressed as a percentage of all patients randomized (in order to avoid confounding by the proportion of patients excluded from surgery). Neoadjuvant RT results in a slight decrease (~5%) in the rate of R_0 resection, whereas neoadjuvant CT or CRT appears to slightly improve (6%–8%) the ability to achieve a complete resection.

A recent meta-analysis of neoadjuvant CT found no evidence of a higher rate of complete resection (relative risk 0.95, 95% CI 0.87–1.03; $P = 0.2$) (20). An earlier meta-analysis that included some of the same studies found a higher R_0 resection rate (odds ratio 0.53, 95% CI 0.33–84; $P = 0.007$) (19). Recent meta-analyses examining this issue in neoadjuvant RT or CRT have not been done.

One of the hopes for neoadjuvant therapy would be to convert large locally advanced tumors into tumors amenable to resection. However, the proportion of unresectable tumors is similar whether neoadjuvant therapy was given (16%) or not (14%) (Table 54.3). A more detailed view suggests that there is little difference in the rate of exploratory thoracotomy among studies of neoadjuvant RT or neoadjuvant CT but is fairly consistently lower with neoadjuvant CRT. In general, the rate of exploratory thoracotomy seems to be related to the proportion of patients in whom surgery was attempted. Among series in whom patients appear to have been chosen more selectively for attempted surgery, the rate of exploratory thoracotomy is lower and vice versa.

A recent meta-analysis of neoadjuvant CT found no evidence of a difference in the rate of resection (relative risk 1.05, 95% CI 0.94–1.18; $P = 0.3$) (20). There was evidence of substantial heterogeneity between trials, possibly implying differences in the willingness of surgeons in different centers to undertake resection. Recent meta-analyses examining the effect of neoadjuvant RT or CRT on the resection rates (R_{0-2}) have not been done.

LONG-TERM SURVIVAL

General Aspects

Several factors make it difficult to define the efficacy of neoadjuvant therapy for esophageal cancer. First of all, esophageal cancer is relatively uncommon and often unresectable at the time of diagnosis. As a result, the published experience of randomized trials of neoadjuvant therapy over the past 30 years includes fewer than 4,000 patients in studies averaging fewer than 200 patients. Second, the survival advantage gained with neoadjuvant therapy appears to be modest, which, in combination with a small sample size, renders survival a challenging endpoint to evaluate. Furthermore, smaller studies are more susceptible to imbalances of prognostic factors between treatment arms, such as the stage. This is a particular issue because determination of the extent of esophageal cancer prior to resection is difficult, and because the majority of studies involved very limited preoperative imaging (Table 54.1). For these reasons it is necessary to examine the body of studies together, to observe the trends that offer guidance where statistics have failed to reach significance.

Neoadjuvant RT and Surgery vs. Surgery Alone

No significant survival differences were seen in any of the studies between RT and surgery versus surgery alone. Three trials suggested a non-significant trend toward a survival advantage with induction RT in short-term survival, but no trend is apparent in long-term survival (Table 54.4). Local control was only reported by 2 of the trials. Gignoux et al. reported significantly fewer local recurrences with neoadjuvant RT in a fairly large trial (35% vs. 54%, P = .05) (6). Furthermore, the duration of survival without local recurrence was significantly longer in the neoadjuvant RT arm (P = .045) (6). No suggestion of a difference in local control was seen in the other trial (34), which also involved a fairly large cohort.

A meta-analysis using updated individual patient data from all of the randomized clinical trials of neoadjuvant RT for esophageal cancer was reported in a Cochrane Review in 2005 (1,147 patients, 5 trials) (37). A hazard ratio of 0.89 was found, which did not quite meet statistical significance (95% Confidence interval [CI] 0.78–1.01, P = 0.06). This represents an 11% reduction in the risk of death, with an absolute survival benefit of 4% at 2 years. However, because of the lack of statistical significance, the benefit of neoadjuvant RT was deemed inconclusive (37).

It is important to note that induction RT was among the first neoadjuvant esophageal cancer strategies to be studied in a randomized fashion, with most patients being accrued between 1973 and 1988. Because the majority of this work predated substantial advances in staging and patient care, the early RT trials contained some of the least accurately staged patients, the lowest resection rates, and the highest operative mortalities. These facts may have limited the ability to demonstrate a significant difference in survival. In addition, the trials of neoadjuvant RT in esophageal cancer were conducted before many of the advances in the delivery of RT, which have improved efficacy and decreased toxicity in many tumors. It is possible that a survival benefit from cancer was offset by an increase in deaths due to late toxicity. It is perhaps notable that the most recent trial (conducted 1983–1985) showed a clear trend toward better survival, although statistical significance was not reached in this small trial. This was the only RT trial that required a CT scan and had one of the lower perioperative mortalities among neoadjuvant RT studies.

One would speculate that the addition of a second local modality would be most likely to affect local control and that this endpoint might be better suited to determine the value of RT; the data, however, conflict and are certainly not convincing of a benefit to RT. In addition, the applicability of these older results to patients seen today can be questioned. However, the possible modest benefit of neoadjuvant RT seems less exciting than other treatment modalities, and there is currently not much interest in examining this approach further.

Neoadjuvant Chemotherapy and Surgery vs. Surgery Alone

Review of Phase III Trial Results

Neoadjuvant CT has been evaluated in 9 randomized trials that are summarized in Table 54.4. Three of the trials found a non-significant trend to better survival, while 3 found a non-significant trend to worse survival and 3 found no difference. A statistically significant survival advantage was only found by the study from the Medical Research Council (MRC) (1). The MRC was by far the largest of the neoadjuvant trials (n = 802) and reported that induction CT led to an increased 5-year survival compared to surgery alone (24% vs. 14%; P = 0.004). However, the next largest trial did not suggest a similar trend (1,8). These latter 2 trials account for more than two-thirds of the randomized patients. It is not readily apparent why these 2 trials found different results. It has been suggested that toxicity offset any survival benefit in the negative trial by Kelsen et al., because a more intense chemotherapy regimen was used (38). However, it is not clear that the toxicity was higher or that there was a difference in treatment-related mortality in the neoadjuvant arm in the trial by Kelsen et al. (1,8), although the rate of resection was lower in the neoadjuvant arm.

No clear pattern emerges with regard to local control. A slight trend to lower local recurrence appears to be suggested as a result of neoadjuvant CT. However, some studies suggested the opposite trend and the largest study found no trend in either direction. A clear trend is apparent with better survival in either arm of

TABLE 54.4

Efficacy of Neoadjuvant Therapy versus Surgery

Study name	N elig	Accrual years	Treatment			% Local recur[a]			MST (mo)[b]		% Two-Year surv[b]		% Five-Year surv[b]		
			Chemo	Sequence	RT(Gy)	Neo	S	p	Neo	S	Neo	S	Neo	S	P
Launois (57)	124	73–76			RT (40)	—	—	—	10	12	20	33	10	12	NS
Gignoux (6)	208	76–82			RT (33)	35	54	.05	11	11	28	31	11	10	NS
Arnott (58)	176	79–83			RT (20)	—	—	—	8	8	22	28	9	17	NS
Wang (34)	206	77–85			RT (40)	13	14	NS	—	—	—	—	35	30	NS
Nygaard (16)	108	83–88			RT (35)	—	—	—	10	7	25	13	(21)[c]	(9)[c]	NS
Average[d]			**RT**			**24**	**34**		**10**	**10**	**24**	**26**	**16**	**17**	
Roth (59)	39	82–86	BVP × 2			—	—	—	9	9	25	14	(25)[c]	(5)[c]	NS
Nygaard (16)	109	83–88	BP × 2			—	—	—	7	7	6	13	(3)[c]	(9)[c]	NS
Maipang (11)	46	88–90	BPV × 2			—	—	.01[e]	17	17	30	40	(31)[c]	(36)[c]	NS
Schlag (15)	46	?	PF × 3			—	—	—	7	6	—	—	—	—	NS
Law (60)	147	89–95	PF × 2			28	45	—	17	13	44	31	(40)[c]	(13)[c]	NS
Baba (12)	42	93–95	PF × 2			33	28	—	(34)[f]	(41)[f]	(40)[f]	(50)[f]	(40)[f]	(50)[f]	NS
Kelsen (8)	440	90–95	PF × 3			32[g]	31	NS	15	16	35	37	19	20	NS
Ancona (10)	94	92–97	PF × 2–3			33[g]	44	NS	25	24	54	56	34	22	NS
MRC (1)	802	92–98	PF × 2			14	13		17	13	43	34	24	14	.004
Average[d]			**Chemo**			**28**	**32**		**15**	**14**	**34**	**32**	**15**	**19**	
Nygaard (16)	103	83–88	BP × 2	seq	RT(35)	—	—	—	8	7	23	13	(17)[c]	(9)[c]	NS
Le Prise (7)	86	88–91	PF × 2	seq	RT (20)	26	26	NS	10	11	26	32	(19)[c]	(14)[c]	NS
Apinop (17)	69	86–92	PF × 2	conc	RT (20)	—	—	—	10	7	30	23	24	10	NS
Urba (13)	100	89–94	PFV × 2	conc	RT (45)	19	42	.02	17	18	40	33	20	10	NS
Walsh (42)	113	90–95	PF× 2	conc	RT (40)	—	—	—	16	11	37	26	(32)[c]	(6)[c]	0.01
Bosset (2)	282	89–95	P× 2	conc	RT[h] (37)	15[i]	25[i]	.01	19	19	41	34	7	9	NS
Burmeister (3)	256	94–00	PF × 1	conc	RT (35)	20	39	—	22	19	47	37	17	13	NS
Lee (4)	101	99–02	PF	conc	RT[j](45)	37	13	NS	28	27	57	55	(49)[c]	(41)[c]	NS
Average[d]			**Chemo/RT**			**23**	**29**		**16**	**15**	**38**	**32**	**17**	**11**	

[a] % of resected patients; [b] % of the total number randomized to the respective arm; [c] 3 year survival; [d] Excluding values in parentheses; [e] post op mortality excluded; [f] Disease Free Survival; [g] includes only R_0 resections; [h] Split course RT; [i] estimated from indirect data provided; [j] hyperfractionated RT (twice daily)

Abbreviations: B = bleomycin; chemo = chemotherapy; conc = concurrent; elig = eligible; F = 5-fluorouracil; Gy = Gray; MST (mo) = median survival time (months); Neo = neoadjuvant arm; NS = Not significant (p > 0.5); p = p value (statistical significance); P = cisplatin; recur = recurrence; RT = radiotherapy; S = Surgery only arm; seq = sequential; surv = survival; V = vinblastine; ? = data not provided.

trials that were conducted in more recent time periods. This likely reflects both improvements in staging as well as improvements in patient care.

It is difficult to draw conclusions with respect to details of the regimens and schedules of chemotherapy. While a number of agents have been evaluated, the largest experience by far has been with cisplatin- and fluorouracil-containing regimens. Other regimens have primarily been used in earlier studies. There is no correlation between the regimen, dose, or number of cycles and the absolute value of endpoints; nor is there a difference between the 2 arms with respect to survival, local control, morbidity, or mortality.

Meta-Analyses

The most recent meta-analysis by Gebski et al. (38) (Figure 54.1) found a survival benefit to neoadjuvant CT (long-term mortality hazard ratio of 0.9) that just reached statistical significance (95% CI 0.81–1.00; $P = 0.05$). This effect was heavily influenced by the large MRC study; however, there was no evidence of heterogeneity between the trials of any temporal effect. The survival benefit was most marked for adenocarcinoma, with only a non-significant trend among squamous cancers (Figure 54.2) (38). Earlier meta-analyses that did not include mature data from the MRC trial generally found little suggestion of an improvement in survival with neoadjuvant CT (18,39), while others that included the MRC study have found a trend to improved survival (20,40).

The study by Gebski et al. (38) estimated the number of patients that would need to be treated (NNT) with neoadjuvant CT in order to cure 1 additional

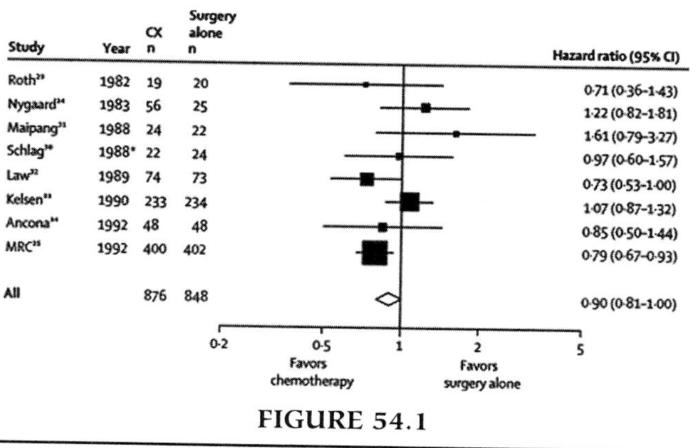

FIGURE 54.1

Meta-analysis of neoadjuvant chemotherapy and surgery versus surgery alone. Figure reproduced from Gebski et al. (38).

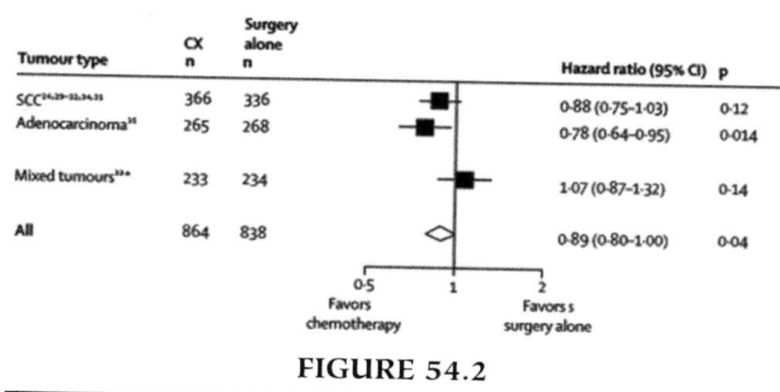

FIGURE 54.2

Meta-analysis of effect of histologic tumor type on results of neoadjuvant chemotherapy and surgery versus surgery alone. Figure reproduced from Gebski et al. (38).

patient. Among patients with a relatively good prognosis (2-year survival of 50%), the NNT was 20 patients, for intermediate-prognosis patients (2-year survival of 35%) the NNT is 15, and for poor-prognosis patients (2-year survival of 20%) an NNT of 8 was estimated (38).

Highlighted Trials of Particular Importance

Kelsen et al. randomized 440 esophageal cancer patients between 1990 and 1995 to induction CT vs. surgery alone (8). A weight loss of ≥ 10% was reported by 23% of the patients in both arms prior to randomization. The total dose of preoperative cisplatin was 50% higher than that of other phase III studies (Table 54.1). This may have contributed to increased toxicity as only 71% of induction patients received the planned regimen and 2% died before surgery. In addition, surgery was not attempted in 20% of the induction patients (compared to only 4% of the surgery-alone patients). The reasons for abstention from surgery were not given.

A clinical response to induction therapy (by barium swallow) was detected in 19% of patients, while a pCR was only found in 2.5%. Patients in the induction arm without evidence of disease progression, who had undergone a curative R_0 resection, were eligible for 2 additional cycles of chemotherapy postoperatively (53% of 126 eligible patients received at least 1 postoperative cycle). No difference in the primary endpoint of overall survival was detected. In fact, when a secondary endpoint of resectability was examined, induction patients were twice as likely to be unresectable (24% vs. 11%). An update of this study published 9 years after the original report likewise failed to demonstrate a survival benefit to induction CT (35). Subset analysis did not show any difference associated with histology.

The MRC Esophageal Working Party coordinated a randomized study involving 42 European centers (1). Between 1992 and 1998, a total of 802 patients were randomized to either preoperative cisplatin and fluorouracil or surgery without induction CT (1). RT was allowed as long as it was given consistently to all patients within a particular institution (9% of the patients in each group were treated). Compliance with chemotherapy was excellent, as 88% of the patients received both scheduled cycles. However, the mortality attributed to this regimen was considerable (3%). That being said, this study represents the largest trial to demonstrate a significant survival benefit associated with induction CT over surgery alone (hazard ratio = 0.79; 95% CI 0.67–0.93, $P = 0.004$) (1).

The most recent support for neoadjuvant CT comes from the Medical Research Council Adjuvant Gastric Infusional Chemotherapy (MAGIC) trial (41). Although the majority of the patients in this study had gastric cancer, 26% of the tumors were esophageal or at the gastroesophageal junction. Perioperative CT (preoperative and postoperative cycles of epirubicin, cisplatin, and fluorouracil) conferred a survival advantage over surgery alone at 5 years (36% vs. 23%; $P = 0.009$).

Neoadjuvant Chemoradiotherapy and Surgery vs. Surgery Alone

Review of Phase III Trial Results

The results of randomized trials involving neoadjuvant CRT are summarized in Table 54.4. A trend to better survival with neoadjuvant CRT was seen in the majority of studies, although the difference was statistically significant only in the study by Walsh et al. (42). On average, neoadjuvant therapy resulted in an improvement in the absolute 2-year and 5-year survival of approximately 6%. The trend is quite consistent and there is no correlation of either the absolute survival results or the difference between arms and either patient characteristics, tumor characteristics or treatment characteristics (i.e., PS, stage, or intensity of chemotherapy). The vast majority of studies have used cisplatin and 5-flouorouracil for the chemotherapy, and RT doses have generally been around 35 to 45 Gy. There is a trend towards better survival in more recent trials. Because many of the neoadjuvant CRT trials have been conducted more recently, these trials involve patients that are staged more accurately preoperatively and have demonstrated some of the lowest operative mortality rates. Local control appears to be better with induction CRT, with 3 trials showing clearly better local control rates (2,3,13). One trial found the opposite trend (4), and 1 trial found no difference (7).

Meta-Analyses

The most recent meta-analysis (38) shows a clear benefit to neoadjuvant CRT vs. surgery alone (Figure 54.3), with a hazard ratio for long-term all-cause mortality of 0.81 (95% CI 0.72–0.92; $P = 0.001$). This result is consistent whether 2 additional studies that have not been formally published are included or omitted. There was no evidence of heterogeneity between trials or any temporal effect. The survival benefit was seen in both squamous carcinoma and adenocarcinoma. The benefit was most clear in concurrent treatment as opposed to sequential treatment strategies (Figure 54.4). Other meta-analyses have shown similar results (18,19,39,40,43), although in several earlier analyses, which did not include some of the more recent trials, only a trend was found that did not reach statistical significance (39,40,43).

The estimated NNT with neoadjuvant CRT in order to cure 1 additional patient is estimated to be relatively low (38). Among patients with a relatively good prognosis (2-year survival of 50%), the NNT is 10 patients; for intermediate-prognosis patients (2-year survival of 35%) the NNT is 8, and for poor-prognosis patients (2-year survival of 20%) an NNT of 7 was estimated (38).

Highlighted Trials of Particular Importance

One of the most controversial neoadjuvant studies was reported by Walsh et al. (42). A total of 113 patients were randomized between 1990 and 1995 to induction therapy (cisplatin + fluorouracil + radiotherapy) followed by surgery vs. surgery alone. The authors describe

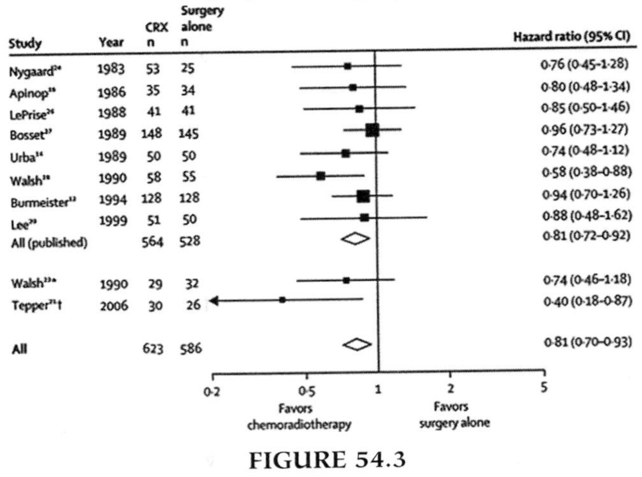

All Cause Mortality of Chemoradiotherapy and Surgery vs. Surgery Alone
Study
Year
CRX n
Surgery alone n
Hazard ratio (95% CI)
Nygaard 1983 53 25 0·76 (0·45–1·28)
Apinop 1986 35 34 0·80 (0·48–1·34)
LePrise 1988 41 41 0·85 (0·50–1·46)
Bosset 1989 148 145 0·96 (0·73–1·27)
Urba 1989 50 50 0·74 (0·48–1·12)
Walsh 1990 58 55 0·58 (0·38–0·88)
Burmeister 1994 128 128 0·94 (0·70–1·26)
Lee 1999 51 50 0·88 (0·48–1·62)
All (published) 564 528 0·81 (0·72–0·92)
Walsh 1990 29 32 0·74 (0·46–1·18)
Tepper 2006 30 26 0·40 (0·18–0·87)
All 623 586 0·81 (0·70–0·93)
0·2
0·5
1
2
5
Favors chemoradiotherapy
Favors surgery alone

FIGURE 54.3

Meta-analysis of neoadjuvant chemoradiotherapy and surgery versus surgery alone. Figure reproduced from Gebski et al. (38).

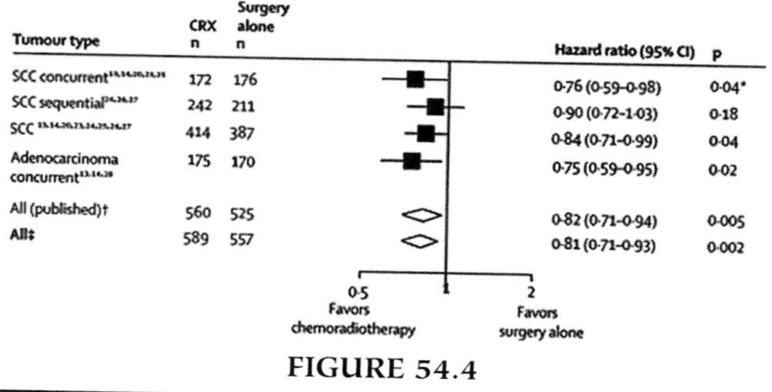

FIGURE 54.4

Meta-analysis of effect of histologic tumor type on results of neoadjuvant chemoradiotherapy and surgery versus surgery alone. Figure reproduced from Gebski et al. (38).

the induction regimen as being well tolerated, although 17% of induction patients were withdrawn from the protocol because of complications or disease progression. Preoperative staging did not routinely include CT scanning and no mention is made of clinical staging in the randomization process. This is particularly relevant to this study as differences in pathologic staging were substantially greater than contemporary protocols. For example, 78% of the patients in the control arm were stage III or IV, compared to only 28% of the induction patients. This disparity is more likely due to preoperative differences in tumor stage than effectiveness of induction therapy, particularly because this level of "down-staging" was not observed in similar induction regimens (7). The median follow-up for this study was short at 10 months, yet the authors found a statistically significant survival advantage with neoadjuvant therapy (median survival 16 vs. 11 months, $P = 0.01$). This study was further criticized by the poor outcome in the surgery-alone group. At 6%, the 3-year survival is approximately 3 times lower than contemporary reports (3,7,13).

Dr. Walsh updated the results of this study in 2002, with a minimum of 5 years' follow-up for each patient (44). A statistically significant survival advantage was again demonstrated among the induction patients (median survival = 17 vs. 12 months, $P = .002$).

Lee et al. reported the results of a single institutional trial that randomized 101 patients between 1999 and 2002 to either induction CRT (cisplatin, fluorouracil, and XRT 45.6 Gy) vs. surgery alone (4). These patients were among the most thoroughly staged preoperatively, as both EUS and CT scanning were performed on all patients. This trial is notable for the majority of patients (65%) having clinically evident nodal metastases, particularly among the induction arm patients (74% vs. 56%, $P = 0.13$). The regimen appeared to be well tolerated, as 96% of the induction patients completed the scheduled therapy. However, only 69% of these patients went on to have surgery, with the most common reason being patient refusal. EUS was used to assess clinical response, and 22% of the induction patients had a complete clinical response. While both T stage and N stage were decreased in the induction group compared to the surgery-alone group, an impressive 43% of the induction patients had a pCR. Patients with stable disease (60% of the induction patients) were given additional chemotherapy after the resection. Despite the most impressive complete response rate among reported randomized trials, the local failure rate following neoadjuvant CRT and surgery was surprisingly high (Table 54.4).

Interim analysis demonstrated no survival difference (median survival 28 vs. 27 months). It is worth pointing out that the patients in the control arm experienced a survival that was superior to contemporary reports (Table 54.4), which may be a reflection of the more accurate staging. The study was terminated over concerns of high drop-out rates among induction patients prior to undergoing surgery.

Most recently the Cancer and Leukemia Group B (CALGB—9781) trial was reported. Although this trial closed early because of poor accrual, 56 patients were randomized to neoadjuvant cisplatin, 5-fluorouracil, and 50.4Gy of radiation or surgery alone. With a median of 6 years of follow-up, the median 5-year survival was 39% among neoadjuvant patients compared to 16% in the surgery-alone group (1).

Specific Issues

Quality of Life Parameters

Most of the randomized studies of neoadjuvant therapy did not assess any quality of life parameters. The study by Le Prise et al. found no difference in symptom-free survival whether or not CRT was given (7). A non-randomized study examined a number of quality of life parameters (dysphagia, fatigue, nausea) and found similarity at 1 year between patients treated with neoadjuvant therapy or surgery alone (45). Thus, the limited available data suggest that neoadjuvant therapy is not associated with a marked difference in quality of life.

Influence of Histologic Subtype

The preponderance of data indicates that there is no difference between squamous carcinoma and adenocarcinoma with respect to neoadjuvant therapy. A review of the tables in this chapter does not indicate any clear correlation between outcomes and the proportion of squamous cancer included. Furthermore, there are multiple confounding factors when comparing one trial to another, including differences in staging, patient selection, and treatment. Two of the CRT trials made a comparison between histologic types and reported a higher pCR rate with squamous carcinoma (38% and 27%) than adenocarcinomas (24% and 9%, respectively for Urba et al. [13] and Burmeister et al. [3]). Furthermore, Burmeister found an increase in progression-free survival associated with induction CRT in patients with squamous cell carcinoma (HR 0.47, 95% CI 0.25–0.86; $P = 0.014$) but not in patients with adenocarcinoma (3). However, the most recent meta-analysis suggested a greater benefit in the hazard rate for adenocarcinoma vs. squamous cancers with both neoadjuvant chemotherapy and chemoradiotherapy (38).

SYNTHESIS OF RESULTS FROM PHASE III TRIALS

Although esophageal cancer is a relatively uncommon cancer, many randomized trials have been conducted over several decades that allow articulation of an evidence-based approach. The approach applies fairly well to the broad population of patients with esophageal cancer who do not have distant metastases, with the exception perhaps of patients who are over age 75 or have a performance status of 2. It is clear that neoadjuvant therapy can be administered safely. Neoadjuvant RT has been extremely well tolerated. Neoadjuvant CT or CRT has also been well tolerated, with very few deaths during the neoadjuvant treatment and an incidence of grade 3,4 toxicity of 25%. Surgical resection can be accomplished after neoadjuvant therapy with essentially the same morbidity and mortality.

Approximately 35% of patients after neoadjuvant CT and 50% after neoadjuvant CRT have a radiographic response. Approximately 50% of patients have significant relief of dysphagia and usually can maintain their weight through the neoadjuvant treatment. Downstaging (by nodal status) does not appreciably occur after neoadjuvant RT, is seen in about 7% of patients after neoadjuvant CT, but occurs in a substantial proportion (25%) after neoadjuvant CRT. Similarly the rate of a pCR is quite low after either neoadjuvant RT or CT (5%–6%) but is consistently seen in approximately 25% after neoadjuvant CRT. However, the rate of a complete (R_0) resection is improved by only about 5%, and is essentially the same for neoadjuvant RT, CT, or CRT. Of all patients, approximately 10% fewer patients eventually undergo resection after either neoadjuvant RT, CT, or CRT. This is due primarily to a higher percentage of patients in whom surgery is not attempted after neoadjuvant therapy, because there are fewer patients who are found to be unresectable at the time of thoracotomy, especially after neoadjuvant CRT.

Neoadjuvant RT has little apparent effect on long-term survival, although there is a suggestion of improved local control. An updated meta-analysis in 2005 found a 9% reduced risk of death that was not statistically significant ($P = 0.2$). The benefit of neoadjuvant CT on survival is marginal. Several meta-analyses support a 10% reduced risk of death with a P value that is just above or below 0.05, depending on the meta-analysis performed. This translates to a 7% absolute increase in 2-year survival, the statistical significance of which is marginal and debatable. On the other hand, a more consistent trend to improved long-term survival is demonstrated by neoadjuvant CRT trials. Meta-analyses clearly demonstrate approximately a 20% reduced risk of death that is statistically significant. This translates to a 13% absolute increase in 2-year survival. Both neoadjuvant CT and CRT appear to result in better local control rates by about 5%. Quality of life does not seem to be affected by neoadjuvant therapy.

In summary, neoadjuvant CRT is reasonably well supported by the available data, with an effect on survival that is more pronounced than neoadjuvant CT or RT alone. This approach is well tolerated, with a treatment-related mortality that is approximately 10% in contemporary series. Nodal downstaging and a pCR are seen in approximately 25% of patients. Fewer patients (~5%) are found at thoracotomy to be unresectable, but more patients (~10%) are excluded from surgery after neoadjuvant CRT. In the final analysis, the rate of complete resection is slightly improved (~5%) by neoadjuvant CRT for all patients (on an intent to treat basis). Chemotherapy has generally involved 2 cycles of cisplatin and 5-FU, and RT doses of 35–45 Gy have been typical. The data appear to weakly support concurrent over sequential treatment, and there appears to be a benefit in both squamous carcinoma and adenocarcinoma.

NEWER APPROACHES

While many of the randomized neoadjuvant chemoradiotherapy trials were finishing accrual, several phase II studies exploring newer approaches were conducted. Interest in the chemotherapeutic agent, paclitaxel, grew considerably after reports of activity in unresectable esophageal cancer patients (partial or complete response of 32%) (46). More recent phase II trials have examined paclitaxel in the neoadjuvant setting (47–52). The largest of these trials was conducted from 1995 to 1999 at 24 sites through the Minnie Pearl Cancer Research Network (51). Neoadjuvant chemoradiotherapy consisting of paclitaxel, carboplatin, fluorouracil, and 45 Gy of RT was given to 129 patients with esophageal cancer. The majority of patients were stage II (17% stage I, 56% stage II, 22% stage III), and harbored an adenocarcinoma (71%). Compliance with paclitaxel and carboplatin was high (96%), as was radiotherapy (98%); however, only 54% of patients received the complete dose of fluorouracil. Although 57% of patients required hospitalization as a result of neoadjuvant therapy, there were no preoperative deaths and 85% of patients went on to surgery. The median survival was 24 months and the 3-year actuarial survival was 41%.

Much of what was found in the Minnie Pearl Cancer Research Network trial was echoed by contemporary phase II trials containing paclitaxel (48,49,52). Although toxicity was common, resection was attempted in 80% of patients, which is similar to the non-paclitaxel trials outlined above. Interestingly, the complete response rates were lower (14%–19%) than either the Minnie Pearl Cancer Research Network trial or the randomized chemoradiotherapy trials. Median survival ranged from 22 to 24 months and actuarial 3-year survival from 36% to 41%.

Comparison of the phase II paclitaxel studies with the more traditional regimens in the randomized chemoradiotherapy trials, however, suggests that the results are fairly comparable. A similar observation has been made by 2 retrospective studies comparing paclitaxel containing regimens to conventional regimens (47,50).

Interest has been growing in the use of irinotecan in esophageal cancer. The combined use of cisplatin and irinotecan is being explored as a neoadjuvant approach with RT because of indications of better tolerability with less gastrointestinal side effects, which is important in this patient population with dysphagia (53–55). More novel regimens include the addition of matrix metalloprotease inhibitors (56).

SUMMARY

Following 3 decades of randomized clinical trials, it is clear that compliance with neoadjuvant therapy is good and that such treatment protocols, including resection, can be carried out safely. Tumor progression does not occur to a significant degree by delaying surgery. Induction therapy, particularly chemoradiotherapy, appears to reduce the likelihood of lymph node metastases and to offer a survival advantage by meta-analysis of the data, although individual studies have generally fallen short of statistically significant differences. Therefore we recommend neoadjuvant chemoradiotherapy for patients with locoregionally confined esophageal cancer and good performance status and who are less than age 75 to 80. Extension beyond this group of patients must be done with care, as a relatively small increase in treatment-related mortality would negate the modest gain from the neoadjuvant approach.

Although the current data support a neoadjuvant approach, there is a lot of room for improvement and many details of the approach remain unclear, making enrollment of patients in clinical trials critical. In addition to evaluating new types of multimodality therapy (novel chemotherapeutics, radiation delivery protocols, surgical approaches), ongoing study of neoadjuvant protocols will clarify the patient population that is best served. Definition of specific patient and tumor characteristics that predict response to particular therapies may allow the treatment strategy to be tailored to an individual patient with less toxicity and greater benefit. Therefore, enrollment of patients with esophageal cancer in a clinical trial should be pursued whenever possible (information can be found at http://www.clinicaltrials.gov).

References

1. Medical Research Council Oesophageal Working Group. Surgical resection with or without preoperative chemotherapy in oesophageal cancer: a randomised controlled trial. *Lancet.* 2002;359(9319):1727–1733.
2. Bosset JF, Gignoux M, Triboulet JP, et al. Chemoradiotherapy followed by surgery compared with surgery alone in squamous-cell cancer of the esophagus. *N Engl J Med.* 1997;337(3):161–167.
3. Burmeister BH, Smithers BM, Gebski V, et al. Surgery alone versus chemoradiotherapy followed by surgery for resectable cancer of the oesophagus: a randomised controlled phase III trial. *Lancet Oncol.* 2005;6(9):659–668.
4. Lee JL, Park SI, Kim SB, et al. A single institutional phase III trial of preoperative chemotherapy with hyperfractionation radiotherapy plus surgery versus surgery alone for resectable esophageal squamous cell carcinoma. *Ann Oncol.* 2004;15(6):947–954.
5. Daly JM, Fry WA, Little AG, et al. Esophageal cancer: results of an American College of Surgeons Patient Care Evaluation Study. *J Am Coll Surg.* 2000;190(5):562–572; discussion 572–573.
6. Gignoux M, Roussel A, Paillot B, et al. The value of preoperative radiotherapy in esophageal cancer: results of a study of the E.O.R.T.C. *World J Surg.* 1987;11(4):426–432.
7. Le Prise E, Etienne PL, Meunier B, et al. A randomized study of chemotherapy, radiation therapy, and surgery versus surgery for localized squamous cell carcinoma of the esophagus. *Cancer.* 1994;73(7):1779–1784.
8. Kelsen DP, Ginsberg R, Pajak TF, et al. Chemotherapy followed by surgery compared with surgery alone for localized esophageal cancer. *N Engl J Med.* 1998; 339(27):1979–1984.
9. Jemal A, Siegel R, Ward E, et al. Cancer statistics, 2007. *CA Cancer J Clin.* 2007; 57(1):43–66.
10. Ancona E, Ruol A, Santi S, et al. Only pathologic complete response to neoadjuvant chemotherapy improves significantly the long term survival of patients with resectable esophageal squamous cell carcinoma: final report of a randomized, controlled trial of preoperative chemotherapy versus surgery alone. *Cancer.* 2001;91(11):2165–2174.
11. Maipang T, Vasinanukorn P, Petpichetchian C, et al. Induction chemotherapy in the treatment of patients with carcinoma of the esophagus. *J Surg Oncol.* 1994;56(3):191–197.
12. Baba M, Natsugoe S, Shimada M, et al. Prospective evaluation of preoperative chemotherapy in resectable squamous cell carcinoma of the thoracic esophagus. *Dis Esophagus.* 2000;13(2):136–141.
13. Urba SG, Orringer MB, Turrisi A, et al. Randomized trial of preoperative chemoradiation versus surgery alone in patients with locoregional esophageal carcinoma. *J Clin Oncol.* 2001;19(2):305–313.
14. Meyers BF, Downey RJ, Decker PA, et al. The utility of positron emission tomography in staging of potentially operable carcinoma of the thoracic esophagus: results of the American College of Surgeons Oncology Group Z0060 trial. *J Thorac Cardiovasc Surg.* 2007;133(3):738–745.
15. Schlag PM. Randomized trial of preoperative chemotherapy for squamous cell cancer of the esophagus. The Chirurgische Arbeitsgemeinschaft Fuer Onkologie der Deutschen Gesellschaft Fuer Chirurgie Study Group. *Arch Surg.* 1992;127(12):1446–1450.
16. Nygaard K, Hagen S, Hansen HS, et al. Pre-operative radiotherapy prolongs survival in operable esophageal carcinoma: a randomized, multicenter study of pre-operative

radiotherapy and chemotherapy. The second Scandinavian trial in esophageal cancer. *World J Surg.* 1992;16(6):1104–1109; discussion 1110.

17. Apinop C, Puttisak P, Preecha N. A prospective study of combined therapy in esophageal cancer. *Hepatogastroenterology.* 1994;41(4):391–393.
18. Urschel JD, Vasan H, Blewett CJ. A meta-analysis of randomized controlled trials that compared neoadjuvant chemotherapy and surgery to surgery alone for resectable esophageal cancer. *Am J Surg.* 2002;183(3):274–279.
19. Urschel JD, Vasan H. A meta-analysis of randomized controlled trials that compared neoadjuvant chemoradiation and surgery to surgery alone for resectable esophageal cancer. *Am J Surg.* 2003;185(6):538–543.
20. Malthaner RA, Collin S, Fenlon D. Preoperative chemotherapy for resectable thoracic esophageal cancer. *Cochrane Database Syst Rev.* 2006;3:CD001556.
21. Rice TW, Blackstone EH, Adelstein DJ, et al. N1 esophageal carcinoma: the importance of staging and downstaging. *J Thorac Cardiovasc Surg.* 2001;121(3):454–464.
22. Berger AC, Farma J, Scott WJ, et al. Complete response to neoadjuvant chemoradiotherapy in esophageal carcinoma is associated with significantly improved survival. *J Clin Oncol.* 2005;23(19):4330–4337.
23. Ribeiro A, Franceschi D, Parra J, et al. Endoscopic ultrasound restaging after neoadjuvant chemotherapy in esophageal cancer. *Am J Gastroenterol.* 2006;101(6):1216–1221.
24. Swisher SG, Maish M, Erasmus JJ, et al. Utility of PET, CT, and EUS to identify pathologic responders in esophageal cancer. *Ann Thorac Surg.* 2004;78(4):1152–1160; discussion 1160.
25. Jones DR, Detterbeck FC, Egan TM, et al. Induction chemoradiotherapy followed by esophagectomy in patients with carcinoma of the esophagus. *Ann Thorac Surg.* 1997;64(1):185–191; discussion 191–192.
26. Jones DR, Parker LA Jr, Detterbeck FC, et al. Inadequacy of computed tomography in assessing patients with esophageal carcinoma after induction chemoradiotherapy. *Cancer.* 1999;85(5):1026–1032.
27. Shaukat A, Mortazavi A, Demmy T, et al. Should preoperative, post-chemoradiotherapy endoscopy be routine for esophageal cancer patients? *Dis Esophagus.* 2004;17(2):129–135.
28. Bates BA, Detterbeck FC, Bernard SA, et al. Concurrent radiation therapy and chemotherapy followed by esophagectomy for localized esophageal carcinoma. *J Clin Oncol.* 1996;14(1):156–163.
29. Mamede M, Abreu ELP, Oliva MR, et al. FDG-PET/CT tumor segmentation-derived indices of metabolic activity to assess response to neoadjuvant therapy and progression-free survival in esophageal cancer: correlation with histopathology results. *Am J Clin Oncol.* 2007;30(4):377–388.
30. Forshaw MJ, Gossage JA, Chrystal K, et al. Symptomatic responses to neoadjuvant chemotherapy for carcinoma of the oesophagus and oesophagogastric junction: are they worth measuring? *Clin Oncol (R Coll Radiol).* 2006;18(4):345–350.
31. Steyn RS, Grenier I, Darnton SJ, et al. Weight gain as an indicator of response to chemotherapy for oesophageal carcinoma. *Clin Oncol (R Coll Radiol).* 1995;7(6):382–384.
32. Margolis M, Alexander P, Trachiotis GD, et al. Percutaneous endoscopic gastrostomy before multimodality therapy in patients with esophageal cancer. *Ann Thorac Surg.* 2003;76(5):1694–1697; discussion 1697–1698.
33. Hammoud ZT, Kesler KA, Ferguson MK, et al. Survival outcomes of resected patients who demonstrate a pathologic complete response after neoadjuvant chemoradiation therapy for locally advanced esophageal cancer. *Dis Esophagus.* 2006;19(2):69–72.
34. Wang M, Gu XZ, Yin WB, et al Randomized clinical trial on the combination of preoperative irradiation and surgery in the treatment of esophageal carcinoma: report on 206 patients. *Int J Radiat Oncol Biol Phys.* 1989;16(2):325–327.
35. Kelsen DP, Winter KA, Gunderson LL, et al. Long-term results of RTOG trial 8911 (USA Intergroup 113): a random assignment trial comparison of chemotherapy followed by surgery compared with surgery alone for esophageal cancer. *J Clin Oncol.* 2007;25(24):3719–3725.
36. Kato H, Tachimori Y, Watanabe H, et al. Anastomotic recurrence of oesophageal squamous cell carcinoma after transthoracic oesophagectomy. *Eur J Surg.* 1998;164(10):759–764.
37. Arnott SJ, Duncan W, Gignoux M, et al. Preoperative radiotherapy for esophageal carcinoma. *Cochrane Database Syst Rev.* 2005(4):CD001799.
38. Gebski V, Burmeister B, Smithers BM, et al. Survival benefits from neoadjuvant chemoradiotherapy or chemotherapy in oesophageal carcinoma: a meta-analysis. *Lancet Oncol.* 2007;8(3):226–234.
39. Malthaner RA, Wong RK, Rumble RB, et al. Neoadjuvant or adjuvant therapy for resectable esophageal cancer: a systematic review and meta-analysis. *BMC Med.* 2004;2(1):35.
40. Kaklamanos IG, Walker GR, Ferry K, et al. Neoadjuvant treatment for resectable cancer of the esophagus and the gastroesophageal junction: a meta-analysis of randomized clinical trials. *Ann Surg Oncol.* 2003;10(7):754–761.
41. Cunningham D, Allum WH, Stenning SP, et al. Perioperative chemotherapy versus surgery alone for resectable gastroesophageal cancer. *N Engl J Med.* 2006;355(1):11–20.
42. Walsh TN, Noonan N, Hollywood D, et al. A comparison of multimodal therapy and surgery for esophageal adenocarcinoma. *N Engl J Med.* 1996;335(7):462–467.
43. Greer SE, Goodney PP, Sutton JE, et al. Neoadjuvant chemoradiotherapy for esophageal carcinoma: a meta-analysis. *Surgery.* 2005;137(2):172–177.
44. Walsh TN, Grennell M, Mansoor S, et al. Neoadjuvant treatment of advanced stage esophageal adenocarcinoma increases survival. *Dis Esophagus.* 2002;15(2):121–124.
45. Blazeby JM, Sanford E, Falk SJ, et al. Health-related quality of life during neoadjuvant treatment and surgery for localized esophageal carcinoma. *Cancer.* 2005;103(9):1791–1799.
46. Ajani JA, Ilson DH, Daugherty K, et al. Activity of Taxol in patients with squamous cell carcinoma and adenocarcinoma of the esophagus. *J Natl Cancer Inst.* 1994;86(14):1086–1091.
47. Kelsey CR, Chino JP, Willett CG, et al. Paclitaxel-based chemoradiotherapy in the treatment of patients with operable esophageal cancer. *Int J Radiat Oncol Biol Phys.* 2007;69(3):770–776.
48. Urba SG, Orringer MB, Ianettonni M, et al. Concurrent cisplatin, paclitaxel, and radiotherapy as preoperative treatment for patients with locoregional esophageal carcinoma. *Cancer.* 2003;98(10):2177–2183.
49. Lowy AM, Firdaus I, Roychowdhury D, et al. A phase II study of sequential neoadjuvant gemcitabine and paclitaxel, radiation therapy with cisplatin and 5-fluorouracil and surgery in locally advanced esophageal carcinoma. *Am J Clin Oncol.* 2006;29(6):555–561.
50. Adelstein DJ, Rice TW, Rybicki LA, et al. Does paclitaxel improve the chemoradiotherapy of locoregionally advanced esophageal cancer? A nonrandomized comparison with fluorouracil-based therapy. *J Clin Oncol.* 2000;18(10):2032–2039.
51. Meluch AA, Greco FA, Gray JR, et al. Preoperative therapy with concurrent paclitaxel/carboplatin/infusional 5-FU and radiation therapy in locoregional esophageal cancer: final results of a Minnie Pearl Cancer Research Network phase II trial. *Cancer J.* 2003;9(4):251–260.
52. Kim DW, Blanke CD, Wu H, et al. Phase II study of preoperative paclitaxel/cisplatin with radiotherapy in locally advanced esophageal cancer. *Int J Radiat Oncol Biol Phys.* 2007;67(2):397–404.
53. Ilson DH. Phase II trial of weekly irinotecan/cisplatin in advanced esophageal cancer. *Oncology (Williston Park).* 2004;18(14 Suppl 14):22–25.
54. Shah MA, Ramanathan RK, Ilson DH, et al. Multicenter phase II study of irinotecan, cisplatin, and bevacizumab in patients with metastatic gastric or gastroesophageal junction adenocarcinoma. *J Clin Oncol.* 2006;24(33):5201–5206.
55. Ajani JA, Faust J, Yao J, et al. Irinotecan/cisplatin followed by 5-FU/paclitaxel/radiotherapy and surgery in esophageal cancer. *Oncology (Williston Park).* 2003;17(9 Suppl 8):20–22.
56. Heath EI, Burtness BA, Kleinberg L, et al. Phase II, parallel-design study of preoperative combined modality therapy and the matrix metalloprotease (mmp) inhibitor prinomastat in patients with esophageal adenocarcinoma. *Invest New Drugs.* 2006;24(2):135–140.
57. Launois B, Delarue D, Campion JP, et al. Preoperative radiotherapy for carcinoma of the esophagus. *Surg Gynecol Obstet.* 1981;153(5):690–692.
58. Arnott SJ, Duncan W, Kerr GR, et al. Low dose preoperative radiotherapy for carcinoma of the oesophagus: results of a randomized clinical trial. *Radiother Oncol.* 1992;24(2):108–113.
59. Roth JA, Pass HI, Flanagan MM, et al. Randomized clinical trial of preoperative and postoperative adjuvant chemotherapy with cisplatin, vindesine, and bleomycin for carcinoma of the esophagus. *J Thorac Cardiovasc Surg.* 1988;96(2):242–248.
60. Law S, Fok M, Chow S, Chu KM, et al. Preoperative chemotherapy versus surgical therapy alone for squamous cell carcinoma of the esophagus: a prospective randomized trial. *J Thorac Cardiovasc Surg.* 1997;114(2):210–217.

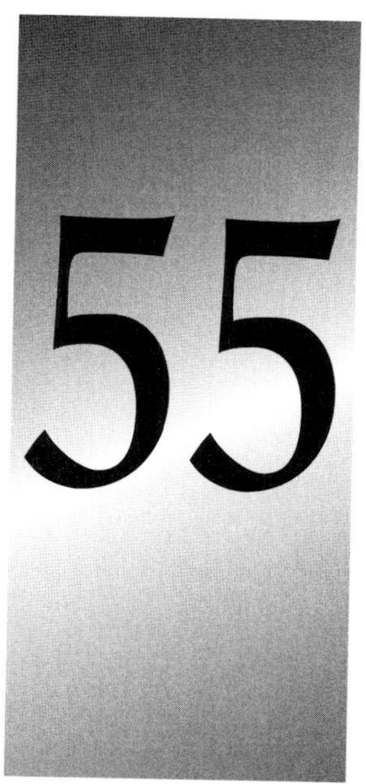

55 Definitive Radiochemotherapy

Ashish Patel
Mohan Suntharalingam

Since the early 1900s, radiation therapy and surgery have played an important role in the management of locally advanced esophageal cancer. Soon after the discovery of radium in 1901, therapeutic applications of radioactivity in esophageal cancer were described (1,2). Contemporary to these reports, surgical literature described transthoracic approaches for resection of esophageal carcinoma, with limited success (3–5). The results of these early studies revealed disappointing 5-year survival rates of approximately 1% to 10%.

The last century has witnessed remarkable advances in the diagnosis and management of cancer; however, esophageal cancer continues to pose a significant therapeutic challenge. In 2007, the American Cancer Society estimates 15,570 new cases of esophageal cancer and 13,940 resultant deaths. The high mortality rate relative to the number of newly diagnosed cases is indicative of the aggressive nature of this disease. The majority of patients present with locally advanced disease, and up to 40% of patients have metastatic disease at presentation (6). Thus, understanding that there is both a high risk of local and systemic failure in patients presenting with locally advanced disease has led to the development of combined-modality treatment approaches. This chapter will focus on the management of esophageal cancer with definitive chemoradiotherapy and will review the biologic rationale for combined-modality treatment, as well as its supporting preclinical and clinical data.

BIOLOGIC RATIONALE FOR CHEMORADIOTHERAPY

Radiation therapy exerts its lethal effects on cells through either direct or indirect interactions that lead to DNA damage. Of the several forms of DNA damage that can result from exposure to ionizing radiation, the DNA double-strand break is biologically the most important. Direct radiation action is the result of an ionizing particle interacting with DNA to cause a double-strand break, while indirect radiation action occurs as a result of hydrolysis of water by an ionizing particle, which leads to the formation of reactive oxygen species. These free radicals then interact with DNA and cause damage. Because water comprises 80% to 90% of the cell, the indirect effect predominates and is ultimately responsible for approximately 70% of DNA damage.

Because the majority of radiation's effect is through indirect action, oxygen is a vital component for free radical–mediated DNA damage. Unfortunately, many tumors exhibit hypoxic regions, which have been shown in vitro and in vivo to be resistant to radiation damage. It is thought that these hypoxic cellular populations proliferate despite exposure to ionizing radiation and

TABLE 55.1
Select Radiosensitizing Chemotherapeutic Agents

Agent	Class	Mechanism of action
5-fluorouracil	Antimetabolite	A pyrimidine analog that acts as a thymidylate synthase inhibitor.
Irinotecan	Topoisomerase Inhibitor	Inhibits deoxyribonucleic acid (DNA) synthesis and replication through the inactivation of topoisomerase I.
Paclitaxel/ Docetaxel	Mitotic Inhibitor	Hyperstabilizes cellular microtubules and prevents their normal function.
Mitomycin C	Antitumor Antibiotic	Inhibits the synthesis of DNA through the formation of crosslinks.
Cisplatin	Platinum Coordination Complex	Causes DNA pruine crosslinks interfering with mitosis and inducing apoptosis.

ultimately contribute to treatment failure. Chemotherapeutic agents, such as 5-fluorouracil (5-FU), mitomycin-c, and cisplatin, have yielded promising preclinical results for increasing the lethality of radiation and sensitizing hypoxic tumor cells (7–9). The interactions between radiation and chemotherapeutic agents are extensive, complex, and not fully understood. Some proposed mechanisms of cell sensitization include: synergistic cell killing, reducing accelerated repopulation, cell cycle arrest in radiosensitive phases, enhancement of radiation injury, and inhibition of sublethal or potentially lethal DNA damage repair. Table 55.1 demonstrates the mechanism of action of several common drugs used in the treatment of esophageal cancer. The results of preclinical work by Zak, Richmond, and Douple led to the development of several phase I/II and eventually phase III trials evaluating the role of combination chemotherapy and radiation therapy.

DEFINITIVE CHEMORADIOTHERAPY

Historic Rationale from Clinical Data for Anal Cancer and Lung Cancer

Contemporary to the laboratory data published in the early 1970s supporting combination chemoradiation, clinical investigators began to report institutional data demonstrating efficacy of this treatment approach. In 1974, Nigro and associates published a small experience of concurrent 5-fluorouracil (5-FU), mitomycin, and irradiation in the treatment of anal cancer (10). The authors reported 3 cases in which varying chemotherapy regimes and radiation doses were delivered, all of which showed clinical and/or pathologic complete response after completion of therapy. These data formed the basis of several important cooperative group studies, which demonstrated the efficacy of definitive chemoradiotherapy in the treatment of anal carcinoma (11–13).

In the 1980s, cisplatin emerged as a chemotherapeutic agent with activity against epithelial cancers and showed synergistic effects with radiation therapy. The European Organization for Research and Treatment of Cancer (EORTC) reported on a phase III trial of split course radiation therapy alone or in combination with chemotherapy in patients with inoperable non-small cell lung cancer (NSCLC) (14). Overall survival and local control were both significantly improved with the addition of cisplatin to thoracic radiation therapy. Similar results were reported by Soresi and associates (15). In this phase III study, 95 patients with locally advanced NSCLC were randomized to radiation therapy alone (50 Gy) or in combination with weekly cisplatin (15 mg/m^2). Again, median survival was improved by 5 months, and local recurrence was decreased in the chemoradiotherapy arm. These studies clearly demonstrate the radiosensitization effects of chemotherapy, which translates to improved local control and overall survival.

Single Institution Clinical Data

Early reports of single modality therapy for esophageal cancer yielded disappointing results, with long-term survival achieved in less than 10% of patients (1–5). The patterns of failure in patients treated with radiation therapy alone have consistently shown poor local control as well as distant failure rates up to 66% even when patients were treated with doses greater than 50 Gy (16). The addition of chemotherapy to radiation therapy was, therefore, a logical next step in the evolution of therapy for esophageal carcinoma. Investigators from Japan were among the first to report results of combined chemoradiotherapy in this disease site. Fujimake and associates reported the pathologic findings of 58 patients treated with bleomycin with and without radiation therapy (17). In this report, a 69% response rate was found with the addition of bleomycin,

TABLE 55.2
Single Institution Results for Definitive Chemoradiation Therapy in Patients with Esophageal Cancer

Trial	Number of patients	Radiation dose (Gy)	Chemotherapeutic agents	Median survival (months)	Two-Year survival (%)
Herskovic, et al. (18)	39	30.0	Cisplatin, 5-FU	9.8	20
	22	50.0	Cisplatin, 5-FU	19.5	36
Coia, et al. (19)	30	60.0	Cisplatin, Mitomycin C	18.0	47
Keane, et al. (45)	20	22.5–25.0	5-FU, Mitomycin C	12	
	15	45.0–50.0		–	48
John, et al. (46)	30	41.4–50.4	Cisplatin, 5-FU, Mitomycin C	11.0	29

Abbreviations: 5-FU = 5-fluorouracil.

suggesting a favorable interaction between chemotherapy and radiation.

In the United States, institutions such as the Fox Chase Cancer Center and Wayne State University pioneered the use of combined modality therapy. Herskovic and associates reported on the Wayne State experience of chemotherapy and radiation with and without surgery in the thoracic esophagus (18). A total of 39 patients were analyzed, all of whom received definitive chemoradiotherapy with cisplatin and 5-FU chemotherapy concurrently with radiation therapy to a total dose of 30 Gy. The median and 2-year survivals in this group of patients were 9.8 months and 20%, respectively. Because of the disappointing results in this early cohort of patients, an additional 22 patients were analyzed as part of a pilot study that increased the radiation dose to 50 Gy. The increased in radiation dose yielded promising results, with median survival of 19 months and 2-year survival of 36%.

One of the largest single institution trials of concurrent chemotherapy and radiation was a phase II study reported by Coia and colleagues from the Fox Chase Cancer Center (19). Ninety patients were enrolled on this study, 57 had stage I/II disease (1983 American Joint Commission on Cancer) and were treated definitively, while the remaining 33 patients with stage III/IV disease received palliative chemoradiotherapy. Among the definitively treated stage I/II patients, radiation therapy was delivered to a total dose of 60 Gy (2 Gy/day) concurrently with 4-day continuous infusion 5-FU (1,000 mg/m^2/24 h) during weeks 1 and 2 and mitomycin C (10 mg/m^2) on day 2. The median survival for this patient subset was 18 months, and the 3- and 5-year overall survival was 29% and 18%, respectively. On multivariate analysis, stage was the most significant prognostic indicator, with a 3-year survival of 73% in stage I patients versus 33% in those with stage II disease (P = 0.01). The acute toxicity of this combined regimen was deemed acceptable with a 56% rate of moderate to severe toxicity, and a low incidence (12%) of late esophageal strictures. Several other institutions (Table 55.2) have reported comparable results with use of platinum-based chemoradiotherapy, which ultimately led to the development of multi-institutional, randomized, phase III trials in both the United States and Europe.

Multi-Institutional Randomized Data

To date, there have been 4 major randomized phase III studies (Table 55.3) comparing definitive chemoradiation with radiation therapy alone. The seminal trial conducted by the Radiation Therapy Oncology Group (RTOG 85–01) has set the standard of care for the definitive treatment of esophageal cancer since its original publication in 1992 (20). This trial randomized patients to treatment with radiation alone (64 Gy) or concurrent chemotherapy (2 cycles of cisplatin/5-FU) and radiation (50 Gy) followed by 2 cycles of adjuvant chemotherapy. From 1986 to 1990, 129 patients were enrolled on this study, and after a planned interim analysis, the study was closed after meeting early stopping rules. An additional 73 patients, who would have been eligible for the study, were prospectively registered and treated with chemoradiotherapy. After a minimum follow-up of 5 years, the median survival was 9.3 months in the radiation alone arm versus 14.1 months in those treated with combined-modality therapy. The 5-year survival was 26% for those who received combination therapy compared to 0% for those treated with radiation alone.

The addition of chemotherapy to radiation improved local control of regional disease and decreased the incidence of distant metastasis as compared to radiation therapy alone. Persistent disease after treatment was found in 37% of patients in the radiation alone

TABLE 55.3
Results from Randomized Trials Evaluating Radiation Therapy Alone versus Chemoradiotherapy in Patients with Esophageal Cancer

Trial	Number of patients	Radiation dose (Gy)	Chemotherapeutic agents	Two-Year survival (%)
Araujo, et al. (21)	28	50.0	None	22
	31	50.0	5-FU, Mitomycin C	38
Smith, et al. (22)	62	40.0	None	12
	65	40.0	5-FU, Mitomycin C	27
Wobbes, et al. (47)	111	40.0[a]	None	15
	110	40.0[a]	Cisplatin	20
Cooper, et al. (48)	62	64.0	None	0[b]
	61	50.0	Cisplatin, 5-FU	26[b]

[a]split course.
[b]3-year survival.
Abbreviations: 5-FU = 5-fluorouracil.

arm, compared to 25% in those treated with chemoradiation ($P < 0.01$). Furthermore, local failure at first site of recurrence also decreased from 24% to 17% with the addition of chemotherapy. One year following therapy, the rate of persistent or recurrent disease remained significantly lower in the chemoradiation arm (62% versus 44%, $P = 0.01$). Finally, a significantly lower rate of distant failure was also associated with combined modality therapy, with a distant failure rate of 38% versus 22% in the chemoradiation arm ($P < 0.005$).

Araujo and associates reported similar results of a phase III trial conducted by the Brazilian National Cancer Institute (21). Fifty-nine patients enrolled between 1982 and 1985 were randomized to either radiation alone (50 Gy) or the same radiation regimen with 1 cycle of concurrent 5-FU and mitomycin C. The 5-year overall survival was improved in the chemoradiation arm (6% versus 16%); however, this did not reach statistical significance ($P = 0.16$). As in the RTOG study, the patterns of failure demonstrate an improvement in local control with the addition of chemotherapy. While these results are not as impressive as the Herskovic data, it should be noted that patients received only 1 cycle of chemotherapy concurrently with radiation and did not receive any adjuvant chemotherapy. Furthermore, this study may have been underpowered to show any significant difference between the 2 arms. Nonetheless, there appears to be a beneficial interaction between the chemotherapy and radiation, which drives the improvement in local control.

More recently, Smith and colleagues published the results of a phase III trial run through the Eastern Oncology Cooperative Group, which randomized patients to radiation therapy (60 Gy) with or without concurrent 5-FU and mitomycin C chemotherapy (22). Patients enrolled in this study had the option to be evaluated for surgical resection after 40 Gy. Ultimately, 54 of 119 patients proceeded to surgery. The median and 2-year overall survivals were both significantly longer for those receiving chemoradiation (14.8 months and 27%, respectively) as compared to the radiation alone arm (9.2 months and 12%, respectively, $P = 0.04$). On multivariate analysis, stage was the only significant predictor for survival; patients with stage I disease had a median survival of 14.8 months compared to 9.4 months in those with stage II disease ($P = 0.01$).

These results have established chemoradiation therapy as the standard of care for locally advanced esophageal carcinoma. However, it is important to note that the benefits of improved local control, decreased distant failure, and longer overall survival associated with the addition of chemotherapy come at the expense of increased acute toxicity. In the RTOG trial, chemoradiotherapy was associated with a 44% and 20% incidence of severe and life-threatening acute toxicities, respectively, versus 25% and 3% in the radiation alone arm. The incidence of late toxicity was similar between both arms. Similar findings were observed in both the ECOG and Brazilian studies. The most significant toxicities encountered in each of these studies included esophagitis and hematologic sequelae.

Despite the significant improvements in outcome associated with chemoradiation therapy, local failure continues to occur in approximately 20% to 50% of patients. Consequently, investigators began to explore radiation dose escalation in the setting of chemoradiation to further improve local control. Building upon the success of RTOG 85–01, the phase III intergroup (INT) trial 0123 was designed to evaluate the efficacy of radiation dose intensification with concurrent chemotherapy (23). Prior to the initiation of this study, modifications had to be made to the original RTOG 85–01 design to account for the expected increased toxicity of dose escalation. Therefore, the daily radiation dose was decreased from 2.0 Gy/day to 1.8 Gy/day, and most importantly, the radiation treatment fields were reduced to 5 cm proximal and distal to the tumor volume and a 2 cm radial margin. The fields used in the previous RTOG study required the entire esophagus to receive 30 Gy followed by a small field boost of an additional 20 Gy with a 5 cm superior and inferior margin. The chemotherapy regimens remained essentially the same in both studies. Patients in this study were randomized to receive cisplatin and 5-FU chemotherapy with either 50.4 Gy or 64.8 Gy of radiation therapy.

After accruing 236 patients, the intergroup study was closed after a planned interim analysis revealed a low probability of finding a statistically significant benefit in the high-dose arm. The median survival was 13 months in the high-dose arm and 18.1 months in the low-dose arm. The locoregional control rates were also similar in both treatment arms (56% versus 52%). The toxicity of treatment, particularly grade V toxicity, was disproportionately higher in the high-dose arm, which had 11 treatment-related deaths versus 2 in the standard arm. However, the majority of deaths (7/11) occurred at doses < 50 Gy, while the remaining 4 occurred during or after the high-dose period. As such, dose escalation should not be interpreted to be associated with higher mortality. Nevertheless, the dose of 50.4 Gy remains the standard of care for combined modality therapy.

Altered Fractionation in Chemoradiation

Throughout the 1980s and 1990s, trials of altered fractionation schemes in sites such as the head and neck and lung demonstrated better rates of local control. Based on these encouraging results, there have been several publications investigating the feasibility and efficacy of this treatment strategy in esophageal cancer. A phase II trial from the Cleveland Clinic evaluated 72 patients treated with induction chemotherapy (cisplatin/5-FU) and concurrent split course of accelerated fractionation radiation (1.5 Gy twice daily to 45 Gy) followed by evaluation for surgical resection (24). The induction therapy was associated with significant toxicity; the most common severe toxicity was mucositis, which occurred in 18% of patients. Sixty-seven patients ultimately underwent surgical resection, and the pathologic complete response rate for induction chemoradiotherapy was 27%. The actuarial 4-year survival for the entire cohort was 44%.

Recently, Choi and associates reported on a phase I/II trial of concurrent chemotherapy (cisplatin, 5-FU, and paclitaxel) and radiation therapy utilizing a concurrent boost technique (25). The radiation was delivered in 1.8 Gy per fraction to a total dose of 45 Gy. A concomitant boost of 1.5 Gy per fraction to a total boost dose of 13.5 Gy was delivered on Days 1 to 5 and 29 to 32 of the chemotherapy cycles. The total dose to the tumor was 58.5 Gy. Patients determined to be resectable after chemoradiotherapy were then offered surgery. Forty-six patients were enrolled on the study from 1995 to 1997. Severe (grade III/IV) esophagitis was reported in 55% of patients. Twenty percent of patients experienced febrile neutropenia requiring hospitalization. Forty patients underwent surgical resection after chemoradiation, and a pathologic complete response was found in 45% of these patients. The median survival time was 34 months, while the 5-year actuarial survival was 37%. While these studies are encouraging, there is clearly a significant increase in treatment-related toxicity associated with altered fractionation regimens. Further investigation is warranted to better delineate suitable candidates and should be done only on a clinical trial.

Definitive Chemoradiation versus Trimodality Therapy

Surgical resection has played a significant role in the management of patients with esophageal cancer since the early 1900s. As newer chemotherapeutic agents and radiation techniques have been developed, surgical resection continues to be incorporated into the management of select patients. While the goal of this strategy is to increase local control, the increase in treatment-related mortality is not inconsequential. Recently, there have been 2 European phase III trials that have randomized patients to definitive chemoradiation versus trimodality therapy.

Bedenne and associates randomized 455 patients with potentially resectable T3 to T4, N0 to N1 esophageal cancer to neoadjuvant chemoradiation or trimodality therapy (26). All patients received 2 cycles of cisplatin and 5-FU chemotherapy concurrently with radiation therapy to a total dose of 46 Gy in 2 Gy per fraction. Patients who achieved a partial response were then randomized to completion of definitive chemoradiation therapy (3 more cycles of chemotherapy and an additional 20 Gy) or surgical resection; 259 patients ultimately underwent randomization, of which the vast majority had squamous type carcinomas (88%). The 2-year survival and local control rates were 34% and 66.4% in the trimodality arm, respectively. This was not significantly different from the chemoradiation alone arm (40% and 57%, respectively). However, the 3-month mortality rate was significantly higher in the trimodality arm (9.3% versus 0.8%, $P = 0.002$). The authors therefore concluded the addition of surgical resection after chemoradiation provides no benefit in the treatment of squamous esophageal carcinomas.

Similarly, Stahl and colleagues published a phase III randomized trial of 172 patients with T3 or T4 and N0 or N1 squamous-cell carcinomas staged by computed tomography and endoscopic ultrasound (27). After randomization, all patients underwent induction chemotherapy with 3 cycles of 5-FU, leucovorin, etoposide, and cisplatin. Patients randomized to the trimodality arm then received concurrent chemoradiotherapy (cisplatin, etoposide, 40 Gy) followed by surgery. Patients assigned to the definitive chemoradiotherapy arm received the same chemotherapy with > 65 Gy. The 3-year overall survival was not statistically different between those who underwent definitive chemoradiation and those who underwent trimodality therapy (20% versus 28%). The 2-year progression-free survival was significant better in the trimodality arm (64% versus 40%). However, treatment-related mortality was also significantly higher in the surgical group. On multivariate analysis, several prognostic factors were evaluated; however, only tumor response after induction chemotherapy proved to be statistically significant. Although an improvement in local control was observed in the trimodality therapy arm, the high postoperative mortality rate counteracts any potential gain in survival associated with the addition of surgery.

The results of these 2 phase III randomized trials comparing trimodality therapy to definitive chemoradiation are strikingly similar in their outcomes. In both trials, the addition of surgery to chemoradiation therapy was associated with increased treatment-related toxicity, which ultimately compromised overall survival. Further investigation is warranted in better delineating factors associated with increased risk of mortality and in the identification of suitable patient populations for trimodality therapy, which may yield more favorable results. In the end, both of these studies reinforce definitive chemoradiation therapy as the standard of care in the management of locally advanced esophageal cancer.

Induction Chemotherapy

One of the more provocative findings in the previously mentioned trimodality study by Stahl et al. was the prognostic significance of response to induction chemotherapy. This treatment strategy has been used in many different disease sites, most notably in head and neck cancer (28,29). The rationale behind incorporating induction chemotherapy into the treatment of locally advanced esophageal cancer include the potential improvement in local control and reduction of distant failure. Investigators from the MD Anderson Cancer Center have reported on this strategy in patients with potentially resectable cancer of the esophagus or gastroesophageal junction. They found a 59% response rate to induction chemotherapy, and with a median follow-up of 20 months, the median survival had not been reached (30). The RTOG recently presented data from a randomized phase II trial (RTOG 0113) that compared 2 paclitaxel-based induction-chemotherapy regimens in non-operative patients and found unacceptably high rates of treatment-related toxicity in both arms (31). Ultimately, the increased toxicity associated with the induction therapy seen in the RTOG study as well as other trials, such as Intergroup 0123, limits the use of this approach in future investigations.

Future Directions: Targeted Therapies

The discovery of growth factors, cell surface receptors, and their resultant signaling cascades has led to a greater understanding of tumorigenesis. Dysregulation of angiogenesis, inflammation, cell cycle control, growth, and cell migration are all essential components of neoplastic transformation that involve growth factors and cell surface receptors. A new class of systemic therapies specifically targeting cellular growth protein receptors and downstream signaling pathways has shown promising results in improving the therapeutic ratio of oncologic treatment.

The epidermal growth factor receptor (EGFR, ErbB-1) is a member of the ErbB family of receptor tyrosine kinases. These receptors combine an extracellular ligand binding domain with an intracellular tyrosine kinase, which, upon activation, initiates cell signaling cascades. Activation of these receptors in cancer cells results several downstream effects, including autocrine stimulation, mutation, and/or overexpression. Approximately 90% of esophageal carcinomas have been shown to overexpress EGFR, which has been correlated with a poor prognosis in several studies (32–35). As a result, several molecular targeting strategies have been developed and include antibodies to the extracellular ligand binding domain or small molecule inhibitors blocking the receptor tyrosine kinase activity. Table 55.4 lists several targeted agents and their mechanisms of action.

Cetuximab, a monoclonal (IgG1) antibody against the extracellular domain of EGFR, has been studied in conjunction with radiation therapy. Preclinical studies have suggested a synergistic effect with the addition of cetuximab to radiation therapy in head and neck squamous-cell carcinoma lines (36). Proposed mechanisms of radiosensitization include: induction of G1 cell cycle arrest, inhibition of cellular proliferation, promotion of radiation-induced apoptosis, inhibition of radiation-induced damage repair, and inhibition of tumor angiogenesis.

TABLE 55.4
Selected Targeted Biologic Agents

Agent	Target	Mechanism of action
Cetuximab	EGFR	Antibody to the extracellular domain that prevents ligand binding and subsequent activation of the receptor.
Erlotinib	EGFR	Small molecule tyrosine kinase inhibitor that prevents kinase activity from initiating downstream signaling cascade.
Trastuzumab	HER-2	Antibody to the extracellular domain that prevents ligand binding and subsequent activation of the receptor.
Laptinib	EGFR/HER-2	Small molecule tyrosine kinase inhibitor that prevents kinase activity from initiating downstream signaling cascade.
Bevacizumab	VEGF	Antibody to the VEGF ligand that prevents its binding to and activation of the VEGFR.
Sorafenib	PDGFR/VEGFR/ Flt-3/c-Kit/Raf	Small molecule tyrosine kinase inhibitor that prevents kinase activity from initiating downstream signaling cascade.

Abbreviations: EGFR = epidermal growth factor receptor; VEGF = vascular endothelial growth factor; VEGFR = vascular endothelial growth factor receptor; PDGFR = platelet derived growth factor receptor.

Recently, a phase III randomized study of radiation therapy versus radiation therapy and cetuximab in patients with locally advanced head and neck cancer demonstrates a local control and overall survival benefit with the addition of cetuximab (37). Notably, there was no increase in treatment-related toxicity in patients who received cetuximab. While cetuximab and radiation therapy has been shown to be tolerable and efficacious, the addition of chemotherapy to this treatment strategy remains investigational.

Two phase II studies incorporating cetuximab with chemoradiation, in esophageal carcinoma, have recently been reported with conflicting results. The first study administered 5,040 cGy/28 fractions of radiation therapy and concurrent weekly cisplatin 30 mg/m^2, irinotecan 65 mg/m^2, and cetuximab 250 mg on weeks 1, 2, 4, and 5, followed by surgery 4 to 8 weeks after completion of RT (38). When compared to similar studies in patients undergoing trimodality therapy, the addition of cetuximab resulted in a lower complete response rate and higher overall toxicity. Conversely, investigators from the Brown University Oncology Group and the University of Maryland Greenebaum Cancer Center found an endoscopic complete response rate of 65% and acceptable toxicity in a phase II trial of cetuximab, carboplatin, paclitaxel, and 50.4 Gy of radiation therapy (39). The Southwest Oncology Group protocol 0414 is a phase II trial of induction cetuximab, cisplatin, and irinotecan, followed by the 3-drug combination and radiotherapy. This protocol closed in the fall of 2007 and results are pending. Ultimately, the role of cetuximab in combination with definitive chemoradiotherapy will be evaluated in an upcoming phase III trial run by the RTOG.

HER-2 (ErbB2), another member of the ErbB receptor family, has also been shown in several studies to be overexpressed in esophageal carcinoma lines (40–42). HER-2 overexpression has been linked to increased tumor invasiveness, lymph node metastasis, and chemoresistance. Traztuzumab is a humanized IgG1 antibody against HER-2 receptor. There appear to be multiple mechanisms through which the antibody exerts its effect, including: G1 cell cycle arrest, downregulation of the HER-2 receptor, disruption of downstream signaling cascades, suppression of angiogenesis, and promotion of apoptosis. Safran and associates recently reported on a phase I/II trial of locally advanced adenocarcinoma treated with traztuzumab, paclitaxel, cisplatin, and radiation therapy in patients with HER-2 overexpression (43). Thirty-three percent of screened patients overexpressed HER-2 by immunohistochemistry. The median survival for the cohort was 18 months, with 42% of patients alive at 2 years. These findings, therefore, warrant further investigation in patients with HER-2 overexpression.

Vascular endothelial growth factor (VEGF) is a family of potent endothelial growth factors that have been extensively investigated in cancer therapy. VEGF has been shown to have apoptotic effects and be involved in the regulation of vascular permeability and proliferation. Bevacizumab, an antibody against VEGF, has been shown to have radiosensitizing effects in preclinical studies with esophageal cancer lines (44). As a result, ongoing trials incorporating bevacizumab into chemoradiation regimens are being evaluated in phase

II trials; however, in light of recent reports of increased associated tracheoesophageal fistula formation in other disease sites, its use may be limited.

CONCLUSION

Over the last 100 years, the management of locally advanced esophageal cancer has evolved from single modality therapy to a combined modality approach. The addition of chemotherapy to radiation therapy has led to a dramatic increase in overall survival when compared to radiation alone; however, 5-year survival of 20% to 25% leaves room for improvement. Increases in distant failure seen over the past 20 years are likely the result of improved local control, therefore, newer strategies should address this changing pattern of failure. The addition of surgery to chemoradiation continues to remain controversial, and ultimately, further investigation is warranted to identify subgroups of patients who are most likely to benefit from this aggressive approach. Recent advances in understanding the molecular biology of cancer have led to the development of targeted systemic therapy. As biologic agents are integrated into chemoradiation regimens, comparisons to standard cisplatin and 5-FU must be performed in phase III trials. As our understanding of the biology of esophageal carcinoma improves, better patient-specific therapies will lead to improved long-term survival.

References

1. Exner A. Veber die Behandlung von Oesophagus Karzinomen mit Ardiumstrahlen. *Wien Klin Wochenschr*. 1904;17:514.
2. Guisez J. Presentation de maladies soignes par la radiumtherapie pour cancer de l'oesophage. *Bull Mem Soc Med Hop Paris*. 1931;47:908–912.
3. Torek F. The first successful case of resection of the thoracic portion of the oesophagus for carcinoma. *Surg Gynecol Obstet*. 1913;16:614–617.
4. Ohsawa T. The surgery of the esophagus. *Arch Jpn Chir*. 1913;16:614–617.
5. Adams W, Phemister D. Carcinoma of the lower thoracic esophagus: report of successful resection and esophagogastrostomy. *J Thoracic Surg*. 1933;7:621–632.
6. Jemal A, Siegel R, Ward E, et al. Cancer statistics, 2006. *CA Cancer J Clin*. 2006;56:106–130.
7. Zak M, Brobnik J. Effect of cis-dichlorodiamine platinum (II) on the post-irradiation lethality in mice after irradiation with X-rays. *Strahlentherapie*. 1971;142:112–115.
8. Richmond RC, Powers EL. Radiation sensitization of bacterial spores by cis-dichlorodiammineplatinum (II). *Radiat Res*. 1976;68:251–257.
9. Douple EB, Richmond RC. Radiosensitization of hypoxic tumor cells by cis- and trans-dichlorodiammineplatinum (II). *Int J Radiat Oncol Biol Phys*. 1979;5:1369–1372.
10. Nigro ND, Vaitkevicius VK, Considine B Jr. Combined therapy for cancer of the anal canal: a preliminary report. *Dis Colon Rectum*. 1974;17:354–356.
11. Sischy B, Doggett RL, Krall JM, et al. Definitive irradiation and chemotherapy for radiosensitization in management of anal carcinoma: interim report on Radiation Therapy Oncology Group study no. 8314. *J Natl Cancer Inst*. 1989;81:850–856.
12. Flam M, John M, Pajak TF, et al. Role of mitomycin in combination with fluorouracil and radiotherapy, and of salvage chemoradiation in the definitive nonsurgical treatment of epidermoid carcinoma of the anal canal: results of a phase III randomized intergroup study. *J Clin Oncol*. 1996;14:2527–2539.
13. Bartelink H, Roelofsen F, Eschwege F, et al. Concomitant radiotherapy and chemotherapy is superior to radiotherapy alone in the treatment of locally advanced anal cancer: results of a phase III randomized trial of the European Organization for Research and Treatment of Cancer Radiotherapy and Gastrointestinal Cooperative Groups. *J Clin Oncol*. 1997;15:2040–2049.
14. Schaake-Koning C, van den Bogaert W, Dalesio O, et al. Effects of concomitant cisplatin and radiotherapy on inoperable non-small-cell lung cancer. *N Engl J Med*. 1992;326:524–530.
15. Soresi E, Clerici M, Grilli R, et al. A randomized clinical trial comparing radiation therapy v radiation therapy plus cis-dichlorodiammine platinum (II) in the treatment of locally advanced non-small cell lung cancer. *Semin Oncol*. 1988;15:20–25.
16. Aisner J, Forastiere A, Aroney R. Patterns of recurrence for cancer of the lung and esophagus. *Cancer Treat Symp*. 1983;2:87.
17. Fujimake M, Soga J, Kawaguchi M, et al. Role of preoperative administration of bleomycin and radiation in the treatment of esophageal cancer. *Jpn J Surg*. 1975;5:48–55.
18. Herskovic A, Leichman L, Lattin P, et al. Chemo/radiation with and without surgery in the thoracic esophagus: the Wayne State experience. *Int J Radiat Oncol Biol Phys*. 1988;15:655–662.
19. Coia LR, Engstrom PF, Paul AR, et al. Long-term results of infusional 5-FU, mitomycin-C and radiation as primary management of esophageal carcinoma. *Int J Radiat Oncol Biol Phys*. 1991;20:29–36.
20. Herskovic A, Martz K, al-Sarraf M, et al. Combined chemotherapy and radiotherapy compared with radiotherapy alone in patients with cancer of the esophagus. *N Engl J Med*. 1992;326:1593–1598.
21. Araujo CM, Souhami L, Gil RA, et al. A randomized trial comparing radiation therapy versus concomitant radiation therapy and chemotherapy in carcinoma of the thoracic esophagus. *Cancer*. 1991;67:2258–2261.
22. Smith TJ, Ryan LM, Douglass HO Jr, et al. Combined chemoradiotherapy vs. radiotherapy alone for early stage squamous cell carcinoma of the esophagus: a study of the Eastern Cooperative Oncology Group. *Int J Radiat Oncol Biol Phys*. 1998;42:269–276.
23. Minsky BD, Pajak TF, Ginsberg RJ, et al. INT 0123 (Radiation Therapy Oncology Group 94–05) phase III trial of combined-modality therapy for esophageal cancer: high-dose versus standard-dose radiation therapy. *J Clin Oncol*. 2002;20:1167–1174.
24. Adelstein DJ, Rice TW, Becker M, et al. Use of concurrent chemotherapy, accelerated fractionation radiation, and surgery for patients with esophageal carcinoma. *Cancer*. 1997;80:1011–1020.
25. Choi N, Park SD, Lynch T, et al. Twice-daily radiotherapy as concurrent boost technique during two chemotherapy cycles in neoadjuvant chemoradiotherapy for resectable esophageal carcinoma: mature results of phase II study. *Int J Radiat Oncol Biol Phys*. 2004;60:111–122.
26. Bedenne L, Michel P, Bouche O, et al. Chemoradiation followed by surgery compared with chemoradiation alone in squamous cancer of the esophagus: FFCD 9102. *J Clin Oncol*. 2007;25:1160–1168.
27. Stahl M, Stuschke M, Lehmann N, et al. Chemoradiation with and without surgery in patients with locally advanced squamous cell carcinoma of the esophagus. *J Clin Oncol*. 2005;23:2310–2317.
28. Vermorken JB, Remenar E, van Herpen C, et al. Cisplatin, fluorouracil, and docetaxel in unresectable head and neck cancer. *N Engl J Med*. 2007;357:1695–1704.
29. Posner MR, Hershock DM, Blajman CR, et al. Cisplatin and fluorouracil alone or with docetaxel in head and neck cancer. *N Engl J Med*. 2007;357:1705–1715.
30. Ajani JA, Komaki R, Putnam JB, et al. A three-step strategy of induction chemotherapy then chemoradiation followed by surgery in patients with potentially resectable carcinoma of the esophagus or gastroesophageal junction. *Cancer*. 2001;92:279–286.
31. Komaki R, Winter K, Ajani A, et al. 142: A randomized phase II study of two paclitaxel-based chemoradiotherapy regimens for patients with the non–operative esophageal carcinoma (RTOG 0113). *Int J Radiat Oncol Biol Phys*. 2006;66:S79–S80.
32. Kitagawa Y, Ueda M, Ando N, et al. Further evidence for prognostic significance of epidermal growth factor receptor gene amplification in patients with esophageal squamous cell carcinoma. *Clin Cancer Res*. 1996;2:909–914.
33. Ozawa S, Ueda M, Ando N, et al. Prognostic significance of epidermal growth factor receptor in esophageal squamous cell carcinomas. *Cancer*. 1989;63:2169–2173.
34. Itakura Y, Sasano H, Shiga C, et al. Epidermal growth factor receptor overexpression in esophageal carcinoma. An immunohistochemical study correlated with clinicopathologic findings and DNA amplification. *Cancer*. 1994;74:795–804.
35. Yoshida K, Kuniyasu H, Yasui W, et al. Expression of growth factors and their receptors in human esophageal carcinomas: regulation of expression by epidermal growth factor and transforming growth factor alpha. *J Cancer Res Clin Oncol*. 1993;119:401–407.
36. Gibson MK, Abraham SC, Wu TT, et al. Epidermal growth factor receptor, p53 mutation, and pathological response predict survival in patients with locally advanced esophageal cancer treated with preoperative chemoradiotherapy. *Clin Cancer Res*. 2003;9:6461–6468.
37. Bonner JA, Harari PM, Giralt J, et al. Radiotherapy plus cetuximab for squamous-cell carcinoma of the head and neck. *N Engl J Med*. 2006;354:567–578.
38. Enzinger PC, Yock T, Suh W, et al. Phase II cisplatin, irinotecan, cetuximab and concurrent radiation therapy followed by surgery for locally advanced esophageal cancer. *J Clin Oncol (Meeting Abstracts)*. 2006;24:4064.
39. Suntharalingam M, Dipetrillo T, Akerman P, et al. Cetuximab, paclitaxel, carboplatin and radiation for esophageal and gastric cancer. *J Clin Oncol (Meeting Abstracts)*. 2006;24:4029.
40. al-Kasspooles M, Moore JH, Orringer MB, et al. Amplification and over-expression of the EGFR and erbB-2 genes in human esophageal adenocarcinomas. *Int J Cancer*. 1993;54:213–219.
41. Dahlberg PS, Jacobson BA, Dahal G, et al. ERBB2 amplifications in esophageal adenocarcinoma. *Ann Thorac Surg*. 2004;78:1790–1800.
42. Shiga K, Shiga C, Sasano H, et al. Expression of c-erbB-2 in human esophageal carcinoma cells: overexpression correlated with gene amplification or with GATA-3 transcription factor expression. *Anticancer Res*. 1993;13:1293–1301.

43. Safran H, DiPetrillo T, Nadeem A, et al. Trastuzumab, paclitaxel, cisplatin, and radiation for adenocarcinoma of the esophagus: a phase I study. *Cancer Invest.* 2004;22:670–677.
44. Gorski DH, Beckett MA, Jaskowiak NT, et al. Blockage of the vascular endothelial growth factor stress response increases the antitumor effects of ionizing radiation. *Cancer Res.* 1999;59:3374–3378.
45. Keane TJ, Harwood AR, Elhakim T, et al. Radical radiation therapy with 5-fluorouracil infusion and mitomycin C for oesophageal squamous carcinoma. *Radiother Oncol.* 1985;4:205–210.
46. John MJ, Flam MS, Mowry PA, et al. Radiotherapy alone and chemoradiation for nonmetastatic esophageal carcinoma. A critical review of chemoradiation. *Cancer.* 1989;63:2397–2403.
47. Wobbes T, Baron B, Paillot B, et al. Prospective randomised study of split-course radiotherapy versus cisplatin plus split-course radiotherapy in inoperable squamous cell carcinoma of the oesophagus. *Eur J Cancer.* 2001;37:470–477.
48. Cooper JS, Guo MD, Herskovic A, et al. Chemoradiotherapy of locally advanced esophageal cancer: long-term follow-up of a prospective randomized trial (RTOG 85–01). Radiation Therapy Oncology Group. *JAMA.* 1999;281:1623–1627.

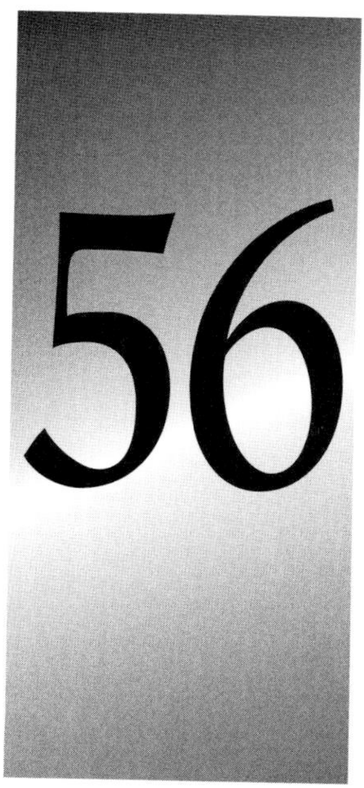

56 Endoscopic Therapies for Barrett's Esophagus

Joep J. Gondrie
F.P. Peters
R.E. Pouw
Jacques J.G.H.M. Bergman

Endoscopic therapy has been proven to be safe and effective for early Barrett's neoplasia, with complete remission rates of 83% to 100%. Achieving such high remission rates depends on adequate patient selection, identifying those patients with only localized disease who have a low- or absent-risk of lymph node metastasis. For adequate patient selection, a systematic endoscopic work-up using high-quality endoscopes and adequate sampling of the Barrett's segment with expert histologic evaluation is necessary. A definitive diagnosis and assessment of the risk of lymph node involvement can be made by endoscopic resection of neoplastic lesions, since it provides a specimen for histologic evaluation. Different endoscopic resection techniques are available, of which the endoscopic cap resection technique after mucosal lifting is the most widely used. The ligate-and-cut technique using the novel multiband mucosectomy kit has made endoscopic resection of large areas of flat mucosa easier, possibly safer and faster. Long-term remission rates are best achieved by eradication of the complete Barrett's segment. Most endoscopic ablation techniques (i.e., photodynamic therapy and argon plasma coagulation) do not achieve complete Barrett's eradication in most patients and are associated with foci of Barrett's glands covered with neosquamous epithelium (a.k.a., buried Barrett's). Persistent genetic abnormalities and recurrences of neoplasia are still frequently seen after ablation. Radical endoscopic resection of the complete Barrett's segment results in complete eradication of all Barrett's mucosa in most patients without persistent genetic abnormalities in the neosquamous epithelium, a lower rate of buried Barrett's, and possibly a lower recurrence rate. This approach, however, also leads to symptomatic esophageal stenosis in a significant percentage of patients. A novel endoscopic ablation technique, making use of radiofrequency energy, may prove to be an effective technique without aforementioned drawbacks.

With the evolution of endoscopic imaging and treatment of Barrett's esophagus and early Barrett's neoplasia, the management of Barrett's esophagus patients has become highly specialized. To be able to determine the optimal endoscopic treatment strategy with good short-term *and* long-term results for patients with early Barrett's neoplasia, systematic prospective registration of treated patients with reporting of long-term follow-up results is imperative. The management of patients with early Barrett's neoplasia and research into management of these patients should, therefore, be performed in expert centers with expert endoscopists, pathologists, and surgeons.

The first report on Barrett's esophagus (BE) was in 1950 by Norman Barrett. Since then, several definitions of BE have been proposed (1). The currently used definition of BE in the United States is that Barrett's esophagus is a change in the esophageal epithelium of any length that can be recognized at endoscopy and is confirmed to have intestinal metaplasia (IM) by biopsy of the tubular esophagus and excludes intestinal metaplasia of the cardia (2–4).

BE is thought to be a result of long-standing severe reflux of gastric and duodenal contents into the esophagus. It is assumed that the normal squamous epithelium is replaced by mucus-secreting columnar mucosa in order to protect the tubular esophagus against the erosive effect of gastroduodenal content.

The typical BE patient is an obese middle-aged Caucasian male. The prevalence of BE is estimated at 10% of patients undergoing upper endoscopy for reflux-associated symptoms (5), whereas a recent large-sized population-based Swedish study showed a population prevalence of 1.6% (6).

A premalignant condition, BE may progress to carcinoma through a metaplasia-neoplasia-carcinoma-pathway in a rate of 0.5% per year (7–9). This pathway is accompanied by several oncogenetic alterations, like numerical chromosomal changes, specific losses of tumor suppressor genes (e.g., p16 and p53), or gains of oncogenes (e.g., HER2/neu) as well as increased expression of certain proteins (e.g., Ki67) (10–21).

The presence of the premalignant Barrett's esophagus, together with this multistep pathway, enables the detection of early neoplastic lesions before an advanced and often incurable adenocarcinoma becomes symptomatic. This is the reason why regular endoscopic surveillance is advised for patients with a known Barrett's esophagus (4). This endoscopic surveillance is aimed at detecting early neoplastic changes in the Barrett's segment, such as high-grade intraepithelial neoplasia (HGIN) or early adenocarcinoma (EAC; i.e., mucosal or superficial submucosal lesions) with a more favorable prognosis (22,23).

The standard treatment of HGIN and EAC used to be surgical esophagectomy. This is an invasive treatment modality with significant morbidity and mortality rates that also reduces quality of life (24,25). These early neoplastic Barrett's lesions have a very low rate (0%–2%) of local lymph node involvement (26–28). Therefore, effective endoscopic therapy of the primary lesion may cure these patients without the need for esophagectomy. A variety of endoscopic resection and ablation techniques are now available for treatment of HGIN and EAC in BE. Studies have shown that in expert hands, endoscopic treatment of early neoplasia in BE is safe and effective in selected patients (29–31).

This review will discuss the adequate selection of BE patients who may be eligible for endoscopic treatment and the different endoscopic techniques available. In addition, we will make recommendations for the (endoscopic) management of Barrett's patients.

PATIENT SELECTION

Most experts consider non-dysplastic BE not an indication for endoscopic resection and ablation. The reason for this is 2-fold:

1. The chances of progression to EAC are small in this category of patients (0.5% per patient year) (5,6);
2. Currently available treatment options are technically demanding, do not result in complete removal of BE or require multiple treatment sessions, are associated with complications, and/or are expensive.

The currently held opinion is therefore that patients with a non-dysplastic BE have little to gain and more to lose by endoscopic treatment. The opposite is true for patients who show unequivocal neoplastic progression (i.e., HGIN or EAC). For these patients, however, proper selection is imperative: basic rule is that only patients with mucosal lesions should be treated endoscopically whereas those with deeper invading lesions are best treated surgically given their chances of local lymph node metastasis. We will discuss the endoscopic work-up of these patients, the histopathologic evaluation of tissue specimens, and procedures required for the staging early neoplastic lesions in BE.

ENDOSCOPIC WORK-UP

During endoscopic work-up, the esophagus of patients with (possible) early Barrett's neoplasia is "mapped." The work-up is aimed at detecting all neoplastic lesions in the Barrett's segment and identifying the most advanced lesion, which is most important to determine the appropriate management strategy. Basic guidelines for optimal endoscopic imaging of Barrett's esophagus encompass 3 variables: the quality of the video-endoscope, the experience of the endoscopist, and a systematic endoscopic approach.

Following the inspection of the Barrett's segment and classification of visible lesions, biopsies should be obtained from all visible lesions, followed by random 4-quadrant biopsies for every 2 centimeters of the Barrett's segment. We follow the principle *"look longer, biopsy less,"* since we believe that thorough inspection followed by targeted biopsies is more important than obtaining random biopsies (32). In the absence of visible lesions, however, random biopsies should still be obtained.

Macroscopically visible lesions are classified according to the Paris classification (33,34), adopted from the Japanese Gastric Cancer Association (35). In this classification type 0 is used for superficial lesions, which is divided into 3 categories. The 0-I and 0-II types are amendable for endoscopic treatment with 0-I and 0-IIc being associated with a higher risk for submucosal invasion. Type 0-III is not suited for endoscopic therapy since these lesions always invade into the submucosa (36).

For optimal endoscopic detection, characterization, and delineation, several advanced imaging techniques are available such as chromoendoscopy, narrow band imaging (NBI), autofluorescence imaging (AFI), and confocal endomicroscopy. The exact role of these techniques has to be defined and none has yet emerged as the imaging technique of choice.

HISTOPATHOLOGIC EVALUATION

The histopathologic evaluation determines the individual patient management, either endoscopic surveillance (non-dysplastic BE and low-grade intestinal neoplasia), endoscopic therapy (HGIN and intramucosal cancer), or surgery (submucosal invading lesions). The histologic evaluation of a biopsy specimen is based on multiple morphologic characteristics, such as (among others) cellularity, presence and distribution of undifferentiated-atypical cells, presence of normal gradual differentiation toward the surface and size, and shape and polarity of nuclei.

The revised Vienna classification is used to classify neoplastic changes in BE (known as intraepithelial neoplasia [IEN]) (37,38). This classification incorporates 5 catergories: non-neoplastic BE, indefinite for neoplasia, low-grade intraepithelial neoplasia (LGIN), high-grade intraepithelial neoplasia (HGIN), and invasive carcinoma. The reliability of the diagnosis appears to increase when an expert pathologist or a second pathologist agrees on the diagnosis. It is therefore strongly advised to have histopathologic specimens reviewed by an expert pathologist before invasive treatment is advised (39). The additional value of molecular markers (e.g., Ki-67, p16, p53, and Her-2/neu) to assist in the grading of IEN will be discussed in other chapters. The histopathologic evaluation of routine tissue slides, however, remains the gold standard for the grading of IEN in BE.

STAGING OF EARLY NEOPLASTIC LESIONS

Infiltration Depth

The most important prerequisite for successful endoscopic treatment is the absence of local lymph node metastases. Lymph node involvement is associated with increasing infiltration depth, a poor differentiation grade and lymphatic vascular involvement (4,27,40,41). Infiltration depth of T1 tumors (i.e., infiltration up to the level of the muscularis propria) in Barrett's esophagus is often classified into 5 to 7 categories. Mucosal lesions are subdivided into 3 or 4 categories, depending on the presence of a double muscularis mucosae, which is often the case in Barrett's esophagus (42). T1m1 indicates that the tumor is limited to the epithelial layer, T1m2 indicates infiltration into the lamina propria, and T1m3/4 indicates infiltration into the (first or second) muscularis mucosae layer. The submucosa is usually divided into 3 equal parts: T1sm1–3. There are strikingly few studies available about risk of lymph node involvement in early Barrett's neoplasia compared to early esophageal squamous cell carcinomas and early gastric carcinomas. With the available data we can conclude that lymph node metastases are never encountered in patients with HGIN (0%: 95% confidence interval [CI]: 0–0) and are only rarely present in patients with mucosal cancers (1.4%; CI:-3.25–6.05) (26–28).

Assessment of infiltration depth is thus important for determining the optimal treatment strategy for the patient. Are there ways to reliably assess this prior to endoscopic or surgical resection? As described earlier, the endoscopic aspect of a lesion may predict its infiltration depth. For Barrett's neoplasia, however, there are not enough data available to determine the depth of infiltration with enough certainty based on the endoscopic view alone.

Endoscopic Ultrasonography

Endoscopic ultrasonography (EUS) is currently the most important and most accurate technique for T and N staging in esophageal cancer and is superior to CT scanning (43). The overall accuracy of standard 7.5–12-MHz EUS in the assessment of infiltration depth, including squamous cell carcinomas and advanced carcinomas, is approximately 75% (44,45). The diagnostic accuracy of EUS pertaining to lymph node involvement (N-stage) has been reported to range from 68% to 86% (46,47). Compared to other imaging techniques, such as CT-scanning, the endosonographic assessment of malignant lymph nodes is clearly superior (47,48), and standard EUS is superior to high frequency miniprobes due to the deeper penetration. With EUS-guided fine needle aspiration (EUS-FNA), suspicious lymph nodes can be sampled to obtain a cytologic diagnosis. EUS-FNA can increase the specificity of EUS N-staging and in advanced cancers the accuracy of EUS N-staging can be increased up to 90%. For the work-up and staging of patients with early lesions, N-staging is of crucial importance: positive lymph nodes will exclude the patient from endoscopic treatment.

Endoscopic Resection as a Staging Tool

For completing and optimizing the T-staging of early Barrett's neoplasia, the lesion can be endoscopically resected. The resection provides a specimen that can be histologically evaluated, leading to an objective T-stage diagnosis (49–52). If the histology of the resection specimen shows a radically removed *mucosal* lesion, the diagnostic endoscopic resection also was the first step in the endoscopic treatment of the patient. The chances of having positive lymph nodes in this patient are then smaller (i.e., < 2%) than the mortality of an esophagectomy justifying subsequent endoscopic management. If the specimen shows a poorly or undifferentiated cancer, if the cancer has a positive vertical resection margin or invades into the submucosa, the patient can still be referred for surgery with no significant delay.

RECOMMENDATIONS FOR WORK-UP AND STAGING OF PATIENTS WITH EARLY BARRETT'S NEOPLASIA

Patients with early Barrett's neoplasia are eligible for endoscopic therapy if they have an endoscopically resectable lesion without (or with a low risk of) lymph node and distant metastases. This is generally the case in patients with a well or moderately differentiated, type 0-I or 0-II lesion, with a maximum infiltration depth of T1m3(-4). In individual cases poorly differentiated and superficial submucosal (T1sm1) lesions can be eligible too (e.g., in case of significant contraindications for surgery).

The work-up of patients with (possible) early Barrett's neoplasia should be performed by an endoscopist with expertise in the endoscopic inspection of Barrett's esophagus using state-of-the-art endoscopic equipment. The endoscopic work-up should be aimed at identification of the most suspicious area and all surrounding additional abnormal areas, after which the infiltration depth of the most suspicious lesion should be determined. EUS can be used for to identify lesions with overt deep (T2–4) invasion but these are usually recognized as such endoscopically. In all other early lesions, infiltration depth can best and objectively be assessed with a diagnostic endoscopic resection.

N- and M-staging plays a minor role in most patients with early Barrett's neoplasia, due to the low risk of lymph node involvement and distant metastasis. Until further evidence, however, N-staging with EUS and, in case of suspicious lymph nodes, EUS-FNA should be performed in patients with early neoplasia. M-staging with CT-scanning of thorax and abdomen and an ultrasound of the neck should be performed in patients with (suspicion of) submucosal infiltration.

In case of deep submucosal infiltration and no contraindications for surgery, the patient should be referred for esophagectomy.

ENDOSCOPIC THERAPY

Endoscopic treatment of early BE neoplasia can be divided into 2 main categories: endoscopic resection and endoscopic ablation techniques. Endoscopic resection (ER) techniques are safe and effective for removal of superficial focal lesions with the advantage of histopathologic correlation (52–56). However, ER is less suitable for the resection of larger lesions since piecemeal resection is often necessary, making it impossible to be conclusive about the radicality of the resection at the lateral margins. Endoscopic ablation therapy, such as photodynamic therapy (PDT), argon plasma coagulation (APC), and radiofrequency ablation (RFA), allows for treatment of larger areas but does not provide a specimen for histopathologic evaluation (31,57–59). In Europe and Japan, endoscopic resection is considered the cornerstone of endoscopic therapy and ablative therapy is mainly used as an adjunct. In the United States, endoscopic resection is less frequently used and ablative therapy is used as the primary endoscopic treatment in most centers.

Endoscopic Resection Techniques

A wide variety of endoscopic resection techniques are available. Most of them have been developed in Japan for treatment of early gastric cancer or squamous cancer of the esophagus. In BE, the endoscopic cap resection technique (ER-cap) (Figure 56.1) (60,61) and the ligate-and-cut-technique (Figure 56.2) (62,63) are most widely used. In both techniques the mucosa is sucked into a cap, placed on the tip of the endoscope thus creating a pseudopolyp. The pseudopolyp is tightened with a snare in the ER cap technique or with a rubber band in the the ligate-and-cut-technique. In both techniques, the pseudopolyp is subsequently resected using electrocoagulation.

Recommendations for When to Use Which ER Technique

May et al. compared 50 ER-cap resections with 50 ligate-and-cut resections in Barrett's esophagus and found both techniques to be equally efficient and safe (64). A number of studies have retrospectively compared the ligate-and-cut technique with the endoscopic cap technique, but there is not enough prospective randomized data available to make an evidence based choice (63,65). For endoscopic resection of small focal lesions (i.e., < 10 mm), en bloc resection with the ligate-and-cut technique is a safe, easy, and effective method. Focal lesions with a diameter between 10 and 20 mm can be best resected using the ER-cap technique with a flexible large caliber cap since this allows for the largest resection specimen increasing the chances of a radical en bloc resection. Focal lesions with a diameter larger than 20 mm will generally require piecemeal resection, which can be performed with the ER-cap technique or the ligate-and-cut technique.

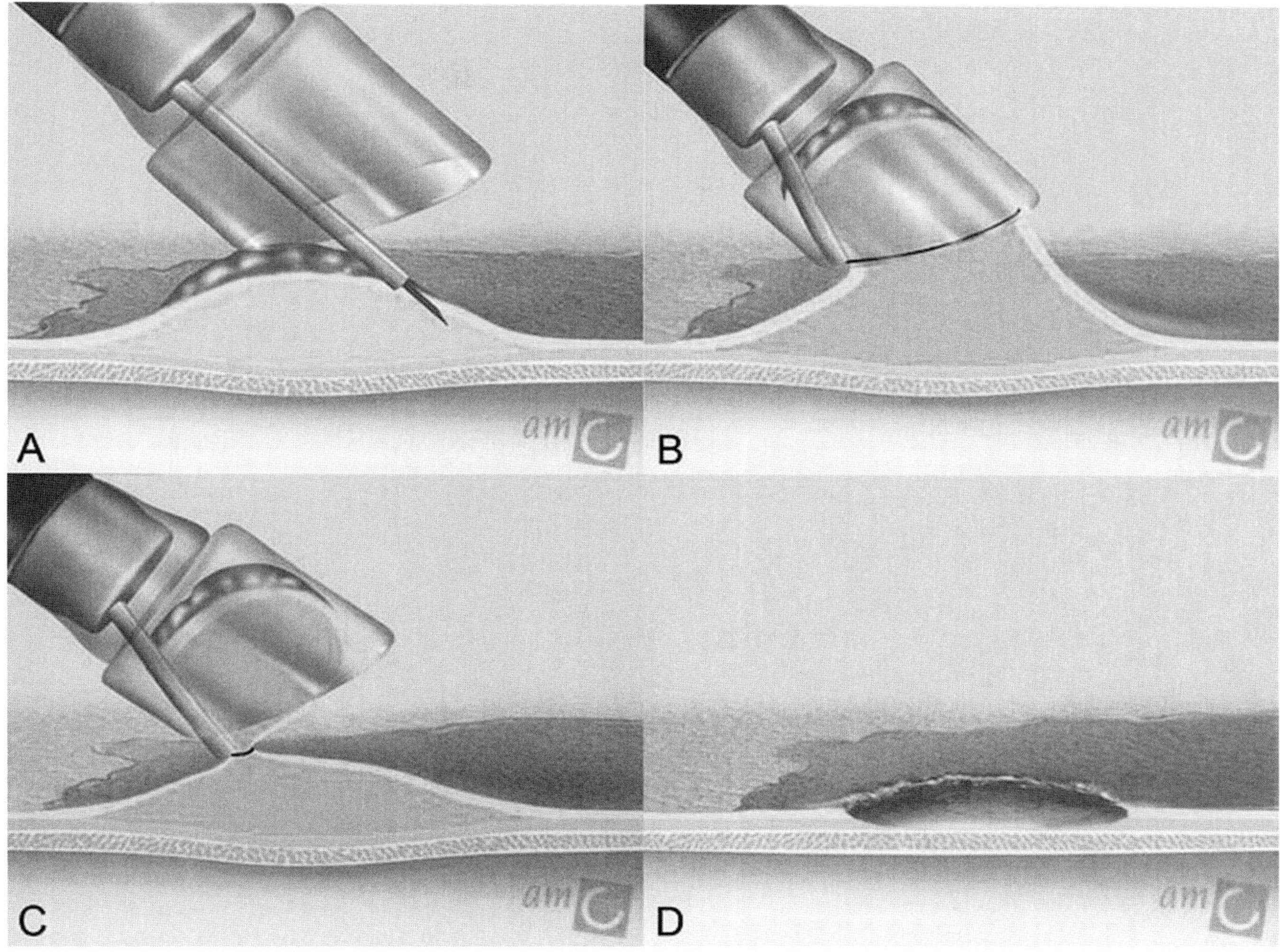

FIGURE 56.1

The endoscopic cap resection technique. The target area is first marked and lifted with submucosal fluid injection before or after placement of a transparent ER-cap (A). After placement of the ER-snare in the ridge of the ER-cap, the target area is aspirated into the ER-cap (B). Subsequently the snare is tightened (C), and the target area is resected (D). Reproduced with permission of http://www.barrett.nl.

Clinical Results with Endoscopic Resection as Monotherapy

Clinical studies of focal Barrett's lesions treated with ER as monotherapy are scarce (29,66). In most centers, patients with residual neoplasia after ER undergo some sort of additional therapy to prevent recurrent or metachronous lesions elsewhere in the Barrett's segment during follow-up (29).

PHOTODYNAMIC THERAPY

Photodynamic therapy (PDT) is the most widely used ablation technique for treatment of early neoplasia in Barrett's esophagus (Figure 56.3). There are 3 essential components in PDT: a drug, light, and oxygen. For PDT a drug is administered that sensitizes (neoplastic) tissue for visible light: a photosensitizer. Illumination of tissues that contain the drug with light of the appropriate wavelength activates the drug. The activated drug absorbs the energy delivered by the light. This energy is transferred to molecular oxygen within the tissue, and this transfer leads to the creation of highly reactive singlet oxygen that produces cell damage. The cell damage subsequently causes delayed cell death by necrosis and apoptosis (67,68). Mainly cellular and mitochondrial membranes are damaged, but nucleic acids and proteins are also affected. To ensure a sufficient oxygen

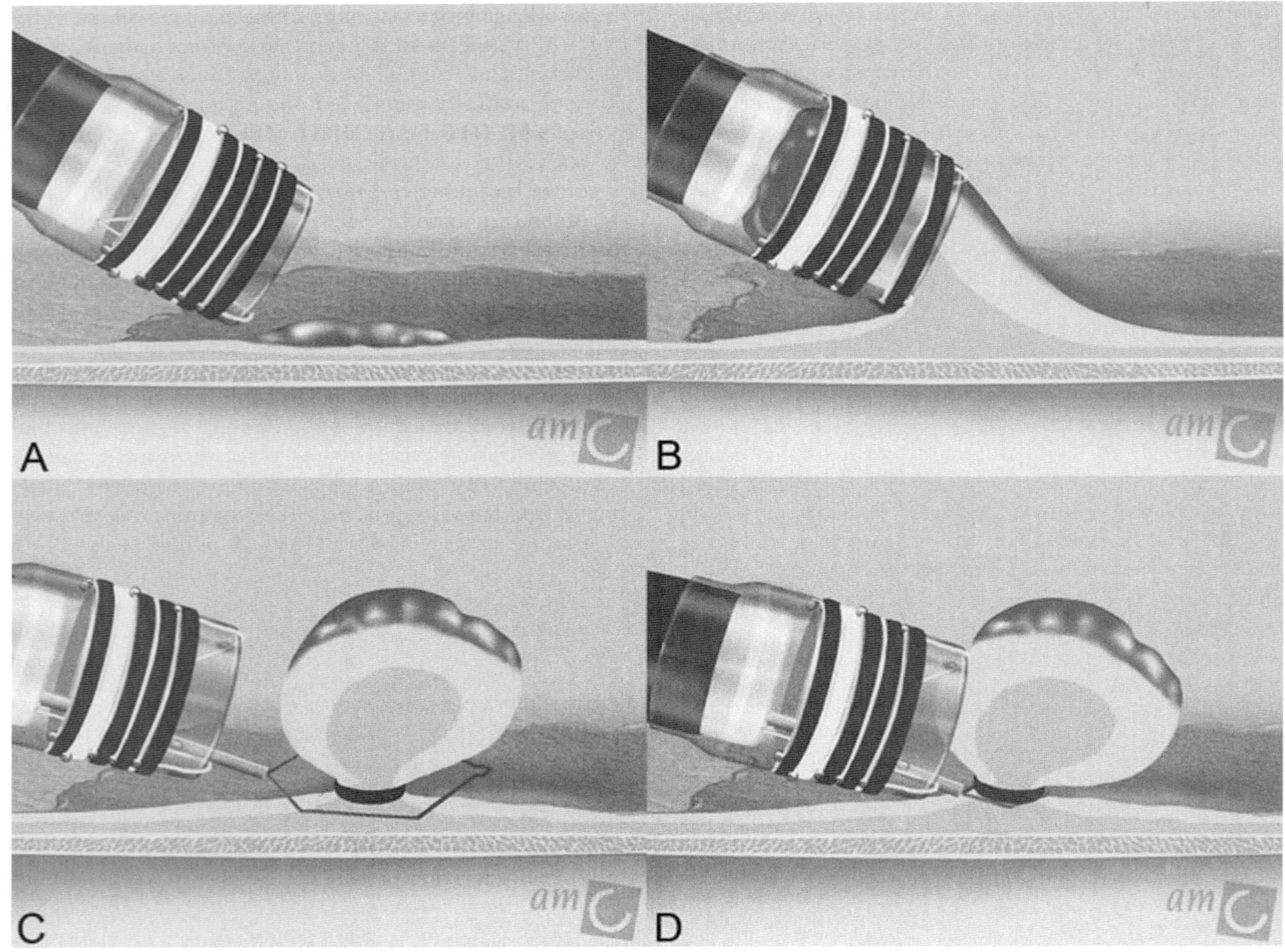

FIGURE 56.2

The ligate-and-cut endoscopic resection technique. With or without (A) prior submucosal lifting, the lesion is sucked into the cap (B) and the rubber band is released, creating a pseudopolyp (C) that is subsequently resected (D). Reproduced with permission of http://www.barrett.nl.

concentration in blood and tissue during treatment patients receive oxygen nasally, and there is some evidence that hyperbaric oxygen may increase the efficacy of PDT (69–71). The tissue damage is delayed and becomes visible 8 to 12 hours after the procedure. This makes the targeted treatment of areas more difficult because there is no direct positional feedback. In many centers, therefore, the patients undergo an endoscopy 24 hours after the treatment to assess the treated area.

The exact method of action, the required wavelength for optimal excitations, and the efficacy and depth of tissue ablation all depend on the type of photosensitizer (e.g., sodium porfimer [Photofrin II], 5-aminolevulinic acid [5-ALA], or meso-tetrahydroxyphenylchlorine [mTHPC]).

Clinical Results of PDT for Early Barrett's Neoplasia

Clinical results obtained in Barrett's esophagus patients with early neoplasia with 5-ALA-PDT, sodium porfimer PDT, and mTHPC are shown in Table 56.1. The initial success rate of 5-ALA-PDT and sodium porfimer PDT for eradication of the neoplastic lesions with both sensitizers is high: 84% for 5-ALA-PDT and 81% for sodium porfimer PDT (not significantly different). The recurrence rates of both techniques are also comparable with 16% for 5-ALA-PDT and 18% for sodium porfimer PDT. Differences between the 2 sensitizers are most pronounced in the stenosis rate, which is 0% for 5-ALA and 33% for sodium porfimer and in the rate of

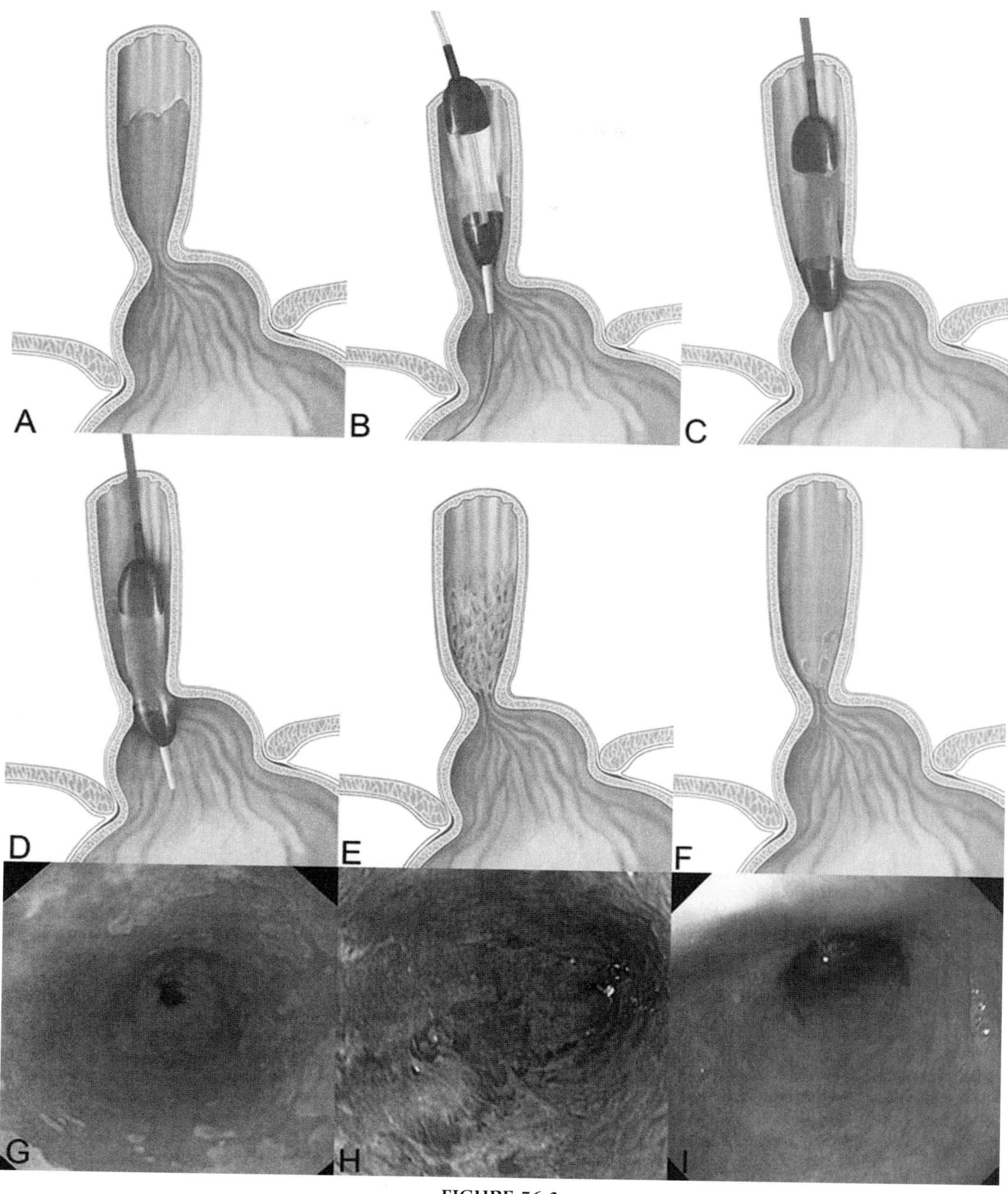

FIGURE 56.3

Photodynamic therapy of Barrett's esophagus. A and G: Pretreatment image of a Barrett's segment, after administration of photosensitizer. B: Insertion of the PDT-balloon over a guidewire. C: Insertion of the laser fiber in the center of the PDT-balloon under guidance of green laser light. D: Treatment of the Barrett's segment with laser light of the appropriate wavelength. E and H: Image of the treated Barrett's segment 24 hours after the procedure, with necrosis of the mucosal layer. F and I: Image of the distal esophagus weeks after the PDT treatment with regeneration with neosquamous mucosa and residual Barrett's islets. Reproduced with permission of http://www.barrett.nl.

development of buried Barrett's (Table 56.1). Although these rates are not statistically different in this limited number of series, there seems to be a trend toward a higher rate in 5-ALA-PDT than in sodium porfimer PDT. This may be explained by the less deep effect that is accomplished with 5-ALA-PDT.

A study by Prasad et al. presented at the Digestive Disease Week (DDW) 2006 showed that the pretreatment presence of a loss of the p16 tumor suppressor gene independently predicted the response to PDT with an odds ratio of 0.12. Assessment of the p16 status before treatment may therefore be used to select patients that may

TABLE 56.1
Clinical Results of Photodynamic Therapy and Argon Plasma Coagulation for the Eradication of Dysplastic Barrett's Esophagus or Early Carcinoma in Barrett's Esophagus

Technique	Author	Patients	Complete eradication neoplasia	Regression BE	Buried Barrett's	Stenosis	Recurrence
5-ALA-PDT	Barr	5	100%	na	40%	na	na
5-ALA-PDT	Gossner	32	84%	68%	7%	na	7%
5-ALA-PDT	Ackroyd	10	70%	Mean 44%	na	na	0%
5-ALA-PDT	Pech	51	100%	na	na	na	24%
5-ALA-PDT	Peters	20	75%	Median 50%	53%	na	27%
			Median: 84% (IQR 73–100)		**Median: 40% (IQR 7–53)**		**Median: 16% (IQR 2–26)**
porphimer-PDT	Overholt	2	50%	50%	na	na	50%
porphimer-PDT	Laukka	5	100%	Mean 24%	yes	na	na
porphimer-PDT	Overholt	8	88%	na	na	38%	13%
porphimer-PDT	Overholt	12	92%	na	8%	33%	17%
porphimer-PDT	Sibille	19	89%	na	na	35%	75%
porphimer-PDT	Overholt	36	81%	75–80%	6%	58%	0%
porphimer-PDT	Overholt	100	80%	75–80%	5%	34%	23%
porphimer-PDT	Overholt	103	77%	na	5%	30%	na
porphimer-PDT	Wolfsen	102	96%	na	4%	20%	na
porphimer-PDT	Overholt	133	77%	72%	na	75%	13%
porphimer-PDT	Foroulis	25	81%	na	20%	6%	18%
			Median: 81% (IQR 77–92)		**Median: 6% (IQR 5–11)**	**Median: 33% (IQR 6–36)**	**Median: 18% (IQR 13–43)**
APC	Pereira-Lima	33	100%	100%	0%	9%	na
APC	Morris	55	96%	na	30%	na	na
APC	Van Laethem	10	80%	na	30%	1%	na
APC	Attwood	29	86%	76%	na	0	na
APC	Ragunath	13	67%	Median 65%	na	15%	na
			Median: 86% (74–98)		**Median: 30% (IQR 0–30)**	**Median: 10% (IQR 2–14)**	

Abbreviations: BE = Barrett's esophagus; NA = not available data; IQR = interquartile range.

benefit most by PDT. This will, however, limit the use of PDT significantly since almost 75% to 90% of patients with early Barrett's neoplasia have a p16 loss (13,72).

Overholt et al. recently published a 5-year follow-up study in patients receiving porfimer PDT for HGIN (73). Initially, in 77% (n = 106) of the PDT-treated patients complete remission of HGIN was achieved. During the 5-year follow-up, 28 patients (26%) had recurrences of HGIN or cancer. In addition, the probability of maintaining complete remission of HGIN after PDT was 48% after 5 years.

Prasad et al. recently published a study in which they compared the long-term survival of patients treated for HGIN with a combination of endoscopic resection and porfimer-PDT or esophagectomy (74). The overall survival between the 2 treatment options was found to be comparable, despite the recurrence of HGIN in the PDT group of 30% and progression to cancer in 5.4% of PDT treated patients. None of the treated patients died from an EAC. The authors, however, contributed this low mortality rate to their precise and accurate follow-up and subsequent endoscopic resection for neoplastic recurrences.

The limited clinical data available on mTHPC-PDT show a varying success rate with a considerable complication rate and up to now no clear advantages over the other 2 photosensitizers.

Complications and Drawbacks of PDT

The most important long-term complication of PDT is the development of symptomatic, often severe esophageal stenosis (Table 56.1). This complication is almost exclusively seen in sodium porfimer PDT since sodium porfimer accumulates in all esophageal wall layers. After sodium porfimer PDT, stenosis is seen in approximately 33% of patients (Table 56.1) and is more frequent after the treatment of more than one area in one procedure, especially when there is overlap of the subsequent areas and with the use of longer PDT balloons (75,76). Lower energy densities are associated with a lower rate of stenosis but, unfortunately, also with lower efficacy (76).

Another drawback of PDT is the presence of small islands of residual Barrett's mucosa (glands with intestinal metaplasia) located underneath the neosquamous mucosa (buried Barrett's). These buried glands are found in a considerable number of patients in published series (Table 56.1) and in papers specifically evaluating the presence of buried Barrett's, the reported rates are even higher, with 33% and 52% (77). The clinical implications of buried Barrett's are not clear. There have been a number of publications on subsquamous carcinomas arising after PDT, supposedly originating from buried Barrett's mucosa (78–80). Some authors, however, suggest that the malignant potential of buried Barrett's is much lower than normal Barrett's mucosa, since the buried mucosa is no longer exposed to the toxic esophageal contents (81,82). Hornick et al. found that in 68% of the biopsies containing buried Barrett's an extension of the Barrett's mucosa to the surface could be detected, questioning the actual percentage of true buried Barrett's, which is, by these authors, supposed to be undetectable due to the lack of any contact with the surface (82). The fact that upon histologic evaluation, areas of subsquamous Barrett's mucosa apparently can be found to communicate with the surface does, however, not imply that the endoscopist can actually detect these areas. To this end, changing the term *buried Barrett's* to *hidden Barrett's* may be more appropriate (83).

Another important problem associated with PDT is that oncogenetic abnormalities as present before PDT are still present in the residual and recurrent Barrett's mucosa after PDT (84–86). In addition, new oncogenetic abnormalities may be actually induced by the oxygen radicals formed by PDT (87,88).

Persistence of oncogenetic abnormalities in the residual Barrett's mucosa implicates that this mucosa still has malignant potential that may be reflected by the recurrence rate of approximately 20% after PDT.

Summary PDT

PDT is mainly used as additional therapy of the residual Barrett's segment after endoscopic resection of focal lesions with HGIN or EC. The purpose of the additional therapy is eradication of any residual neoplastic changes and prevention of recurrent neoplasia. The initial success rate of PDT in eradicating HGIN and EC is acceptable. The recurrence rates, however, are substantial and are hardly better than the recurrence rates after treatment with endoscopic resection of neoplastic lesions as monotherapy. Considering the primary purposes of PDT, treatment of neoplasia, *and* prevention of recurrences, PDT does not seem to live up to these expectations. This disappointing recurrence rate in combination with the problems of buried Barrett's and persistent and induced genetic abnormalities limits the indications for PDT significantly, and alternatives are desirable.

ARGON PLASMA COAGULATION

Argon plasma coagulation (APC) is another endoscopic ablation technique that is used for treatment of early Barrett's neoplasia and larger areas of (non-)dysplastic Barrett's mucosa (Figure 56.4).

APC is a modality that applies high-frequency electric current to tissue causing its thermal ablation. The

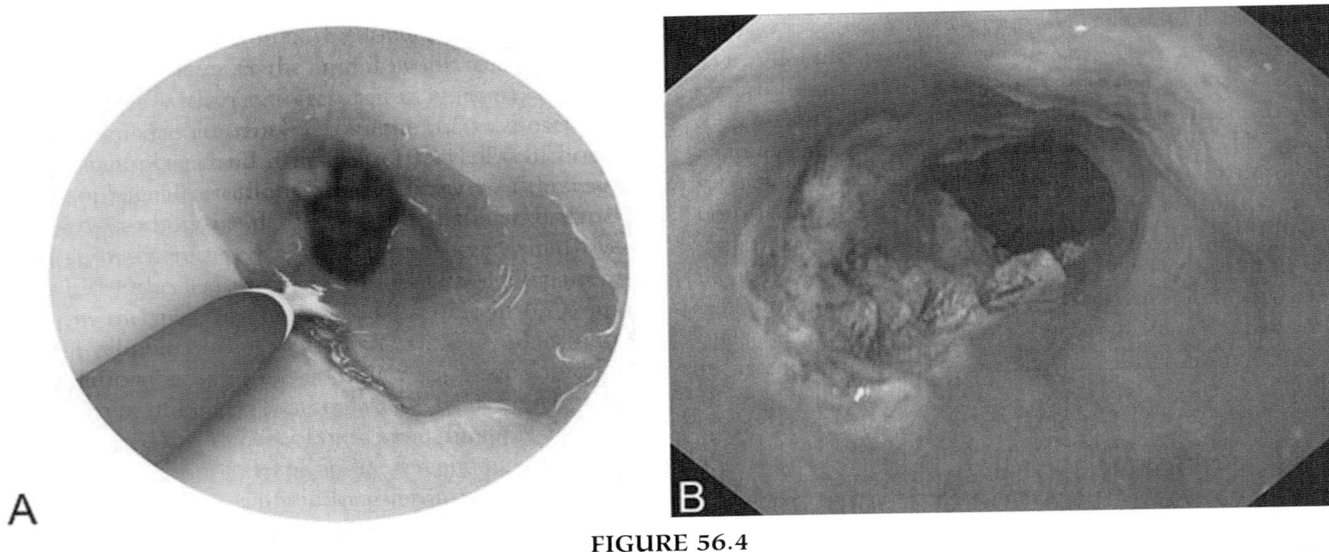

FIGURE 56.4

Argon plasma coagulation ablation. A: Image of argon plasma coagulation of Barrett's mucosa. B: Endoscopic image of the continuous golden-brown coagulum after argon plasma coagulation of Barrett's mucosa. Reproduced with permission of http://www.barrett.nl.

high-frequency current is conducted to the tissue via ionized and therefore electrically conductive argon gas. The current generates heat, causing different thermal effects in zones with different distance to the location of application. In the zone where the current first reaches the tissue, the tissue is devitalized; in the second zone, the tissue is coagulated; in the third zone, the tissue is desiccated; and in the fourth zone, the tissue shrinks. When a location on the tissue surface loses its electric conductivity due to desiccation, the beam automatically changes its direction to a location that still is electrically conductive. This results in a relatively uniform depth of the different zones: the maximum depth of the thermal effects is automatically limited, decreasing the risk of perforation. The maximum depth of the thermal effects is determined by the power settings and the duration of application.

APC requires an argon gas source, high frequency current source, and an applicator to deliver the argon and current to the tissue. The APC probe used in gastrointestinal endoscopy consists of a flexible tube with a lumen for the argon gas flow and a wire connected to an electrode at the tip of the probe for conducting the current (APC-Sonde 2200A, Erbe Elektromedizin GmbH, Tübingen, Germany). The probes fit through the accessory channel of the endoscope and are connected to the APC source and generator (Erbotom ICC 200 and Erbe APC 300, Erbe Elektromedizin GmbH). By placing a neutral electrode on the patient, an electric field is created between the tissue and the electrode in the probe that ionizes the argon gas and creates the high-frequency current to the tissue. The probe should not make contact with the tissue, since the current travels through the gas. In general, low-power settings are safer but less effective than higher settings. For adequate treatment with a treatment depth of approximately 2–3 mm a power of 60–80W is used with an argon gas flow of 1.6–2 L/min. The tissue should be targeted until a homogenous and continuous coagulum has developed there should be no separate patches of coagulum. Care should be taken not to target one location too long and not to make contact between the probe and the tissue, since this could cause a microperforation that can be fatal (89). Besides pain and odynophagia, perforation and stenosis after large-area ablation are the only reported complications of APC. Late perforations may theoretically occur due to transmural necrosis, although this has not been reported in clinical series. It is important to make sure that all the mucosa of the target area is homogeneously ablated, since any residual Barrett's mucosa could give rise to residual Barrett's mucosa after healing or buried Barrett's underneath the regenerated neosquamous mucosa (see PDT section). Buried Barrett's is seen in approximately 15% of the patients treated with APC (Table 56.1) (90–92) and subsquamous carcinoma arising in these buried glands has been reported (93). Technical drawbacks of APC are that the flow of argon gas causes inflation of the stomach, which is uncomfortable for the patient and causes retching and hiccups, complicating the procedure. Second, coagulum can accumulate on the tip of the probe, making, in some cases, repeated cleaning of the probe necessary. Another important drawback of APC is that, in line with PDT, some preexisting genetic abnormalities of the Barrett's epithelium are not completely eradicated by APC. Lopes et al. found overexpression of p53 protein in the neosquamous mucosa after APC (94), and Hage et al. found persistent genetic abnormalities in the persistent Barrett's mucosa after APC (95).

Clinical Results of APC for Treatment of Early Neoplasia in Barrett's Esophagus

Clinical results obtained in the few series of APC ablation of large areas of Barrett's mucosa in patients with early neoplasia are shown in Table 56.1. The median percentage of successful eradication of neoplasia is reasonable with 86% (IQR 73–97) and comparable to that of PDT but with fewer complications and less stenosis. During follow-up, recurrences of neoplastic lesions have not been reported, but few studies with significant follow-up are available. Complete ablation of all Barrett's mucosa is reached in only a minority of patients or requires multiple treatment sessions. Recurrence of Barrett's mucosa is seen in a median of 8% (IQR 5–30) of patients (90,93,96–99). One prospective randomized trial has been performed comparing APC with sodium porfimer PDT for eradication of HGIN (80). This trial showed that sodium porfimer PDT was more effective for eradicating neoplasia (77% vs. 67%, $P = 0.03$) and equally efficient for eradicating Barrett's mucosa. PDT was more expensive than APC. Four prospective randomized trials have been performed comparing APC with either 5-ALA-PDT or multipolar electrocoagulation (MPEC) for ablation of BE without dysplasia or with LGIN (58,95,100,101). One study found APC to be more effective than 5-ALA-PDT in eradication of Barrett's mucosa (100); the other studies showed no significant differences in efficacy of the different treatment modalities.

A German group has recently published a prospective feasibility study in which they treated 131 BE patients with high power APC (30–80W) (VIO APC, Erbe Electromedizin, Tübingen, Germany) with or without prior ER or PDT for HGIN or EAC (102). They reported an overall complication rate of 11% for minor complications (e.g., chest pain, odynophagy) and 1% for major complications (e.g., stricture) at 30W. The minor complication rate increased, however, to 43% if the power was raised to 70W.

In Summary

For eradication of early Barrett's neoplasia, APC has an acceptable success rate comparable with PDT and seems to be associated with fewer recurrences during follow-up (Table 56.1). It is also associated with only partial ablation of BE in most patients with again a significant percentage of buried Barrett's, persistent genetic abnormalities, and recurrence of Barrett's mucosa during follow-up. The technique is time consuming when used for large areas, and it is uncomfortable for the patient. Therefore, we believe that APC is not suitable for ablation of large areas of Barrett's mucosa. It can, however, in some cases be useful for ablation of small residual isles of Barrett's mucosa for example after piecemeal endoscopic resection for eradication of small residual bridges between the resections.

STEPWISE RADICAL ENDOSCOPIC RESECTION

Given the aforementioned limitations of PDT and APC, some centers have treated patients with complete endoscopic resection of the Barrett's segment in multiple sessions. With this stepwise radical endoscopic resection (SRER), all premalignant tissue is completely resected *with* histologic correlation (Figure 56.5). It is expected to induce less buried Barrett's, since endoscopic resection usually extends into the submucosa, leaving no residual Barrett's mucosa behind to be buried. SRER may therefore lead to a permanent cure of Barrett's esophagus and its associated neoplasia.

Seewald et al. published a series of 12 patients with a median Barrett's length of 5 cm (30). They performed endoscopic resections using the simple-snare technique and required a median number of 2.5 sessions with a median of 5 resections per session. There were no severe complications and no recurrence of Barrett's mucosa or neoplasia during a median follow-up of 9 months was observed. Two of 12 patients (17%) developed stenosis managed by bougienage.

The Amsterdam group has reported their SRER experience in 56 patients (103). In the first SRER session, 50% of the BE was removed including the most suspicious area. Subsequent SRER sessions were performed with an interval of 6 to 8 weeks until eradication of all Barrett's mucosa and all neoplasia was achieved. Complete eradication of early neoplasia was achieved in all 56 treated patients (100%). Acute complications occurred in 4 of 165 (2%) endoscopic resection procedures: 1 asymptomatic perforation and 3 delayed bleedings. Stenosis occurred in 24 of 58 (41%) patients but this was effectively treated by endoscopic bougienage.

During a median follow-up of 24 months, only 1 patient showed recurrence of HGIN: after a 17-month follow-up, a 2-mm island of Barrett's mucosa with HGIN was detected and then resected endoscopically. From these data we can conclude that SRER is safe and

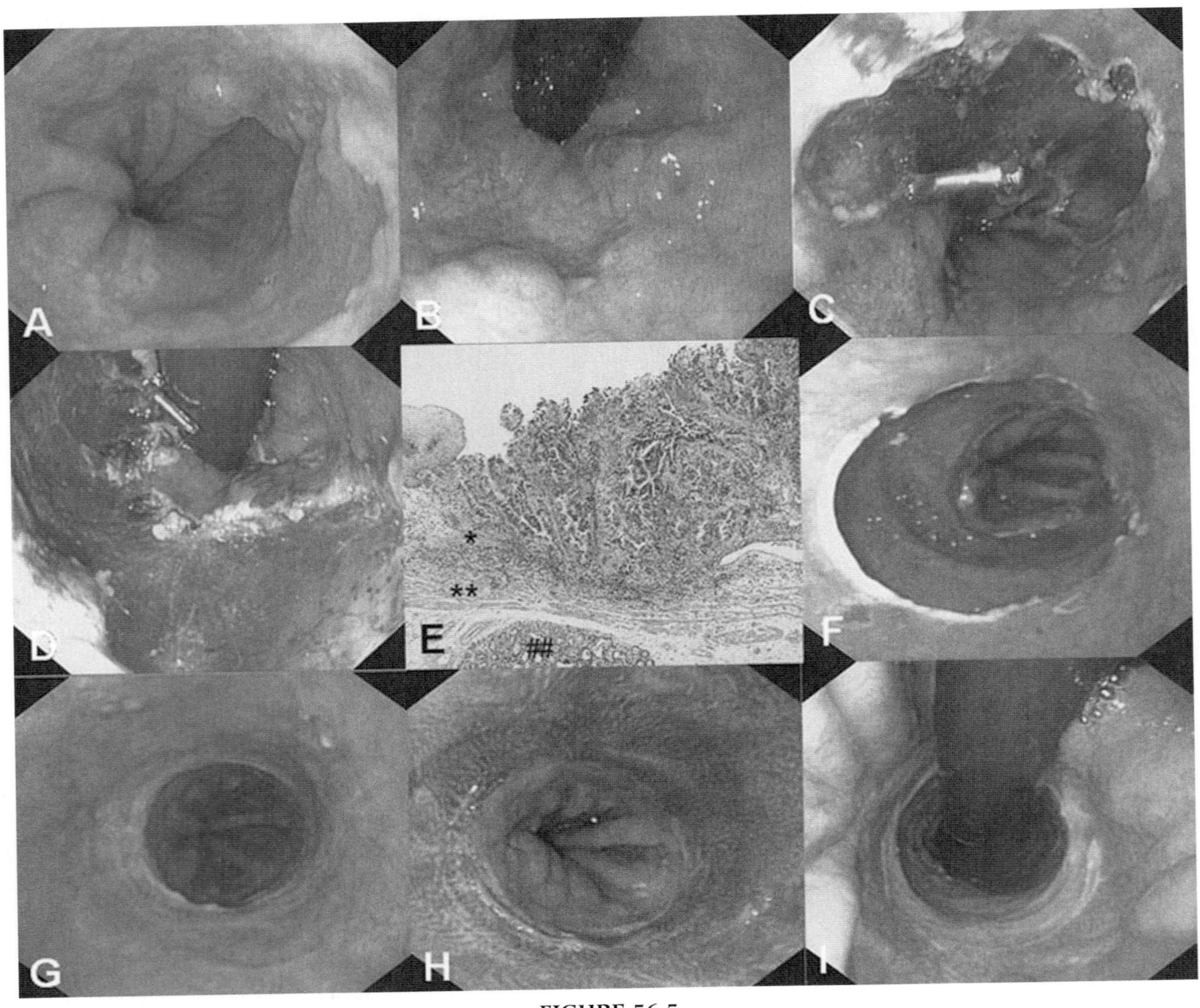

FIGURE 56.5

Stepwise radical endoscopic resection. A: A 2-cm Barrett's segment with a 25-mm type 0-IIa-IIc lesion at the 11–3 o'clock position, biopsies from the area showed carcinoma. B: In retrograde position, the lesion is visible at the 3–7 o'clock position. C: Situation after diagnostic piecemeal resection (3 pieces); argon plasma coagulation was used for small residual Barrett's isles and a hemoclip was necessary for hemostasis. D: As C, view in retrograde position. E: Histopathologic image of the ER specimen (H&E staining) showing a mucosal cancer and part of the squamocolumnar junction (left-hand side). The lesion infiltrates through the first layer of the muscularis mucosae (*), but not through the second muscularis mucosae layer (**). A submucosal periesophageal gland is clearly visible (##). F: Second endoscopic resection performed after 8 weeks for removal of the remainder of the Barrett's segment. G: Situation after 6 months' follow-up: the distal esophagus is completely lined with neosquamous epithelium. H: As in G, after lugol staining. I: As in G, retrograde view. Reproduced with permission of http://www.barrett.nl.

effective for eradication of early Barrett's neoplasia. Recurrence of neoplasia is rare (2%) and can be retreated endoscopically.

A limitation is that SRER is technically demanding. Judgement of whether the resection has extended deep enough into the hiatal hernia may be difficult. It requires experience to adequately resect the target area in a piecemeal resection and to avoid leaving residual Barrett's mucosa between the resection wounds that may require the use of APC. Furthermore, with every endoscopic resection, fibrous tissue is induced, making subsequent submucosal lifting and resections more difficult. It is therefore important that the first endoscopic resection is targeted to the area in the Barrett's segment with the highest grade of neoplasia. The development of scar tissue is, unfortunately, also the cause of the most significant late complication encountered with this treatment protocol: the development of symptomatic stenosis in up to 41% of patients, a rate comparable to that of sodium porfimer PDT.

In summary, SRER is safe and effective for the treatment of selected patients with early neoplasia in Barrett's esophagus. Compared to most endoscopic ablation modalities, SRER appears to achieve a higher rate of eradication of neoplasia and of Barrett's mucosa. In addition, SRER may give fewer recurrences during follow-up, since all the mucosa at risk is effectively removed *with* histologic correlation. A significant number of patients, however, develop a symptomatic stenosis after SRER and the procedure is technically complicated.

RADIOFREQUENCY ABLATION

The newest ablation technique used for complete ablation in Barrett's esophagus is stepwise circumferential and focal ablation using the HALO system (Figure 56.6). This techniques uses radiofrequency energy generated by a special RF generator and applied to the tissue by a balloon-based electrode (HALO^{360}) that contains multiple tightly spaced bipolar electrodes that alternate in polarity (BARRx, Sunnyvale, CA, USA). The electrode is 3 cm in length, and a variety of different diameters is available (22–34 mm). The total energy (J) delivered to the tissue is controlled by the generator and determines the depth of injury. The energy is adjusted to the balloon diameter, thereby delivering a standardized energy density (J/cm^2) to the tissue. The energy amount can be selected and is delivered in less than 1 second at 300 W (104). In an experimental study, energy densities of 8–20 J/cm^2 resulted in complete epithelial ablation without inducing esophageal stenosis (104).

The device has first been tested in a large U.S. multicenter trial for ablation of intestinal metaplasia (AIM-study) (105). In the study, 102 patients with a BE of a length of 2–6 cm were treated at 10 J/cm^2 delivered twice in 1 session (105). Complete remission for Barrett's esophagus was achieved in 70% of patients after 2 treatment sessions using the balloon-based HALO360 system. There were no severe complications, the procedures were well tolerated, and none of the patients developed an esophageal stenosis. The residual Barrett's mucosa was typically in the form of small, visible islands. A focal ablation device was subsequently used for targeted ablation of islands of Barrett's mucosa that remained after the HALO360 treatment. This HALO^{90} system consists of a cap-based device that is mounted on the distal tip of an endoscope. The device has a 20 mm x 15 mm articulated platform on its upper surface with an electrode array identical to that of HALO^{360}. After treatment with the HALO90, 98% of patients in the AIM-study had complete endoscopic and histologic removal of all intestinal metaplasia. In addition, no buried Barrett's was observed in all biopsies obtained from the neosquamous mucosa during follow-up.

The Amsterdam group has performed 2 cohort studies in which RFA was used to treat flat HGIN (n = 10) or residual LGIN/HGIN after endoscopic resection of HGIN/EAC (n = 13) (31,106). Patients were treated with stepwise circumferential and focal ablation using the HALO360 and the HALO90 system, respectively. In all patients complete eradication of neoplasia was achieved; 2 patients required an endoscopic resection for residual Barrett's mucosa with LGIN/HGIN after the ablation. Complete endoscopic and histologic eradication of BE was achieved in all patients. No buried Barrett's was detected in over 850 biopsies from the neosquamous epithelium obtained during follow-up endoscopies, and none of the patients developed an ablation-related stenosis.

Summarizing, stepwise circumferential and focal ablation using the HALO system appears to be an effective treatment modality for flat HGIN, LGIN, and complete Barrett's eradication. No ablation-related stenoses have been described over 200 patients treated, and no buried Barrett's has been detected in, overall, more than 5,000 biopsies. This suggests that this ablation technique is the first to find the right trade-off between effectiveness on one hand (causing complete removal of all Barrett's with no buried Barrett's) and the avoidance of damage to the deeper layers causing complications, such as stenosis. Long-term follow-up results are eagerly awaited and large multicenter randomized trials are currently being conducted in the United States and Europe.

CLINICAL RESULTS OF ENDOSCOPIC RESECTION COMBINED WITH ABLATION

As mentioned earlier, endoscopic ablation is mainly used as an adjunct to endoscopic resection. Focal lesions are first endoscopically resected, followed by ablation of the residual Barrett's segment with an endoscopic ablation modality for treatment of any residual flat neoplasia and to prevent recurrences by eradicating all Barrett's epithelium. Only a small number of series reporting the success of such combined treatment protocols have been published.

The short-term success rates for complete elimination of all neoplasia after PDT are high, ranging from 83% to 98% (66,107–109), but complete eradication of all Barrett's mucosa is rarely achieved, as could be

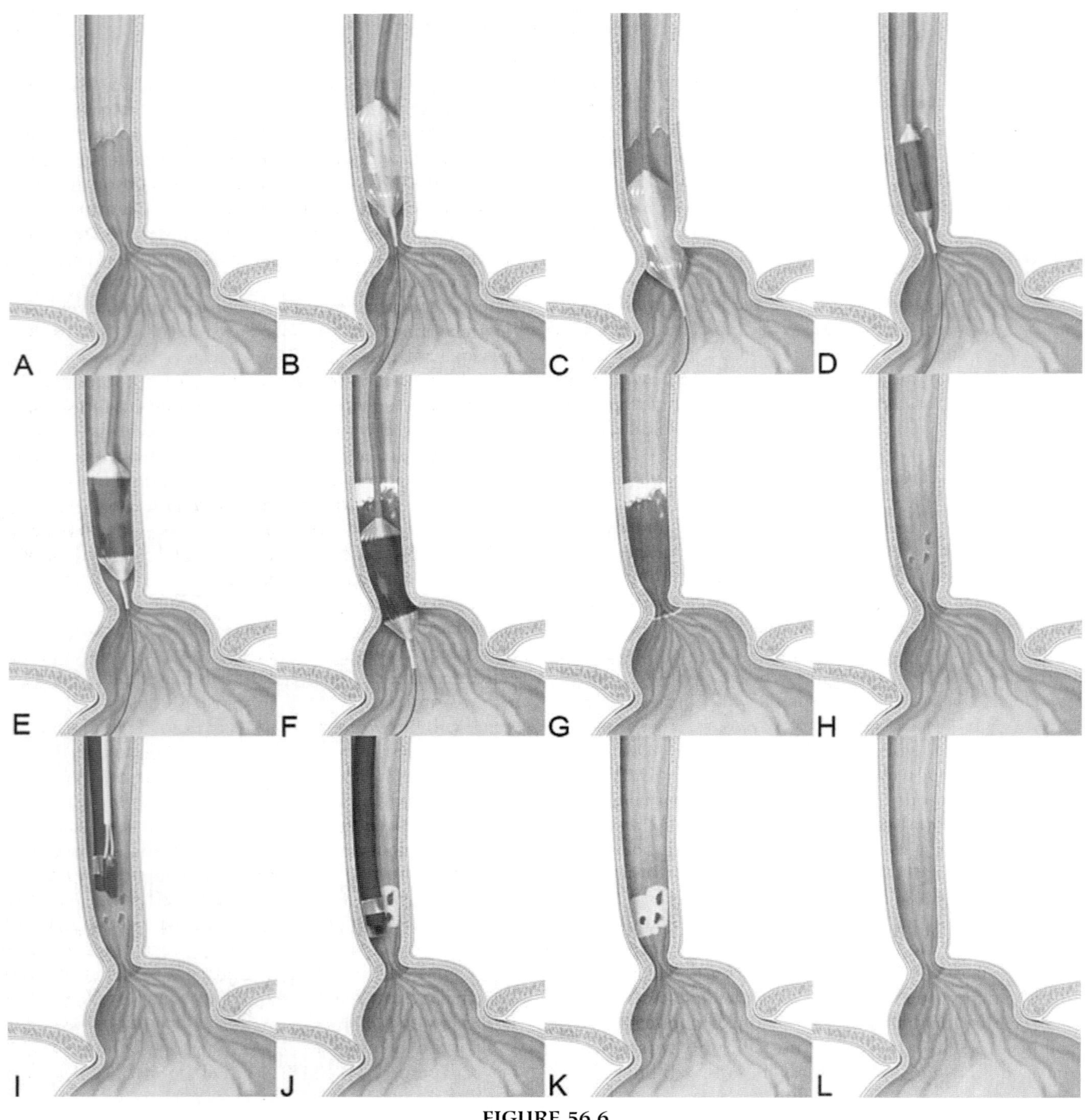

FIGURE 56.6

Radiofrequency ablation. A: Pretreatment image of a Barrett's segment. B and C: the esophageal diameter is measured at 1-cm intervals with a sizing balloon placed over a guidewire. D: Introduction of the RFA balloon catheter with the appropriate diameter over the guidewire. E: The inflated RFA balloon positioned 1 cm above the top of the Barrett's segment. F: The RFA balloon repositioned for ablation of the second zone after ablation of the first zone with an overlap of 1 cm with the first ablation zone. G: Image of the treated Barrett's segment immediately after the RFA ablation with visible necrosis of the superficial mucosa. H: Image of the healed distal esophagus 3 months after RFA treatment with regeneration with neosquamous mucosa and 3 small isles with residual Barrett's mucosa. I: Introduction of the endoscope with the HALO90. cap for focal ablation placed at the tip. J: Ablation of the third isle of Barrett's mucosa. The necrosis caused by ablation of the first 2 isles visible. K: Image of the distal esophagus immediately after ablation of the 3 residual isles of Barrett's mucosa. L: Image of the healed distal esophagus, showing complete regeneration with neosquamous mucosa. Reproduced with permission of http://www.barrett.nl.

expected from results that are achieved with the use of ablation modalities as monotherapy (see above). In addition, the known drawbacks of ablative treatment (e.g., buried Barrett's, stenosis) also hold for the combination treatment of ER and ablation. The development of new or recurrent lesions during follow-up is, therefore, still seen in a considerable number of patients (0%–39%) (66,107–109). The goal of treatment of neoplasia and prevention of recurrences through the combined treatment with endoscopic resection and ablation (PDT) is thus only partly reached.

The success rate for complete eradication of neoplasia, as welll as removal of all Barrett's mucosa after combined treatment with ER and HALO ablation, are excellent (31,106). An advantage of HALO ablation is the possibility to use ER as "an escape treatment" after ablation, since it does not results in significant scarring of the esophageal wall.

POSTENDOSCOPIC TREATMENT ACID-SUPPRESSION THERAPY

Injury to the Barrett's epithelium followed by healing in an acid-controlled environment reverses the Barrett's epithelium into squamous epithelium (110–113). Therefore, all endoscopic treatment sessions in Barrett's esophagus should be accompanied by strong acid-suppressant therapy. There is no consensus on the type and duration of the acid-suppressant therapy. We treat all our patients with ranitidine 300 mg at bedtime and sucralfate 1 g four times a day for 2 weeks after treatment, added to the maintenance dosage of esomeprazole 40 mg twice a day.

FUTURE PROSPECTS IN ENDOSCOPIC TREATMENT

It is now believed that the complete Barrett's segment should be eradicated to achieve long-term remission in patients with early Barrett's neoplasia. Developments in endoscopic resection techniques are, therefore, focused on easier and faster techniques for resection of large areas and techniques that allow safe en bloc resection of lesions larger than 2 cm in diameter. The ligate-and-cut technique using the multiband mucosectomy kit may be such an easy and fast technique for resection of large areas of flat mucosa. Endoscopic resection of complete Barrett's segments is, however, accompanied with a high percentage of symptomatic esophageal stenosis. Methods to prevent the development of esophageal stenosis would be of great value, and more research should be performed in this area.

A promising new development is the ablation of Barrett's mucosa using the HALO system. The first results that are achieved with this technique show a high efficacy in eradicating HGIN, LGIN, and (non dysplastic) Barrett's mucosa, without the threats of buried Barrett's mucosa or esophageal stenosis. Long-term results will have to prove whether this technique is all it promises to be.

References

1. Barrett NR. Chronic peptic ulcer of the oesophagus and 'oesophagitis'. *Br J Surg.* 1950;38(150):175–182.
2. Haggitt RC. Barrett's esophagus, dysplasia, and adenocarcinoma. *Hum Pathol.* 1994;25(10):982–993.
3. Reid BJ, Weinstein WM. Barrett's esophagus and adenocarcinoma. *Annu Rev Med.* 1987;38:477–492.
4. Sampliner RE. Updated guidelines for the diagnosis, surveillance, and therapy of Barrett's esophagus. *Am J Gastroenterol.* 2002;97(8):1888–1895.
5. Sharma P, Sidorenko EI. Are screening and surveillance for Barrett's oesophagus really worthwhile? *Gut.* 2005;54 Suppl 1:i27–i32.
6. Ronkainen J, Aro P, Storskrubb T, et al. Prevalence of Barrett's esophagus in the general population: an endoscopic study. *Gastroenterology.* 2005;129(6):1825–1831.
7. Cameron AJ, Ott BJ, Payne WS. The incidence of adenocarcinoma in columnar-lined (Barrett's) esophagus. *N Engl J Med.* 1985;313(14):857–859.
8. Lagergren J, Bergstrom R, Lindgren A, et al. Symptomatic gastroesophageal reflux as a risk factor for esophageal adenocarcinoma. *N Engl J Med.* 1999;340(11):825–831.
9. Bytzer P, Christensen PB, Damkier P, et al. Adenocarcinoma of the esophagus and Barrett's esophagus: a population-based study. *Am J Gastroenterol.* 1999;94(1):86–91.
10. Krishnadath KK, Tilanus HW, van Blankenstein M, et al. Accumulation of p53 protein in normal, dysplastic, and neoplastic Barrett's oesophagus. *J Pathol.* 1995;175(2):175–180.
11. Skacel M, Petras RE, Gramlich TL, et al. The diagnosis of low-grade dysplasia in Barrett's esophagus and its implications for disease progression. *Am J Gastroenterol.* 2000;95(12):3383–3387.
12. Younes M, Ertan A, Lechago LV, et al. p53 Protein accumulation is a specific marker of malignant potential in Barrett's metaplasia. *Dig Dis Sci.* 1997;42(4):697–701.
13. Barrett MT, Sanchez CA, Galipeau PC, et al. Allelic loss of 9p21 and mutation of the CDKN2/p16 gene develop as early lesions during neoplastic progression in Barrett's esophagus. *Oncogene.* 1996;13(9):1867–1873.
14. Reid BJ. p53 and neoplastic progression in Barrett's esophagus. *Am J Gastroenterol.* 2001;96(5):1321–1323.
15. Rygiel AM, van Baal JW, Milano F, et al. Efficient automated assessment of genetic abnormalities detected by fluorescence in situ hybridization on brush cytology in a Barrett esophagus surveillance population. *Cancer.* 2007;109(10):1980–1988.
16. Ross JS, McKenna BJ. The HER-2/neu oncogene in tumors of the gastrointestinal tract. *Cancer Invest.* 2001;19(5):554–568.
17. Brien TP, Odze RD, Sheehan CE, et al. HER-2/neu gene amplification by FISH predicts poor survival in Barrett's esophagus-associated adenocarcinoma. *Hum Pathol.* 2000;31(1):35–39.
18. Halm U, Tannapfel A, Breitung B, et al. Apoptosis and cell proliferation in the metaplasia-dysplasia-carcinoma-sequence of Barrett's esophagus. *Hepatogastroenterology.* 2000;47(34):962–966.
19. Going JJ, Keith WN, Neilson L, et al. Aberrant expression of minichromosome maintenance proteins 2 and 5, and Ki-67 in dysplastic squamous oesophageal epithelium and Barrett's mucosa. *Gut.* 2002;50(3):373–377.
20. Polkowski W, Van Lanschot JJ, ten Kate FJ, et al. The value of p53 and Ki67 as markers for tumour progression in the Barrett's dysplasia-carcinoma sequence. *Surg Oncol.* 1995;4(3):163–171.
21. Koppert LB, Wijnhoven BP, van DH, et al. The molecular biology of esophageal adenocarcinoma. *J Surg Oncol.* 2005;92(3):169–190.
22. Sharma P, Sidorenko EI. Are screening and surveillance for Barrett's oesophagus really worthwhile? *Gut.* 2005;54 Suppl 1:i27–i32.
23. Aldulaimi DM, Cox M, Nwokolo CU, et al. Barrett's surveillance is worthwhile and detects curable cancers. A prospective cohort study addressing cancer incidence, treatment outcome and survival. *Eur J Gastroenterol Hepatol.* 2005;17(9):943–950.
24. de Boer AG, van Lanschot JJ, van Sandick JW, et al. Quality of life after transhiatal compared with extended transthoracic resection for adenocarcinoma of the esophagus. *J Clin Oncol.* 2004;22(20):4202–4208.

25. Blazeby JM, Alderson D, Farndon JR. Quality of life in patients with oesophageal cancer. *Recent Results Cancer Res.* 2000;155:193–204.
26. Westerterp M, Koppert LB, Buskens CJ, et al. Outcome of surgical treatment for early adenocarcinoma of the esophagus or gastro-esophageal junction. *Virchows Arch.* 2005;446(5):497–504.
27. Liu JF, Wang QZ, Hou J. Surgical treatment for cancer of the oesophagus and gastric cardia in Hebei, China. *Br J Surg.* 2004;91(1):90–98.
28. Bollschweiler E, Baldus SE, Schroder W, et al. High rate of lymph-node metastasis in submucosal esophageal squamous-cell carcinomas and adenocarcinomas. *Endoscopy.* 2006;38(2):149–156.
29. Peters FP, Kara MA, Rosmolen WD, et al. Endoscopic treatment of high-grade dysplasia and early stage cancer in Barrett's esophagus. *Gastrointest Endosc.* 2005;61(4):506–514.
30. Seewald S, Akaraviputh T, Seitz U, et al. Circumferential EMR and complete removal of Barrett's epithelium: a new approach to management of Barrett's esophagus containing high-grade intraepithelial neoplasia and intramucosal carcinoma. *Gastrointest Endosc.* 2003;57(7):854–859.
31. Gondrie JJ, Pouw RE, Sondermeijer CM, et al. Effective treatment of early Barrett's neoplasia with stepwise circumferential and focal ablation using the HALO system. *Endoscopy.* 2008 May;40(5):370–9.
32. Kara MA, Peters FP, Rosmolen WD, et al. High-resolution endoscopy plus chromoendoscopy or narrow-band imaging in Barrett's esophagus: a prospective randomized crossover study. *Endoscopy.* 2005;37(10):929–936.
33. The Paris endoscopic classification of superficial neoplastic lesions: esophagus, stomach, and colon: November 30 to December 1, 2002. *Gastrointest Endosc.* 2003;58(6 Suppl):S3–S43.
34. Update on the Paris classification of superficial neoplastic lesions in the digestive tract. *Endoscopy.* 2005;37(6):570–578.
35. Japanese Gastric Cancer Association. Japanese Classification of Gastric Carcinoma—2nd English Edition. *Gastric Cancer.* 1998;1(1):10–24.
36. Tani M, Sakai P, Kondo H. Endoscopic mucosal resection of superficial cancer in the stomach using the cap technique. *Endoscopy.* 2003;35(4):348–355.
37. Schlemper RJ, Riddell RH, Kato Y, et al. The Vienna classification of gastrointestinal epithelial neoplasia. *Gut.* 2000;47(2):251–255.
38. Schlemper RJ, Kato Y, Stolte M. Diagnostic criteria for gastrointestinal carcinomas in Japan and Western countries: proposal for a new classification system of gastrointestinal epithelial neoplasia. *J Gastroenterol Hepatol.* 2000;15 Suppl:G49–G57.
39. Hulscher JB, Haringsma J, Benraadt J, et al. Comprehensive Cancer Centre Amsterdam Barrett Advisory Committee: first results. *Neth J Med.* 2001;58(1):3–8.
40. Westerterp M, Koppert LB, Buskens CJ, et al. Outcome of surgical treatment for early adenocarcinoma of the esophagus or gastro-esophageal junction. *Virchows Arch.* 2005;446(5):497–504.
41. Bollschweiler E, Baldus SE, Schroder W, et al. High rate of lymph-node metastasis in submucosal esophageal squamous-cell carcinomas and adenocarcinomas. *Endoscopy.* 2006;38(2):149–156.
42. Takubo K, Sasajima K, Yamashita K, et al. Double muscularis mucosae in Barrett's esophagus. *Hum Pathol.* 1991;22(11):1158–1161.
43. Pech O, May A, Gunter E, et al. The impact of endoscopic ultrasound and computed tomography on the TNM staging of early cancer in Barrett's esophagus. *Am J Gastroenterol.* 2006;101(10):2223–2229.
44. Meining A, Dittler HJ, Wolf A, et al. You get what you expect? A critical appraisal of imaging methodology in endosonographic cancer staging. *Gut.* 2002;50(5):599–603.
45. Heeren PA, van Westreenen HL, Geersing GJ, et al. Influence of tumor characteristics on the accuracy of endoscopic ultrasonography in staging cancer of the esophagus and esophagogastric junction. *Endoscopy.* 2004;36(11):966–971.
46. Van DJ. Endosonographic evaluation of the patient with esophageal cancer. *Chest.* 1997;112(4 Suppl):184S–190S.
47. Caletti G, Bocus P, Fusaroli P, et al. Cancer of the esophagus—endoscopic ultrasound: selection for cure. *Can J Gastroenterol.* 1998;12(5):341–346.
48. Van DJ. Endosonographic evaluation of the patient with esophageal cancer. *Chest.* 1997;112(4 Suppl):184S–190S.
49. Mino-Kenudson M, Brugge WR, Puricelli WP, et al. Management of superficial Barrett's epithelium-related neoplasms by endoscopic mucosal resection: clinicopathologic analysis of 27 cases. *Am J Surg Pathol.* 2005;29(5):680–686.
50. Maish MS, DeMeester SR. Endoscopic mucosal resection as a staging technique to determine the depth of invasion of esophageal adenocarcinoma. *Ann Thorac Surg.* 2004;78(5):1777–1782.
51. Larghi A, Lightdale CJ, Memeo L, et al. EUS followed by EMR for staging of high-grade dysplasia and early cancer in Barrett's esophagus. *Gastrointest Endosc.* 2005;62(1):16–23.
52. Peters FP, Brakenhoff KP, Curvers WL, et al. Histologic evaluation of resection specimens obtained at 293 endoscopic resections in Barrett's esophagus. *Gastrointest Endosc.* 2008 Apr;67(4):604–9.
53. Mino-Kenudson M, Brugge WR, Puricelli WP, et al. Management of superficial Barrett's epithelium-related neoplasms by endoscopic mucosal resection: clinicopathologic analysis of 27 cases. *Am J Surg Pathol.* 2005;29(5):680–686.
54. Ell C, May A, Pech O, et al. Curative endoscopic resection of early esophageal adenocarcinomas (Barrett's cancer). *Gastrointest Endosc.* 2007;65(1):3–10.
55. Bergman JJ. Endoscopic treatment of high-grade intraepithelial neoplasia and early cancer in Barrett's oesophagus. *Best Pract Res Clin Gastroenterol.* 2005;19(6):889–207.
56. Bergman JJ. Endoscopic resection for treatment of mucosal Barrett's cancer: time to swing the pendulum. *Gastrointest Endosc.* 2007;65(1):11–13.
57. Ackroyd R, Brown NJ, Davis MF, et al. Photodynamic therapy for dysplastic Barrett's oesophagus: a prospective, double blind, randomised, placebo controlled trial. *Gut.* 2000;47(5):612–617.
58. Dulai GS, Jensen DM, Cortina G, et al. Randomized trial of argon plasma coagulation vs. multipolar electrocoagulation for ablation of Barrett's esophagus. *Gastrointest Endosc.* 2005;61(2):232–240.
59. Overholt BF, Panjehpour M, Halberg DL. Photodynamic therapy for Barrett's esophagus with dysplasia and/or early stage carcinoma: long-term results. *Gastrointest Endosc.* 2003;58(2):183–188.
60. Inoue H, Takeshita K, Hori H, et al. Endoscopic mucosal resection with a cap-fitted panendoscope for esophagus, stomach, and colon mucosal lesions. *Gastrointest Endosc.* 1993;39(1):58–62.
61. Inoue H, Noguchi O, Saito N, et al. Endoscopic mucosectomy for early cancer using a pre-looped plastic cap. *Gastrointest Endosc.* 1994;40(2 Pt 1):263–264.
62. Ell C, May A, Wurster H. The first reusable multiple-band ligator for endoscopic hemostasis of variceal bleeding, nonvariceal bleeding and mucosal resection. *Endoscopy.* 1999;31(9):738–740.
63. Peters FP, Kara MA, Curvers WL, et al. Multiband mucosectomy for endoscopic resection of Barrett's esophagus: feasibility study with matched historical controls. *Eur J Gastroenterol Hepatol.* 2007;19(4):311–315.
64. May A, Gossner L, Behrens A, et al. A prospective randomized trial of two different endoscopic resection techniques for early stage cancer of the esophagus. *Gastrointest Endosc.* 2003;58(2):167–175.
65. Tanabe S, Koizumi W, Mitomi H, et al. Usefulness of EMR with an oblique aspiration mucosectomy device compared with strip biopsy in patients with superficial esophageal cancer. *Gastrointest Endosc.* 2004;59(4):558–563.
66. May A, Gossner L, Pech O, et al. Local endoscopic therapy for intraepithelial high-grade neoplasia and early adenocarcinoma in Barrett's oesophagus: acute-phase and intermediate results of a new treatment approach. *Eur J Gastroenterol Hepatol.* 2002;14(10):1085–1091.
67. Agarwal ML, Clay ME, Harvey EJ, et al. Photodynamic therapy induces rapid cell death by apoptosis in L5178Y mouse lymphoma cells. *Cancer Res.* 1991;51(21):5993–5996.
68. Webber J, Luo Y, Crilly R, et al. An apoptotic response to photodynamic therapy with endogenous protoporphyrin in vivo. *J Photochem Photobiol B.* 1996; 35(3):209–211.
69. Maier A, Tomaselli F, Anegg U, et al. Combined photodynamic therapy and hyperbaric oxygenation in carcinoma of the esophagus and the esophago-gastric junction. *Eur J Cardiothorac Surg.* 2000;18(6):649–654.
70. Maier A, Anegg U, Fell B, et al. Effect of photodynamic therapy in a multimodal approach for advanced carcinoma of the gastro-esophageal junction. *Lasers Surg Med.* 2000;26(5):461–466.
71. Maier A, Anegg U, Fell B, et al. Hyperbaric oxygen and photodynamic therapy in the treatment of advanced carcinoma of the cardia and the esophagus. *Lasers Surg Med.* 2000;26(3):308–315.
72. Peters FP, Krishnadath KK, Rygiel AM, et al. Stepwise radical endoscopic resection of the complete Barrett's esophagus with early neoplasia successfully eradicates pre-existing genetic abnormalities. *Am J Gastroenterol.* 2007 Sep;102(9):1853–61.
73. Overholt BF, Wang KK, Burdick JS, et al. Five-year efficacy and safety of photodynamic therapy with Photofrin in Barrett's high-grade dysplasia. *Gastrointest Endosc.* 2007;66(3):460–468.
74. Prasad GA, Wang KK, Buttar NS et al. Long-term survival following endoscopic and surgical treatment of high-grade dysplasia in Barrett's esophagus. *Gastroenterology.* 2007;132(4):1226–1233.
75. Panjehpour M, Overholt BF, Haydek JM, Lee SG. Results of photodynamic therapy for ablation of dysplasia and early cancer in Barrett's esophagus and effect of oral steroids on stricture formation. *Am J Gastroenterol.* 2000;95(9):2177–2184.
76. Panjehpour M, Overholt BF, Phan MN, et al. Optimization of light dosimetry for photodynamic therapy of Barrett's esophagus: efficacy vs. incidence of stricture after treatment. *Gastrointest Endosc.* 2005;61(1):13–18.
77. Ban S, Mino M, Nishioka NS, et al. Histopathologic aspects of photodynamic therapy for dysplasia and early adenocarcinoma arising in Barrett's esophagus. *Am J Surg Pathol.* 2004;28(11):1466–1473.
78. Van Laethem JL, Peny MO, Salmon I, et al. Intramucosal adenocarcinoma arising under squamous re-epithelialisation of Barrett's oesophagus. *Gut.* 2000;46(4):574–577.
79. van Hillegersberg R, Haringsma J, ten Kate FJ, et al. Invasive carcinoma after endoscopic ablative therapy for high-grade dysplasia in Barrett's oesophagus. *Dig Surg.* 2003;20(5):440–444.
80. Ragunath K, Krasner N, Raman VS, et al. Endoscopic ablation of dysplastic Barrett's oesophagus comparing argon plasma coagulation and photodynamic therapy: a randomized prospective trial assessing efficacy and cost-effectiveness. *Scand J Gastroenterol.* 2005;40(7):750–758.
81. Kelty C, Ackroyd R. Re-epithelialisation of Barrett's oesophagus. *Gut.* 2000;47(5):741.
82. Hornick JL, Blount PL, Sanchez CA, et al. Biologic properties of columnar epithelium underneath reepithelialized squamous mucosa in Barrett's esophagus. *Am J Surg Pathol.* 2005;29(3):372–380.
83. Bergman JJ, Fockens P. Ablating Barrett's metaplastic epithelium: are the techniques ready for clinical use? *Gut.* 2006;55(9):1222–1223.
84. Krishnadath KK, Wang KK, Taniguchi K, et al. Persistent genetic abnormalities in Barrett's esophagus after photodynamic therapy. *Gastroenterology.* 2000;119(3):624–630.
85. Hage M, Siersema PD, Vissers KJ, et al. Molecular evaluation of ablative therapy of Barrett's oesophagus. *J Pathol.* 2005;205(1):57–64.

86. Hage M, Siersema PD, Vissers KJ, et al. Genomic analysis of Barrett's esophagus after ablative therapy: persistence of genetic alterations at tumor suppressor loci. *Int J Cancer.* 2006;118(1):155–160.
87. Farhadi A, Fields J, Banan A, et al. Reactive oxygen species: are they involved in the pathogenesis of GERD, Barrett's esophagus, and the latter's progression toward esophageal cancer? *Am J Gastroenterol.* 2002;97(1):22–26.
88. Chen X, Ding YW, Yang G, et al. Oxidative damage in an esophageal adenocarcinoma model with rats. *Carcinogenesis.* 2000;21(2):257–263.
89. Byrne JP, Armstrong GR, Attwood SE. Restoration of the normal squamous lining in Barrett's esophagus by argon beam plasma coagulation. *Am J Gastroenterol.* 1998;93(10):1810–1815.
90. Ackroyd R, Tam W, Schoeman M, et al. Prospective randomized controlled trial of argon plasma coagulation ablation vs. endoscopic surveillance of patients with Barrett's esophagus after antireflux surgery. *Gastrointest Endosc.* 2004;59(1):1–7.
91. Morris CD, Byrne JP, Armstrong GR, et al. Prevention of the neoplastic progression of Barrett's oesophagus by endoscopic argon beam plasma ablation. *Br J Surg.* 2001;88(10):1357–1362.
92. Van Laethem JL, Jagodzinski R, Peny MO, et al. Argon plasma coagulation in the treatment of Barrett's high-grade dysplasia and in situ adenocarcinoma. *Endoscopy.* 2001;33(3):257–261.
93. Kahaleh M, Van Laethem JL, Nagy N, Cremer M, Deviere J. Long-term follow-up and factors predictive of recurrence in Barrett's esophagus treated by argon plasma coagulation and acid suppression. *Endoscopy.* 2002;34(12):950–955.
94. Lopes CV, Pereira-Lima J, Hartmann AA. p53 immunohistochemical expression in Barrett's esophagus before and after endoscopic ablation by argon plasma coagulation. *Scand J Gastroenterol.* 2005;40(3):259–263.
95. Hage M, Siersema PD, van Dekken H, et al. 5-Aminolevulinic acid photodynamic therapy versus argon plasma coagulation for ablation of Barrett's oesophagus: a randomised trial. *Gut.* 2004;53(6):785–790.
96. Mork H, Barth T, Kreipe HH, et al. Reconstitution of squamous epithelium in Barrett's oesophagus with endoscopic argon plasma coagulation: a prospective study. *Scand J Gastroenterol.* 1998;33(11):1130–1134.
97. Van Laethem JL, Cremer M, Peny MO, et al. Eradication of Barrett's mucosa with argon plasma coagulation and acid suppression: immediate and mid term results. *Gut.* 1998;43(6):747–751.
98. Basu KK, Pick B, Bale R, et al. Efficacy and one year follow up of argon plasma coagulation therapy for ablation of Barrett's oesophagus: factors determining persistence and recurrence of Barrett's epithelium. *Gut.* 2002;51(6):776–780.
99. Pinotti AC, Cecconello I, Filho FM, et al. Endoscopic ablation of Barrett's esophagus using argon plasma coagulation: a prospective study after fundoplication. *Dis Esophagus.* 2004;17(3):243–246.
100. Kelty C, Ackroyd R, Brown NJ, et al. Endoscopic ablation of Barrett's esophagus: a randomized trial of photodynamic therapy (PDT) versus argon plasma coagulation (APC) [abstract]. *Gastrointest Endosc.* 2004;59(5):AB250.
101. Sharma P, Wani S, Weston AP, et al. A randomised controlled trial of ablation of Barrett's oesophagus with multipolar electrocoagulation versus argon plasma coagulation in combination with acid suppression: long term results. *Gut.* 2006;55(9):1233–1239.
102. Manner H, May A, Rabenstein T, et al. Prospective evaluation of a new high-power argon plasma coagulation system (hp-APC) in therapeutic gastrointestinal endoscopy. *Scand J Gastroenterol.* 2007;42(3):397–405.
103. Peters FP, Kara MA, Rosmolen WD, et al. Stepwise radical endoscopic resection is effective for complete removal of Barrett's esophagus with early neoplasia: a prospective study. *Am J Gastroenterol.* 2006;101(7):1449–1457.
104. Ganz RA, Utley DS, Stern RA, et al. Complete ablation of esophageal epithelium with a balloon-based bipolar electrode: a phased evaluation in the porcine and in the human esophagus. *Gastrointest Endosc.* 2004;60(6):1002–1010.
105. Sharma VK, Wang KK, Overholt BF, et al. Balloon-based, circumferential, endoscopic radiofrequency ablation of Barrett's esophagus: 1-year follow-up of 100 patients. *Gastrointest Endosc.* 2007;65(2):185–195.
106. Rosmolen WD, Krishnadath KK, Ten Kate F, et al. Stepwise circumferential and focal ablation of Barrett's esophagus with high-grade dysplasia: results of the first prospective series of 11 patients. *Endoscopy.* 2008 May;40(5):359–69.
107. Buttar NS, Wang KK, Lutzke LS, et al. Combined endoscopic mucosal resection and photodynamic therapy for esophageal neoplasia within Barrett's esophagus. *Gastrointest Endosc.* 2001;54(6):682–688.
108. Pacifico RJ, Wang KK, Wongkeesong LM, et al. Combined endoscopic mucosal resection and photodynamic therapy versus esophagectomy for management of early adenocarcinoma in Barrett's esophagus. *Clin Gastroenterol Hepatol.* 2003;1(4):252–257.
109. Peters F, Kara M, Rosmolen W, et al. Poor results of 5-aminolevulinic acid-photodynamic therapy for residual high-grade dysplasia and early cancer in barrett esophagus after endoscopic resection. *Endoscopy.* 2005;37(5):418–424.
110. Sampliner RE, Hixson LJ, Fennerty MB, Garewal HS. Regression of Barrett's esophagus by laser ablation in an anacid environment. *Dig Dis Sci.* 1993;38(2):365–368.
111. Sampliner RE, Fennerty B, Garewal HS. Reversal of Barrett's esophagus with acid suppression and multipolar electrocoagulation: preliminary results. *Gastrointest Endosc.* 1996;44(5):532–535.
112. Barham CP, Jones RL, Biddlestone LR, et al. Photothermal laser ablation of Barrett's oesophagus: endoscopic and histological evidence of squamous re-epithelialisation. *Gut.* 1997;41(3):281–284.
113. Berenson MM, Johnson TD, Markowitz NR, et al. Restoration of squamous mucosa after ablation of Barrett's esophageal epithelium. *Gastroenterology.* 1993;104(6):1686–1691.

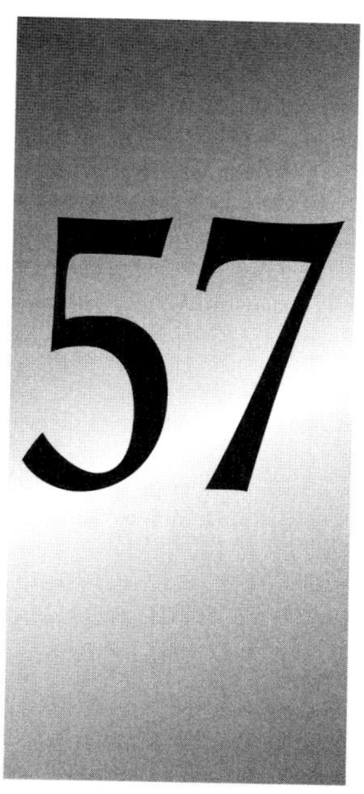

57 Endoscopic Therapy for Superficial Cancer

Sarah A. Rodriguez

The management of high-grade dysplasia (HGD) in Barrett's esophagus has long been a controversial area. The traditional approach and still-accepted standard of care for HGD is esophagectomy. This is based on surgical literature showing that the rate of unsuspected cancer in esophagectomy specimens of patients only thought to have HGD preoperatively is as high as 30% to 40% (1–3). Additionally, patients with HGD have a high rate of progression to cancer; a study of 15 patients with unifocal HGD who were followed for 37 months found that 53% of patients progressed to cancer or multifocal HGD (4). Notably, 47% of patients regressed to either no dysplasia or low-grade dysplasia. Although the natural history of HGD is not entirely clear and progression is not inevitable, patients with HGD are at substantial risk for the development of cancer (5). Treatment is generally recommended for HGD, although some authors advocate intensive, frequent endoscopic surveillance with treatment only if cancer develops (6). Esophageal cancer is a highly lethal malignancy with a poor 5-year survival rate, in part due to the usually advanced stage at time of diagnosis (7). When cancer is detected early, however, therapy can often be curative.

Currently, options for management of HGD include intensive surveillance with definitive therapy if cancer is detected, endoscopic therapy, or esophagectomy. For patients with early cancer (EC), defined as carcinoma limited to the mucosal layer of the esophagus, continued surveillance alone is not recommended.

Esophagectomy is the only treatment that clearly ensures complete removal of all dysplastic Barrett's mucosa, although recurrent BE has been reported after subtotal esophagectomy (8). However, esophagectomy is associated with mortality rates of 3% to 5% and morbidity rates of 20% to 50%, even in experienced hands (9,10). Additionally, many patients with HGD and EC have multiple medical comorbidities that make them less than ideal candidates for surgery. Endoscopic therapy has been developed as an esophagus-sparing method of treatment for patients with HGD or EC who are felt to be at low risk for lymph node metastases based on pretreatment staging. The goals of endoscopic therapy are to provide definitive treatment for patients with low-risk lesions while avoiding the short- and long-term morbidity of esophagectomy. Despite a lack of long-term efficacy data on endoscopic therapies, it appears that many gastroenterologists are already offering it to patients (11).

Endoscopic therapy is based on the principle that if neoplastic Barrett's mucosa is ablated and the area is allowed to heal in a non-acidic environment, the new esophageal lining may be normal squamous epithelium (12). The available endoscopic therapies that will be discussed in this chapter include endoscopic mucosal resection (EMR) and various mucosal ablative therapies including photodynamic therapy, balloon-based radiofrequency ablation, argon plasma coagulation (APC), and laser treatment.

PATIENT SELECTION

Accurate endoscopic evaluation and staging is essential in order to choose patients who are appropriate candidates for endoscopic therapy. All patients should undergo diagnostic upper endoscopy with extensive biopsies; some authors advocate the use of enhanced endoscopic imaging including narrow band imaging and chromoendoscopy to adequately detect all foci of dysplasia (13). In general, visible lesions must be less than 20 mm in diameter in order to be resected en bloc, which allows for adequate assessment of margins. Additionally, cancers should be limited to the mucosa because of the risk of lymph node metastases with tumors that invade more deeply into the submucosa. For staging purposes, the mucosal layer and submucosal layer have been subdivided into thirds with each third going deeper into the esophageal wall, such that T1 tumors now have 6 different layers of invasion: T1m_1–m_3 (m_1 = limited to the epithelial layer, m_2 = invades lamina propria, m_3 = invades into but not through muscularis mucosae) and T1sm_1–sm_3 (different thirds of the submucosa). The risk of lymphatic spread in patients with tumors limited to the mucosa (pathologic stage T1a) appears to be very low. In a series of patients with T1 adenocarcinoma who underwent esophagectomy and regional lymphadenectomy, none of 38 with pT1a disease had lymph node involvement (14). In contrast, 10/56 (17.9%) of patients with tumors invading the submucosa (T1b) had lymph node metastases. Another study of 77 patients found that zero of 20 patients with tumors limited to the mucosa or the first third of the submucosal layer (pTm_{1-3} or pTsm_1) had lymph node metastases, while 23% of patients with pTsm_2 tumors and 69% of patients with pTsm_3 tumors had lymph node involvement (15). In studies of early squamous cell cancers, the risk of nodal metastases with stage T1m_3 cancer was 6% to 8% (16,17). Finally, recurrence rates for cancers limited to the mucosa are significantly less than for those invading the submucosa. A study of patients who had undergone esophagectomy found that 1 out of 79 (1.2%) patients with cancer limited to the mucosa or first layer of the submucosa had a local recurrence at 5 years, versus 8 out of 41 (19.5%) patients with invasion into the second and third layers of the submucosa (18). Therefore, patients whose cancers are found to invade the submucosa on final pathologic analysis should be considered for curative surgery.

Modalities for staging include cross-sectional imaging (primarily CT scan) and endoscopic ultrasound (EUS). EUS provides the most accurate local staging for tumor depth (T-stage) and regional lymph node metastases (N-stage), with T-stage accuracy rates of 85% overall and 81% for locoregional lymph nodes (19–21). The T-stage accuracy may be less for superficial cancers. One earlier study suggested that EUS was insensitive for evaluation of invasion into the submucosa (22). In a larger series, EUS correctly predicted T-stage in only 55% of patients overall, in only 29% of patients with T1 cancers, and in 42% of patients with T2 lesions (23). N-stage was also misdiagnosed in 25% of patients, with 41% of patients with N1 disease classified as N0. However, this study included data from as far back as 1987, when endosonographic equipment did not have the same resolution as current instruments. A more recent study of 42 patients who were staged with EUS and subsequently underwent esophagectomy found that EUS was 76% accurate for T-stage and 89% accurate for N-stage (24). In this study, there were no significant differences between different T-stages and overall accuracy. The error in 4 early stage tumors in this study was overstaging rather than understaging. The addition of fine-needle aspiration biopsies of suspicious lymph nodes may increase the accuracy of EUS for N-staging compared to endosonographic characteristics alone (25–27).

Despite the above limitations, EUS remains the most accurate modality for locoregional staging. It is important to note that EUS, like any imaging technique, is operator-dependent. Staging of esophageal cancer is discussed in more detail in chapters 21–25.

Because EUS may not be sufficiently reliable to exclude submucosal invasion in ECs, removal of the lesion via EMR can also be a useful adjunct for staging purposes. During the staging evaluation, if a lesion is found to be limited to the mucosa by EUS, it can be often removed via EMR, which is discussed again later in the chapter. A pathologic analysis can then be done to assess for margin adequacy as well as depth of invasion. As mentioned above, there has been some importance attached to the different layers of the mucosa and submucosa (m_{1-3}, sm_{1-3}) because of the risk of lymph node involvement with deeper invasion of the mucosa and submucosa. However, it can be difficult to distinguish between these different layers with EUS, even using high frequency probes (28), although use of a high-frequency 20 mHz ultrasound probe correctly identified the depth of 25/26 superficial lesions in one study (29). By removing the entire lesion, pathologic analysis can help determine more precisely the level of invasion and guide subsequent therapy. This was shown in a study of 48 patients who underwent staging with EUS, followed by EMR of the lesion (30). EUS staged 85% of patients correctly, with 1 overstaged and 6 understaged. The EMR specimen in the 6 patients felt to have mucosal invasion only by EUS showed submucosal invasion, which potentially could have led to a change in management if those patients were surgical candidates.

TABLE 57.1
Patient Factors to Consider When Offering Endoscopic Therapy

- HGD only
- Early cancer limited to the mucosa; no submucosal invasion
- Visible lesions are less than 20 mm in diameter
- Tumor histology is moderately to well differentiated rather than poorly differentiated
- EUS shows no lymph node involvement
- CT scan shows no distant metastases
- Patient desires endoscopic therapy rather than surgery and is willing to be compliant with follow-up endoscopy

Additionally, pathologists have better agreement regarding depth of invasion when evaluating EMR specimens compared to biopsy specimens, presumably due to having a larger tissue specimen leading to better ability to identify anatomic landmarks (31).

In summary, patients with HGD or EC who are not surgical candidates or who wish to undergo endoscopic therapy as an alternative to surgery must be carefully selected in order to minimize the risk of recurrent or residual disease. Patients should be counseled that esophagectomy is still the current standard of care and that although favorable data exist for some endoscopic therapies, long-term data are lacking at this time. All patients considering endoscopic therapy should undergo EUS followed by EMR of visible lesions less than 20 mm, with pathologic analysis dictating the subsequent therapy. If lesions are found to invade deeper than the mucosa, surgery should be recommended, providing the patient is a surgical candidate. Table 57.1 summarizes factors that make patients appropriate for consideration for endoscopic therapy.

ABLATIVE THERAPIES

Ablative therapies are methods of destroying the epithelial or mucosal layer of the esophagus. The therapy is applied in the region of the abnormal Barrett's epithelium, which is then replaced by normal "neosquamous" lining when healing occurs, especially if healing occurs in a non-acidic environment. There are several different ablative therapies, including APC, laser therapy, multipolar electric coagulation, and newer modalities such as photodynamic therapy and balloon-based radiofrequency ablation.

After ablation therapy, studies have generally used proton-pump inhibitor therapy to allow healing to occur in a non-acid environment. The amount and duration of acid-inhibition necessary has not been defined.

Photodynamic Therapy

Photodynamic therapy (PDT) is a nonthermal ablative technique that involves administering a photosensitizing agent either orally or intravenously. This agent is absorbed by all tissues but is selectively concentrated into neoplastic tissues such as Barrett's esophagus (32). Stimulation by light of a certain wavelength activates the photosensitizer, causing formation of singlet oxygen molecules and mediating cell death. Figure 57.1 displays the catheters used in PDT. Forty-eight hours after administration of the photosensitizer, the drug reaches maximal tissue concentration and red light is applied by a laser in the region of the Barrett's, usually at a wavelength of 630 nm, causing destruction of the mucosa. The only photosensitizer with current FDA approval in the United States is porfimer sodium (Photofrin, Lederle Parenterals), which is administered intravenously. Another photosensitizer used in Europe is 5-aminolevulinic acid (5-ALA, Levulan kerastick). This agent is given orally and appears to concentrate more superficially in the Barrett's mucosa, unlike porfimer which accumulates in the submucosa as well. 5-ALA may result in a shallower injury to the esophagus and therefore fewer potentially complications, but a deeper injury may be desired in order to ablate all the Barrett's glands. There are no trials comparing the 2 agents, and there have been no randomized trials of 5-ALA in Barrett's with HGD.

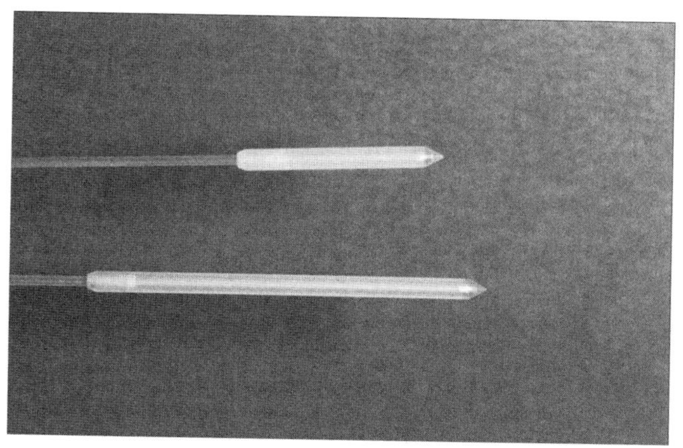

FIGURE 57.1

Catheters used in photodynamic therapy.

Outcomes in HGD and EC

PDT for treatment of Barrett's esophagus with HGD and early carcinoma was first reported in 1993 (33). A number of observational, nonrandomized studies have since reported HGD ablation rates ranging from 88% to 95% and elimination of superficial cancer in 72% in one study (34–36). A study of 103 patients, 65 of whom had HGD, reported long-term follow-up of 5 years. In the intention-to-treat analysis, eradication of HGD and EC was successful in 78% and 44.4%, respectively (37). Three patients (4.6%) developed adenocarcinoma underneath the neosquamous lining; 2 of these patients developed cancer 5 years after treatment. In some of these patients, residual Barrett's was treated with an Nd:YAG laser. One recent series included 6 patients with T1b (submucosal invasion) or limited T2 adenocarcinoma who were treated with PDT (38). The long-term results were not encouraging for these deeper cancers: 2 out of 6 patients died from cancer at 24 and 46 months, tumor recurred in 2 out of 6 at 15 and 17 months, and 2 out of 6 had no evidence of tumor at 12 and 19 months following treatment.

PDT using 5-aminolevulinic acid (5-ALA) has also been successful in observational studies of patients with HGD and EC. A study of 66 patients (n = 35 HGD and n = 31 EC) were treated; disease-free survival in the HGD group was 89% at 5 years and 68% in the EC group (39).

These observational studies suggest that PDT is a viable endoscopic option for treatment of HGD, but the risk of recurrence is a definite concern. For ECs, PDT alone may not be adequate treatment, in part because the lack of a surgical specimen makes it more difficult to determine if an EC is actually more invasive. It is important to note that PDT has not been compared to surgery in a prospective fashion. It is, however, the only ablative therapy with randomized trial data for treatment of HGD. There are 4 published randomized trials of PDT and Barrett's, only one of which included patients with HGD. This multicenter, randomized trial of 208 patients with HGD compared PDT plus omeprazole to omeprazole alone (40). The main outcome measure was complete ablation of HGD. In the PDT group, 77% had complete resolution of HGD versus 39% in the omeprazole arm at 18 months of follow-up, $P < 0.0001$. In the PDT group, 13% developed adenocarcinoma vs. 20% in the omeprazole arm, $P < 0.006$.

Although PDT has not been compared to surgery in a prospective fashion, a retrospective study did compare these treatments in 199 patients with HGD and found similar 5-year survival (41). The mortality rate in PDT patients was 9% at 5 years versus 8.5% in surgical patients at 5 years, a nonsignificant difference.

A major concern with PDT, as with all mucosal ablative therapies, is that islands of Barrett's tissue will persist underneath the neosquamous lining after healing has occurred, termed *buried glands*. These have been observed with other types of ablative therapies and may be more common in those with more superficial injury and less uniform application, such as APC. Ban et al. studied biopsy specimens on 33 patients who had undergone PDT for HGD and/or early adenocarcinoma and found buried glands in 17 (51%) as well as foci of HGD or cancer in 27% (42). These studies highlight the importance of repeat endoscopy with intensive surveillance biopsies following any ablative therapy. Patients must be counseled prior to endoscopic therapy that they will need to return for surveillance endoscopy. The optimal timing and duration of intensive surveillance following endoscopic therapy has not been defined.

Apart from the possibility of incomplete eradication of dysplasia, there are a few important limitations to discuss with use of PDT. Acute complications include chest pain, odynophagia, nausea, and cutaneous photosensitivity. Patients must avoid sunlight for up to a month following treatment with porfimer to avoid sunburn. Arrhythmias have also been reported during and after PDT (43,44).

The main long-term complication following PDT is stricture formation, which has been a serious concern with this therapy. Strictures are reported in 30% to 40% of patients and usually present with solid food dysphagia within a few weeks of treatment. One study examined risk factors for stricture formation after PDT. This retrospective study evaluated 131 patients who had undergone PDT at a single institution. Thirty-five (27%) patients developed strictures; risk factors included EMR prior to PDT and prior esophageal stricture; there was also an increased risk with increased numbers of PDT applications (45). The use of centering balloons for PDT delivery was not protective. Although most PDT-induced strictures are reported to be successfully treated by endoscopic therapy, these strictures may be more difficult to palliate than benign peptic strictures or rings. Patients in one series required an average of 4 dilations (44); another series reported the need for "multiple" dilations, use of intralesional steroid injections, and long duration of treatment up to 104 weeks (34). Use of 5-ALA rather than porphyrin appears to cause less stricturing, presumably because of more shallow tissue injury with this agent. 5-ALA is not used in the United States.

In summary, PDT appears to be more effective at eliminating HGD than acid suppression alone, and reduces the risk of cancer (39). Overall, there is a recurrence rate of BE or dysplasia of about 20% at follow-up. Although this is the ablative therapy with the most comprehensive data (and thus far the best outcomes), major concerns still exist, including incomplete eradication of HGD; incomplete treatment of cancer; the presence of buried glands, which may make subsequent surveillance difficult; lack of a surgical specimen; and a high rate of stricture formation. These are concerns with all ablative therapies. PDT has not been compared to surgery, and patients should be counseled that there is a risk of recurrence of dysplasia and cancer with any ablative therapy. However, many patients with HGD and EC are elderly and have comorbid illnesses, making them ineligible for surgery, and some patients with HGD may not wish to undergo the substantial risk associated with surgery in the absence of frank carcinoma. In this group of patients, PDT and other ablative therapies may be offered in those who want more therapy than continued surveillance or in those who already have EC. Available data suggest that PDT alone may be inadequate treatment for EC. Combination therapy with EMR of visible lesions followed by ablative therapy may be considered in this case. This type of approach is discussed below. Additionally, as more data become available on balloon-based radiofrequency ablation, that therapy may supplant PDT as the ablative therapy of choice when surgery is not desired, because thus far it appears that stricture formation and buried glands seem to occur less frequently with balloon-based radiofrequency ablation therapy than with PDT.

Balloon-Based Radiofrequency Ablation

Background

Some limitations of ablative therapies include nonuniform application as well as incomplete depth of tissue destruction. A new technology using a balloon specifically sized to the individual esophagus followed by radiofrequency ablation has been designed to overcome these limitations. This procedure was first described in a dosimetry and efficacy phased study of porcine esophagus followed by a small number of human patients with adenocarcinoma who had the treatment just prior to esophagectomy (46). After the appropriate energy density was determined, there were no strictures reported. A limited amount of data has since been published using this device in nondysplastic BE as well as HGD.

Technique

The device consists of a sizing balloon catheter, a set of ablation balloon catheters, and a high-power radiofrequency generator. After the patient's esophagus is measured with the sizing balloon, the appropriately sized ablation balloon is placed into the area of Barrett's mucosa. The balloon has a wire port allowing it to be placed beside (rather than through) the endoscope for direct visualization during the procedure. The ablation balloon is placed into the proximal region of the Barrett's esophagus, with the top end of the balloon extending 1 cm above the proximal extent of the Barrett's mucosa. High energy radiofrequency is applied via the generator. The radiofrequency ablation portion of the process takes less than 1 second. The balloon is then moved distally and the energy is again applied, creating a zone of overlap to ensure no areas are missed. This is repeated until the gastroesophageal junction is identified by visualization of the gastric folds. The key features of this device compared to other ablative technologies such as APC are that it is designed to achieve a uniform ablation depth and wide-field, uniform treatment because of the specifically sized balloons. Figure 57.2 displays an endoscope-mounted RFA paddle that can be used to target islands of Barrett's.

Efficacy in HGD and EC

To date, limited data on the efficacy of a balloon-based radiofrequency ablation system (HALO^{360}, Barrx Medical, Inc., Sunnyvale, CA) for treatment of HGD have been accumulated. A dose-response and efficacy study of this device with 1-year follow-up was recently published in patients with nondysplastic Barrett's esophagus. This multicenter study involved 32 patients for the dosimetry phase and 70 patients for the effectiveness phase (47). At 1 year of follow-up, BE was completely eliminated in 70% of patients, there were no strictures reported, and the procedure was well tolerated. Importantly, no buried glands were seen in 4,306 biopsy fragments following treatment.

A smaller study using the HALO^{360} system in patients with HGD was performed to determine the depth of tissue injury and the efficacy of the device in HGD. Eight patients with HGD underwent treatment with the device immediately prior to esophagectomy, and

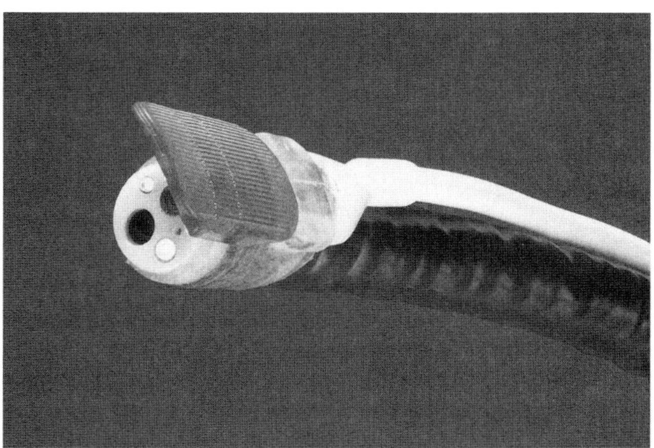

FIGURE 57.2

An endoscope-mounted RFA paddle.

the esophagectomy specimens were analyzed to determine maximal ablation depth and whether all HGD had been ablated (48). The maximal ablation depth was the muscularis mucosae, and complete ablation of intestinal metaplasia and HGD occurred in 9 out of 10 ablation zones (90%). One focus of HGD remained in an area of incomplete overlap.

A multicenter U.S. registry of patients with HGD who undergo treatment with the HALO^{360} system has been established. The initial experience of these 9 centers was published in April 2007 in abstract form and included 40 patients (49). Follow-up was available for 22 patients, ranging from 3 to 15 months. No HGD was seen in 73% of patients on follow-up biopsies; 5 had HGD remaining; and 1 had an intramucosal adenocarcinoma 1 month post ablation. No strictures were noted and there were no serious adverse events.

These preliminary studies suggest that balloon-based radiofrequency ablation may be an ideal ablative therapy. The depth of tissue destruction seems to be deep enough to eliminate Barrett's mucosa but not so deep as to cause stricture formation. Figure 57.3 demonstrates a patient before (A), immediately after (B), and 6 weeks (C) following RFA balloon ablation. The low incidence of buried glands also seems promising. However, until data are available, especially with regard to efficacy in HGD, it should only be used in a research setting. A randomized, multicenter, sham-controlled trial using this device in patients with LGD and HGD is currently underway in the United States and should provide more definitive evidence of the efficacy and safety of this type of treatment.

Ablation with Argon Plasma Coagulation, Lasers, Multipolar Electrocoagulation, and Cryotherapy

The argon plasma coagulator is used for destruction of mucosa via thermal coagulation. Initially created for use in surgical procedures, it has now been used in a variety of GI tract conditions, including destruction of arteriovenous malformation and radiation proctitis. A monopolar current is applied to argon gas, which travels through a probe placed through an endoscope. The probe does not need to come into direct contact with the mucosa to provide tissue destruction. Because of widespread availability and relative ease of use, APC for the treatment of BE has been extensively reported, mainly in nondysplastic Barrett's mucosa.

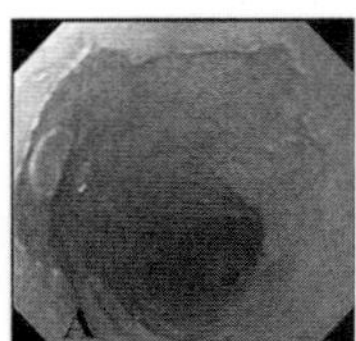

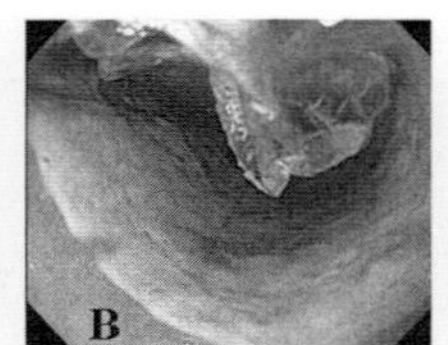

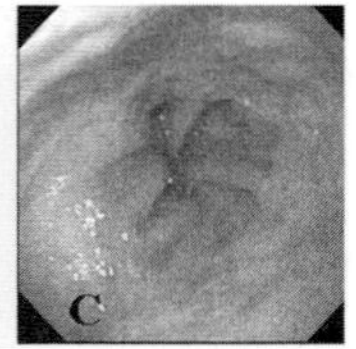

FIGURE 57.3

A patient (A) before, (B) immediately after, and (C) 6 weeks following RFA-balloon ablation.

Multiple trials have shown that it is feasible and safe to eradicate nondysplastic Barrett's esophagus with APC, but recurrence following therapy is common. For example, a study with follow-up of 1 year showed that although 68% of patients with nondysplastic BE treated with APC had initial eradication of BE, only 32% of these had continued eradication at 1 year (50). There have been only small series published with use of APC in HGD or EC. One study of 10 patients (7 HGD, 3 EC) used APC and found that 1 patient had persistent HGD and 1 progressed to cancer at a mean of 24 months of follow-up (51). Another small series of 3 patients with EC limited to the mucosa found that 1 patient had recurrent cancer at 2 years. Although data are limited, these results suggest that APC is insufficient treatment for patients with HGD or EC. It might be useful as an ablative therapy following EMR, but this approach cannot be recommended as it has not been of proven benefit. Use of APC is limited not only by a lack of data but also by difficulty in obtaining uniform, wide field application. Although APC is generally regarded as safe, reported complications occur in up to 24% of patients and include bleeding, chest pain, perforation, stricture formation, and pneumatosis. Additionally, buried glands have been reported in up to 40% of patients (52), presumably due to the shallow depth of tissue injury. For example, a study of 50 patients with nondysplastic BE who underwent multiple treatments with APC found that 68% of patients had complete macroscopic ablation of BE at 1 year (53). Nearly half (44%) of those patients with successful macroscopic clearance of BE had buried glands.

The use of lasers in treatment of HGD and EC has been studied in a limited fashion; most studies are small and had only short-term follow-up. The KTP laser was used to treat 10 patients in one study: 4 patients had HGD; 4 had LGD; and 2 had no dysplasia (54). After a mean follow-up of 10.6 months, 20% of patients had residual BE but there was no dysplasia or cancer. Another study of 14 patients with either HGD or EC underwent treatment with the Nd:YAG laser; this study found 22% had residual BE but no dysplasia or cancer at 12.8 months of follow-up (55).

Multipolar electrocoagulation causes thermal injury to mucosa and is applied via a probe that is passed through the accessory channel of an endoscope. Heater probes or bipolar electrocautery probes may be used. This therapy has been studied mainly in nondysplastic BE. Overall, about 75% of Barrett's mucosa was eradicated in these studies, with residual BE in 0% to 27%

at 4 to 36 months of follow-up (56–58). Several sessions are usually necessary to achieve endoscopic eradication of BE, and it can be difficult to cover all the surface area necessary due to the small size of the probe. This technique is not recommended for use in HGD or EC, as it has not been studied in this setting.

Cryoablation is a method of causing tissue destruction by application of liquid nitrogen through a catheter that is inserted through the accessory channel of an endoscope. A pilot study of 11 patients with BE, including 5 with LGD and 1 with HGD, showed no dysplasia in any biopsy specimen post treatment at 1 and 6 months (59). Complications included esophageal ulcerations (n = 2), chest pain (n = 1), and solid food dysphagia (n = 1). Another study published in abstract form examined the results of cryoablation in patients with LGD (n = 5), HGD (n = 3), adenocarcinoma (n = 1), and squamous cell cancer (n = 1) (60). No dysplasia was found in the majority of patients at a mean follow-up of 16.3 months; the patient with squamous cell cancer, which was a T2 lesion, has LGD remaining. Although these preliminary results are encouraging, cryoablation remains an untested strategy in the treatment of HGD and EC. A potential problem similar to that seen with APC is nonuniform application, as this is a handheld catheter and control of the application rests with the endoscopist.

In summary, the limited available data suggest that APC and laser therapy are insufficient treatments for HGD and EC. There is insufficient evidence to recommend the use of cryoablation until further data are published.

ENDOSCOPIC MUCOSAL RESECTION

The concept of using EMR to remove superficial cancers originated in Japan, where ECs are more commonly found due to screening programs for early gastric cancer. Instead of using ablation techniques, EMR excises neoplastic tissue endoscopically. As discussed previously, EMR can be used as a staging tool. The entire lesion can be submitted for pathologic analysis to determine the depth of invasion of an EC. If the lesion is found to be limited to the mucosa, with no submucosal invasion, EMR is potentially curative, providing there is no evidence of lymph node involvement on staging EUS. Therefore, EMR can be used as both a diagnostic tool as well as a therapeutic option. The ability to provide a surgical specimen for pathologic analysis is one of the main advantages of EMR over ablative therapies.

EMR can be accomplished by 2 different methods: the cap and snare technique and the variceal ligation device with snare. These are described in detail in chapter 56. The 2 methods were found to be similarly efficacious in a randomized trial (61).

Outcomes in HGD and Superficial Cancer

Several prospective observational studies have been published on outcomes in HGD and EC after EMR. A prospective, nonrandomized study of 64 patients with HGD (n = 3) or EC (n = 61, limited to T1 lesions) studied the efficacy and safety of EMR (62); 120 resections were performed, and patients were followed for a mean of 12 months. Patients were separated into a low-risk group (n = 35) for HGD or cancer limited to the mucosa and lesion < 2 cm, and a high-risk group (n = 29) for lesion > 2 cm, invasion into submucosa, or poorly differentiated histology. In the low-risk group 97% of patients had a complete local remission (no HGD or cancer) at 12 months, although 6 patients required repeat EMR during the 12 months for recurrent or metachronous cancer. In the high-risk group, 59% of patients achieved complete local remission at 12 months, and during follow-up, recurrent or metachronous cancers were found in 14% of patients.

A follow-up to this study was recently published by the same authors. In addition to the original 35 patients in the low-risk group previously published, 65 more patients with HGD or low-risk early adenocarcinoma underwent treatment with EMR and were followed for a mean of 37 months (63); 99% of the patients achieved complete local remission initially. During follow-up, metachronous lesions (HGD or EC) were found in 11 patients (11%), all of whom had repeat local therapy successfully. The calculated 5-year survival rate was 98%. Nearly half of the patients underwent some form of ablative therapy of the nondysplastic remaining Barrett's at the endoscopist's discretion.

Another study of 70 patients with HGD or EC who underwent EMR demonstrated a local remission rate of 98%, but recurrent metachronous lesions were found in 30% at 34 months of follow-up (64).

EMR of a visible lesion removes the dysplastic tissue, and margin adequacy can be assessed. However, this method leaves the remaining Barrett's esophagus behind, with the potential for recurrent dysplasia or cancer. Therefore, removal of the entire field of Barrett's with multiple EMRs (mucosectomy) has been attempted to minimize this problem. Complete, circumferential removal of all Barrett's esophagus with EC by EMR was first described in a case report in 2003 (65), followed by a case series of 12 patients with multifocal HGD, with EC with visible lesions, or with early stage malignant changes in flat mucosa who underwent circumferential EMR over a median 2.5 sessions (66). The median length of Barrett's removed was 5 cm. At 9 months, no patients had recurrence of BE or malignancy on surveillance biopsy. Two patients (20%) developed strictures that were successfully managed with endoscopic dilation.

TABLE 57.2
Selected Studies of Efficacy of EMR for HGD and EC

Type	HGD (n)	EC (n)	Eradication	Recurrent cancer	Follow-Up (months)
EMR (63)[a]	0	100	99%	11%	37
Circ. EMR (67)	18	23	76%	12.2%	32
Circ. EMR (66)	3	9	100%	0%	9
EMR (70)	28 pts HGD or EC	96.5%	0% (19.2%HGD)	19	
EMR+PDT (71)	0	24	16.6%	12	

Abbreviations: EMR = endoscopic mucosal resection; Circ. EMR = circumferential EMR of entire Barrett's; HGD = high grade dysplasia; EC = early adenocarcinoma.
[a] Some patients in this study received PDT or APC at the endoscopist's discretion.

A larger study with longer follow-up of 41 patients with HGD, some of whom had early adenocarcinoma (n = 23), found similar initial results with circumferential EMR. All patients underwent EMR of visible lesions followed by EMR of the remaining Barrett's (67). At a mean follow-up of 31.6 months, there was no remaining Barrett's in 76% of patients. However, recurrent BE was found in 24% and recurrent or metachronous EC was found in 5 (12.2%) patients. Table 57.2 summarizes outcomes in EMR for HGD and EC.

Complications of EMR include stricture formation, bleeding, and perforation. Rates of stricture formation may be higher in patients in whom circumferential EMR is performed in an attempt to remove all the Barrett's. A retrospective study of 137 patients who underwent EMR found that risk factors for stricture formation included removal of greater than 75% circumference of the mucosa as well as removal of greater than 3 cm of length (68). However, the previously mentioned study of 41 patients with HGD or EC who underwent circumferential EMR reported stricture formation in only one of 41 patients (2.4%) (66). Another study reported strictures in 2 out of 12 (17%) patients after circumferential EMR (65). EMR preceding the use of PDT was found to be an independent risk factor for subsequent strictures in one retrospective study (44).

The major complications of EMR include bleeding and perforation. Bleeding is usually reported as an immediate complication and can generally be dealt with by usual endoscopic methods. Perforation is a more serious complication but it appears that the risk is low with use of the variceal ligation device.

In summary, EMR has been increasingly used as a diagnostic and therapeutic tool. Studies of EMR monotherapy have reported recurrent neoplasia in up to 20% of patients (69) because the remaining field of neoplastic mucosa at risk remains intact. Because of this limitation, many endoscopists now use EMR to remove visible lesions and either completion EMR of the remaining Barrett's or an ablative therapy.

COMBINED THERAPY

Circumferential EMR is used to remove visible lesions and to remove the remainder of the mucosa at risk for dysplasia. In patients with long segment Barrett's esophagus, complete removal via EMR is not feasible. Combination therapy with EMR and ablation therapy to treat the remainder of the Barrett's mucosa has been studied in nonrandomized trials. A single center study of 28 patients who underwent EMR of visible lesions (HGD or EC) followed by observation only (n = 5) or ablative therapy with PDT using 5-ALA or APC found that local remission was obtained in 26 out of 28 patients at 4.5 months of therapy (70). During median follow-up of 19 months, 19% of patients treated with EMR/PDT had recurrent HGD, and 7 were found to have buried glands. This approach was also compared to surgical outcomes in a retrospective study of 24 patients with EC treated with EMR/PDT versus 64 patients treated with esophagectomy (71). Of patients in the EMR group, 83% were cancer free at 12 months versus 100% of patients in the surgery group at 19 months. Major complications were significantly higher in the surgery group.

TREATMENT OF BARRETT'S ESOPHAGUS WITH NO DYSPLASIA OR WITH LOW-GRADE DYSPLASIA

The risk of adenocarcinoma development in patients with BE is 0.5% per year (72). There is currently little evidence that nondysplastic BE or BE with LGD should

TABLE 57.3
Comparison of Endoscopic Therapies

Therapy	Advantages	Disadvantages	Approximate recurrence rate (dysplasia/cancer)
PDT	One to few sessions required, uniform application with centering balloon, treat wide field.	Stricture formation in 30–40%. Photosensitivity. Buried glands. Not widely available.	0–20%
EMR	Removes lesion for staging and may be curative. Often only one or two sessions needed.	Advanced endoscopic skill needed. Strictures reported with circumferential use. EMR of lesion only leaves behind field of BE at risk.	0–16.6%
Laser, APC	Widely available, easy to use, most endoscopists familiar with technique, treat wide field.	Shallow burn with APC leading to buried glands in many, nonuniform application ("point and shoot"), not much data in HGD or EC.	20–68% (residual BE)
Balloon RFA	Uniform, wide field ablation. No strictures or buried glands reported yet. Ease of use.	Very limited data available; essentially no outcomes in HGD or EC to date.	?

be treated because the risk of malignant transformation is sufficiently low enough to outweigh the potential benefit of treatment.

SUMMARY

The goal of endoscopic therapy for HGD or EC is to provide definitive therapy while sparing the esophagus and avoiding the morbidity of esophagectomy. Patients with HGD and EC should be counseled that esophagectomy remains the current standard of care and is the only treatment that definitively removes all neoplastic esophageal tissue. However, for patients with only HGD or EC, endoscopic therapy may be offered as a reasonable esophagus-sparing treatment in carefully selected, willing patients or in patients who are poor surgical candidates, although it must be emphasized that it is not known at this time whether long-term outcomes will be comparable to surgical outcomes. Accurate pretreatment staging is crucial to avoid endoscopic treatment in patients who have a higher risk of lymph node involvement. A complete staging evaluation should include EUS followed by EMR of visible lesions, with pathologic analysis guiding the subsequent approach. Although randomized trials comparing various endoscopic treatments to each other (and to surgery) are lacking, the best approach may ultimately prove to be EMR of visible lesions followed by either completion EMR of the remaining Barrett's esophagus, an ablative therapy, or continued surveillance, providing the remaining Barrett's is not dysplastic. The optimal ablative therapy, one which provides adequate depth of treatment with low rates of stricture formation, has not yet been developed, although early data on balloon-based radiofrequency ablation are promising. Table 57.3 summarizes the advantages and disadvantages of the various ablative therapies.

After endoscopic treatment for HGD or EC, patients must be willing to return for surveillance endoscopy on a regular basis. The optimal protocol for surveillance after endoscopic therapy has not been defined, although many endoscopists perform EGD with intensive surveillance biopsies every 3 months following treatment, at least in the short term. Other unanswered questions include long-term efficacy, outcomes compared to surgery, the best method of endoscopic treatment, the required duration of acid inhibition, and the optimal endpoint of therapy.

In summary, endoscopic therapy appears to be safe and efficacious for treatment of HGD and EC, at least in the short term, and spares patients the substantial morbidity and mortality of esophagectomy. There is no study comparing the endoscopic therapies to each other or to surgery for HGD or EC. Long-term follow-up data on recurrence rates after endoscopic treatment are mostly limited to 3 years or less at this time, although some long-term data are available for PDT (37). As newer methods continue to be developed and further data are accumulated, endoscopic therapy may move to the forefront of treatment of HGD and EC, provided that recurrence rates are acceptably low. Randomized trials are needed to determine the best approach to these patients.

References

1. Collard J. High-grade dysplasia in Barrett's esophagus. The case for esophagectomy. *Chest Surg Clin N Am.* 2002;12:77.
2. Reed M, Tolis G, Edil B, et al. Surgical treatment of esophageal high-grade dysplasia. *Ann Thorac Surg.* 2005;79:1110.
3. Pera M, Trastek V, Carpenter H, et al. Barrett's esophagus with high-grade dysplasia: an indication for esophagectomy? *Ann Thorac Surg.* 1992;54:199–204.
4. Weston A, Sharma P, Topalovski M, et al. Long-term follow-up of Barrett's high grade dysplasia. *Am J Gastroenterol.* 2000;95:1888–1893.
5. Puli S, Rastogi A, Mathur S, et al. Development of esophageal adenocarcinoma in patients with Barrett's esophagus and high grade dysplasia undergoing surveillance: a meta-analysis and systematic review [abstract]. *Gastrointest Endosc.* 2006;63:AB83.
6. Schnell T, Sontag S, Chejfec G, et al. Long-term nonsurgical management of Barrett's esophagus with high-grade dysplasia. *Gastroenterology.* 2001;120:1607–1619.
7. Sihvo E, Luostarienen M, Salo J. Fate of patients with adenocarcinoma of the esophagus and the esophagogastric junction: a population-based analysis. *Am J Gastroenterol.* 2004;99:419–424.
8. O'Riordan JM, Tucker ON, Byrne PJ, et al. Factors influencing the development of Barrett's epithelium in the esophageal remnant postesophagectomy. *Am J Gastroenterol.* 2004;99:205–211.
9. Hulscher JB, van Sandick JW, de Boer AG, et al. Extended transthoracic resection compared with limited transhiatal resection for adenocarcinoma of the esophagus. *N Engl J Med.* 2002;347:1662–1669.
10. Van Lanschot J, Hulscher J, Buskens C, et al. Hospital volume and hospital mortality for esophagectomy. *Cancer.* 2001;91:1574–1578.
11. Gross CP, Cruz-Correa M, Canto MI, et al. The adoption of ablation therapy for Barrett's esophagus: a cohort study of gastroenterologists. *Am J Gastroenterol.* 2002;97:279–286.
12. Sampliner RE, Hixson LJ, Fennerty MB, et al. Regression of Barrett's esophagus by laser ablation in an anacid environment. *Dig Dis Sci.* 1993; 38:365–368.
13. Sharna P, Wani S, Rastogi A. Endoscopic therapy for high-grade dysplasia in Barrett's esophagus: ablate, resect, or both? *Gastrointest Endosc.* 2007;66:469–474
14. Stein H, Feith M, Mueller J, et al. Limited resection for early adenocarcinoma in Barrett's esophagus. *Ann Surg.* 2000;232:733–742.
15. Buskens C, Westerterp M, Lagarde S, et al. Prediction of appropriateness of local endoscopic treatment for high-grade dysplasia and early adenocarcinoma by EUS and histopathologic features. *Gastrointest Endosc.* 2004;60:703–710.
16. Endo M, Yoshino K, Kawano T, et al. Clinicopathologic analysis of lymph node metastasis in surgically resected superficial cancer of the thoracic esophagus. *Dis Esophagus.* 2000;13:125.
17. Shimada H, Nabeya Y, Matsubara H, et al. Prediction of lymph node status in patients with superficial esophageal carcinoma: analysis of 160 surgically resected cancers. *Am J Surg.* 2006;191:250.
18. Westerterp M, Koppert L, Buskens C, et al. Outcome of surgical treatment of early adenocarcinoma of the esophagus or gastroesophageal junction. *Virchows Arch.* 2005;446:497.
19. Mallrey S, Van Dam J. EUS in the evaluation of esophageal carcinoma. *Gastrointest Endosc.* 2000;52:(Suppl):S6–S11.
20. Kelly S, Harris K, Berry E, et al. A systematic review of the staging performance of endoscopic ultrasound in gastro-oesopheageal carcinoma. *Gut*2001;49(4):534–539.
21. Grimm H, Binjoeller K, Hamper K, et al. Endosconography for preoperative locoregional staging of esophageal and gastric cancer. *Endoscopy.* 1993;25:224–230.
22. Falk GW, Catalano ME, Sivak MV Jr, et al. Endosonography in the evaluation of patients with Barrett's esophagus and high-grade dysplasia. *Gastrointest Endosc.* 1994;40:207–212.
23. Zuccaro G, Rice T, Vargo J, et al. Endoscopic ultrasound errors in esophageal cancer. *Am J Gastroenterol.* 2005;100:601–606.
24. Shimpi R, George J, Jowell P, et al. Staging of esophageal cancer by EUS: staging accuracy revisited. *Gastrointest Endosc.* 2007;66:475–482.
25. Vazquez-Sequeiros E, Wiersema M, Clain J, et al. Impact of lymph node staging on esophageal carcinoma therapy. *Gastroenterology.* 2003;125:1626–1635.
26. Reed C, Mishra G, Sahai A, et al. Esophageal cancer staging: improved accuracy by endoscopic ultrasound of celiac lymph nodes. *Ann Thorac Surg.* 1999;67:319–322.
27. Wallace M, Hawes R, Sahai A, et al. Dilation of malignant esophageal stenosis to allow EUS guided fine-needle aspiration; safety and effect on patient management. *Gastrointest Endosc.* 2000;51:309–313.
28. Chak A, Canto M, Stevens Pd, et al. Clinical applications of a new through-the-scope ultrasound probe: prospective comparison with an ultrasound endoscope. *Gastrointest Endosc.* 1997:45:291–295.
29. Waxman I, Saitoh Y. Clinical outcome of endoscopic mucosal resection for superficial GI lesions and the role of high-frequency US probe sonography in an American population. *Gastrointest Endosc.* 2000;52:322–327.
30. Larghi A, Lightdale C, Memeo L, et al. EUS followed by EMR for staging of high-grade dysplasia and early cancer in Barrett's esophagus. *Gastrointest Endosc.* 2005;62:16–23.
31. Mino-Kenudson M, Hull M, Brown I, et al. EMR for Barrett's esophagus-related superficial neoplasms offers better diagnostic reproducibility than mucosal biopsy. *Gastrointest Endosc.* 2007:66:660–666.
32. Nishioka N. Drug, light, and oxygen: a dynamic combination in the clinic. *Gastroenterology.* 1998;114:604.
33. Overholt B, Panjehpour M, Teffetellar E, et al. Photodynamic therapy for treatment of early adenocarcinoma in Barrett's esophagus. *Gastrointest Endosc.* 1993;39:73–76.
34. Overholt B, Panjehpour M, Haydek J. Photodynamic therapy for Barrett's esophagus: follow-up in 100 patients. *Gastrointest Endosc.* 1999;49:1–7.
35. Panjehpour M, Overholt B, Haydek J, et al. Results of photodynamic therapy for ablation of dysplasia and early cancer in Barrett's esophagus and effect of oral steroids on stricture formation. *Am J Gastroenterol.* 2000;95:2177–2184.
36. Wolfson H, Hemminger L, Wallace M, et al. Clinical experience of patients undergoing photodynamic therapy for Barrett's dysplasia or cancer. *Aliment Pharmacol Ther.* 2004;20:1125–1131.
37. Overholt B, Panjehpour M, Halberg D. Photodynamic therapy for Barrett's esophagus with dysplasia and early carcinoma: long-term results. *Gastrointest Endosc.* 2003;58:183–188.
38. Foroulis C, Thorpe J. Photodynamic therapy (PDT) in Barrett's esophagus with dysplasia or early cancer. *Eur J Cardiothorac Surg.* 2006;29:30–34.
39. Pech O, Gossner L, May A, et al. Long-term results of photodynamic therapy with 5-aminolevulinic acid for superficial Barrett's cancer and high-grade intraepithelial neoplasia. *Gastrointest Endosc.* 2005;62:24–30.
40. Overholt B, Lightdale C, Wang K, et al. Photodynamic therapy with porfimer sodium for ablation of high-grade dysplasia in Barrett's esophagus: international, partially blinded, randomized phase III trial. *Gastrointest Endosc.* 2005;62:488–498.
41. Prasad G, Wang K, Buttar N, et al. Long-term survival following endoscopic and surgical treatment of high-grade dysplasia in Barrett's esophagus. *Gastroenterology.* 2007;132:1226–1233.
42. Ban S, Mino M, Nishioka N, et al. Histopathologic aspects of photodynamic therapy for dysplasia and early adenocarcinoma arising in Barrett's esophagus. *Am J Surg Pathol.* 2004;28:1466–1473.
43. Overholt B, Panjehpour M, Ayres M. Photodynamic therapy for Barrett's oesophagus: cardiac effects. *Lasers Surg Med.* 1997;21:317–320.
44. Wolfsen H, Woodward T, Raimondo M. Photodynamic therapy for dysplasia and early oesophageal adenocarcinoma. *Mayo Clin Proc.* 2002;77:1176–1181.
45. Prasad G, Wang K, Buttar N, et al. Predictors of stricture formation after photodynamic therapy for high-grade dysplasia in Barrett's esophagus. *Gastrointest Endosc.* 2007;65:60–66.
46. Ganz R, Utley D, Stern R, et a. Complete ablation of esophageal epithelium with a balloon-based bipolar electrode: a phased evaluation in the porcine and in the human esophagus. *Gastrointest Endosc.* 2004;60:1002–1010.
47. Sharma V, Wang K, Overholt B, et al. Balloon-based, circumferential, endoscopic radiofrequency ablation of Barrett's esophagus: 1-year follow-up of 100 patients. *Gastrointest Endosc.* 2007;65:185–195.
48. Smith C, Bejarano P, Melvin W, et al. Endoscopic ablation of intestinal metaplasia containing high-grade dysplasia in esophagectomy patients using a balloon-based ablation system. *Surg Endosc.* 2007;21:560–569.
49. Ganz R, Overholt G, Panjehpour M, et al. Treatment of Barrett's esophagus and high-grade dysplasia using the HALO-360 ablation system: a multi-center experience. *Gastrointest Endosc.* 2006;63:AB124.
50. Basu K, Pick B, Bale R, et al. Efficacy and one year follow-up of argon plasma coagulation therapy for ablation of Barrett's oesophagus: factors determining persistence and recurrence of Barrett's epithelium. *Gut.* 2002;51:776–780.
51. Van Laethem JL, Jagodzinski R, Peny MO, et al. Argon plasma coagulation in the treatment of Barrett's high grade dysplasia and in situ adenocarcinoma. *Endoscopy.* 2001;33:257–261.
52. Grade AJ, Shah IA, Medlin SM, et al. The efficacy and safety of argon plasma coagulation therapy in Barrett's esophagus. *Gastrointest Endosc.* 1999;50:18–22.
53. Basu K, Pick B, Bale R, et al. Efficacy and one year follow-up of argon plasma coagulation therapy for ablation of Barrett's oesophagus: factors determining persistence and recurrence of Barrett's epithelium. *Gut.* 2002;51:776–780.
54. Gossner L, May A, Stolte M, et al. KTP laser destruction of dysplasia and early cancer in columnar-lined Barrett's esophagus. *Gastrointest Endosc.* 1999;49:8–12.
55. Weston AP, Sharma P. Neodymium:yttrium-aluminum garnet contact laser ablation of Barrett's high grade dysplasia and early adenocarcinoma. *Am J Gastroenterol.* 2002;97:2998–3006.
56. Montes CG, Brandalise NA, Deliza R, et al. Antireflux surgery followed by bipolar electrocoagulation in the treatment of Barrett's esophagus. *Gastrointest Endosc.* 1999;50:173–177.
57. Micholpoulos S, Tsibouris P, Bouzakis H, et al. Complete regression of Barrett's esophagus with heat probe thermocoagulation: mid-term results. *Gastrointest Endosc.* 1999;50:165–172.
58. Sampliner RE, Faigel D, Fennerty MB, et al. Effective and safe endoscopic reversal of nondysplastic Barrett's esophagus with thermal electrocoagulation combined with high-dose acid inhibition: a multicenter study. *Gastrointest Endosc.* 2001;53:554–558.
59. Johnston, M, Eastone J, Horwhat J, et al. Cryoablation of Barrett's esophagus: a pilot study. *Gastrointest Endosc.* 2005;62(6):842–848.
60. Johnston M, Cash B, Dykes C, et al. Cryoablation of dysplasia in Barrett's esophagus (BE) and early stage esophageal cancer. *Gastrointest Endosc.* 2006;63(5):AB223.
61. May A, Gossner L, Behrens A, et al. A prospective randomized trial of two different endoscopic resection techniques in 100 consecutive resections in patients with early cancer of the esophagus. *Gastrointest Endosc.* 2003;58:167–175.
62. Ell C, May A, Gossner L, et al. Endoscopic mucosal resection of early cancer and high-grade dysplasia in Barrett's esophagus. *Gastroenterology.* 2000;118:670–677.

63. Ell C, May A, Pech O, et al. Curative endoscopic resection of early esophageal adenocarcinomas (Barrett's cancer). *Gastrointest Endosc.* 2007;65:3–10.
64. May A, Gossner L, Pech O, et al. Local endoscopic therapy for intraepithelial high-grade neoplasia and early adenocarcinoma in Barrett's oesophagus: acute-phase and intermediate results of a new treatment approach. *Eur J Gastroenterol Hepatol.* 2002;14:1085–1091.
65. Satodate H, Inoue H, Yoshida T, et al. Circumferential EMR of carcinoma arising in Barrett's esophagus: case report. *Gastrointest Endosc.* 2003;58:288–292.
66. Seewald S, Akaraviputh T, Seitz U, et al. Circumferential EMR and complete removal of Barrett's epithelium: a new approach to management of Barrett's esophagus containing high-grade intraepithelial neoplasia and intramucosal carcinoma. *Gastrointest Endosc.* 2003;57:854–859.
67. Lopes C, Hela M, Pesenti C, et al. Circumferential endoscopic resection of Barrett's esophagus with high-grade dysplasia or early adenocarcinoma. *Surg Endosc.* 2007;21:820–824.
68. Katada C, Muto M, Manabe T, et al. Esophageal stenosis after endoscopic mucosal resection of superficial esophageal lesions.*Gastrointest Endosc.* 2003;57:165–169.
69. Peters FP, Kara MA, Rosmolen WD, et al. Endoscopic treatment of high-grade dysplasia and early stage cancer in Barrett's esophagus. *Gastrointest Endosc.* 2005;61:506–514.
70. Peters F, Kara M, Rosmolen W, et al. Endoscopic treatment of high-grade dysplasia and early cancer in Barrett's esophagus. *Gastrointest Endosc.* 2005;61:506–514.
71. Pacifico R, Wang K, Wongkeesong L, et al. Combined endoscopic mucosal resection and photodynamic therapy versus esophagectomy for management of early adenocarcinoma in Barrett's esophagus. *Clin Gastroenterol Hepatol.* 2003;1:252–257.
72. Sharma P, Falk GW, Weston AP, et al. Dysplasia and cancer in a large multicenter cohort of patients with Barrett's esophagus. *Clin Gastroenterol Hepatol.* 2006;4:566–572.

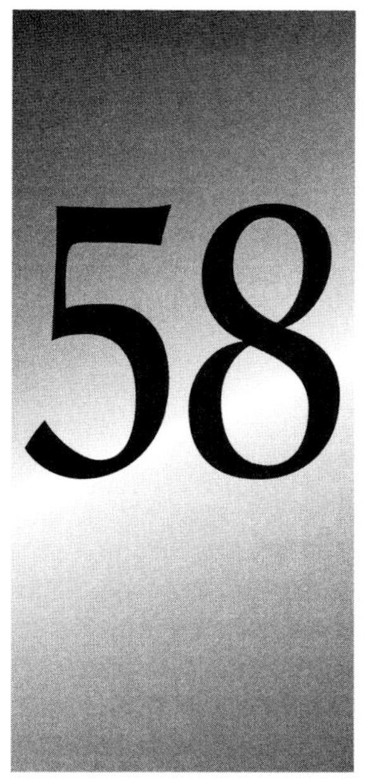

58 Therapy for Advanced Locoregional Cancer

Subroto Paul
Nasser K. Altorki

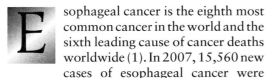

Esophageal cancer is the eighth most common cancer in the world and the sixth leading cause of cancer deaths worldwide (1). In 2007, 15,560 new cases of esophageal cancer were diagnosed and 13,940 patients died of esophageal cancer in the United States alone (2). Although the incidence of squamous cell carcinoma of the esophagus has declined in the past decades in the Western world, rates of adenocarcinoma of the distal esophagus and gastroesophageal junction have steadily risen. In the United States, the majority of patients present with adenocarcinoma (2–5). The cause of this increased incidence is unclear. Several postulates have been suggested, including the increased prevalence of gastroesophageal reflux, the treatment of *Helicobacter pylori* and the increasing obesity epidemic (3,5–7).

Despite advances in treatment, the mortality associated with esophageal cancer remains high, with overall survival rates between 15% and 25% (1,5). Poor outcomes reflect locoregionally advanced disease (T3–4N0–1 or T1–2N1, stages IIB, III) and metastatic disease (M1) at initial presentation with over 50% of patients having metastatic disease at diagnosis. Among patients who undergo surgical resection, 7% to 16% have stage IIB (T1N1, T2N1) disease and 40% to 54% have stage III (T3N1, T4N0–1) disease (1,5). Surgery alone results in poor local control and long-term outcomes. Multimodality therapy combining surgery with chemotherapy and/or radiotherapy therapy attempts to improve outcomes in these patients. In this review, we will examine the merits of multimodality therapy for patients with locally advanced esophageal cancer.

SINGLE MODALITY TREATMENT FOR LOCALLY ADVANCED ESOPHAGEAL CANCER

Surgery Alone

Although surgical resection is widely regarded as the only chance for cure in early stage esophageal cancer, it is vastly inadequate for patients with locally advanced disease. Five-year survival rates with surgery alone have varied from 10% to 30% for those with stage IIB or stage III disease in contrast to 50% to 80% survival for stage I disease and 30% to 40% for stage IIA disease (8–13). Debate over the optimal surgical approach remains unresolved. The prevailing view (represented by transhiatal or conventional transthoracic esophagectomy) holds that the disease is systemic at the time of diagnosis and that extended or en bloc resection techniques add to the morbidity and possibly the mortality of the operation without a meaningful improvement in survival. Surgical practice influenced by this view limits nodal clearance to easily accessible periesophageal and perigastric nodes. Proponents of more radical resection strategies argue that en bloc or 3-field dissections reduce or eliminate locoregional tumor burden thus improving local disease control and possibly enhancing survival (14,15).

The 2 surgical approaches were compared in a recent randomized trial by Hulscher et al. where 220 patients with adenocarcinoma of the esophagus or gastroesophageal junction were randomly assigned to either a transhiatal resection or a transthoracic en bloc esophagectomy (16). Although the difference in overall and disease-free survival between the 2 arms of the study did not achieve statistical significance, there appeared to be a trend favoring improvement in survival following transthoracic esophagectomy (39% vs. 29%) (16). Regardless of how this controversy about surgical techniques is ultimately resolved, it is clear that surgical resection alone is not adequate for the treatment of locally advanced disease.

Radiotherapy Alone

Radiotherapy is ineffective as the sole treatment modality for esophageal cancer. Overall 5-year survival rates have been between 0% and 30% in most studies (1,17–21). Herskovic et al. reported on a randomized trial conducted by the Radiation Therapy Oncology Group (RTOG) where patients with squamous cell cancer or adenocarcinoma of the thoracic esophagus were randomly assigned to 6,400 cGy of radiation alone or to concurrent fluorouracil and cisplatin plus 5,000 cGy of radiation (22). Median survival and 2-year survival in the radiotherapy arm was 8.9 months and 10% respectively compared to 12.5 months and 33% in the combined modality arm. This study has effectively discounted the benefit of radiotherapy alone as definitive therapy for esophageal cancer (22).

Chemotherapy Alone

When treated with fluorouracil, a taxane (paclitaxel or docetaxel), or irinotecan, 15% to 30% of patients have a better than 50% reduction in tumor mass. Cisplatin can also be used in combination with these agents (4,7,23–28). Both adenocarcinoma and squamous cell carcinomas of the esophagus respond to chemotherapy though squamous cell carcinomas are slightly more responsive. Chemotherapy can palliate symptoms with responses lasting a few months, but survival rarely exceeds 1 year (4,7,23–28).

RATIONALE FOR NEOADJUVANT THERAPY

Surgery, radiotherapy, or chemotherapy alone, as discussed above, are poor primary treatment modalities for locally advanced esophageal cancer with treatment failures associated with local and/or distant progression of disease. The putative objective of neoadjuvant therapy is to improve overall and disease-free survival by enhancing locoregional disease control through tumor downstaging; and by decreasing the probability of systemic failure through earlier treatment of micrometastatic disease. It also provides an in vivo test of the tumor behavior, since patients with a significant response to neoadjuvant therapy often have improved survival indicating more favorable tumor biology. Various modalities have been employed prior to surgery including preoperative radiotherapy, chemotherapy, or both.

Preoperative Radiotherapy Followed by Surgery

Radiotherapy was the first modality given in a neoadjuvant setting with the promise that using 2 modalities of local therapy may improve resectabilty and hence survival. Table 58.1 lists the results of 6 randomized trials that compared preoperative radiotherapy followed by surgical resection to surgery alone (29,17–19,30). The full radiation dose varies from 20 Gy to 53 Gy in these studies as does the temporal interval between last radiation dose and surgical resection (1–6 weeks) (29,17–19,30). In none of these trials was a survival benefit conferred by preoperative radiation therapy. The Esophageal Cancer Collaborative Group reported a meta-analysis of 5 of these trials (Fok et al. was excluded) using individual updated data from 1,147 patients who had a median follow-up of 9 years. The results suggested a small absolute improvement in survival of 4% at 5 years. A second meta-analysis reported in Malthaner et al. using 1-year survival data from all of these trials found no benefit from preoperative radiotherapy compared to surgery alone with a hazard ratio of 1.01 (95% confidence interval [CI] 0.88–1.16) (31–34). Given that no single randomized trial demonstrated any benefit to preoperative radiotherapy and the conflicting results of the meta-analyses, preoperative radiotherapy is not advocated as a treatment option for esophageal cancer.

Preoperative Chemotherapy Followed by Surgery

At least 10 randomized trials performed since 1980 have compared preoperative chemotherapy with surgery alone (Table 58.2). The following discussion will focus on the largest and most mature trials reported to date (35–37). The U.S. intergroup trial (INT113) compared the outcomes of 440 patients with either adenocarcinoma or squamous cell carcinoma of the esophagus, stages I to III, who were randomized to receive either 3 cycles of cisplatin and 5-fluorouracil (5-FU) followed by surgery (213 patients) or surgery

TABLE 58.1
Neoadjuvant Radiotherapy Randomized Trials

Study	Patients		Dose of RT	Median survival (mo)	Five-Year survival (%)	*P* value
Launois (1981)[4]	RT + S	62	40 Gy	10	10	NS
	S	47		12	12	
Gignoux (1988)[6]	RT + S	115	33 Gy	48	10	NS
	S	114		45	9	
Wang (1989)[8]	RT + S	104	40 Gy	NA	35	NS
	S	102		NA	30	
Arnott (1992)[11]	RT + S	90	20 Gy	8	9	NS
	S	86		8	17	
Fok (1994)[1]	RT + S	58	35–53 Gy	11	10	NS
	S	50		22	16	

alone (227 patients) (Table 58.2) (36). Patients randomized to preoperative chemotherapy followed by surgery received an additional 2 cycles of the same chemotherapy postoperatively. The complete pathologic response rate was only 2.5% for those receiving at least 1 cycle of preoperative chemotherapy with no differences in the curative resection rate between the 2 trial arms. There was no significant difference in either median or 2-year survival between the 2 arms of the study (14.9 months and 35% for chemotherapy and surgery [C+S] vs. 16.1 months and 37% for surgery alone [S], $P = 0.53$) (36). The authors concluded that preoperative chemotherapy provides no additional benefit over surgery alone for esophageal cancer.

This stands in contrast to results from the United Kingdom Medical Research Council (MRC OEO-2) trial, which included 802 patients with either squamous cell carcinoma or adenocarcinoma of the esophagus. Eligible patients were randomly assigned to either surgery alone or 2 preoperative cycles of cisplatin and 5-FU followed by surgical resection. This trial demonstrated that preoperative chemotherapy significantly improved both median survival as well as 2-year overall survival (16.8 months vs. 13.3 months, $P < 0.004$: 43% vs. 34%, $P < 0.004$, respectively) (35). The discrepancy between INT113 and the MRC trial may be due to the larger sample size in the European trial and the fact that fewer patients proceeded to surgical resection in the U.S. trial compared to the MRC trial (80% and 92% respectively) (4,7,35,36,38–40).

The Medical Research Council Adjuvant Gastric Infusional Chemotherapy (MAGIC) trial also attempted to ascertain the efficacy of neoadjuvant chemotherapy. This randomized trial included 503 patients with gastric cancer and adenocarcinoma of the esophagus and gastroesophageal junction, stage II or higher, who were randomized to surgery alone (253 patients) or 3 cycles of epirubicin, cisplatin, and 5-FU, followed by surgery and an additional 3 cycles of chemotherapy postoperatively (250 patients) (37). Only 42% of the patients completed postoperative chemotherapy, and any benefit from chemotherapy is attributed to its preoperative use. Although the majority of the patients had gastric cancer, 26% of patients in both arms had tumors of the lower esophagus or lower gastroesophageal junction (7,37–41).

The MAGIC trial demonstrated that preoperative chemotherapy was associated with a significant improvement in median survival (24 months vs. 20 months, $P < 0.009$) and 5-year overall survival (36% vs. 23%, $P < 0.009$) (7,37–41). Multivariate analysis showed that the treatment effect was unchanged after adjustment for primary tumor site. However, it should be noted that unlike the prior studies, which had patients with both adenocarcinoma and squamous cell carcinoma of the esophagus, the MAGIC trial included exclusively patients with adenocarcinoma and therefore its results may not be necessarily applicable to patients with squamous cell cancer.

A recently reported French Intergroup Trial (FFCD and FNLCC) randomized 224 patients with adenocarcinoma of the distal esophagus, gastroesophageal junction, and stomach, stage II or greater, to either surgery alone or 2 to 3 cycles of fluorouracil and cisplatin followed by surgery and 1 to 4 additional cycles of the same chemotherapy (42). Unlike the MAGIC trial, 75% of patients in this trial had adenocarcinoma of the distal esophagus and gastroesophageal junction. The preoperative chemotherapy arm showed a statistically significant improvement in R0 resection rate (87% vs. 74%, $P = 0.04$), 5-year disease-free survival (34% vs. 21%, $P = 0.003$) and overall survival (38% vs. 24%, $P = 0.02$) (42).

Further support for the use of preoperative chemotherapy comes from meta-analysis data. In a Cochrane review reported in 2003, 11 randomized trials with a total of 2,051 patients were analyzed (31). Clinical relevance was based on median survival and survival from years 1 to 5. When specific survival was not available, it

TABLE 58.2
Neoadjuvant Chemotherapy Randomized Trials

Study		Patients	Chemotherapy	pCR (%)	Median survival (mo)	Five-Year survival (%)	*P* value
Roth (1988)[13]	C + S	19	Neo: Cis,Vin, Bleo	NA	9	NA	NS
	S	20	Adjuvant: Cis, Vin		9	NA	
Nygaard (1992)[16]	C + S	50	Cis, Bleo	NA	8	3-y 3	NS
	S	41			8	9	
Ancona (2001)[19]	C + S	47	Cis, 5-FU X 2 or 3	13%	25	34	NS
	S	47			24	22	
Schlag (1992)[9]	C + S	22	Cis, 5-FU X 3	NA	10	NA	NS
	S	24			10		
Kelsen - INT113 (1998)[14]	C + S	213	Neo Cis, 5-FU X 3	2.5%	14.9	2 y 35	NS
	S	227	Adj Cis, 5-FU X 2		16.1	37	
MRC (2002)[7]	C + S	400	Cis, 5-FU X 2	4%	16.8	2 y 43	$P = 0.004$
	S	402			13.3	34	
Cuningham (2006)[21]	C + S	250	Cis, 5-FU, Epi X 3	0%	24	36.3	$P = 0.009$
	S	253	Adj Cis, 5-FU, Epi X 3		20	23.0	

was calculated from the published survival curves. The pooled response rate to chemotherapy was 36%, with 3% of patients having a complete pathologic response. Although there was no difference in survival at 1 and 2 years, a survival advantage was seen at 3 years and achieved statistical significance at 5 years (31). A more recent meta-analysis was presented by Thirion et al. at the American Society of Clinical Oncology meeting 2007 (43). The particular strength of this meta-analysis is its reliance on individual patient data that were checked and reanalyzed. The study encompassed 9 randomized trials performed from the early 1980s to the mid-1990s. Slightly more than half the patients had squamous cell carcinoma. The results showed that preoperative chemotherapy resulted in a modest but statistically significant improvement in disease-free and overall survival (4.3% and 4.1% respectively) without adversely affecting perioperative mortality (43).

Based on the results of at least 3 well-powered randomized trials and the meta-analysis by Thirion et al., there appears to be level 1 evidence for a modest benefit of preoperative chemotherapy in esophageal and gastroesophageal junction adenocarcinoma. The effect of preoperative chemotherapy in squamous cell cancer appears less certain at this time.

Preoperative Chemoradiation Followed by Surgery

Concurrent chemotherapy and radiotherapy given in the neoadjuvant setting has been the subject of numerous clinical trials. The addition of radiotherapy to preoperative chemotherapy regimens was thought to be an effective means of increasing pathologic complete response rates and thereby improve survival. There have been 46 non-randomized trials evaluating neoadjuvant therapy from 1981 to 1999. Geh et al. examined the results of the 2,704 patients enrolled in these trials. Of these patients, 69% had squamous cell carcinoma, and 31% had adenocarcinoma of the esophagus (44). The radiation dose varied from 30 to 60 Gy with the majority of the patients receiving 5-FU and cisplatin for chemotherapy. Collectively, the resection rate was 74% with a complete pathologic response in 24% of patients (44).

Eight randomized trials evaluating neoadjuvant chemoradiation were done from 1992 to 2002 (20–21, 45–51). These studies are listed in Table 58.3. Interpretation of the results from these trials is difficult, primarily due to small sample sizes, as well as incomplete staging procedures employed in many of these trials. Most of these trials used cisplatin- and 5-FU–based chemotherapy with radiotherapy doses varying from 20 to 40 Gy. A few of the sentinel and larger more recent trials will be discussed in depth.

The study by Walsh et al. randomized 113 patients with esophageal adenocarcinoma to either 2 cycles of cisplatin and 5-FU and 40 Gy of radiotherapy (58 patients) or surgery alone (55 patients). Nodal disease was seen in 42% of patients who received preoperative chemoradiation compared to 82% of the patients who underwent surgery alone ($P = 0.001$). A complete pathologic response was seen in 25% of the patients who underwent

TABLE 58.3
Neoadjuvant Chemoradiotherapy Randomized Trials

Study	Patients		Histology	Chemotherapy RT	Surgical mortality	pCR (%)	Median survival (mo)	Three-Year survival (%)	*P* value
Nygaard (1992)[16]	S	41	S	Cis + Bleo	13	NA	7.5	9	NS
	CRT +S	47		35 Gy	24		7.5	17	
Le Prise (1994)[20]	S	45	S	Cis + 5-FU	7	10	10	14	NS
	CRT +S	41		20 Gy	8.5		10	19	
Apinop (1994)[5]	S	34	S	Cis + 5-FU	15	NA	7	20	NS
	CRT +S	35		40 Gy	14		10	26	
Walsh (1996)[10]	S	55	A	Cis + FU	4	25	11	6	*P* = 0.01
	CRT +S	58		40 Gy	8		16	32	
Law (1998)[3]	S	30	S	Cis + 5-FU	0	25	27	NA	NS
	CRT +S	30		40 Gy	0		26	NA	
Bosset (1997)[12]	S	139	S	Cis	4	26	19	37	NS
	CRT +S	143		37 Gy	12.3		19	39	
Urba (2001)[17]	S	50	S (25%)	Cis + 5-Fu + Vin	2	28	18	16	NS
	CRT +S	50	A (75%)	45 Gy	7		17	30	
Burmeister (2002)[18]	S	128	S (36%)	Cis + 5-FU	NA	16%	22	NA	NS
	CRT +S	128	A (61%)	35 Gy			19	NA	
Tepper (2005)[2]	S	26	S (25%)	Cis + 5-FU	7.7	40%	54	39	*P*<0.008
	CRT +S	30	A (75%)	50.4 Gy	0		22	16	

surgery after chemoradiotherapy. Three-year survival was significantly better in the multimodality arm compared to surgery alone (32% vs. 6%; $P < 0.01$). Median survival also increased to 16 months from 11 months with neoadjuvant chemoradiation ($P < 0.01$) (10). Criticism of this trial includes inadequate preoperative staging and unusually poor survival in the surgery-alone arm (6% at 3 years). Most surgical series, including those from the study center itself, showed a 3-year survival of at least 20% with surgery alone. These results suggest a potential critical imbalance between the 2 arms of the trial favoring the trimodality arm (4,38–40,48). Despite these limitations, this study remains the only completed randomized trial demonstrating a survival benefit from preoperative chemoradiation (4,38–41,48).

Other randomized studies, including those by Urba et al., Nygaard et al., Le Prise et al., Burmeister et al., Bosset et al. and Aninop et al., were unable to demonstrate a statistically significant survival benefit from neoadjuvant chemoradiation (Table 58.3) (20,21,47,49–51). However, most of these trials presented evidence based on secondary end-point or post-hoc subgroup analysis that suggests a potential benefit from preoperative chemoradiation.

For example, in one of the largest trials to date, Burmeister et al. randomized 256 patients with esophageal carcinoma to either surgery alone or neoadjuvant cisplatin and 5-FU and concurrent 35 Gy of radiotherapy followed by surgery. Roughly 60% of patients in each group had adenocarcinoma and all had resectable disease (stage I to III) as staged by endoscopy and computed tomography. A complete pathologic response was seen in 27% of the patients (16% overall, 10% for those with adenocarcinoma). Although neither overall survival nor disease-free survival differed between the 2 study arms, this study reported that neoadjuvant chemoradiation improved disease-free survival in patients with squamous cell carcinoma (hazard ratio [HR] 0.47; 95% CI 0.25–0.86, $P = 0.014$) with a trend toward improved recurrence-free survival for those with adenocarcinoma (21).

Bosset et al. also showed a similar improvement in 3-year disease-free but not overall survival in patients receiving neoadjuvant therapy (40% vs. 28%, $P = 0.003$) (49). In this study, 282 patients with squamous cell carcinoma, stage I and II, were randomized to cisplatin and 37 Gy of radiotherapy split over two 1-week courses followed by surgery (143 patients) or surgery alone (139 patients). A complete pathologic response was seen in 26% patients receiving neoadjuvant therapy. Although no significant difference in median or overall survival was observed, there was a significant difference in disease-free survival (a secondary end-point) favoring the combined modality arm. In this trial, neoadjuvant therapy was associated with a significantly higher postoperative mortality (17 of 138 deaths in the neoadjuvant chemotherapy arm vs. 5 of 137 in the surgery-alone arm, $P = 0.012$).

The lack of any observed survival benefit in these 2 trials may be due to the suboptimal chemotherapy regimens given in each trial. In the Bosset et al. trial, cisplatin was administered 0 to 2 days before radiation as a single dose in two 1-week courses, while in the Burmeister et al. study a single cycle of cisplatin and 5-FU was given. Single agent or single cycle of chemotherapy may not be sufficient to provide a survival benefit (4,21,38–41,49).

The American Cancer and Acute Leukemia Group B (CALGB)-9781 trial evaluating neoadjuvant chemoradiation for esophageal cancer was closed prematurely due to poor accrual of patients with only 56 patients, out of a planned accrual of 500 patients, enrolled prior to closure. The majority of the patients had esophageal adenocarcinoma (75%) and all had resectable disease (stages I to III). Patients were randomized to either 2 cycles of chemotherapy with 5-FU and 50.4 Gy of radiation prior to surgery (30 patients) or surgery (26 patients) alone (4,45). Despite the small numbers, this trial demonstrated an overall median survival benefit for preoperative chemoradiation followed by surgery (4.5 years vs. 1.8 years, $P = 0.02$) with a 10% rate of complete pathologic response. Five-year survival was also improved from 16% to 39% ($P < 0.008$) after preoperative therapy (4,45). As this trial was closed prematurely due to poor accrual, it is difficult to completely validate the results of this trial.

Four recent meta-analyses evaluating neoadjuvant chemoradiotherapy have been reported by Malthaner et al., Urschel et al., Fiorica et al., and Greer et al. (32,52–54). Each of these studies reported a small survival benefit from preoperative chemoradiation but only after 3 years. However, there was a trend toward higher post-operative mortality after chemoradiation (32, 52–54).

Fiorica et al. pooled 6 randomized controlled trials comparing preoperative chemoradiation and surgery vs. surgery alone (20,47–51) encompassing 764 patients (53). Trials were restricted to include only patients with resectable esophageal carcinoma and no metastatic disease. Only 1 of the 6 trials (48) showed a statistically significant survival benefit after preoperative chemoradiation. Three-year mortality was lower after chemoradiation and surgery compared to surgery alone (odds ratio [OR] 0.53; 95% CI 0.31–0.92; $P = 0.025$). However, the postoperative mortality was almost doubled after chemoradiation and surgery (OR 2.10; 95% CI 1.18–3.73; $P = 0.01$) (53). Greer et al. pooled the same trials and reached similar conclusions although their results did not reach statistical significance (OR 0.86; 95% CI, 0.74–1.01; $P = 0.07$) (54). Both of these meta-analyses did not analyze individual patient data but rather group averages. Hence, any small therapeutic benefit from chemoradiation may have been lost in the statistical analysis depending on the modeling methods used.

Urschel et al. combined data from 9 randomized controlled trials. The 6 trials analyzed by Fiorica et al. and Greer et al. were included, as well as 3 additional trials (21,46,55). These trials included the results of 1,116 patients and were graded for quality using the 5-point Jadad scale (52). No additional benefit was found to the addition of preoperative chemoradiation to surgery until 3 years were reached (OR 0.66; 95% CI 0.47–0.92; $P = 0.016$). A nonsignificant trend toward increased postoperative mortality with preoperative chemoradiation was seen (OR 1.63; 95% CI 0.99–2.68; $P = 0.053$). Another meta-analysis pooled the data from 8 trials (20,21,47–51,56) and compared survival at 3 years. As reported by Malthaner et al., 3-year mortality was lower for patients receiving preoperative chemoradiation (OR 0.87; 95% CI 0.80–0.96; $P = 0.004$) (32). Although individual patient data were obtained to some extent in both of these meta-analyses, this was not possible for most of the trials analyzed. The majority of the results in both of these studies is therefore based on summary estimates, which seriously limits the strength of the conclusions reached by Urschel et al. and Malthaner et al.

Preoperative Chemotherapy Followed by Surgery vs. Preoperative Chemoradiation Followed by Surgery

Despite the lack of evidence supporting the use of preoperative chemoradiotherapy, trimodality regimens have gained popularity, especially in the United States and parts of Europe. The question remains, however, whether chemotherapy or chemoradiotherapy constitutes the optimal preoperative regimen. A direct attempt to answer this question was conducted by the German Esophageal Cancer Study Group in their Preoperative Chemotherapy or Radiochemotherapy in Esophagogastric Adenocarcinoma Trial (POET) trial (57).

In this trial, patients with stage T3–4NxM0 adenocarcinoma of the esophagus were randomly assigned to either preoperative chemotherapy only with 2.5 cycles of cisplatin and 5-FU or 2 courses of cisplatin and 5-FU followed by 3 weeks of chemoradiotherapy (30 Gy, cisplatin, and etoposide) (57). Surgical resection was planned 3 to 4 weeks after the end of preoperative therapy in each arm. The study was closed early due to poor accrual with only 126 out of the planned 394 patients accrued. A total of 120 eligible patients were randomly assigned; 90 patients underwent surgical resection. As reported by Stahl et al., a complete pathologic response was found in 2.5% of patients who received neoadjuvant chemotherapy in comparison to 17% of patients who received neoadjuvant chemoradiation (P = 0.06) (57). However, this did not translate into a statistically significant survival benefit (median survival 32.8 vs. 21.1 months, 3-year survival 43% vs. 27%, logrank P = 0.14 for chemoradiation vs. chemotherapy). Although this study was underpowered due to poor patient accrual, extrapolation of these results suggests that preoperative chemoradiation may be marginally superior to preoperative chemotherapy in treating locally advanced esophageal cancer. However, this benefit may come at the cost of an increased postoperative mortality (8.3% vs. 3.3% postoperative mortality for preoperative chemoradiation vs. preoperative chemotherapy, respectively).

Based on the results of this trial as well as the previously discussed randomized trials, there are sparse data supporting the routine use of neoadjuvant chemoradiation as a treatment modality for locally advanced esophageal cancer. The randomized trials are either underpowered or have shortcomings such as inadequate staging or high operative mortality. The single trial to date that showed a survival advantage for preoperative chemoradiation, Walsh et al. (48), has multiple shortcomings, as previously discussed. Even the results of the meta-analyses demonstrate only a marginal survival benefit, if at all, from neoadjuvant chemoradiation, often achieved at the expense of increased postoperative morbidity. Collectively, these results do not provide level 1 evidence to support the routine use of preoperative chemoradiotherapy. Hence, neoadjuvant chemoradiation regimens should be deemed investigational in nature and limited to the context of clinical trials.

Definitive Chemoradiation

Two recent randomized trials have compared the efficacy of chemoradiation and surgery to chemoradiation alone (58,59). All patients in these trials had locally advanced carcinoma of the esophagus (T3N0–1M0). In the French 9102 trial, Bedenne et al. evaluated 444 patients (90% squamous cell carcinoma) who received 2 cycles of 5-FU and cisplatin with radiation (concurrent 46 Gy on the fourth, fifth weeks or a split course of 15 Gy on days 1–5 and 22–26). Of these 444 patients, 259 patients had a partial response and were then randomized to additional chemoradiation (130 patients) or surgery (129 patients). Neither median survival nor 2-year survival were statistically different between the 2 groups: 17.7 months (chemoradiation [CRT] + surgery [S]) vs. 19.3 months (CRT); and 34% (CRT + S) vs. 40% (CRT), P = 0.56 (59). However, those who underwent surgery had improved 2-year local control rates with less dysphagia and need for stents: 66.4% (CRT + S) vs. 57.0% (CRT) local control rate, P = 0.0014; 5% (CRT + S) vs. 32% (CRT) stent usage, P < 0.001. Although the authors concluded that surgery is not necessary for those with locally advanced esophageal cancer, there are important limitations in the study design. Since only patients who responded to chemoradiation were included, the question of whether surgery is beneficial in nonresponders cannot be answered. Hence, this trial is inherently biased against surgery (4,38–40,59). Furthermore, 6-month mortality in the chemoradiation and surgery arm was 16% and only 6% in the chemoradiation only arm (P = 0.15). The authors concluded that the addition of surgery to chemoradiation simply increases 6 months mortality without improving survival. An alternative explanation is that the high postoperative mortality likely reflects the multicenter nature of the trial underscoring the need to limit such complex treatment designs to high-volume centers thus reducing surgical mortality and thereby identifying any possible benefit from surgical resection.

In another trial reported by Stahl et al., 172 patients with squamous cell carcinoma of the esophagus (T3–4N0–1M0) were randomized after 3 cycles of induction chemotherapy with 5-FU, leucovorin, and cisplatin to either definitive chemoradiation with cisplatin, etoposide, and 65 Gy of radiation (86 patients) or more chemoradiation with cisplatin, etoposide, and 40 Gy followed by surgery in 4 to 6 weeks (86 patients) (58). This trial also demonstrated no survival difference between the 2 study arms in median survival and 2-year survival (16.4 months [CRT + S] vs. 14.9 months [CRT]; and 31% [CRT + S] vs. 24% [CRT], P = 0.007 for equivalence), despite demonstrating a difference in local progression-free survival (64.3% [CRT + S] vs. 40.7% [CRT], P = 0.003) (58). Mortality was significantly increased in those who had surgery than those who had chemoradiotherapy (12.8% vs. 3.5%, respectively, P = 0.03). However, the chemoradiotherapy regimen given was unconventional making the results of this trial difficult to interpret. Both trials had patients with predominantly squamous cell histology, which is known to be slightly more responsive to chemotherapy than adenocarcinoma. Hence, these results may not be applicable to those with esophageal adenocarcinoma. As in Bedenne et al., the authors of this study similarly concluded that the addition of surgery to chemoradiation increases mortality without a survival benefit. However, this trial was a multicenter trial with 11 participating centers, 5 of which contributed less than 10 patients. Hence, the high postoperative mortality once again underscores the need to restrict these trials to high-volume centers in order to remove any confounding from surgical morbidity and mortality. Given these shortcomings and the fact that the trial was underpowered to prove equivalence, the trial results are not conclusive (4,38–40). In fact, Stahl et al. suggest that surgery may benefit those who fail to respond to chemotherapy since this group of patients had a 32% 3-year survival with a R0 resection. These trials, like other studies evaluating therapies for esophageal cancer, invites further randomized trials (4,38–40,59).

BRIEF WORD ON ADJUVANT THERAPY

Several randomized trials have been published evaluating the use of postoperative chemotherapy or chemoradiation after esophagectomy. Two randomized Japanese trials have compared the benefit of adjuvant chemotherapy for squamous cell carcinoma of the esophagus after esophagectomy with patients receiving cisplatin and vindesine in one trial and cisplatin and 5-FU in another over surgery alone (41,60,61). Each of these trials had randomized 100 patients to each arm. No difference in overall survival was detected in either trial. The trial evaluating postoperative cisplatin and 5-FU did, however, show an improved disease-free survival at 5 years (55% vs. 45%, $P = 0.37$) (41,60,61).

Data are sparse for the use of postoperative chemoradiotherapy in patients with adenocarcinoma of the esophagus. MacDonald et al. reported the results of intergroup trial 0116 in which 556 patients with gastric and gastroesophageal cancer were randomized to surgery followed by postoperative 5-FU and leucovorin combined with 45 Gy of radiotherapy or surgery alone. Improved median survival was seen in the adjuvant treatment group (36 months vs. 27 months, $P = 0.005$) (62). However, it is unclear if this trial is applicable to esophageal cancer, as patients with predominantly gastric and gastroesophageal junction cancers were evaluated. Yet this trial and the previous trials do suggest that adjuvant therapies may be provide a survival benefit. More conclusive data are needed to answer such questions, but trials may be limited by the fact that there is little theoretical support to favor adjuvant over neoadjuvant therapies for esophageal cancer (4,40,62).

References

1. Enzinger PC, Mayer RJ. Esophageal cancer. *N Engl J Med.* 2003;349:2241–2252.
2. Jemal A, Siegel R, Ward E, et al. Cancer statistics, 2007. *CA Cancer J Clin.* 2007; 57:43–66.
3. Jemal A, Ward E, Hao Y, et al. Trends in the leading causes of death in the United States, 1970–2002. *JAMA.* 2005;294:1255–1259.
4. Ilson DH. Cancer of the gastroesophageal junction: combined modality therapy. *Surg Oncol Clin N Am.* 2006;15:803–824.
5. Devesa SS, Blot WJ, Fraumeni JF, Jr. Changing patterns in the incidence of esophageal and gastric carcinoma in the United States. *Cancer.* 1998;83:2049–2053.
6. Jemal A, Murray T, Ward E, et al. Cancer statistics, 2005. *CA Cancer J Clin.* 2005; 55:10–30.
7. Ilson DH. Cancer of the gastroesophageal junction: current therapy options. *Curr Treat Options Oncol.* 2006;7:410–423.
8. Pera M, Trastek VF, Carpenter HA, et al. Barrett's esophagus with high-grade dysplasia: an indication for esophagectomy? *Ann Thorac Surg.* 1992;54:199–204.
9. Headrick JR, Nichols FC III, Miller DL, et al. High-grade esophageal dysplasia: long-term survival and quality of life after esophagectomy. *Ann Thorac Surg.* 2002;73:1697–1702; discussion 1702–1693.
10. Reed CE. Surgical management of esophageal carcinoma. *Oncologist* 1999;4:95–105.
11. Siewert JR, Stein HJ, Feith M, et al. Histologic tumor type is an independent prognostic parameter in esophageal cancer: lessons from more than 1,000 consecutive resections at a single center in the Western world. *Ann Surg.* 2001;234:360–367; discussion 368–369.
12. Collard JM, Otte JB, Fiasse R, et al. Skeletonizing en bloc esophagectomy for cancer. *Ann Surg.* 2001;234:25–32.
13. Greene FL, Page DL, Fleming ID. *AJCC Cancer Staging Manual.* 6th edition. New York: Springer-Verlag, 2002.
14. Altorki N. En-bloc esophagectomy—the three-field dissection. *Surg Clin North Am.* 2005;85:611–619, xi.
15. Altorki NK, Girardi L, Skinner DB. En bloc esophagectomy improves survival for stage III esophageal cancer. *J Thorac Cardiovasc Surg.* 1997;114:948–955; discussion 955–946.
16. Hulscher JB, van Sandick JW, de Boer AG, et al. Extended transthoracic resection compared with limited transhiatal resection for adenocarcinoma of the esophagus. *N Engl J Med.* 2002;347:1662–1669.
17. Launois B, Delarue D, Campion JP, et al. Preoperative radiotherapy for carcinoma of the esophagus. *Surg Gynecol Obstet.* 1981;153:690–692.
18. Gignoux M, Roussel A, Paillot B, et al. The value of preoperative radiotherapy in esophageal cancer: results of a study by the EORTC. *Recent Results Cancer Res.* 1988; 110:1–13.
19. Wang M, Gu XZ, Yin WB, et al. Randomized clinical trial on the combination of preoperative irradiation and surgery in the treatment of esophageal carcinoma: report on 206 patients. *Int J Radiat Oncol Biol Phys.* 1989;16:325–327.
20. Urba SG, Orringer MB, Turrisi A, et al. Randomized trial of preoperative chemoradiation versus surgery alone in patients with locoregional esophageal carcinoma. *J Clin Oncol.* 2001;19:305–313.
21. Burmeister BH, Smithers BM, Gebski V, et al. Surgery alone versus chemoradiotherapy followed by surgery for resectable cancer of the oesophagus: a randomised controlled phase III trial. *Lancet Oncol.* 2005;6:659–668.
22. Herskovic A, Martz K, al-Sarraf M, et al. Combined chemotherapy and radiotherapy compared with radiotherapy alone in patients with cancer of the esophagus. *N Engl J Med.* 1992;326:1593–1598.
23. Enzinger PC, Ilson DH, Saltz LB, et al. Phase II clinical trial of 13-cis-retinoic acid and interferon-alpha-2a in patients with advanced esophageal carcinoma. *Cancer.* 1999; 85:1213–1217.
24. Ilson DH, Saltz L, Enzinger P, et al. Phase II trial of weekly irinotecan plus cisplatin in advanced esophageal cancer. *J Clin Oncol.* 1999;17:3270–3275.
25. Enzinger PC, Ilson DH, Kelsen DP. Chemotherapy in esophageal cancer. *Semin Oncol.* 1999;26:12–20.
26. Enzinger PC, Ilson DH, Saltz LB, et al. Irinotecan and cisplatin in upper gastrointestinal malignancies. *Oncology (Williston Park).* 1998;12:110–113.
27. Mooney MM. Neoadjuvant and adjuvant chemotherapy for esophageal adenocarcinoma. *J Surg Oncol.* 2005;92:230–238.
28. von Rahden BH, Stein HJ. Therapy of advanced esophageal malignancy. *Curr Opin Gastroenterol.* 2004;20:391–396.
29. Fok M, McShane J, Law S, et al. Prospective randomised study in the treatment of oesophageal carcinoma. *Asian J Surg.* 1994;17:223–229.
30. Arnott SJ, Duncan W, Kerr GR, et al. Low dose preoperative radiotherapy for carcinoma of the oesophagus: results of a randomized clinical trial. *Radiother Oncol.* 1992;24:108–113.
31. Malthaner R, Fenlon D. Preoperative chemotherapy for resectable thoracic esophageal cancer. *Cochrane Database Syst Rev.* 2003:CD001556.
32. Malthaner RA, Wong RK, Rumble RB, et al. Neoadjuvant or adjuvant therapy for resectable esophageal cancer: a systematic review and meta-analysis. *BMC Med.* 2004; 2:35.
33. Arnott SJ, Duncan W, Gignoux M, et al. Preoperative radiotherapy in esophageal carcinoma: a meta-analysis using individual patient data (Oesophageal Cancer Collaborative Group). *Int J Radiat Oncol Biol Phys.* 1998;41:579–583.
34. Arnott SJ, Duncan W, Gignoux M, et al. Preoperative radiotherapy for esophageal carcinoma. *Cochrane Database Syst Rev.* 2005:CD001799.
35. Medical Research Council Oesophageal Cancer Working Group. Surgical resection with or without preoperative chemotherapy in oesophageal cancer: a randomised controlled trial. *Lancet.* 2002;359:1727–1733.
36. Kelsen DP, Ginsberg R, Pajak TF, et al. Chemotherapy followed by surgery compared with surgery alone for localized esophageal cancer. *N Engl J Med.* 1998;339: 1979–1984.
37. Cunningham D, Allum WH, Stenning SP, et al. Perioperative chemotherapy versus surgery alone for resectable gastroesophageal cancer. *N Engl J Med.* 2006;355:11–20.
38. Piraino A, Vita ML, Tessitore A, et al. Neoadjuvant therapy for esophageal cancer: surgical considerations. *Rays.* 2006;31:37–45.
39. Yoon HH, Gibson MK. Combined-modality therapy for esophageal and gastroesophageal junction cancers. *Curr Oncol Rep.* 2007;9:184–192.

40. McKian KP, Miller RC, Cassivi SD, et al. Curing patients with locally advanced esophageal cancer: an update on multimodality therapy. *Dis Esophagus.* 2006;19:448–453.
41. Shinoda M, Hatooka S, Mori S, et al. Clinical aspects of multimodality therapy for resectable locoregional esophageal cancer. *Ann Thorac Cardiovasc Surg.* 2006;12: 234–241.
42. Boige V, Pignon J, Saint-Aubert B, et al. Final results of a randomized trial comparing preoperative 5-fluorouracil (F)/cisplatin (P) to surgery alone in adenocarcinoma of stomach and lower esophagus (ASLE): FNLCC ACCORD07-FFCD 9703 trial. *J Clin Oncol.* 2007;25:4510.
43. Thirion PG, Michiels S, Le Maitre A, et al. Individual patient data-based meta-analysis assessing pre-operative chemotherapy in resectable oesophageal adenocarcinoma. *J Clin Oncol.* 2007;25:4512.
44. Geh JI, Crellin AM, Glynne-Jones R. Preoperative (neoadjuvant) chemoradiotherapy in oesophageal cancer. *Br J Surg.* 2001;88:338–356.
45. Tepper J, Krasna MJ, Niedzwicki D. Superiority of trimodality therapy to surgery alone in esophageal cancer: results of CALGB 9781. *J Clin Oncol.* 2006;24:181.
46. Law S, Kwong DLW, Tung HM. Preoperative chemoradiation for squamous cell esophageal cancer: a prospective randomized trial [abstract]. *Can J Gastroenterology.* 1998;12(Suppl B):161.
47. Apinop C, Puttisak P, Preecha N. A prospective study of combined therapy in esophageal cancer. *Hepatogastroenterology.* 1994;41:391–393.
48. Walsh TN, Noonan N, Hollywood D, et al. A comparison of multimodal therapy and surgery for esophageal adenocarcinoma. *N Engl J Med.* 1996;335:462–467.
49. Bosset JF, Gignoux M, Triboulet JP, et al. Chemoradiotherapy followed by surgery compared with surgery alone in squamous-cell cancer of the esophagus. *N Engl J Med.* 1997;337:161–167.
50. Nygaard K, Hagen S, Hansen HS, et al. Pre-operative radiotherapy prolongs survival in operable esophageal carcinoma: a randomized, multicenter study of pre-operative radiotherapy and chemotherapy. The second Scandinavian trial in esophageal cancer. *World J Surg.* 1992;16:1104–1109; discussion 1110.
51. Le Prise E, Etienne PL, Meunier B, et al. A randomized study of chemotherapy, radiation therapy, and surgery versus surgery for localized squamous cell carcinoma of the esophagus. *Cancer.* 1994;73:1779–1784.
52. Urschel JD, Vasan H. A meta-analysis of randomized controlled trials that compared neoadjuvant chemoradiation and surgery to surgery alone for resectable esophageal cancer. *Am J Surg.* 2003;185:538–543.
53. Fiorica F, Di Bona D, Schepis F, et al. Preoperative chemoradiotherapy for oesophageal cancer: a systematic review and meta-analysis. *Gut.* 2004;53:925–930.
54. Greer SE, Goodney PP, Sutton JE, et al. Neoadjuvant chemoradiotherapy for esophageal carcinoma: a meta-analysis. *Surgery.* 2005;137:172–177.
55. Walsh TN, McDonnell CO, Mulligan ED. Multimodal therapy versus surgery alone for squamous call carcinoma of esophagus. *Gastroenterology.* 2000;118 (suppl 2): A1008.
56. Lee JL, Kim SB, Jung HY, et al. A single institutional phase III trial of preoperative chemotherapy with hyperfractionation radiotherapy plus surgery (CRT-S) versus surgery (S) alone for stage II, III resectable esophageal squamous cell carcinoma (SCC): an interim analysis [abstract 1043]. *Proc Annu Meet Am Soc Clin Oncol.* 2003;22.
57. Stahl M, Walz MK, Stuschke M, et al. Preoperative chemotherapy (CTX) versus preoperative chemoradiotherapy (CRTZ) in locally advanced esophagogastric adenocarcinomas: First results of a randomized phase III trial. *J Clin Oncol.* 2007;25:4511.
58. Stahl M, Stuschke M, Lehmann N, et al. Chemoradiation with and without surgery in patients with locally advanced squamous cell carcinoma of the esophagus. *J Clin Oncol.* 2005;23:2310–2317.
59. Bedenne L, Michel P, Bouche O, et al. Chemoradiation followed by surgery compared with chemoradiation alone in squamous cancer of the esophagus: FFCD 9102. *J Clin Oncol.* 2007;25:1160–1168.
60. Ando N, Iizuka T, Ide H, et al. Surgery plus chemotherapy compared with surgery alone for localized squamous cell carcinoma of the thoracic esophagus: a Japan Clinical Oncology Group Study—JCOG9204. *J Clin Oncol.* 2003;21:4592–4596.
61. Ando N, Iizuka T, Kakegawa T, et al. A randomized trial of surgery with and without chemotherapy for localized squamous carcinoma of the thoracic esophagus: the Japan Clinical Oncology Group Study. *J Thorac Cardiovasc Surg.* 1997;114:205–209.
62. Macdonald JS, Smalley SR, Benedetti J, et al. Chemoradiotherapy after surgery compared with surgery alone for adenocarcinoma of the stomach or gastroesophageal junction. *N Engl J Med.* 2001;345:725–730.
63. Roth JA, Pass HI, Flanagan MM, et al. Randomized clinical trial of preoperative and postoperative adjuvant chemotherapy with cisplatin, vindesine, and bleomycin for carcinoma of the esophagus. *J Thorac Cardiovasc Surg.* 1988;96:242–248.
64. Ancona E, Ruol A, Santi S, et al. Only pathologic complete response to neoadjuvant chemotherapy improves significantly the long term survival of patients with resectable esophageal squamous cell carcinoma: final report of a randomized, controlled trial of preoperative chemotherapy versus surgery alone. *Cancer.* 2001;91:2165–2174.
65. Schlag PM. Randomized trial of preoperative chemotherapy for squamous cell cancer of the esophagus. The Chirurgische Arbeitsgemeinschaft Fuer Onkologie der Deutschen Gesellschaft Fuer Chirurgie Study Group. *Arch Surg.* 1992; 27:1446–1450.

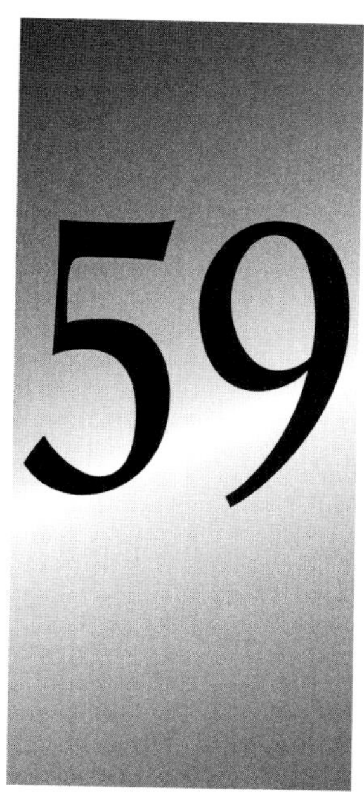

Treatment Options for Locally Recurrent Esophageal Cancer

Wilson B. Tsai
Arman Kilica
Matthew J. Schuchert
James D. Luketich
Sebastien Gilbert

Although esophageal carcinoma is a relatively uncommon malignancy, its incidence and prevalence have been dramatically increasing in the Western countries. Squamous cell cancer represents 95% of all esophageal cancer and is the seventh-leading cause of cancer death worldwide. Its incidence varies between 30 and 800 cases per 100,000 in parts of northern Iran, southern Russia, and northern China (1). Environmental teratogens such as smoking and alcohol have been implicated in the development of squamous cell carcinoma. Other definite risk factors include chronic achalasia, lye-induced strictures, tylosis, and human papilloma virus. Although adenocarcinomas make up only 5% of the worldwide esophageal cancer cases, they account for more than 50% of the esophageal malignancies in Western civilizations (1). Unlike squamous cell cancer, which is seen in association with a history of smoking and alcohol use, adenocarcinoma has been linked gastroesophageal reflux and Barrett's epithelium (1).

Regardless of histology and despite best medical and surgical care, esophageal cancer continues to carry a dismal prognosis. According to the Surveillance, Epidemiology, and End-Results Program from the National Cancer Institute, there will be 15,560 new cases of esophageal cancer in 2007, and out of those patients, 13,940 patients will die from this disease. At diagnosis, less than 5% of patients will have localized disease without regional lymph node involvement, 50% of patients will present with locoregional involvement, and the rest will present with distant metastasis (1).

PATTERNS OF RECURRENCE

The optimal treatment for resectable esophageal cancer is still the subject of debate. Some advocate surgical resection, either as the sole treatment or in combination with neoadjuvant or adjuvant therapy. Other groups recommend a nonsurgical approach and treat patients with definitive chemoradiation alone (2–6). Despite the different combinations of therapeutic regimens and the extent of esophageal resection, 36.1% to 64.2% of esophagectomy patients will develop recurrent disease (7–9). In patients who undergo complete surgical resection, recurrent disease can present as either local recurrence at the anastomotic site, recurrence in regional lymph nodes, distant recurrence (i.e., liver, bone), or a mixed recurrence, which is a combination of any of the above. Another unique type of recurrence is Barrett's esophagus, which develops in the postesophagectomy. This problem may be more likely to develop in esophagectomy patients who have been reconstructed with a thoracic anastomosis and have a longer proximal esophageal remnant. Even if the initial esophageal resection was complete with negative surgical margins, ongoing reflux of gastric contents across the anastomosis may lead to metaplasia and dysplasia (10,11). Even though most esophageal resections involve division of the vagal trunks, Gutschow et al. demonstrated that the denervated stomach recovers its ability to secrete acid over time (12). Other investigators observed a significant increase in the median acid and bile scores in 63% and 80% of esophagectomy patients (13). They also found a correlation between gastroesophageal reflux and the development of Barrett's metaplasia. Given the relatively high reported incidence of intestinal metaplasia after esophagectomy (50%), periodic screening endoscopy may be justified especially in long-term survivors.

Mariette et al. retrospectively reviewed the patterns of recurrence following complete resection of esophageal carcinoma and the factors predictive of recurrent disease in 230 out of 439 consecutive patients (14). From 1982 to 2002, 460 patients underwent subtotal esophagectomy with 2-field lymphadenectomy and complete resections. The predominant histologic type was squamous cell carcinoma over adenocarcinoma in a ratio of 4.7:1. Even with an extensive and potentially curative resection, the French group observed a 52.4% (230 of 439) recurrence rate. Local recurrence, defined as anastomotic recurrence, occurred in 53 patients (12.1%). Regional recurrence was observed in 90 patients (20.5%), and this was defined as mediastinal or upper abdomen at the site of previous resection and nodal clearance or recurrence in the cervical area, where no lymphadenectomy was performed. Finally, distant recurrence occurred in 87 patients (19.8%), with the predominant sites being liver (35 patients), lung (21 patients), bone (18 patients), and brain (7 patients). The mean time to recurrence after the operation was 17.8 months with 45.7% (105 of 230) recurrences developing within 12 months of surgery. The median time to recurrence was 12 months, and the median survival after recurrence was 7 months. There was no significance difference in median disease-free survival between patients with adenocarcinoma and squamous cell carcinoma. Tumor location (i.e., upper, middle, lower esophagus) did not have a significant impact on survival. In a multivariate analysis, the only factor that was predictive of recurrent disease was the depth of invasion of the tumor (T stage) on initial pathologic assessment.

Hulscher et al. also evaluated the recurrence pattern of esophageal cancer after transhiatal resection. In their patient population, the most common histology was adenocarcinoma (15). Of the 149 patients, 72 (52.6%) developed a recurrence. Thirty-two patients (23.4%) developed locoregional recurrence, 21 patients (15.3%) developed distant recurrence, and 19 patients (13.9%) presented with both locoregional and distant recurrence. Only 1 patient recurred with stage I cancer (5.9%), while the recurrence rates for stages IIa, IIb, III, and IV were 42.4%, 63.6%, 69.8%, and 76.9%, respectively. Lymph node status was an independent prognostic factor for recurrence. The other predictor of recurrence was the completeness of resection (R0 vs. R1). R0 refers to complete surgical resection with negative microscopic margins, and R1 signifies documented microscopic residual disease after surgery. Of the 109 patients who had an R0 resection, 50 (45.9%) developed a recurrence, while the R1 group had a 78.6% overall recurrence rate.

SURGICAL OPTIONS FOR LOCALLY RECURRENT ESOPHAGEAL CANCER

Salvage Esophagectomy for Recurrence after Surgical Resection

Despite the generally poor survival in recurrent esophageal cancer, there may be a benefit from repeat resection in patients with local recurrence (16–19). The largest published series originated from Japan and retrospectively analyzed 131 out of 367 consecutive patients with postsurgical recurrence (16). Out of 131 patients, 94 patients underwent some form of treatment that included chemotherapy (n = 35), radiation ± chemotherapy (n = 35), and surgery ± other therapy in the form of chemotherapy, radiation, or both (n = 24). There were no significant differences observed in pathological stage among the treatment groups. The 5-year survival rate in the chemotherapy, radiation ± chemotherapy, surgical resection ± other treatment, and no-treatment groups were 0%, 11.8%, 29.2%, and 0%, respectively. The 5-year survival rate was significantly improved in patients who had recurrent disease amenable to surgical resection. Another group from the Mayo Clinic evaluated the role of re-resection for locally recurrent esophageal cancer (20). They analyzed 27 consecutive patients who presented with locally recurrent esophageal carcinoma after surgical resection. Of the 27, 19 (70%) were re-resected, while the other 8 were deemed unresectable at the time of surgical exploration. Complete R0 resection was achieved in 15 out of the 19 patients (79%), and the other 4 patients had microscopic margins. The most common postoperative complications were arrhythmias (26%), anastomotic leaks (26%), and sepsis (19%). The total rate of complications was 59% with an operative mortality rate of 7.4% (n = 2). In completely resected patients, the survival rates at 1, 3, and 5 years were 62%, 44%, and 35%, respectively. The corresponding survival rates for incompletely re-resected patients were lower at 27%, 18%, and 0%, respectively. Prognostic factors associated with an improvement in survival were disease-free interval greater than 2 years and complete resection. Age, neoadjuvant therapy, presence or absence of symptoms, complications, and site of local recurrence did not significantly affect survival. In a recent study by Nemoto et al., patients with locally recurrent esophageal cancer after curative resection were treated with external beam radiation and had 1-year and 3-year survival rates of 33% and 12% (21). Patients treated with combined chemotherapy and radiotherapy similarly had lower survival rates as compared to surgical re-resection of 47% at 1 year and 4% at 3 years (22). The authors concluded that, although technically challenging and associated with significant morbidity, complete surgical resection of locally recurrent esophageal cancer may result in prolonged survival when compared to other forms of nonoperative therapy. However, the results should be interpreted in context of the biases attributed to retrospective study designs.

Salvage Esophagectomy for Recurrence after Definitive Chemoradiation

Definitive chemoradiation without surgery is an acceptable form of treatment for esophageal cancer. One randomized, prospective trial from Hong Kong compared surgery to definitive chemoradiation in 80 patients with squamous cell esophageal cancer and found no significant difference in early, cumulative survival, and disease-free survival (23). It has been suggested that radical surgical intervention offers no significant survival benefit over definitive chemoradiation in the treatment of stages II to III esophageal cancer (24). Despite maximum doses of chemoradiation, a significant proportion of patients recur, and there is relatively limited information on the role of salvage esophagectomy in this clinical scenario.

At the M. D. Anderson Cancer Center, 13 patients were treated with salvage esophagectomy after chemoradiation over a 13-year period (25). These patients were compared to a control group (n = 99) who had a planned esophagectomy after neoadjuvant chemoradiation. The patients undergoing the salvage procedure generally had a significantly higher dose of radiotherapy as compared to the control group (56.7 Gy vs. 41.4 Gy). The salvage group was reconstructed mainly with a cervical anastomosis. The operative time, blood loss, and units of packed red blood cells transfused were significantly higher in these patients. There was a trend toward a longer period of ventilator dependence and a higher operative mortality after salvage esophagectomy. The length of hospital stay (29.4 days vs. 18.4 days) and the anastomotic leak rate (38% vs. 7%) were significantly higher in patients who received a higher preoperative radiation dose. Despite differences in short-term complication rates, the 5-year survival rate was similar between the groups. Although the numbers are too small to make generalizations, salvage esophagectomy appeared to benefit 4 patients who lived longer than 2 years and 2 others who were still alive without any evidence of disease 5.7 years and 12.2 years. In their multivariate analysis, the authors stated that there was a trend toward improved long-term survival in early-stage, node-negative tumors (T1–2 N0) (25).

Complications of Salvage Esophagectomy

The complications of salvage esophagectomy for recurrence after any form of treatment are high. The 2 major complications are respiratory failure from acute respiratory distress syndrome (ARDS) and/or pneumonia and sepsis from anastomotic leaks (26). These adverse events can potentially be lethal. Other morbidities include airway necrosis and fistula formation, recurrent laryngeal nerve injury, chylothorax, and pericardial effusion (26–28).

Respiratory Failure

Respiratory failure is a generalized condition without any precise criteria, but ARDS, acute lung injury, and pneumonia are the most common variants. Keller et al. demonstrated that high-dose radiation therapy and concurrent chemotherapy for esophageal cancer are associated with significant life-threatening injury to the lungs (29). Radiation to the mediastinal area can also cause pneumonitis, and surgery releases a myriad of cytokines that can also result in acute lung injury. Mechanical ventilation may also perpetuate the inflammatory cascade and cause acute lung injury by exposing the lungs to prolonged periods of intraoperative single lung ventilation, high lung volumes, and high oxygen concentrations. Moreover, the pulmonary lymphatic obstruction resulting from mediastinal lymph node dissection and mediastinal radiation therapy may also contribute to acute lung injury (30,31). These factors may explain the increased morbidity and mortality from respiratory failure after esophagectomy with neoadjuvant or adjuvant chemoradiation (30–34).

Respiratory complications are very common after esophagectomy and range from 18% to 57% (35,36). Ferguson and Durkin reviewed 292 patients who underwent an esophagectomy for cancer and identified age, spirometry function (i.e., percent predicted FEV_1), and performance status as 3 preoperative risk factors for pulmonary complications (37). Other independent risk factors include chronic lung disease, malnutrition, immunosuppression, and swallowing dysfunction. Avendano et al. confirmed that besides advanced age and immunosuppression from neoadjuvant therapy, one of the most important risk factors leading to pneumonia was previous chronic lung disease (FEV1 < 65% predicted) (38).

Anastomotic Failure

A leak occurring at the esophagogastric anastomosis is a dreaded complication associated with a significant risk of sepsis and death (39). Urschel et al. observed a 35% mortality rate in a retrospective review of 23 anastomotic leaks in 307 patients undergoing esophagectomy. They postulated that although not statistically significant, factors that contributed to an increased mortality were advanced age, early postoperative leaks, and clinically significant anastomotic leak (40). The etiology of anastomotic breakdown is multifactorial but can usually be attributed to technical errors and/or poor gastric tissue perfusion (41,42,43). The perfusion of the gastric conduit depends on intact right gastroepiploic vessels and the submucosal vascular plexus, which allows for collateral blood to the proximal fundus even after ligation of the left gastric, left gastroepiploic, and short gastric vessels. Improper surgical technique in preserving the right gastroepiploic vessels during dissection, aggressive transthoracic mobilization of the conduit, excessive tubularization, and imprecise alignment of the anastomosis leading to tension and tissue trauma are the primary technical culprits leading to anastomotic leaks (41,42). Preoperative radiation may also increase the risk of anastomotic dehiscence by obliterating the submucosal collateral vessels of the proximal stomach and the vessels supplying the esophageal portion of the anastomosis as well. Improvements in the rates of mortality and leaks after esophagectomy have been attributed to improved surgical techniques, mechanical stapling devices, earlier recognition of the problem, and increased surgical experience (41,42,44–47).

Malignant and Nonmalignant Fistulae

Fistulae from the trachea or bronchus to the esophagus or pleura are serious complications of salvage esophagectomy. Radiation therapy, anastomotic leaks, extensive intrathoracic dissection and mobilization, and residual or recurrent malignancy are all factors that increase the probability of developing a fistula to the airways or major blood vessels. Fistulae to the airways are clinically challenging and are associated with a mortality rate of 29% to 47% (48). These fistulae can be divided into nonmalignant and malignant in origin. Unfortunately, the only treatment option for malignant tracheoesophageal fistula is palliation because the underlying process is usually incurable (48,49). Malignant tracheoesophageal fistulae are best palliated by exclusion from the alimentary tract using either endoscopic stents or surgery (48,49). The perioperative mortality rate of surgical bypasses for malignant fistulae is 25% to 61%, while the mortality from endoscopic stent insertion ranges from 0% to 15%. With supportive measures alone, the survival rate is dismal at 1 to 6 weeks (48). Therefore, endoscopic palliation is probably the preferred palliative option in most cases (50,51).

Bartels et al. described the prevalence, predisposing factors, and outcomes of 31 out of 785 patients who developed tracheobronchial fistulae after esophagectomy. Fistulae were more prevalent in transthoracic than transhiatal resections, in tumors located at or above the tracheal bifurcation, with substernal gastric conduit placement, and in patients treated with neoadjuvant chemoradiation (52). All patients had a more extensive resection that may have resulted in increased esophagogastric devascularization and ischemia. Ten out of the 31 patients (32%) died during the first postoperative month from respiratory failure, multiorgan failure secondary to sepsis, or bleeding secondary to erosion into the aorta. The authors also noted that a reduction in tidal volume and increase in respiratory rate in their ventilator management dramatically reduced the air leak rate from 2.8 L/min to 1.1 L/min. This, in turn, resulted in earlier extubation and complete healing or decrease in size of the fistulae in 23 patients (53). The principles of treatment for nonmalignant tracheoesophageal fistulae are nutritional support and exclusion of the airways from the alimentary tract. Available treatment options to achieve exclusion include esophageal stents, tracheal stents, fibrin-based sealants, and surgical repair with pedicled muscle flaps (48–58).

CHEMOTHERAPY AND RADIATION FOR RECURRENT ESOPHAGEAL CANCER

Another treatment modality for patients with recurrent esophageal cancer is chemotherapy, radiotherapy, or a combination of both. The response rates for first-line single-agent chemotherapy in esophageal cancer patients range from 16% to 33% (63–68). According to the literature, the combination of cisplatin, 5-fluorouracil, and radiotherapy has resulted in complete response rates ranging from 35% to 50%; however, the associated toxicities have led researchers to evaluate newer compounds, such as taxanes and irinotecan (59–63). It is important, however, to keep in mind that a good response does not necessarily equate to an improved survival and that in patients with metastatic esophageal cancer, the median survival is still only 4 to 8 months despite the use of such therapeutic modalities (61).

In 1985, the Radiation Therapy Oncology Group initiated a randomized, prospective phase III trial (RTOG 81-01) to evaluate the benefit of multimodality treatment (concurrent chemotherapy with radiation) over single-agent radiation treatment in the long-term survival of patients with esophageal cancer (65). Patients that were included had squamous cell or adenocarcinoma, T 1–3,

N 0–1, M 0, and Karnofsky scores of at least 50. An interim analysis in 1990 caused an early termination in the study when it showed a staggering difference in 5-year survival between those patients receiving chemotherapy plus radiation versus radiation alone in both randomized (26% vs. 0%, respectively) and nonrandomized groups (14% vs. 0%). On further follow-up, it was observed that 22% (n = 10) were still alive 8 years and that 20% (n = 3) were alive at 10 years after initiation of treatment. The authors therefore concluded that nonoperative multimodality treatment could potentially cure selected patients with esophageal cancer (65).

Ultimately, patients with recurrent or metastatic esophageal cancer have a poor prognosis, and the role of chemotherapy should be directed toward palliation rather than cure. The combination of cisplatin and 5-FU is still the most commonly prescribed regimen, with documented rates of response nearing 35% and median survival durations of 6 to 8 months (61,65,67,69). As stated before, though, an improvement in response rate may not correlate with an increased survival. For instance, Mariette et al. observed a median survival of 7 months in patients with untreated recurrent esophageal cancer (14). From 1986 to 1993, Raoul et al. evaluated 31 patients with recurrent esophageal cancer after surgical resection and treated them with combined chemoradiation (22). The chemotherapy regimen included cisplatin and 5-FU, and radiation therapy was administered to a total dose of 60 Gy. The French group observed symptomatic relief that lasted for a median of 6.3 months in 74% (n = 23) of their patients. Tumor response was observed in 65% of the patients, and among these patients, 26% achieved complete response according to clinical evaluation and radiographic imaging. The survival rates at 1, 2, and 3 years were 47%, 17%, and 4%, respectively, and median duration of survival was 10.7 months from the initial diagnosis of recurrence. The authors stated that a combination of chemotherapy and radiation was beneficial in treating recurrent esophageal cancer, in improving in the quality of life, and in accomplishing the goals of palliation (22). Other investigators have also reported similar results after chemoradiation in a small group (n = 33) of patients with locoregional recurrence (21).

ENDOSCOPIC PALLIATION FOR RECURRENT LOCALLY RECURRENT ESOPHAGEAL CANCER

Endoscopic Palliation

The focus of treatment shifts from curative to palliative intent in patients with inoperable recurrent disease. Because of the dismal prognosis associated with unresectable esophageal cancer, the primary goal becomes rapid relief of dysphagia with minimal hospital stay in the remaining days of life. Endoscopic palliation may help to achieve this goal with the use of stents, dilation, brachytherapy, neodymium:yttrium-aluminum garnet (Nd:YAG) laser, and photodynamic therapy (PDT).

Endoscopic dilation is a widely available and relatively safe means to provide short-term relief of dysphagia. In their retrospective study of 26 patients undergoing 616 palliative dilations, Moses and colleagues reported that 92% of patients were able to resume a soft or regular diet with minimal procedural morbidity and no mortality (72). The large number of repeat dilations in this series points to the temporary nature of the improvement in swallowing afforded by this modality. Lundell et al. reviewed 41 patients undergoing 128 dilations and noted a significant improvement in dysphagia, but repeat dilations were required at approximately 4-week intervals (71). The procedure was also associated with a 5% perforation rate. Similar to these reports, a third series evaluating 46 patients reported dysphagia relief in 90% with a complication rate of 8% (73). Because of its wide availability, low cost, and relative technical ease, dilation may be a reasonable palliative option in selected patients with a very limited life expectancy. However, expandable metal stents (EMS) are still preferred because they provide longer lasting relief and require less re-interventions.

Stenting is the most frequently employed modality for palliation of esophageal cancer (74). Silicon stents were originally used but were associated with a high rate of obstruction, perforation, and migration as well as a high procedural mortality (75,76). EMS were introduced to offer a potentially safer palliative approach. Two randomized trials conducted in the 1990s compared silicon and metal stents. Knyrim and colleagues evaluated 42 patients with esophageal cancer and found that technical success (95%–100%), relief of dysphagia (95%), improvement in Karnofsky performance score, reintervention rate (33%), and 30-day mortality (EMS = 14%; silicon = 29%) were statistically similar between the two groups (76). However, 2 important differences were noted: complications were more frequent in the silicon stent group (43% vs. 0%), and the mean length of hospitalization after stent placement was longer in the silicon cohort (12.5 vs. 5.4 days). These two factors led the authors to conclude that metal stents were more cost effective despite a higher initial purchase price. Siersema et al. randomized 75 patients to receive either latex-based or coated metal stent (77). As in the previous trial, successful placement of the stent (97%–100%), improvement in mean dysphagia score (3.1–0.75), and rate of recurrent dysphagia (25%) were similar between the two groups. Those with a latex prosthesis had a longer hospital stay (6.3 vs. 4.3 days) and higher complication rate (47% vs. 16%). Several large series, each evaluating over 100 patients with EMS, have consistently demonstrated successful stent placement and improvement of dysphagia in over 85% of patients along with a low procedural mortality of 0% to 2.5% (79–84). Procedural complications of EMS placement are limited to 5% to 15% of patients and include perforation, bleeding, aspiration pneumonia, and chest pain. Delayed complications such as fistulization, bleeding, obstruction, stent migration, and tumor ingrowth or overgrowth occur in 30% to 45% (85). Other benefits of EMS are relatively easier insertion, as well as no requirement for expertise in rigid endoscopy. Additionally, newer generation EMS can be fully or partially covered with polyurethane or silicone, allowing for less tumor ingrowth at the cost of an increased migration rate (86). In the case of tracheoesophageal fistulae, covered EMS are the preferred treatment as closure may be achieved in up to 70% to 100% of patients (87–89).

Brachytherapy allows local delivery of radiation and can also be utilized to palliate obstructing esophageal cancer. In a multicenter randomized trial comparing outcomes of stent placement (n = 108) and brachytherapy (n = 101), dysphagia was relieved more rapidly with stenting, but brachytherapy was associated with superior relief after 30 days (90). Dysphagia improved in 73% of patients receiving brachytherapy, and there were no significant differences in rate of recurrent dysphagia or survival between the cohorts. In their 10-year retrospective analysis of 149 patients receiving high-dose-rate brachytherapy, Homs et al. noted improvement in dysphagia in 51% of patients with a 12% major complication rate, including bleeding (5%) and fistula formation (4%), as well as a 2% mortality rate (91). Another study evaluating 197 patients reported a similar rate (54%) of dysphagia improvement with brachytherapy (92). The major disadvantage of brachytherapy is the relatively prolonged time necessary to afford relief. This becomes an important issue in palliative care where survival is limited and rapid symptomatic relief a priority.

Nd:YAG laser therapy is another option that can offer temporary relief of malignant dysphagia. Small exophytic tumors (< 6 cm) in the middle third of the esophagus are most suitable for this type of treatment (12). In a randomized trial comparing alcohol injection (n = 23) with Nd:YAG (n = 24), 78% and 88% of patients had a substantial improvement in dysphagia, respectively. There was 1 (4.3%) esophageal perforation that occurred during the preliminary dilation in the ethanol injection group. No complications were encountered with Nd:YAG, and there were no procedure-related deaths in either group (93). Another prospective randomized trial of laser therapy (n = 18) and metal stents (covered, n = 23; uncovered, n = 19) concluded that stents were more effective at relieving dysphagia (94). A potential disadvantage of Nd:YAG laser treatment is the need for repeated sessions, as dysphagia tends to recur within 4 to 6 weeks (84). The addition of external beam radiotherapy prolongs the dysphagia-free interval in patients treated with this modality (95). Additional limitations include availability and cost of the necessary equipment as well as the technical expertise required.

Photodynamic therapy (PDT) is another modality that offers palliative benefits by utilizing a photosensitizing agent followed by nonthermal ablation. In a review of 215 patients undergoing palliation with PDT at our institution, 85% of patients had an improvement in swallowing with a mean dysphagia-free interval of 66 days (96). Additionally, the perforation rate was 2% and procedural mortality was 1.8%. In a multicenter randomized trial including 218 patients (PDT = 110; Nd:YAG = 108), the proportion of patients with relief of dysphagia was similar between the 2 groups at 1-week (PDT = 40%, Nd:YAG = 44%) and 1-month follow-up (PDT = 32%, Nd:YAG = 27%). Termination of therapy secondary to side effects was less frequent in those receiving PDT (3% vs. 19%), and the rate of perforation was higher in the laser group (7% vs. 1%). Adverse effects following PDT in this trial included sunburn (19%), fever (16%), pleural effusion (10%), and nausea (8%).

Judicious patient selection is an important factor in determining the appropriate plan of care for patients with recurrent esophageal cancer. Only a careful, comprehensive clinical evaluation will identify patients who are fit enough to potentially benefit from surgery, chemotherapy, or radiation despite associated complications and toxicities. Therefore, surgeons and physicians must be prepared to offer patients additional options, such as esophageal dilation and stent insertion, laser therapy with Nd:YAG or photodynamic therapy, and brachytherapy, for more immediate and effective means of palliation.

References

1. Polednak AP. Trends in survival for both histologic types of esophageal cancer in US surveillance, epidemiology and end results areas. *Int J Cancer.* 2003;105(1):98–100.
2. Herskovic A, Martz K, al-Sarraf M, et al. Combined chemotherapy and radiotherapy compared with radiotherapy alone in patients with cancer of the esophagus. *N Engl J Med.* 1992;326(24):1593–1598.
3. Cooper JS, Guo MD, Herskovic A, et al. Chemoradiotherapy of locally advanced esophageal cancer: long-term follow-up of a prospective randomized trial (RTOG 85-01). Radiation Therapy Oncology Group. *JAMA.* 1999;281(17):1623–1627.
4. Araújo CM, Souhami L, Gil RA, et al. A randomized trial comparing radiation therapy versus concomitant radiation therapy and chemotherapy in carcinoma of the thoracic esophagus. *Cancer.* 1991;67(9):2258–2261.
5. Wilson KS, Lim JT. Primary chemo-radiotherapy and selective oesophagectomy for oesophageal cancer: goal of cure with organ preservation. *Radiother Oncol.* 2000;54(2):129–134.
6. Algan O, Coia LR, Keller SM et al. Management of adenocarcinoma of the esophagus with chemoradiation alone or chemoradiation followed by esophagectomy:

results of sequential nonrandomized phase II studies. *Int J Radiat Oncol Biol Phys.* 1995;32(3):753–761.
7. Matsubara T, Ueda M, Takahashi T, et al. Localization of recurrent disease after extended lymph node dissection for carcinoma of the thoracic esophagus. *J Am Coll Surg.* 1996;182(4):340–346.
8. Bhansali MS, Fujita H, Kakegawa T, et al. Pattern of recurrence after extended radical esophagectomy with three-field lymph node dissection for squamous cell carcinoma in the thoracic esophagus. *World J Surg.* 1997;21(3):275–281.
9. Dresner SM, Griffin SM. Pattern of recurrence following radical oesophagectomy with two-field lymphadenectomy. *Br J Surg.* 2000;87(10):1426–1433.
10. Lindahl H, Rintala R, Sariola H, et al. Cervical Barrett's esophagus: a common complication of gastric tube reconstruction. *J Pediatr Surg.* 1990;25(4):446–448.
11. Hamilton SR, Yardley JH. Regeneration of cardiac type mucosa and acquisition of Barrett's mucosa after esophagogastostomy. *Gastroenterology.* 1977;72:669–675.
12. Gutschow C, Collard JM, Romagnoli R, et al. Denervated stomach as an esophageal substitute recovers intraluminal acidity with time. *Ann Surg.* 2001;233(4):509–514.
13. O'Riordan JM, Tucker ON, Byrne PJ, et al. Factors influencing the development of Barrett's epithelium in the esophageal remnant postesophagectomy. *Am J Gastroenterol.* 2004;99(2):205–211.
14. Mariette C, Balon JM, Piessen G, et al. Pattern of recurrence following complete resection of esophageal carcinoma and factors predictive of recurrent disease. *Cancer.* 2003;97(7):1616–1623.
15. Hulscher JB, van Sandick JW, Tijssen JG, et al. The recurrence pattern of esophageal carcinoma after transhiatal resection. *J Am Coll Surg.* 2000;191(2):143–148.
16. Kato H, Tachimori Y, Watanabe H, et al. Anastomotic recurrence of oesophageal squamous cell carcinoma after transthoracic oesophagectomy. *Eur J Surg.* 1998;164(10):759–764.
17. Karin E, Haddad R, Kashtan H. Segmental resection for recurrent carcinoma of the esophagus. *Isr Med Assoc J.* 2001;3(3):228–229.
18. Kurtzman SH, Turnbull AD, Burt M, et al. Recurrence of resected esophagogastric adenocarcinoma: results of re-resection. *J Surg Oncol.* 1990;45(4):224–226.
19. Pichlmayr R, Büttner D. Reoperation in recurrence of carcinoma of the esophagus, cardia and stomach. *Langenbecks Arch Chir.* 1976;342:227–235.
20. Schipper PH, Cassivi SD, Deschamps C, et al. Locally recurrent esophageal carcinoma: when is re-resection indicated? *Ann Thorac Surg.* 2005;80(3):1001–1005.
21. Nemoto K, Ariga H, Kakuto Y, et al. Radiation therapy for loco-regionally recurrent esophageal cancer after surgery. *Radiother Oncol.* 2001;61(2):165–168.
22. Raoul JL, Le Prisé E, Meunier B, et al. Combined radiochemotherapy for postoperative recurrence of oesophageal cancer. *Gut.* 1995;37(2):174–176.
23. Chiu PW, Chan AC, Leung SF, et al. Multicenter prospective randomized trial comparing standard esophagectomy with chemoradiotherapy for treatment of squamous esophageal cancer: early results from the Chinese University Research Group for Esophageal Cancer (CURE). *J Gastrointest Surg.* 2005;9(6):794–802.
24. Hironaka S, Ohtsu A, Boku N, et al. Nonrandomized comparison between definitive chemoradiotherapy and radical surgery in patients with T(2–3)N(any) M(0) squamous cell carcinoma of the esophagus. *Int J Radiat Oncol Biol Phys.* 2003;57(2):425–33.
25. Swisher SG, Wynn P, Putnam JB, et al. Salvage esophagectomy for recurrent tumors after definitive chemotherapy and radiotherapy. *J Thorac Cardiovasc Surg.* 2002;123(1):175–183.
26. Urschel JD, Ashiku S, Thurer R, et al. Salvage or planned esophagectomy after chemoradiation therapy for locally advanced esophageal cancer—a review. *Dis Esophagus.* 2003;16(2):60–65.
27. Stahl M, Stuschke M, Lehmann N, et al. Chemoradiation with and without surgery in patients with locally advanced squamous cell carcinoma of the esophagus. *J Clin Oncol.* 2005;23(10):2310–2317.
28. Chidel MA, Rice TW, Adelstein DJ, et al. Resectable esophageal carcinoma: local control with neoadjuvant chemotherapy and radiation therapy. *Radiology.* 1999;213(1):67–72.
29. Keller SM, Ryan LM, Coia LR, et al. High dose chemoradiotherapy followed by esophagectomy for adenocarcinoma of the esophagus and gastroesophageal junction: results of a phase II study of the Eastern Cooperative Oncology Group. *Cancer.* 1998;83(9):1908–1916.
30. Williams EA, Quinlan GJ, Anning PB, et al. Lung injury following pulmonary resection in the isolated, blood-perfused rat lung. *Eur Respir J.* 1999;14(4):745–750.
31. Jordan S, Mitchell JA, Quinlan GJ, et al. The pathogenesis of lung injury following pulmonary resection. *Eur Respir J.* 2000;15(4):790–799.
32. Reid PT, Donnelly SC, MacGregor IR, et al. Pulmonary endothelial permeability and circulating neutrophil-endothelial markers in patients undergoing esophagogastrectomy. *Crit Care Med.* 2000;28(9):3161–3165.
33. Katsuta T, Saito T, Shigemitsu Y, et al. Relation between tumour necrosis factor alpha and interleukin 1beta producing capacity of peripheral monocytes and pulmonary complications following oesophagectomy. *Br J Surg.* 1998;85(4):548–553.
34. Schilling MK, Gassmann N, Sigurdsson GH, et al. Role of thromboxane and leukotriene B4 in patients with acute respiratory distress syndrome after oesophagectomy. *Br J Anaesth.* 1998;80(1):36–40.
35. Luketich JD, Alvelo-Rivera M, Buenaventura PO, et al. Minimally invasive esophagectomy: outcomes in 222 patients. *Ann Surg.* 2003;238(4):486–494.
36. Hulscher JB, van Sandick JW, de Boer AG, et al. Extended transthoracic resection compared with limited transhiatal resection for adenocarcinoma of the esophagus. *N Engl J Med.* 2002;347(21):1662–1669.
37. Ferguson MK, Durkin AE. Preoperative prediction of the risk of pulmonary complications after esophagectomy for cancer. *J Thorac Cardiovasc Surg.* 2002;123(4):661–669.
38. Avendano CE, Flume PA, Silvestri GA, et al. Pulmonary complications after esophagectomy. *Ann Thorac Surg.* 2002;73(3):922–926.
39. Alanezi K, Urschel JD. Mortality secondary to esophageal anastomotic leak. *Ann Thorac Cardiovasc Surg.* 2004;10(2):71–75.
40. Urschel JD, Sellke FW. Complications of salvage esophagectomy. *Med Sci Monit.* 2003;9(7):RA173–RA180.
41. Santos RS, Raftopoulos Y, Singh D, et al. Utility of total mechanical stapled cervical esophagogastric anastomosis after esophagectomy: a comparison to conventional anastomotic techniques. *Surgery.* 2004; 136(4):917–925.
42. Rizk NP, Bach PB, Schrag D, et al. The impact of complications on outcomes after resection for esophageal and gastroesophageal junction carcinoma. *J Am Coll Surg.* 2004;198(1):42–50.
43. Patil PK, Patel SG, Mistry RC, et al. Cancer of the esophagus: esophagogastric anastomotic leak—a retrospective study of predisposing factors. *J Surg Oncol.* 1992;49(3):163–167.
44. Blewett CJ, Miller JD, Young JE, et al. Anastomotic leaks after esophagectomy for esophageal cancer: a comparison of thoracic and cervical anastomoses. *Ann Thorac Cardiovasc Surg.* 2001;7(2):75–78.
45. Orringer MB, Marshall B, Chang AC, et al. Two thousand transhiatal esophagectomies: changing trends, lessons learned. *Ann Surg.* 2007;246(3):363–372; discussion 372–374.
46. Orringer MB, Marshall B, Iannettoni MD. Transhiatal esophagectomy: clinical experience and refinements. *Ann Surg.* 1999;230(3):392–400; discussion 400–403.
47. Luketich JD, Landreneau RJ. Minimally invasive resection and mechanical cervical esophagogastric anastomotic techniques in the management of esophageal cancer. *J Gastrointest Surg.* 2004;8(8):927–929.
48. Spivak H, Katariya K, Lo AY, et al. Malignant tracheo-esophageal fistula: use of esophageal endoprosthesis. *J Surg Oncol.* 1996;63(1):65–70.
49. Ross WA, Alkassab F, Lynch PM, et al. Evolving role of self-expanding metal stents in the treatment of malignant dysphagia and fistulas. *Gastrointest Endosc.* 2007;65(1):70–76.
50. Reed MF, Mathisen DJ. Tracheoesophageal fistula. *Chest Surg Clin N Am.* 2003;13(2):271–289.
51. Duranceau A, Jamieson GG. Malignant tracheoesophageal fistula. *Ann Thorac Surg.* 1984;37(4):346–354.
52. Bartels HE, Stein HJ, Siewert JR. Tracheobronchial lesions following oesophagectomy: prevalence, predisposing factors and outcome. *Br J Surg.* 1998;85(3):403–406.
53. Bartels HE, Stein HJ, Siewert JR. Respiratory management and outcome of non-malignant tracheo-bronchial fistula following esophagectomy. *Dis Esophagus.* 1998;11(2):125–129.
54. Belleguic C, Lena H, Briens E, et al. Tracheobronchial stenting in patients with esophageal cancer involving the central airways. *Endoscopy.* 1999;31(3):232–236.
55. Murthy S, Gonzalez-Stawinski GV, Rozas MS, et al. Palliation of malignant aerodigestive fistulae with self-expanding metallic stents. *Dis Esophagus.* 2007;20(5):386–389.
56. Al-Haddad M, Craig CA, Odell J, et al. The use of self-expandable plastic stents for non-malignant esophago-pleural fistulas. *Dis Esophagus.* 2007;20(6):538–541.
57. Keckler SJ, Spilde TL, St Peter SD, et al. Treatment of bronchopleural fistula with small intestinal mucosa and fibrin glue sealant. *Ann Thorac Surg.* 2007;84(4):1383–1386.
58. Takanami I. Closure of a bronchopleural fistula using a fibrin-glue coated collagen patch. *Interact Cardiovasc Thorac Surg.* 2003;2(3):387–388.
59. Enzinger PC, Ilson DH, Kelsen DP. Chemotherapy in esophageal cancer. *Semin Oncol.* 1999;26(5 suppl 15):12–20.
60. Jatoi A, Martenson JA, Foster NR, et al.Paclitaxel, carboplatin, 5-fluorouracil, and radiation for locally advanced esophageal cancer: phase II results of preliminary pharmacologic and molecular efforts to mitigate toxicity and predict outcomes: North Central Cancer Treatment Group (N0044). *Am J Clin Oncol.* 2007;30(5):507–513.
61. Kleinberg L, Forastiere AA. Chemoradiation in the management of esophageal cancer. *J Clin Oncol.* 2007;25(26):4110–4117.
62. Ilson DH, Ajani J, Bhalla K, et al. Phase II trial of paclitaxel, fluorouracil, and cisplatin in patients with advanced carcinoma of the esophagus. *J Clin Oncol.* 1998;16(5):1826–1834.
63. Enzinger PC, Kulke MH, Clark JW, et al. A phase II trial of irinotecan in patients with previously untreated advanced esophageal and gastric adenocarcinoma. *Dig Dis Sci.* 2005;50(12):2218–2223.
64. Ilson DH, Saltz L, Enzinger P, et al. Phase II trial of weekly irinotecan plus cisplatin in advanced esophageal cancer. *J Clin Oncol.* 1999;17(10):3270–3275.
65. Cooper JS, Guo MD, Herskovic A, et al. Chemoradiotherapy of locally advanced esophageal cancer: long-term follow-up of a prospective randomized trial (RTOG 85-01). Radiation Therapy Oncology Group. *JAMA.* 1999;281(17):1623–1627.
66. Panettiere FJ, Leichman LP, Tilchen EJ, et al. Chemotherapy for advanced epidermoid carcinoma of the esophagus with single-agent cisplatin: final report on a Southwest Oncology Group study. *Cancer Treat Rep.* 1984;68(7–8):1023–1024.
67. Ezdinli EZ, Gelber R, Desai DV, et al. Chemotherapy of advanced esophageal carcinoma: Eastern Cooperative Oncology Group experience. *Cancer.* 1980;46(10):2149–2153.
68. Ajani JA, Ilson DH, Daugherty K, et al. Activity of taxol in patients with squamous cell carcinoma and adenocarcinoma of the esophagus. *J Natl Cancer Inst.* 1994;86(14):1086–1091.
69. Bleiberg H, Conroy T, Paillot B, et al. Randomised phase II study of cisplatin and 5-fluorouracil (5-FU) versus cisplatin alone in advanced squamous cell oesophageal cancer. *Eur J Cancer.* 1997;33(8):1216–1220.
70. Yamashita H, Nakagawa K, Tago M, et al. Salvage radiotherapy for postoperative loco-regional recurrence of esophageal cancer. *Dis Esophagus.* 2005;18(4):215–220.

71. Lundell L, Leth R, Lind T, et al. Palliative endoscopic dilation in carcinoma of the esophagus and esophagogastric junction. *Acta Chir Scand.* 1989;155(3):179–184.
72. Moses FM, Peura DA, Wong RK, et al. Palliative dilation of esophageal carcinoma. *Gastrointest Endosc.* 1985;31(2):61–63.
73. Siersema PD. New developments in palliative therapy. *Best Pract Res Clin Gastroenterol.* 2006;20(5):959–978.
74. Gasparri G, Casalegno PA, Camandona M, et al. Endoscopic insertion of 248 prostheses in inoperable carcinoma of the esophagus and cardia: short-term and long-term results. *Gastrointest Endosc.* 1987;33(5):354–356.
75. Tytgat GN. Endoscopic therapy of esophageal cancer: possibilities and limitations. *Endoscopy.* 1990;22(6):263–267.
76. Knyrim K, Wagner HJ, Bethge N, et al. A controlled trial of an expansile metal stent for palliation of esophageal obstruction due to inoperable cancer. *N Engl J Med.* 1993;329(18):1302–1307.
77. Siersema PD, Hop WC, Dees J, et al. Coated self-expanding metal stents versus latex prostheses for esophagogastric cancer with special reference to prior radiation and chemotherapy: a controlled, prospective study. *Gastrointest Endosc.* 1998;47(2):113–120.
78. Cwikiel W, Tranberg KG, Cwikiel M, et al. Malignant dysphagia: palliation with esophageal stents—long-term results in 100 patients. *Radiology.* 1998;207(2):513–518.
79. O'Sullivan GJ, Grundy A. Palliation of malignant dysphagia with expanding metallic stents. *J Vasc Interv Radiol.* 1999;10(3):346–351.
80. Raijman I, Siddique I, Ajani J, et al. Palliation of malignant dysphagia and fistulae with coated expandable metal stents: experience with 101 patients. *Gastrointest Endosc.* 1998;48(2):172–179.
81. Song HY, Do YS, Han YM, et al. Covered, expandable esophageal metallic stent tubes: experiences in 119 patients. *Radiology.* 1994;193(3):689–695.
82. Christie NA, Buenaventura PO, Fernando HC, et al. Results of expandable metal stents for malignant esophageal obstruction in 100 patients: short-term and long-term follow-up. *Ann Thorac Surg.* 2001;71(6):1797–1801.
83. Song HY, Lee DH, Seo TS, et al. Retrievable covered nitinol stents: experiences in 108 patients with malignant esophageal strictures. *J Vasc Interv Radiol.* 2002;13(3):285–293.
84. Homs MY, Kuipers EJ, Siersema PD. Palliative therapy. *J Surg Oncol.* 2005;92(3):246–256.
85. Angueira CE, Kadakia SC. Esophageal stents for inoperable esophageal cancer: which to use? *Am J Gastroenterol.* 1997;92(3):373–376.
86. Morgan RA, Ellul JP, Denton ER, et al. Malignant esophageal fistulas and perforations: management with plastic-covered metallic endoprostheses. *Radiology.* 1997;204(2):527–532.
87. Low DE, Kozarek RA. Comparison of conventional and wire mesh expandable prostheses and surgical bypass in patients with malignant esophagorespiratory fistulas. *Ann Thorac Surg.* 1998;65(4):919–923.
88. May A, Ell C. Palliative treatment of malignant esophagorespiratory fistulas with Gianturco-Z stents: a prospective clinical trial and review of the literature on covered metal stents. *Am J Gastroenterol.* 1998;93(4):532–535.
89. Homs MY, Steyerberg EW, Eijkenboom WM, et al. Single-dose brachytherapy versus metal stent placement for the palliation of dysphagia from oesophageal cancer: multicentre randomized trial. *Lancet.* 2004;364(9444):1497–1504.
90. Homs MY, Eijkenboom WM, Coen VL, et al. High dose rate brachytherapy for the palliation of malignant dysphagia. *Radiother Oncol.* 2003;66(3):327–332.
91. Brewster AE, Davidson SE, Makin WP, et al. Intraluminal brachytherapy using the high dose rate microselectron in the palliation of carcinoma of the oesophagus. *Clin Oncol (R Coll Radiol).* 1995;7(2):102–105.
92. Carazzone A, Bonavina L, Segalin A, et al. Endoscopic palliation of oesophageal cancer: results of a prospective comparison of Nd:YAG laser and ethanol injection. *Eur J Surg.* 1999;165(4):351–356.
93. Adam A, Ellul J, Watkinson AF, et al. Palliation of inoperable esophageal carcinoma: a prospective randomized trial of laser therapy and stent placement. *Radiology.* 1997;202(2):344–348.
94. Sargeant IR, Tobias JS, Blackman G, et al. Radiotherapy enhances laser palliation of malignant dysphagia: a randomised study. *Gut.* 1997;40(3):362–369.
95. Litle VA, Luketich JD, Christie NA, et al. Photodynamic therapy as palliation for esophageal cancer: experience in 215 patients. *Ann Thorac Surg.* 2003;76(5):1687–1692.
96. Lightdale CJ, Heier SK, Marcon NE, et al. Photodynamic therapy with porfimer sodium versus thermal ablation therapy with Nd:YAG laser for palliation of esophageal cancer: a multicenter randomized trial. *Gastrointest Endosc.* 1995;42(6):507–512.

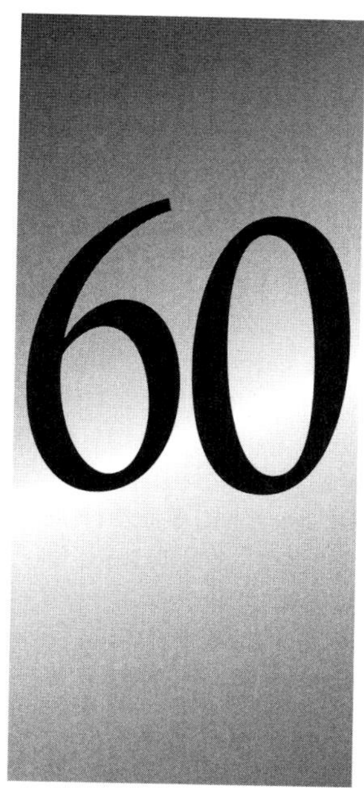

60 Preoperative Immunonutrition

Malissa Warren
Robert G. Martindale
Natalia Bailey

Esophageal cancer has significant nutritional implications with at least 40% of patients being malnourished at the time of diagnosis (1). Unintentional weight loss > 5% in 1 month or > 10% over 6 months, low body mass index, and declining oral intake is suggestive of malnutrition or increased nutritional risk (2–4). Malnutrition results in diminished lean body mass, impaired immune function, and adverse effects on wound healing. It is associated with a significant increase in perioperative morbidity and mortality (2,5). Signs of malnutrition are listed in Table 60.1.

Poor preoperative nutrition status of esophagectomy patients has been correlated with increased complications postoperatively. Even when compared to other major gastrointestinal surgeries, esophagectomy patients appear to be at highest risk (6,7). Tashiro et al. investigated the metabolic changes following esophagectomy in comparison to gastric or colorectal cancer surgery. Esophageal cancer patients undergoing surgery had the greatest increase in protein loss over both gastric and colorectal surgery (7).

TABLE 60.1
Signs of Malnutrition

BMI < 18.5 kg/m²
Unintentional weight loss > 10% in 3 to 6 months.
BMI < 20 kg/m² + unintentional weight loss > 5% in 3 to 6 months
Minimal to zero oral intake > 5 days
Disease or altered functional status (cancer, dysphagia)

The etiology of malnutrition in esophageal cancer is multifactorial. Tumor location, stage, tissue type, and timing of presentation, as well as the metabolic alterations related to the tumor burden have a role in the high frequency of malnutrition observed in this population. Dysphagia, altered taste, severe reflux, anorexia, and altered gastric motility also contribute to a malnourished state secondary to diminished food intake (3). Nutrient metabolism and appetite are negatively influenced by altered proinflammatory and catabolic hormone levels, neuropeptides, cytokines, and neurotransmitters that are associated with the tumor burden (3,5). In addition to the local and systemic effects of esophageal tumors, treatment of esophageal cancer also adversely affects nutrition status. Neoadjuvant therapy often results in food aversions, odynophagia with mucositis, xerostomia, nausea, vomiting, diarrhea, dehydration, and pain. Surgery commonly results in altered gastric motility, early satiety, odynophagia, and pain (3). Because of the high risk of malnutrition developing during the treatment of esophageal cancer, pretreatment nutrition screening and assessment is recommended to optimize the patients' response to treatment and minimize perioperative morbidity and mortality.

NUTRITION ASSESSMENT

Nutrition Screening

The purpose of nutrition screening is to identify patients with nutrition risk who are more likely to benefit from nutrition assessment and intervention (8). More than 50 published screening tools are available that evaluate and score a variety of criteria, such as weight loss, changes in appetite, gastrointestinal complaints, chewing or swallowing dysfunction, lab parameters, and psychological and functional status (8–10). The patients' scores from the screening tools identify their nutrition risk, and a referral for nutrition assessment of those deemed moderate to high risk for malnutrition is strongly recommended. The Nutritional Risk Screening incorporates measures of potential undernutrition and disease severity (major surgery, malignancy, chronic disease, and so on) and is the preferred screening tool for hospitalized patients in Europe (4,11). The Subjective Global Assessment (SGA) has also been investigated as a viable nutrition screening tool in the surgical population (12). The components of the SGA include weight changes, changes in dietary intake, gastrointestinal symptoms, and functional capacity (9,12). The Nutrition Risk Index (NRI) is a simple equation using albumin and weight loss. The NRI and the SGA have been shown to be predictive for malnutrition and postoperative complications in patients undergoing major abdominal surgery (12,13).

Recently revised Joint Commission on Accreditation of Healthcare Organizations (JCAHO) standards require all hospitalized patients to be screened for nutrition risk within 24 hours of admission. However, the standards clearly do not apply to the complex gastrointestinal (GI) surgical patient where perioperative nutrition therapy is often necessary to optimize outcome and reduce risk (14,15). Despite emphasis on nutrition screening related to the standards of the JCAHO, there is no consensus on the best method for screening at-risk patients (5,9,10–16). Table 60.2 provides examples of commonly used nutrition screening tools in surgical populations.

TABLE 60.2
Nutrition Screening Tools

Malnutrition Universal Screening Tool (MUST)
Mini Nutritional Assessment (MNA)
Nutritional Risk Index (NRI)
Nutritional Risk Screening (NRS)

Nutrition Assessment

Nutrition assessment is a comprehensive evaluation of patient data, including nutritional adequacy, health status, and functional and behavioral status (Table 60.3), for those patients who are identified at nutrition risk (8). Nutritional adequacy data describe dietary habits and adequacy of nutrient intake (3,8). Appropriate evaluation of the health status provides information regarding anthropometric data, laboratory data, and physical and clinical information. Examples of physical information include the severity of symptoms related to tumor or treatment and its impact on nutritional status (3). Clinical data include pertinent medical history or medications that also impact nutritional status (3). Biochemical parameters or laboratory data are particularly significant in preoperative nutrition assessment (3). Studies have demonstrated that in the preoperative setting serum albumin remains the single best indicator of postoperative complications (2,6,17,18). Kudsk et al. used albumin levels to stratify nutritional risk. In this retrospective cohort study, the authors reported that albumin levels are relatively accurate and inexpensive indicator of potential morbidity (6). They also noted that the significance of preexisting hypoalbuminemia is underrecognized and therefore undertreated. They recommended that in esophageal, gastric, and pancreatic surgery, when albumin is below 3.25 g/dL, the operation should be postponed whenever possible for additional nutritional and metabolic support (2,6,14). Although albumin is a valuable marker for preoperative assessment and postoperative outcomes, a valid interpretation of serum proteins requires careful consideration of all the factors that may influence their result, particularly in the postoperative period. The decreased serum albumin

TABLE 60.3
Features of Nutrition Assessment[a]

Nutritional adequacy
- Dietary history/detailed nutrient intake

Health status
- Anthropometric measurements (height, weight, and weight changes)
- Biochemical measurements (visceral proteins, lymphocyte count, and liver function tests)
- Physical and clinical conditions (physiological and disease status)

Functional and behavioral status
- Social and cognitive function
- Psychological and emotional factors
- Quality-of-life measures
- Change readiness

[a]Adapted from Lacey and Pritchett (8).

and prealbumin levels observed immediately following esophagectomy or any major insult are due to hepatic reprioritization of protein synthesis, volume shifts, and the associated inflammatory response rather than malnutrition (2,3,16). Hydration status, renal function, liver function, and corticosteroids can influence serum protein levels separately from nutrition status as well (2,3,16). Despite the availability of numerous global assessment tools, visceral proteins, and various combinations of the two, no single tool or laboratory value consistently yields information that would alter nutritional practice in the acute setting (14).

CANDIDATES FOR NUTRITION THERAPY

Nutrition intervention is recommended for patients identified at nutrition risk or those who will undergo treatments that may potentially contribute to malnutrition. In addition to the criteria previously mentioned (unintentional weight loss [Table 60.1] and serum proteins), stages 3 to 4 disease, poor performance status, and advanced age (> 70) are additional factors that may indicate the need for nutrition support (1). Nutrition therapy should also be considered when neoadjuvant treatment is planned prior to surgery in patients with preexisting malnutrition.

Recent studies have reported that appropriate nutritional therapy preceding neoadjuvant treatment minimized weight loss, improved treatment tolerance, and was associated with fewer hospital admissions (19–22). The American Society for Parenteral and Enteral Nutrition (A.S.P.E.N.) practice guidelines for nutrition support of adults with cancer is described in Table 60.4.

TABLE 60.4
A.S.P.E.N. Guidelines for Nutrition Support of Adults With Cancer (33)[a]

1. Specialized nutrition support (SNS) should not be used routinely in patients undergoing major cancer operations.
2. Preoperative SNS may be beneficial in moderately or severely malnourished patients if administered for 7 to 14 days preoperatively, but the potential benefits of nutrition support must be weighed against the potential risk of the SNS itself and of delaying the operation.
3. SNS should not be used routinely as an adjunct to chemotherapy.
4. SNS should not be used routinely in patients undergoing head and neck, abdominal, or pelvic irradiation.
5. SNS is appropriate in patients receiving active anticancer treatment who are malnourished and who are anticipated to be unable to ingest and/or absorb adequate nutrients for a prolonged period of time.

[a]Adapted from A.S.P.E.N. Board of Directors and the Clinical Guidelines Task Force. Guidelines for the use of parenteral and enteral nutrition in adult and pediatric patients. *J Parenter Enteral Nutr.* 2002;26:1SA–137SA.

NUTRIENT REQUIREMENTS

Indirect calorimetry is considered the gold standard for determining calorie requirements; however, it is not widely available. General A.S.P.E.N. guidelines recommend 25 to 35 kcal/kg/d and 1.75 to 2.25 g protein/kg in cancer patients. The upper end of the range is recommended for patients who are hypermetabolic, are severely stressed, have wounds, or need to gain weight (3). Cancer cachexia, which is commonly present in the malnourished esophageal cancer patient with advanced disease, significantly alters nutrient metabolism and requirements. Cancer cachexia is the result of poorly understood complex catabolic processes. It is described by loss of lean body tissue, adipose tissue, and metabolic reserves. Nutrient repletion and/or reversal of lean body mass is nearly impossible with nutrition alone (23). The nutrition-specific treatments for patients with cancer cachexia are beyond the scope of this chapter, but several nutrients and protocols have shown potential benefit. These include appetite regulatory hormone manipulation and the use of an enteral formula containing omega-3 fatty acids (EPA and DHA) with various proteins and amino acid combinations (24–29).

NUTRITION THERAPY IN ESOPHAGEAL CANCER

Nutrition therapy may include oral nutrition supplements, enteral tube feeding, or parenteral nutrition. A regimen for nutrition therapy in malnourished patients should be considered in the initial stages of treatment planning. Appropriate perioperative nutrition therapy can reduce postoperative complications (30). Although minimal, nutrition support therapies are not without risk, these risks must also be considered when planning nutrition therapy.

ORAL NUTRITION SUPPLEMENTS

Standard oral nutrition supplements are generally the first choice for those patients able to tolerate oral intake. Oral supplements range from commercially prepared products, some containing immune modulating nutrients, to homemade shakes and fortified foods. In recent randomized control trials, severely malnourished surgical patients that received standard oral nutrition supplements preoperatively experienced less weight loss and suffered fewer minor postoperative complications than those who were not supplemented (31,32). Little evidence supports the use of standard oral nutrition supplements for preoperative patients who are not malnourished.

Adequate volitional oral intake is generally not resumed for 7 to 10 days following esophagectomy. Once oral intake is tolerated after esophagectomy, oral supplements may have a role in providing adequate nutrition postoperatively.

ENTERAL NUTRITION

Enteral nutrition (EN) is preferred in malnourished patients who are unable to meet their needs through oral intake, so they can successfully obtain enteral access and have a functioning gastrointestinal tract. Few absolute contraindications exist for enteral feeding. Thorough assessment of the patient's medical status and anatomy is required to decipher absolute and/or relative contraindications for enteral feeding. Contraindications to enteral feeding in the esophageal cancer patient are commonly associated with the inability to access the GI tract. Timing, formula selection, and dosing of EN have become key concepts when considering nutrition therapy (2,13). Standardized enteral feeding protocols have emerged to successfully guide these nutrition therapy concepts (33–36).

Timing

EN should be initiated as soon as appropriate prior to neoadjuvant therapy and/or surgery for patients who are unable to meet nutrition needs through oral intake. Postoperatively, feeding should be started as soon as the patient is hemodynamically stable and adequately resuscitated. Most protocols reporting benefit start enteral feeds at low rates (10–20 cc/h) within 48 hours of surgery and slowly advance feeds by 10 to 20 cc/h every 12 to 24 hours until goal rates are obtained. Randomized controlled trials have clearly shown that early (within 24–48 hours postoperatively) EN decreases infectious complications and lengths of stay (37,38). Favorable effects of early EN include improved immune competence, improved nitrogen balance and wound healing, better substrate utilization, decreased hypermetabolic response to injury, prevention of mucosal atrophy, and preservation of gut flora (2,13,37–41). Enteral feeding should not be started in the hemodynamically unstable patient.

Formula Selection and Dosing

Formula selection is dependent on the patient's nutrient requirements, digestive and absorptive capacity, disease state, organ function, and the route of administration of enteral feeding (3). Generally a standard high protein enteral formula (1 cal/mL) is used for patients needing enteral support prior to neoadjuvant treatment prescribed at 25 to 35 kcal/kg. The current literature would support the use of preemptive immune or metabolic modulating therapy for 5 to 7 days preoperatively (3 servings, or ~750 mL of an immune-modulating formula containing arginine and omega-3 fatty acids from fish oil sources) is preferred (42). Immune and metabolic modulating formulas and nutrients are described in detail later in this chapter. If an immune modulating formula is not available preoperatively, then an immune modulating formula can be used in the immediate (within 24–48 hours) postoperative period for approximately 7 to 10 days (40,42). If the immune-modulating formulas are not available, a standard complete high-protein tube feeding with adequate vitamins and trace elements should be used. Initial postoperative calorie recommendations are conservative, ~20 to 25 kcal/kg for the first 5 to 7 days. During the initial days postoperatively, the primary goal is not caloric adequacy but delivery of nutrients that enhance immune and metabolic function as well as maintain the mucosal barrier and gut-associated lymphoid tissue (11,37,39,43). Calories from EN are titrated toward 30 to 35 kcal/kg as appropriate for anabolism and postoperative healing following the first week.

Enteral Feeding Protocols

Standardized enteral feeding protocols guide appropriate selection, timing, dosing, and monitoring of EN. A well-designed enteral feeding protocol will provide consistency in nutrition therapy and aid in eliminating barriers to feeding, such as delayed initiation and unnecessary holding or stopping. Enteral feeding protocols also act to heighten awareness regarding possible signs of intolerance (33–36). Recent studies of patients in an intensive care unit (ICU) in which a standardized, evidence-based feeding protocol was implemented reported shortened duration of mechanical ventilation and a reduced morality (35,36). EN may be initiated once the patient is fully resuscitated and is hemodynamically stable, within 24 to 48 hours postoperatively. Giuseppe et al. published their protocol in 2005 for jejunostomy feedings following esophagectomy (44). Standard tube feeding is started 12 hours postoperatively at 30mL/h advancing 20mL/h every 5 hours to a max rate of 110mL/h (44). Published protocols vary in rate of advancing feeds postoperatively. The authors of this chapter take a more conservative approach in the early postoperative period and start feeding within 24 to 48 hours, following adequate stabilization and resuscitation, at 10 mL/h and then advance infusion rates slowly over 2 to 5 days to reach protein and caloric goals. Caloric delivery is not the prime objective with early postoperative feeding. The feeding is done primarily to help maintain the mucosal border integrity and gut-associated immune function (39). Careful patient assessment and evaluation is required for the appropriateness of feeding advancement regardless of protocol guidelines.

IMMUNE/METABOLISM-MODULATING ENTERAL FORMULAS

Over the past several decades, numerous animal and human models have shown that certain individual nutrients are able to modulate immune function. These specific nutrients have been shown to provide added benefit above and beyond their role in routine metabolism. Most of the current focus appears to involve the nutrients arginine, glutamine, omega-3 fatty acids, and nucleotides (40). As a result of these promising animal and now multiple clinical studies, several enteral formula manufacturers have developed and are marketing immune-modulated enteral formulas. These formulas have been shown to improve clinical outcomes by decreasing infectious complications, shortening hospital length of stay, and minimizing wound complications. These benefits have been shown in high-risk surgical and/or critically ill patients (41,42,45–47). The immune-modulating formulas commercially available all vary slightly in the quantity and quality of the "neutraceuticals" they contain. More than 36 human studies have been conducted to determine if surgical, medical, or critically ill patients experience risk reduction or beneficial outcomes as a result of receiving these formulations (48,49). Results of these studies vary, but the general consensus of all 5 meta-analysis done to date in surgical patients is that they have benefit (50). These studies have been extensively scrutinized for variables including lack of feeding comparisons, lack of homogeneous study population, and the manner in which the data were analyzed. Despite the minor study design variations, most of these studies show clear benefit of reduced rates of infection, decreased antibiotic use, lowered incidence of intra-abdominal abscesses, and reduced ICU and hospital length of stay (40). The vast majority of the 36 currently published peer-reviewed studies report benefit in the surgical population with only a few reporting no significant change (51,52). In addition to the more than 36 individual studies, 5 meta-analyses have now been completed, all showing similar outcome benefit in the surgical population (48,49,51,53).

SPECIFIC NUTRIENTS OF INTEREST

The exact nutrient makeup for the ICU and immediate postoperative period remains a relatively controversial topic. More than 200 enteral formulas are currently available for use, and several are considered appropriate for the ICU and postoperative esophageal surgical patient.

Arginine

Arginine is classified as a conditionally essential amino acid, indicating that in stress situations inadequate amounts are available to meet the accelerated demand. Studies indicate that supplemental arginine is beneficial in wound healing, immune response, and enhancing net nitrogen balance (54). The exact mechanism for these benefits remains open for some speculation. Arginine has been reported to influence several systems from vasomotor tone to maintaining immune function through its action in lymphocytes. Arginine is also a potent stimulant of growth hormone, glucagon, prolactin, and insulin release (55). Arginine is also the only precursor for nitric oxide, a highly reactive molecule synthesized from arginine by the action of 1 of the 3 isoforms of nitric oxide synthase resulting in the formation of nitric oxide and citrulline (55). Nitric oxide is a ubiquitous molecule with important roles in the maintenance of vascular tone, coagulation, the immune system, and the GI tract and has been implicated as a factor in disease states as diverse as sepsis, hypertension, and cirrhosis (55).

Glutamine

Glutamine is the other conditionally essential amino acid that has recently gained even greater support in the surgical and critical care arena. Over the past 20 years, glutamine has been reported to offer a myriad of benefits in surgical patients, including maintenance of acid/base balance, provision of primary fuel for rapidly proliferating cells (i.e., enterocytes and lymphocytes), being a precursor in the synthesis of glutathione and arginine, attenuation of the oxidant stress, decreasing peripheral insulin resistance, enhanced stress protein response, attenuation of the inflammatory response, and its function as a key substrate for gluconeogenesis (56). Recent evidence that glutamine can induce heat-shock protein is yet another beneficial molecular effect of this amino acid (57). The heat-shock proteins are a class of cellular chaperone proteins that support appropriate protein folding (58). With glutamine-enhancing heat-shock protein, the cell is able to better protect itself from subsequent stress.

Lipids

Understanding lipid modulation of the metabolic response in the surgical and critical care setting is hampered by the fact that lipids are traditionally given as one of many active components of an immune-enhancing formula. When delivered with multiple other immune-modulating nutrients, determining the exact contribution of the lipid component is virtually impossible. This is made even more confusing by recent data demonstrating that the omega-3 fatty acid eicosapentaenoic acid modulates arginine metabolism (59). The omega-3 fats found in fish oil (DHA and EPA) have multiple beneficial effects in the perioperative period, including modulation of leukocyte function and regulation of inflammatory cytokine release through nuclear signaling and gene expression (60). Leukotrienes, thromboxane, and prostaglandins derived from omega-6 lipids have demonstrated a much higher proinflammatory response than that associated with the omega-3 class (61). The omega-3 lipids have recently been reported to enhance the production of a new group of prostaglandin derivatives called resolvins and neuroprotectins (62). These new compounds play a role in accelerating the resolution of the proinflammatory state (63). Abundant data report the influence of omega-3 fats on nuclear signaling and gene expression (60). For example, polyunsaturated fatty acids interact with various nuclear receptor proteins, such as peroxisome proliferator–activated receptor, which then influence nuclear factor kappa B and gene expression. In effect, by decreasing nuclear factor kappa B migration into the nucleus, omega-3 fats down-regulate the proinflammatory response to stressful stimuli (61). Heller et al. (64) recently reported that omega-3 fatty acids given intravenously at a dose of 0.11 g/kg/d for a mean of 8.7 days demonstrated a decrease in mortality in 661 surgical and ICU patients, many of which were esophageal surgery patients. The route of delivery of omega-3 fats is important to keep in mind; when given enterally, it takes approximately 3 days to achieve adequate omega-3 fat levels in the cellular membrane. However, when given parenterally, a clinically relevant response can be achieved in 1 to 3 hours (60).

In summary, the literature strongly supports the concept that immune-modulated formulas may be beneficial in esophageal surgery patients. The patients who appear to benefit the most are those who will undergo or have undergone complicated esophageal resections, who are malnourished preoperatively, or who have a history of previous major GI surgery (40). Although these formulas have shown consistent reduction in length of ICU and hospital stay and reduction in infectious complications, they have not shown a decrease in mortality in all populations.

ENTERAL VERSUS PARENTERAL NUTRITION THERAPY

EN offers multiple structural, functional, and metabolic benefits compared to parenteral nutrition (PN) (Table 60.5). Current literature supports the use of PN only when EN is not feasible or has failed. However, esophageal cancer and its treatment, either surgical or medical, sometimes results in the need for supplemental total PN to supply timely adequate nutrition support.

Randomized controlled trials evaluating perioperative PN and EN have generally reported fewer infections and reduced hospital stays in the EN-fed groups (30,65,66). Takagi et al. (67) evaluated isocaloric PN versus EN in esophagectomy patients from 1 week prior to 2 weeks following surgery. Serum IL-6, IL-10, and endotoxin concentration were measured before, during, and at 2 h and 1, 3, and 7 days after the operation. Serum IL-6 and endotoxin concentration were significantly lower in the EN group than in the PN groups on the third and seventh days (67). In another study of esophagectomy patients, early postoperative EN was compared to PN. EN patients had shorter lengths of stay and recovered bowel function more quickly than PN patients (66). Although the results of these studies are comparable to other randomized controlled trials in surgical populations, the small sample sizes and methods lead to study limitations. Clearly the enteral route of nutrition is the preferred method whenever possible.

TUBE FEEDING ACCESS

The appropriate access device is dependent on the patient's medical and surgical history, anatomy and function of the digestive tract, and expected duration of therapy. Multiple tube feeding devices are available; however, the most commonly used will be described.

TABLE 60.5
Benefits of Enteral Nutrition (4)[a]

Helps maintains normal gastrointestinal function and flora
Maintains mucosal barrier
Provides physiological nutrients not available in PN
Improves immune response
Reduced cost compared to PN

[a]Adapted from *A.S.P.E.N. Nutrition Support Core Curriculum: A Case-Based Approach*. A.S.P.E.N., 2007.

Nasoenteric Feeding Tube Placement

Nasoenteric feeding tubes can be placed at the bedside using standardized protocols, endoscopically, or under fluoroscopic guidance to the stomach or small intestine (duodenum or jejunum) (68). Nasoenteric feeding tube placement is the preferred method when duration of nutrition therapy is expected to be less than 4 weeks and the esophagus is not completely occluded. A recent study showed successful placement of nasoenteric feeding tube placement by using an ultrathin transnasal endoscope in esophageal cancer patients when traditional methods failed (69). Nasoenteric feeding tube placement is generally the preferred access device by surgeons for appropriate patients awaiting esophagectomy. Nasoenteric feeding tubes are not without disadvantages, as they can be inconvenient for the patient, cause nasal irritation, slightly increase the risk of sinusitis, and clog frequently because of the small tube size and can be easily dislodged (70).

Percutaneous Endoscopic Gastrostomy

Percutaneous endoscopic gastrostomy (PEG) is not widely used in esophageal cancer because of concerns about altering the stomach as a suitable esophageal replacement, transversing the esophageal tumor with the endoscope, and potentially inoculating tumor metastasis to the abdominal wall. Despite these concerns, Margolis et al. showed that PEG placement in patients with esophageal cancer receiving neoadjuvant therapy followed by surgical resection may be safe and does not compromise the stomach as a conduit (70). Sixty-one patients received PEG placement prior to surgical resection without evidence of compromise to the gastric conduit. Of significance was the ability of the PEG patient to attain target doses of chemotherapy and radiation prior to surgical resection better than the non-PEG patients (70). Another retrospective review of patients with upper aerodigestive tract cancer also showed improved outcome for patients with early nutrition via PEG at the start of cancer treatment (71). Eighty out of 85 PEGs were successfully placed by Hujala et al. in early stages of treatment planning for esophageal cancer (72). The majority of these PEGs were placed by an otorhinolaryngologist who performed additional diagnostic procedures during the pretreatment work-up, such as open biopsy and panendoscopy (72).

A suitable gastric conduit appears a valid concern; however, the benefits of enhancing perioperative nutrition and attainment of target neoadjuvant therapy may outweigh the risk of PEG placement. An interdisciplinary approach is imperative to highlight the patient's medical background and surgical plan prior to PEG placement to optimize location and avoid compromise of the conduit.

Jejunostomy

In certain circumstances, nasoenteric or PEG feeding tube placements are not possible in esophageal cancer preoperatively because of esophageal obstruction. Jenkinson et al. places laparoscopic feeding tubes at the time of standard laparoscopic staging with success resulting in minimal complications or added cost (22).

Nearly 50% to 60% of esophagectomy patients require nutrition support for more than 10 days following surgery (67). For this reason, as well as the multiple benefits of EN discussed earlier in this chapter (Table 60.5), feeding jejunostomy or feeding access to the small bowel at the time of esophagectomy is strongly recommended.

In 1994, Gerndt and Orringer described successful placement of jejunostomy feeding tubes in a large retrospective review with a low complication rate of 2.1% (73). Giuseppe et al. also described safe and successful jejunostomy feeding tube placement in 262 patients with a comparably low complication rate of 1.5% (44). In a recent population-based study, patients receiving postoperative jejunostomy feeding tube placement had a reduced risk of postoperative weight loss compared to the group without jejunostomy feeding tube placement (74). Although the general consensus in the literature favors feeding tube placement at the time of open esophagectomy, the use of jejunostomy feeding tube placement as routine practice still varies among institutions. The growing trend toward laparoscopic esophagectomy may decrease the need for small-bowel feeding access at the time of surgery as these patients appear to have earlier return of bowel function and fewer postoperative nutritional issues, from early personal observations at our institution.

POSTOPERATIVE DIET ADVANCEMENT

The typical diet advancement following esophagectomy begins with liquids and transitions to soft semisolids or pureed diet over the course of 4 to 6 weeks. Eventually, the esophagectomy patient may be able to tolerate a near normal diet. Small frequent meals and remaining upright following mealtime are key recommendations to promote adaptation in the postoperative period. Table 60.6 provides general diet recommendations following esophagectomy. Dysphagia, reflux, appetite loss, and postoperative dumping are symptoms that often occur postoperatively and can adversely affect postoperative nutrition status (75). A speech language pathologist as

TABLE 60.6
General Diet Guidelines Following Esophagectomy

1. Eat 5 to 6 small meals per day
2. Sit upright while eating
3. Remain upright for 45 to 60 minutes after eating
4. Take small bites and chew food thoroughly
5. Drink no more than ½ cup of liquid with meals
6. Avoid concentrated sweets
7. Supplement meals with high-calorie milkshakes if having difficulty maintaining weight

well as the dietitian play an integral role in modifying the diet according to food texture and nutrient needs throughout the course of recovery.

CONCLUSION

The importance of nutrition in the perioperative management of the esophageal cancer patient cannot be understated. It is now abundantly clear that EN is the preferred route of nutrition therapy in the perioperative period for esophageal cancer patients. Studies suggest that immune-modulating formulas may provide significant benefit over standard formulas for patients undergoing esophagectomy. Several studies now support the concept "preoperative loading of the cell" with metabolically active nutrients may offer additional benefit in optimizing outcomes. Early identification of malnourished esophageal cancer patients and a multidisciplinary approach to treatment will optimize outcomes.

References

1. Mangar S, Slevin N, Mais K, et al. Evaluating predictive factors for determining enteral nutrition in patients receiving radical radiotherapy for head and neck cancer: a retrospective review. *Radiother Oncol.* 2006;78:152–158.
2. Martindale RG, Zhou M. Nutrition and metabolism. In: O'Leary P, ed. *The Physiologic Basis of Surgery.* 4th ed. Philadelphia: Lippincott Williams & Wilkins; 2008:112–149.
3. Roberts S, Mattox R. Cancer. In: Gottschlich M, ed. *The A.S.P.E.N. Nutrition Support Core Curriculum: A Case-Based Approach—The Adult Patient.* Silver Spring, MD: American Society for Parenteral and Enteral Nutrition; 2007:649–675.
4. Kondrup J, Rasmussen H, Hamburg O, et al. Nutritional risk screening (NRS 2002): a new method based on an analysis of controlled clinical trials. *Clin Nutr.* 2003;22:321–336.
5. Kuzu MA, Terzioglu H, Genc V, et al. Preoperative nutritional risk assessment in predicting postoperative outcome in patients undergoing major surgery. *World J Surg.* 2006;30:378–390.
6. Kudsk KA, Tolley EA, DeWitt C, et al. Preoperative albumin and surgical site identify surgical risk for major postoperative complications. *J Parenter Enteral Nutr.* 2003;27:1–9.
7. Tashiro T, Yamamori H, Takagi K, et al. Changes in immune function following surgery for esophageal carcinoma. *Nutrition.* 1999;15:760–766.
8. Lacey K, Pritchett E. Nutrition care process and model: ADA adopts road map to quality care and outcomes management. *J Am Diet Assoc.* 2003;103:1061–1072.
9. Krystofiak R, Mueller C. Nutrition screening and assessment. In: Gottschlich M, ed. *The A.S.P.E.N. Nutrition Support Core Curriculum: A Case-Based Approach—The Adult Patient.* Silver Spring, MD: American Society for Parenteral and Enteral Nutrition; 2007:163–186.
10. Elia M, ed. *Development and use of the "Malnutrition Universal Screening Tool" ("MUST") for adults.* A report by the Malnutrition Advisory Group of the British Association for Parenteral and Enteral Nutrition. Reddtich, Worcestershire: British Association for Parenteral and Enteral Nutrition; 2003.
11. Kondrup J, Allison P, Elia M, et al. ESPEN guidelines for nutrition screening. *Clin Nutr.* 2003;22:415–421.
12. Sungurtekin H, Sungertekin U, Balci C, et al. The influence of nutritional status on complications after major intraabdominal surgery. *Am J Clin Nutr.* 2004;23:227–232.
13. Kudsk K, Reddy S, Sacks G, et al. Joint Commission for Accreditation of Health Care Organizations Guidelines: Too late to intervene for nutritional at risk surgical patients. *J Parenter Enteral Nutr.* 2003;27:288–290.
14. Martindale RG, Maerz L. Management of perioperative nutrition support. *Curr Opin Crit Care.* 2006;12:290–294.
15. Hall JC. Nutritional assessment of surgery patients. *J Am Coll Surg.* 2006;202: 837–843.
16. Gibbs J, Cull W, Henderson W, et al. Preoperative serum albumin as a predictor of operative mortality and morbidity: results from the National VA Surgical Risk Study. *Arch Surg.* 1999;134:36–42.
17. Daley J, Forbes M, Young G, et al. Validating risk-adjusted surgical outcomes: site visit assessment of process and structure. National VA Surgical Risk Study. *J Am Coll Surg.* 1997;185:341–351.
18. Ryan A, Hearty A, Prichard R, et al. Association of hypoalbuminemia on the first postoperative day and complications following esophagectomy. *J Gastrointest Surg.* 2007;10:1355–1360.
19. Cheng S, Terrell J, Bradford C, et al. Variables associated with feeding tube placement in head and neck cancer. *Arch Otolaryngol Head Neck Surg.* 2006;132:655–661.
20. Odelli C, Burgess D, Bateman L, et al. Nutrition support improves patient outcomes, treatment tolerance and admission characteristics in oesophageal cancer. *Clin Oncol (R Coll Radiol).* 2005;17:639–645.
21. Bertrand P, Piquet M, Bordier I, et al. Preoperative nutritional support at home in head and neck cancer patients. *Curr Opin Clin Nutr Metab Care.* 2002;5:435–440.
22. Jenkinson A, Lim J, Agrawal N, et al. Laparascopic feeding jejunostomy in esophagogastric cancer. *Surg Endosc.* 2007;21:299–302.
23. Senior K. Why is progress in treatment of cancer cachexia so slow? *Lancet Oncol.* 2007;8:671–672.
24. Fearon K, Barber M, Moses A, et al. Double-blind, placebo-controlled, randomized study of ecaisopentenoic acid diester in patients with cancer cachexia. *J Clin Oncol.* 2006;24:3401–3407.
25. Fearon K, Voss A, Hustead D. Definition of cancer cachexia: effect of weight loss, reduced food intake and systemic inflammation on functional status and prognosis. *Am J Clin Nutr.* 2006;83:1345–1350.
26. Barber M, Ross J, Fearon K. Disordered metabolic response with cancer and its management. *World J Surg.* 2000;24:681–689.
27. Skipworth R, Fearon K. The scientific rationale for optimizing nutritional support in cancer. *Eur J Gastro Hepatol.* 2007;19:371–377.
28. Mottershead M, Karteris E, Barclay J, et al. Immunohistochemical and quantitative mRNA assessment of ghrelin expression in gastric and oesophageal adenocarcinoma. *J Clin Pathol.* 2007;60:405–409.
29. Vissers Y, Dejong C, Luiking Y, et al. Plasma arginine concentrations are reduced in cancer patients: evidence for arginine deficiency? *Am J Clin Nutr.* 2005;81:1142–1146.
30. Bozzetti F, Gavazzi C, Miceli R, et al. Perioperative total parenteral nutrition in malnourished, gastrointestinal cancer patients: a randomized, clinical trial. *J Parenter Enteral Nutr.* 2000; 24:7–14.
31. MacFie J, Woodcock NP, Palmer MD, et al. Oral dietary supplements in pre- and postoperative surgical patients: a prospective and randomized clinical trial. *Nutrition.* 2000;16:723–728.
32. Smedley F, Bowling T, James M, et al. Randomized clinical trial of the effects of preoperative and postoperative oral nutritional supplements on clinical course and cost of care. *Br J Surg.* 2004;91:983–990.
33. Arabi Y, Haddad S, Sakkijha M, et al. the impact of implementing and enteral tube feeding protocol on calorie and protein delivery in intensive care unit patients. *Nutr Clin Pract.* 2004;19:523–530.
34. Barr A, McQuiggan M, Kozar R, et al. Gastric feeding as an extension of an established enteral nutrition protocol. *J Parenter Enteral Nutr.* 2004;19:504–510.
35. Kozar R, McQuiggan M, Moore F, et al. Postinjury enteral tolerance is reliably achieved by a standardized protocol. *J Surg Res.* 2002;104:70–75.
36. Barr J, Hecht M, Flavin K, et al. Outcomes in critically ill patients before and after the implementation of an evidence-based nutritional management protocol. *Chest.* 2004;4:1446–1457.
37. Marik P, Zaloga G. Early enteral nutrition in acutely ill patients: a systematic review. *Crit Care Med.* 2001;29:2264–2270.
38. Gabor S, Renner H, Matzi V, et al. Early enteral feeding compared with parenteral nutrition after oesophageal or oesophagogastric resection and reconstruction. *Br J Nutr.* 2005,93:509–513.
39. Kang W, Kudsk K. Is there evidence that the gut contributes to mucosal immunity in humans? *J Parenter Enteral Nutr.* 2007;31:246–258.

40. Consensus recommendations from the US summit on immune-enhancing enteral therapy. *J Parenter Enteral Nutr.* 2001;25:S1–S63.
41. Braga M, Gianotti L, Nespoli L, et al. Nutritional approach in malnourished surgical patients: a prospective randomized study. *Arch Surg.* 2002;137:174–180.
42. Gianotti L , Braga M, Nespoli L, et al. A randomized controlled trial of preoperative oral supplementation with a specialized diet in patients with gastrointestinal cancer. *Gastroenterology.* 2002;122:1763–1770.
43. Hise M, Halterman K, Gajewski B, et al. Feeding practices of severely ill intensive care unit patients: an evaluation of energy sources and clinical outcomes. *J Am Diet Assoc.* 2007;107:458–465.
44. Giuseppe S, Sujendran V, Wheeler J, et al. Needle catheter jejunostomy at esophagectomy for cancer: how I do it. *J Surg Oncol.* 2005;91:276–279.
45. Takeuchi H, Ikeuchi S, Kawaguchi Y, et al. Clinical significance of perioperative immunonutrition for patients with esophageal cancer. *World J Surg.* 2007;31:2160–2167.
46. Xu J, Zhong Y, Jing D, et al. Preoperative enteral immunonutrition improves postoperative outcome in patients with gastrointestinal cancer. *World J Surg.* 2006;30:1284–1289.
47. Daley J, Khuri S, Henderson W, et al. Risk adjustment of the postoperative morbidity rate for the comparative assessment of the quality of surgical care: results of the National Veterans Affairs Surgical Risk Study. *J Am Coll Surg.* 1997;185:328–340.
48. Beale RJ, Bryg DJ, Bihari DJ. Immunonutrition in the critically ill: a systematic review of clinical outcome. *Crit Care Med.* 1999;27:2799–2805.
49. Heys SD, Walker LG, Smith I, et al. Enteral nutritional supplementation with key nutrients in patients with critical illness and cancer: a meta-analysis of randomized controlled clinical trials. *Ann Surg.* 1999;229:467–477.
50. Waitzberg DL, Saito H, Plank LD, et al. Postsurgical infections are reduced with specialized nutrition support. *World J Surg.* 2006;30:1592–1604.
51. Saffle JR, Wiebke G, Jennings K, et al. Randomized trial of immune-enhancing enteral nutrition in burn patients. *J Trauma.* 1997;42:793–800. discussion 800–802.
52. Heyland DK, Novak F, Drover JW, et al. Should immunonutrition become routine in critically ill patients? A systematic review of the evidence. *JAMA.* 2001;286:944–953.
53. Zhou M, Martindale RG. Arginine in the critical care setting. *J Nutr.* 2007;137: S1687–S1692.
54. Zhou M, Martindale RG. Immune modulating enteral formulations: optimum components, appropriate patients, and controversial use of arginine in sepsis. *Curr Gastroenterol Rep.* 2007;9:329–374.
55. Coeffier M, Dechelotte P. The role of glutamine in intensive care unit patients: mechanisms of action and clinical outcome. *Nutr Rev.* 2005;63:65–69.
56. Ziegler TR, Ogden LG, Singleton KD, et al. Parenteral glutamine increases serum heat shock protein 70 in critically ill patients. *Intensive Care Med.* 2005;31:1079–1086.
57. Macario AJ, Conway de Macario E. Sick chaperones, cellular stress, and disease. *N Engl J Med.* 2005;353:1489–1501.
58. Bansal V, Syres KM, Makarenkova V, et al. Interactions between fatty acids and arginine metabolism: implications for the design of immune-enhancing diets. *J Parenter Enteral Nutr.* 2005;29:S75–S80.
59. Calder PC. Fatty acids and gene expression related to inflammation. *Nestlé Nutr Workshop Ser.* 2002;7:19–40.
60. Ferrucci L, Cherubini A, Bandinelli S, et al. Relationship of plasma polyunsaturated fatty acids to circulating inflammatory markers. *J Clin Endocrinol Metab.* 2006; 91:439–446.
61. Campbell EL, Louis Na, Tomasetti SE, et al. Resolvin E1 promotes mucosal surface clearance of neutrophils: a new paradigm for inflammatory resolution. *FASEB J.* 2007;12:3162–3170.
62. Serhan CN. Novel eicosanoid and docosanoid mediators: resolvins, docosatrienes, and neuroprotectins. *Curr Opin Clin Nutr Metab Care.* 2005;8:115–121.
63. Li H, Ruan XZ, Powis SH, et al. EPA and DHA reduce LPS-induced inflammation responses in HK-2 cells: evidence for a PPAR-gamma-dependent mechanism. *Kidney Int.* 2005;67:867–874.
64. Heller AR, Rossler S, Litz RJ, et al. Omega-3 fatty acids improve the diagnosis related clinical outcome. *Crit Care Med.* 2006;34:972–979.
65. Veterans Affairs Total Parenteral Nutrition Cooperative Study Group. Perioperative total parenteral nutrition in surgical patients. *N Engl J Med.* 1991;325:525–532.
66. Elia M, Van Bokhorst-de van der Schueren MA, Garvey J, et al. Enteral (oral or tube administration) nutritional support and eicosapentaenoic acid in patients with cancer: a systematic review. *Int J Oncol.* 2006;28:5–23.
67. Takagi K, Yamamori H, Toyoda Y, et al. Modulating effects of the feeding route on stress response and endotoxin translocation in severely stressed patients receiving thoracic esophagectomy. *Nutrition.* 2000;16:355–360.
68. Bankhead R, Fang J. Enteral access devices. In: Gottschlich M, ed. *The A.S.P.E.N. Nutrition Support Core Curriculum: A Case-Based Approach—The Adult Patient.* Silver Spring, MD: American Society for Enteral and Parenteral Nutrition; 2007:233–245.
69. De Aguilar-Nascimento JE, Kudsk KA. Use of small-bore feeding tubes: successes and failures. *Curr Opin Clin Nutr Metab Care.* 2007;10:291–296.
70. Margolis M, Alexander P, Trachiotis G, et al. Percutaneous endoscopic gastrostomy before multimodality therapy in patients with esophageal cancer. *Ann Thorac Surg.* 2003;76:1694–1698.
71. Beer K, Krause K, Zuercher T, et al. Early percutaneous endoscopic gastrostomy insertion maintains nutritional state in patients with aerodigestive tract cancer. *Nutr Cancer.* 2005;52:29–34.
72. Hujala K, Sipila J, Pulkkinen J, et al. Early percutaneous endoscopic gastrostomy nutrition in head and neck cancer patients. *Acta Otolaryngol.* 2004;124:847–850.
73. Gerndt S, Orringer M. Tube jejunostomy as an adjunct to esophagectomy. *Surgery.* 1994;115:164–169.
74. Martin L, Lagergren J, Jia C, et al. The influence of needle catheter jejunostomy on weight evelopment after oesophageal cancer surgery in a population-based study. *EJSO.* 2007;33:713–717.
75. Viklund P, Wengstrom Y, Rouvelas I, et al. Quality of life and persisting symptoms after oesophageal cancer surgery. *Eur J Cancer.* 2007;42:1407–1414.

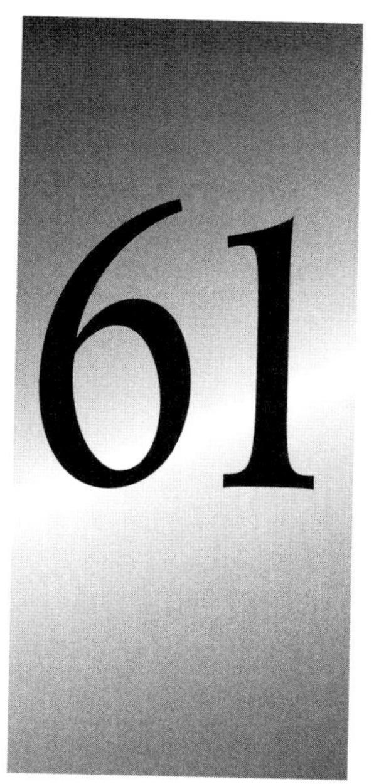

Surgery Techniques: Management of Benign Esophageal Tumors

Sajida Ahad
Roger P. Tatum
Carlos A. Pellegrini

Benign tumors of the esophagus are on the whole rather rare, making up only approximately 1% of all esophageal tumors. These tumors are a heterogeneous group, and as such the surgical management, when indicated, may take a variety of approaches. The choice of these depends on factors such as whether they are symptomatic and their type, size, and location, and they range from endoscopic resection to esophagectomy. Because of this, it will be most useful to discuss the surgical techniques in the context of the different types of benign esophageal tumor that may be encountered.

LEIOMYOMA

Esophageal leiomyomas are the most common benign intramural esophageal tumors. These are rare and account for only 0.4% of all esophageal tumors (1). They represent about 10% of all gastrointestinal leiomyomas. In autopsy series, their incidence is reported to be between 0.006% and 0.1%. They are more common in men (ratio of 2:1), they are mostly solitary, and 90% of them occur in the lower two-thirds of the esophagus (1). Diffuse esophageal leiomyomatosis is uncommon (2,3). Malignant transformation of leiomyomas has been reported rarely (0.2%) (4). These tumors are typically asymptomatic and are discovered incidentally. They generally tend to cause symptoms when the size reaches 5 cm or more.

PREOPERATIVE WORK-UP

Imaging

Asymptomatic leiomyomas are usually discovered when an abnormal chest radiograph prompts further work-up. However, chest X-rays are neither sensitive nor specific enough to detect leiomyomas.

Because of its inexpensive and noninvasive nature, barium swallow is the most commonly used imaging modality for esophageal leiomyomas as well as other benign esophageal tumors. These tumors usually appear as round, elevated filling defects with clearly demarcated margins between esophagus and tumor. There is usually no ulceration of overlying mucosa (Figure 61.1).

Computed tomography (CT) scanning can be helpful in planning surgical therapy. CT demonstrates the relationship of the mass with surrounding organs; yields information regarding tumor size, location, and invasion into surrounding structures; and differentiates between extrinsic compression and masses intrinsic to the esophagus. However, CT does not as readily differentiate between solid and cystic masses and cannot image the layers of the esophageal wall.

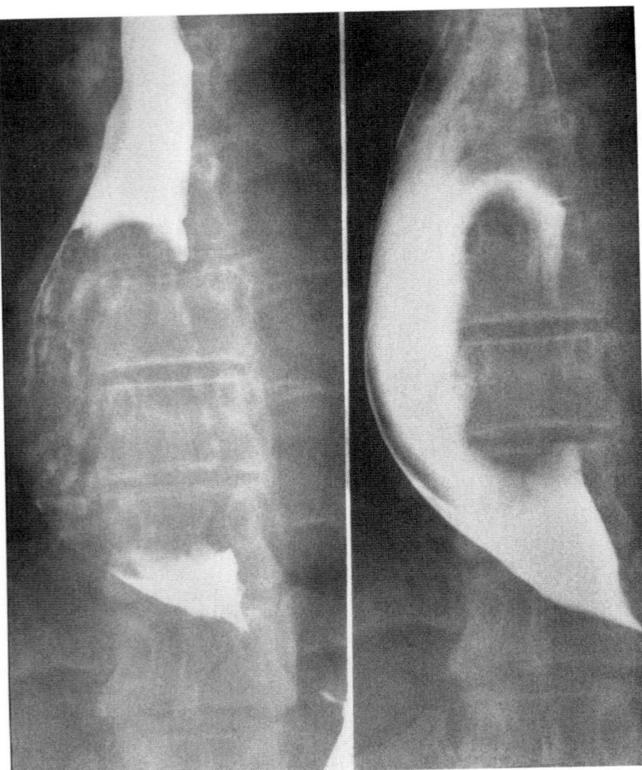

FIGURE 61.1

Barium radiograph of a large distal esophageal leiomyoma.

Endoscopy and Endosonography

Endoscopy should be performed in all patients suspected of harboring this lesion to better ascertain the diagnosis, define its characteristics, and determine the exact location. The 4 endoscopic findings characteristic of leiomyoma include the following: the overlying mucosa appears normal and intact, the tumor projects into the lumen of the esophagus, the tumor is freely mobile as is the overlying mucosa over the lesion, and no stenosis or obstruction of the lumen is present. Biopsy of a leiomyoma is not necessary and may increase the chance of perforation (at the time of operation), bleeding and infection (5,6).

Endoscopic ultrasound (EUS) may be employed to ascertain the layer of origin of the tumor. On EUS, leiomyomas appear as well circumscribed, homogeneous, hypoechoic masses with smooth borders. However, EUS does not differentiate between benign and malignant masses. Some researches have advocated the use of EUS-guided fine-needle aspiration (EUS-FNA) of the mass to determine its malignant nature. A multicenter prospective trial that included a series of 115 gastrointestinal (GI) tract lesions reported that the sensitivity, specificity, and accuracy of EUS-FNA in diagnosing neoplastic GI tract lesions were 61%, 79%, and 67%, respectively (7). While EUS-FNA potentially adds to the diagnostic accuracy of EUS alone, further studies are needed to evaluate the utility of this technique.

THERAPY

Treatment options for esophageal leiomyomas include endoscopic resection, minimally invasive surgical approaches, and open resection. Each is discussed next.

Endoscopic Resection

Endoscopic approaches utilized in the treatment of esophageal leiomyomas include polypectomy, rubber band ligation, and tumor ablation (8). However, these treatment options are constrained by a number of technical factors, such as tumor size, origin, and shape. The advent of EUS allows for more precise characterization of esophageal lesions. Esophageal leiomyomas can originate from either the muscularis mucosa or the muscularis propria. Leiomyomas originating from the former are usually small protruding masses like a polyp, less than 2 cm in size, and usually discovered incidentally. These are the most amenable to endoscopic techniques. Therefore, most agree that EUS is necessary to confirm the origin of these tumors from the muscularis mucosa rather than the muscularis in order to attempt endoscopic resection (9,10).

Kajiyama et al. first described the use of endoscopic techniques in the treatment of esophageal leiomyomas in 1995 (11). Two years later, Hyun et al. reported their series of 62 patients who underwent endoscopic resection by either polypectomy or incisional enucleation (12). The mean tumor diameter was 19 mm with one tumor reported to be 7 cm. Wehrmann et al. reported their experience with endoscopic resection in 20 patients with biopsy-proven benign esophageal tumors. The mean tumor size was 17 ± 8 mm. In the majority of patients, the tumor was ligated with a rubber band and resected with a snare (n = 11), while others required simple snare resection (n = 7) or cap resection (n = 2). In all but 2 patients was a complete resection (R0) possible. None of the patients had significant bleeding after the procedure (13).

To perform polypectomy, the tumor is first separated from the submucosal layer by injection of a hypertonic solution of 10% glycerol, 5% fructose, and saline. The tumor is then suctioned into a transparent cylinder, and a snare wire is closed around the lesion. Alternatively, ethanol injections can be employed to cause necrotic exfoliation of the tumor.

Although they are the least invasive, endoscopic approaches are not widely used. Most of these tumors do not lend themselves to endoscopic resection, as they span the entire wall, tend to protrude outside as well as inside, and there is a potential risk of hemorrhage and perforation. Ultimately it is indicated only for those tumors originating from the muscularis mucosa, and therefore this technique cannot be advocated for all esophageal leiomyomas.

Minimally Invasive Surgery

Tumors less than 7 cm in size can be resected through either a thoracoscopic or laparoscopic approach. Usually, tumors in the distal third of esophagus and the gastroesophageal junction (GEJ) are approached laparoscopically, while tumors in the middle third of the esophagus are approached thoracoscopically via the right chest. The thoracoscopic approach requires intubation with a double-lumen tube to exclude the right lung by selective ventilation. An on-table endoscopy should be performed to confirm the location of the tumor by transillumination. It is also useful to perform endoscopy after resection to confirm the integrity of the esophageal mucosa.

The patient is placed in a left lateral decubitus position with the surgeon standing behind the patient and the assistant in front. Four ports are placed as follows: a 10-mm camera port in the eighth intercostal space in the midaxillary line, another 10-mm port in the fourth intercostal space in the anterior axillary line, and 2 5-mm "working ports" posterior to the posterior axillary line.

The inferior pulmonary ligament is divided by ultrasonic shears, and the lung is retracted anteriorly and away from the esophagus. The mediastinal pleura overlying the esophagus is now exposed and divided (Figure 61.2). To facilitate intraoperative localization of the tumor, a flexible endoscope or an esophageal bougie can be used. Another alternative is to use a balloon-mounted endoscope to facilitate protrusion of the tumor from the esophageal wall. The longitudinal fibers of the muscularis propria overlying the tumor are then divided with electrocautery (Figure 61.3). The plane between the tumor and the esophagus is developed using a combination of blunt and sharp dissection (Figure 61.4). Once the tumor is completely enucleated, it is removed using a retrieval bag. The tumor bed is then inspected to assess the integrity of the mucosa. Insufflation of the esophageal lumen with air while it is submerged under water may help identify small leaks. Any gaps in the mucosa are repaired primarily. The muscle layer is then reapproximated with a nonabsorbable suture (Figure 61.5). Occasionally one may find that the tumor is not just round but has horseshoe-type extensions around one side or the other of the esophagus. While these tumors can still be resected using minimally invasive approaches, the dissection is much more complex. After removing the tumor, a 28-Fr chest tube is left in place through one of the port sites. This tube is removed the following day. A contrast study

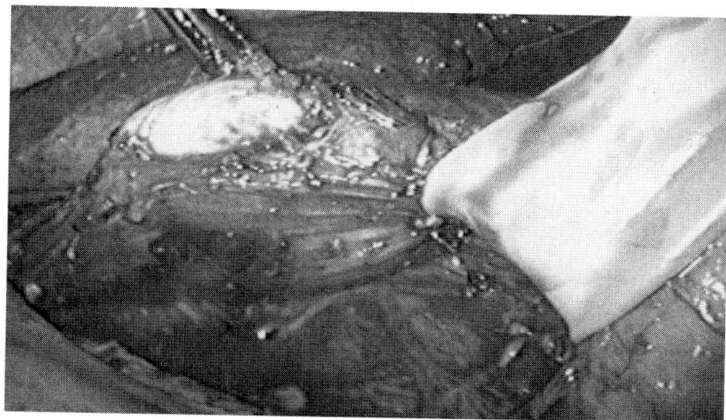

FIGURE 61.3

Myotomy made to expose esophageal leiomyoma and begin enucleation.

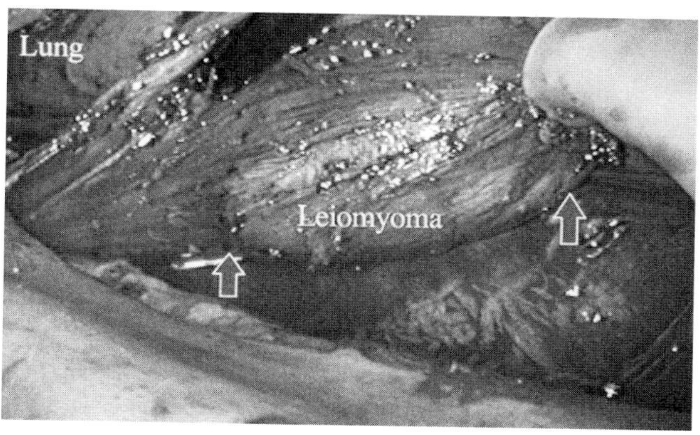

FIGURE 61.2

Thoracoscopic view of esophageal leiomyoma after exposure and mobilization of the esophagus.

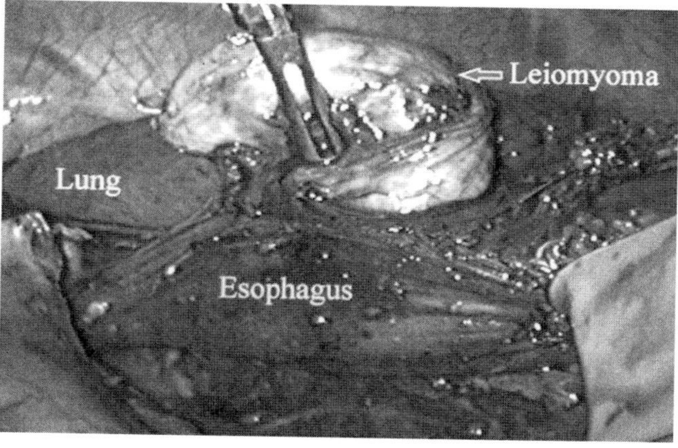

FIGURE 61.4

Thoracoscopic enucleation of esophageal leiomyoma.

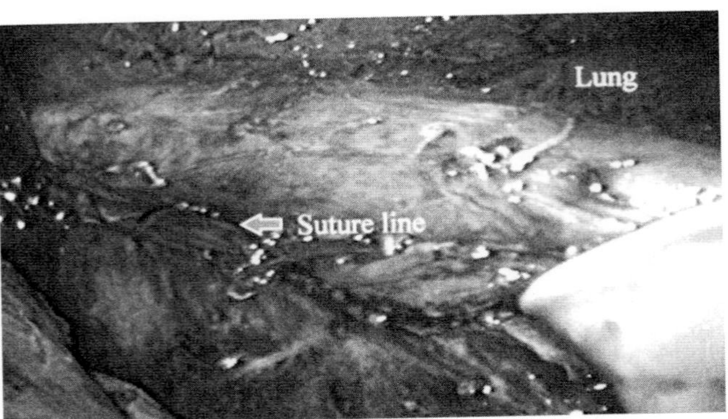

FIGURE 61.5

Closure of myotomy after enucleation of leiomyoma.

of the esophagus is obtained on postoperative day 1 to rule out any leak.

Kent et al. reported their experience of 20 patients who underwent minimally invasive surgery for benign esophageal tumors. Mean tumor size was 3.5 cm, while the median length of stay was 2.75 days. They found worsening (n = 3) or new onset (n = 2) reflux in 5 patients requiring fundoplication (5). Whether the myotomy should be resutured after enucleation is also a subject of controversy. Some authors maintain that if the integrity of the mucosa is not compromised, then the muscle need not be reapproximated. Yet other surgeons believe that suturing the muscularis is essential in order to prevent mucosal bulging and development of a pseudodiverticulum (14,15). Further, reapproximation of the esophageal wall likely maintains the continuity of peristalsis and prevents esophageal dysmotility; thus, it is our preferred technique (6,16).

The laparoscopic approach is more commonly used for tumors at or near the GEJ. The patient is placed in a modified, low lithotomy position. A beanbag is used to create a "seat" for the patient, which avoids patient slippage when placing the patient in the steep reverse Trendlenburg position. The surgeon stands between the patient's legs and operates in the most ideal ergonomic position, while the assistant stands on the left side of the patient.

Ports are placed similarly to the technique used to perform a laparoscopic Nissen fundoplication. A 1-cm transverse incision is made over the left costal margin lateral to the midclavicular line, and a Veress needle is introduced through this incision and carbon dioxide pnuemoperitoneum established. An optical trocar is then advanced through the planes of the abdominal wall. Four additional ports are placed: a 10-mm periumblical port to the left of midline (for the camera), a 10-mm left-sided port approximately 10 cm below and to the left of the subcostal port, another 10-mm port on the right side for the liver retractor, and a 10-mm port at the right costal margin. The phrenoesophageal membrane is divided and the esophagus mobilized. A Penrose drain is placed around the esophagus to aid in retraction. Extensive mobilization of the esophagus and dissection of the posterior mediastinum are necessary to permit adequate visualization of distal esophageal and GEJ tumors. Once the tumor is identified, enucleation and completion of the procedure are performed in an identical manner to that described for the thoracoscopic approach as detailed previously.

Open Surgical Excision

The principles guiding the open technique are the same as those outlined for minimally invasive procedures. The choice of surgical approach depends on the size and location of tumor, suspicion for malignant potential, surgeon preference, and surgeon experience. Studies have demonstrated shorter hospital stays, less pulmonary complications, and less postoperative pain with minimally invasive techniques compared with open approaches (5,17).

The location of the tumor along the esophageal body dictates whether a right (middle third) or a left (lower third) thoracotomy is performed. An upper midline laparotomy may also be utilized for very low (near GEJ) tumors. Once the tumor is identified, the longitudinal fibers are split, and the tumor bluntly dissected away from surrounding structures. Recurrence after surgical resection is extremely rare (18).

Esophagectomy

Esophagectomy may be necessary for tumors that are large (more than 8 cm), adherent to overlying mucosa, or when diffuse leiomyomatosis of the esophagus is present. However, there is significant postoperative morbidity associated with esophagectomy, including reflux esophagitis, anastomotic strictures, dumping syndrome, diarrhea, and weight loss. Many of these complications are thought to be caused when vagal nerves are sacrificed during surgery. To avoid these complications, some authors have advocated the use of a vagal-sparing technique. After vagal-sparing esophagectomy was performed for a number of benign esophageal diseases including leiomyoma, Banki et al. found that patients were free of dumping and diarrhea and had normal bowel function (19).

GASTROINTESTINAL STROMAL TUMOR

Over the past 2 decades, a mesenchymal tumor type known as a gastrointestinal stromal tumor (GIST) has been recognized. Many of these were previously thought to be leiomyomas, but in fact they are distinct from these tumors and appear to derive from the interstitial cells of Cajal (20–22). They are defined pathologically by positivity on immunostaining for the KIT antibody (CD117) (20). Only 5% or less of all GISTs occur in the esophagus (22,23).

The biologic behavior of GISTs is difficult to predict. Whereas some will pursue a benign and indolent course, approximately 10% to 30% may ultimately metastasize or locally recur (24), and this incidence is likely higher for GISTs in the esophagus (25). The risk for malignant potential is determined primarily by size and mitotic rate. Small tumors (less than 2 cm in greatest dimension) and those with less than 5 mitotic figures per 50 high-power fields are considered low risk; however, occasionally metastases have been seen associated with tumors having these characteristics (20).

Although many esophageal GISTs may be discovered incidentally, frequently patients with these tumors will present with dysphagia (25). In addition, upper GI bleeding as the presenting symptom has been described (25,26). The work-up is the same as that described previously for leiomyomas and typically includes upper endoscopy and computed tomography. Endosonography is also quite helpful in determining the layer of origin of the tumor within the esophageal wall. Unfortunately, none of these methods are able to distinguish GIST from leiomyoma (22).

Management for esophageal GISTs without evidence of metastasis involves complete surgical excision. This can be accomplished by enucleation using thoracoscopic or laparoscopic techniques as described for leiomyoma (22,27). For larger tumors (> 8 cm), however, esophagectomy will be necessary (23). A tyrosine kinase inhibitor, imatinib mesylate (Gleevec), has been used with significant benefit in the treatment of metastatic or unresectable GIST and will likely have a role in the adjuvant therapy of those tumors with higher risk of malignant behavior after surgical resection (21,23). Imatinib has also been used in the neoadjuvant setting to decrease tumor volume and enhance resectability for GISTs at various sites, including the esophagus (28).

OTHER BENIGN TUMORS

Benign esophageal tumors are a miscellaneous group that includes leiomyomas, fibrovascular polyps, angiolipomas, granular cell tumors, hemangiomas, and schwannomas. Because of the rarity of these tumors, the exact incidence is unknown. Management reported in the literature has ranged from endoscopic polypectomy to simple enucleation to esophagectomy as dictated by tumor location, size, and preoperative assessment of the potential for malignancy.

Schwannoma

Neurogenic tumors of the esophagus are very rare, and only a few are reported in the literature. These lesions are located mostly within the muscularis propria. They are usually round or oval and tend to protrude into the esophageal lumen. Reported schwannomas have ranged in size from 0.5 to 14 cm in greatest diameter and are commonly located in the upper esophagus. Tumors less than 2 cm can be resected endoscopically; however, larger tumors may have a cervical blood supply that can result in significant hemorrhage if bleeding vessels are not directly controlled (29,30).

Fibrovascular Polyp

These tumors are very rare, slow-growing tumors. They most commonly originate in the cervical esophagus and are usually pedunculated. Patients present with dysphagia and weight loss (31,32). In some cases, the polypoid mass can also be regurgitated into the oral cavity, causing airway obstruction (32). Because of the propensity for fibrovascular polyps to occur in the proximal esophagus, this tumor is usually approached through a left cervical esophagotomy (33) (Figure 61.6).

Angiolipoma

Angiolipomas of the esophagus have been rarely reported. The typical presentation includes dysphagia and weight loss. These tumors are usually more hypodense on CT than are leiomyomas. Depending on the location

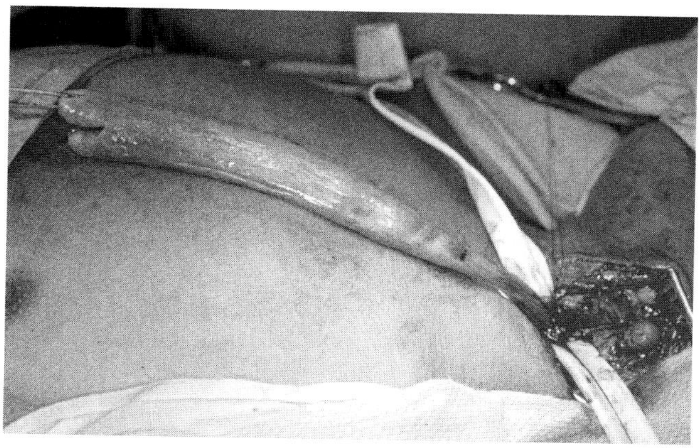

FIGURE 61.6

Excision of a fibrovascular polyp via the cervical approach. Note the very long stalk of this polyp.

within the esophagus and the size of the lesion, endoscopic as well as open resection techniques have been employed (34).

Granular Cell Tumor

This lesion is usually restricted to the submucosa, but occasionally it can be seen arising from the muscularis. The lesions are located in the distal third of esophagus. There is a higher incidence in women. It is estimated that between 1.5% and 2.7 % of these tumors are malignant (35).

Most of these tumors are asymptomatic and are diagnosed incidentally. When symptoms do arise, they are nonspecific and include epigastric pain, dyspepsia, and thoracic pain. On endoscopy, they appear as small sessile submucosal nodules with a firm consistency. The overlying mucosa is usually intact but can be ulcerated as well (36). Microscopically, they comprise epitheloid cells with eosinophilic cytoplasm and hyperchromatic nuclei. They stain positively for S100, vimentin, neuron specific enolase, and laminin on immunohistochemistry.

EUS is useful for diagnosis. Palazzo et al. reported their experience with 21 lesions suspected to be granular cell tumors on endoscopy. Twenty were removed endoscopically, with only 1 requiring open surgery (37). For tumors with a high suspicion for malignancy, open resection may be considered.

Hemangioma

With the widespread use of endoscopy, the incidental discovery of asymptomatic esophageal hemangiomas is increasing. When symptomatic, they can cause dysphagia, weight loss, or upper gastrointestinal hemorrhage. On endoscopy they are purplish-red tumors confined to the submucosa. These are most commonly seen in the middle and lower thirds of the esophagus. While endoscopic biopsy secures the diagnosis, it also carries the risk of hemorrhage. Like other benign esophageal tumors, hemangiomas can be removed endoscopically or via minimally invasive and open approaches (38).

CONCLUSION

While there are several widely different types of benign esophageal tumor, the incidence of each is relatively rare. A variety of approaches may be employed in resecting these lesions, including endoscopic removal, enucleation by thoracoscopy or laparoscopy, open enucleation, and occasionally esophagectomy. The choice of approach primarily depends on the size and location of the lesion as well as the tissue of origin (mucosa, submucosa, muscularis) and is less dependent on the type of lesion. Most can be removed with little to no residual deficit in esophageal function, and, with the exception of GIST, recurrence is extremely uncommon.

References

1. Seremetis MG, Lyons WS, deGuzman VC, et al. Leiomyomata of the esophagus: an analysis of 838 cases. *Cancer.* 1976;38:2166–2177.
2. Fernandes JP, Mascarenhas MJ, Costa CD, et al. Diffuse leiomyomatosis of the esophagus: a case report and review of the literature. *Am J Dig Dis.* 1975;20:684–690.
3. Cheng YL, Hsu JY, Hsu HH, et al. Diffuse leiomyomatosis of the esophagus. *Dig Surg.* 2000;17:528–531.
4. Arnorsson T, Aberg C, Aberg T. Benign tumours of the oesophagus and oesophageal cysts. *Scand J Thorac Cardiovasc Surg.* 1984;18:145–150.
5. Kent M, d'Amato T, Nordman C, et al. Minimally invasive resection of benign esophageal tumors. *J Thorac Cardiovasc Surg.* 2007;134:176–181.
6. Bonavina L, Segalin A, Rosati R, et al. Surgical therapy of esophageal leiomyoma. *J Am Coll Surg.* 1995;181:257–262.
7. Wiersema MJ, Vilmann P, Giovannini M, et al. Endosonography-guided fine-needle aspiration biopsy: diagnostic accuracy and complication assessment. *Gastroenterology.* 1997;112:1087–1095.
8. Bolzan H, Spatola J, Chiarenza C. [Endoscopic resection of esophageal leiomyoma with elastic band ligation]. *Acta Gastroenterol Latinoam.* 2005;35:165–168.
9. Kawamoto K, Yamada Y, Furukawa N, et al. Endoscopic submucosal tumorectomy for gastrointestinal submucosal tumors restricted to the submucosa: a new form of endoscopic minimal surgery. *Gastrointest Endosc.* 1997;46:311–317.
10. Dorais J, Marcon N. Endoscopic resection of gastrointestinal tumors: how far can the endoscopist go? *Endoscopy.* 1997;29:192–195.
11. Kajiyama T, Sakai M, Torii A, et al. Endoscopic aspiration lumpectomy of esophageal leiomyomas derived from the muscularis mucosae. *Am J Gastroenterol.* 1995;90:417–422.
12. Hyun JH, Jeen YT, Chun HJ, et al. Endoscopic resection of submucosal tumor of the esophagus: results in 62 patients. *Endoscopy.* 1997;29:165–170.
13. Wehrmann T, Martchenko K, Nakamura M, et al. Endoscopic resection of submucosal esophageal tumors: a prospective case series. *Endoscopy.* 2004;36:802–807.
14. Bardini R, Segalin A, Ruol A, et al. Videothoracoscopic enucleation of esophageal leiomyoma. *Ann Thorac Surg.* 1992;54:576–577.
15. Roviaro GC, Maciocco M, Varoli F, et al. Videothoracoscopic treatment of oesophageal leiomyoma. *Thorax.* 1998;53:190–192.
16. Gossot D, Fourquier P, el Meteini M, et al. Technical aspects of endoscopic removal of benign tumors of the esophagus. *Surg Endosc.* 1993;7:102–103.
17. von Rahden BH, Stein HJ, Feussner H, et al. Enucleation of submucosal tumors of the esophagus: minimally invasive versus open approach. *Surg Endosc.* 2004;18:924–930.
18. Hatch GF III, Wertheimer-Hatch L, Hatch KF, et al. Tumors of the esophagus. *World J Surg.* 2000;24:401–411.
19. Banki F, Mason RJ, DeMeester SR, et al. Vagal-sparing esophagectomy: a more physiologic alternative. *Ann Surg.* 2002;236:324–335; discussion 35–36.
20. Fletcher CD, Berman JJ, Corless C, et al. Diagnosis of gastrointestinal stromal tumors: a consensus approach. *Hum Pathol.* 2002;33:459–465.
21. Wu PC, Langerman A, Ryan CW, et al. Surgical treatment of gastrointestinal stromal tumors in the imatinib (STI-571) era. *Surgery.* 2003;134:656–665; discussion 65–66.
22. Portale G, Zaninotto G, Costantini M, et al. Esophageal GIST: case report of surgical enucleation and update on current diagnostic and therapeutic options. *Int J Surg Pathol.* 2007;15:393–396.
23. Gouveia AM, Pimenta AP, Lopes JM, et al. Esophageal GIST: therapeutic implications of an uncommon presentation of a rare tumor. *Dis Esophagus.* 2005;18:70–73.
24. Miettinen M, Sarlomo-Rikala M, Lasota J. Gastrointestinal stromal tumors: recent advances in understanding of their biology. *Hum Pathol.* 1999;30:1213–1220.
25. Miettinen M, Sarlomo-Rikala M, Sobin LH, et al. Esophageal stromal tumors: a clinicopathologic, immunohistochemical, and molecular genetic study of 17 cases and comparison with esophageal leiomyomas and leiomyosarcomas. *Am J Surg Pathol.* 2000;24:211–222.
26. Manu N, Richard P, Howard S. Bleeding esophageal GIST. *Dis Esophagus.* 2005;18: 281–282.
27. Ertem M, Baca B, Dogusoy G, et al. Thoracoscopic enucleation of a giant submucosal tumor of the esophagus. *Surg Laparosc Endosc Percutan Tech.* 2004;14:87–90.
28. Andtbacka RH, Nq CS, Scaife CL, et al. Surgical resection of gastrointestinal stromal tumors after treatment with imatinib. *Ann Surg Oncol.* 2007;14:14–24.
29. Madrid G, Pardo J, Perez C, et al. The neurofibroma of the oesophagus: case report. *Eur J Radiol.* 1986;6:67–69.
30. Eberlein TJ, Hannan R, Josa M, et al. Benign schwannoma of the esophagus presenting as a giant fibrovascular polyp. *Ann Thorac Surg.* 1992;53:343–345.

31. Schuhmacher C, Becker K, Dittler HJ, et al. Fibrovascular esophageal polyp as a diagnostic challenge. *Dis Esophagus.* 2000;13:324–327.
32. Minutolo V, Rinzivillo C, Li Destri G, et al. Giant esophageal polyp: a rare and benign neoplasm. *Chir Ital.* 1999;51:313–316.
33. Solerio D, Gasparri G, Ruffini E, et al. Giant fibrovascular polyp of the esophagus. *Dis Esophagus.* 2005;18:410–412.
34. Jensen EH, Klapman JB, Kelley ST. Angiolipoma of the esophagus: a rare clinical dilemma. *Dis Esophagus.* 2006;19:203–207.
35. David O, Jakate S. Multifocal granular cell tumor of the esophagus and proximal stomach with infiltrative pattern: a case report and review of the literature. *Arch Pathol Lab Med.* 1999;123:967–973.
36. De Rezende L, Lucendo AJ, Alvarez-Arguelles H. Granular cell tumors of the esophagus: report of five cases and review of diagnostic and therapeutic techniques. *Dis Esophagus.* 2007;20:436–443.
37. Palazzo L, Landi B, Cellier C, et al. Endosonographic features of esophageal granular cell tumors. *Endoscopy.* 1997;29:850–853.
38. Sogabe M, Taniki T, Fukui Y, et al. A patient with esophageal hemangioma treated by endoscopic mucosal resection: a case report and review of the literature. *J Med Invest.* 2006; 53:177–182.

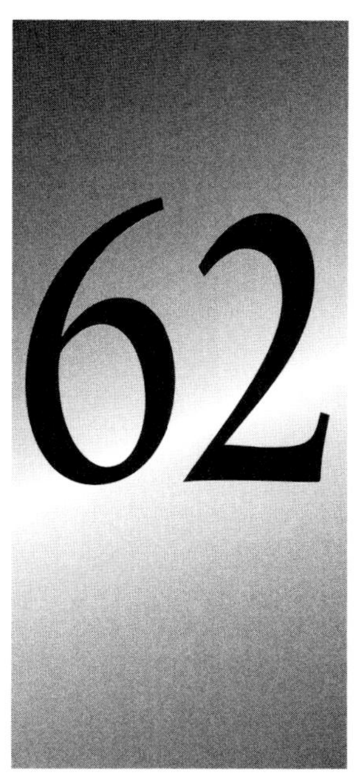

62 Surgery Techniques: Patient Preparation and Surgical Approach in Cancer Treatment

Thomas J. Watson
Victor Maevsky

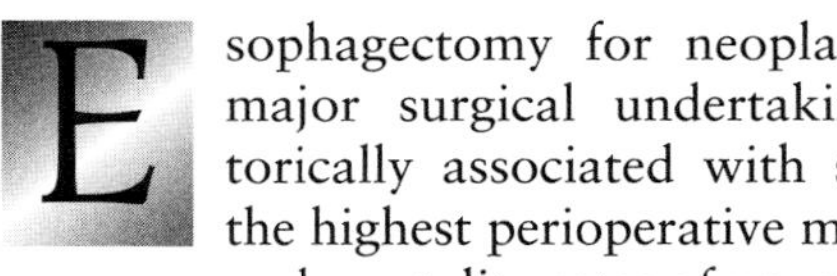

Esophagectomy for neoplasia is a major surgical undertaking, historically associated with some of the highest perioperative morbidity and mortality rates of any routinely performed elective surgical procedure. In the decades leading up to and including the 1970s, esophagectomy carried with it a mortality rate of greater than 25% (1). With advances in patient selection and preparation for surgery, perioperative care, and surgical technique, the rate of complications and death resulting from esophagectomy has been improving, particularly in high-volume institutions. Recent U.S. results analyzed from large administrative databases reveal perioperative mortality rates far below what had been previously reported. A 2007 publication utilized the Nationwide Inpatient Sample to assess esophagectomy outcomes in 17,395 patients over the years 1999–2003 (2). Overall mortality after esophagectomy was 8.7% and high-volume centers (performing more than 10 esophagectomies per year) had significantly lower mortality rates compared to lower-volume institutions. In a prior report reviewing complications in U.S. Veterans Administration hospitals, 1,777 esophagectomies were performed in 109 facilities during the years 1991–2000 and 30-day postoperative mortality was 9.8% (3). Many of the procedures, however, were undertaken in hospitals with a small institutional or surgeon experience in performing esophagectomy, as only 1.6 esophagectomies were done per year in the average facility. The importance of institutional volume also was demonstrated in a study derived from a Medicare database that analyzed esophagectomy outcomes during the time period 1994–1999 (4). Mortality after esophagectomy was 20.3% in hospitals where fewer than 2 esophagectomies were performed, compared to 8.4% in hospitals performing more than 19 esophagectomies per year. Of all operations assessed, esophagectomy was found to be among the most sensitive to the influence of institutional procedural volume on operative mortality.

In comparison, data derived from high-volume facilities in the United States specializing in esophageal surgery suggest operative mortality rates in the range of 3%–5% following esophagectomy for cancer (Table 62.1). In addition, when surgery is performed in specialty centers and is undertaken in selected patients for a specific indication (Barrett's esophagus with high-grade dysplasia [HGD]), esophagectomy can be performed with a mortality approximating 1% (8). A number of plausible factors explain the apparent improvement in outcomes following esophagectomy for HGD. Of most significance, perhaps, is the ability to select appropriate patients for esophagectomy in this setting, given alternative management strategies for HGD in the high-risk patient.

Considerable judgment must be exercised on the part of the operating surgeon in deciding upon whom to

TABLE 62.1
Modern Mortality after Esophagectomy for Cancer in U.S. Specialty Centers

Institution	Resection type	Year	Number	Mortality (%)
Brigham (5)	TTE	2001	250	3.6
Cornell (6)	3-field	2002	80	5
USC (7)	THE/TTE	2004	263	4.5
Rochester (8)	THE/TTE	2007	244	4.1
MSKCC (9)	THE/TTE	2007	352	4.5
Michigan (10)	THE	2007	1,525	3

Abbreviations: TTE = transthoracic esophagectomy; THE = transhiatal esophagectomy; USC = University of Southern California; MSKCC = Memorial Sloan-Kettering Cancer Center.

operate, the optimal timing of surgical intervention, and the best match of surgical approach to the given patient and their disease. Given the extensive array of esophagectomy techniques, the surgeon must be knowledgeable about their appropriate application and be technically adept at a number of different foregut resective and reconstructive procedures. Unlike resections for many gastrointestinal malignancies where surgical options are limited and decision making is straightforward, esophagectomy carries with it a litany of decisions and the need for flexibility; a "one size fits all" approach is generally not applicable.

PATIENT SELECTION AND PREPARATION

The epidemiology of esophageal cancer has changed over the past 3 decades, from predominantly squamous cell carcinoma associated with alcohol consumption and tobacco use to adenocarcinoma associated with gastroesophageal reflux disease. With this change in risk factors for these 2 diseases, and with improvements in screening and surveillance of the major precursor of esophageal adenocarcinoma, Barrett's esophagus, the potential to detect esophageal neoplasia at an early, or even preinvasive, stage has improved. Despite this fact, esophageal cancer too commonly presents in an advanced stage and frequently remains a disease of the elderly. According to the Surveillance Epidemiology and End Results (SEER) database of the National Cancer Institute, the median age at diagnosis for all esophageal cancer patients was 69 years over the time period 2001–2005, 67 years in men, and 73 years in women (11). Surgeons performing esophagectomy often must decide, therefore, whether to subject an elderly individual to a major and potentially morbid or mortal procedure.

Assessment of Cardiopulmonary Function

An assessment of the patient's cardiopulmonary reserve is essential prior to any major surgical undertaking such as esophagectomy. Evaluation commences with a thorough history, concentrating on respiratory difficulties at rest or with exertion, exercise tolerance, chest pain, or fatigability. Physical examination should concentrate on cardiopulmonary findings. When questions exist about coexistent cardiac or pulmonary disease based on the patient's age, comorbidities, physical signs, or symptoms, formal physiologic testing should be pursued. Cardiac imaging and stress testing can elicit subtle changes in cardiac function suggestive of ischemia, cardiomyopathy, or valvular heart disease. It has been estimated that approximately 20%–30% of patients with esophageal cancer present with evidence of cardiovascular disease. Prophylactic perioperative beta-blocker therapy is effective in reducing perioperative cardiac complications (death or myocardial infarction) in the population at risk (12,13).

When coronary artery or valvular pathology is deemed significant, interventions such as angioplasty, coronary stenting, or even open heart surgery should be completed prior to elective esophageal surgery in an effort to minimize perioperative risk at the time of esophagectomy. Recent data suggest that angioplasty alone should be performed when major surgery must be carried out within approximately 2 months (14). If surgery can be postponed for a period of at least 2 months, which is often the case when considering esophagectomy, then placement of a bare metal stent becomes an option. Drug-eluting stents (DES) should only be used if surgery can be postponed for at least 1 year, given the risk of early stent thrombosis and the need for aggressive antiplatelet therapy in the period immediately following stent placement (14). Thus, in general, DES placement should be avoided when an esophagectomy for cancer is being planned.

For patients with a history of smoking or chronic obstructive pulmonary disease, preoperative pulmonary function testing and arterial blood gas analysis should be performed. Patients with significant impairment in the forced expiratory volume at 1 second (FEV1 < 1.2 liters), the presence of hypercapnia ($PaCO_2$ > 45 mm Hg) or hypoxemia (PaO_2 < 55 mm Hg), maximum voluntary ventilation < 35% of predicted normal values, mid-expiratory flow (forced expiratory flow 25%–75%) of < 0.6 to 1 liters/second, or diffusion capacity <35% of predicted normal values are at increased risk for respiratory complications after surgery (15). Preoperative optimization through smoking cessation, bronchodilators, expectorants, antibiotics, or steroids (inhaled or systemic) is prudent. For more severe cases, consideration should be given to a formal pulmonary rehabilitation program. Patient education should commence before surgery about the importance of postoperative incentive spirometry, ambulation, and pulmonary toilet.

Recent smoking exposes patients to a variety of potential postoperative pulmonary complications ranging from increased production and reduced clearance of sputum to atelectasis, pneumonia, and respiratory failure requiring intubation (16). The association between cigarette smoking and delayed wound healing is well recognized in clinical practice (17,18). Nicotine increases platelet adhesiveness, thrombotic microvascular occlusion and vasoconstriction resulting in reduction of blood flow, tissue ischemia, and impaired healing. Smoking cessation should occur several weeks prior to surgery in order to achieve the maximum reversal of smoking-induced reduction in lung function and impairment of immune function (19).

Nutritional Assessment and Support

Nutritional assessment, education, and support have become a part of routine patient preparation in most high-volume esophageal surgery centers. The quantification of weight loss, physical examination, and albumin/prealbumin assays are helpful in the prediction of patient recovery, morbidity and mortality after surgery, as well as the possibility of prolonged mechanical respiratory support. A correlation exists between preoperative values of prognostic nutritional indices and the incidence of postoperative complications (20). In addition, the rate of esophageal tumor resectability in patients with anorexia is significantly decreased (21). Nutritional supplementation is crucial in any cancer patient with 10% or greater weight loss or an abnormally low serum albumin level (22). The exact timing, duration, and mode of preoperative nutritional support are matters of controversy and are discussed more thoroughly in another chapter, though enteral nutrition appears preferable. Finally, patients receiving neoadjuvant chemotherapy or radiation are at substantially higher risk for preoperative malnutrition.

Prophylaxis against Venous Thrombosis and Thromboembolism

Pulmonary embolism (PE) and deep venous thrombosis (DVT) prophylaxis is a standard of care in all cancer patients, particularly during the perioperative period, due to the possibility of cancer-induced hypercoagulability, the pro-coagulable effects of general anesthesia, and the potential for insufficient ambulation after surgery. Patients undergoing major surgery have an approximately 6-fold increase in risk of PE (23). Cancer patients undergoing surgery have twice the risk of developing DVT and a 3-fold increase in risk of fatal PE compared with patients without cancer (24,25). The presence of malignancy is associated with an impaired response to thromboprophylaxis (25). Patient education, pain control, early use of TED stockings, lower extremity intermittent pneumatic compression (IPC) devices, preoperative and perioperative use of prophylactic anticoagulation (low-dose unfractionated heparin 5000 units 2 or 3 times daily or its equivalent of lower molecular weight heparin), and early ambulation all play an important role in PE/DVT prevention.

Anesthetic Assessment and Postoperative Analgesia

The importance of an evaluation by an anesthesiologist in advance of esophagectomy cannot be overemphasized. Such an encounter serves many purposes, including risk stratification based on the American Society of Anesthesiologists (ASA) classification system, a review of comorbidities and medications and how they might affect anesthetic management, a detailing of prior surgeries and exposures to anesthetic agents, a pertinent family history of adverse anesthetic effects (e.g., malignant hyperthermia), and a discussion of the options for postoperative pain control.

Three widely utilized modalities for postoperative pain control following esophagectomy are regional epidural catheter placement, intercostal nerve block, and intravenous patient-controlled analgesia. Such methods can be used alone or in combination. Preoperative insertion of epidural catheters in patients undergoing esophageal resection has become common practice unless medically contraindicated. Epidural analgesia, when accomplished correctly, provides excellent pain control with decreased need for systemic narcotics, effective pulmonary toilet, return of ambulation, and a decreased incidence and severity of postoperative ileus. Objective improvements have been found in functional vital capacity as a result of epidural placement, leading to a reduced risk of pulmonary complications (26). The use of epidural analgesia has also contributed to a decrease in length of stay (27). Epidural medication usage must be judicious, particularly with regard to instillation of local anesthetic agents, to prevent systemic hypotension and the potential for profound adverse effects on the esophageal replacement conduit. Of course, an eventual and adequate transition to intravenous and oral analgesics is necessary. The success of epidural analgesia is only as good as the competency of the anesthesiologist in accurate catheter placement and management, as well as the ability of a pain team to provide continuous, around-the-clock monitoring and care of the patient. If not all elements of the pain service are adequate, the benefits of epidural use may be outweighed by the shortcomings.

Patient Education and General Preparation

Preoperative patient education is an important part of the preparation for esophageal cancer surgery. The complexity of the surgical approach and perioperative care, the expected postoperative course and length of stay, possible adverse effects and complications of the procedure, discharge planning and postoperative recovery should be explained to the patient and their family in detail. An accurate set of expectations is paramount to an outcome perceived as successful by the patient and their referring physicians. Issues that deserve specific emphasis in the preoperative discussions include the high incidence of at least minor morbidity following surgery and the surgeon's or institution's mortality rate for the procedure. Esophagectomy-specific perioperative complications include the potential for pneumonia and/or respiratory failure, bleeding requiring transfusion, chylothorax requiring subsequent thoracic duct ligation, recurrent laryngeal nerve injury leading to transient or permanent hoarseness, injury to the membranous airway, anastomotic leakage, and anastomotic stricture requiring (serial) dilatation. If placement of a feeding jejunostomy tube is opted at the time of surgery, the plans for its use should be outlined. Finally, the expectations for long-term functional outcomes should be reviewed in terms of meal capacity and frequency, as well as the potential for gastroesophageal reflux, dysphagia, choking, diarrhea, cramping, and dumping.

Though the patient and his/her physicians may feel time pressure to treat an esophageal malignancy, a successful surgical outcome depends upon a thorough work-up, adequate assessment of risk factors, and optimization of comorbidities. While no absolute thresholds exist for abandoning surgery due to nutritional, pulmonary, or cardiac compromise, such objective information often can assist the surgeon quite significantly in making a decision for or against esophagectomy and in the type of operation chosen.

Evaluation of the Colon for Use as an Esophageal Substitute

When the colon is being considered as a potential esophageal substitute, colonoscopy or barium radiography is performed to evaluate the status of the colonic mucosa. Mild diverticular disease is generally not a contraindication to the use of colon as an esophageal replacement, though extensive diverticulosis, frank diverticulitis, or inflammatory fibrosis may preclude colon interposition. Similarly, the presence of a few colonic polyps, whether hyperplastic or adenomatous, that can be removed before surgery does not preclude the use of colon. The presence of extensive polyposis or malignancy, however, is an absolute contraindication.

Some controversy exists around the necessity of routine preoperative mesenteric arteriography when colonic interposition is planned. As the successful use of colon critically depends upon an adequate vasculature, the surgeon should have a low threshold to perform such studies. When arteriography is performed, selective injections of the celiac, superior mesenteric (SMA), and inferior mesenteric (IMA) arteries should be undertaken, including lateral views, and paying particular attention to any anatomic aberrancy. When the left colon is to be utilized for interposition, the most important angiographic finding is the status of the IMA, particularly at its origin, which can be stenosed in elderly individuals or in those with peripheral vascular disease. As the blood supply of a left colon interposition critically depends upon adequate inflow from the IMA, a significant stenosis of this vessel is a contraindication to the use of the left colon for esophageal reconstruction (28). A right colon interposition, based on the middle colic branches of the SMA, can be used in this situation, as it is not dependent upon IMA inflow. Other angiographic features thought important to the successful use of left colon for interposition include a visible ascending branch of the left colic artery, a well-defined anastomosis between the left colic and middle colic systems (along the marginal artery of Drummond) and a single middle colic trunk prior to division into right and left branches. Because of its more reliable and predictable arterial inflow and venous outflow, not to mention its better size match to the native esophagus, the left colon is generally preferred over the right colon for esophageal replacement.

As patients undergoing foregut reconstruction have not uncommonly undergone multiple prior abdominal operations, mesenteric arteriography can help to define the resultant vascular anatomy and ascertain that vessels supplying planned esophageal substitutes are patent and not disrupted by prior surgeries. In particular, prior operations involving the greater curvature of the stomach may have disrupted the right gastroepiploic artery, critical to the blood supply of a planned gastric pull-up, or the middle colic artery and marginal artery of Drummond, critical to the blood supply of a planned colon interposition. Preoperative knowledge of such vascular abnormalities can help the surgeon plan surgery and save considerable time and effort during the procedure.

APPROACHES TO ESOPHAGECTOMY FOR CANCER

The first attempts at cervical esophagectomy were undertaken by Billroth in the late 19th century. The first successful cervical esophagectomy for carcinoma in a human was credited to Czerny in 1877, while the first successful transthoracic esophagectomy (TTE) was performed by Torek in 1913. Since these initial efforts, a wide spectrum of esophagectomy procedures and reconstructive options has arisen. As long ago as 1928, the observation was made that "judging from the literature, it would seem that every method which ingenuity can invent has been practiced for the purpose of reestablishing the continuity of the esophagus after resection" (29).

At present, a number of techniques are commonly employed for resection of esophageal cancer (Table 62.2). The surgeon must choose, therefore, from such a menu of procedures when deciding upon the optimum approach for a given individual, both in terms of the strategy for resection as well as for plans for reconstruction. Mobilization of the esophagus can be accomplished successfully by open transthoracic, thoracoscopic, or transhiatal (open or minimally invasive) approaches. The route chosen depends, in part, upon surgeon experience and preference. Certain principles, however, favor one approach over another (Table 62.3).

TABLE 62.2
Esophagectomy Options

- *"Minimally invasive"* (thoracoscopic, laparoscopic, robotic)
- Transhiatal with cervical esophagogastrostomy +/– vagal-sparing
- Transhiatal with jejunal interposition
- Right thoracotomy, laparotomy, intrathoracic esophagogastrostomy
- Right thoracotomy, laparotomy, cervical esophagogastrostomy
- Left thoracotomy/thoracoabdominal with intrathoracic esophagogastrostomy
- Radical (en bloc) esophagectomy
    - with 2-field lymphadenectomy
    - with 3-field lymphadenectomy
    - using gastric pull-up
    - using colon interposition
- Others

TABLE 62.3
Factors Influencing Type of Esophagectomy

1. Surgeon training and experience
2. Tumor location and size
3. Patient comorbidities and performance status
4. Availability and suitability of esophageal replacement conduits (stomach, jejunum, colon)
5. Prior thoracic or upper abdominal operations
6. Goals of surgery (cure, palliation)

Factors Favoring Transthoracic Resection

Factors favoring a transthoracic resection, whether open or thoracoscopic, include any situation that make a safe blunt resection potentially difficult or hazardous, such as large tumors abutting the membranous airway, azygos vein, or aorta where resectability may be an issue. In the setting of prior surgery involving the intrathoracic esophagus, such as a myotomy, diverticulectomy, or repair of an esophageal perforation, periesophageal fibrosis may require direct transthoracic visualization to allow safe resection. When esophageal squamous cell carcinoma arises within the background of achalasia and a megaesophagus, extensive esophageal neovascularization can complicate dissection and lead to significant hemorrhage if a blunt resection is attempted. While safe transhiatal esophagectomy (THE) has been undertaken in the setting of a megaesophagus, considerable judgment and experience are required and the surgeon must exercise a low threshold for conversion to a transthoracic approach if the dissection proves difficult (30,31).

A TTE allows for a more thorough and complete mediastinal lymphadenectomy than is afforded by a transhiatal approach. An en bloc resection of the esophagus with the adjacent periesophageal and subcarinal lymph nodes, azygos vein and its tributaries, thoracic duct and mediastinal pleura can be accomplished via either a right or left transthoracic approach. Paratracheal lymph nodes and recurrent laryngeal nerve nodes, if desired, can be resected as well, particularly from the right.

If the available esophageal replacement conduits are of limited length, a considerable segment of intrathoracic esophagus may need to be preserved in order to reestablish alimentary continuity after esophagectomy. In addition, such a situation mandates an intrathoracic (posterior mediastinal or retrosternal) anastomosis. Of course, a limited esophageal resection can only occur in the setting of distal esophageal or gastroesophageal junction tumors, in that resection margins will be compromised for more proximal malignancies.

Finally, some surgeons prefer routine placement of an esophagogastric anastomosis in an intrathoracic position, citing the lower incidence of symptomatic anastomotic strictures compared to cervical esophagogastrostomy. General thought holds that such anastomoses should be placed high in the chest, at or above the level of the azygos arch, to minimize the potential for postoperative gastroesophageal reflux. The extent of reflux, however, based upon the position of an esophagogastric anastomosis has never been subject to careful objective scrutiny. Some centers have reported extensive experiences with low intrathoracic anastomoses after esophagectomy for cancer, though the long-term symptomatic outcomes are not well characterized.

Factors Favoring Transhiatal Resection

Factors favoring a transhiatal resection include situations where much of the intrathoracic esophagus is uninvolved with tumor, particularly if an extensive lymphadenectomy is not required. Examples include pharyngeal neoplasms as well as Barrett's esophagus with HGD. In the latter case, some centers have advocated a vagal-sparing transhiatal operation without deliberate lymphadenectomy in order to preserve gastrointestinal function (32,33). In the setting of HGD without an endoscopically visible esophageal mucosal nodule or ulcer, the likelihood of encountering an occult invasive carcinoma that penetrates deeper than the muscularis mucosa and, therefore, may have metastasized to regional lymph nodes is quite low.

An obvious advantage of THE is the avoidance of a thoracic incision or incisions with their potential for pain, postoperative respiratory compromise, and the need for single-lung ventilation during surgery. For patients deemed at high risk for operation because of underlying pulmonary comorbidities, a transhiatal approach holds intuitive appeal for these reasons. When deciding upon a tailored approach to surgery based on individual patient factors, many surgeons will choose a transhiatal operation in the setting of the frail or elderly patient or those with significant respiratory embarrassment prior to surgery.

Some surgeons will choose a THE as their procedure of choice for most esophageal or esophagogastric junction cancer resections, barring the presence of a specific contraindication as listed above. Advocates cite the ability to perform a mediastinal lymphadenectomy through the esophageal hiatus, particularly if maneuvers are undertaken to open the space in a wide fashion, and the advantages inherent to avoidance of a thoracotomy in terms of operative time, pain, cosmesis, and pulmonary sequelae.

Transhiatal esophagectomy requires placement of the subsequent esophageal anastomosis in the neck or upper thorax. While the consequences of an intrathoracic leak are generally worse than those in the neck, the leak rate reported after cervical esophagogastrostomy is generally higher. The University of Michigan group recently reported a cervical anastomotic leak rate of 12% (10). The incidence has fallen in recent years, however, with improvements in anastomotic techniques. In their hands, the clinically significant leak rate now falls in the range of 3%, with an additional 2% rate of gastric tip necrosis (10,34).

Also of tremendous significance is the incidence of esophagogastric anastomotic strictures developing after cervical esophagogastrostomy. The need for postoperative dilation has been reported to be as high as 55% after THE, though rarely represents a disabling, long-term complication (10). Considering that many patients are referred for foregut reconstruction due to severe dysphagia, the persistence of dysphagia after surgery, however, can be a significant adverse outcome.

Outcomes after Transthoracic and Transhiatal Esophagectomy for Cancer

A number of large series from single institutions have reported outcomes after transthoracic, transhiatal, or minimally invasive esophagectomies and will be covered in separate chapters. Limitations of much of the available data, however, include the fact that such reports are generally nonrandomized, retrospective case series. Stage-for-stage outcomes comparisons are difficult, given the potential for stage migration when a more thorough lymphadenectomy is undertaken via a transthoracic approach. In addition, some centers have relegated transhiatal esophagectomy to older, sicker patients with more advanced disease, utilizing a more extensive en bloc resection for more physiologically fit individuals with a higher chance of cure. Such reports also inherently reflect surgeon or institutional bias in terms of the optimal treatment approach, not only regarding surgical resection but also relative to multimodality therapy such as neoadjuvant or adjuvant chemotherapy or combined chemoradiation.

A number of studies have compared results between THE and en bloc resections and a few deserve further mention (Table 62.4). A recent report assessed perioperative outcomes after transthoracic and transhiatal esophagectomy over the years 1999 through 2003 utilizing the Nationwide Inpatient Sample (NIS) (2). The NIS contains data representing approximately 20% of all hospital discharges from nonfederal U.S. facilities. The database included 17,395 patients undergoing esophagectomy, 11,914 of them undergoing THE, and 5,481 undergoing TTE. Thus, in the United States, recent practice patterns demonstrate an approximately 2:1 utilization of THE compared to TTE. The 2 groups were evenly matched for age (61.9 versus 62.0 years in the THE and TTE groups, respectively). Overall morbidity was 50.7%, consistent with prior reports. In-hospital mortality after THE was 8.91% and 8.47% after TTE (P = 0.642). Multivariate logistic regression analysis demonstrated no significant differences in the incidence of pulmonary, cardiovascular, infectious, or overall complications or hospital length of stay between the 2 groups. High-volume centers (performing more than 10 esophagectomies per year) had significantly lower mortality rates compared to low-volume centers. In addition, a higher incidence of gastrointestinal and systemic complications was seen after TTE in low-volume centers. The authors concluded that perioperative outcomes after THE and TTE were equivalent, though higher volume institutions demonstrated lower morbidity and mortality.

Care must be taken in interpreting these data. Such an analysis cannot control for surgeon bias in selection of patients for the various operations. Conceivably, THE was chosen for sicker individuals with more comorbidities. Also, no information is available regarding tumor stage or location, completeness of resection, use of neoadjuvant therapy, or long-term follow-up.

In a population-based, retrospective, case-control study from Finland, the long-term cure rate of 42 patients undergoing esophagectomy with 2-field lymphadenectomy was compared to 129 patients following standard esophagectomy (35). The 5-year survival was significantly better following 2-field lymphadenectomy than with a less extensive resection (50% versus 23.2%, respectively; P = 0.005). This survival advantage held up at 8 years of follow-up as well (43% versus 21%), suggesting a durable effect.

The only prospective randomized controlled study to date comparing simple to extended esophagectomy was performed in the Netherlands by Hulscher and colleagues (36,37). The initial results in 220 patients at a median follow-up of 4.7 years demonstrated a trend toward improved survival with the en bloc resection, which did not reach statistical significance (P = 0.08) (36). The study has been faulted, however, for being underpowered (38). The calculations for sample size were

TABLE 62.4
Comparison Trials between Transhiatal Esophagectomy and Transthoracic En Bloc Esophagectomy of Long-Term Survival[a]

Source	Type of trial	Resections, no.	Survival, %		Follow-up, y	P value
			THE group	EBE group		
Hagen et al, (51) 1993	Retro	30 EBE 39 THE	14	41	5	<.001
Putnam et al, (52) 1994	Retro	102 EBE 30 THE	12	30	4	.02
Horstmann et al, (53) 1995	Retro	41 EBE 46 THE	18	17	3	NS
Altorki et al, (54) 1997	Retro	78 EBE 50 THE	11	35	4	.007
Hulscher et al, (36) 2002	RCT	114 EBE 106 THE	27	39	5	.08

Abbreviations: EBE = en bloc esophagectomy; NS = not significant; RCT = randomized controlled trial; Retro = retrospective clinical study; THE = transhiatal esophagectomy.
[a] Adapted with permission from *Archives of Surgery* 2004, Vol. 138, 627–633 (39).

based on a survival of 30% following simple transhiatal resection, whereas the available literature would support a 25% survival rate even in specialty centers. In addition, the authors estimated a 15% difference in survival between the 2 arms but observed a difference of only 10%. Given these data and corrected assumptions, the sample size necessary to detect a statistically significant difference is 260 patients per arm, while the study enrolled only approximately 110 patients per arm.

A follow-up report to this trial was published in 2007 and contained complete 5-year survival data (37). After transhiatal and transthoracic resection, 5-year survival was 34% and 36%, respectively ($P = 0.71$) (Figure 62.1). In the 90 patients found to have a Siewert type I tumor, a statistically significant survival benefit of 14% was seen with TTE (Figure 62.2). In addition, patients found to have 1 to 8 positive regional lymph nodes in the resection specimen demonstrated a 5-year locoregional disease-free survival advantage following TTE, whereas patients with fewer or greater numbers of positive nodes showed no such benefit (Figure 62.3). Based on their analysis, the authors favored an extended TTE for type I esophageal carcinoma, especially in the setting of a limited number of clinically suspicious lymph nodes, and a limited THE for type II carcinoma of the gastroesophageal junction.

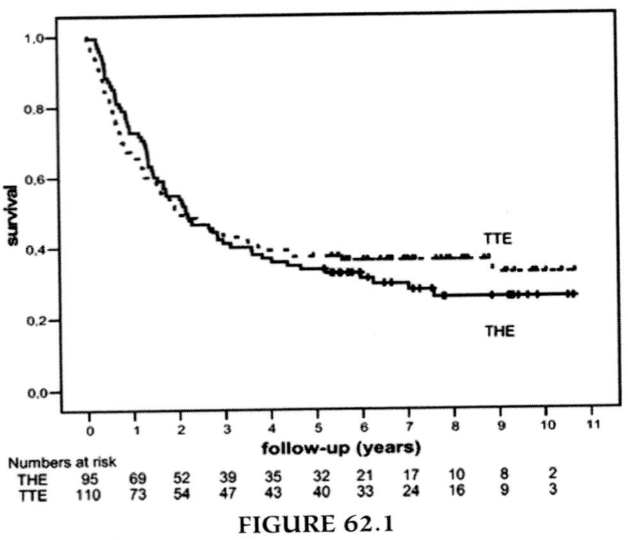

FIGURE 62.1

Overall survival of all patients after transhiatal (THE) or transthoracic (TTE) esophagectomy ($P = 0.71$) based on per protocol analysis and after exclusion of patients who did not undergo surgical resection. Adapted with permission from Omloo JMT, Lagarde SM, Hulscher JBF, et al., Extended transthoracic resection compared with limited transhiatal resection for adenocarcinoma of the mid/distal esophagus: five-year survival of a randomized clinical trial. *Annals of Surgery*, 2007, 246, 992–1001 (37).

Critics of an extended lymphadenectomy claim that although a more extensive resection may improve survival, any apparent advantages are offset by the increased morbidity and mortality inherent to a more invasive operation. The Netherlands trial showed a higher incidence of pulmonary complications, a longer mechanical ventilation time, a longer intensive care stay, and a longer overall hospitalization in patients undergoing a TTE compared to THE (36). Reports assessing early postoperative morbidity and mortality after

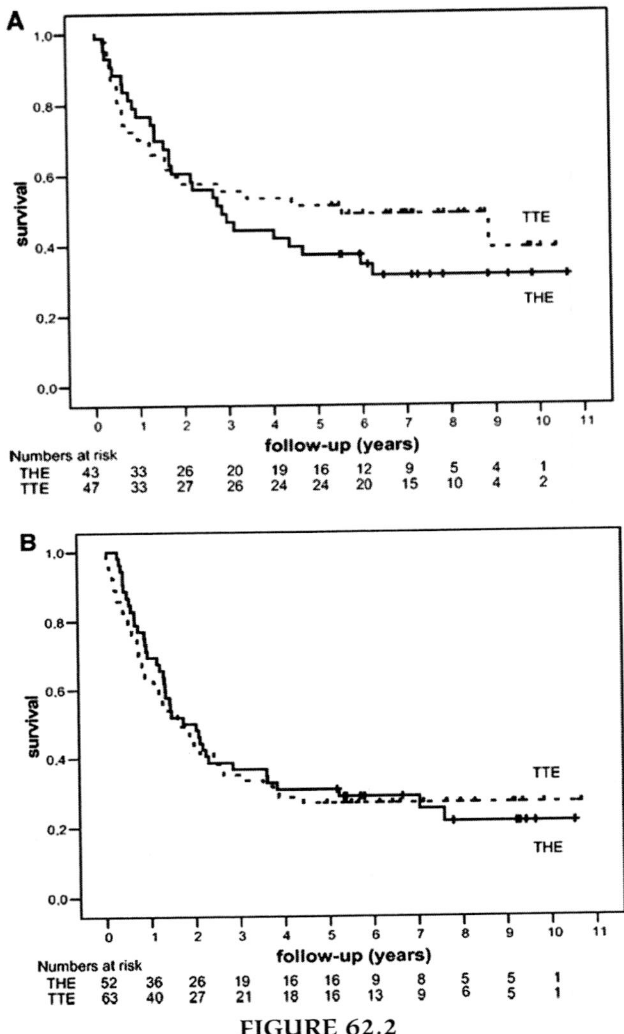

FIGURE 62.2

(A) Overall survival of patients with type I adenocarcinoma of the esophagus after transhiatal (THE) or transthoracic esophagectomy (TTE) ($P = 0.33$). (B) Overall survival of patients with type II adenocarcinoma of the gastric cardia after transhiatal or transthoracic esophagectomy. Adapted with permission from Omloo JMT, Lagarde SM, Hulscher JBF, et al., Extended transthoracic resection compared with limited transhiatal resection for adenocarcinoma of the mid/distal esophagus: five-year survival of a randomized clinical trial. *Annals of Surgery*, 2007, 246, 992–1001 (37).

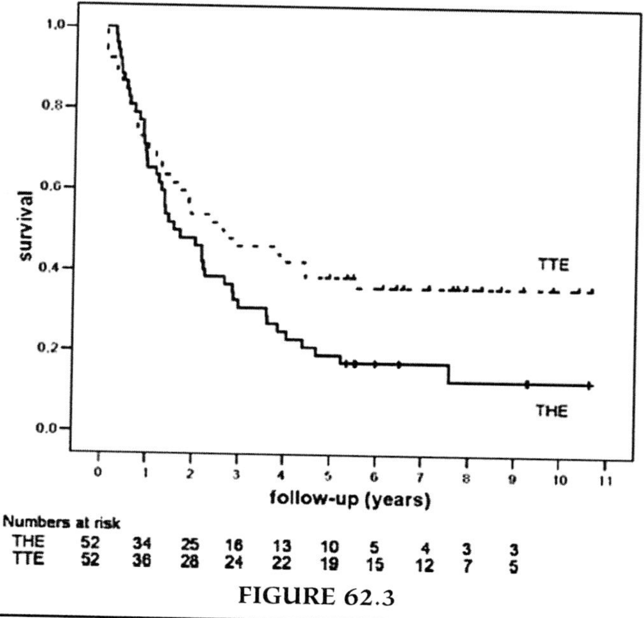

FIGURE 62.3

Overall survival of all patients with 1 to 8 positive lymph nodes in the resection specimen after transhiatal (THE) or transthoracic (TTE) esophagectomy. Adapted with permission from Omloo JMT, Lagarde SM, Hulscher JBF, et al., Extended transthoracic resection compared with limited transhiatal resection for adenocarcinoma of the mid/distal esophagus: five-year survival of a randomized clinical trial. *Annals of Surgery*, 2007, 246, 992–1001 (37).

TTE and THE do not, in general, show an appreciable difference between the two approaches, though such a retrospective analysis cannot assess the severity of complications or patient selection biases (Table 62.5). Finally, given the limitations in current preoperative staging techniques, particularly relative to the number and location of involved lymph nodes, selection of appropriate candidates likely to be benefited by en bloc resections remains difficult as well.

Esophageal Replacement Conduit

The preferred esophageal substitute is a widely discussed and debated issue. Historically, esophagectomy for carcinoma was associated with a poor long-term survival (1). Outcomes assessment after surgery, therefore, focused on operative mortality and early postoperative morbidity. More recently, with changes in the epidemiology of esophageal cancer and the screening and surveillance of malignant precursors (e.g., Barrett's esophagus), patients have been detected with earlier stage cancer. Due to this fact, as well as to improvements in operative techniques and perioperative management, an increasing number of patients are surviving surgery and are cured after esophagectomy for carcinoma. Long-term symptomatic outcomes, therefore, are assuming increasing importance. In the case of foregut reconstruction for benign disease or early stage malignancy, where life expectancy may be

TABLE 62.5
Mortality and Morbidity Rates for Transthoracic En Bloc Esophagectomy and Transhiatal Esophagectomy[a]

Source	Patients, no.	Mortality, %	Morbidity, %	LOS, d
EBE				
Putnam et al, (52) 1994*	134	8	75	20
Horstmann et al, (53) 1995*	41	10	NA	23
Altorki et al, (54) 1997*	78	5	24	NA
Hulscher et al, (36) 2002*	114	4	57	19
Swanson et al, (5) 2001	250	4	33	13
Hagen et al, (55) 2001	100	6	71	14
Overall range		4–10	24–75	13–23
THE				
Putnam et al, (52) 1994*	42	5	69	19
Horstmann et al, (53) 1995*	46	11	NA	26
Altorki et al, (54) 1997*	50	6	26	NA
Hulscher et al, (36) 2002*	106	2	27	15
Orringer et al, (56) 1993	417	5	32	11–14
Rentz et al, (57) 2003	385	10	49	NA
Overall range		2–11	26–69	11–26

Abbreviations: EBE = en bloc esophagectomy; LOS = length of hospital stay; NS = not significant; THE = transhiatal esophagectomy.
*Both EBE and THE are included in the study.
[a] Adapted with permission from *Archives of Surgery* 2004, Vol. 138, 627–633 (39).

measured in many years or decades, the issue of the best esophageal substitute remains controversial.

The 2 most commonly utilized conduits for esophageal replacement are the stomach and the colon. Each organ has been extensively evaluated and each has its proponents. A closer analysis demonstrates that the stomach and colon possess several theoretic advantages and disadvantages compared to each other and to the jejunum.

Proponents of esophageal replacement via gastric pull-up tout the relative ease of gastric mobilization, the need for only a single (esophagogastric) anastomosis, as well as the relatively quick operative time and return of alimentation. In addition, where expertise exists, the operation can be completed through minimally invasive means, with laparoscopic gastric mobilization and cervical esophagogastrostomy or intrathoracic anastomosis accomplished via thoracoscopy.

Disadvantages of the stomach include the loss of the gastric reservoir with the potential for early satiety and dumping, and the potential for gastroesophageal reflux into the remaining esophageal remnant or pharynx. The placement of the stomach within the negative pressure environment of the thorax, coupled with the loss of the normal GEJ anti-reflux barriers, predisposes the patient to reflux, regurgitation, and aspiration. Although there is general acceptance of the concept that a cervical esophagogastrostomy is less prone to reflux than an intrathoracic anastomosis, particularly when placed low in the chest, reflux can occur in either scenario and may cause significant symptomatology or induce complications. The placement of gastric mucosa in juxtaposition to squamous esophageal mucosa predisposes the patient to proximal esophagitis, stricture, or Barrett's esophagus, resulting from the chronic exposure of the remaining esophageal mucosa to gastric and/or duodenal content. A series from Japan demonstrated reflux esophagitis in 44% of patients and Barrett's metaplasia in 12% of patients followed for more than 2 years after a cervical esophagogastrostomy (40). Several other reports have shown the risk of development of columnar metaplasia in the esophageal remnant over the years following esophagectomy and primary esophagogastrostomy (Table 62.6). Of note, esophageal columnar metaplasia appears more likely to occur in those with Barrett's mucosa resected at the time of esophagectomy than in those without, suggesting an underlying genetic predisposition to the development of metaplasia in susceptible individuals. The clinical significance of this metaplastic response, however, is uncertain in that the incidence of cancer in the esophageal remnant after esophagectomy and gastric pull-up is unknown and likely quite low. In contrast, the esophageal mucosa in patients undergoing colon interposition appears to undergo few histologic changes.

The blood supply to the proximal tip of the gastric conduit can be quite tenuous. The incidence of ischemic complications, such as esophagogastric anastomotic leaks or strictures, is relatively high as a result. The anastomotic leak rate after cervical esophagogastrostomy ranges between 3% and 20% in large surgical series. (34,45–47).

TABLE 62.6
Occurrence of Intestinal Metaplasia after Esophagectomy and Primary Esophagogastrostomy

Author	# Patients	% IM	Time until IM (yrs)
Hamilton (41)	17	18%	6.3–8.8
Oberg (42)	32	9%	8.5–10.4
Dresner (43)	40	22%	1.0–9.8
Lord (44)	20	20%	N/A

Abbreviations: IM = intestinal metaplasia within esophageal remnant.

With regard to colon interposition, several theoretical advantages have been suggested. The interposed colonic segment separates the remaining esophageal mucosa from acid-producing gastric mucosa and duodenal content, as previously stated. The incidence of reflux-induced complications, such as esophagitis, stricture, or Barrett's esophagus, is low. The blood supply to the colon, when mobilized appropriately, is generally quite robust. The incidence of ischemic complications at the esophageal anastomosis, such as leaks or strictures, is also quite low. Watson et al. reported on 85 patients undergoing colonic interposition for benign disease, with an esophagocolonic leak rate of 3.5% and a need for postoperative anastomotic dilation in 5% (48). Both of these rates were much less than those after cervical esophagogastrostomy in their series, where anastomotic leaks occurred in 20% and the need for dilation in 30% of patients. Similarly, Briel et al. reported on 395 consecutive patients undergoing esophagectomy for both malignant and benign disease (45). The development of either anastomotic leak or stricture was analyzed in patients undergoing gastric pull-up compared to colonic interposition. Leaks and strictures were more common (14.3% versus 6.1%, $P = 0.013$, 31.3% versus 8.7%, $P < 0.0001$, respectively), and strictures were more severe after gastric pull-up.

The colon possesses a reservoir function, allowing for a more normal meal capacity. The distal colonic segment and residual stomach remain in the positive pressure environment of the abdomen, helping to guard against reflux. In some individuals, the stomach is not suitable or available for use as an esophageal substitute. In such cases, the colon may serve the purpose quite well and can be anastomosed distally to a Roux limb of jejunum if the antrum has been resected or there is a significant gastric outlet obstruction. Finally, if the interposed colon becomes dilated or tortuous over the long term, it often can be successfully revised via a tailoring coloplasty or segmental resection (48,49). A dilated, tortuous, or poorly emptying gastric pull-up, on the other hand, cannot be similarly remediated and requires replacement should significant dysfunction develop.

Disadvantages of the colon as an esophageal substitute are most apparent. The colon must be free of significant pathology such as extensive diverticulosis, polyposis, or frank malignancy, and must be adequately evaluated and prepared for use, as for elective colon resection. Along with the need for 3 anastomoses (esophagocolonic, cologastric, and colocolonic), there is an inherently longer operative time, with a greater extent of mobilization and dissection compared to gastric pull-up. The operation may be technically challenging, especially in terms of preserving the arterial inflow and venous drainage of the conduit. Seemingly minor mistakes in judgment or technique can have disastrous consequences with regard to maintenance of adequate vascularity. Leaks and/or strictures can occur at any of the anastomoses, and bowel obstruction can occur if the colonic mesentery is not adequately closed. Minimally invasive techniques for completion of the operation have yet to be mastered. The colon is generally thought to be slower to allow resumption of alimentation compared to the stomach. Finally, and of great importance, is the fact that colon interpositions are known to become dilated and/or tortuous when in place for many years. Such redundancy can lead to problems with dysphagia, regurgitation, and/or aspiration, though surgical remediation is often feasible, as stated above.

Clinical experience with the jejunum as an esophageal substitute is much less than with either stomach or colon. This fact is largely due to the limited extent to which the jejunum can be brought into the thorax, either as a Roux limb or a jejunal interposition, because of its short mesentery and tethered blood supply. Supercharged pedicled jejunum has been used with success for total esophageal replacement in esophageal cancer patients with limited reconstructive options (50). Of course, a free jejunal interposition can be placed wherever there is a suitable arterial inflow and venous outflow, though it is a technically more demanding procedure than the other options due to the need for microvascular anastomoses.

The many published reports on esophageal replacement inherently reflect an institutional or surgeon-specific bias in terms of the types of reconstructions performed. Randomized trials comparing the different reconstructive options are lacking. Analysis of the published reports reveals that they suffer from a lack of uniform assessment of long-term symptomatic and functional outcomes. The long time periods covered in the various reports also make results difficult to interpret in the setting of changing surgeons, refinements in operative technique, and advancements in perioperative care. Firm conclusions, therefore, regarding the optimal operative approach and esophageal replacement conduit for a given patient are lacking. Be that as it may, current practice patterns reveal that the stomach is the most widely utilized esophageal substitute.

CONCLUSIONS

Esophagectomy for carcinoma remains a significant surgical undertaking best performed in high-volume centers with considerable experience and a well-established multidisciplinary team. Despite the magnitude of the operation and the comorbidities inherent to the cohort of patients presenting with esophageal cancer, esophageal resection can be accomplished successfully in selected patients with low mortality and acceptable morbidity. Considerable judgment is required on the part of the surgeon in deciding upon an overall treatment strategy, appropriate candidates for surgery, assessment and optimization of comorbidities, choice of operative approach, timing of intervention, selection and preparation of an esophageal replacement conduit, and perioperative management. Experience in the technical details and nuances of the various operative approaches is also critical to a successful outcome. Considerable controversy continues regarding the best operation for a given patient, though a procedure that the surgeon can perform safely is certainly best.

References

1. Earlam R, Cunha-Melo JR. Oesophageal squamous cell carcinoma: I. a critical review of surgery. *Br J Surg.* 1980;67:381–390.
2. Connors RC, Reuben BC, Neumayer LA, Bull DA. Comparing outcomes after transthoracic and transhiatal esophagectomy: a 5-year prospective cohort of 17,395 patients. *J Am Coll Surg.* 2007;205:735–740.
3. Bailey SH, Bull DA, Harpole DH, et al. Outcomes after esophagectomy: a ten-year prospective cohort. *Ann Thorac Surg.* 2003;75:217–222.
4. Birkmeyer JD, Siewers AE, Finlayson EV, et al. Hospital volume and surgical mortality in the United States. *N Eng J Med.* 2002;346(15):1128–1137.
5. Swanson SJ, Batirel HF, Bueno R, et al. Transthoracic esophagectomy with radical mediastinal and abdominal lymph node dissection and cervical esophagogastrostomy for esophageal carcinoma. *Ann Thorac Surg.* 2001;72:1918–1925.
6. Altorki N, Kent M, Ferrara C, Port J. Three-field lymph node dissection for squamous cell and adenocarcinoma of the esophagus. *Ann Surg.* 2002;236(2):177–183.
7. Portale G, Hagen JA, Peters JH, et al. Modern 5-year survival of resectable esophageal adenocarcinoma: single institution experience with 263 patients. *J Am Coll Surg.* 2006;202(4):588–596.
8. Williams VA, Watson TJ, Herbella FA, et al. Esophagectomy for high grade dysplasia is safe, curative, and results in good alimentary outcome. *J Gastrointest Surg.* 2007;11:1589–1597.
9. Barbour AP, Rizk NP, Gonen M, et al. Adenocarcinoma of the gastroesophageal junction: influence of resection margin and operative approach on outcome. *Ann Surg.* 2007;246:1–8.
10. Orringer MB, Marshall B, Chang AC, Lee J, Pickens A, Lau CL. Two thousand transhiatal esophagectomies: changing trends, lessons learned. *Ann Surg.* 2007;246(3):363–374.
11. National Cancer Institute Surveillance Epidemiology and End Results Database. http://seer.cancer.gov/statfacts/html/esoph.html. Accessed January 18, 2009.

12. Mangano DT, Layug EL, Wallace A, Tateo I. Effect of atenolol on mortality and cardiovascular morbidity after noncardiac surgery: multicenter study of Peri-Operative Ischemia Research Group. *N Eng J Med.* 1996;335:1713–1720.
13. Wallace A, Layug B, Tateo I. Prophylactic atenolol reduces postoperative myocardial ischemia. *Anesthesiology.* 1998;88:7–17.
14. Grines CL, Bonow RO, Casey DE, et al. Prevention of premature discontinuation of dual antiplatelet therapy in patients with coronary artery stents. *Circulation.* 2007;115:813–818.
15. Szelky LA, Oelberg DA, Wright C, et al. Preoperative predictors of operative morbidity and mortality in COPD patients undergoing bilateral lung volume reduction surgery. *Chest.* 1998;113:883–889.
16. Moores LK. Smoking and postoperative pulmonary complications: an evidence-based review of the recent literature. *Clin Chest Med.* 2000;21:139–146.
17. Silverstein P. Smoking and wound healing. *Am J Med.* 1992;93:22–24.
18. Sorensen LT, Jorgensen T, Kirkeby LT, Skovdal J, Vennits B, Wille-Jorgensen P. Smoking and alcohol abuse are major risk factors for anastomotic leakage in colorectal surgery. *Br J Surg.* 1999;86:927–931.
19. Warner MA, Offord KP, Lennon RL, Conover MA, Jansson-Schumacher U. Role of preoperative cessation of smoking and other factors in postoperative pulmonary complications: a blinded prospective study of coronary bypass patients. *Mayo Clin Proc.* 1989;64:609–616.
20. Nozoe T, Kimura Y, Ishida M, Saeki H, Korenaga D, Sugimachi K. Correlation of preoperative nutritional condition with postoperative complications in surgical treatment for oesophageal carcinoma. *Eur J Surg Oncol.* 2002;28:396–400.
21. Belghiti J, Langonnet F, Bourstyn E, Fekete F. Surgical implications of malnutrition and immunodeficiency in patients with carcinoma of the oesophagus. *Br J Surg.* 1983;70:339–341.
22. Reed CE. Surgical management of esophageal carcinoma. *Oncologist.* 1999;4: 95–105.
23. Geerts WH, Pineo GF, Heit JA, et al. Prevention of venous thromboembolism: the seventh ACCP conference on antithrombotic and thrombolytic therapy. *Chest.* 2004;126:338S–400S.
24. White RH, Zhou H, Romano PS. Incidence of symptomatic venous thromboembolism after different elective or urgent surgical procedures. *Thromb Haemost.* 2003;90:446–455.
25. Gallus AS. Prevention of postoperative deep leg vein thrombosis in patients with cancer. *Thromb Haemost.* 1997;78:126–132.
26. Wahba WM, Don HF, Craig DB. Postoperative epidural analgesia: effect on lung volumes. *Can Anaesth Soc J.* 1975;22:519–527.
27. Lima NF, Carvalho AL. Early discharge following major thoracic surgery: identification of related factors. *Rev Port Pneumol.* 2003;9:205–213.
28. Peters JH, Kronson J, Katz M, DeMeester TR. Arterial anatomic considerations in colon interposition for esophageal replacement. *Arch Surg.* 1995;130(8):858–862.
29. Saint JH. Surgery of the esophagus. *Arch Surg.* 1929;19(1):53–128.
30. Banbury MK, Rice TW, Goldblum JR, et al. Esophagectomy with gastric reconstruction for achalasia. *J Thorac Cardiovasc Surg.* 1999;117(6):1077–1084.
31. Devaney EJ, Iannettoni MD, Orringer MB, Marshall B. Esophagectomy for achalasia: patient selection and clinical experience. *Ann Thorac Surg.* 2001;72:854–858.
32. Banki F, Mason RJ, DeMeester SR, et al. Vagal-sparing esophagectomy: a more physiologic alternative. *Ann Surg.* 2002;236(3):324–336.
33. Peyre CG, DeMeester SR, Rizzetto C, et al. Vagal-sparing esophagectomy: the ideal operation for intramucosal adenocarcinoma and Barrett with high-grade dysplasia. *Ann Surg.* 2007;246(4):665–671.
34. Orringer MB, Marshall B, Iannettoni MD. Eliminating the cervical esophagogastric anastomotic leak with a side-to-side stapled anastomosis. *J Thorac Cardiovasc Surg.* 2000;119:277–288.
35. Sihvo EIT, Luostarinen ME, Salo JA. Fate of patients with adenocarcinoma of the esophagus and the esophagogastric junction: a population-based analysis. *Am J Gastroenterol.* 2004;99:419–424.
36. Hulscher JBF, van Sandick JW, de Boer AGEM, et al. Extended transthoracic resection compared with limited transhiatal resection for adenocarcinoma of the esophagus. *N Eng J Med.* 2002;347:1662–1669.
37. Omloo JMT, Lagarde SM, Hulscher JBF, et al. Extended transthoracic resection compared with limited transhiatal resection for adenocarcinoma of the mid/distal esophagus: five-year survival of a randomized clinical trial. *Ann Surg.* 2007;246:992–1001.
38. Williams VA, Peters JH. Adenocarcinoma of the gastroesophageal junction: benefits of an extended lymphadenectomy. *Surg Oncol Clin N Am.* 2006;15:765–780.
39. Johansson JJ, DeMeester TR, Hagen JA, et al. En bloc vs. transhiatal esophagectomy for stage T3N1 adenocarcinoma of the distal esophagus. *Arch Surg.* 2004;139:627–633.
40. Ide H, Nakamura T, Okamoto F, et al. Reflux esophagitis after reconstruction of the esophagus using gastric tube: factors for occurrence of reflux esophagitis and Barrett's epithelium. Paper presented at: The International Society of Surgery Conference; 1997; Acapulco, Mexico, August 24–30, 1997.
41. Hamilton SR, Yardley JH. Regeneration of cardiac type mucosa and acquisition of Barrett mucosa after esophagogastrostomy. *Gastroenterology.* 1977;72:669–675.
42. Oberg S, Johansson J, Wenner J, Walther B. Metaplastic columnar mucosa in the cervical esophagus after esophagectomy. *Ann Surg.* 2002;235(3):338–345.
43. Dresner SM, Griffin SM, Wayman J, Bennett MK, Hayes N, Raimes, SA. Human model of duodenogastro-oesophageal reflux in the development of Barrett's metaplasia. *Br J Surg.* 2003;90:1120–1128.
44. Lord RVN, Wickramasinghe K, Johansson JJ, DeMeester SR, Brabender J, DeMeester TR. Cardiac mucosa in the remnant esophagus after esophagectomy is an acquired epithelium with Barrett's-like features. *Surgery.* 2004;136:633–640.
45. Briel JW, Tamhankar AP, Hagen JA, et al: Prevalence and risk factors for ischemia, leak and stricture of esophageal anastomosis: gastric pull-up versus colon interposition. *J Am Coll Surg.* 2004;198:536–542.
46. Dewar L, Gelfand G, Finley RJ, et al. Factors affecting cervical anastomotic leak and stricture formation following esophagogastrectomy and gastric tube interposition. *Am J Surg.* 1992;163:484–489.
47. Blackmon SH, Correa AM, Wynn B, et al. Propensity-matched analysis of three techniques for intrathoracic esophagogastric anastomosis. *Ann Thorac Surg.* 2007;83:1805–1813.
48. Watson TJ, DeMeester TR, Kauer WK, Peters JH, Hagen JA. Esophageal replacement for end-stage benign esophageal disease. *J Thorac Cardiovasc Surg.* 1998;115:1241–1247.
49. Schein M, Conlan AA, Hatchuel MD: Surgical management of the redundant transposed colon. *Am J Surg.* 1990;160(5):529–530.
50. Ascioti AJ, Hofstetter WL, Miller ML, et al. Long-segment, supercharged, pedicled jejunal flap for total esophageal reconstruction. *J Thorac Cardiovasc Surg.* 2005;130:1391–1398.
51. Hagen JA, Peters JH, DeMeester TR. Superiority of extended en bloc esophagogastrectomy for carcinoma of the lower esophagus and cardia. *J Thorac Cardiovasc Surg.* 1993;106:850–858.
52. Putnam JB Jr, Suell DM, McMurtrey MJ, et al. Comparison of three techniques of esophagectomy within a residency training program. *Ann Thorac Surg.* 1994;57:319–325.
53. Horstmann O, Verreet PR, Becker H, Ohmann C, Roher HD. Transhiatal oesophagectomy compared with transthoracic resection and systematic lymphadenectomy for the treatment of oesophageal cancer. *Eur J Surg.* 1995;161:557–567.
54. Altorki NK, Girardi L, Skinner DB. En bloc esophagectomy improves survival for Stage III esophageal cancer. *J Thorac Cardiovasc Surg.* 1997;114:948–955.
55. Hagen JA, DeMeester SR, Peters JH, Chandrasoma P, DeMeester TR. Curative resection for esophageal adenocarcinoma: analysis of 100 en bloc esophagectomies. *Ann Surg.* 2001;234:520–530.
56. Orringer MB, Marshall B, Stirling MC. Transhiatal esophagectomy for benign and malignant disease. *J Thorac Cardiovasc Surg.* 1993;105:265–276.
57. Rentz J, Bull D, Harpole D, et al. Transthoracic versus transhiatal esophagectomy: a prospective study of 945 patients. *J Thorac Cardiovasc Surg.* 2003;125:1114–1120.

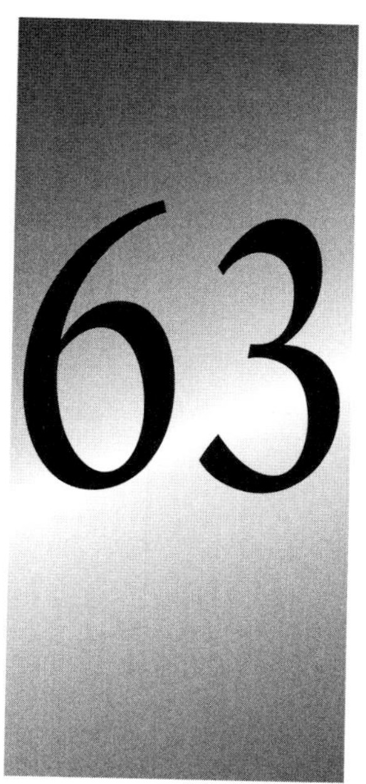

63 Surgery Techniques: Anesthesia in the Esophageal Cancer Patient

Norman A. Cohen
Jeffrey R. Kirsch

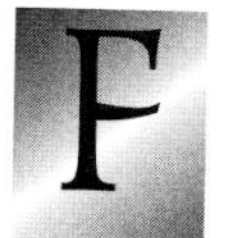

For those providing an anesthetic service, the primary goal is to maintain and, where possible, improve the safety and health of the patient undergoing a surgical intervention. Esophageal surgery presents special challenges to the anesthesiologist because of the comorbidities of the typical patient and the significant risk of morbidity and mortality related to this class of surgery. Preanesthetic preparation focuses on identifying and optimizing the patient's other medical conditions. Intraoperative management includes selection of anesthetic techniques and agents that will maintain homeostasis; provide amnesia, analgesia, and muscle relaxation; and ensure an optimal operating environment for the surgeon. Postoperative care addresses management of postsurgical pain and treatment of pulmonary, cardiac, and other system derangements often associated with esophageal surgery. The anesthesiologist works closely with the surgeon, oncologist, critical care team, and other consultants to achieve these goals. This chapter provides the nonanesthesiologist physician involved in the surgical care of esophageal cancer an overview of the anesthesia management for these patients.

GENERAL ANESTHETIC CONSIDERATIONS

Over the past several decades, the risk of significant morbidity and mortality associated with anesthesia has decreased dramatically. The development of new anesthetic agents with improved therapeutic margins, the introduction of monitoring devices to quickly identify hypoxemia and inadequate ventilation, and enhanced understanding of the effects of anesthetic agents and surgical interventions on the patient have all contributed to these improvements in care. In the 1999 Institute of Medicine (IOM) publication *To Err Is Human: Building a Safer Health System,* the IOM specifically recognized the specialty itself, the American Society of Anesthesiologists and the Anesthesia Patient Safety Foundation as having a visible commitment to reducing errors and improving patient safety (1). These advances have changed the risk-to-benefit equation, allowing patients who were never before considered surgical candidates to undergo highly invasive and complex procedures. Esophageal surgery for cancer management clearly falls into this procedural category.

PREANESTHESIA EVALUATION

Patients receiving anesthesia care undergo a preanesthetic evaluation that is very similar to a new-patient visit evaluation and management service (2). The elements of the evaluation include identification of the patient, a history of present illness, past medical and surgical history, identification of prior anesthetic difficulties, delineation of medications and allergies, a personal and social history, family history of conditions relevant to anesthesia care such as malignant hyperthermia or pseudocholinesterase deficiency, a thorough review of systems, and a physical examination to identify integumentary, airway, cardiac, pulmonary, and neurological anomalies as well as potential difficulty with vascular access.

The anesthesiologist carefully reviews available medical records, confirms the surgical consent with the patient, interprets available laboratory and diagnostic studies, reviews any medication orders from the surgical team, and, where indicated, discusses any special anesthetic requests or requirements with the surgical team. Based on the entirety of the evaluation, the anesthesiologist develops an anesthetic plan that includes the chosen technique, medications to be used or avoided, determination of the need for invasive monitoring, and vascular access requirements. Discussion of the anesthetic procedure, alternatives where available, common and serious risks associated with the selected anesthetic technique, and solicitation and answering of any patient questions make up the anesthetic informed consent. The anesthesiologist enters the findings, assessment, and plan into the medical record before providing anesthesia care.

Proper evaluation leads to the development of an anesthetic plan that meets the specific needs of the individual patient. From addressing the needs of the chronic pain patient to identifying patients who may be difficult to intubate with an endotracheal tube, the preanesthetic evaluation is a crucial and indispensable element in the safe delivery of anesthesia.

Comorbidities

Anesthesia morbidity ranges in severity from the minor to the serious. Minor morbidity is time limited and does not create permanent injury. This may include sore throat, hoarse voice, nausea, and postdural puncture headache. Serious anesthesia morbidity may involve respiratory or cardiac adverse events, airway misadventures, or drug reactions or interactions. Often the final common expression for these incidents is brain injury, ranging from mild cognitive impairment through persistent vegetative state or even brain death. Certain coexisting disease states present preoperatively may increase the frequency and severity of anesthesia morbidity.

Patients with esophageal cancer frequently have coexisting medical conditions that may affect anesthesia risk, alter anesthesia planning, or both. These conditions may be risk factors for the development of this cancer, frequently presenting comorbidities, or consequences of the disease itself. The following sections cover each category in turn, with attention to the need for further evaluation before surgery and implications for anesthesia care.

Risk Factors for the Development of Esophageal Cancer

Smoking, heavy alcohol consumption, achalasia, esophageal diverticuli, and human papilloma virus infection appear to be risk factors for squamous cell carcinoma of the esophagus, while smoking, chronic gastroesophageal reflux disease (GERD) including Barrett's esophagitis, and risk factors for GERD such as obesity and certain medications that affect lower esophageal sphincter tone are risk factors for esophageal adenocarcinoma.

Tobacco

Tobacco use has been found to increase perioperative morbidity in a number of ways (3). In addition to development of chronic obstructive pulmonary disease, the risk of myocardial infarction and thromboembolism increases, as does pulmonary complications such as failure to wean from the ventilator in bariatric surgery patients (4). Recent exposure to cigarette smoke increases carboxyhemoglobin levels because of the presence of carbon monoxide in smoke. Carboxyhemoglobin reduces oxygen delivery to end organs, leading to increased risk for coronary ischemia (5) and ventricular arrythmias (6).

Smokers undergoing ventral hernia repair (7) but not total hip arthroplasty have an increased risk of wound infection (8). Interestingly, smoking does not appear to affect the viability of vascular or free flaps, perhaps because of preferential blood flow to skeletal muscle caused by nicotine (9–11).

The influence of tobacco use on pain perception appears to be complex, with chronic pain more frequently seen in smokers and postoperative analgesic requirements being greater; however, acute tobacco use appears to increase the pain threshold, possibly because of the analgesic effects of nicotine itself (12). Smokers have a reduced incidence of nausea and vomiting postoperatively. Tobacco use does have measurable effects on drug metabolism because of induction of the cytochrome P450 system and may also affect central nervous system response to benzodiazepines and other anesthetics. Propofol requirements for induction of anesthesia do appear to be increased; however, the effect is small (13).

Alcohol

Chronic alcohol use can create pathophysiological changes of importance to anesthesia care. In excess, this drug can alter hepatic function, induce hematological changes, contribute to coagulopathy, and potentiate the risk for postoperative cognitive dysfunction (14). Cirrhosis and portal hypertension can lead to increased perioperative bleeding from esophageal varices, platelet dysfunction, and coagulation factor deficiencies.

Alcohol appears to have only minimal effect on propofol drug pharmacokinetics and pharmacodynamics (15). Conversely, the depressant affects of alcohol when combined with opioids increases the potential for respiratory depression.

Unrecognized or underappreciated chronic alcohol abuse may lead to the development of acute alcohol withdrawal in the postoperative period. Alcohol withdrawal syndrome is a highly morbid condition, with a 9.7% risk of mortality in intensive care unit (ICU) patients; furthermore, alcohol dependence is an independent predictor of organ failure, sepsis, and septic shock in those admitted to the ICU (16).

The anesthesiologist may consider interventions to reduce the potential for alcohol withdrawal syndrome. Regional anesthetic techniques to reduce postoperative analgesic needs and use of alpha 2 agonist therapy with agents such as clonidine and dexmedetomidine may be beneficial in managing this syndrome (17).

GERD

In addition to being a predisposing factor for the development of esophageal adenocarcinoma, reduced lower esophageal sphincter tone may increase the risk for pulmonary aspiration of gastric contents during surgery, particularly during induction of and emergence from anesthesia. Aspiration is relatively infrequent, occurring in 3.1 to 10.2 patients per 10,000 anesthetics in the United States (18). While pulmonary morbidity may be significant, mortality is fairly low, ranging from 0% to 4.6% of patients who aspirate during anesthesia. Furthermore, chronic reflux may lead to chronic and recurrent pulmonary aspiration, with deleterious affects on pulmonary gas exchange.

Techniques to reduce the risk of aspiration during anesthesia induction include treatment with nonparticulate antacids shortly before surgery (e.g., sodium citrate), maintenance of the patient on their chronic medications for GERD (e.g., ranitidine and pantoprazole) or treatment with these agents for untreated GERD patients, and a period of fasting before surgery to allow for maximal gastric emptying (19). Yamanaka et al. (20) demonstrated that oral omeprazole 20 mg significantly decreased gastric acidity and volume in 13 patients undergoing a rapid sequence induction, with a history of gastric tube reconstruction for esophageal cancer.

With symptomatic GERD, most anesthesiologists will elect to perform a "rapid-sequence induction" of anesthesia, first described by Sellick in 1961 (21). This technique incorporates posterior cricoid pressure during anesthesia induction. Since the cricoid consists of a circumferential ring of cartilage, pressure applied to the cricoid may help occlude the esophagus, thus reducing the possibility of gastric reflux and pulmonary aspiration once the patient loses his or her protective airway reflexes. In addition to cricoid pressure, the anesthesiologist will typically not ventilate the patient from the time that the induction drugs and rapid acting muscle relaxant are administered, until the endotracheal tube has been placed into the trachea and the cuff has been inflated. This technique requires ventilation with a 100% oxygen mixture for several minutes before induction. This period of preoxygenation usually provides a several-minute window of adequate arterial oxygen levels during the apneic period.

Some controversy exists as to the efficacy of cricoid pressure in reducing aspiration risk. Smith et al. (22), in a study evaluating anatomic changes via magnetic resonance imaging, demonstrated that, before application of cricoid pressure, the esophagus is lateral to the trachea more than 50% of the time and that both lateral laryngeal displacement (67%) and airway compression (81%) occur with application of such pressure. In awake patients, cricoid pressure actually reduces lower esophageal sphincter tone; however, administration of remifentanil with or without propofol attenuates this relaxation (23).

When considering mask ventilation, cricoid pressure does appear to reduce insufflation of air into the stomach (24). Butler and Sen (25) reviewed 241 papers published between 1950 and 2005, addressing emergent airway management. They ultimately focused on 3 papers that addressed whether cricoid pressure reduced the incidence of aspiration in patients undergoing emergency rapid sequence induction. They concluded that "there is little evidence to support the widely held belief that the application of cricoid pressure reduces the incidence of aspiration during a rapid sequence intubation," noting that cricoid pressure may interfere with airway management, create difficulties with passing the endotracheal tube, and worsen the view on direct laryngoscopy. In addition, maintenance of cricoid pressure during active regurgitation could result in esophageal rupture, requiring that cricoid pressure be discontinued if the patient begins to vomit (e.g., secondary to inadequate muscle relaxation).

Frequently Presenting Comorbidities

Esophageal cancer patients commonly present with other coexisting medical conditions that are not specifically risk factors for their cancer but that do significantly contribute to perioperative morbidity. In the case of esophageal resection surgery, differentiating whether anesthesia, surgery, or both are the cause of serious morbidity may be very difficult; therefore, this discussion will discuss the implications of coexisting disease on morbidity without focusing on causation.

Analysis of tumor registries demonstrate that approximately 20% of esophageal cancer patients have pulmonary disease, cardiac disease, or diabetes; each occur in about 10% of patients, and 4% to 7% of patients present with 2 or more major comorbidities. Presence of comorbidities predict an increase in the 30-day postsurgical mortality, with an odds ratio of 1.5 to 1.6 per comorbid condition (26). Given the fairly high prevalence of comorbid conditions, the anesthetic evaluation will focus on establishing the severity of the condition including other related systemic derangements, determining the condition's stability, identifying conditions that may impact perioperative morbidity, and determining strategies to improve the patient's health status before and throughout the perioperative period.

Managing cardiac risk is challenging because of variations in patient condition, lack of an accurate prediction tool, and limited randomized controlled trials evaluating management strategies. The combination of patient-specific factors such as the extent of atherosclerotic disease, surgical-specific elements including the risk for mechanical injury to the heart, and the patient's functional status have all been shown via multivariate analysis to predict the need for further investigation; however, guidelines for the use of specific studies (e.g., exercise or dobutamine echocardiography) most appropriate for the patient remain in question. When the patients do have significant atherosclerotic disease, the most appropriate management strategies, such as percutaneous coronary interventions, statin therapy, beta receptor blockade, or the use of alpha-2 agonists, should be tailored to the individual patient's needs and preexisting conditions and therapies (27,28).

Historically, anesthesiologists have believed that severe arterial hypertension significantly increases the risk of perioperative morbidity. Practitioners often establish limits for elective surgery, such as a systolic blood pressure over 200 or a diastolic blood pressure over 100. In the absence of other conditions, Howell et al. demonstrated that isolated arterial hypertension has only a mild but statistically significant risk for perioperative cardiac morbidity in patients undergoing surgery, with an odds ratio of 1.35 (29).

The development of atrial fibrillation (AF) perioperatively dramatically increases the incidence of a number of undesired outcomes, including stroke, mortality, length of stay, and overall cost of hospitalization. In an analysis of more than 2,500 thoracic surgery patients tracked via database prospectively, Vaporciyan et al. identified risk factors for the development of AF using multivariate analysis. Esophageal resection had a significant association with AF, with an odds ratio of 2.95. Other factors with positive predictive value included increasing age, male sex, intraoperative transfusion, history of congestive heart failure, arrhythmias, and peripheral vascular disease (30).

The American College of Physicians (ACP) recently published a practice guideline on risk assessment and management strategies to reduce perioperative pulmonary complications (PPC) (31). The authors noted that PPC are as common as cardiac complications and contribute equally to morbidity, mortality, and extended lengths of stay.

Many patients undergoing esophageal surgery for cancer have a number of characteristics identified by the ACP as risk factors for pulmonary complications. These include American Society of Anesthesiologists (ASA) physical status (32) of 2 or greater, age greater than 60, chronic obstructive pulmonary disease, abdominal surgery, thoracic surgery, use of general anesthesia, and a low serum albumin level. Other less common but equally worrisome predictors for PPC include congestive heart failure and functional dependence (being either partially or completely dependent on others for performance of normal activities of daily living); however, obesity and asthma do not appear to be reliable indicators. Other factors that may increase risk for PPC include obstructive sleep apnea, impaired level of consciousness, alcohol use, abnormalities on chest examination, and weight loss.

Advanced age is an independent predictor of increased morbidity and mortality. Moskovitz et al. reported that octogenarians have a surgical mortality from esophageal resection 3.9 fold greater than cohorts in the 50–79 age-group after correcting for comorbidities (33).

Recently, researchers have focused increasing attention on the relationship between anesthesia, surgery, age, and postprocedure cognitive dysfunction (POCD). Newman and colleagues' recent systematic review of the literature (34) demonstrated "relatively clear evidence" of cognitive impairment 1 week after major (but not minor) surgical procedures and that this result appears to be more common in the elderly. Incidence did not significantly differ by anesthetic technique. The studies currently available show "a little evidence" for long-term cognitive dysfunction. The authors do caution that many of the studies looking at POCD lacked sufficient numbers of subjects to demonstrate statistically significant differences and also suffered from other methodological confounding factors, including neither control over types of surgery studied nor types of tests used for evaluating cognitive performance.

Sequelae of Esophageal Cancer Present at Surgery

Sequelae of esophageal cancer itself are often present at the time of surgery. These include malnutrition, anemia, chronic pain, recurrent laryngeal nerve injury, and hypercalcemia associated with paraneoplastic syndrome.

Malnutrition has a number of deleterious effects on anesthesia care, warranting careful preanesthesia evaluation. These effects include altered drug bioavailability, reduced colloid oncotic pressure, increased potential for coagulation disorders, and general functional impairment. ASA physical status scoring proves to be a poor predictor of nutritional status and should be separately evaluated (35) using tools such as the Mini Nutritional Assessment (36). In addition to determining functional capacity, the anesthesiologist may consider additional preoperative testing to help assess and modify the sequelae of malnutrition preoperatively.

Esophageal resection may be associated with sufficient intraoperative blood loss to require transfusion of red blood cells in the perioperative period. The presence of preoperative anemia may lead the anesthesiologist to have additional blood products available for the planned surgical procedure. The decision to transfuse preoperatively weighs the patient's health status against the risks of transfusion. For example, moderate anemia, with a hemoglobin of 8 to 9 g/dL in a patient with stable but symptomatic ischemic heart disease, is more likely to lead to preoperative transfusion than the same values in an otherwise healthy patient. The risks of transfusion are numerous and include transfusion reaction, infection, transfusion-related lung injury, and increased risk of cancer reoccurrence through immune system modulation.

The presence of chronic pain alters anesthetic planning. Multimodal analgesic therapies remain the cornerstone of managing this difficult problem. Use of nonopioid analgesics including NMDA antagonists (ketamine), alpha-2 agonists (clonidine, dexmedetomidine), nonsteroidal agents (acetaminophen, ketorolac, celecoxib), and certain anticonvulsants (gabapentin, pregabelin) have all been shown to reduce postprocedural pain and intraoperative anesthetic requirements in major surgical procedures. In addition, thoracic epidural anesthesia (TEA) as an adjunct to general anesthesia reduces the need for postoperative ventilation and attenuates the endocrine and metabolic components of the surgical stress response, in addition to its analgesic role (see the following discussion) (37,38). TEA does not appear to attenuate immune system suppression that occurs with upper abdominal surgery (39).

Preoperative recurrent laryngeal nerve injury is an important finding. Its presence may alter decision making regarding timing of extubation. Contralateral injury intraoperatively may lead to prolonged ventilator dependence (40).

Hypercalcemia may present with anorexia, nausea, vomiting, weakness, and polyuria. In severe cases, ataxia, lethargy, confusion, and even coma may occur. Because of the potential for major morbidity, treatment with intravenous hydration with saline followed by diuresis with a loop diuretic should occur as an initial step and should precede elective surgery. If anesthesia commences shortly after initiation of treatment, invasive assessment of fluid status with central venous or pulmonary artery pressure monitoring may be useful. Also, one should test for iatrogenic hypokalemia and hypomagnesemia intraoperatively.

INTRAOPERATIVE MANAGEMENT

During the intraoperative phase of the surgical intervention, the anesthesiologist functions as the internist/intensivist in the operating room, managing acute perturbations of chronic conditions and the pathophysiological sequelae of the surgical intervention itself, all while making the patient insensible to pain and supporting vital cardiac and pulmonary function. These responsibilities extend far beyond the classic anesthetic triad of amnesia, analgesia, and muscle relaxation. In the case of patients undergoing esophageal surgery for cancer, the anesthetic plan typically involves a general anesthetic with monitoring appropriate to the patient's condition and the surgical approach. Rather than providing a primer on anesthesia, the following sections discuss the typical anesthetic management for esophageal cancer surgery and touch on anesthetic decision making that may play a role in improving outcome.

Anesthetic Management

The intraoperative phase of anesthesia management consists of induction of anesthesia, maintenance of the anesthetic state, and emergence from the effects of anesthesia medications sufficient to allow the patient to regain consciousness, reacquire protective airway and other reflexes, and no longer require support of vital physiological functions. The primary anesthetic technique for esophageal resection operations is "general anesthesia" in which the anesthesiologist employs a combination of medications, typically via the intravenous and inhalational routes, to produce unconsciousness, pain relief, amnesia, muscle relaxation, and blunt the physiological response to noxious stimuli. Table 63.1 contains a listing of medications commonly administered during anesthesia organized by their pharmacological class.

Monitoring

In addition to standard monitors, which include electrocardiogram, pulse oximetry, capnography, noninvasive blood pressure, and temperature (41), the anesthesiologist may employ additional tools to assess and manage

TABLE 63.1
Commonly Used Anesthesia Medications and Their Classes

Medication class	Agents used in anesthesia
Volatile inhalational agents	Isoflurane Sevoflurane Desflurane
Induction agents	Propofol Thiopental Etomidate Ketamine
Intravenous anesthetics	Propofol Dexmedatomidine
Opiates	Fentanyl Sufentanil Hydromorphone
Amnestics/anxiolytics	Midazolam Diazepam Dexmedatomidine
Depolarizing neuromuscular blockers	Succinylcholine
Nondepolarizing neuromuscular blockers	Vecuronium Rocuronium Pancuronium Cis-atracurium Mivacurium
Neuromuscular reversal agents	Neostigmine (usually with glycopyrrolate) Edrophonium (usually with atropine) Sugammadex

the patient during the anesthetic. These include invasive monitoring lines, such as arterial, central venous, or pulmonary artery catheters, and minimally invasive or noninvasive techniques, such as processed electroencephalographic monitoring to help assess likelihood of amnesia for intraoperative care and esophageal Doppler to optimize fluid management (42).

Induction

On arrival in the surgical suite, the operating room team assists the patient in transferring to the surgical table and places monitoring devices as described here, and the patient breathes 100% oxygen for several minutes before induction of anesthesia. This period of preoxygenation/denitrogenization helps prevent hypoxemia during anesthesia induction, even with a period of hypoventilation or apnea.

Induction of anesthesia usually involves administration of an intravenous agent to produce unconsciousness, a neuromuscular blocking agent to facilitate endotracheal intubation, and often other adjunctive agents. Currently, the most commonly used induction agent is propofol, and other frequently used agents include sodium thiopental and etomidate. The choice of agent depends on a combination of personal preference, consideration of cost, and assessment of patient condition. In patients where development of hypotension is of great concern, etomidate may be the drug of choice, as it produces significantly less venodilatation and cardiac depression than either thiopental or propofol. Inhalational induction of anesthesia is also an option in some patients, with sevoflurane being the preferred agent currently because of its low pungency and rapid onset of effect.

For rapid sequence intubation (see the previous discussion of GERD), the rapidly acting depolarizing muscle relaxant succinylcholine is often chosen; however, certain characteristics of this drug, such as causing a transient increase in potassium levels, the high rate of postoperative myalgias, and being a triggering agent for malignant hyperthermia, are contraindications in some patients. One may use nondepolarizing muscle relaxants at induction as well as during anesthetic maintenance. These drugs fall into 2 general categories: steroid-based (vecuronium, rocuronium, and pancuronium) and curariform (atracurium, cis-atricurium, and mivacurium) agents. Side effects of the drugs, duration of action, metabolic pathways, and patient conditions all play a role in drug selection. For example, the mild increase in heart rate seen with pancuronium may be sufficient to counteract the bradycardia induced by the synthetic opiates such as fentanyl, helping to maintain stable hemodynamics; however, pancuronium's duration is significantly prolonged in patients with renal insufficiency (43), thus making its use in this setting less desirable.

After successful anesthetic induction, patients undergoing esophageal cancer surgery require endotracheal intubation. While abdominal and abdominal-cervical surgical approaches do not typically require 1-lung ventilation, most procedures with an intrathoracic component do. If the surgery requires selective lung ventilation, the anesthesiologist will typically place either a double-lumen endobronchial tube (Figure 63.1) or a bronchial blocker device (Figure 63.2). When the surgeon requests, the anesthesiologist will cease ventilation on the operative side, allowing the lung to deflate via gas absorption and passive exhalation. This technique improves surgical exposure and reduces the risk of traumatic injury to the lung. The endobronchial tube has 2 lumens: one extends into the mainstem bronchus on either the right or the left side, and the other is shorter, ending in the trachea.

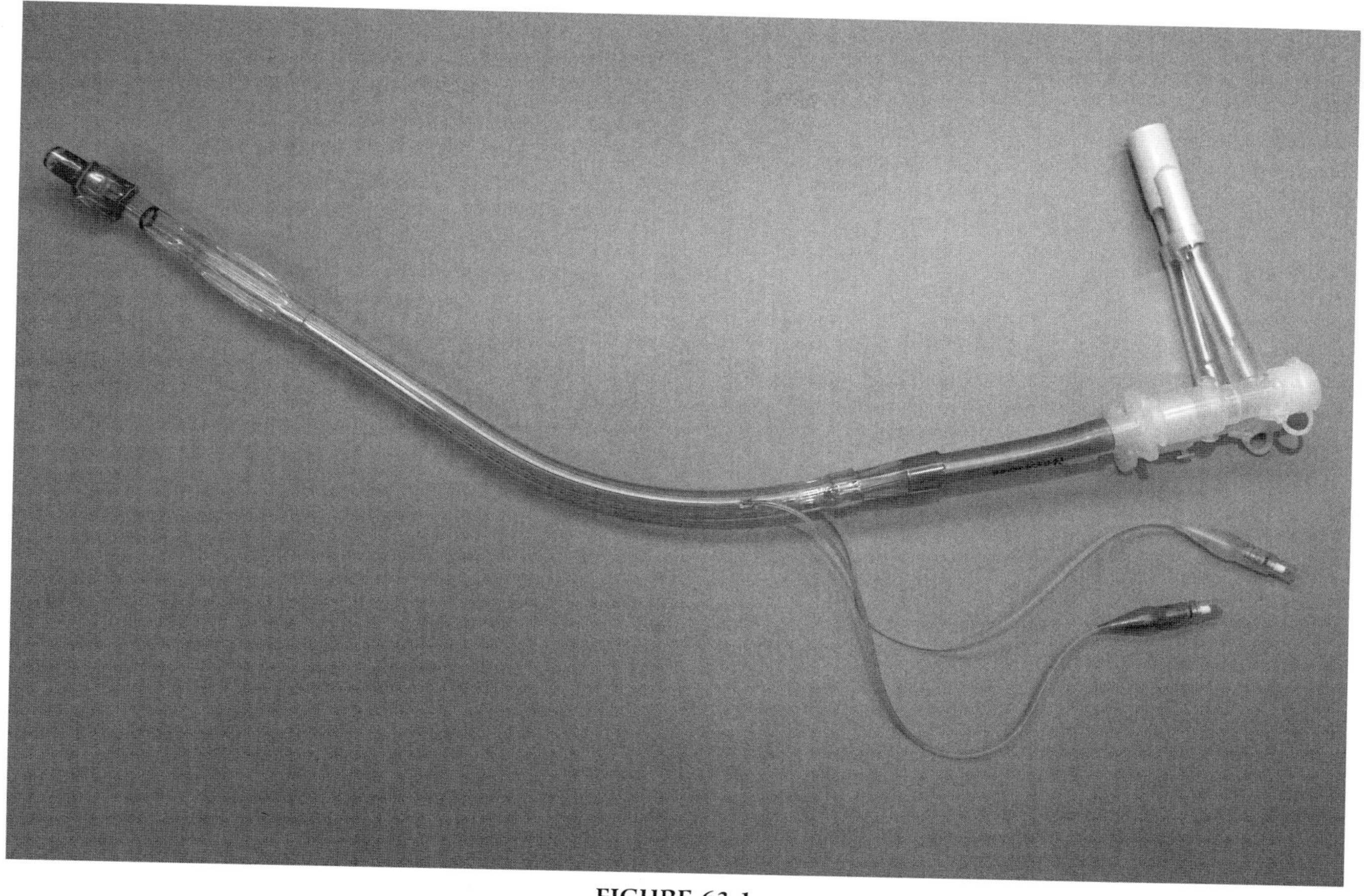

FIGURE 63.1

Double-lumen endobronchial tube.

A bronchial blocker is typically a balloon-tip catheter that is advanced into the desired mainstem bronchus through the endotracheal tube. To initiate selective ventilation, the anesthesiologist inflates the balloon, thereby blocking ventilation to that lung. With both endobronchial tubes and bronchial blockers, the anesthesiologist typically uses a flexible fiber-optic bronchoscope to visually confirm correct positioning. With correct placement, the endobronchial lumen extends far enough into the right or left main stem bronchus to allow cuff inflation without herniation into the trachea while not occluding the left or right upper lobe bronchus. The left-sided endobronchial tube is often used in preference to a right-sided endobroncial tube because the right-sided endobronchial tube often occludes the right upper lobe bronchus, due to its close proximity to the carina. Although 1-lung ventilation improves surgical exposure, it also worsens ventilation-perfusion mismatch and can cause intraoperative hypoxemia, particularly in patients with preexisting pulmonary dysfunction.

Maintenance

The period of time between induction into and emergence from anesthesia is known as the maintenance phase. During this period, the anesthesiologist maintains the anesthetic state, monitors for potentially adverse changes in the patient's condition, and intervenes to return the patient to a state of homeostasis. The medications used to maintain anesthesia are numerous and include the volatile inhalational agents, intravenous anesthetics, opiates, amnestics, and the neuromuscular blocking agents previously mentioned. Anesthesiologists typically use a combination of medications that produce desired effects while minimizing the often dose-dependent, undesirable side effects. While inhalational agents provide fine control over anesthetic depth and possess cardioprotective properties (44), higher doses lead to cardiac depression and hypotension and potentiate ventilation-perfusion mismatching (45). Similarly, a primary opioid anesthetic technique delivers excellent hemodynamic stability and

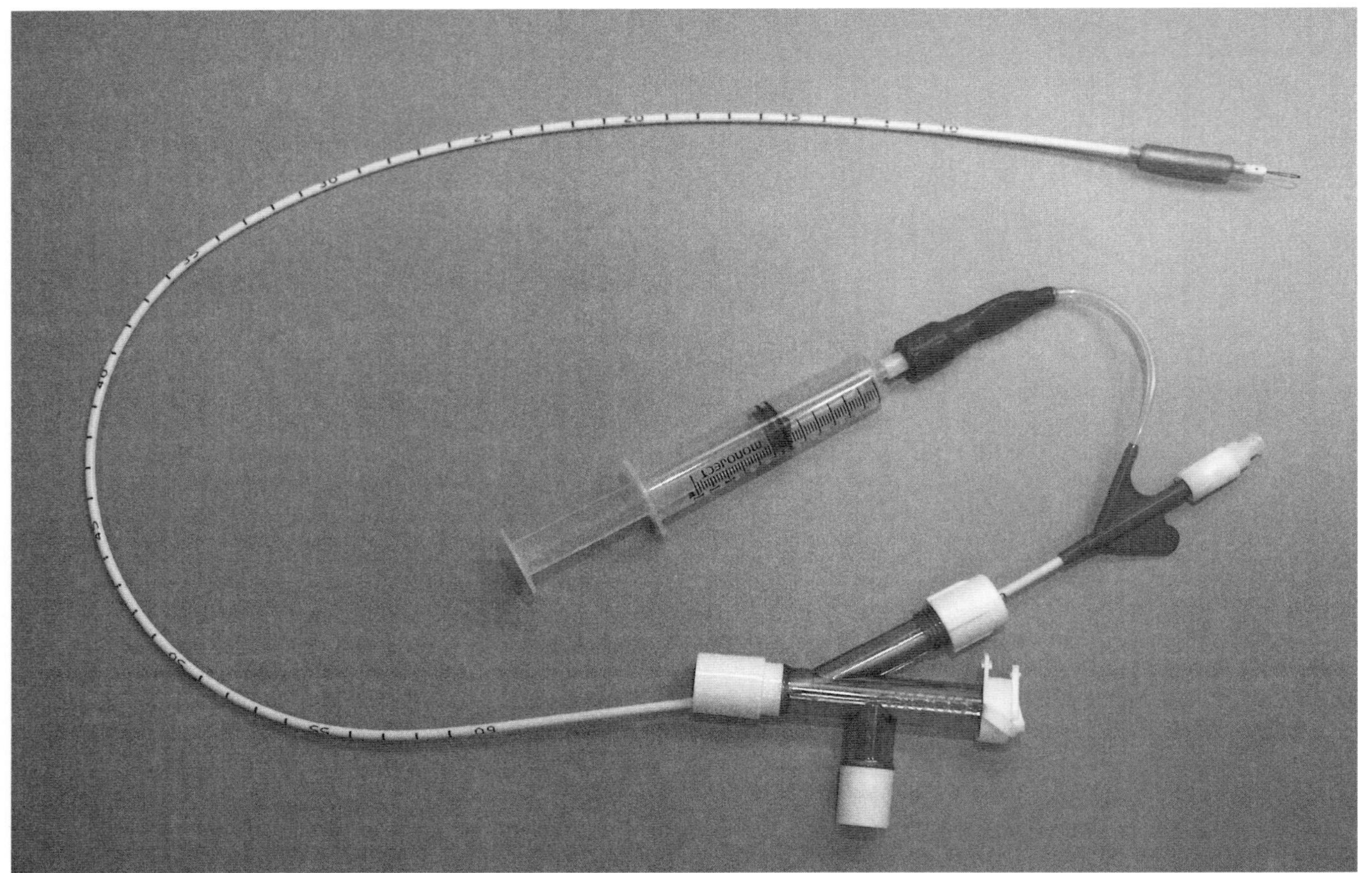

FIGURE 63.2

Bronchial blocker device.

analgesia while sometimes leading to prolonged depression of ventilation, inadequate amnesia, and the potential development of opioid-induced hyperalgesia (46).

In addition to undesirable effects of anesthesia medications, surgery itself often creates local tissue injury and systemic effects. Esophageal resection creates a number of anesthetic challenges. In addition to the frequent requirement for 1-lung ventilation, lung and heart injury can occur secondary to surgical manipulation, leading to hypoxemia, ventilatory insufficiency, arrhythmias, and impaired cardiac function. When performing surgery near vital structures, surgical hemorrhage is always a possibility, and optimizing fluid administration to maintain cardiovascular function without creating compromising tissue edema is a challenge in these patients.

Hemodynamic Management

During the process of surgical exposure, resection and reanastomosis of the esophagus, injury to the heart may occur. Cardiac contusion can cause impaired contractility, diminished cardiac output, and hypotension. This outcome is possibly more likely in transhiatal resections because of the need for blind dissection near the heart. Treatment consists of fluid optimization and addition of inotropes as indicated.

Even without injury, surgical manipulation can cause impaired cardiac venous return and, as a consequence, hypotension. The anesthesiologist must consider operative interventions as causes for the acute development of hemodynamic instability; furthermore, the anesthesiologist should keep the surgeon apprised of any significant changes in vital signs, as the simple repositioning of a retractor, movement of a sponge, or other minor action may be corrective.

Anesthetic Strategies to Reduce Pulmonary Morbidity

Esophagectomy has been shown to cause a profound inflammatory response (47). The magnitude of the inflammatory response and the presence of perioperative hypoxemia are predictors of postoperative pulmonary complications. Tandon and colleagues retrospectively reviewed the risk factors for acute lung injury following esophagectomy, finding an association between adult respiratory distress syndrome (ARDS) and "a low pre-operative body mass index, a history of cigarette smoking, the experience of the surgeon, the duration of both the operation and of one-lung ventilation, and the occurrence of a post-operative anastomotic leak." Additionally, perioperative hypoxemia, hypotension, fluid and blood administration, and anastomotic leaks also predicted ARDS (48).

Noting that ARDS patients benefit from ventilation with low tidal volumes and positive end-expiratory pressure (PEEP) by demonstrating improved gas exchange and overall outcomes and that this strategy appears to reduce levels of inflammation as measured by cytokine levels, Michelet and colleagues prospectively evaluated a "protective ventilatory strategy" in esophagectomy patients without preexisting lung disease, receiving intraoperative 1-lung ventilation (49). The authors randomized patients to receive either conventional ventilation strategies (9 mL/kg tidal volume and no PEEP during both 1- and 2-lung ventilation) or the low tidal volume + PEEP strategy (9 mL/kg 2-lung, 5 mL/kg 1-lung, and 5 cm H_20 PEEP throughout). The protective strategy demonstrated reduced systemic inflammation from the end of 1-lung ventilation through the postoperative period, improved oxygenation, reduced lung water, attenuation of the increase in airway plateau pressure, and duration of postoperative ventilation in the ICU. The groups did not differ in postoperative morbidity or ICU length of stay.

These studies suggest that simple alterations in intraoperative ventilatory management may have significant implications for postsurgical outcome. At the very least, it has engendered significant debate and is an active area of exploration (50–53).

Blood and Fluid Management

On occasion, intraoperative bleeding can be brisk, frequently requiring transfusion of red blood cells and other blood products. In deciding to transfuse, the anesthesiologist must clinically assess, using indirect measures, whether oxygen delivery to the tissues is adequate and whether clotting factors and platelet levels are sufficient. In collaboration with the surgeon, the decision whether to transfuse must then balance the known risks, including infection, transfusion reaction, lung injury, and immunomodulation, against the clinical factors indicating a need for transfusion.

Even without bleeding, surgical dissection and tissue manipulation create a fluid shift from the intravascular to interstitial compartments. Relative hypovolemia is common, with the extent of edema formation often enhanced because of lowered plasma oncotic pressure found in this malnourished patient population. Most anesthetic agents produce hypotension in the setting of hypovolemia. Brandstrup et al. recently demonstrated that fluid restriction appears to reduce postoperative complications in colorectal surgery (54).

However, Wakeling et al. and Noblett et al. provided results that conflict with those of Brandstrup. These researchers demonstrated that, in colorectal surgeries, fluid optimization guided by Doppler ultrasound assessment of cardiac output, when compared to conventional management, resulted in *increased* colloid fluid administration, reduced time to return of bowel function, reduced gastrointestinal morbidity, reduced time to discharge readiness, reduced ICU admission rate, and reduced levels of the cytokine IL-6 (55,56). IL-6 is a marker of inflammation. Although provocative, the role of Doppler assessment of fluid management in esophageal surgery has not yet been reported, at least in part because of the requirement for probe placement in the esophagus.

Emergence and Postprocedure Care

A major part of the art of anesthesia is providing a smooth transition from a level of surgical anesthesia to the awake state. This occurs over a relatively brief period of time and must be timed to avoid premature arousal so as to avoid disrupting the final stages of the surgical procedure.

The process of emergence from anesthesia involves ceasing anesthetic medication administration, antagonizing neuromuscular blockade, facilitating the return to spontaneous ventilation, ensuring return of protective airway reflexes, and allowing the patient to return to consciousness. The anesthesiologist must accomplish these tasks while maintaining adequate analgesia and blunting the potentially dangerous sympathetically mediated hyperdynamic response to emergence. Emergence is a continuum that begins shortly before the conclusion of the surgical procedure and continues into and beyond the patient's stay in the postanesthesia care unit (PACU).

Emerging from anesthesia is a relatively risky period of anesthesia. In a French survey investigating the incidence of mortality secondary to anesthesia, 22% of all deaths attributed to anesthesia occurred in the PACU (57). Arbous and colleagues also carefully evaluated anesthesia related morbidity and mortality in a case control study involving all patients undergoing anesthesia in the Netherlands during 1995–1997 (58). In this study, reversal of neuromuscular blockade (odds ratio [OR] 0.10) and opioids (OR 0.29), having 2 anesthesia providers present at emergence (OR 0.69), and postoperative provision of opiates (OR 0.165), local anesthetics (OR 0.06), or both (OR 0.324) for analgesia were predictors of better outcomes.

Removal of the endotracheal tube at the conclusion of surgery is desirable whenever possible and can occur after most esophagectomies (59). Adequate pain relief, often due to an effective epidural infusion (see the following section), and an uneventful surgical procedure, effective management of the patient's comorbidities in the perioperative period, fluid balance optimization, full reversal of neuromuscular blockade, hemodynamic stability, and minimal intraoperative lung injury usually lead to early extubation.

Medical decision making becomes much more challenging when one or more of these criteria are not fully met. The anesthesiologist seeks objective findings of adequate ventilation and oxygenation with spirometry, capnography, and pulse oximetry. Evidence for return of muscle strength (e.g., at least 4 seconds of head lift, leg lift, or hand grasp) indicate fairly complete reversal of neuromuscular blockade. The anesthesiologist determines the level of consciousness, assesses the respiratory pattern, and evaluates for evidence of inadequately treated pain. Considering the subjective and objective findings, the anesthesiologist uses clinical experience and judgment to determine the need for early postoperative ventilatory or circulatory support.

Transport to the PACU or ICU occurs with supplemental oxygenation, elevation of the head of the bed as the patient tolerates to reduce aspiration risk (60,61) and to improve gas exchange, and monitoring of vital signs for longer transports or when the patient has shown hemodynamic instability.

On arrival in the PACU or ICU, the anesthesiologist reports pertinent historical findings, reviews the anesthetic course with the nurse receiving the patient, and provides orders for analgesics, the epidural (if placed), antiemetics, and oxygen and ventilator settings as necessary. Report is also given to the intensivist. The anesthesiologist remains available for consultation in the PACU and will ensure coverage for the epidural infusion.

THORACIC EPIDURAL ANALGESIA

Thoracic epidural analgesia (TEA) for postoperative pain treatment has become a mainstay of therapy for surgical esophagectomy. Those involved in the care of these patients should understand the benefits, risks, and clinical management of TEA. It is imperative that the anesthesiologist place the catheter in the midthoracic area to maximize efficacy and minimize side effects.

Efficacy

The widespread introduction of TEA in the 1990s has led to earlier endotracheal extubation, earlier ambulation, reduced ICU and hospital length of stay, and improved postoperative pulmonary function in esophagectomy patients (62,63). Brodner and colleagues evaluated a multimodal approach that included TEA to control complications and enhance rehabilitation. After introduction of this modality, these researchers found that extubation, mobilization, ICU discharge, and intermediate care discharge occurred earlier compared to a retrospective analysis of patients at the same institution prior to the protocol's introduction (64).

Recently, Cense et al. demonstrated reduced pneumonia, reintubation, and postsurgical mortality rates as well as reduced ICU and hospital stays when comparing transthoracic esophagectomy patients who either received epidural analgesia for at least 2 days versus those who did not (65).

A retrospective study of patients undergoing single-stage, en bloc esophagectomy with 2-field lymphadenectomy at a single center evaluated risk factors for anastomotic leak. While cervical location of the anastomosis (OR 5.5) and development of ARDS (OR 21.3) were independent predictors of developing a leak, TEA reduced the likelihood (OR 0.13) (66). In an animal model, Lázár and colleagues demonstrated that TEA improves gastric microcirculation in the setting of experimental gastric tube formation, perhaps providing some explanation for the finding of reduced anastomotic failures in patients receiving epidural analgesia (67).

Explanations for improved outcome with epidural analgesia may include enhanced tissue oxygenation (68), reduced sympathetic tone, and an attenuation but not complete ablation of the stress response (69). TEA does not appear to alter immune response compared to general anesthesia alone. In addition, earlier extubation and initiation of pulmonary physiotherapy may contribute to improved outcomes with TEA.

Risk

TEA is a fairly safe, minimally invasive method of pain control. Minor risks include tenderness at the insertion site, local inflammation, dural puncture with possible postural headache, hypotension, pruritus, muscle weakness, excessive numbness, failure to successfully place the catheter, and failure to provide adequate analgesia. Major risks include toxicity from intravascular or subarachnoid injection, respiratory depression, local infection, epidural abscess, epidural hematoma, spinal cord injury, other nerve injury, and rarely death. In a meta-analysis of studies comparing parenteral to lumbar or thoracic epidural analgesia, Block and colleagues (70) found that the "rates for all complications were relatively low."

Wheatley et al. reviewed relevant studies published between 1976 and 2000 to determine the efficacy and safety of postoperative epidural analgesia (71), and the authors concluded that the risks of serious neurological injury is quite low: 0.005% to 0.006% in retrospective studies and 0.03% in prospective analyses. While epidural hematoma is also a rare occurrence, the increasing use of anticoagulants, such as warfarin and low-molecular-weight heparin (LMWH), in the perioperative period has led to an increased incidence of this complication. Current recommendations include 24-hour dosing of LMWH and insertion or removal of the epidural at least 12 hours after the last dose. Antiplatelet medications do not appear to increase the risk of epidural hematoma.

Epidural abscess is exceedingly rare with 2 reviews, totaling around 60,000 patients, showing no episodes at all (72,73). More recent studies demonstrate an incidence of around 0.05% of catheter placements, with immunocompromised status (cancer, diabetes, chronic obstructive pulmonary disease, and so on), perioperative anticoagulation, and duration of catheter placement (mean 11 days, median 6 days) being associated with this complication (74).

With a reasonably high benefit-to-risk ratio, epidural analgesia has proven to be a useful adjunct to the management of patients undergoing esophageal cancer surgery. Based on the evidence available, surgeons increasingly request this modality, provided that their patients have reasonably normal coagulation function and no evidence of local or systemic infection. The physician placing the epidural should use strict aseptic technique, and the total period for an epidural to remain in place should be kept to a minimum because of the association between duration of catheter being in situ and epidural abscess formation.

Process

Typically, the anesthesiologist places the epidural preoperatively, usually in the midthoracic region, using strict aseptic technique. The anesthesiologist must test the catheter to confirm that the catheter tip is not in a blood vessel or the subarachnoid space by injecting a small volume of a local anesthetic and epinephrine mixture. If the catheter is subarachnoid, a spinal block will quickly develop, and if the catheter is in a blood vessel, the epinephrine will usually cause the patient's heart rate to increase significantly. This local anesthetic test dose will usually create a sensory block several dermatomes wide when administered epidurally, with the block centered at the level of the catheter tip position.

During the surgical procedure, the anesthesiologist may inject or infuse medications through the epidural catheter as an adjunct to general anesthesia. Whether or not this occurs, it is desirable to have created a sensory block before emergence, as this will reduce the need for additional analgesics, blunt the hyperdynamic response to anesthetic emergence, and help provide a smooth transition to the initial stages of surgical recovery. There is inconclusive evidence to support benefit from preemptive analgesia with epidural dosing before skin incision.

The anesthesiologist, potentially working with an acute pain management team, will initiate an infusion of medications through the epidural. The goals are to provide analgesia while minimizing side effects. These side effects include drowsiness, muscular weakness, nausea, and respiratory depression. The infusion mixture usually consists of a local anesthetic, such as ropivacaine or bupivacaine, and an opioid, such as fentanyl, sufentanil, morphine, or hydromorphone. The physician managing the epidural adjusts the infusion to provide a sensory block sufficient to cover the incision and innervation to the involved organs. The patient typically receives an infusion for several days, provided that analgesia remains adequate and there is no evidence of epidural site infection. The physician will adjust the epidural infusion rate and/or the concentration of agents being administered so that the patient can transition to less invasive means of pain control at the earliest reasonable opportunity.

CONCLUSION

Anesthetic management of patients undergoing esophageal resection is challenging. Patients often have multiple comorbidities that increase the risk related to anesthesia. The surgery requires special ventilatory techniques. The patients usually require invasive monitoring. Surgical manipulation can create hemodynamic instability through bleeding, fluid shifts, and direct effects on the heart and major vessels. The surgery itself has a high potential for inducing patient injury.

Anesthesia care is more than just keeping the patient still, free of pain, and unaware. By careful attention to preoperative assessment, a thorough understanding of the effects of anesthetic agents on these patients, technical proficiency in placing invasive lines and epidural catheters, appropriate selection of ventilation parameters, and continuous optimization of fluid status, the anesthesiologist can play a significant role in improving outcomes for these patients.

References

1. Kohn LT, Corrigan J, Donaldson MS. *To Err Is Human: Building a Safer Health System.* Washington, DC: National Academies Press, 1999.
2. American Society of Anesthesiologists. *Basic Standards for Preanesthesia Care.* Park Ridge, IL: American Society of Anethesiologist; 2005.
3. Warner DO. Tobacco dependence in surgical patients. *Curr Opin Anaesthesiol.* 2007;20:279–283.
4. Livingston EH, Arterburn D, Schifftner TL, et al. National Surgical Quality Improvement Program analysis of bariatric operations: modifiable risk factors contribute to bariatric surgical adverse outcomes. *J Am Coll Surg.* 2006;203:625–633.
5. Aronow WS, Cassidy J, Vangrow JS, et al. Effect of cigarette smoking and breathing carbon monoxide on cardiovascular hemodynamics in anginal patients. *Circulation.* 1974;50:340–347.
6. Sheps DS, Herbst MC, Hinderliter AL, et al. Production of arrhythmias by elevated carboxyhemoglobin in patients with coronary artery disease. *Ann Intern Med.* 1990;113:343–351.
7. Finan KR, Vick CC, Kiefe CI, et al. Predictors of wound infection in ventral hernia repair. *Am J Surg.* 2005;190:676–681.
8. Sadr Azodi O, Bellocco R, Eriksson K, et al. The impact of tobacco use and body mass index on the length of stay in hospital and the risk of post-operative complications among patients undergoing total hip replacement. *J Bone Joint Surg Br.* 2006;88:1316–1320.
9. Khouri RK, Cooley BC, Kunselman AR, et al. A prospective study of microvascular free-flap surgery and outcome. *Plast Reconstr Surg.* 1998;102:711–721.
10. Mehrara BJ, Santoro TD, Arcilla E, et al. Complications after microvascular breast reconstruction: experience with 1195 flaps. *Plast Reconstr Surg.* 2006;118:1100–1109; discussion 1110–1111.
11. Fleming BP, Barron KW, Heesch CM, et al. Response of the arteriolar network in rat cremaster muscle to intraarterial infusion of nicotine. *Int J Microcirc Clin Exp.* 1989;8:275–292.
12. Flood P, Daniel D. Intranasal nicotine for postoperative pain treatment. *Anesthesiology.* 2004;101:1417–1421.
13. Lysakowski C, Dumont L, Czarnetzki C, et al. The effect of cigarette smoking on the hypnotic efficacy of propofol. *Anaesthesia.* 2006;61:826–831.
14. Hudetz JA, Iqbal Z, Gandhi SD, et al. Postoperative cognitive dysfunction in older patients with a history of alcohol abuse. *Anesthesiology.* 2007;106:423–430.
15. Servin FS, Bougeois B, Gomeni R, et al. Pharmacokinetics of propofol administered by target-controlled infusion to alcoholic patients. *Anesthesiology.* 2003;99:576–585.
16. O'Brien JMJ, Lu B, Ali NA, et al. Alcohol dependence is independently associated with sepsis, septic shock, and hospital mortality among adult intensive care unit patients. *Crit Care Med.* 2007;35:345–350.
17. Maccioli GA. Dexmedetomidine to facilitate drug withdrawal. *Anesthesiology.* 2003;98:575–577.
18. Ng A, Smith G. Gastroesophageal reflux and aspiration of gastric contents in anesthetic practice. *Anesth Analg.* 2001;93:494–513.
19. Practice guidelines for preoperative fasting and the use of pharmacologic agents to reduce the risk of pulmonary aspiration: application to healthy patients undergoing elective procedures: a report by the American Society of Anesthesiologist Task Force on Preoperative Fasting. *Anesthesiology.* 1999;90:896–905.
20. Yamanaka Y, Mammoto T, Kita T, et al. A study of 13 patients with gastric tube in place after esophageal resection: use of omeprazole to decrease gastric acidity and volume. *J Clin Anesth.* 2001;13:370–373.
21. Sellick BA. Cricoid pressure to control regurgitation of stomach contents during induction of anaesthesia. *Lancet.* 1961;2:404–406.
22. Smith KJ, Dobranowski J, Yip G, et al. Cricoid pressure displaces the esophagus: an observational study using magnetic resonance imaging. *Anesthesiology.* 2003;99: 60–64.
23. Thorn K, Thorn SE, Wattwil M. The effects of cricoid pressure, remifentanil, and propofol on esophageal motility and the lower esophageal sphincter. *Anesth Analg.* 2005;100:1200–1203.
24. Lawes EG, Campbell I, Mercer D. Inflation pressure, gastric insufflation and rapid sequence induction. *Br J Anaesth.* 1987;59:315–318.
25. Butler J, Sen A. Best evidence topic report. Cricoid pressure in emergency rapid sequence induction. *Emerg Med J.* 2005;22:815–816.
26. Steyerberg EW, Neville BA, Koppert LB, et al. Surgical mortality in patients with esophageal cancer: development and validation of a simple risk score. *J Clin Oncol.* 2006;24:4277–4284.
27. Ashley EA, Vagelos RH. Preoperative cardiac evaluation: mechanisms, assessment, and reduction of risk. *Thorac Surg Clin.* 2005;15:263–275.
28. Auerbach AD, Goldman L. Beta-blockers and reduction of cardiac events in noncardiac surgery: scientific review. *JAMA.* 2002;287:1435–1444.
29. Howell SJ, Sear JW, Foex P. Hypertension, hypertensive heart disease and perioperative cardiac risk. *Br J Anaesth.* 2004;92:570–583.
30. Vaporciyan AA, Correa AM, Rice DC, et al. Risk factors associated with atrial fibrillation after noncardiac thoracic surgery: analysis of 2588 patients. *J Thorac Cardiovasc Surg.* 2004;127:779–786.
31. Qaseem A, Snow V, Fitterman N, et al. Risk assessment for and strategies to reduce perioperative pulmonary complications for patients undergoing noncardiothoracic surgery: a guideline from the American College of Physicians. *Ann Intern Med.* 2006;144:575–580.
32. Owens WD, Felts JA, Spitznagel ELJ. ASA physical status classifications: a study of consistency of ratings. *Anesthesiology.* 1978;49:239–243.
33. Moskovitz AH, Rizk NP, Venkatraman E, et al. Mortality increases for octogenarians undergoing esophagogastrectomy for esophageal cancer. *Ann Thorac Surg.* 2006;82:2031–2036; discussion 2036.
34. Newman S, Stygall J, Hirani S, et al. Postoperative cognitive dysfunction after noncardiac surgery: a systematic review. *Anesthesiology.* 2007;106:572–590.
35. Sakarya M, Karadag F, Luleci N, et al. [Relationship between nutrition and ASA-classification in the elderly]. *Anasthesiol Intensivmed Notfallmed Schmerzther.* 2004;39:400–405.
36. Cohendy R, Rubenstein LZ, Eledjam JJ. The Mini Nutritional Assessment—Short Form for preoperative nutritional evaluation of elderly patients. *Aging (Milano).* 2001;13:293–297.
37. Scott NB, Turfrey DJ, Ray DA, et al. A prospective randomized study of the potential benefits of thoracic epidural anesthesia and analgesia in patients undergoing coronary artery bypass grafting. *Anesth Analg.* 2001;93:528–535.
38. Bakhtiary F, Therapidis P, Dzemali O, et al. Impact of high thoracic epidural anesthesia on incidence of perioperative atrial fibrillation in off-pump coronary bypass grafting: a prospective randomized study. *J Thorac Cardiovasc Surg.* 2007;134:460–464.
39. Kawasaki T, Ogata M, Kawasaki C, et al. Effects of epidural anaesthesia on surgical stress-induced immunosuppression during upper abdominal surgery. *Br J Anaesth.* 2007;98:196–203.
40. Wright CD, Zeitels SM. Recurrent laryngeal nerve injuries after esophagectomy. *Thorac Surg Clin.* 2006;16:23–33, v.
41. American Society of Anesthesiologists. *Standards for Basic Anesthetic Monitoring.* Park Ridge, IL: American Society of Anethesiologist; 2005.
42. Pub 100–03 Medicare National Coverage Determinations, Transmittal 76. 2007. http://www.cms.hhs.gov/transmittals/downloads/R76NCD.pdf. Accessed November 4, 2008.
43. Somogyi AA, Shanks CA, Triggs EJ. The effect of renal failure on the disposition and neuromuscular blocking action of pancuronium bromide. *Eur J Clin Pharmacol.* 1977;12:23–29.
44. Zaugg M, Schaub MC, Foex P. Myocardial injury and its prevention in the perioperative setting. *Br J Anaesth.* 2004;93:21–33.
45. Dembinski R, Rossaint R, Kuhlen R. Modulating the pulmonary circulation: an update. *Curr Opin Anaesthesiol.* 2003;16:59–64.
46. Wilder-Smith OH, Arendt-Nielsen L. Postoperative hyperalgesia: its clinical importance and relevance. *Anesthesiology.* 2006;104:601–607.
47. Kooguchi K, Kobayashi A, Kitamura Y, et al. Elevated expression of inducible nitric oxide synthase and inflammatory cytokines in the alveolar macrophages after esophagectomy. *Crit Care Med.* 2002;30:71–76.
48. Tandon S, Batchelor A, Bullock R, et al. Peri-operative risk factors for acute lung injury after elective oesophagectomy. *Br J Anaesth.* 2001;86:633–638.
49. Michelet P, D'Journo XB, Roch A, et al. Protective ventilation influences systemic inflammation after esophagectomy: a randomized controlled study. *Anesthesiology.* 2006;105:911–919.
50. Choi G, Wolthuis EK, Bresser P, et al. Mechanical ventilation with lower tidal volumes and positive end-expiratory pressure prevents alveolar coagulation in patients without lung injury. *Anesthesiology.* 2006;105:689–695.
51. Richard JC, Brochard L, Vandelet P, et al. Respective effects of end-expiratory and end-inspiratory pressures on alveolar recruitment in acute lung injury. *Crit Care Med.* 2003;31:89–92.
52. Senturk M. Protective ventilation during one-lung ventilation. *Anesthesiology.* 2007;107:176–177; author reply 177.
53. Schultz MJ, Haitsma JJ, Slutsky AS, et al. What tidal volumes should be used in patients without acute lung injury? *Anesthesiology.* 2007;106:1226–1231.
54. Brandstrup B, Tonnesen H, Beier-Holgersen R, et al. Effects of intravenous fluid restriction on postoperative complications: comparison of two perioperative fluid regimens: a randomized assessor-blinded multicenter trial. *Ann Surg.* 2003;238:641–648.
55. Wakeling HG, McFall MR, Jenkins CS, et al. Intraoperative oesophageal Doppler guided fluid management shortens postoperative hospital stay after major bowel surgery. *Br J Anaesth.* 2005;95:634–642.
56. Noblett SE, Snowden CP, Shenton BK, et al. Randomized clinical trial assessing the effect of Doppler-optimized fluid management on outcome after elective colorectal resection. *Br J Surg.* 2006;93:1069–1076.
57. Lienhart A, Auroy Y, Pequignot F, et al. Survey of anesthesia-related mortality in France. *Anesthesiology.* 2006;105:1087–1097.
58. Arbous MS, Meursing AE, van Kleef JW, et al. Impact of anesthesia management characteristics on severe morbidity and mortality. *Anesthesiology.* 2005;102:257–268; quiz 491–492.
59. Chandrashekar MV, Irving M, Wayman J, et al. Immediate extubation and epidural analgesia allow safe management in a high-dependency unit after two-stage oesophagectomy: results of eight years of experience in a specialized upper gastrointestinal unit in a district general hospital. *Br J Anaesth.* 2003; 90:474–479.
60. Torres A, Serra-Batlles J, Ros E, et al. Pulmonary aspiration of gastric contents in patients receiving mechanical ventilation: the effect of body position. *Ann Intern Med.* 1992;116:540–543.
61. Drakulovic MB, Torres A, Bauer TT, et al. Supine body position as a risk factor for nosocomial pneumonia in mechanically ventilated patients: a randomised trial. *Lancet.* 1999;354:1851–1858.

62. Orringer MB, Marshall B, Iannettoni MD. Transhiatal esophagectomy: clinical experience and refinements. *Ann Surg.* 1999;230:392–400; discussion 400–403.
63. Whooley BP, Law S, Murthy SC, et al. Analysis of reduced death and complication rates after esophageal resection. *Ann Surg.* 2001;233:338–344.
64. Brodner G, Pogatzki E, Van Aken H, et al. A multimodal approach to control postoperative pathophysiology and rehabilitation in patients undergoing abdominothoracic esophagectomy. *Anesth Analg.* 1998;86:228–234.
65. Cense HA, Lagarde SM, de Jong K, et al. Association of no epidural analgesia with postoperative morbidity and mortality after transthoracic esophageal cancer resection. *J Am Coll Surg.* 2006;202:395–400.
66. Michelet P, D'Journo XB, Roch A, et al. Perioperative risk factors for anastomotic leakage after esophagectomy: influence of thoracic epidural analgesia. *Chest.* 2005;128:3461–3466.
67. Lázár G, Kaszaki J, Abraham S, et al. Thoracic epidural anesthesia improves the gastric microcirculation during experimental gastric tube formation. *Surgery.* 2003;134:799–805.
68. Kabon B, Fleischmann E, Treschan T, et al. Thoracic epidural anesthesia increases tissue oxygenation during major abdominal surgery. *Anesth Analg.* 2003;97:1812–1817.
69. Yokoyama M, Itano Y, Katayama H, et al. The effects of continuous epidural anesthesia and analgesia on stress response and immune function in patients undergoing radical esophagectomy. *Anesth Analg.* 2005;101:1521–1527.
70. Block BM, Liu SS, Rowlingson AJ, et al. Efficacy of postoperative epidural analgesia: a meta-analysis. *JAMA.* 2003;290:2455–2463.
71. Wheatley RG, Schug SA, Watson D. Safety and efficacy of postoperative epidural analgesia. *Br J Anaesth.* 2001;87:47–61.
72. Kane RE. Neurologic deficits following epidural or spinal anesthesia. *Anesth Analg.* 1981;60:150–161.
73. Dahlgren N, Tornebrandt K. Neurological complications after anaesthesia: a follow-up of 18,000 spinal and epidural anaesthetics performed over three years. *Acta Anaesthesiol Scand.* 1995;39:872–880.
74. Wang LP, Hauerberg J, Schmidt JF. Incidence of spinal epidural abscess after epidural analgesia: a national 1-year survey. *Anesthesiology.* 1999;91:1928–1936.

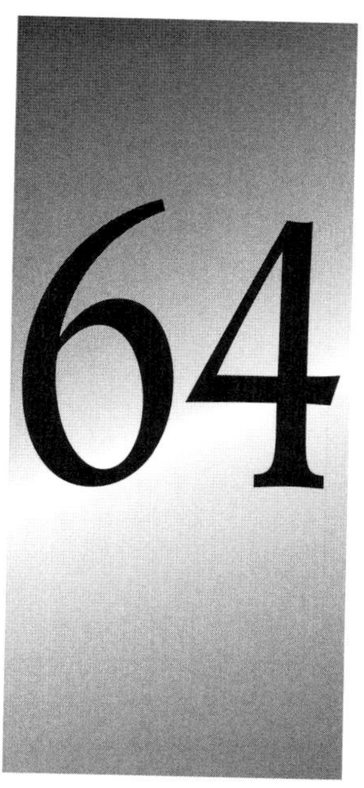

64 Surgery Techniques: Anastomotic Technique and Selection of Location

Simon Law

The technique of esophageal anastomosis seems a subject close to the heart of many surgeons. This may be related mainly to its propensity to leakage. Anastomotic leakage between the esophagus and the conduit used for esophageal replacement is the highest among any surgical anastomosis and is a dreaded complication because of its consequence. It remains a principal cause of surgical sepsis, and its associated morbidity and mortality is high. The incidence of this complication varies widely. A review of surgical series reported in the 1980s revealed an average leakage rate of 12% (1), but even in the modern era in specialized centers, rates of around 10% is sometimes seen (2).

Many aspects of esophagectomy are interrelated and influence the technique and the location of the esophageal anastomosis, such as whether a thoracotomy is used for resection; the intended proximal surgical margin, which in turn is related to the location of the primary tumor; the preferred actual method of construction of the anastomosis; the philosophy toward lymphadenectomy; and so forth. Improvement in surgical techniques is likely to reduce the incidence of leaks, while better management strategy may lead to a reduction in leak-related morbidity and mortality. Other anastomotic problems that are encountered in surgical practice are occurrence of anastomotic stricture and recurrences. Both complications defeat one of the main aims of surgical resection: the relief of dysphagia. It is the purpose of this chapter to apprise some of these problems associated with the esophageal anastomosis. A section specifically on anastomotic leak is described, and aspects on stricture and recurrences are discussed where relevant.

TECHNIQUE OF ESOPHAGEAL ANASTOMOSIS

The esophageal anastomosis can be constructed with either a hand-sewn technique or by using the stapler, which can be a circular or a linear stapler. Individual surgeon preference determines what method of hand-sewn anastomosis and which suture material are used. Careful preparation of the organs for anastomosis, meticulous attention to technical details, and ensuring that the union is tension free result in a very low occurrence of anastomotic leakage. The method of anastomosis is perhaps less important than its proper application. This applies whether the method of anastomosis is 1 or 2 layered, interrupted or continuous, hand-sewn, or stapled.

In the author's practice, all hand-sewn anastomoses are performed in a standard manner regardless of the location of anastomosis or type of substitute used. The circular stapler can be used for anastomosis in the chest or abdomen, but it is awkward to use in the neck because of limited bowel length and confined space. In general, in experienced hands, the stapled and hand-sewn techniques give equivalent leakage rates. The stapled method may be less operator dependent. Long-term follow-up yields more stricture formation for the stapled method (3). The following describes the stapled anastomosis in an intrathoracic anastomosis (both using a circular and a linear side-to-side stapler) and the hand-sewn method suitable for any site.

Anastomosis with a Circular Stapler

For an intrathoracic anastomosis, the esophagus is usually transected at the apex of the thoracic cavity. With the esophagus slightly stretched, a Satinsky clamp is placed across the freed esophagus. The esophagus is divided below the Satinsky clamp by electrocautery. When the Satinsky clamp on the proximal divided esophagus is released, the esophagus retracts upward. Its wall is gently picked up with blunt forceps, and 6 fine stay sutures are placed at equal distances from each other, incorporating all layers of the esophagus and at a depth of 1 cm from the divided margin. It is best if the mucosa is flush with the muscular wall so that no excessive mucosal protrusion or retraction occurs.

An appropriate size stapler is chosen (Figure 64.1). The largest-size stapler that can be inserted safely into the esophagus is chosen because of the increased incidence of anastomotic stricture associated with the smaller-size staplers (3). A purse string is placed around the proximal esophagus using a strong monofilament suture such as 0-Prolene (polypropylene). This is chosen for its sliding property and strength. The purse string suture is placed from adventitia to mucosa starting at the middle of the anterior lip of the esophagus 5 mm from the edge. It is then brought out (mucosa to adventitia), and the subsequent suturing follows this direction over the edge of the esophagus to complete the circle, ending with both ends of the purse string on the outside (Figure 64.2). The stay sutures are kept tight during the placement of the purse string to ensure that each bite takes in an adequate tissue depth and is of full thickness.

For the insertion of the stapler shaft into the stomach, a 2-cm anterior gastrotomy is made in its midbody with electrocautery. Held apart by Babcock forceps, the gastrotomy is dilated with the chosen sizer. The stapling instrument (without the anvil) is inserted into the stomach toward the gastric fundus. The center rod of the stapler shaft is advanced through a clear area on the back of the fundus near the apex, away from blood vessels and the linear staple line. Once the center rod has perforated the gastric wall, the anvil nut is securely fitted and the center rod advanced. No purse string is necessary on the gastric side.

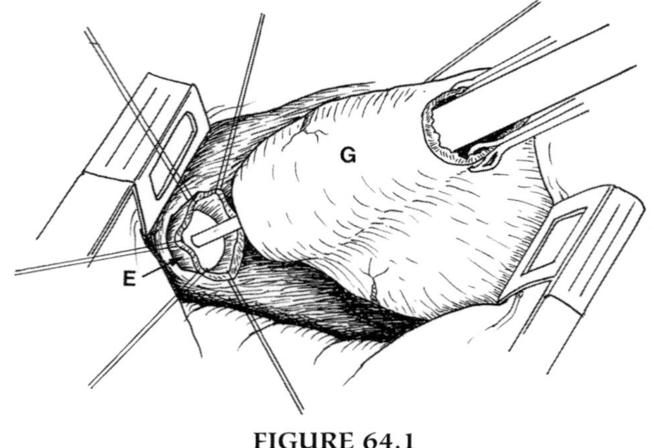

FIGURE 64.1

The stapled anastomosis. After the stapling instrument without the anvil is introduced into the stomach via an anterior gastrotomy, the center rod is advanced through a clear area at the back of the gastric fundus near the apex. With the anvil securely fitted into the center rod, it is placed into the esophagus. E = esophagus; G = gastrotomy.

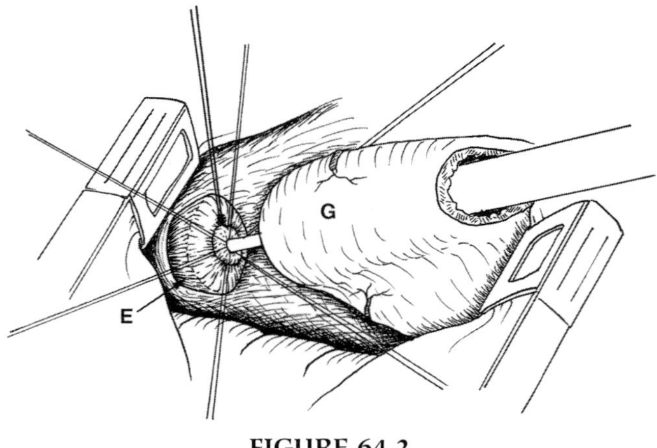

FIGURE 64.2

Appearance of the esophagus after tying the purse string around the anvil of the stapler; the whole device and the esophagus are gently pulled downward and outward, away from the back of the trachea and the mediastinum to avoid accidental inclusion of these structures. The stay sutures are cut and removed at this point.

With the stay sutures held tightly apart, the anvil is inserted into the esophageal lumen. To facilitate insertion, the anvil is first tilted under the anterior lip of the esophageal wall, followed by the posterior lip. The alternate pulling of the anterior stay sutures and the posterior stay sutures will make placement of the esophageal circumference around the anvil easier and minimizes the risk of splitting the esophagus. After the placement of the entire anvil into the esophageal lumen, the purse string is tightened by sliding the monofilament suture back and forth to close the edge of the esophagus around the center rod. The suture is securely fastened around the anvil. The stay sutures should be relaxed when the purse string is being tied and can be removed after the knot is secured.

Before closure of the anvil onto the stapler shaft, the anvil with the proximal esophagus is pulled downward and outward to avoid incorporating the membranous portion of the trachea. The wall of the stomach is also examined to ensure a smooth gastric surface on stapling. The anvil is then apposed to the shaft and fired. The stapler is disengaged and removed by first tilting the posterior part of the anvil through the anastomosis ring. Doughnuts of the esophagus and stomach are recovered from within the shaft and examined for completeness. The integrity of the anastomosis is inspected on the outside and also from the inside by placing 2 small retractors into the stomach. The anterior gastrotomy is closed with a continuous layer of fine monofilament suture after advancement of the nasogastric tube into the stomach.

Anastomosis with a Side-to-Side Linear Stapler

This method is modified from that reported by Collard (4) or Orringer (5). The gastric conduit is brought up to the thoracic cavity. The esophagus is divided, and stay stitches are applied. The stomach is transected with linear staplers and the specimen removed. The divided esophagus is placed medial to the stomach tube. A small gastrotomy is made near the greater curvature and a linear stapler introduced (Antosuture Endo GIA 30–3.5; United States Surgical Corp., Norwalk, CT); the other limb of the stapler is inserted into the esophagus. The stapler is then fired. The remaining opening is either closed with sutures or another stapler (Figures 64.3 and 64.4). This method creates a larger diameter anastomosis compared to an end-to-end or end-to-side anastomosis. In this method, a longer esophageal stump is generally necessary; thus, it may not be very suitable for patients with superior mediastinal segment tumor, when the length of the proximal resection margin may be compromised. Similarly, when used in the neck, a longer esophageal stump and a sufficiently long enough stomach protruding into the neck are required for comfortable introduction of the linear stapler.

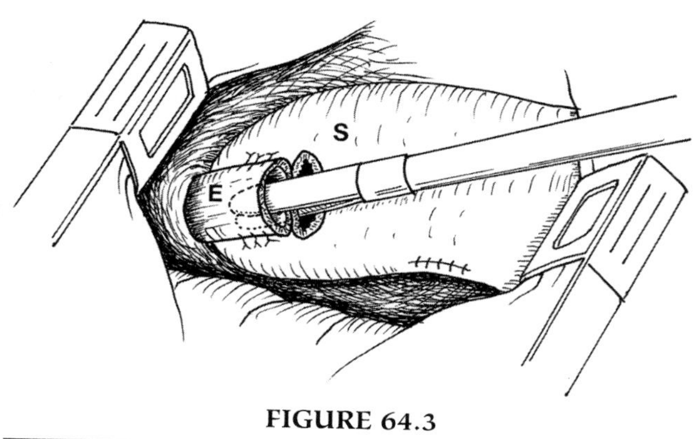

FIGURE 64.3

One lip of the linear stapler is placed through the gastrotomy into the stomach, while the other lip is in the divided esophagus placed next to the greater curvature of the stomach.

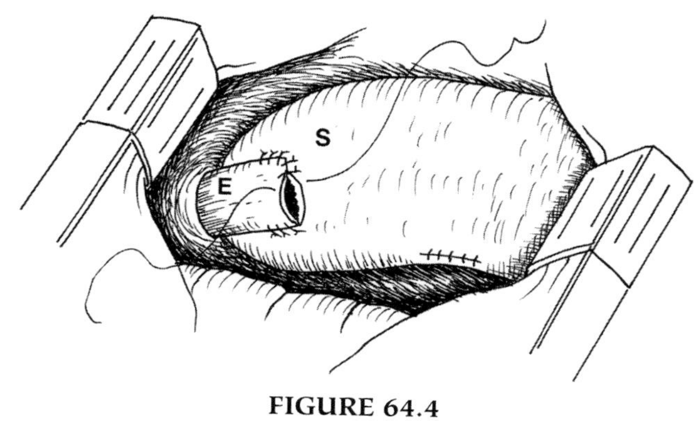

FIGURE 64.4

The stapler has been fired, and the opening is closed by suturing.

The Hand-Sewn Anastomosis

For the hand-sewn anastomosis, the steps in the preparation of the proximal esophagus are the same as described for the stapled anastomosis. Usually only 4 fine stay sutures are placed on the proximal esophagus. For a grossly dilated esophagus, more stay sutures are needed.

Whatever is used as the esophageal substitute, the technique for the anastomosis is the same. When the stomach is used, we commonly used the tip of the linear gastric stapled line where the stomach has been transected, as the gastric tube is usually made small, having resected the redundant fundus. The tip of this stapled line will finally be incorporated into the esophageal anastomosis. Initially a ring of seromuscular wall on the stomach is cut with electrocautery; the size can be adjusted to match the divided esophagus, although the stomach can usually be made smaller, as it tends to enlarge when stretched. The exposed but undivided mucosa is then grasped with another pair of forceps and divided flush with the previous cut on the serosa. This step allows a greater ring of mucosa to be removed, reducing excessive mucosal eversion. It is more convenient to have the stapled line facing anteriorly when the anastomosis is made. This makes a later step of incorporating the apex of this stapled line into the anastomosis easier.

The hand-sewn anastomosis is performed with a single layer of continuous monofilament absorbable sutures, such as 4–0 polyglyconate (Maxon; Davis and Geck, Danbury, CT). This method of anastomosis requires 2 single-armed sutures to be securely tied at the ends (Figure 64.5). The knot is used to anchor inside the bowel lumen, and also 2 lengths are available for use. Depending on the location of the anastomosis and where the surgeon is standing, the first stitch can take the stomach or the esophagus. Thus, for a right-sided intrathoracic anastomosis with the surgeon standing at the back of the patient, the first step is to pass 1 needle from the inside of the stomach to the outside and from the outside of the esophagus into its lumen, beginning on the left border with the surgeon standing on the right side. By pulling the suture on the esophageal side, the knot brings the substitute to the esophagus. Using the needle from the esophageal side, this suture is then continued in an over-and-over manner to complete the posterior wall anastomosis. Full thickness bites of the substitute of at least 5 mm and full thickness of the esophageal wall at 5-mm depth and 5 mm apart are incorporated in the suture. When the posterior wall is completed (Figure 64.6), the suture is continued around the corner in a similar manner to approximately one-third the way across the anterior wall. At the right lateral angle, the suture takes the full thickness of the esophagus with a minimum of mucosa, and on the substitute only the seromuscular layer is incorporated, thus inverting the mucosa on both sides. When this part is completed, the suture is brought from within the lumen to the outside of the stomach.

The rest of the anterior wall anastomosis is begun on the left side with the other needle, which is first brought to the outside through the esophageal wall. The anterior wall is then completed by taking only the seromuscular wall of the substitute but a full thickness of the esophagus with minimal mucosa. Once again, each needle pass should include 5 mm of each side. When the gastric stapled line is incorporated into the anastomosis in a T configuration, it is inverted into the anastomosis. This can be achieved by taking slightly smaller bites of the seromuscular wall only on either sides of the staple line. This step is easier with the stapled line facing anteriorly. Before the anterior layer is finished, a radiopaque nasogastric tube is advanced through the anastomosis into the substitute by the anesthetist. Alternatively, a sterile tube is introduced into the substitute by the surgeon, and the proximal end of the tube is passed upward into the pharynx and brought out through the nose by the anesthetist. At the end of the anastomosis, the 2 sutures should be on opposite sides and can be simply tied (Figure 64.7). After tying, a metal clip is placed near the knot to mark the site of the anastomosis, which helps its identification when a contrast study is performed later

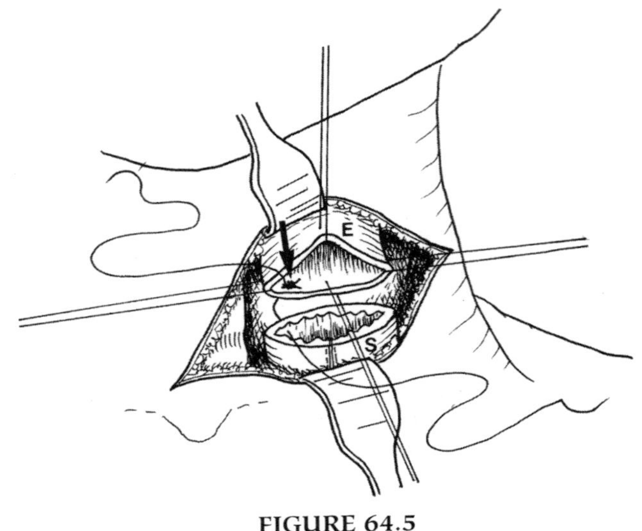

FIGURE 64.5

A left cervical esophagogastrostomy. The anastomosis is made using a continuous single-layer technique with 2 single-armed monofilament absorbable sutures tied at the ends. The esophageal lumen is opened up by 4 stay sutures. The first step is to pass 1 needle from the inside of the esophagus to the outside and from the outside of the stomach into its lumen. The posterior layer can then be completed using a continuous technique. Note that in this case the stapled line of the stomach is facing anteriorly; this will make later inversion of this junction easier. Arrow pointing at the knot of the 2 sutures: this serves as an "anchor" inside the stomach lumen. E = esophagus; S = stomach.

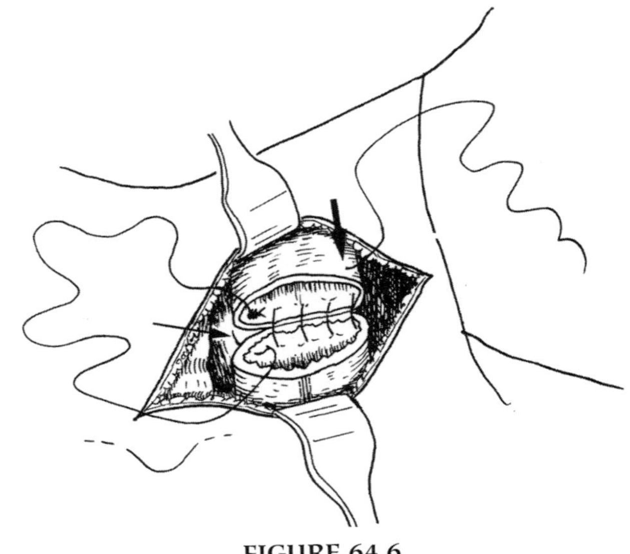

FIGURE 64.6

The posterior wall of the anastomosis is completed. The suture is seen emerging from the lumen of the esophagus after the posterior wall has been completed (large arrow). The other needle is passed from within the stomach wall to the outside (small arrow).

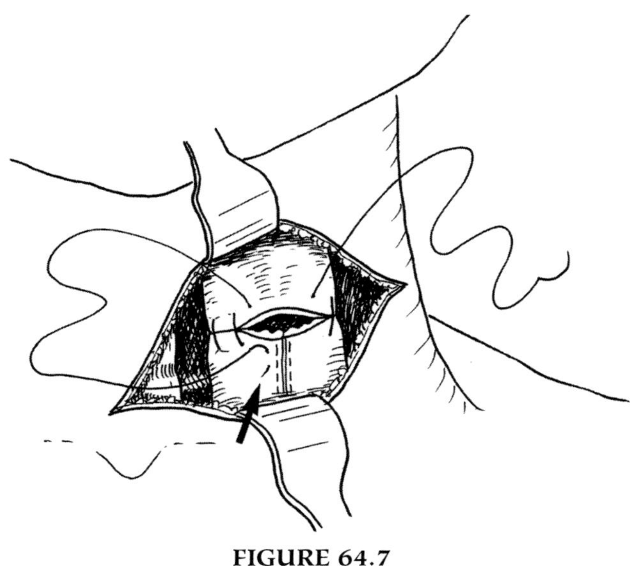

FIGURE 64.7

The anterior wall of the esophagus can be sutured to the stomach. When the stapled line of the stomach is incorporated into the anastomosis, making a T junction, the tip of the stapled line should be inverted into the anastomosis. This is accomplished by taking a small bite of the stomach adjacent to the stapled line at approximately 3 mm from the edge (large arrow). This will invert the stapled line when the suture is tightened. When the left side is reached, the 2 sutures are tied together to complete the anastomosis.

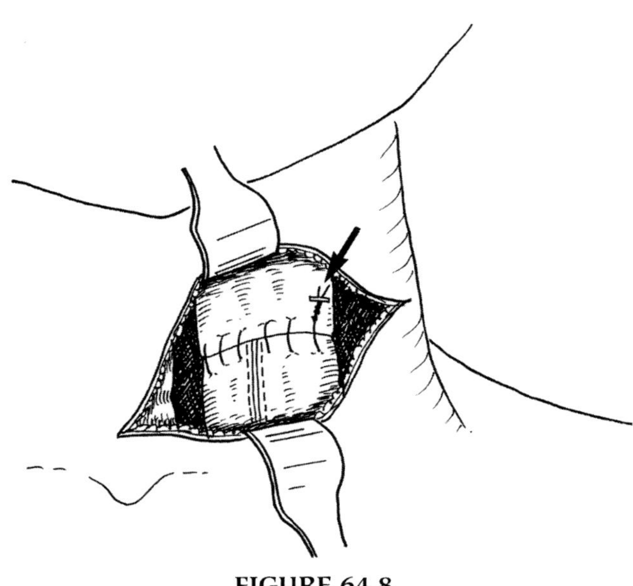

FIGURE 64.8

The completed anastomosis. A metal clip (arrow) is placed near the knot to mark the site of the anastomosis for identification in chest radiograph and subsequent contrast study.

(Figure 64.8). It is important to stress that the esophagus and the substitute are merely apposed by the sutures with minimal tension. Excessive tension will result in tissue strangulation.

Postoperative Management

It is the author's experience that the nasogastric tube can be removed 3 to 4 days after surgery. Early removal also improves patient discomfort and encourages coughing. A meglumine diatrizoate (Gastrografin) contrast swallow is performed 1 week after surgery for documentation, but this may be optional since anastomotic leakage is now a very rare occurrence and in any event is relevant only when leakage is clinically evident. The decision to advance oral diet is based on clinical parameters and not radiological appearance.

SELECTION OF LOCATION OF ANASTOMOSIS

Many considerations determine the location of the esophageal anastomosis. The location of the primary tumor is important. An inadequate resection margin may result in a histologically involved margin and hence subsequent recurrence. The reported prevalence of anastomotic tumor recurrence varied from 2% (6) to 32% (7). The propensity of esophageal cancer to spread intramurally and to have multiple disparate tumors is well recognized and contributes in part to such recurrence. The prevalence of intraepithelial or subepithelial spread was as high as 46% and 54% in 1 report (8). Our own pathologic study by serial sectioning of resected specimens showed a 26% incidence of intramural metastasis (9). The pattern of spread may vary with the depth of invasion of the primary lesion. Contiguous intraepithelial spread frequently exists in early-stage cancer, whereas subepithelial lesions are found in advanced cancer. The deeper the wall penetration of the primary tumor, the further away such spread can take place (8). Some surgeons advocate routine subtotal esophagectomy with cervical anastomosis to attain the longest resection margin regardless of the site of the primary cancer. For tumors located in the superior mediastinal segment, a cervical anastomosis is mandatory. For tumors in the middle and lower esophagus, a choice exists. We have shown previously that the chance of anastomotic recurrence is a function of the length of proximal resection margin obtained at operation. In our patients, all patients who developed recurrences had a proximal margin of less than 5 cm (10). Taking into account shrinkage of the specimen after resection (11), as a guide to surgery, an in situ margin of approximately 10 cm should be the aim (10,12).

The choice of surgical approach is another factor. Proponents of transhiatal resection would routinely perform cervical anastomosis (2). If thoracoscopic or laparoscopic esophagectomy is carried out, then it makes sense again for cervical anastomosis because of the relatively difficult intrathoracic anastomosis by minimally invasive methods, such as the application of the purse-string suture and introduction of the stapler, although some investigators have overcome this problem with innovative modifications of technique (13). When a transthoracic open resection is performed, then either an intrathoracic anastomosis (Lewis-Tanner esopahgectomy) or a cervical esophagectomy (3-phase esophagectomy) can be done. In general, when an intrathoracic anastomosis is performed, the higher the level of anastomosis, the more desirable it is because of the increased resection margin, and also less gastroesophageal reflux symptoms result. In this regard, a narrower gastric tube makes "gastric retention" less likely and thus less reflux.

Another consideration is the sequence of resection and reconstruction. For instance, the situation may arise when a previous gastrectomy exists in a patient and an open thoracotomy resection is planned. A laparotomy may be required first to ensure that a vascularized conduit (such as a colonic loop) of adequate length is available for reconstruction. It is then customary to perform the reconstruction first via the retrosternal route to the neck, followed by an open thoracotomy for tumor resection. In this manner, only 1 patient position change is required. When a 3-phase esophagectomy is performed beginning with a thoracotomy, again a cervical anastomosis is easier to avoid a second position change.

The organ used for esophageal substitution influences the location of the anastomosis. When a gastroesophageal junction tumor involving the gastric cardia is resected with a substantial portion of the proximal stomach, the "distal" stomach when used as the conduit may not be able to reach the neck, thus dictating an intrathoracic esophagogastrostomy. When a colonic interposition is carried out, the anastomosis is usually in the neck to allow a straighter path. When a jejunal conduit is used, an intrathoracic (via a thoracotomy) or low mediastinal (using a stapler via a widened abdominal diaphragmatic hiatus) anastomosis is preferred because of the tedious and often difficult preparation of the loop to reach the neck, risking ischemia.

The surgeon's own anastomotic leakage rate is also a determinant of the anastomotic location because it is generally perceived that a cervical leak is easier to manage and is less lethal compared with a thoracic leak (14). Mortality rates associated with cervical and thoracic leaks were estimated to be around 20% and 60%, respectively (1,15,16), although modern management has improved on this death rate. But if a surgeon is plagued by a high leakage rate, a cervical anastomosis seems more appropriate. Unfortunately, the site of the esophageal anastomosis is also implicated as an important factor predisposing to leakage. Cervical anastomoses seem to have a higher tendency to leak compared with intrathoracic anastomoses. Less than 10% of thoracic anastomoses and 10% to 25% of cervical anastomoses develop insufficiency (14,17–19). A higher leakage rate in the neck may be due to a longer route used (and hence tension created) and compression of the conduit at the thoracic inlet. In this respect the retrosternal route has higher leakage rates compared with the orthotopic route (20).

This higher leak rate in the neck, however, is not universal. It was reported by us and others that similar leakage rates occurred at the 2 sites (10,21,22). In addition, a cervical leak may not be truly confined to the neck since mediastinal contamination from above is common. However, multivariate analysis in our patients did show a higher anastomotic stricture rate with cervical anastomosis (10).

ETIOLOGY AND PREVENTION OF LEAKS

There are many theoretical reasons for why the esophageal anastomosis is so prone to failure (17). The esophagus is believed to be unfavorable anatomically for suturing; it has no serosa like the rest of the gastrointestinal tract, its longitudinal muscle holds sutures poorly, and the anastomosis is carried out in poorly exposed, awkward positions. Other local factors include vascular (both arterial and venous) insufficiency to the gastric fundus (the most commonly used esophageal substitute), tension at the anastomosis, gastric distention in the early postoperative period, and compression at the thoracic inlet compromising a cervical anastomosis. Systemic factors include severe malnutrition, hypoalbuminemia, perioperative hypoxia, or hypotension.

That the esophageal wall is weak and does not hold sutures probably is not the main factor accounting for most anastomotic leaks. In the absence of tension at the anastomosis, its apparent "weakness" is not significant. The stomach is usually of ample length to reach the neck, except perhaps when pharyngogastric anastomosis is performed after pharyngolaryngoesophagectomy for cervical or hypopharyngeal cancers. It is claimed by some investigators that the generally higher leakage rates reported in surgical series from the West compared to that in the East is due to a lower gastric to thoracic length ratio in the former; it is 1.5 to 1.6 in the American population and 2.5 to 2.9 in Japanese (23). The technique of "fundus rotation gastroplasty" is used by some surgeons in order to preserve length as well as vascular supply from the left gastric vessels, and an extra 30% length can be added to the stomach (24,25). The method may well be useful in some situations but oncological clearance may be compromised because of the high incidence of metastatic lymph nodes along the left gastric vessels and lesser curvature of the stomach (26–28). These may not be adequately cleared.

One important factor that contributes to leakage is tissue ischemia; this is more likely from the conduit than the esophagus. The esophagus has a rich submucosal vascular network; this is evident from brisk bleeding often encountered at the esophageal edge when it is cut. The stomach usually has an adequate blood supply if it is prepared with care. Corrosion casts study of the gastric conduit showed that the stomach blood flow can rely on the right gastroepiploic artery alone, with the best blood supply to a 4-cm gastric tube on the greater curvature (29). The right gastric artery can be divided if preservation results in tension to the esophagogastric anastomosis (30). The colon's blood supply is more variable, but preoperative arteriogram may help in identifying reliable vasculature and lessen the risk of graft failure. Arterial anatomic features are favorable in at least 80% of patients with arteriogram examination, and anastomotic leakage rate and graft failure can be less than 2% (31,32).

Vascular insufficiency of the conduit may result if its preparation results in bruising or kinking of the supplying vessels resulting in ischemia, often from inexperience. Clinically inapparent ischemia of the gastric fundus probably contributes to anastomotic failure. The degree of gastric fundal oxygenation measured by oximetry after stomach mobilization correlated with anastomosis healing (33). Others have measured tissue blood flow using laser Doppler flowmetry and intramucosal pH, and these were shown to play some role in predicting anastomotic leaks (34–36). Various innovative methods were proposed to improve vascular supply to the stomach tube. Some authors recommended using the splenic hilar vasculature following a splenectomy to preserve blood supply to the gastric fundus (37); other techniques include additional grafting of the vessel arcades of the substitute organ using microvascular techniques (38), preoperative embolization of the left gastric and splenic artery to "open up" vascular supply via the right gastroepiploic artery (39), and laparoscopic mobilization of the stomach followed by a staged-transthoracic resection a few days later with an aim at "ischemic conditioning" the gastric fundus to improve oxygenation (40). These methods are complicated and remain investigational. Their value in routine use seems limited since a low leakage rate can be obtained using conventional anastomotic techniques anyway.

The advent of the stapling device has lowered the incidence of leakage and was advocated as the preferred method of anastomosis (41–43). The result of circular stapling is certainly less operator dependent. Most surgeons prefer to staple high thoracic anastomosis and suture cervical anastomosis. The linear stapler has also been used with success in some centers for anastomosis in the neck. One group reduced their cervical anastomotic leakage rate from 10% to 15% using a hand-sewn technique to 2.7% using linear staples with a side-to-side anastomosis (5). With experience, however, the hand-sewn method is as safe, if not more so, and certainly less expensive. In the author's unit, leak rates used to be nearly 25% between 1964 and 1982, which has improved to less than 5% and is at present 3% (10,44,45).

For hand anastomosis, a variety of methods are favored. The use of absorbable or nonabsorbable, 1- or 2-layered, continuous, or interrupted sutures remain controversial (20,46–49). The results of most of these techniques are comparable. Other methods have been designed to lower leak rates. These include covering the anastomoses with omentum, pleura, or pericardial fat and using fibrin glue to spray the anastomosis (42, 50–52). None of these are of proven value. A study showed that a larger cross-sectional area of anastomosis resulted in a lower leakage and stricture rate. One hundred patients who underwent transhiatal resections were randomized; in the first group a crescent was excised from the anterior wall of the gastric fundus, and in the second group the fundus was merely opened transversely for esophagogastric anastomosis. The leak rate was 4.3% in the first group compared to 20.8% in the second (53). It is an interesting finding, though the reason is not readily apparent. Pooled data from randomized trials comparing stapled with hand-sewn esophagogastric anastomoses, however, showed no significant difference for leaks (stapled 9%, hand-sewn 8%) but a higher incidence of strictures in stapled anastomoses (stapled 27%, hand-sewn 16%) (54). We had similar findings in our own randomized trial (3). All our anastomoses are now hand-sewn regardless of anatomic sites. On the contrary, an interesting recent study compared 3 techniques of anastomosis: hand-sewn, circular stapler, and side-to-side stapled anastomosis. With careful propensity matching, the investigators showed that leakage rates were similar for all 3 groups (4.3%, 4.3%, and 8.7%, respectively), but postoperative stricture rate was higher for the hand-sewn method (34.8% for the hand-sewn group vs. 8.7% for both the circular and the side-to-side method). The hand-sewn technique employed, however, was mostly a 2-layered interrupted method with silk sutures. Our own 1-layer technique with monofilament suture has a stricture rate of 11% (10).

A drainage procedure in the form of a pyloroplasty or pyloromyotomy of the vagotomized stomach and the placement of a nasogastric tube help decompression of the gastric conduit in the early postoperative period. This reduces distention and hence tension at the anastomosis. Furthermore, delayed gastric emptying is averted (55–57).

Avoiding excessive blood loss during surgery, good pulmonary and cardiovascular support postoperatively to avoid hypoxia and hypotension are also important. Other inconstant factors predisposing to leakage include radiotherapy, chemotherapy, diabetes, age of patient, cirrhosis, and cardiopulmonary diseases (17). Malignant infiltration of the esophageal resection margin was implicated in some studies (15,17) but not in others (48,58). In our own study, a positive resection margin did not predispose to anastomotic leakage (12).

Technical errors probably account for most cases of anastomotic leaks (48,49,59). A recent analysis of our patients who underwent transthoracic resection over a 16-year period showed that of 17 leaks, at least 1 technical or surgical factor was identifiable that had the potential to contribute to leakage. For example, patients in the leak group were significantly more likely to have documented anastomotic technical difficulty, damage to tracheobronchial tree, postoperative gastric outlet obstruction, and reexploration for mediastinal hemorrhage (45). The higher propensity of cervical anastomosis to leak compared to its intrathoracic counterpart has already been mentioned. Many of the finer points in the construction of the esophageal anastomosis were described in the previous section.

ANASTOMOTIC LEAK: DIAGNOSIS AND MANAGEMENT

Early fulminant leaks within the first 48 hours are usually due to punctate necrosis or gangrene of the conduit. The patient may present with septicemia, and a large volume of foul chest tube discharge may be evident. Operative intervention is mandatory. The conduit should be taken down, appropriate debridement and drainage of the thoracic cavity and mediastinum established, a cervical esophagostomy performed, and a feeding enterostomy done for nutritional support. Maximum esophageal length should be preserved to ease future reconstruction.

Clinically apparent thoracic leaks usually take place within the first week. It should be suspected in any patient who is not recovering adequately, such as in those who develop fever, tachycardia, arrhythmia, or poor arterial oxygenation. In our experience, onset of atrial arrhythmia may be an early indication of surgical sepsis, and a proactive search for a source, including anastomotic leak, is mandatory (60). This may be confirmed by excessive output from the chest tube, which may be turbid in color or bile stained. Pleural collections on chest radiograph or computed tomography scans may be evident. Confirmation can be obtained by giving the patient methylene blue dye orally and observing this dye appearing in the chest drainage. The location and magnitude of the leak can be visualized by a water-soluble contrast study. A carefully performed flexible endoscopic examination is also helpful to appreciate the site and size of leakage and should not aggravate the leak if done carefully. The treatment of anastomotic leaks should be individualized. For small contained leaks, conservative observation may suffice. In septic patients with a sizable leak, exploration is warranted. In selected patients, a combination of endoscopically guided nasogastric tube placement for decompression, nasocavity drain for collection drainage, and nasojejunal tube for nutritional support, with or without radiologically guided percutaneous drainage, can be successful without the need for surgical reexploration. Direct repair is seldom possible or effective.

For a cervical anastomosis, leakage is suspected when there is inflammation and pain of the neck wound. Turbid infected discharge is found when the skin stitches are removed. Leaks truly confined to the neck are simply treated by laying the wound open with daily washing and frequent change of dressing. The patient is usually not septic. Leaks that communicate with the mediastinum may require formal exploration and placement of mediastinal drains.

A more recently employed technique is the use of covered stents to occlude the fistula. These can be metallic (40,61,62) or plastic stents (63,64–66). Success in fistula occlusion is generally high (> 90%), with control of sepsis, earlier alimentation, and shorter intensive care and hospital stay (63), although misplacement of stent may worsen the clinical situation, such as enlarging the leak (65). Depending on the type of stent used, subsequent removal may be difficult. Argon beam coagulation was reported as necessary to remove some stents (62). Removal of plastic stent seems easier. On the contrary, stent migration is also another concern. Migration rate can be up to 40%. Stent harvesting from the patients' excrement has been reported (61). Certainly stent insertion for leak occlusion is an attractive minimally invasive option. It is more suitable for intrathoracic compared to cervical leaks; the short proximal esophagus in the latter situation does not provide enough room for stent purchase, and in theory migration is more likely. Some investigators have also reported on the use of a vicryl plug plus fibrin glue injection to hasten healing (67,68). This technique remains investigational.

Subclinical leaks detected by contrast study only may be treated conservatively. Follow-up contrast study is done to monitor healing. Treatment is modified if clinical sepsis occurs or radiologic progression takes place. Drainage should also be considered in leaks close to the trachea or aorta, as bronchogastric fistulation has been reported (69,70).

Treatment of anastomotic leaks has improved over the years. At the author's institute, leakage rate from 1964 to 1982 was 16%; 61% of these patients died, making an overall leak-related mortality rate of 9.8% (44). From 1982 to 1998, leakage rate was 3.5%; 35% of patients died, and leak-related mortality rate was 1.2% (45). In recent years (1996–2002), the corresponding figures were 3.2%, 0% and 0%. Surgical experience should lead to lower leakage rates. A high index of suspicion, timely diagnosis, and intervention will lower the mortality rate from this feared complication of esophageal surgery.

References

1. Muller JM, Erasmi H, Stelzner M, et al. Surgical therapy of oesophageal carcinoma. *Br J Surg.* 1990;77:845–857.
2. Orringer MB, Marshall B, Chang AC, et al. Two thousand transhiatal esophagectomies: changing trends, lessons learned. *Ann Surg.* 2007;246(3):363–372.
3. Law S, Fok M, Chu KM, et al. Comparison of hand-sewn and stapled esophagogastric anastomosis after esophageal resection for cancer: a prospective randomized controlled trial. *Ann Surg.* 1997;226(2):169–173.
4. Collard JM, Romagnoli R, Goncette L, et al. Terminalized semimechanical side-to-side suture technique for cervical esophagogastrostomy. *Ann Thorac Surg.* 1998;65(3):814–817.
5. Orringer MB, Marshall B, Iannettoni MD. Eliminating the cervical esophagogastric anastomotic leak with a side-to-side stapled anastomosis. *J Thorac Cardiovasc Surg.* 2000;119(2):277–288.
6. McKeown KC. The surgical treatment of carcinoma of the oesophagus: a review of the results in 478 cases. *J R Coll Surg Edinb.* 1985;30(1):1–14.
7. Miller C. Carcinoma of the thoracic esophagus and cardia: a review of 405 cases. *Br J Surg.* 1962;49:507–522.
8. Tsutsui S, Kuwano H, Watanabe M, et al. Resection margin for squamous cell carcinoma of the esophagus. *Ann Surg.* 1995;222(2):193–202.
9. Lam KY, Ma LT, Wong J. Measurement of extent of spread of oesophageal squamous carcinoma by serial sectioning. *J Clin Pathol.* 1996;49:124–129.
10. Law S, Suen DT, Wong KH, et al. A single-layer, continuous, hand-sewn method for esophageal anastomosis: prospective evaluation in 218 patients. *Arch Surg.* 2005;140(1):33–39.
11. Siu KF, Cheung HC, Wong J. Shrinkage of the esophagus after resection for carcinoma. *Ann Surg.* 1986;203(2):173–176.
12. Law S, Arcilla C, Chu KM, et al. The significance of histologically infiltrated resection margin after esophagectomy for esophageal cancer. *Am J Surg.* 1998;176:286–290.
13. Misawa K, Hachisuka T, Kuno Y, et al. New procedure for purse-string suture in thoracoscopic esophagectomy with intrathoracic anastomosis. *Surg Endosc.* 2005;19(1):40–42.
14. Chasseray VM, Kiroff GK, Buard JL, et al. Cervical or thoracic anastomisis for esophagectomy for carcinoma. *Surg Gynecol Obstet.* 1989;169:55–62.
15. Patil PK, Patel SG, Mistry RC, et al. Cancer of the esophagus: esophagogastric anastomotic leak—a retrospective study of predisposing factors. *J Surg Oncol.* 1992;49(3):163–167.
16. Giuli R, Gignoux M. Treatment of carcinoma of the esophagus: retrospective study of 2400 patients. *Ann Surg.* 1980;192:44–52.
17. Urschel JD. Esophagogastrostomy anastomotic leaks complicating esophagectomy: a review. *Am J Surg.* 1995;169:634–640.
18. Hankins JR, Attar S, Coughlin TR Jr, et al. Carcinoma of the esophagus: a comparison of the results of transhiatal versus transthoracic resection. *Ann Thorac Surg.* 1989;47:700–705.
19. Shahian DM, Neptune WB, Ellis FH Jr, et al. Transthoracic versus extrathoracic esophagectomy: mortality, morbidity, and long term survival. *Ann Thorac Surg.* 1986;41:237–246.
20. Zieren HU, Muller JM, Pichlmaier H. Prospective randomized study of one- or two-layer anastomosis following oesophageal resection and cervical oesophagogastrostomy. *Br J Surg.* 1993;80(5):608–611.
21. Goldfaden D, Orringer MB, Appelman HD, et al. Adenocarcinoma of the distal esophagus and gastric cardia: comparison of results of transhiatal esophagectomy and thoracoabdominal esophagogastrectomy. *J Thorac Cardiovasc Surg.* 1986;91:242–247.
22. Lam TC, Fok M, Cheng SW, et al. Anastomotic complications after esophagectomy for cancer. A comparison of neck and chest anastomoses. *J Thorac Cardiovasc Surg.* 1992;104(2):395–400.
23. Goldsmith HS, Akiyama H. A comparative study of Japanese and American gastric dimensions. *Ann Surg.* 1979;190(6):690–693.
24. Schilling MK, Mettler D, Redaelli C, et al. Circulatory and anatomic differences among experimental gastric tubes as esophageal replacement. *World J Surg.* 1997;21(9):992–997.
25. Schilling MK, Eichenberger M, Wagener V, et al. Impact of fundus rotation gastroplasty on anastomotic complications after cervical and thoracic oesophagogastrostomies: a prospective non-randomised study. *Eur J Surg.* 2001;167(2):110–114.
26. Law S, Wong J. Commentary on "Circulatory and anatomical differences between experimental gastric tubes as esophageal replacement." *World J Surg.* 1997;21:998.
27. Schroder W, Baldus SE, Monig SP, et al. Lesser curvature lymph node metastases with esophageal squamous cell carcinoma: implications for gastroplasty. *World J Surg.* 2001;25(9):1125–1128.
28. Akiyama H, Tsurumaru M, Udagawa H, et al. Radical lymph node dissection for cancer of the thoracic esophagus. *Ann Surg.* 1994;220(3):364–372.
29. Liebermann-Meffert DMI, Meier R, Siewert JR. Vascular anatomy of the gastric tube used for esophageal reconstruction. *Ann Thorac Surg.* 1992;54:1110–1115.
30. Siewert JR, Stein HJ, Liebermann-Meffert D, et al. Esophageal reconstruction: the gastric tube as esophageal substitute. *Dis Esophagus.* 1995;8:11–19.
31. Peters JH, Kronson JW, Katz M, et al. Arterial anatomic considerations in colon interposition for esophageal replacement. *Arch Surg.* 1995;130:858–863.
32. Davis PA, Law S, Wong J. Colonic interposition after esophagectomy for cancer. *Arch Surg.* 2003;138(3):303–308.
33. Salo JA, Perhoniemi VJ, Heikkinen LO. Pulse oximetry for the assessment of gastric tube circulation in esophageal replacements. *Am J Surg.* 1992;163:446–447.
34. Tarui T, Murata A, Watanabe Y, et al. Earlier prediction of anastomotic insufficiency after thoracic esophagectomy by intramucosal pH. *Crit Care Med.* 1999; 27(9):1824–1831.
35. Pierie JP, de Graaf PW, Poen H, et al. Impaired healing of cervical oesophagogastrostomies can be predicted by estimation of gastric serosal blood perfusion by laser Doppler flowmetry. *Eur J Surg.* 1994;160(11):599–603.
36. Ikeda Y, Niimi M, Kan S, et al. Clinical significance of tissue blood flow during esophagectomy by laser Doppler flowmetry. *J Thorac Cardiovasc Surg.* 2001;122(6):1101–1106.
37. Ueo H, Abe R, Takeuchi H, et al. A reliable operative precedure for preparing a sufficiently nourished gastric tube for esophageal reconstruction. *Am J Surg.* 1993;165:273–276.
38. Hirabayashi S, Miyata M, Shoji M, et al. Reconstruction of the thoracic esophagus, with extended jejunum used as a substitute, with the aid of microvascular anastomosis. *Surgery.* 1993;113:515–519.
39. Akiyama S, Ito S, Sekiguchi H, et al. Preoperative embolization of gastric arteries for esophageal cancer. *Surgery.* 1996;120:542–546.
40. Holscher AH, Schneider PM, Gutschow C, et al. Laparoscopic ischemic conditioning of the stomach for esophageal replacement. *Ann Surg.* 2007;245(2):241–246.
41. Hopkins RA, Alexander JC, Postlethwait RW. Stapled esophagogastric anastomosis. *Am J Surg.* 1984;147:283–287.
42. Fekete F, Breil PH, Ronsse H, et al. EEA stapler and omental graft in esophagogastrectomy: experience with 30 intrathoracic anastomoses for cancer. *Ann Surg.* 1981;193:825–830.
43. Wong J, Cheung HC, Lui R, et al. Esophagogastric anastomosis performed with a stapler: the occurence of leakage and stricture. *Surgery.* 1987;101:408–415.
44. Lorentz T, Fok M, Wong J. Anastomotic leakage after resection and bypass for esophageal cancer: lessons learned from the past. *World J Surg.* 1989;13(4):472–477.
45. Whooley BP, Law S, Alexandrou A, et al. Critical appraisal of the significance of intrathoracic anastomotic leakage after esophagectomy for cancer. *Am J Surg.* 2001;181(3):198–203.
46. Bardini R, Bonavina L, Asolati M, et al. Single-layered cervical esophageal anastomoses: a prospective study of two suturing techniques. *Ann Thorac Surg.* 1994;58:1087–1090.
47. Fok M, Ah Chong AK, Cheng SW, et al. Comparison of a single layer continuous hand-sewn method and circular stapling in 580 oesophageal anastomoses. *Br J Surg.* 1991;78(3):342–345.
48. Peracchia A, Bardini R, Ruol A, et al. Esophagovisceral anastomotic leak: a prospective statistical study of predisposing factors. *J Thorac Cardiovasc Surg.* 1988;95(4):685–691.
49. Dewar L, Gelfand G, Finley RJ, et al. Factors affecting cervical anastomotic leak and stricture formation following esophagogastrectomy and gastric tube interposition. *Am J Surg.* 1992;163:484–489.
50. Mathisen DJ, Grillo HC, Wilkins E Jr, et al. Transthoracic esophagectomy: a safe approach to carcinoma of the esophagus. *Ann Thorac Surg.* 1988;45:137–143.
51. Goldsmith HS, Kiely AA, Randall HT. Protection of intrathoracic esophageal anastomoses by omentum. *Surgery.* 1968;63:464–468.
52. Hsu HK, Hsu WH, Huang MH. Prospective study of using fibrin glue to prevent leak from esophagogastric anastomosis. *J Surg Assoc ROC.* 1992;25:1248–1252.
53. Gupta NM, Gupta R, Rao MS, et al. Minimizing cervical esophageal anastomotic complications by a modified technique. *Am J Surg.* 2001;181(6):534–539.
54. Urschel JD, Blewett CJ, Bennett WF, et al. Handsewn or stapled esophagogastric anastomoses after esophagectomy for cancer: meta-analysis of randomized controlled trials. *Dis Esophagus.* 2001;14(3–4):212–217.
55. Fok M, Cheng SW, Wong J. Pyloroplasty versus no drainage in gastric replacement of the esophagus. *Am J Surg.* 1991;162(5):447–452.

56. Law S, Cheung MC, Fok M, et al. Pyloroplasty and pyloromyotomy in gastric replacement of the esophagus after esophagectomy: a randomized controlled trial. *J Am Coll Surg.* 1997;184(6):630–636.
57. Lee YM, Law S, Chu KM, et al. Pyloroplasty in gastric replacement of the esophagus after esophagectomy: one-layer or two-layer technique? *Dis Esophagus.* 2000;13(3):203–206.
58. Wilson SE, Stone R, Scully M, et al. Modern management of anastomotic leak after esophagogastrectomy. *Am J Surg.* 1982;144:95–101.
59. Law SY, Fok M, Wong J. Risk analysis in resection of squamous cell carcinoma of the esophagus. *World J Surg.* 1994;18(3):339–346.
60. Murthy SC, Law S, Whooley BP, et al. Atrial fibrillation after esophagectomy is a marker for postoperative morbidity and mortality. *J Thorac Cardiovasc Surg.* 2003;126(4):1162–1167.
61. Kauer WK, Stein HJ, Dittler HJ, et al. Stent implantation as a treatment option in patients with thoracic anastomotic leaks after esophagectomy. *Surg Endosc.* 2008;22(1):50–53.
62. Doniec JM, Schniewind B, Kahlke V, et al. Therapy of anastomotic leaks by means of covered self-expanding metallic stents after esophagogastrectomy. *Endoscopy.* 2003;35(8):652–658.
63. Hunerbein M, Stroszczynski C, Moesta KT, et al. Treatment of thoracic anastomotic leaks after esophagectomy with self-expanding plastic stents. *Ann Surg.* 2004;240(5):801–807.
64. Gelbmann CM, Ratiu NL, Rath HC, et al. Use of self-expandable plastic stents for the treatment of esophageal perforations and symptomatic anastomotic leaks. *Endoscopy.* 2004;36(8):695–699.
65. Langer FB, Wenzl E, Prager G, T et al. Management of postoperative esophageal leaks with the Polyflex self-expanding covered plastic stent. *Ann Thorac Surg.* 2005;79(2):398–403.
66. Schubert D, Scheidbach H, Kuhn R, et al. Endoscopic treatment of thoracic esophageal anastomotic leaks by using silicone-covered, self-expanding polyester stents. *Gastrointest Endosc.* 2005;61(7):891–896.
67. Pross M, Manger T, Reinheckel T, et al. Endoscopic treatment of clinically symptomatic leaks of thoracic esophageal anastomoses. *Gastrointest Endosc.* 2000; 51(1):73–76.
68. Truong S, Bohm G, Klinge U, et al. Results after endoscopic treatment of postoperative upper gastrointestinal fistulas and leaks using combined Vicryl plug and fibrin glue. *Surg Endosc.* 2004;18(7):1105–1108.
69. Bona D, Sarli D, Saino G, et al. Successful conservative management of benign gastro-bronchial fistula after intrathoracic esophagogastrostomy. *Ann Thorac Surg.* 2007;84(3):1036–1038.
70. Mok VW, Ting AC, Law S, et al. Combined endovascular stent grafting and endoscopic injection of fibrin sealant for aortoenteric fistula complicating esophagectomy. *J Vasc Surg.* 2004;40(6):1234–1237.

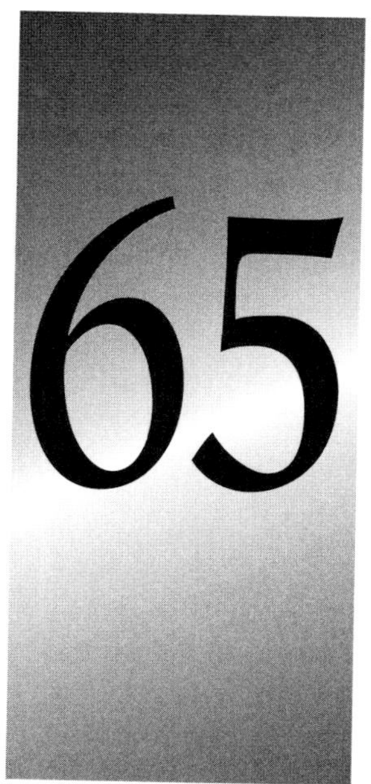

65 Surgery Techniques: Conduit Preparation and Route of Reconstruction

Arnulf H. Hölscher

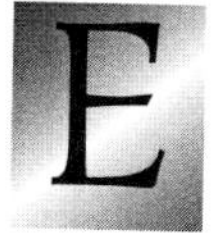

Esophageal replacement after subtotal esophagectomy can be performed using stomach or colon. The small bowel is rarely suitable for total substitution of the esophagus. Jejunal interposition does have a place, however, for partial esophageal replacement of both proximal and distal esophagus. The construction of a gastric conduit and its pull-up is the technically simplest form for esophageal replacement. Furthermore, as it guarantees good long-term functional results, it has become the method of first choice, especially after esophagectomy for cancer. It is only when the stomach is not available because of previous gastric surgery or after esophagogastrectomy or in benign esophageal diseases that colonic interposition is used.

Further, the location of the anastomosis (see the following chapter) and the route of the reconstruction have to be selected. Basically, the posterior or the anterior mediastinum can be used for the pull-up of the conduit. The antesternal subcutaneous route is usually not indicated. The time of reconstruction can be chosen as either directly after esophageal resection as a 1-stage procedure or delayed.

STOMACH CONDUIT

History

The use of the stomach as esophageal replacement has been introduced by Kirschner in 1920 as a nonresectional operative bypass. He mobilized the stomach and brought it antesternal subcutaneously up to the divided cervical esophagus. The application of gastric pull-up using either the orthotopic route in the posterior mediastinum or the retrosternal space after esophagectomy was introduced and standardized by Ong, Nakayama, and Akiyama.

Preoperative Examinations

The stomach may be used as an esophageal substitute only if it has not previously been operated on. Following gastric resections, the length will be insufficient, and after vagotomy procedures the vascularization is doubtful. If lesser procedures such as suturing of a bleeding ulcer or closure of a perforation have been performed, then a transposition of the stomach may be possible, but the vascularity should be checked at the beginning of the operation. A preoperative gastroscopy should be carried out to exclude any mucosal pathology and to confirm the borders of the esophageal tumor. If the cancer is infiltrating the cardia or the subcardial area, the safety margin between the lower edge of the tumor and the resection line of the gastric conduit may not be sufficient. In this case, a narrow gastric tube can be constructed, or alternative methods of esophageal replacement have to be applied. In all cases in which the use of the stomach is doubtful, the colon should be prepared by preoperative bowel lavage and colonoscopy.

Vascularization of the Stomach

The knowledge of the arterial blood supply of the stomach is essential for the preparation of a well-vascularized gastric conduit (1). The arterial supply of the stomach originates from the celiac trunc. Four vessels are important (Figure 65.1):

- Left gastric artery
- Right gastric artery
- Right gastroepiploic artery
- Left gastroepiploic artery

The *left gastric artery* comes mostly from the celiac trunk and runs to the subcardial lesser curvature. There it turns in an aboral direction and supplies the anterior and posterior gastric wall by small branches.

The *right gastric artery* originates from the proper hepatic artery and proceeds to the lesser curvature from the pylorus in an oral direction. By those means, an arterial ring along the lesser curvature is completed with its strongest inflow being from the left gastric artery.

The *right gastroepiploic artery* arises from the gastroduodenal artery and runs along the greater curvature in an oral direction. It is the most important artery for the conduit.

The *left gastroepiploic artery* originates from the splenic artery and runs through the gastrocolic ligament parallel to the greater curvature in an aboral direction. This artery gives gastric branches to both walls of the stomach and anastomosis mostly with the right gastroepiploic artery. This arterial ring, however, can have considerable arterial variations. The upper part of the greater curvature and the fundus are further supplied from the short gastric arteries, which arise from the splenic artery at the splenic hilus.

All 4 gastric arteries anastomosis between themselves directly or indirectly by intra- or extramural branches. This phenomenon preserves the vascularization of the gastric conduit, which affords the division of the left gastric and left gastroepiploic artery.

The veins of the stomach lead the blood to the portal vein and are of similar importance for a good conduit as the arteries. With only minor exceptions, they correspond in their names and their course to the 4 gastric arteries. The left gastric vein, or so-called coronary vein, and the left gastroepiploic vein as well as the short gastric veins have to be divided for mobilization of the conduit.

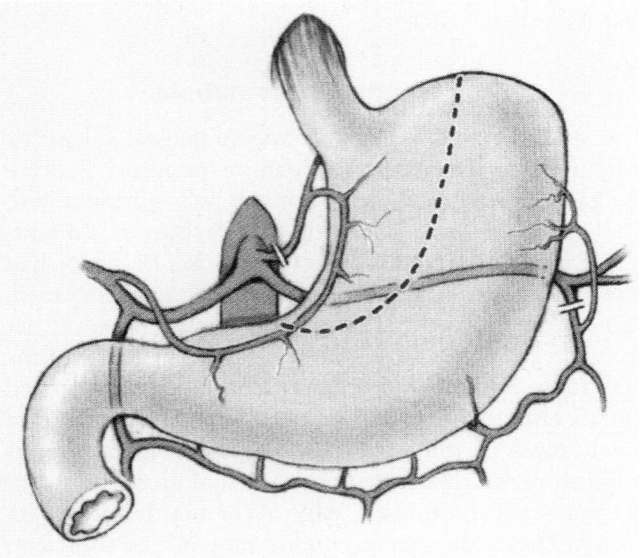

FIGURE 65.1

Normal vascular anatomy of the stomach and outline of conduit preparation.

Open Surgical Technique

General Remarks

The patient lies in a supine position, and if a cervical esophagogastrostomy is planned, the head is turned to the right for an easy approach to the left side of the neck. The abdomen is opened by an upper midline incision in direction of the xiphoid process. An alternative is the combination of an upper midline and a transverse incision, which ensures a very good overview of the upper abdomen. The revision of the abdomen is important to rule out distant metastases and to clarify a possible tumor infiltration of the cardia or the subcardial region. This has to be taken into account for tailoring the gastric conduit.

Preparation of the Stomach

The first step is the dissection of the lesser omentum and the preparation of the right diaphragmatic crus (1). After incision of the peritoneal coverage of the abdominal esophagus, the hiatus is prepared and the esophagus taped (Figure 65.2). If an advanced distal tumor is infiltrating the cardia, a cuff of the crura of the diaphragm may be resected en bloc with the esophagus in order to increase radicality. The left crus is prepared, and neighbored easily accessible upper short gastric vessels can also be dissected at this stage. The skeletonization of the stomach begins along the greater curvature outside the gastroepiploic arch in a thin transparent part of the gastrocolonic ligament. This can be facilitated by lifting the stomach up with a forceps or the hand through the omental bursa along the lesser curvature. The skeletonization is performed stepwise first in direction to the fundus and then to the pylorus (Figure 65.3). After dividing the left gastroepiploic artery and vein, the preparation of the short gastric vessels may be performed close to the gastric wall. The dissection of the gastrosplenic and the gastrocolic ligament is easiest with an "ultrasonic sheers" or "Ligasure" device but can also be done using ligations or suture ligations. As the gastroepiploic arch together with the right gastric artery will be the only contributors to the gastric tube, their preparation calls for the utmost care in order to guarantee their potency. Especially the origin of the right gastroepiploic artery and vein has to be handled with care (Figure 65.4). Adhesions of the stomach and the duodenum to the gallbladder have to be dissected. The right colonic flexure must be freed, and the duodenum should be mobilized with a Kocher maneuver so that the pylorus can move upward during the gastric pull-up. However, for an intrathoracic anastomosis of the gastric conduit, the complete Kocher maneuver mostly is not necessary.

Lymph Node Dissection

Now the stomach can be lifted up, and a good access to the omental burse is possible for the lymphadenectomy (Figure 65.5). The lymph nodes are dissected in a manner similar to that which is carried out in gastric cancer. This means that all lymph nodes along the common hepatic artery, the celiac trunc, and the medial part of the splenic artery are dissected and taken with the specimen.

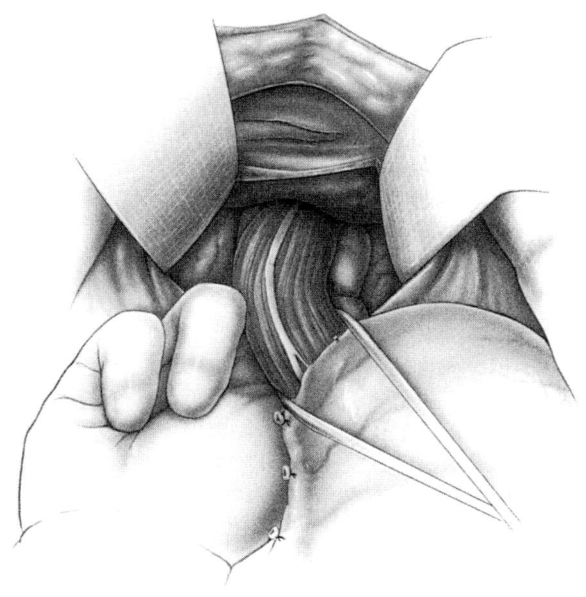

FIGURE 65.2

Preparation of the distal esophagus in the lower mediastinum.

FIGURE 65.3

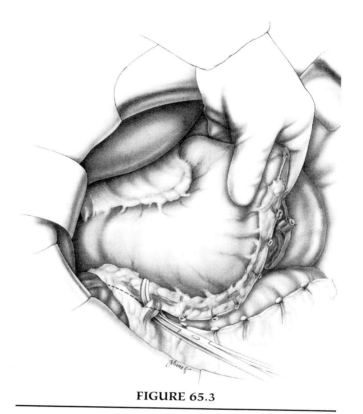

Skeletonization of the stomach outside the gastroepiploic arch.

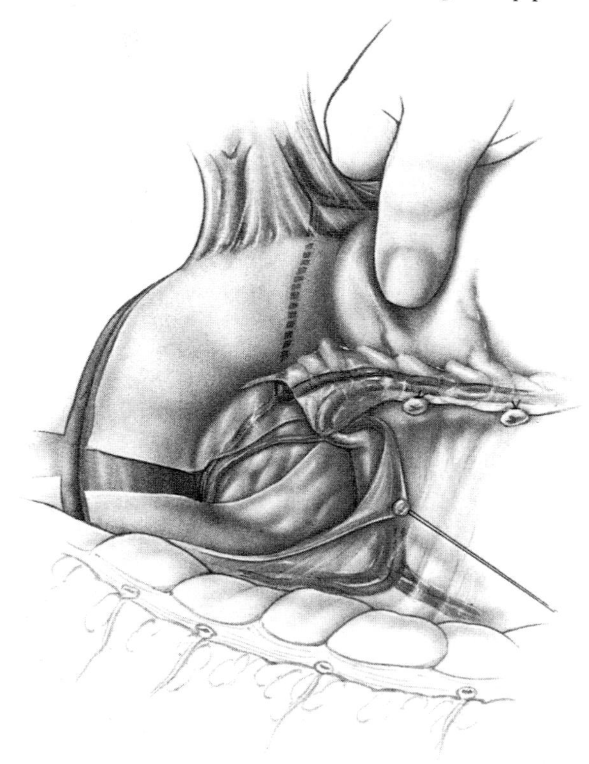

FIGURE 65.4

Preservation of the right gastroepiploic artery and vein.

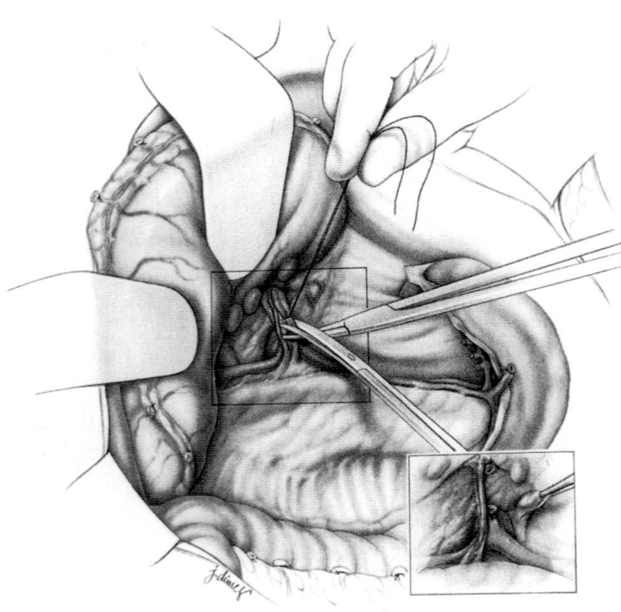

FIGURE 65.5

Dissection and suture ligation of the left gastric artery and vein and lymph node dissection at the common hepatic and splenic artery.

The ligation of the left gastric artery and vein is performed near its trunk of origin. After dissecting final adhesions between the lesser curvature and the right and left crus, the stomach is completely freed except its connection to the esophagus and duodenum.

Formation of the Gastric Conduit

Choice of Procedure

The formation of the conduit depends on the location of the tumor, on the type of anastomosis (cervical or intrathoracic), and on whether the reconstruction is performed with a gastric tube or the whole stomach. If an esophageal adenocarcinoma is infiltrating the cardia or even the subcardial region, the safety margin toward the cardia has to be larger compared to a mid-esophageal squamous cell carcinoma. If an intrathoracic anastomosis is planned, the final tailoring of the conduit can be done in the chest, whereas for a cervical anastomosis, the conduit has to be finished in the abdomen.

The great majority of esophageal surgeons today use a gastric conduit of 4 to 5 cm in diameter (1,2). The arguments for the whole stomach are the preservation of the intramural vascular network and the greater reservoir (3). Another issue is the necessity of a pyloroplasty. Prospective randomized trials have shown that a pyloroplasty does not lead to significantly better results than no pyloroplasty. Patients without pyloroplasty and delayed gastric emptying in the postoperative phase usually recover or can have endoscopic pyloric balloon dilatation. As an advantage, their long-term pyloric sphincter function is preserved, avoiding bile reflux. If there are special indications, a Heinecke-Mikulicz procedure can be performed during conduit preparation in the typical way. However, leakages of this suture line can happen because of the stress after gastric pull-up. An alternative is the pyloric dilatation with a large forceps via an incision at the lesser curvature (1). This is the preferred method of the author in open surgery. The incision of the lesser curvature can be closed and stapled off with the resection of the lesser curvature later.

Intrathoracic Final Conduit Formation

If an intrathoracic esophagogastrostomy is planned, which is preferred by the author, the fat tissue of the lesser curvature between the middle and distal third is dissected in oral direction for 2 cm. After closure of the abdomen and right thoracotomy, the en bloc esophagectomy is performed with dissection of the esophagus high up in the thorax. The entire stomach is pulled up in the right pleural cavity, and the circular stapler is inserted through an incision at the upper third of the lesser curvature (Figure 65.6[a]). The sharp tip of the stapler is perforated through the left anterior wall of the fundus, and after connection and closure of the stapler, the anastomosis is performed. Now the esophagus, the right part of the fundus, and the upper two-thirds of the lesser curvature, including the former introduction site of the stapler, are resected en bloc after placing 1 or 2 TA 90 linear staplers (Autosuture Covidien) (Figure 65.6[b]). The lesser curvature stapler line is oversewn with interrupted 3.0 Vicryl sutures to avoid bleeding. This leaves a gastric conduit of 4 to 5 cm in diameter behind (Figure 65.7). If the diaphragmatic hiatus is too wide f.e., in case of hiatal hernia the crus are narrowed by nonresorbable sutures but without stenosing the conduit.

Conduit for Cervical Anastomosis

This type of anastomosis affords the complete finishing of the conduit in the abdomen before gastric pull-up and esophagogastrostomy in the neck. The esophagus, which has previously been dissected by a transthoracic or transmediastinal approach, is pulled out of the esophageal hiatus for the final preparation of the gastric tube. After dissecting the fat tissue and the vessels at the lesser curvature between the middle and distal third for 2 cm, the stomach is stretched by careful pulling at the highest point, which is quite a distance to the left of the cardia. One or 2 TA 90 stapler lines (Covidien) are now placed

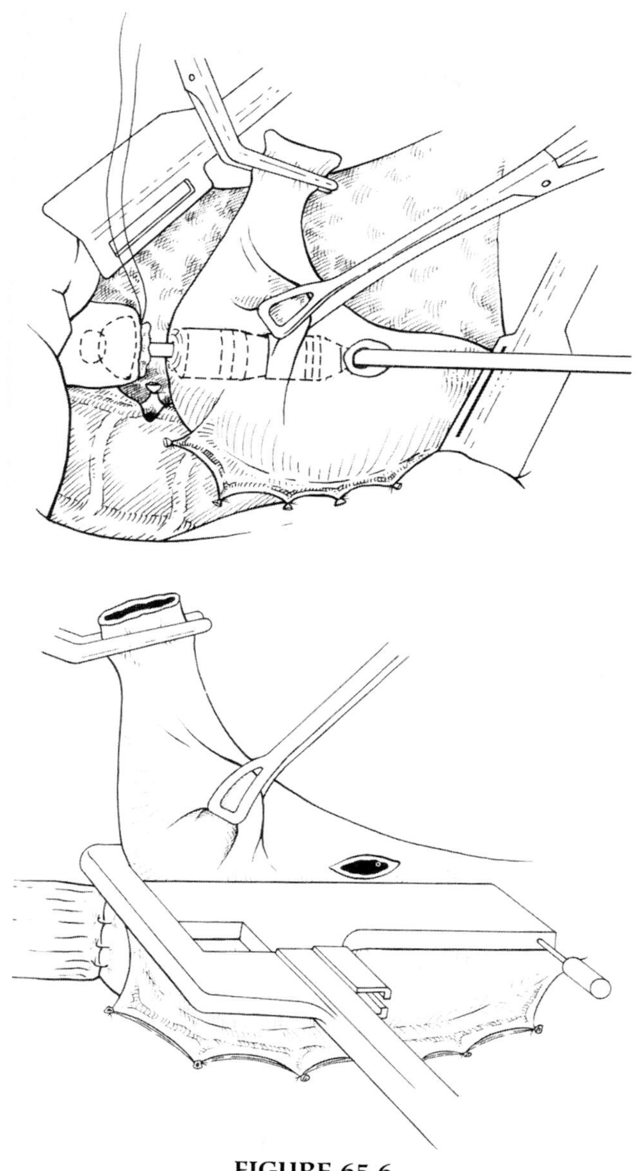

FIGURE 65.6

Gastric pull-up into the right pleural cavity after esophagectomy. (a) The stapler is pushed through an opening of the subcardial lesser curvature, and after perforation of the central rod at the anterior wall of the fundus, it is connected with the purse string sutured anvil in the esophageal stump. (b) Resection of the lesser curvature and the gastrostomy en bloc with the esophagus by applying the TA 90 stapler and final formation of the gastric conduit.

between the area of skeletonization at the lesser curvature and right to the highest point of the gastric fundus (Figure 65.8). Before complete stapling, the pylorus dilatation can be performed with a long forceps inserted via the nonstapled area at the lesser curvature (see the previous discussion). The staple line can be oversewn by interrupted sutures in case of bleeding because electric coagulation should be avoided on the staples. The pull-up of the gastric conduit should be done with special carefulness in order to avoid serosal tears and disturbance of intramural vascularization. Therefore, the procedure should be a combination of pushing and careful pulling under protection of a plastic bag.

Whole Stomach Conduit

It is possible to use the whole stomach rather than a gastric tube as the esophageal interposition. This can be performed only if the tumor is not infiltrating the gastroesophageal junction. The skeletonization should start at the same point and in the same manner as for the formation of the gastric tube. However, it is continued along the lesser curvature up to the cardia as for highly selective vagotomy. The staple line using a TA 55 stapler (Covidien) is then placed directly below the cardia to preserve the whole gastric fundus. Pyloric dilatation should be performed through an additional incision in the subcardial stomach, which is closed afterward by stapler. The alternative is a Heinecke-Mikulicz pyloroplasty. The advantage of using the whole stomach as the esophageal substitute is that the intramural vascular network at the lesser curvature is preserved and that the gastroesophageal anastomosis does not include the tangential staple line at the highest point of the gastric fundus (3,4). This may avoid a "locus minoris resistentiae" of such an anastomosis.

Laparoscopic Technique

The minimal invasive technique in conduit preparation follows the same rules as the open technique mentioned previously. The laparoscopic procedure is performed in supine position of the patient with straddled legs (2,5). The surgeon stands between the patient's legs. Five abdominal ports (9 × 5 mm and 4 × 11 mm) are used for the dissection. The gastrohepatic ligament is divided, and the right and left crura of the diaphragm are dissected. The phrenoesophageal membrane is divided, and the lower mediastinum is entered to dissect the lower esophagus. In case of distal esophageal carcinoma in advanced stage, superficial parts of the right and left crura are dissected and remain as a cover of the esophagus. The pericardium is prepared, and the right and left pleura are not opened. If the pleura is opened on 1 side, a chest tube is inserted. The stomach is freed by dividing the short gastric vessels using the Ligasure device (Autosuture, Covidien). The gastrocolic omentum is carefully divided, preserving the right gastroepiploic arcade. The right colonic flexure is detached, and a Kocher maneuver is performed. Retrogastric adhesions are dissected, and the gastroduodenal

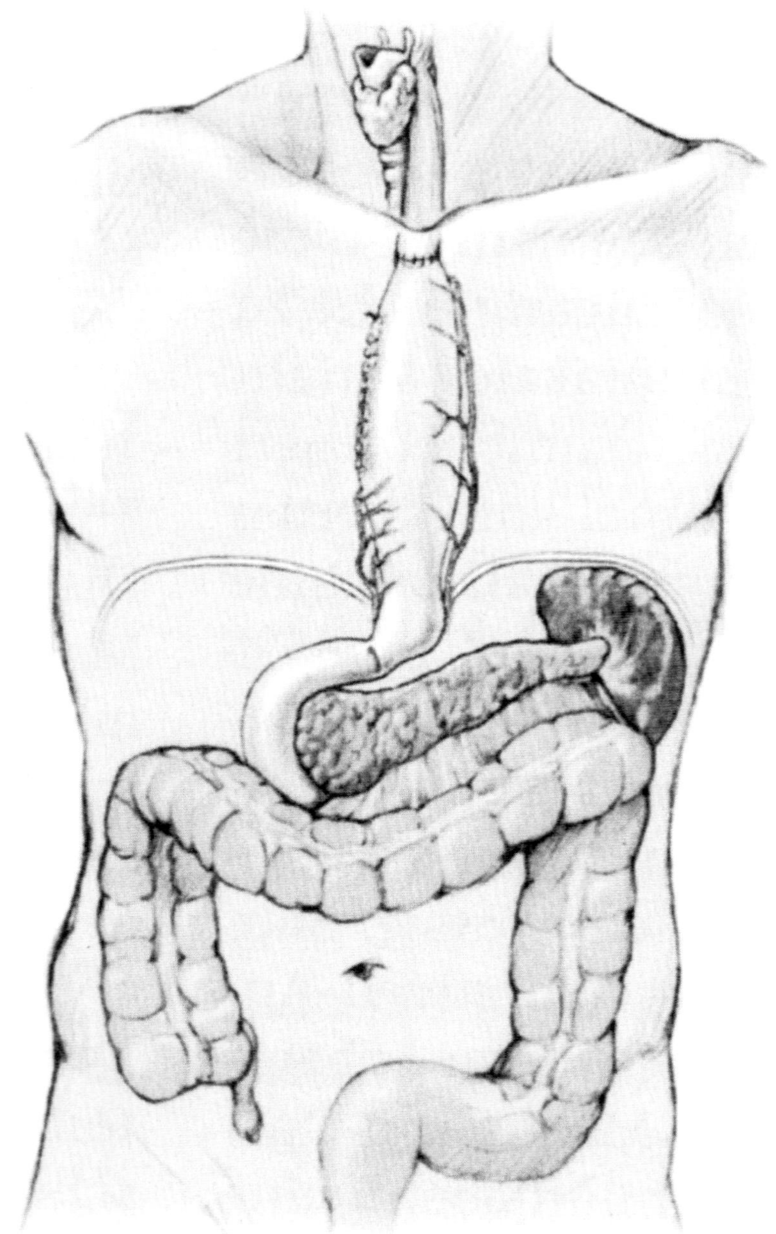

FIGURE 65.7

Final aspect after gastric pull-up and high intrathoracic esophagogastrostomy.

artery as well as the right gastroepiploic artery and vein are visualized. The stomach is retracted superiorly, and the superior edge of the pancreas is exposed. The common hepatic artery and the central part of the splenic artery are cleared of the surrounding lymphatic tissue. The fatty tissue around the origin of the left gastric artery and vein is dissected so that the lymph nodes of group 7 remain at the left gastric artery. The left gastric vein is closed with the Ligasure. The left gastric artery is closed with 2 laparoclips and cut in between. The right gastric

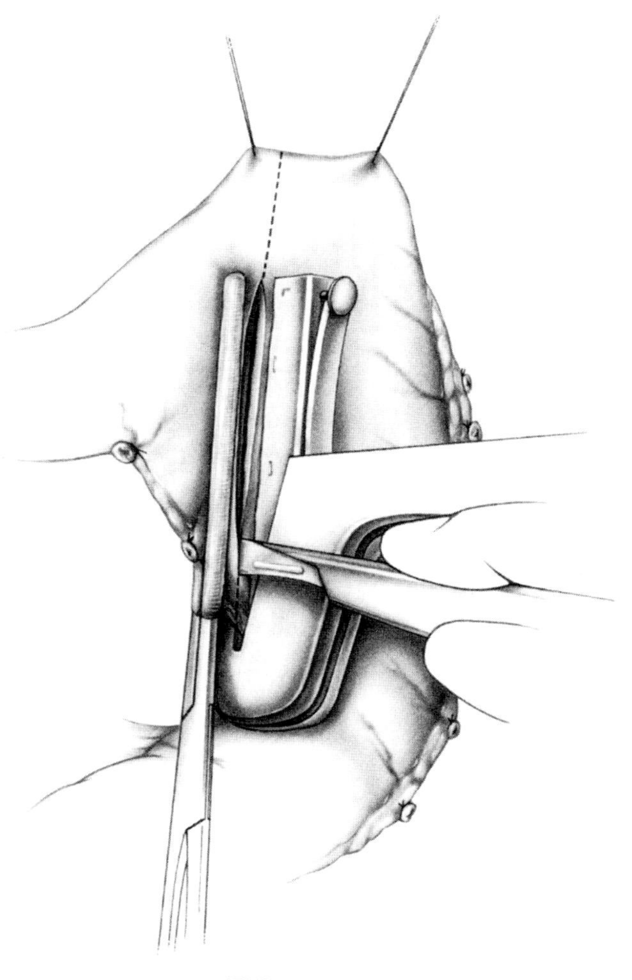

FIGURE 65.8

Resection of the lesser curvature, the right part of the fundus en bloc with the esophagus and formation of a 4 to 5 wide gastric conduit by stapler.

artery is preserved. The fat tissue of the lesser curvature between the middle and distal third is dissected with the Ligasure in an oral direction of 2–3 cm. No pyloroplasty is performed during laparoscopy. In case of a narrow hiatus, the right crura are partially divided to allow an easy passage later of the gastric tube through the hiatus and to prevent gastric outlet obstruction. The 5 port sites are closed.

Ischemic Conditioning

Anatomic studies focusing on the gastric vascularization demonstrated a rarefaction of the intramural vessels of the upper part of the gastric conduit (4). Experiments in animals and clinical studies have shown that, after ligation of the left gastric and the left gastroepiploic artery, mucosal pCO_2 as indicator of microcirculation significantly rises and gastric blood flow is reduced to about 50% (6). Ischemic conditioning, also described as a delay phenomenon, is derived from the creation of skin flaps. In animal experiments, the effect of conditioning is also well analyzed for the gastric conduit and esophagogastrostomy (7). The theoretical background is that after partial devascularization, the gastric conduit should recover, and tissue perfusion should be improved prior to gastric pull-up and anastomosis to the esophagus. This should result in better prerequisites for anastomotic healing. Our own studies demonstrated that mucosal pCO_2 of the stomach initially rises and declines to basic values 4 to 5 days after devascularization and gastric pull-up (6). Therefore, the concept is laparoscopic preparation of the gastric conduit and delayed esophagectomy and reconstruction at the fifth postoperative day (5). The patient is usually extubated in the operation room and transferred to the normal ward. He or she is allowed to drink liquids and soup as well as caloric drinks starting on the evening of the day of operation. Five days after the laparoscopic procedure, a right-sided transthoracic en bloc esophagectomy and esophagogastrostomy is performed. In a first series of 83 patients, it was shown that laparoscopic ischemic conditioning of the stomach for esophageal replacement is feasible and safe. There was no 90-day mortality in this group of patients (5). The real indication for this procedure has to be defined in further studies; however, especially for risky patients, it can be an advantage.

COLON CONDUIT

Vascularization of the Colon

The arterial blood supply of the colon comes from the superior as well as the inferior mesenteric artery (Figure 65.9). The requirements for a successful colon interposition are an artery and vein of adequate caliber extending continuously along a sufficient length of colon (8). It is nearly always possible to prepare such a conduit of about 40 cm for esophageal replacement. The prerequisite is a careful complete mobilization of both colonic flexures, the ascending, transverse, descending, and also, partially, sigmoid colon. By these means, the colon can be eventerated, and a diaphanoscopy of the mesentery can help clarify the vascularization.

Preoperative Examinations and Approach

Preoperative cleansing of the bowel and colonoscopy is suggested to detect and remove polyps. However, there are no evidence-based data showing that this is beneficial (9). The patient should be placed in a supine position, and a long median laparotomy is most appropriate.

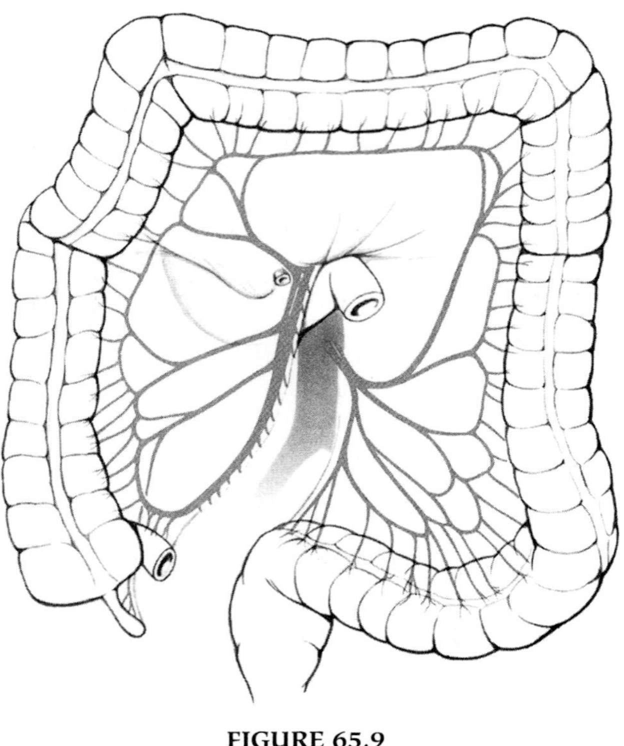

FIGURE 65.9

Vascular anatomy of the colon.

Isoperistaltic Conduit

Standardized techniques of isoperistaltic colon conduit preparation should be preferred. Accumulated experience has resulted in the consensus that an isoperistaltic transplant is preferable to an anisoperistaltic graft, as reflux and regurgitation are less and swallowing better (8). Therefore, this technique will be the major focus of discussion (1).

Transverse Colon

Remarks

According to our opinion, the best form of colon interposition is the transverse colon, including the right and left colonic flexure pedicled on the ascending branch of the left colic artery (Figure 65.10). An advantage of this form is the good venous drainage from the left colic vein directly into the inferior mesenteric vein. For patients of normal size, the necessary length of the conduit is about 40 cm for a cervical anastomosis. This can easily be achieved with the transverse colon and both flexures. It is always better to have a certain reserve in length and shorten the conduit later than to face the problem of missing length.

Preparation

The greater omentum is detached from the transverse colon, and both flexures as well as the fetal adhesions of the cecum and the ascending, descending, and sigmoid colon are mobilized. Under diaphany of the colic mesentery, the following vessels are identified and prepared (Figure 65.9):

1. Middle colic artery and its left and right branch
2. Left colic artery and its ascending branch
3. Descending branch of the left colic artery
4. Marginal artery between the middle colic artery and the right colic artery

The veins accompanying these arteries are also detected. The length of the necessary colon conduit is measured between neck and upper abdomen with a sterile centimeter scale, and this extent is marked with stay sutures on the colon. In order to simulate the later conduit vascularization, artery number 1 is clamped at its origin with a bulldog, and also numbers 3 and 4 are interrupted by bulldog clamps. If the vascularization remains undisturbed, these clamped arteries and their veins can be suture ligated and cut.

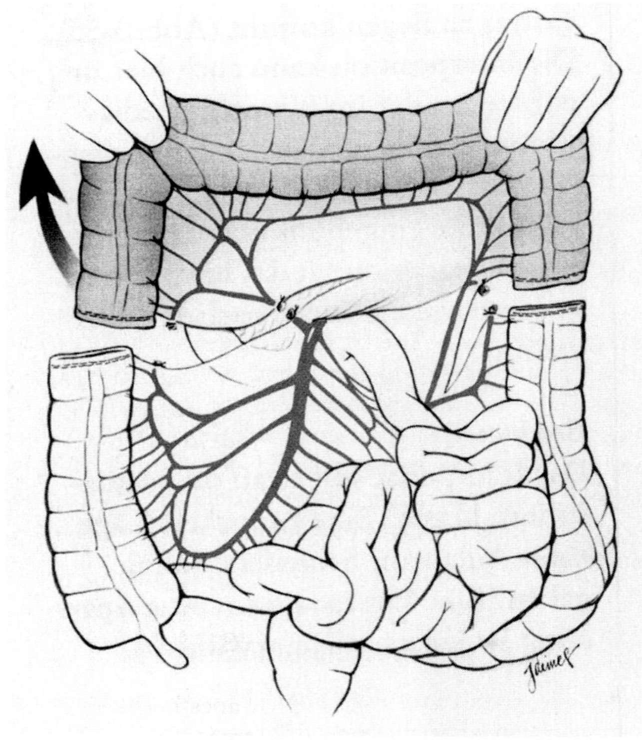

FIGURE 65.10

Conduit of the transverse colon pedicled on the ascending branch of the left colic artery.

The vascular parts of the mesentery are dissected, and the colon is stapled and cut with a GIA 60 (Covidien) according to the extent of Figure 65.10. The oral part of the conduit is moved to the neck and placed on a sterile towel in front of the thorax. The pulsation of the marginal arteries and the adequate vascularization of the bowel are reconfirmed. The ascending and descending colon are anastomosed end to end by 1 layer interrupted or running sutures, and the mesenteric gap is closed. The pedicle of conduit must be handled with special care to avoid strangulation or twisting.

Interposition

If the stomach is still in place, the colon conduit is pulled up behind the stomach so that the vascular pedicle is located retrogastric. If a cervical anastomosis is planned, the conduit is inserted in a plastic bag and carefully pulled to the neck through the posterior or anterior mediastinum (see the section "Route of Reconstruction" later in this chapter). The conduit should be extended in the mediastinum to avoid kinking (Figure 65.11). Redundant colonic length can be resected, but tension should also be avoided.

The cervical anastomosis should be performed end to end and splinted by a gastric tube (Figure 65.11). The gastrocolic anastomosis is performed to the front wall of the stomach most easily by circular stapler. A pyloroplasty *or pyloric dilatation* should be added in order to achieve adequate gastric emptying after esophagectomy with truncal vagotomy. If the stomach is also resected, the aboral end of the colon can be connected end to end to the duodenum or to the first jejunal loop end to side by stapler or by suturing. In this case, bile reflux into the colon conduit can be avoided by side-to-side Braun anastomosis at the basis of the jejunal loop or by formation of a jejunal Roux-en-Y loop.

If an intrathoracic anastomosis is planned, the conduit can first be connected to the stomach and placed with the closed oral part through the hiatus into the right pleural cavity. After closure of the abdomen and right thoracotomy, the esophageal stump high up in the thorax can be anastomosed with the colon conduit end to side f.e. by stapler or end to end by sutures (see the anastomotic techniques discussed later). However, the length of the conduit has to be adapted to the individual circumstances eventually by segmental resection of the oral part. The conduit should lie straight in the mediastinum but without tension on the anastomosis.

Right Hemicolon

Some authors favor the isoperistaltic interposition of the right hemicolon up to the cecum or together with the terminal ileum (Figure 65.12). The arterial blood supply comes from the middle colic artery, and the venous drainage results from the middle colic vein. As the middle colic artery is mostly large in diameter, this transplant is very well vascularized. However, the middle colic artery and vein originate right of the midline, and after lifting up, the interponat kinking of this vessel to the left could be a problem for vascularization. If the distal ileum is preserved in continuity with the right hemicolon, the advantage is the same-size diameter for the anastomosis to the cervical esophagus. In this case, an appendectomy has to be added (Figure 65.13). The interposition of the prepared graft follows the same rules as mentioned for the transverse colon conduit (see the previous discussion).

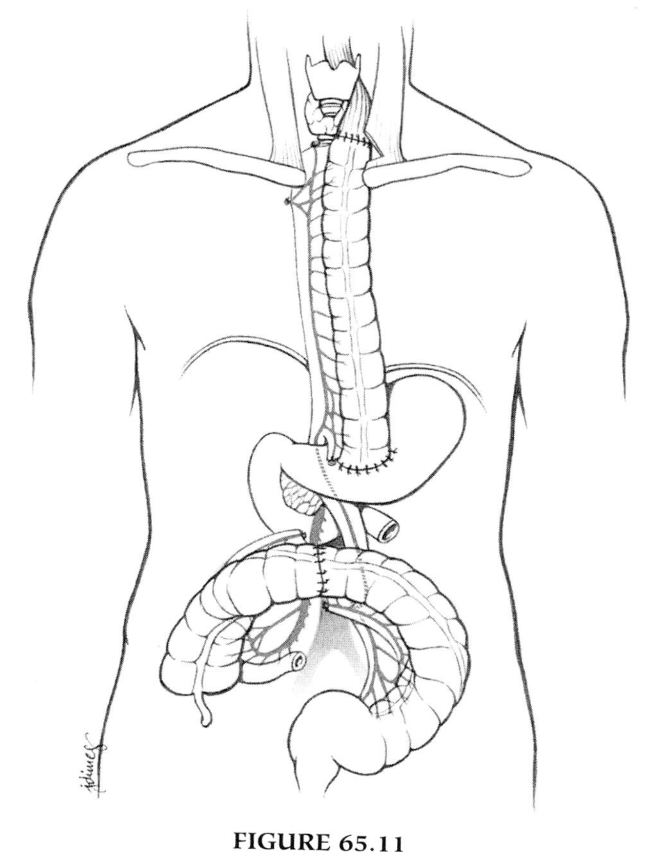

FIGURE 65.11

Isoperistaltic interposition of the transverse colon between the cervical esophagus and the stomach. Reconstruction of the colon by ascendodescendostomy.

Anisoperistaltic Conduit

As mentioned previously, anisoperistaltic grafts should be avoided. However, in the case of vascular anatomic variations or previous colon operations, preparation of

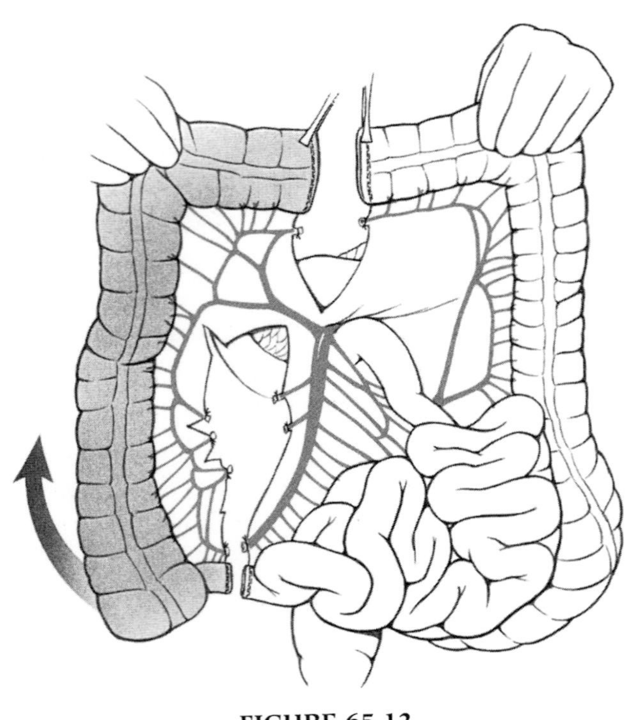

FIGURE 65.12

Conduit of the right hemicolon with distal ileum pedicled on the right colic artery.

an isoperistaltic conduit can be impossible. In this situation, a transverse colon conduit can also be pedicled on the middle colic artery. The ascending colon is then dissected about 10 cm orad of the right colonic flexure and the left hemicolon in the area of the left colonic flexure or more aborad according to the needed length (Figure 65.14). The interposition is performed corresponding to the same technical criteria as described for the isoperistaltic colon interposition (Figure 65.15).

Cervical Supercharge

If the vascularization of the upper part of the transverse colon conduit after isoperistaltic pull-up to the neck seems insufficient, an additional vascular anastomosis can be performed between the stump of the middle colic artery with the inferior thyroid artery or branches of the carotid artery (10,11). A venous anastomosis can be constructed between the middle colic vein and the internal jugular vein or its branches. For this purpose, it is necessary to leave long stumps of these colonic vessels during conduit preparation and to spare a long f.e. inferior thyroid artery during preparation of the cervical esophagus. The vascular anastomosis are sutured in microsurgical technique (see the section "Free Jejunal Interposition After Cervical Esophagectomy" later in this chapter).

JEJUNUM CONDUIT

Replacement after Distal Esophageal Resection

Replacement of the distal esophagus can be necessary in 2 situations:

1. After extended total gastrectomy with transhiatal distal esophageal resection for advanced adenocarcinoma of the gastroesophageal junction
2. After vagal sparing transhiatal distal esophageal resection with upper gastric resection (Merendino operation) for mucosal Barrett's or cardia carcinoma or chronic peptic stenosis

In the first situation, the best reconstruction is performed with a long Roux-en-Y loop and transhiatal end-to-side esophagojejunostomy by stapler (see the chapter on adenocarcinoma of the gastroesophageal junction).

In the second situation, a 15-cm segment of the upper jejunum is prepared with a long vascular pedicle of good arterial inflow and adequate venous drainage

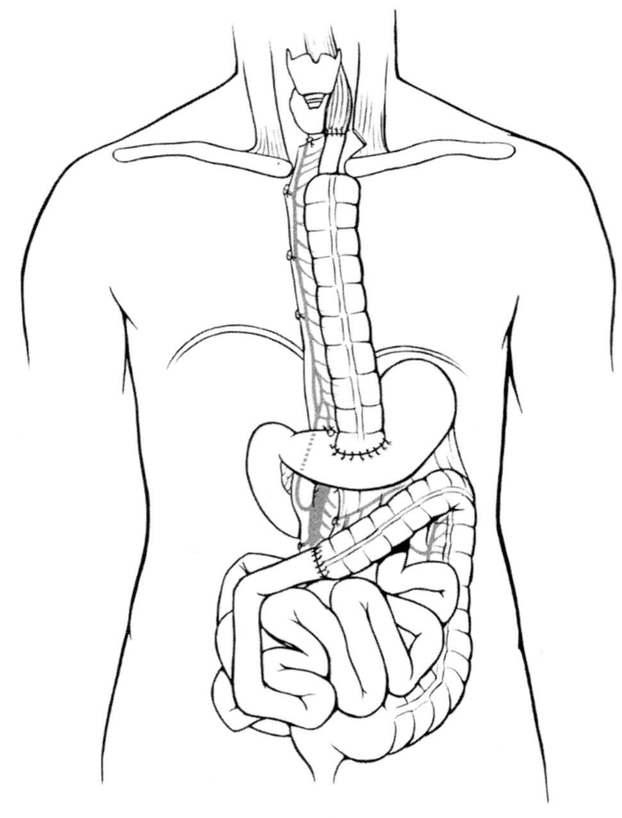

FIGURE 65.13

Isoperistaltic interposition of the right hemicolon. Cervical anastomosis between esophagus and ileum.

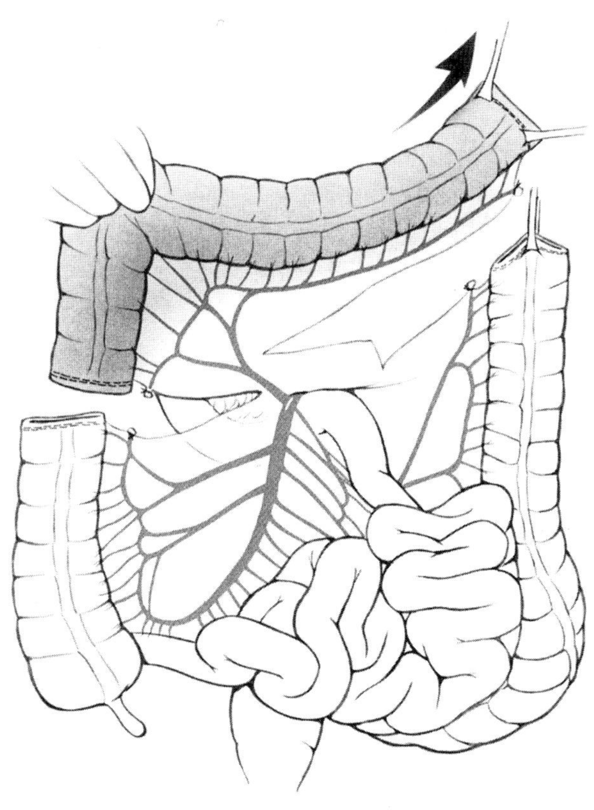

FIGURE 65.14

Anisoperistaltic conduit of the transverse colon and right colonic flexure pedicled on the middle colic artery and vein.

(12,13). This loop is elevated in isoperistaltic manner into the lower mediastinum with retrocolic and retrogastric guidance of the pedicle (Figure 65.16). The transhiatal esophagojejunostomy is performed end to side and the jejunogastrostomy to the fundus via gastrotomy end to side each by circular stapler. The jejunum is reconstructed by end-to-end anastomosis.

Replacement after Subtotal Esophagectomy

The reconstruction of the whole esophagus by jejunum is considered only if the stomach or colon is not available because of previous operations or specific diseases. The reason is the limitation of the mesenteric blood supply. Only in special cases do the mesenteric arcades of the jejunum show an anatomy that allows the construction of a well-vascularized loop of sufficient length (Figure 65.17). However, advances in microsurgical technique have expanded the significance of the jejunum in esophageal replacement by the creation of longer loops through supercharging (14,15). This means microvascular augmentation of the proximal mesenteric circulation of a jejunal conduit through arterial or venous anastomoses to internal thoracic or cervical vessels. The safety of this procedure is increased by a monitor flap that is left attached to the proximal revascularized mesenteric arcade and then externalized through the cervical wound. After 7 to 10 days postoperative and proven viable jejunal loop, the monitor flap can be removed by ligating and dividing its pedicle at the skin level.

Free Jejunal Interposition after Cervical Esophagectomy

After resection of the cervical esophagus via a left cervical incision and upper sternotomy, the reconstruction can be performed with a free jejunal transplant (1,11,16). This affords microvascular arterial and venous anastomoses between the mesenteric vessels and appropriate cervical vessels like the inferior or superior thyroid artery and the internal jugular vein (Figure 65.18).

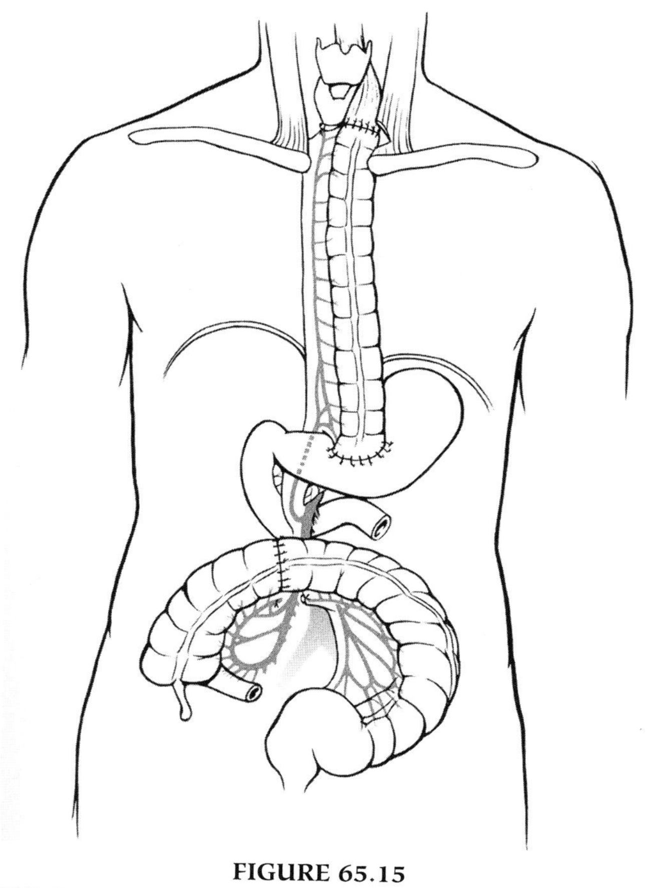

FIGURE 65.15

Anisoperistaltic colon interposition of the transverse colon and the right colonic flexure.

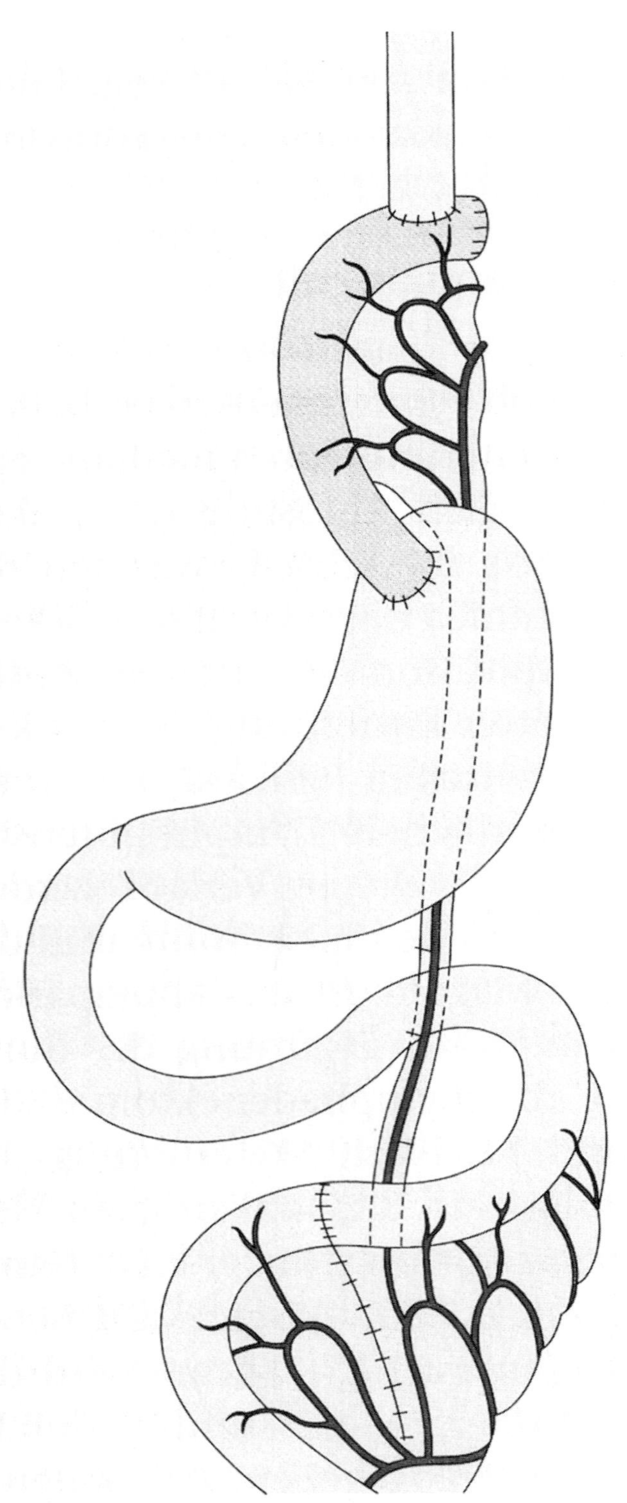

FIGURE 65.16

Merendino operation: resection of the distal esophagus and cardia and isoperistaltic jejunal interposition.

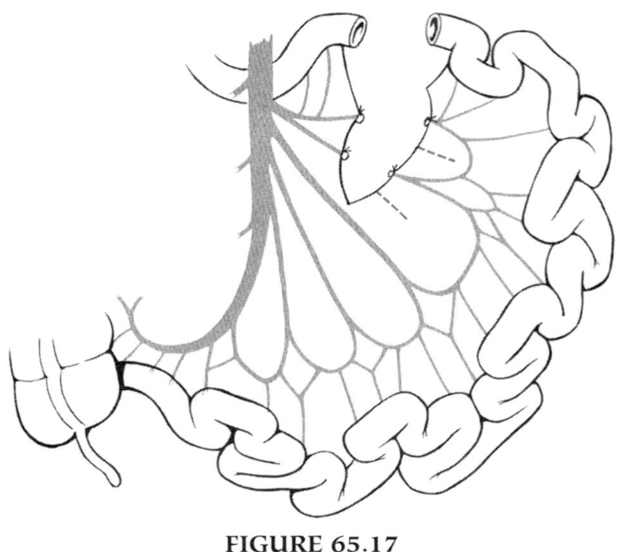

FIGURE 65.17

Technique of jejunal loop preparation for replacement after subtotal esophagectomy.

The hypopharynx is anastomosed end to side to the upper part of the isoperistaltic jejunum and its lower part end to end or side to end to the esophagus. The jejunal segment of about 15 cm has to be chosen and prepared with special care, especially concerning adequate diameter and length of the vessels. An alternative is a segment of the distal ileum pedicled on the distal part of the ileocolic artery. A temporary monitor flap as mentioned for the cervical supercharge of a long jejunal graft is also recommended for the free jejunal interposition.

ROUTE OF RECONSTRUCTION

Posterior Mediastinum

The best route of reconstruction after subtotal esophagectomy is the orthotopic one because it is the most physiologic and the shortest way. However, this route can be disadvantageous because of local tumor recurrence, especially in case of incomplete resection of the esophageal cancer. Further postoperative irradiation of the former esophageal bed may be harmful to the conduit in the posterior mediastinum.

Retrosternal

An alternative is the retrosternal route in the anterior mediastinum. On average, this way is 5 cm longer than the orthotopic one and leads to a little kinking of the

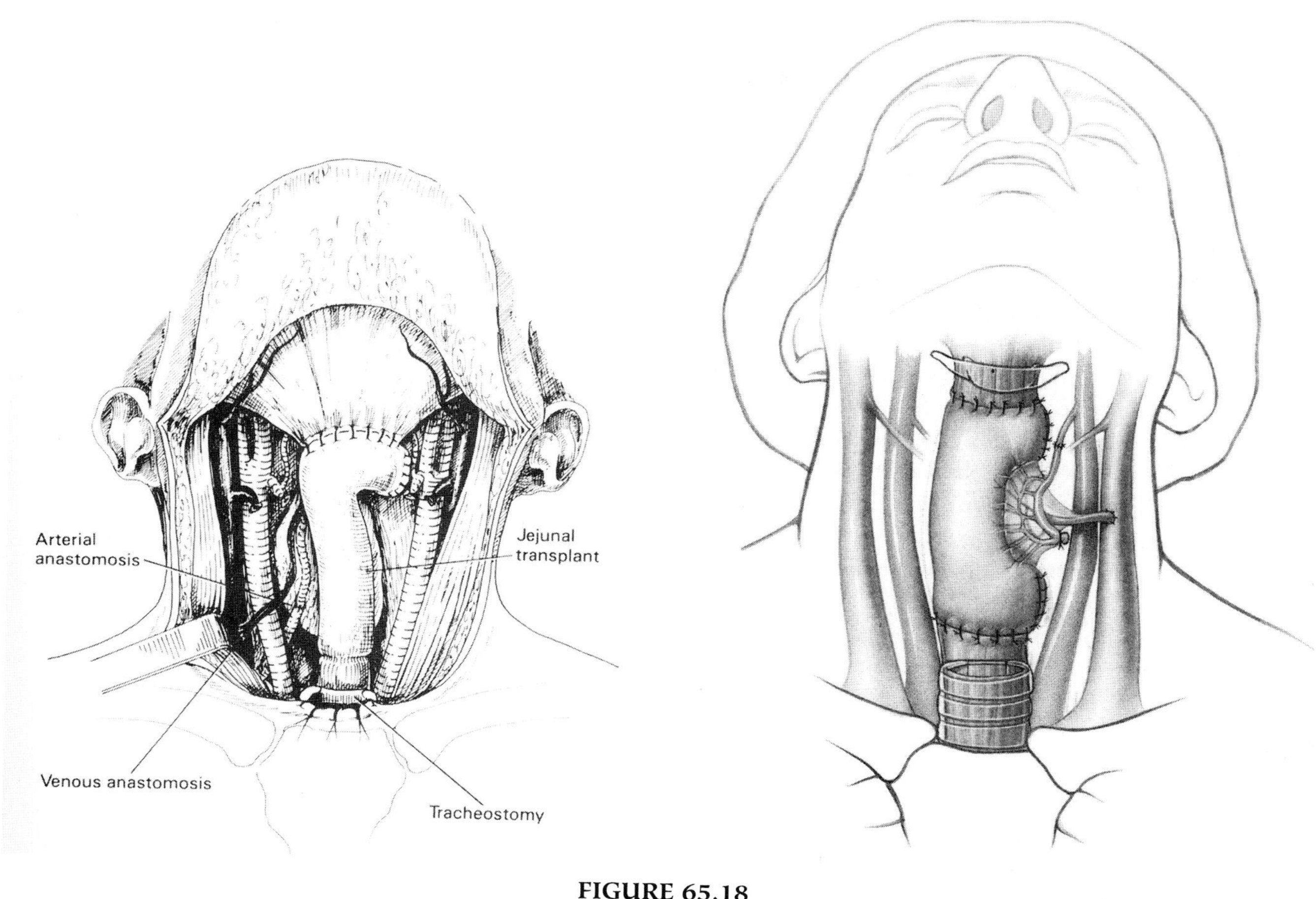

FIGURE 65.18

(A) Free jejunal transfer between hypopharynx end to side. Thoracic esophagus end to end or side to end (B) with microvascular arterial and venous anastomosis.

conduit at the junction between the thoracic inlet and the neck. This can cause problems of vascularization of the oral part of the conduit and in long-run swallowing disorders.

Antesternal

Today the antesternal subcutaneous route is nearly out of use because it is even more longer, functionally difficult, and cosmetically inappropriate. This route should be considered only in cases without alternatives.

TIME OF RECONSTRUCTION

One Stage

The standard is the 1-stage procedure of esophagectomy and immediate replacement mostly by gastric conduit.

Conditioning of the Conduit

However, the conditioning of the stomach after laparoscopic mobilization and reconstruction after a 5-day interval to improve gastric vascularization may have some indications (see the previous discussion) (5).

Esophagectomy with Delayed Reconstruction

An alternative concept with intention to reduce morbidity and mortality after esophagectomy is the initial transthoracic esophagectomy and delayed reconstruction after 10 to 14 days. This 2-stage procedure has been described for high-risk patients especially with poor functional status after neoadjuvant chemoradiation (17,18). However, the disadvantages of this principle are the need for a temporary cervical esophagostoma, no possibility of intrathoracic anastomosis, and the reconstruction always through the longer route of the anterior mediastinum.

References

1. Siewert, JR, Hölscher AH. Eingriffe beim Ösophaguskarzinom und Eingriffe beim Adenokarzinom des gastroösophagealen Übergangs. In: Gschnitzer F, Kern E, Schweiberer L, eds. *Breitner: Chirurgische Operationslehre, 2.A. Band IV,* Siewert JR, ed. *Chirurgie des Abdomens 2* (pp. 9–119). Munich: Urban & Schwarzenberg; 1994.
2. Luketich JD, Alvelo-Rivera M, Buenaventura O, et al. Minimal-invasive esophagectomy: outcomes in 222 patients. *Ann Surg.* 2003;238:486–495.
3. Collard JM, Romagnoli R, Goncette L, et al. Whole stomach with antro-pyloric nerve preservation as an esophageal substitute: an original technique. *Dis. Esophagus.* 2004;17:164–167.
4. Liebermann-Meffert DMI, Meier R, Siewert JR. Vascular anatomy of the gastric tube used for the esophageal reconstruction. *Ann Thorac Surg.* 1992;54:1110–1115.
5. Hölscher AH, Schneider PM, Gutschow C, et al. Laparoscopic ischemic conditioning of the stomach for esophageal replacement. *Ann Surg.* 2007;245:241–246.
6. Schröder W, Stippel D, Hölscher AH, et al. Postoperative recovery of microcirculation after gastric tube formation. *Langenbecks Arch Surg.* 2004;389:267–271.
7. Reavis KM, Chang EY, Hunter JG, et al. Utilization of the delay phenomenon improves blood flow and reduces collagen deposition in esophagogastric anastomosis. *Ann Surg.* 2005;241:736–747.
8. DeMeester TR, Johansson KE, Franze I, et al. Indications, surgical technique and long-term functional results of colon interposition or bypass. *Ann Surg.* 1988;208:460–474.
9. Leers JM, Schröder W, Hölscher AH, et al. Preoperative colonoscopy before esophageal replacement. *Chirurg.* 2004;75:1210–1214.
10. Fujita H, Yamana H, Sueyoshi S, et al. Impact on outcome of additional microvascular anastomosis-supercharge-on colon interposition for esophageal replacement: comparative and multivariate analysis. *World J Surg.* 1997;21:998–1003.
11. Sekido M, Yamamoto Y, Minakawa H, et al. Use of the "supercharge" technique in esophageal and pharyngeal reconstruction to augment microvascular blood flow. *Surgery.* 2003;134:420–424.
12. Gutschow C, Schröder W, Hölscher AH, et al. Merendino procedure with preservation of the vagus for early carcinoma of the gastroesophageal junction. *Zentralbl Chir.* 2004;129:276–281.
13. Linke GR, Borovicka J, Tutuian R, et al. Altered esophageal motility and gastroesophageal barrier in patients with jejunal interposition after distal esophageal resection for early stage adenocarcinoma. *J Gastrointest Surg.* 2007;1262–1267.
14. Ascioti AJ, Hofstetter WL, Miller MJ, et al. Long-segment, supercharged, pedicled jejunal flap for total esophageal reconstruction. *J Thorac Cardiovasc Surg.* 2005;130:1391–1398.
15. Hirabayashi S, Miyata M, Shoji M, et al. Reconstruction of the thoracic esophagus, with extended jejunum used as a substitute, with the aid of microvascular anastomosis. *Surgery.* 1993;113:515–519.
16. Chen HC, Tang YB. Microsurgical reconstruction of the esophagus. *Semin Surg Oncol.* 2000;19:235–245.
17. Sugimachi K, Kitamura M, Maekawa S, et al. Two-stage operation for poor risk patients with carcinoma of the esophagus. *J Surg Oncol.* 1987;36:105.
18. Saito T, Shimoda K, Shigemitsu Y, et al. Extensive lymphadenectomy for thoracic esophageal carcinoma: a two-stage operation for high risk patients. *Surg Today.* 1994;24:610.

66 Surgery Techniques: Vagal-Sparing Esophagectomy

Steven R. DeMeester

Adenocarcinoma of the esophagus has the fastest-rising incidence of any cancer in the United States and develops as a consequence of chronic gastroesophageal reflux disease (1). Barrett's esophagus is the precursor lesion from which adenocarcinoma develops, and surveillance programs have led to the detection of high-grade dysplasia and early-stage adenocarcinoma in an increasing number of patients. Both high-grade dysplasia and intramucosal adenocarcinoma, while potentially lethal, are curable lesions in most patients (2–4). Although new technologies allow some patients to be treated endoscopically, esophagectomy remains the standard of care for the definitive management of these lesions.

Patients with only high-grade dysplasia are uniformly cured with esophagectomy since invasive cancer has not developed and will not after removal of all the Barrett's mucosa. However, a number of surgical series have demonstrated that despite extensive preresection biopsies, 30% to 50% of patients thought only to have high-grade dysplasia will in fact have an invasive cancer in the resected specimen (5,6). In the absence of a visible ulcer or nodule on endoscopy, these occult adenocarcinomas have always been limited to the mucosa in our experience (5). In contrast, if a lesion of any sort is seen endoscopically within the columnar-lined portion of the esophagus, that lesion is at high risk to be a cancer. Further, any visible lesion that on biopsy shows adenocarcinoma cannot be assumed to be limited to the mucosa, regardless of the size or appearance of the lesion. Even very small lesions may penetrate into the submucosa; thus, the endoscopic appearance of the lesion can not be used to determine the "T" stage. It was hoped that endoscopic ultrasound would allow accurate determination of intramucosal versus submucosal tumor invasion, but even high-frequency 20-MHz probes have not provided acceptable differentiation of these lesions (7). Currently the only method able to accurately determine the depth of invasion of a small visible lesion is endoscopic mucosal resection (EMR). This technique enables endoscopic excision of lesions up to 1.5 cm in size along with the adjacent mucosa and submucosa down to the muscularis propria and thereby allows the precise depth of invasion of the tumor to be pathologically determined. The accuracy of EMR as a staging procedure for early esophageal cancer has been established, and we use it routinely for patients with a visible lesion within the Barrett's mucosa (8,9).

The critical importance of accurately determining the depth of invasion of a small esophageal adenocarcinoma is the direct link between depth of invasion and the likelihood of lymph node metastases. While intramucosal tumors rarely metastasize to lymph nodes, submucosal invasion is associated with lymph node metastases in 30% to 50% of patients (10,11). Consequently, in patients with submucosal invasion endoscopic or other therapies that do not address potential lymph node metastases are not appropriate. In contrast, the likelihood of nodal metastases is low (< 5%) in patients with a tumor confined to the mucosa (2,10). Recently we assessed the importance of a lymph node dissection in these patients. We reviewed the outcome of 85 patients with an intramucosal adenocarcinoma that we treated with a transthoracic en bloc, transhiatal, or vagal-sparing esophagectomy. The importance of this comparison is that while each operation removes the diseased esophagus, there is a substantial difference in the lymphadenectomy that accompanies each approach. In particular, no formal node dissection accompanies a vagal-sparing esophagectomy, and typically none or only a few nodes are removed. Our results confirmed that cancer related survival is excellent in these patients (95% at 5 years) and was independent of the type of resection and extent of lymphadenectomy (12). Thus, a vagal-sparing esophagectomy is an excellent option for patients with high-grade dysplasia or intramucosal adenocarcinoma.

In an era of potential endoscopic therapy for early esophageal lesions, a critical issue frequently mentioned by both patients and physicians is the procedure-related morbidity and mortality for an esophagectomy. Traditional esophagectomy includes a vagotomy and pyloroplasty and can be associated with troublesome postoperative dumping and diarrhea symptoms. Further, mortality for an esophagectomy is often quoted as nearly 10%, based largely on old literature in malnourished patients with large tumors. Recent series of esophagectomy in patients with high-grade dysplasia or early-stage esophageal adenocarcinoma present a completely different picture, with mortality rates of 1% or less. Further, many centers now offer a minimally invasive procedure to further minimize the impact of the operation and reduce long-term morbidity (13–15).

In appropriate patients with high-grade dysplasia or intramucosal cancer, I favor a laparoscopic vagal-sparing esophagectomy with gastric pull-up. The vagal-sparing esophagectomy was first described by Akiyama in Japan, and we subsequently adopted it as a means to remove the diseased esophagus in situations where a lymph node dissection was not necessary (16). This operation preserves the vagal innervation to the pylorus and the remaining gastrointestinal tract and is associated with reduced morbidity, including avoidance of postvagotomy dumping and diarrhea, while maintaining the advantages of complete removal of the diseased esophagus. No lymph node dissection is possible without potentially injuring the vagus nerves and branches along the lesser curve, and therefore the procedure is an option only for patients with benign conditions and for those with Barrett's and high-grade dysplasia or intramucosal adenocarcinoma.

A vagal-sparing esophagectomy is performed by stripping the esophagus out of the mediastinum using a vein stripper. For potentially malignant lesions, the entire esophagus is stripped out by inverting it on itself. In patients with achalasia, it is also possible to strip out only the mucosa and leave the muscular wall of the esophagus in place, but this would be inappropriate for Barrett's or early adenocarcinoma. Reconstruction can be with either a gastric pull-up or a colon interposition. No pyloroplasty is performed since pyloric innervation is preserved. When using a gastric pull-up, the lesser curve is dissected immediately adjacent to the gastric wall, and the left gastric artery is not divided. This preserves the vagal branches as well as left gastric arterial branches to the antrum and contributes to the excellent blood supply of the gastric graft with this procedure. If a colon interposition is selected, it is done to the posterior wall of the intact stomach after dividing the cardia with a stapler; thus, the normal gastric reservoir is maintained. These patients eat exceptionally well, but with longer follow-up some patients develop troublesome regurgitation symptoms, and we therefore favor the gastric pull-up procedure in most circumstances.

Previously we verified that vagal preservation is realistic with an esophagectomy using the stripping technique and showed that the incidence of dumping and diarrhea as well as the extent of postoperative weight loss were all reduced with a vagal-sparing compared to a standard esophagectomy (17). In a recent update of our experience with vagal-sparing esophagectomy for Barrett's and intramucosal adenocarcinoma, we again confirmed that preservation of the vagal nerves is feasible during esophagectomy and is associated with reduced morbidity. Specifically, we showed that infectious, respiratory, and anastomotic complications were all reduced in patients that had a vagal-sparing compared to a transhiatal esophagectomy (12). Given the equivalent oncologic result, the reduction in morbidity with the vagal-sparing technique should make this the esophagectomy of choice for patients who do not require a lymphadenectomy.

The combination of endoscopic mucosal resection for a nodule or intramucosal cancer and ablation of any residual Barrett's is being evaluated at a number of centers for the treatment of patients with high-grade dysplasia or intramucosal adenocarcinoma as an alternative to esophagectomy. The enthusiasm for this approach is fueled in part by the excellent 5-year survival reported by Ell and colleagues, who treated 100 patients with intramucosal adenocarcinoma by EMR alone (18). However, there are several important considerations that are worth reviewing before this approach is widely accepted as a therapeutic option for these patients, and these issues are covered fully in the chapter on EMR as therapy for esophageal lesions.

In light of the recent advances in endoscopic procedures that allow esophageal preservation and the new, less invasive and potentially less morbid surgical techniques to remove the esophagus, I propose that it is time to alter our approach to the evaluation of patients with high-grade dysplasia and early esophageal adenocarcinoma. In addition to determining the stage of the cancer and assessing the overall health of the patient, we should also evaluate the pathophysiologic abnormalities associated with the patient's reflux disease. In particular, an assessment should be made of the function of the stomach, lower esophageal sphincter, and esophageal body as well as the size of the hiatal hernia, length of Barrett's, and presence and severity of reflux symptoms. Esophageal preservation might be the preferred therapy in a patient with few symptoms, a small hiatal hernia, normal esophageal body function, and a short segment of Barrett's with a low-risk intramucosal carcinoma. In contrast, patients who are poor candidates for esophageal preservation are those who present with high-grade dysplasia or an intramucosal adenocarcinoma and have severe reflux symptoms or dysphagia; long-segment Barrett's with a large, fixed hiatal hernia; and poor esophageal body motility. These patients are best treated with a vagal-sparing esophagectomy since in my opinion esophageal preservation makes sense only if the esophagus is worth preserving based on physiologic evaluation. Vagal-sparing esophagectomy is also indicated for patients with multiple lesions within long-segment Barrett's or lesions with positive lateral margins after endoscopic mucosal resection. Thus, the decision to treat high-grade dysplasia or intramucosal cancer endoscopically or with an esophagectomy takes into consideration not just the stage of the lesion but also the pathophysiology of the esophagus and the severity of the underlying reflux disease. In this way, outcomes can be optimized not only for the dysplasia or cancer but for the patient's reflux disease and long-term quality of life as well.

References

1. Pohl H, Welch HG. The role of overdiagnosis and reclassification in the marked increase of esophageal adenocarcinoma incidence. *J Natl Cancer Inst.* 2005;97(2): 142–146.
2. Oh DS, Hagen JA, Chandrasoma PT, et al. Clinical biology and surgical therapy of intramucosal adenocarcinoma of the esophagus. *J Am Coll Surg.* 2006;203(2):152–161.
3. Rice TW, Blackstone EH, Goldblum JR, et al. Superficial adenocarcinoma of the esophagus. *J Thorac Cardiovasc Surg.* 2001;122(6):1077–1090.
4. Stein HJ, Feith M, Bruecher BL, et al. Early esophageal cancer: pattern of lymphatic spread and prognostic factors for long-term survival after surgical resection. *Ann Surg.* 2005;242(4):566–573; discussion 573–575.
5. Nigro JJ, Hagen JA, DeMeester TR, et al. Occult esophageal adenocarcinoma: extent of disease and implications for effective therapy. *Ann Surg.* 1999;230(3):433–440.
6. Dar MS, Goldblum JR, Rice TW, et al. Can extent of high grade dysplasia in Barrett's oesophagus predict the presence of adenocarcinoma at oesophagectomy? *Gut.* 2003;52(4):486–489.
7. May A, Gunter E, Roth F, et al. Accuracy of staging in early esophageal cancer using high resolution endoscopy and high resolution endosonography: a comparative, prospective, and blinded trial. *Gut.* 2004;53:634–640.
8. Maish MS, DeMeester SR. Endoscopic mucosal resection as a staging technique to determine the depth of invasion of esophageal adenocarcinoma. *Ann Thorac Surg.* 2004;78:1777–1782.
9. Prasad GA, Buttar NS, Wongkeesong LM, et al. Significance of neoplastic involvement of margins obtained by endoscopic mucosal resection in Barrett's esophagus. *Am J Gastroenterol.* 2007;102(11):2380–2386.
10. Rice TW, Zuccaro G Jr, Adelstein DJ, et al. Esophageal carcinoma: depth of tumor invasion is predictive of regional lymph node status. *Ann Thorac Surg.* 1998;65(3): 787–792.
11. Nigro JJ, Hagen JA, DeMeester TR, et al. Prevalence and location of nodal metastases in distal esophageal adenocarcinoma confined to the wall: implications for therapy [see comments]. *J Thorac Cardiovasc Surg.* 1999;117(1):16–23; discussion 23–25.
12. Peyre C, DeMeester SR, Rizzetto C, et al. Vagal-sparing esophagectomy: the ideal operation for intramucosal adenocarcinoma and Barrett's with high-grade dysplasia. *Ann Surg.* 2007;246:665–674.
13. DeMeester SR. Endoscopic mucosal resection and vagal-sparing esophagectomy for high-grade dysplasia and adenocarcinoma of the esophagus. *Semin Thorac Cardiovasc Surg.* 2005;17(4):320–325.
14. Moraca RJ, Low DE. Outcomes and health-related quality of life after esophagectomy for high-grade dysplasia and intramucosal cancer. *Arch Surg.* 2006;141(6):545–549; discussion 549–551.
15. Luketich JD, Alvelo-Rivera M, Buenaventura PO, et al. Minimally invasive esophagectomy: outcomes in 222 patients. *Ann Surg.* 2003;238(4):486–494; discussion 494–495.
16. Akiyama H, Tsurumaru M, Udagawa H, et al. Radical lymph node dissection for cancer of the thoracic esophagus. *Ann Surg.* 1994;220(3):364–372; discussion 372–373.
17. Banki F, Mason RJ, DeMeester SR, et al. Vagal-sparing esophagectomy: a more physiologic alternative. *Ann Surg.* 2002;236(3):324–335; discussion 335–336.
18. Ell C, May A, Pech O, et al. Curative endoscopic resection of early esophageal adenocarcinomas (Barrett's cancer) [see comment]. *Gastrointest Endosc.* 2007;65(1):3–10.

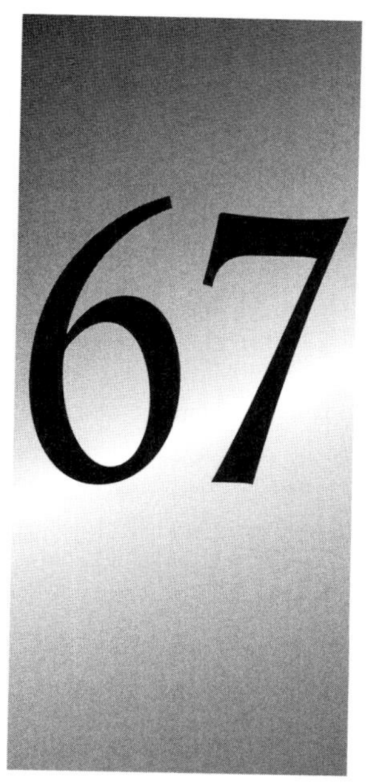

Surgery Techniques: Minimally Invasive Esophagectomy

Harmik Soukiasian
Blair A. Jobe
James D. Luketich

There continues to be a natural progression toward smaller incisions and minimally invasive approaches in all fields of surgery. Open cholecystecomy has been replaced by laparoscopic cholecystectomy. Open gastric bypass has been replaced by laparoscopic Roux-en-Y gastric bypass. Open prostatectomy is being replaced with laparoscopic, robotic-assisted prostatectomy, and open lung resections are trending toward minimally invasive video-assisted thoracic surgery techniques. Similarly, open esophagectomy is seeing the early phases of minimally invasive approaches.

At the current time, minimally invasive esophagectomy (MIE) is not performed in most medical centers, primarily because it is a complex and technically challenging procedure. However, open operations are associated with significant morbidity and mortality rates (6%–7%), even in experienced centers (1,2). Continued improvement in instrumentation and optics and increased surgeon familiarity with thoracoscopy and laparoscopy have resulted in the development of advanced minimally invasive techniques for the treatment of complex esophageal diseases, including thoracoscopic and laparoscopic staging of esophageal cancer and laparoscopic repair of paraesophageal hernia (3–7). This prior work has paved the way for the widespread introduction of the totally minimally invasive esophagectomy.

In 1998, one of us (JD Luketich) and his colleagues (8) reported a combined thoracoscopic and laparoscopic approach to esophagectomy. They combined thoracoscopic esophageal mobilization with laparoscopic construction of the gastric conduit via gastric pull-up with a cervical anastomosis. In 1999, Watson et al. reported a minimally invasive Ivor Lewis technique (9) in which a laparoscopic gastric mobilization and tubularization was followed by thoracoscopic esophagectomy with construction of a hand-sewn, intrathoracic esophagogastric anastomosis. Based on these early experiences, it was felt that combined 2-cavity esophageal mobilization provided superior safety, exposure, and lymphadenectomy when compared to an entirely transhiatal approach.

The first large series of MIE was reported by Luketich et al. and included thoracoscopic esophageal mobilization, laparoscopic gastric tubularization, and cervical anastomosis (10). In this series of 222 patients, MIE was successfully performed in a completely minimally invasive manner in 206 (92.8%) patients. The median intensive care unit stay was 1 day, and hospital stay was 7 days. Operative mortality was 1.4%, and the anastomotic leak rate was 11.7%. At a mean follow-up of 19 months, quality of life scores were similar to preoperative values and population norms. Tumor stage-specific survival was similar to that published for open esophagectomy series. We have now performed MIE on more than 500 patients with high-grade dysplasia or cancer (8,10–16).

Our technique has evolved over time, and we now most frequently employ an Ivor Lewis esophagectomy, which incorporates a thoracoscopic, circular, stapled esophagogastrostomy immediately superior to the divided azygos arch. The proposed advantages of this approach over the McKeown MIE include a reduction in the incidence of recurrent laryngeal nerve injury, improved conduit perfusion with a subsequent decrease in dehiscence rate, and the absence of anastomotic tension (17).

MIE is a technically demanding operation and should be performed by surgeons who have extensive experience in minimally invasive esophageal surgery. To help build experience in the safest manner, surgeons should perform cases in less challenging patients when starting out, including patients with high-grade dysplasia or small tumors. The beginning surgeon should try to avoid attempting MIE in obese patients and those with previous upper abdominal and/or right thoracic operations. We believe that patients with previous neoadjuvant chemotherapy, radiation, or even previous operations, either thoracic or abdominal, are still candidates for both staging laparoscopy and MIE.

TECHNIQUE: MIE

There are 2 options available in performing MIE: thoracoscopic and laparoscopic esophagectomy with a cervical anastomosis (McKeown MIE) and thoracoscopic and laparoscopic Ivor Lewis resection. The choice of surgical approach is based on surgeon preference and, in some cases, on the location of the tumor. At the current time, we prefer the Ivor Lewis resection technique in most cases; however, for historical reasons and because of considerable technical overlap in the procedures, MIE with cervical anastomosis is discussed first.

Thoracoscopic and Laparoscopic Esophagectomy with a Cervical Anastomosis (McKeown MIE)

In general, the use of both laparoscopy and thoracoscopy allows for better visualization of the esophagus and surrounding structures, such as the thoracic duct. We feel that this approach affords safe mobilization of the esophagus and allows a complete mediastinal lymphadenectomy to be performed as well. Thoracoscopic and laparoscopic esophagectomy is performed in 3 stages. In the first stage, the patient is positioned in the left lateral decubitus position for thoracoscopic mobilization of the intrathoracic esophagus. In the second stage, the patient is placed in a supine position for construction of the gastric conduit. In the third stage, the patient remains in the supine position for mobilization of the cervical esophagus via the left neck, removal of the surgical specimen, gastric pull-up, and construction of an esophagogastric anastomosis.

Before the procedure is started, an esophagogastroduodenoscopy (EGD) is performed in order to assess the tumor size and location prior to gastric tubularization. If the EGD, endoscopic ultrasound, or computed tomography scan findings suggest gastric extension, T4 local invasion, or possible metastases, we perform a staging laparoscopy, thoracoscopy, or both in order to determine resectability and to rule out distant disease.

Chest. The patient is positioned in the left lateral decubitus position. The surgeon stands posterior to the patient. With the right lung collapsed, 4 ports are placed for thoracoscopy (Figure 67.1). The camera port (30°, 5 or 10 mm) is placed in the seventh or eighth intercostal space just anterior to the midaxillary line. Next, a 10-mm port is placed in the eighth or ninth intercostal space 1 to 2 cm behind the posterior axillary line and is used mainly for the Autosonic coagulating shears (United States Surgical Corp., Norwalk, CT). A 10-mm port is then placed in the anterior axillary line at the level of the fourth intercostal space and is used for placement of a retractor to assist with exposure of the esophageal bed, usually with anterior and medial reflection of the lung. A 5-mm port is placed posterior to the tip of the scapula. A heavy traction suture, usually 1–0 (0-Surgidac; United States Surgical Corp.), is placed in the central tendon of the diaphragm exiting close to the costophrenic reflection through a stab incision in the inferior anterior chest wall using the Endo Close device (United States Surgical Corp.). When placed at the proper angle, this traction suture will apply constant downward retraction on the diaphragm aiding with exposure of the distal esophagus.

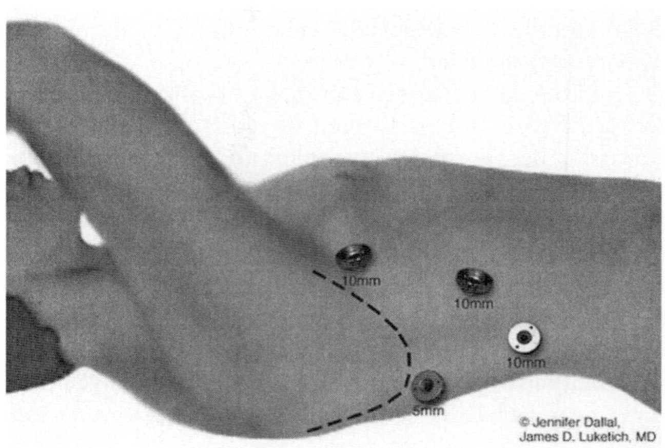

FIGURE 67.1

Thoracoscopic ports for minimally invasive esophagectomy.

The thoracic cavity is inspected for metastatic disease. The lung is retracted anteromedially to expose the esophagus. The inferior pulmonary ligament is divided using Autosonic coagulating shears (United States Surgical Corp.). The pleura overlying the esophagus is divided, and the entire thoracic esophagus is exposed. It is best to start in a plane distant to the tumor while dissecting around the esophagus circumferentially. A Penrose drain can be placed around the esophagus to facilitate traction and exposure (Figure 67.2). When possible, we begin anteriorly by lifting the mediastinal pleura directly off of the pericardium overlying the left atrium. This plane is carried superiorly to the level VII lymph node packet, which is maintained with the specimen. Great care is taken to avoid injury to the right and left bronchi and membranous trachea. We then move superiorly and the azygos vein is isolated and divided using the Endo GIA cutting stapler loaded with a vascular cartridge (United States Surgical Corp.). Preservation of the pleural layer superior to the azygos may seal the plane around the gastric tube near the thoracic inlet, thereby minimizing the extension of a cervical leak downward into the chest.

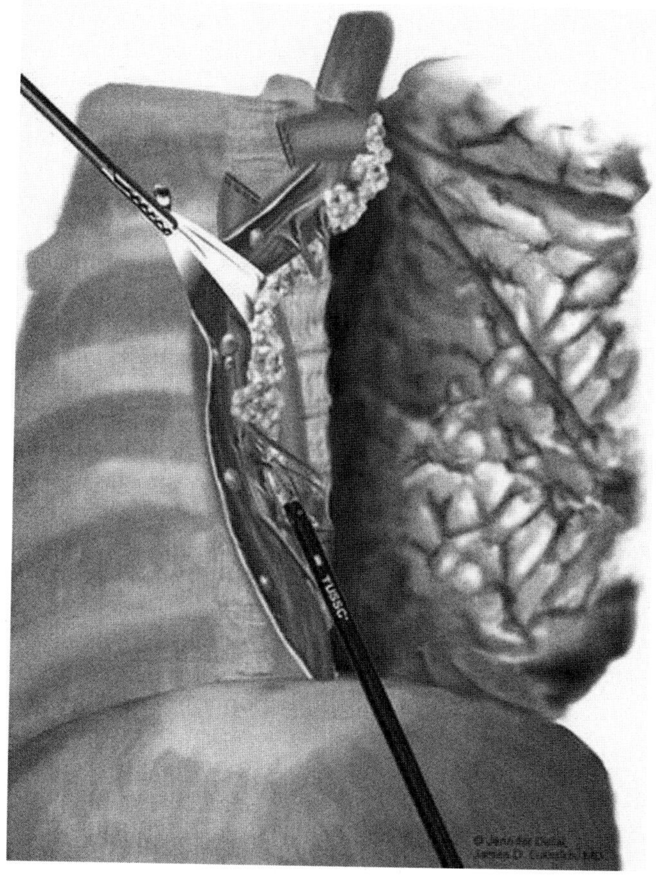

FIGURE 67.2

Thoracoscopic esophageal mobilization with en bloc lymphadenectomy.

The mediastinal pleura is opened anterior to the azygos vein, and all periesophageal fat and lymphatics overlying the aorta and contralateral pleura are maintained en bloc with the esophagus as the dissection is carried inferiorly. Aortoesophageal blood vessels are divided under direct vision after dissection. Care is taken to avoid injury to the thoracic duct, which remains in situ. The vagus nerve is transected immediately superior to the azygos vein. We do not routinely dissect the recurrent laryngeal or cervical lymph nodes. Above the level of the azygos vein, the dissection is continued directly on the esophagus to avoid potential injury to the airway or the recurrent nerves. At the completion of the mobilization, the Penrose drain is left in the thoracic inlet around the cervical esophagus and will be retrieved during the cervical dissection of the esophagus. Care is taken to identify and clip any lymphatic branches coming off the thoracic duct. The intercostal nerves are then blocked with 1 to 2 cc of bupivicaine (0.5%) in dilute epinephrine for control of immediate postoperative pain. A single 28-F chest tube is inserted in the camera port, the right lung is reinflated, and the port sites are closed.

Abdomen. After completing the thoracic esophageal mobilization, the patient is turned to the supine position. A standard 5-port approach is used to access to the abdomen. The placement of these ports is similar to the port placement used for laparoscopic Nissen fundoplication (Figure 67.3). A liver retractor is used to anteriorly reflect the left lateral segment of the liver providing exposure to the esophageal hiatus (Diamond-Flex, Snowden-Pencer, Tucker, GA). The retractor is then secured into position with a Mediflex self-retaining system (Velmed, Wexford, PA). First, the gastrohepatic ligament is divided, allowing exposure of the right crus of the diaphragm (Figure 67.4). The phrenoesophageal membrane is not divided at this time, as early entry into the mediastinum may lead to loss of pneumoperitoneum into the chest cavity and difficulty with exposure. The dissection is continued over the anterior surface of the esophagus. Next, the diaphragmatic attachments of the spleen are removed at the level of the left crus, allowing the spleen to fall away, which facilitates the dissection of the retroesophageal space and the left crus. Next, the short gastric vessels are divided with the Autosonic coagulating shears (United States Surgical Corp.). The dissection is carried along the greater curvature of the stomach, being careful to identify and preserve the right gastroepiploic vessels (Figure 67.5). A communication between the right and left gastroepiploic arcades should be preserved. The retrogastric area is then dissected by folding the stomach over and reflecting it superiorly. This allows dissection of the undersurface of the stomach and en bloc mobilization of the celiac and gastric vessel lymph nodes. The left gastric artery and vein are then exposed and divided at their base using the Endo GIA cutting vascular stapler.

Once gastric mobilization is completed, a pyloroplasty is performed using the Autosonic coagulating shears (United States Surgical Corp.) and closed transversely with interrupted 2–0 sutures using the Endo Stitch device (United States Surgical Corp.) (Figure 67.6). The fat and lymph nodes on the lesser curve are dissected en bloc with the stomach, taking care to preserve the right gastric vessels.

The gastric tube is then fashioned using the Endo GIA 3.5- or 4.8-mm stapler (United States Surgical Corp.) (Figures 67.7 and 67.8). There may be some variability in the length of the gastric tube based on intraoperative and EGD findings. In cases where the tumor has significant gastric extension, the surgeon must be prepared to resect a significant portion of the proximal stomach. In these cases, an intrathoracic anastomosis may need to be performed. We prefer to fashion a tube measuring 5 to 6 cm in diameter. Extreme care must be taken to ensure that the conduit is not traumatized and to avoid spiraling during stapling. Once the tube is fashioned, it is attached to the esophagogastric specimen using two 2–0 sutures (Figure 67.9).

We recommend placement of a laparoscopic feeding jejunostomy tube during MIE. Usually, an additional 10-mm port is inserted in the right lower quadrant to

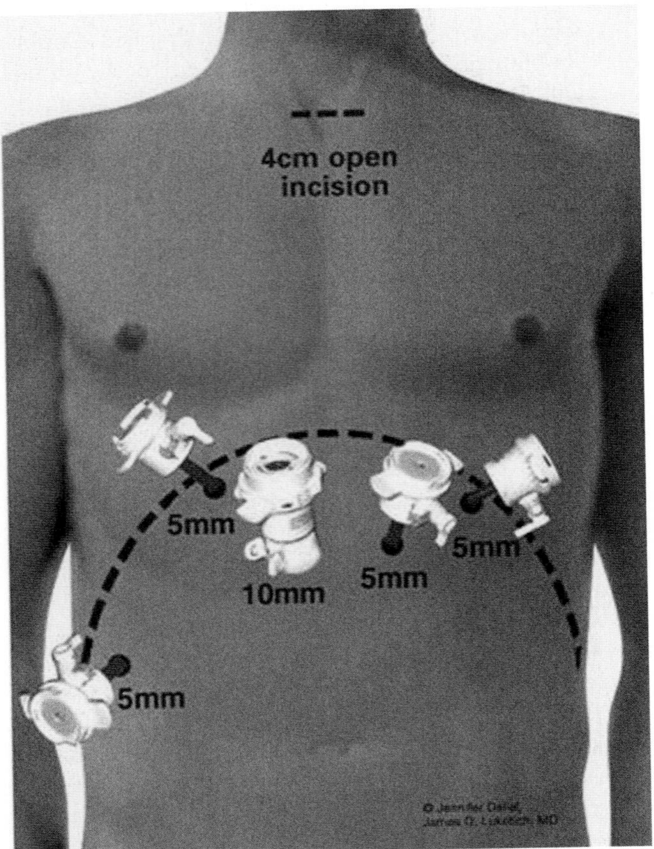

FIGURE 67.3

Laparoscopic ports for minimally invasive esophagectomy.

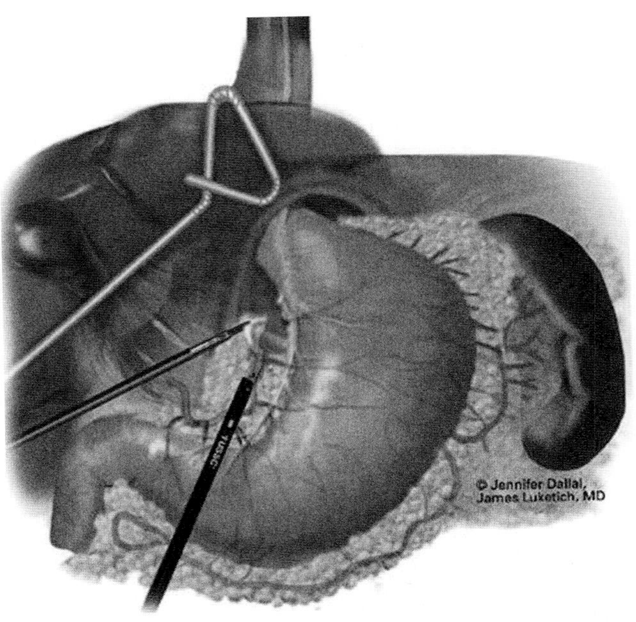

FIGURE 67.4

Abdominal dissection of the gastrohepatic ligament, allowing exposure of the right crus of the diaphragm.

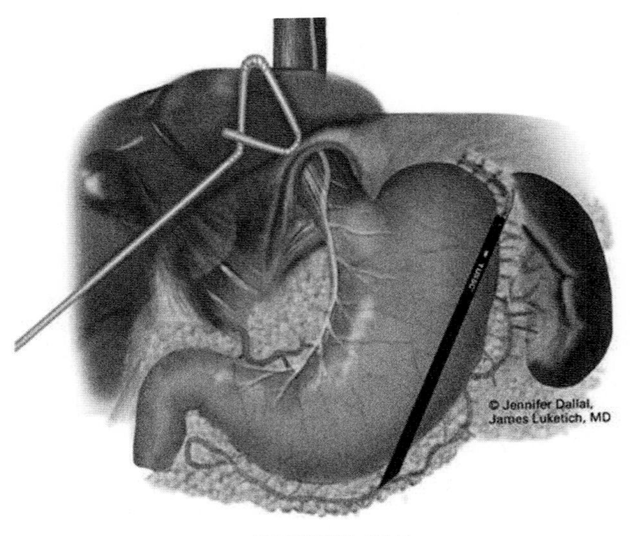

FIGURE 67.5

Laparoscopic gastric mobilization with division of short gastric vessels.

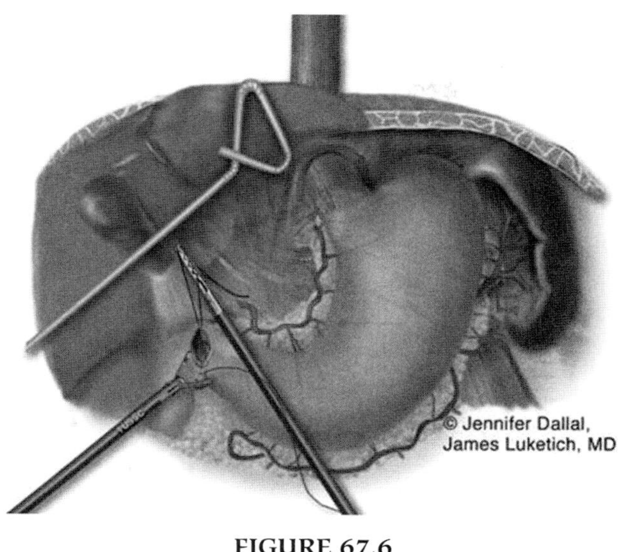

FIGURE 67.6

Laparoscopic pyloroplasty.

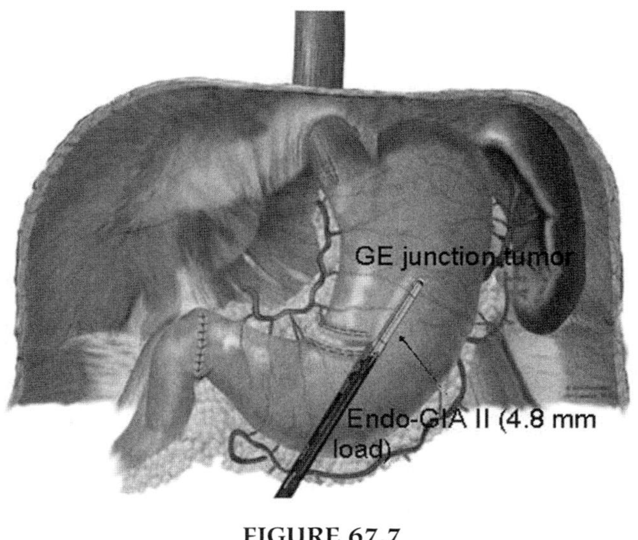

FIGURE 67.7

Laparoscopic construction of gastric conduit.

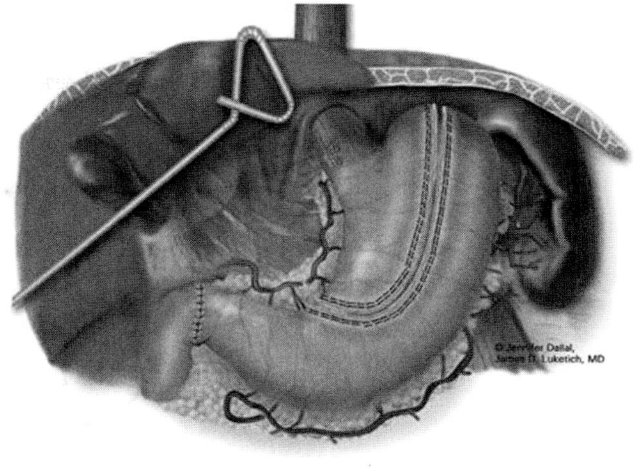

FIGURE 67.8

Laparoscopic construction of gastric conduit.

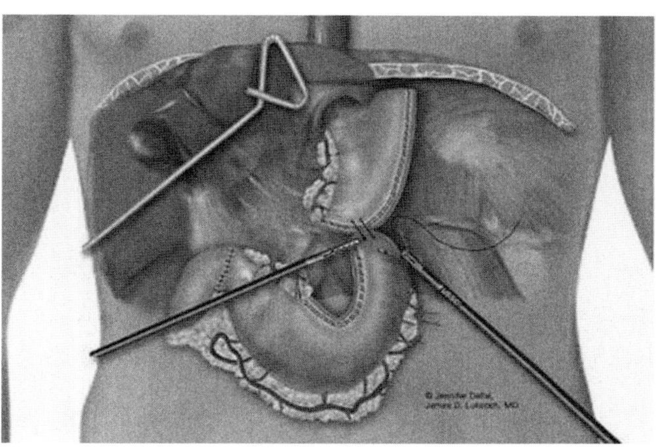

FIGURE 67.9

Attachment of the gastric tube to the esophagogastric specimen.

facilitate suturing of the jejunum to the anterior abdominal wall. The colon is retracted superiorly, the ligament of Treitz is identified, and the jejunum is traced distally for a distance of 50 cm. The jejunum is fixed to the left anterior abdominal wall with 2–0 suture. We prefer to use a needle jejunostomy feeding catheter kit (Compat Biosystems, Minneapolis, MN) that is placed percutaneously into the peritoneal cavity under direct laparoscopic visualization and is directed into the selected portion of jejunum. Using the Seldinger technique, a guide wire is advanced through the introducer needle and into the lumen of the jejunum, and the catheter is then threaded over the guide wire. To ensure intralumenal placement of the catheter, a small amount of air is injected into the lumen to confirm positioning. The puncture site is then sealed either with a purse-string suture or with 3 tacking sutures positioned circumferentially between the jejunal entry site and anterior abdominal wall. Another suture is placed 3 to 4 cm distally to prevent torsion.

After the feeding jejunostomy tube is placed, the phrenoesophageal membrane is divided to complete the esophageal mobilization. If necessary, the right and left crura can be divided with the coagulating shears to widen the hiatus and allow passage of the gastric tube into the chest. This maneuver helps minimize diaphragmatic compression of the gastric conduit, a potential cause of delayed gastric emptying postoperatively.

Neck. We then turn our attention to the neck. A 4- to 6-cm horizontal left neck incision is made 2 cm above the sternal notch. After dividing the subcutaneous tissue and platysma muscle, the plane between the carotid sheath and trachea is opened sharply. The omohyoid muscle is divided. The strap muscles are most often retracted medially but also can be partially divided. A finger or sponge stick is used to retract the thyroid, avoiding retraction of the recurrent laryngeal nerve. The deep cervical fascia is opened, and the posterior mediastinal space is entered bluntly directly over the anterior aspect of the spine. This maneuver places the surgeon in direct continuity with the mobilized thoracic portion of the esophagus. The Penrose drain, which was placed thoracoscopically, is then retrieved through the neck incision (Figure 67.10). The esophagus is divided 3 cm distal to the cricopharyngeus, and the esophagogastric specimen is carefully pulled out of the wound while the laparoscopic assistant carefully delivers the conduit into proper alignment in the mediastinum. Care is taken to prevent trauma to the ascending gastroepiploic arcade and avoid spiraling of the stomach (Figure 67.10). Tissue is sent for frozen section analysis of the surgical margins. An anastomosis is then performed between the esophagus and gastric tube using a hand-sewn technique (Figure 67.11). A nasogastric tube is passed distally through the anastomosis into the gastric tube for postoperative decompression.

The gastric antrum is grasped carefully, and gentle caudal retraction is applied to remove any redundant gastric tube that may have been pulled above the diaphragm during pull-up. The gastric tube is sutured in proper orientation to the right and left crura and anteriorly to the diaphragmatic hiatus to prevent hiatal herniation. The neck is irrigated with antibiotic solution and the skin of the neck closed, loosely approximated,

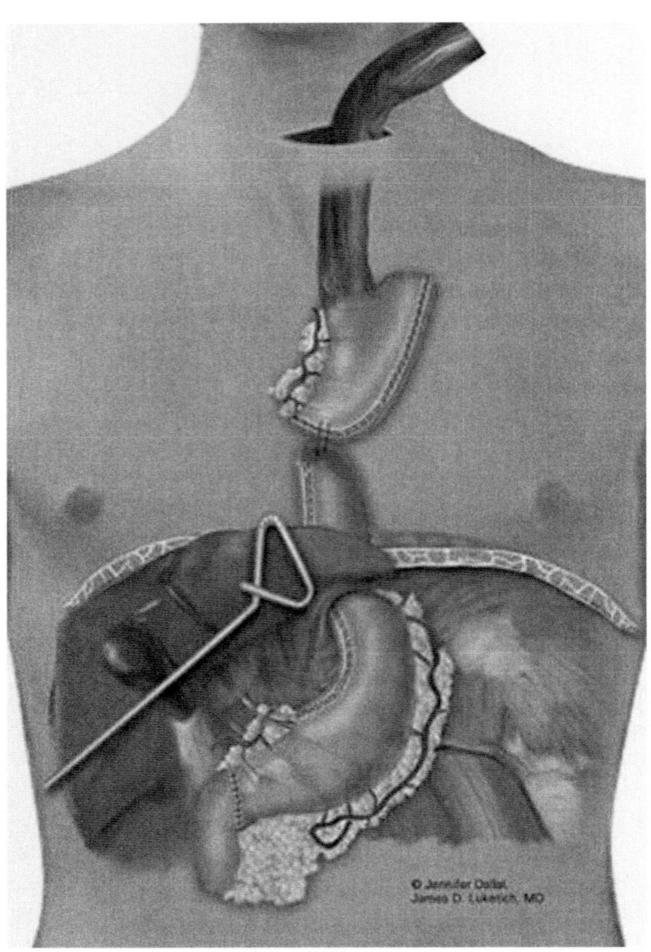

FIGURE 67.10

Retrieval of surgical specimen through a neck incision and gastric pull-up.

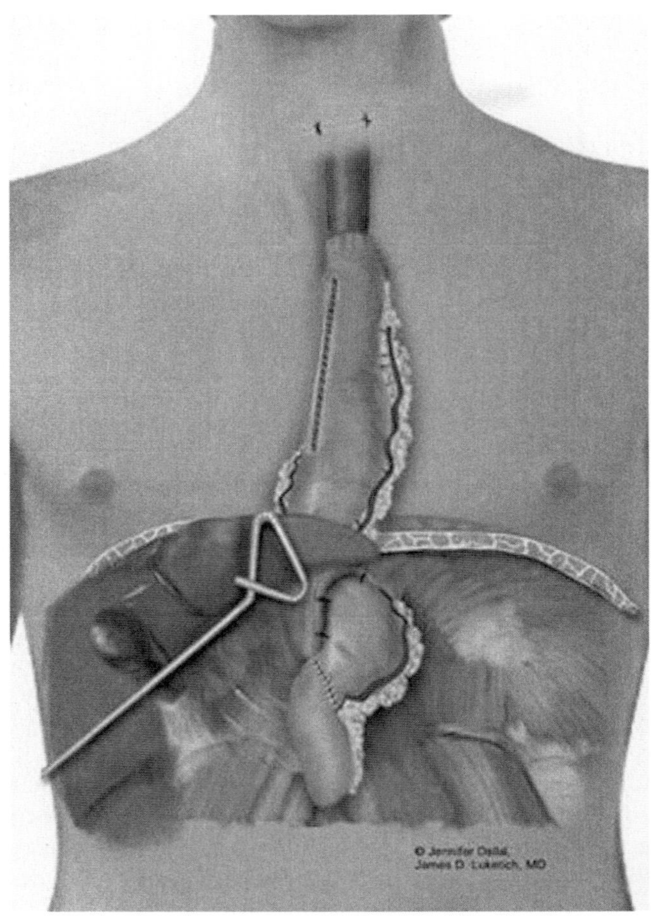

FIGURE 67.11

Completed schematic view of thoracoscopic and laparoscopic esophagectomy with cervical anastomosis.

with staples or sutures. The completed reconstruction is shown in Figure 67.11.

Laparoscopic and Thoracoscopic Ivor Lewis Resection

The Ivor Lewis MIE is performed in 2 stages. In the first stage, the patient is supine for laparoscopic construction of the gastric conduit, pyloroplasty, and feeding jejunostomy tube placement. In the second stage, the patient is repositioned to a left lateral decubitus position for mobilization of the thoracic esophagus, removal of the esophageal specimen, gastric pull-up, and construction of an intrathoracic esophagogastric anastomosis. All technical aspects of this procedure prior to construction of the intrathoracic anastomosis are as described in the previous procedure.

Intrathoracic anastomosis. We use the port sites for thoracoscopy that were described earlier. The only modification is to enlarge the posterior eighth intercostal port site to 4 cm to allow the introduction of the end-to-end anastomosis (EEA) stapler (United States Surgical Corp.) and removal of the specimen. A laparoscopic wound protector is used at this site to minimize the risk of port site contamination. Once the esophagus has been mobilized to a level 4 to 5 cm above the azygos vein, the distal esophagus and stomach are brought through the hiatus into the chest, along with the gastric tube that has been sutured to the specimen. The esophagus is elevated and transected 2 to 3 cm above the level of the azygos vein. The tumor specimen is removed using an Endo Catch bag (United States Surgical Corp.). The anvil of a 25 mm EEA stapler is then placed into the proximal esophagus and secured using a purse string. The stapler is then placed through the enlarged port, introduced into the tip of the newly created gastric conduit, and a circular anastomosis (side of gastric conduit to end of esophagus) is created at the level of the azygos vein (Figure 67.12). The redundant portion of the gastric conduit is trimmed using an articulating, linear stapler (Endo GIA II, U.S. Surgical), and a 28-F chest tube and 10-mm closed-suction drain are placed near the anastomosis. The potential space between the conduit and the right crus of the diaphragm is then closed with interrupted stitches to prevent delayed herniation.

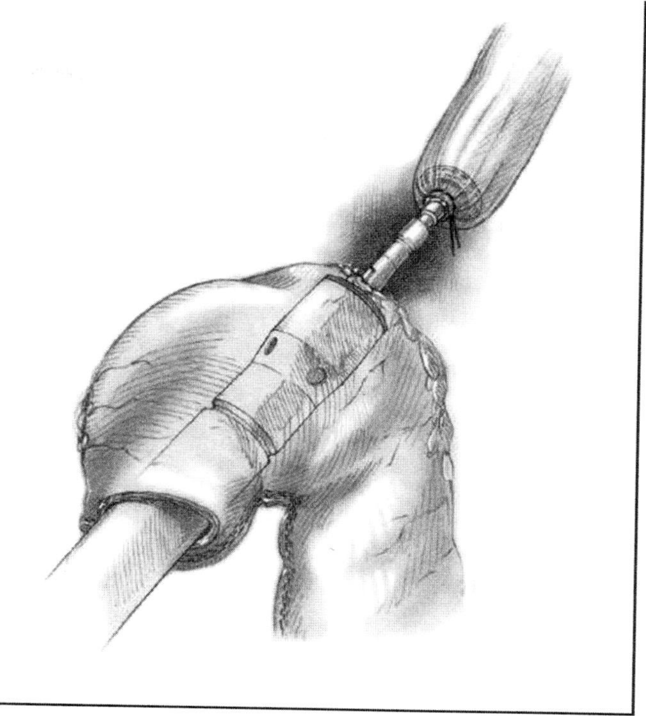

FIGURE 67.12

The handle of the EEA stapler is brought out along the greater curve and joined with the anvil in the proximal esophagus. Prior to bringing the stapler out along the greater curve, the amount of conduit in the chest is assessed to prevent redundancy of the stomach above the diaphragm. © Heart, Lung and Esophageal Surgery Institute; University of Pittsburgh Medical Center.

CONCLUSION

MIE is technically demanding with a long learning curve. The outcomes from MIE match and, in many instances, surpass those of most open esophagectomy series. The successful outcomes encountered with the use of MIE will help broaden the applicability of this technique to higher-risk patient groups, such as the elderly (18). Currently, a Phase II Eastern Cooperative Oncology Group Intergroup Study (E2202) is underway to evaluate the clinical outcomes of MIE in patients with high-grade dysplasia of the esophagus or stages I to III esophageal cancer as compared with traditional, open surgery. The objectives of the study are to determine the feasibility of performing MIE in patients with high-grade dysplasia or stages I to III esophageal cancer using 30-day mortality as the primary end point, determine the complications associated with this procedure, determine the rate at which conversion to open operation is required, and determine the length of the operation, duration of intensive care unit stay, and length of hospital stay. This large study should help define optimal MIE surgical protocols based on patient criteria. Until a consensus is reached, however, the surgeon must tailor the surgical approach for each patient, taking into account tumor size, location, and patient characteristics, as well as the surgeon's own comfort and level of expertise with the chosen approach.

References

1. Kelsen DP Ginsberg R, Pajak TF, et al. Chemotherapy followed by surgery compared with surgery alone for localized esophageal cancer. *N Engl J Med.* 1998;339(27):1979–1984.
2. Birkmeyer JD, Siewers AE, Finlayson EV, et al. Hospital volume and surgical mortality in the United States. *N Engl J Med.* 2002;346(15):1128–1137.
3. Luketich JD, Fernando HC, Christie NA, et al. Outcomes after minimally invasive esophagomyotomy. *Ann Thorac Surg.* 2001;72:1909–1913. [PubMed]
4. Pierre A, Luketich JD, Fernando HC, et al. Results of laparoscopic repair of giant para-esophageal hernia: 200 consecutive patients. *Ann Thorac Surg.* 2002;74:1909–1915.
5. Krasna MJ, Jiao X. Thoracoscopic and laparoscopic staging for esophageal cancer. *Sem Thorac Cardiovasc Surg.* 2000;12:186–194.
6. Luketich JD, Schauer P, Landreneau R, et al. Minimally invasive surgical staging is superior to endoscopic ultrasound in detecting lymph node metastases in esophageal cancer. *J Thorac Cardiovasc Surg.* 1997;114:817–823.
7. Luketich JD, Schauer PR, Christie NA, et al. Minimally invasive esophagectomy. *Ann Thorac Surg.* 2000;70:906–912.
8. Luketich JD, Nguyen NT, Weigel T, et al. Minimally invasive approach to esophagectomy. *J Soc Laparoendosc Surg.* 1998;2(3):243–247.
9. Watson DI, Davies N, Jamieson GG. Totally endoscopic Ivor Lewis esophagectomy. *Surg Endosc.* 1999;13:293–297.
10. Luketich JD, Alvelo-Rivera M, Buenaventura PO, et al. Minimally invasive esophagectomy: outcomes in 222 patients. *Ann Surg.* 2003;238(4):486–494.
11. Fernando HC, Christie NA, Luketich JD. Thoracoscopic and laparoscopic esophagectomy. *Semin Thorac Cardiovasc Surg.* 2000;12(3):195–200.
12. Fernando HC, Luketich JD, Buenaventura PO, et al. Outcomes of minimally invasive esophagectomy (MIE) for high-grade dysplasia of the esophagus. *Eur J Cardiothorac Surg.* 2002;22(1):1–6.
13. Nguyen NT, Schauer PR, Luketich JD. Combined laparoscopic and thoracoscopic approach to esophagectomy. *J Am Coll Surg.* 1999;188(3):328–332.
14. Nguyen NT, Schauer P, Luketich JD. Minimally-invasive esophagectomy for Barrett's esophagus with high-grade dysplasia. *Surgery.* 2000;127(3):284–290.
15. Pierre AF, Luketich JD. Technique and role of minimally invasive esophagectomy for premalignant and malignant diseases of the esophagus. *Surg Oncol Clin N Am.* 2002;11(2):337–350.
16. Litle VR, Buenaventura PO, Luketich JD. Minimally invasive resection for esophageal cancer. *Surg Clin N Am.* 2002;82(4):711–728.
17. Bizekis C, Kent MS, Luketich JD, et al. Initial experience with minimally invasive Ivor Lewis esophagectomy. *Ann Thorac Surg.* 2006;82(2):402–406; discussion 406–407.
18. Perry Y, Fernando HC, Buenaventura PO, et al. Minimally invasive esophagectomy in the elderly. *J Soc Laparoendoscop Surg.* 2002;6(4):299–304.

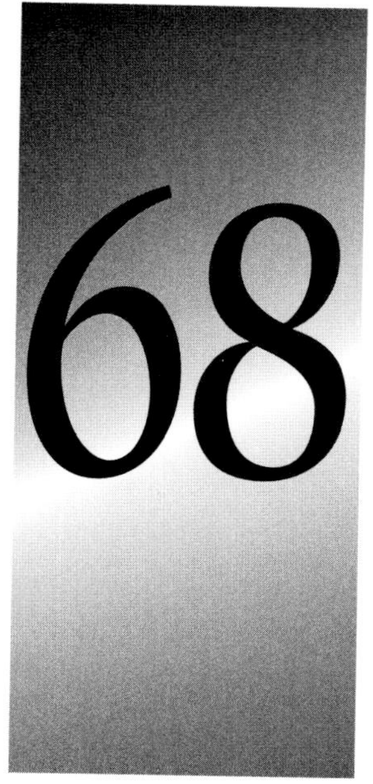

68 Surgery Techniques: Ivor-Lewis Esophagectomy

Xavier Benoit D'Journo
Pascal Ferraro
Jocelyne Martin
André Duranceau

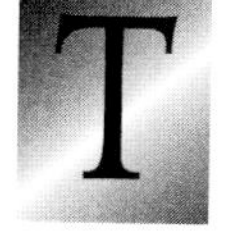

The Ivor-Lewis esophagectomy is used for patients with tumors of the middle or lower third of the esophagus. Originally described in 1946, the operation then involved a 2-stage approach in 2 separate settings (1). A laparotomy with gastric mobilization was completed initially, and 2 weeks later, a right thoracotomy allowed the completion of the operation. The current technique has evolved into a single-stage operation with its abdominal component, followed by a right chest approach for removal of the diseased esophagus and reconstruction using the mobilized stomach. A number of reports have now documented consecutive series of more than 100 patients without mortality and with minimum morbidity (2–4).

When treating cancer, the Ivor-Lewis esophagectomy must respect 3 main objectives:

1. Offer a complete resection of the tumor with an extended lymphadenectomy.
2. Prevent complications with a safe and simple technique of dissection and reconstruction.
3. Provide excellent and satisfactory digestive comfort with a high intrathoracic anastomosis.

THE PROCEDURE

Anesthesia

The use of a double-lumen endotracheal tube allows the lung to be collapsed and affords excellent exposure for the esophageal dissection and subsequent anastomosis. Epidural analgesia is essential to obtain satisfactory levels of analgesia postoperatively, thereby facilitating physiotherapy and enhancing respiratory function. Moreover, epidural analgesia has been shown to improve the microcirculation in the gastric tube in the early postesophagectomy period (5,6). The level of epidural anesthesia should be to T5–6. Arterial and central venous pressure lines are inserted, and the patient is installed with bladder drainage.

During the thoracic approach, a single lung ventilation is useful to obtain proper exposure for a systematic dissection of the esophagus and adjacent structures (7). Warming of the patient during the operation should allow early extubation (8).

Surgical Approach

The Ivor-Lewis esophagectomy is a 2-stage operation where the abdominal approach gives the advantage of a meticulous abdominal exploration and dissection to exclude any subdiaphragmatic spread undiagnosed by the preoperative clinical staging, to mobilize the stomach on its vascular pedicles so that it can be transposed as an esophageal replacement into the chest, and to resect all lymphatic drainage from the paraesophageal and cardiac nodes, as well as those of the lesser curvature and left gastric nodes (9,10). This is followed by a right thoracotomy with esophageal resection and reconstruction.

Abdominal Operation

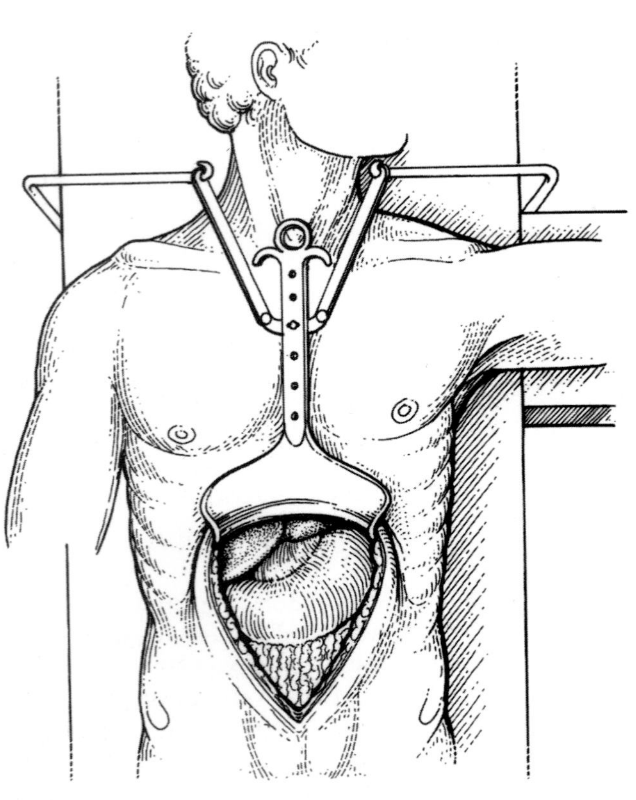

FIGURE 68.1

The operation is started with a midline epigastric incision extending to the right paraombilical region. From Chapman F. Surgery of the upper digestive tract. In: Rob & Smith, eds. *Operative Surgery*. Launois B. London: Chapman & Hall Medical; 1994:179.

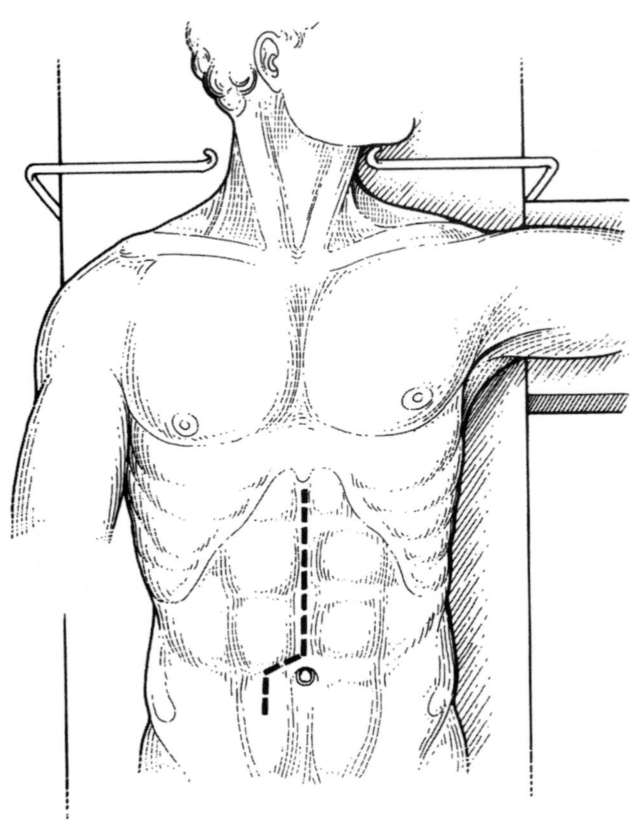

FIGURE 68.2

Assessment of the supramesocolic area as well as of the remaining abdominal cavity is completed to rule out liver metastases, extensive lymph node disease, or peritoneal seedings. An upper hand retractor is installed after resection of the xyphoid process, and a Balfour self-retractable system provides ample access to the stomach, transverse colon, and the hiatus and intra-abdominal esophagus. From Chapman F. Surgery of the upper digestive tract. In: Rob & Smith, eds. *Operative Surgery*. Launois B. London: Chapman & Hall Medical; 1994:179.

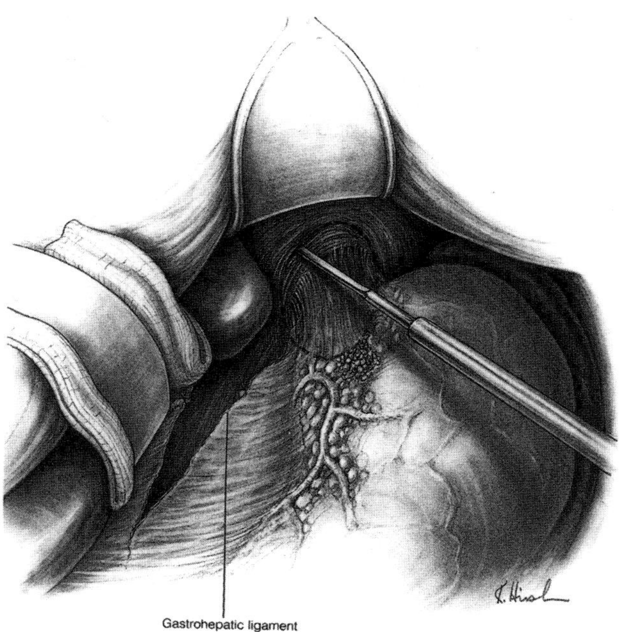

FIGURE 68.3

The triangular ligament of the left lobe of the liver is divided and the lobe retracted to the right, exposing the left lobe vein and the connecting infradiaphragmatic vein. The gastrohepatic ligament is sectioned with ligation of an occasional arterial branch from the left gastric artery to the left lobe of the liver. The right crus of the diaphragmatic hiatus is thus exposed. The right gastric artery is protected to the level of the second branch above the incisura. The hiatus is exposed without trying to dissect the esophagus, and resection of the hiatus will be left in continuity with the esophagogastric junction. From Skinner DB. Esophagectomy without thoracotomy. In: Skinner DB, ed. *Atlas of Esophageal Surgery.* New York: Churchill Livingstone; 1991:43.

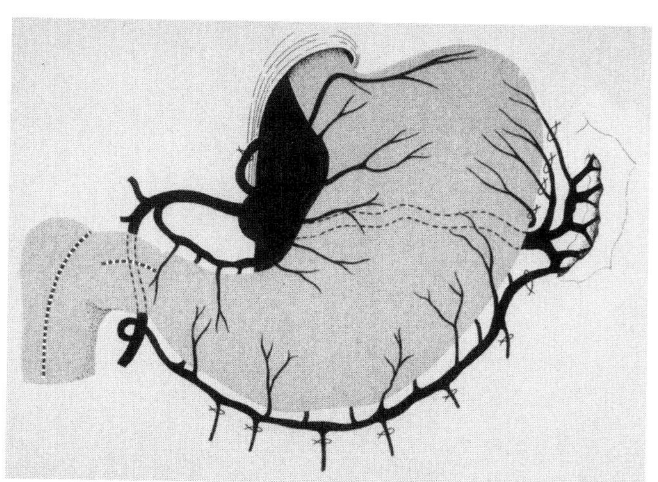

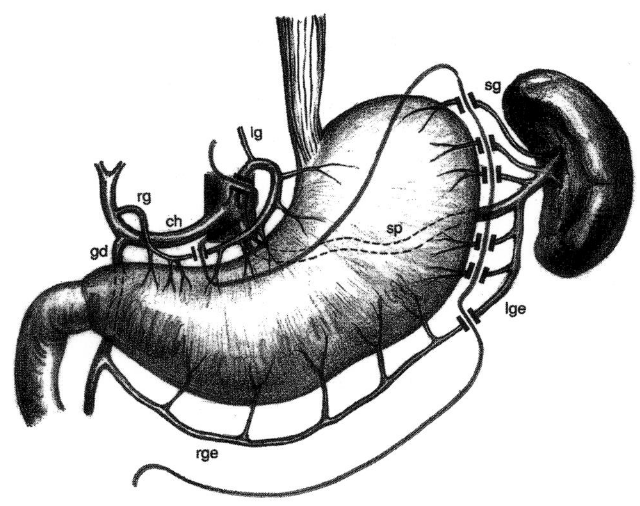

FIGURE 68.4

Mobilization of the greater curve of the stomach is made with careful protection of the right gastroepiploic vessel. This is done by opening the lesser sac: the retrogastric space is accessed directly or by freeing the greater omentum from the transverse colon. The gastroepiploic artery is identified on its entire bourse, until its last branch enters the greater curvature of the stomach. The right gastroepiploic arcade is interrupted where it meets the left gastroepiploic artery, usually at the level of the spleen-inferior pole. The short gastrosplenic vessels are clipped and divided as far laterally as possible. Once freed from the spleen, the retracted fundus exposes the left crus of the diaphragmatic hiatus. From Akiyama H. *Surgery for Cancer of the Esophagus.* In: Akiyama H, eds. Philadelphia: Williams and Wilkins; 1990:56.

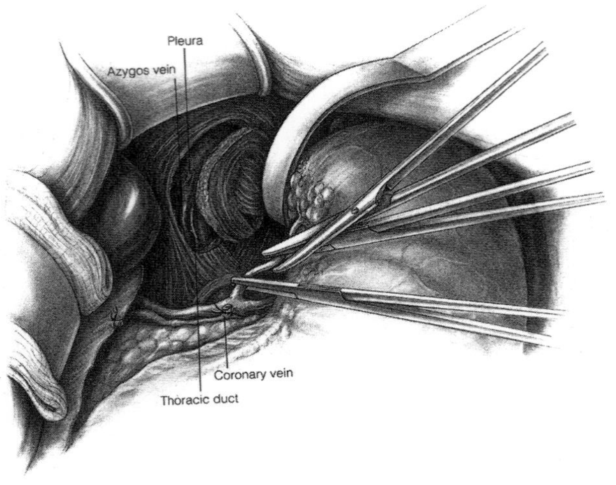

FIGURE 68.5

Once the hiatus is completely exposed, a cuff of diaphragm including part of the right and left crura is divided and left in continuity with the esophagus, providing a healthy tissue margin around the tumor. The mediastinum becomes widely accessible, and the distal esophagus is dissected above the diaphragm. A tape is passed around it. From Skinner DB. Esophagectomy without thoracotomy. In: Skinner DB, ed. *Atlas of Esophageal Surgery*. New York: Churchill Livingstone; 1991:45.

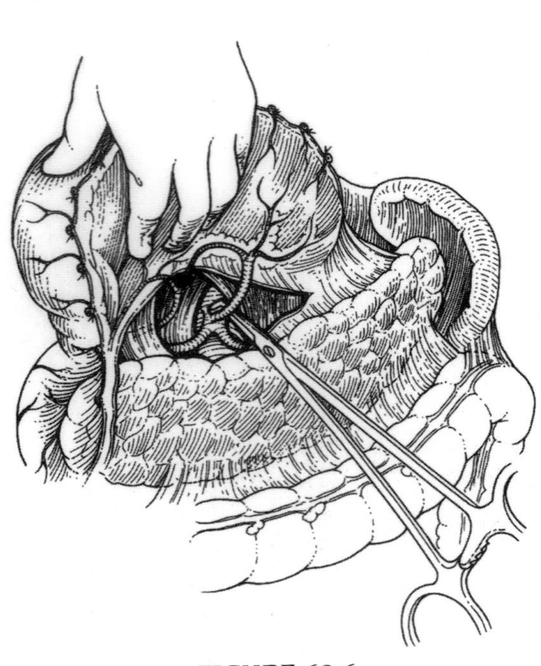

FIGURE 68.6

With the mobilized greater curve and fundus, the stomach is held upward, and the left gastric vessels are exposed. The left gastric vein and artery are individually ligated and divided. Posterior mobilization of the hiatus is completed. The distal esophagus and stomach are completely free. From Chapman F. Surgery of the upper digestive tract. In: Rob & Smith, eds. *Operative Surgery*. Launois B. London: Chapman & Hall Medical; 1994:179.

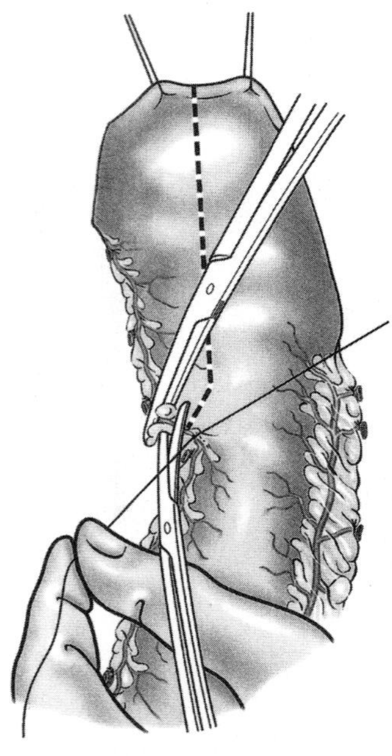

FIGURE 68.7

The smaller curvature transection line on the stomach is prepared during the abdominal part of the operation. Anterior and posterior right gastric vessels to the smaller curvature are ligated above the second branches proximal to incisura, over a distance of 4 cm. The denuded smaller curvature allows for an easier stapler application when the resection is completed in the right chest. From Holsher AF. Use the stomach as an esophageal substitute. In: Jamieson G, Kaiser LR, eds. *Operative Thoracic Surgery*. London: HodderArnold; 2006:357.

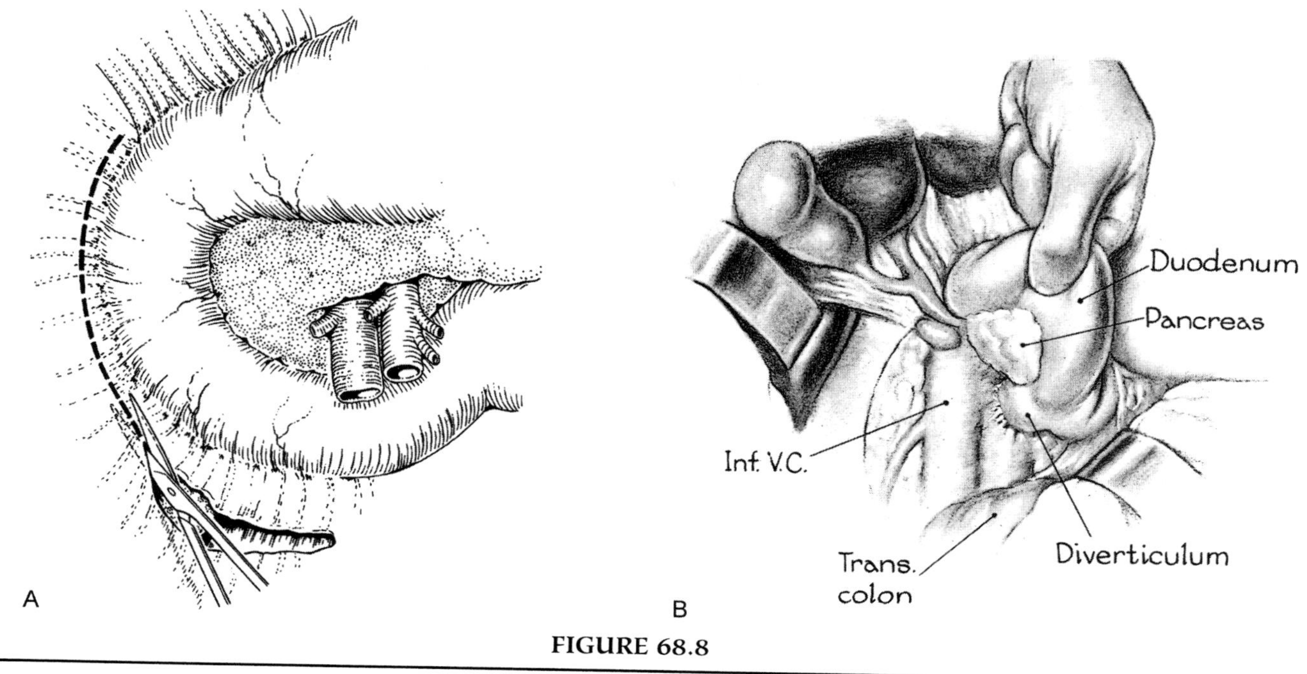

FIGURE 68.8

Mobilization of the duodenum to the margin of the third portion (Kocher maneuver) is then performed to provide increased gastric mobility (A). (From Chapman F. Surgery of the upper digestive tract. In: Rob & Smith, eds. *Operative Surgery*. Kluwer; 1994:539 with permission) The head of the pancreas is freed from the interior vena cava, and the left renal vein is visualized where it enters the vena cava. With this mobilization, the pylorus should reach the midline, in proximity to the hiatus (B). (From Madden's J. Esophagectomy. In: Madden's J, ed. *Atlas of Technics in Surgery*. Bloomington: Appleton Country Crofts; 1958:325).

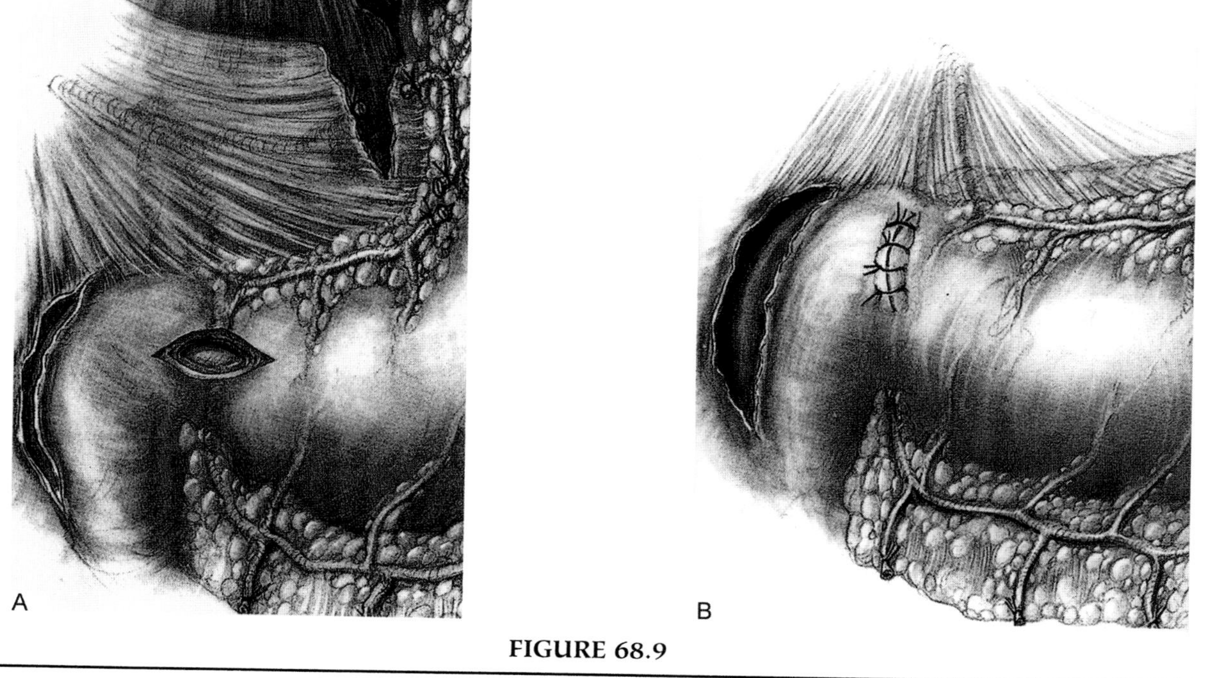

FIGURE 68.9

A pyloromyotomy is added to allow easier gastric emptying. A 3-cm horizontal incision is completed, 1 cm on the duodenum and 2 cm on the anterior antrum (A). The pyloric muscle is divided as for the Fredet-Ramstedt operation, and the muscle is closed vertically as for a Heineke-Mikulicz pyloroplasty. If entry into the duodenal mucosa occurs, a standard pyloroplasty closure is completed with an added omentum coverage for safety (B). From Skinner DB. Esophagectomy without thoracotomy. In: Skinner DB, ed. *Atlas of Esophageal Surgery*. New York: Churchill Livingstone; 1991:57.

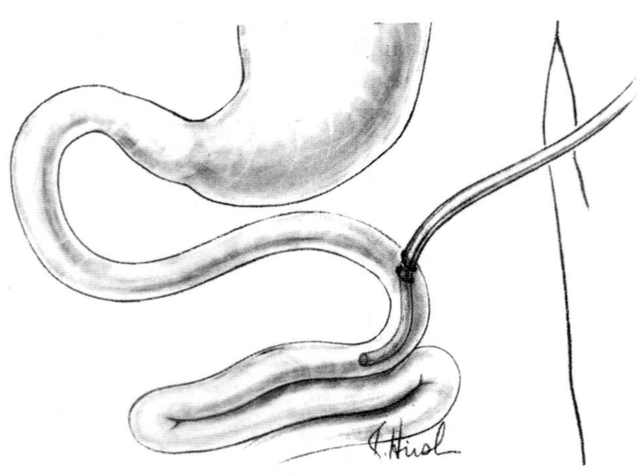

FIGURE 68.10

A feeding jejunostomy is installed routinely to provide proper caloric intake early in the postoperative period. It also provides a enteral approach in the event of unexpected major morbidity. A double purse-string suture is positioned on the antimesenteric wall of the first jejunal loop. A no. 18 T tube is installed and exteriorized in a left paraombilical position. Several interrupted sutures then anchor the perijejunostomy serosa to the peritoneum, and the tube is fixed at skin level. From Skinner DB. Esophagectomy without thoracotomy. In: Skinner DB, ed. *Atlas of Esophageal Surgery*. New York: Churchill Livingstone; 1991:181.

Thoracic Operation

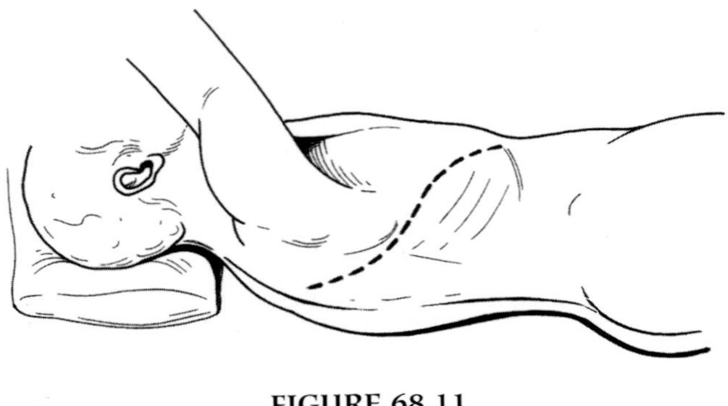

FIGURE 68.11

The right thoracotomy is completed above the sixth rib with division of the rib posteriorly. This allows exposure of the esophagus without interference of the aortic arch. If needed, a second distal thoracotomy may be carried out over the eighth or ninth rib by the same incision. This permits exposure and dissection of the distal esophagus with the azygos and the thoracic duct under direct vision. From Belsey RH, Stipa G, eds. *La chirurgia dell'esophago*. Padova: Piccin Editore; 1980:444.

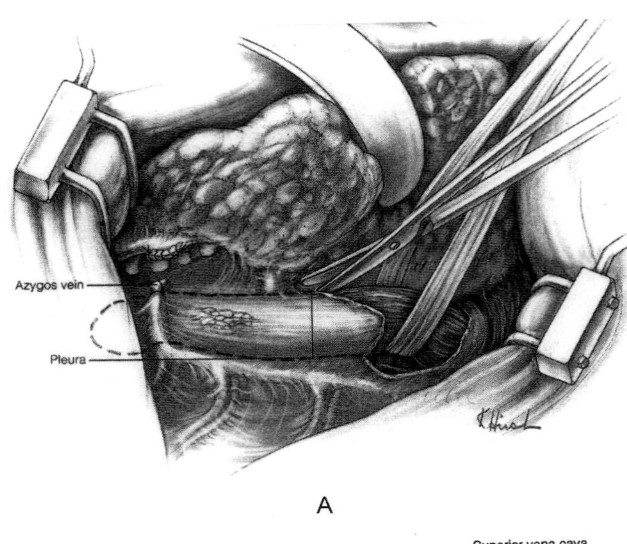

A

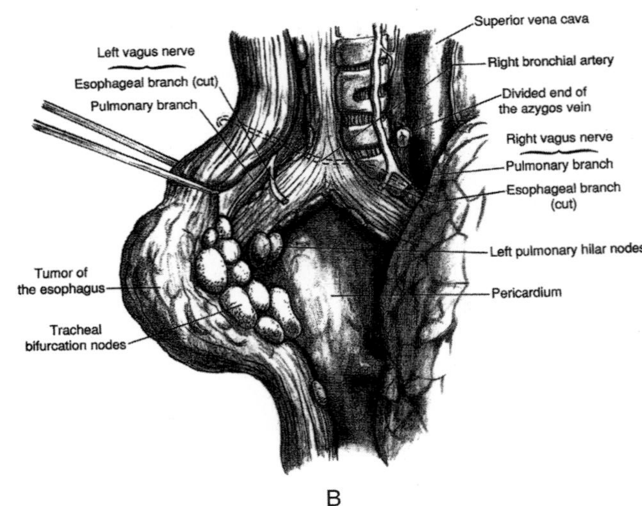

B

FIGURE 68.12

Once the chest opened, the lung is collapsed and retracted anteriorly. The esophagus, with the resected hiatus, is surrounded with a penrose drain. The inferior pulmonary ligament is divided to the inferior pulmonary vein and the mediastinal pleura divided along the posterior limits of the pericardium (A). The dissection follows the vascular plane behind the posterior pericardium toward the tracheal bifurcation. The subcarinal nodes are dissected free and left in continuity with the esophagus. The pleura is left in continuity with the esophagus. The azygos vein is ligated and divided near its insertion in the vena cava (B). From Skinner DB. Esophagectomy without thoracotomy. In: Skinner DB, ed. *Atlas of Esophageal Surgery*. New York: Churchill Livingstone; 1991:37.

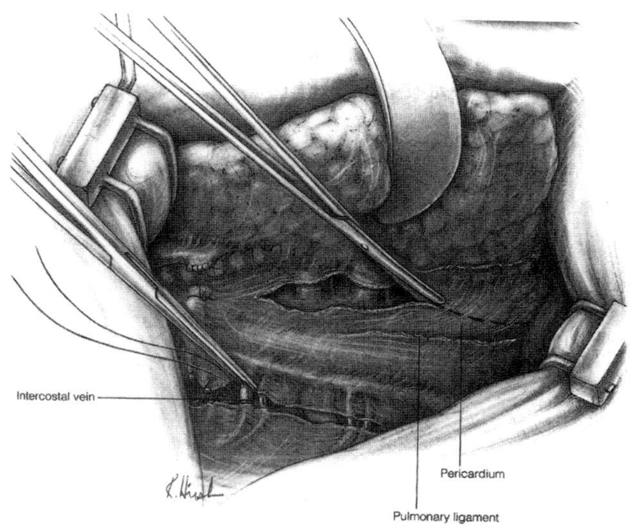

FIGURE 68.13

Posteriorly, the third and fourth intercostal veins are also tied and divided to free the upper part of the azygos arch. For an en bloc resection of the esophagus, all the intercostal veins are ligated and divided, and the aortic adventitia is opened and dissected to expose and ligate all the esophageal arteries penetrating the posterior mesoesophagus. At the level of the right crus of the diaphragm, a mass ligation of the azygos and thoracic duct allows the esophagus to be completely free from its mediastinal attachments between the diaphragm to the level immediately above the azygos arch. From Skinner DB. Esophagectomy without thoracotomy. In: Skinner DB, ed. *Atlas of Esophageal Surgery.* New York: Churchill Livingstone; 1991:33.

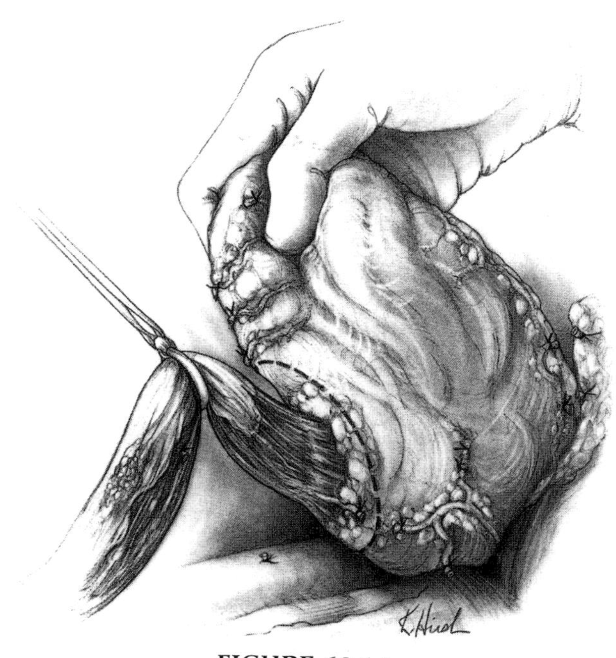

FIGURE 68.14

The stomach and gastroesophageal junction are freed after the abdominal dissection. Through the open hiatus, the entire stomach can be brought carefully in the chest cavity, taking care of keeping the smaller curvature toward the right side of the vertebral bodies, leaving the fundus and greater curvature toward the mediastinum. From Skinner DB. Esophagectomy without thoracotomy. In: Skinner DB, ed. *Atlas of Esophageal Surgery.* New York: Churchill Livingstone; 1991:41.

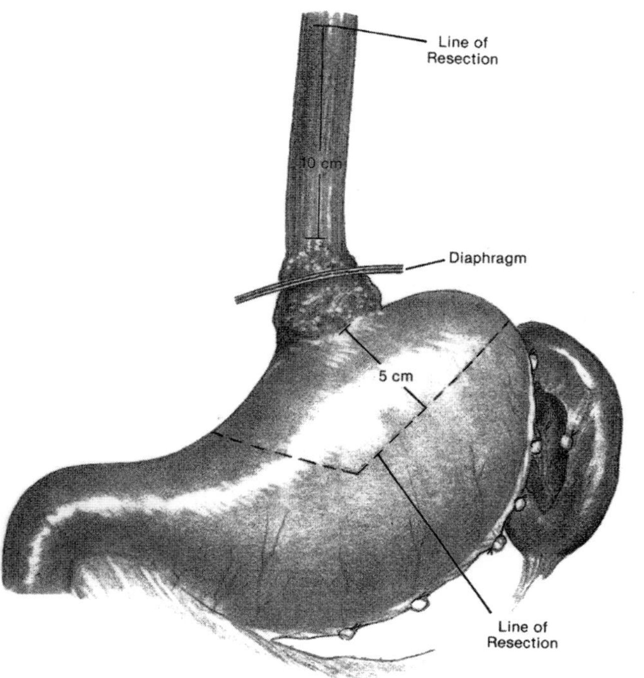

FIGURE 68.15

Once the stomach is properly positioned, the resection line is planned on the stomach: a distance of 5 cm should be kept from the macroscopic margin of the tumor when it is a cardia lesion. The stapling instrument is initially applied on the proximal greater curvature. The resection line is then oriented toward the previously prepared smaller curvature. The gastric tube is completed. (A) Transection of the esophagus is preferably made 10 cm above the proximal margin of the tumor. (B) When the tumor is located in the middle or distal esophagus, only the cardia is resected with the lymphatic drainage of the smaller curvature. From Hood RM, ed. *Techniques in General Thoracic Surgery.* Philadelphia: W. B. Saunders; 1985:202.

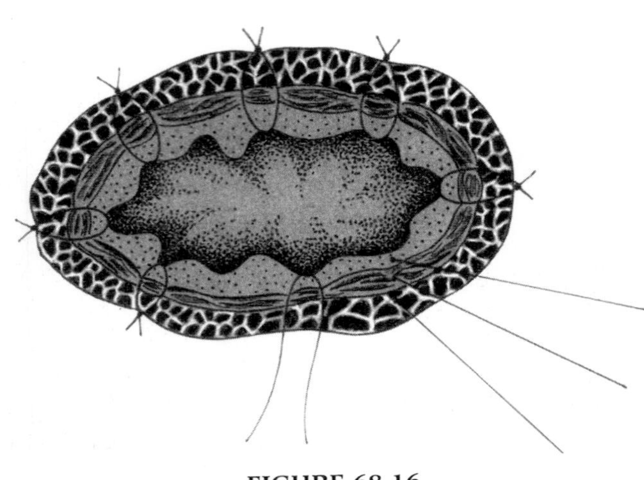

FIGURE 68.16

The esophageal remnant is prepared for the anastomosis once the pathologist has excluded residual disease on the transection line. Using small resorbable sutures (4–0), the esophageal wall layers are assembled together to create a single layer, preventing retraction of the mucosal and muscular planes. The position of the anastomosis is then selected on the anterior wall of the gastric tube, near the greater curvature.

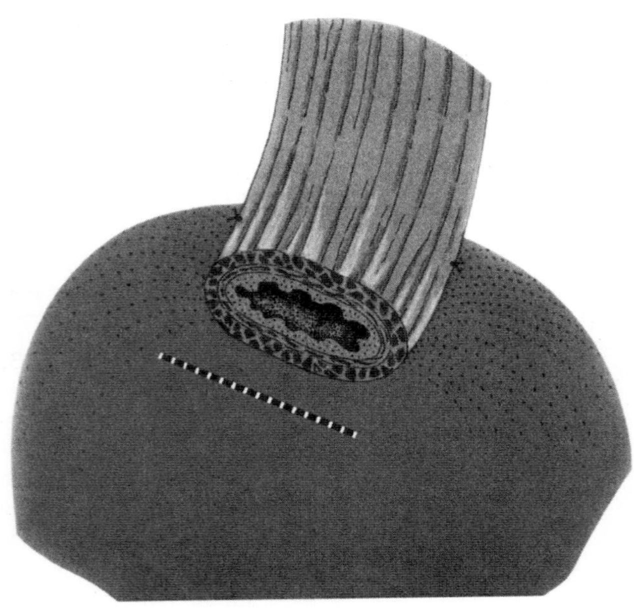

FIGURE 68.17

The position of the anastomosis is selected on the anterior wall of the gastric tube near the greater curvature. The proximal tip of the stomach tube is fixed by 4 silk sutures to the posterior wall of the esophagus, 4 to 5 cm above the transection line.

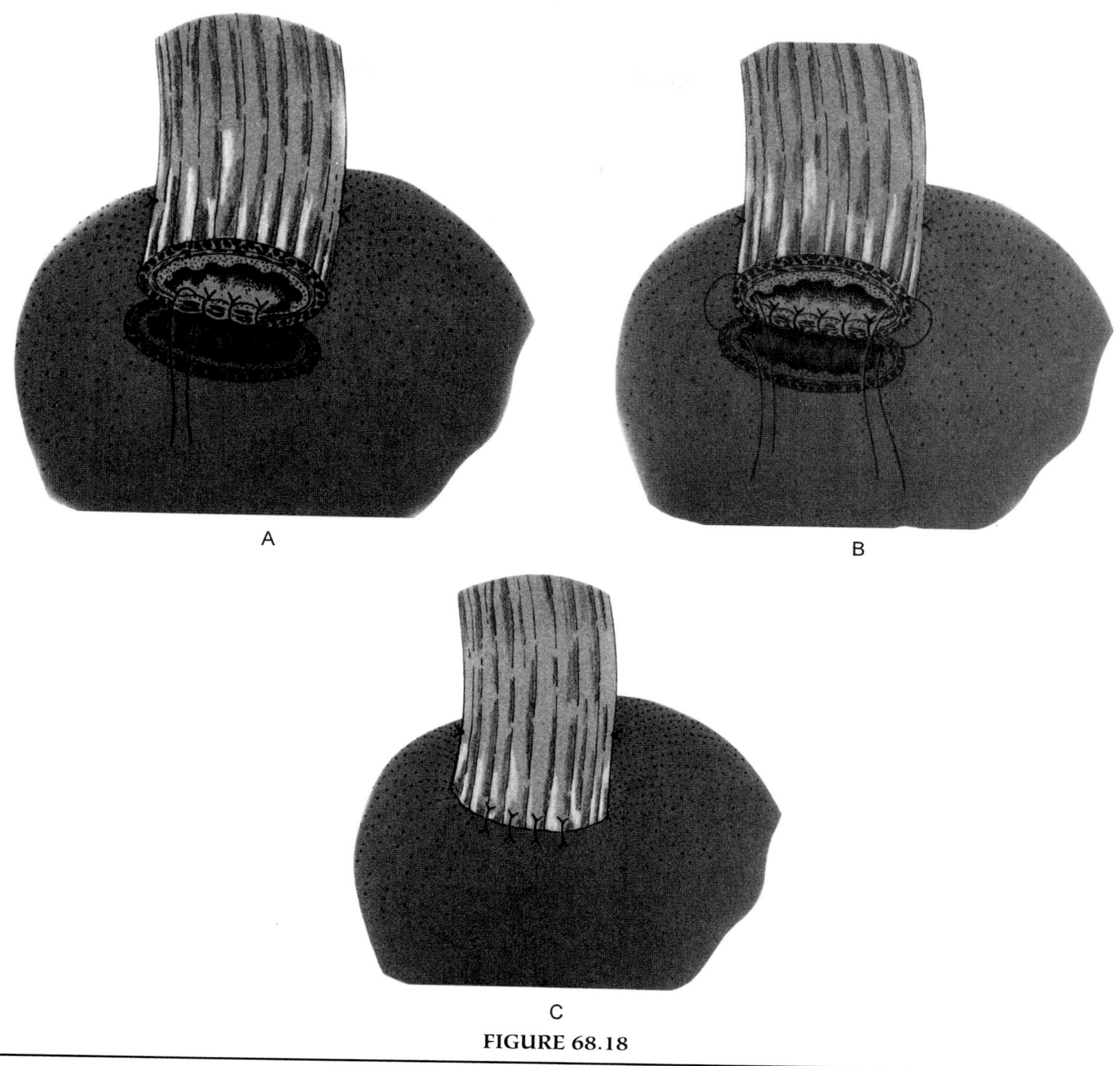

FIGURE 68.18

The stomach cavity is opened and a single layer anastomosis is created with separate 3–0 polyglycolic acid sutures on the posterior wall. (A) Inverting sutures are continued on the lateral limits of the anastomosis (B), and the anterior wall is closed with 5 to 6 separate stitches tied on the outside (C). A double-lumen (sump-type) nasogastric tube is positioned in the stomach cavity under direct vision before closing the anterior anastomosis. Gastrocolic omentum is brought to cover the completed reconstruction.

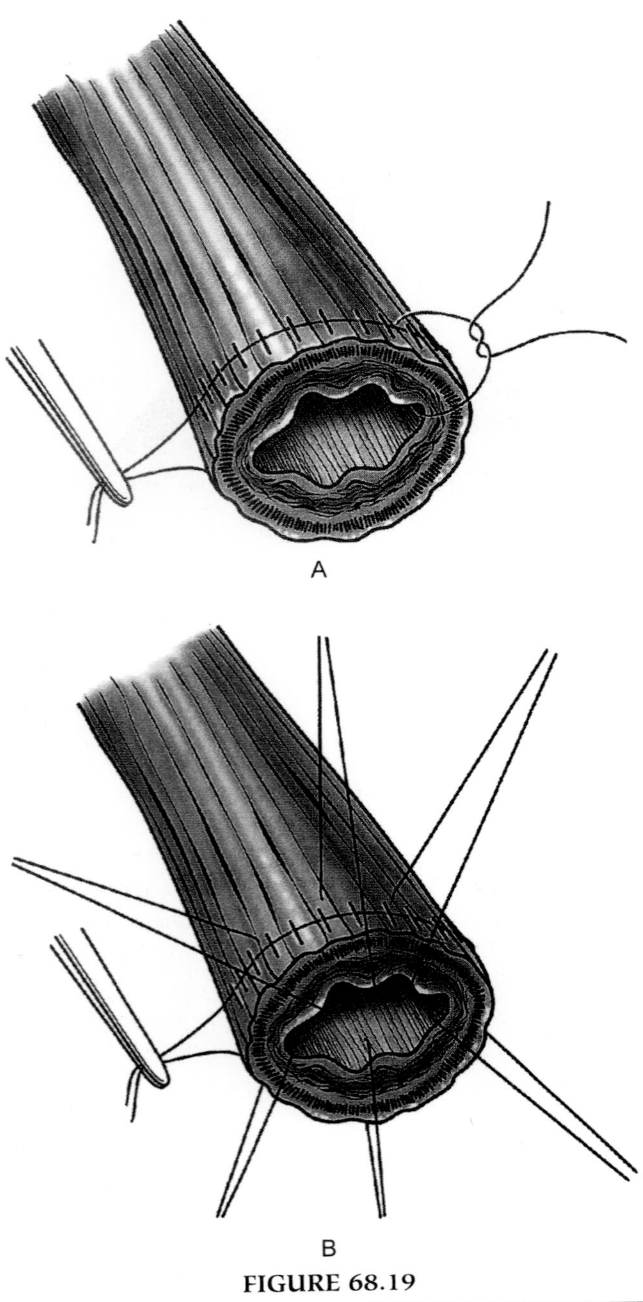

FIGURE 68.19

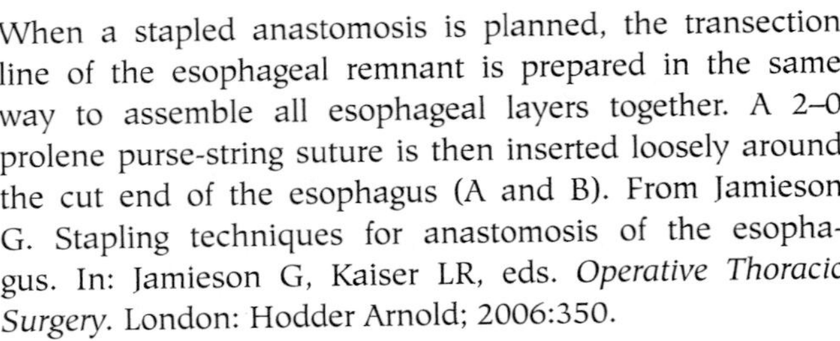

When a stapled anastomosis is planned, the transection line of the esophageal remnant is prepared in the same way to assemble all esophageal layers together. A 2–0 prolene purse-string suture is then inserted loosely around the cut end of the esophagus (A and B). From Jamieson G. Stapling techniques for anastomosis of the esophagus. In: Jamieson G, Kaiser LR, eds. *Operative Thoracic Surgery*. London: Hodder Arnold; 2006:350.

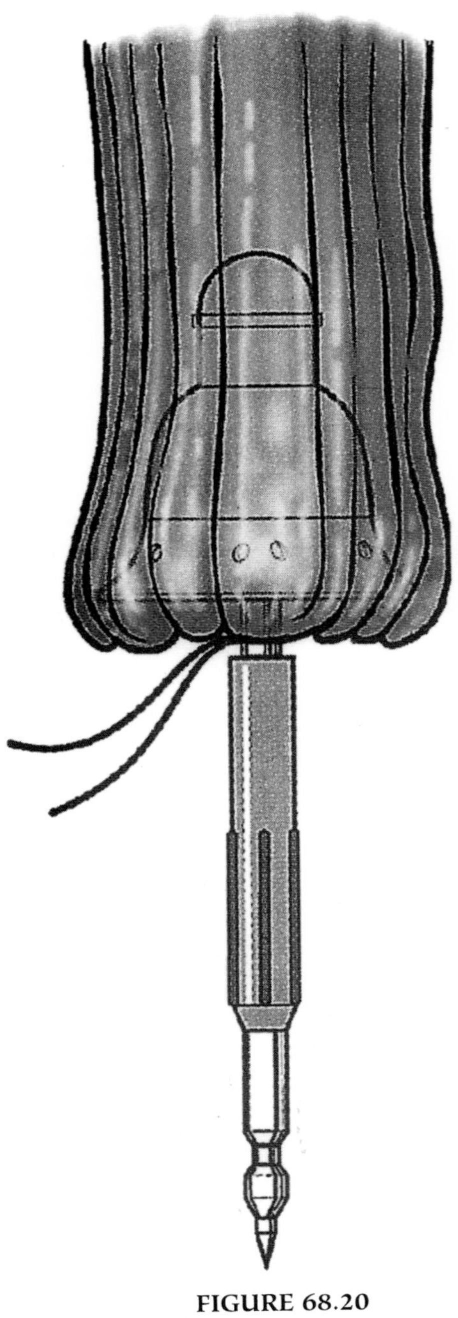

FIGURE 68.20

The 25- or 28-mm anvil head is detached from the stapling gun and positioned into the esophageal remnant. The purse-string suture is tied snugly around the shaft of the anvil head. From Kelly J. Sutured anastomoses. In: Jamieson G, Kaiser LR, eds. *Operative Thoracic Surgery*. London: Hodder Arnold; 2006:352.

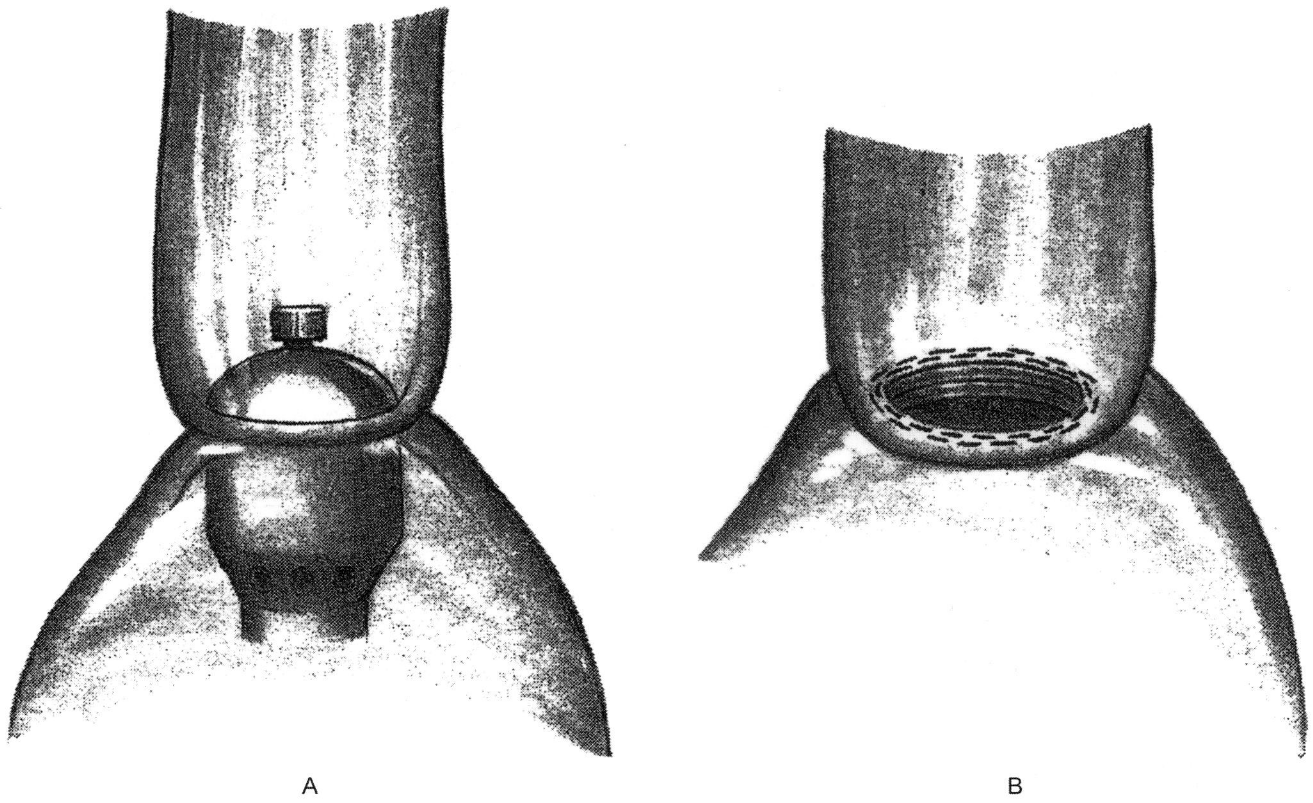

A B

FIGURE 68.21

Two to 3 cm of the stapled line of the gastric tube are removed, and the stapling gun is inserted into the cavity of the stomach tube. Its pointed shaft is fully retracted until the exact position of the gun for the anastomosis has been identified. This is usually on the posterior wall of the gastric tube near the greater curvature but with protection of its blood supply (A). The gun shaft is exteriorized to penetrate the gastric wall. It is then connected with the protruding shaft of the anvil head, which has been inserted into the remaining esophagus. The gun is fired and removed, and the esophageal and gastric doughnuts are inspected to ensure their circumferential integrity (B). From Hood M, ed. *Techniques in General Thoracic Surgery.* Philadelphia: W. B. Saunders; 1985:206.

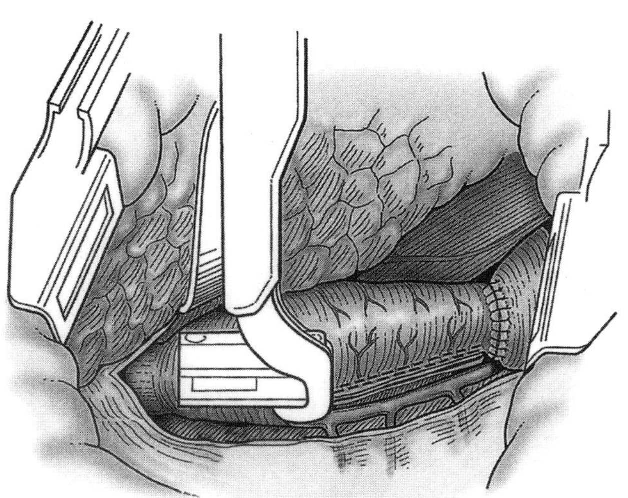

FIGURE 68.22

A linear stapler (TA 60) completes the reclosure of the gastric tube on the smaller curvature. The tip of the anterior gastric tube is fixed to the esophagus, covering the anastomosis area. From Launois B. Abdominal and right thoracic subtotal esophagectomy. In: Jamieson G, Kaiser LR, eds. *Operative Thoracic Surgery.* London: Hodder Arnold; 2006:377).

POSTOPERATIVE MANAGEMENT

After extubation, the patient is usually transferred to the step-down unit of the Thoracic Surgery Division, where optimal monitoring is maintained for the initial postoperative 72 hours. A chest radiograph confirms normal lung reexpansion, and intravenous fluids are administrated to maintain appropriate hematocrit and intravascular volume. Prophylactic antibiotics covering aerobes and anaerobes are used before the operation, and an additional 2 doses are administered after completion of the surgery. Epidural analgesia usually enables good pain control and early ambulation with the help of the physiotherapist. Thromboembolic prophylaxis is provided with elastic stockings and subcutaneous heparin injections.

Nasogastric tube suction is maintained until appropriate gastric emptying is documented. With return of normal peristalsis, jejunostomy feeding is started, usually on the third or fourth postoperative day. Enteral feeding is maintained until appropriate caloric intake is quantified.

The chest tube is removed when no air leak has been observed and drainage is less than 200 mL in a 24-hour period. The integrity of the anastomosis is controlled radiologically 7 or 8 days after the operation.

COMPLICATIONS

Specific major complications in patients undergoing esophagectomy and reconstruction with the stomach include respiratory failure, anastomotic leakage, and delayed gastric emptying. Gastroesophageal reflux damage is frequent and does not correlate with the usual reflux symptom.

Atelectasis and Respiratory Failure

Their prevalence is high after transthoracic esophagectomy (11–13). Good analgesia, physiotherapy, appropriate hydration, nasogastric drainage (14), and early mobilization are all essential to minimize respiratory complications.

Anastomotic Leakage

This may occur in the early postoperative period (2–3 days). It then should be attributed to a technical failure. A later leak (6–8 days) is thought more likely to be due to ischemic changes in the stomach. The most common area for gastric tube ischemia is between the anastomosis and the resection line on the smaller curvature. If the leak is small and contained or if it is well drained by the chest tube, a conservative management is in order. Gastric ischemia may be associated with profound acidosis, pulmonary patchy infiltrates, and respiratory distress. Such signs should alert the team to the possibilities of gastric necrosis. Endoscopy may help in this setting, but early reexploration and appropriate resection is mandatory. If necrosis of the stomach is documented, resection to viable tissue with a cervical esophagostome and gastrostomy on the remaining stomach repositioned in the abdomen should be done. If local repair or reanastomosis is attempted, devitalized tissue should be debrided, and the repair should be buttressed with healthy tissue, such as omentum, pericardial flap, or pedicled muscle. A cervical esophagostome is preferred with gastric decompression if any concern exists about the repair.

Delayed Gastric Emptying

There are a number of reasons for delayed gastric emptying: the stomach is denervated, the pylorus may cause functional obstruction, angulation may occur at the level of the hiatus, or the intrathoracic stomach may be redundant, especially if a total gastric replacement has been used. A pyloromyotomy or pyloroplasty may help prevent gastric retention but allows for mixed reflux to occur. Delayed gastric emptying may be helped by metoclopramide domperidone or by erythromycin. Failure of conservative management requires reoperation and an appropriate drainage procedure.

Gastroesophageal Reflux

Intrathoracic esophagogastric reconstruction induces gastroesophageal reflux. The severity of mucosal damage in the esophageal remnant is influenced by the level of reconstruction by the duration of evolution after the operation and by the gastric emptying capacity. Symptoms are not reliable, and endoscopic follow-up is the most reliable method for an objective diagnosis and appropriate management.

CONCLUSION

The Ivor-Lewis esophagectomy is an excellent operation for lesions of the middle and lower third of the esophagus (15). The long-term functional results are good. It provides, when curative, excellent staging information while usually insuring a safe reconstruction without tension and with the use of a well vascularized gastric transplant.

References

1. Lewis I. The surgical treatment of carcinoma of the esophagus with special reference to a new operation for growths of the middle third. *Br J Surg.* 1946;34:18.
2. Visbal AL, Allen MS, Miller DL, et al. Ivor Lewis esophagogastrectomy for esophageal cancer. *Ann Thorac Surg.* 2001;71:1803–1808.
3. Karl RC, Schreiber R, Boulware D, et al. Factors affecting morbidity, mortality, and survival in patients undergoing Ivor Lewis esophagogastrectomy. *Ann Surg.* 2000;231:635–643.
4. Cerfolio RJ, Bryant AS, Bass CS, et al. Fast tracking after Ivor Lewis esophagogastrectomy. *Chest.* 2004;126:1187–1194.
5. Michelet P, Roch A, D'Journo XB, et al. Effect of thoracic epidural analgesia on gastric blood flow after oesophagectomy. *Acta Anaesthesiol Scand.* 2007;51:587–594.
6. Michelet P, D'Journo XB, Roch A, et al. Perioperative risk factors for anastomotic leakage after esophagectomy: influence of thoracic epidural analgesia. *Chest.* 2005; 128:3461–3466.
7. Michelet P, D'Journo XB, Roch A, et al. Protective ventilation influences systemic inflammation after esophagectomy: a randomized controlled study. *Anesthesiology.* 2006; 105:911–919.
8. Chandrashekar MV, Irving M, Wayman J, et al. Immediate extubation and epidural analgesia allow safe management in a high-dependency unit after two-stage oesophagectomy: results of eight years of experience in a specialized upper gastrointestinal unit in a district general hospital. *Br J Anaesth.* 2003;90:474–479.
9. Mathisen DJ. Ivor Lewis procedure. In: Griffith Pearson F, et al, eds. *Esophageal Surgery.* New York: Churchill Livingstone; 1995:669.
10. Fumagalli U, Akiyama H, DeMeester TR, et al. Resective surgery for cancer of the thoracic esophagus: results of a consensus conference held at the VIth World Congress of the International Society for Diseases of the Esophagus. *Dis Esophagus.* 1996; 9:30–38.
11. Avendano CE, Flume PA, Silvestri GA, et al. Pulmonary complications after esophagectomy. *Ann Thorac Surg.* 2002;73:922–926.
12. Ferguson MK, Durkin AE. Preoperative prediction of the risk of pulmonary complications after esophagectomy for cancer. *J Thorac Cardiovasc Surg.* 2002;123:661–669.
13. Karl RC, Schreiber R, Boulware D, et al. Factors affecting morbidity, mortality, and survival in patients undergoing Ivor Lewis esophagogastrectomy. *Ann Surg.* 2000; 231:635–643.
14. Shackcloth MJ, McCarron E, Kendall J, et al. Randomized clinical trial to determine the effect of nasogastric drainage on tracheal acid aspiration following oesophagectomy. *Br J Surg.* 2006;93:547–552.
15. Hulscher JB, van Sandick JW, de Boer AG, et al. Extended transthoracic resection compared with limited transhiatal resection for adenocarcinoma of the esophagus. *N Engl J Med.* 2002;347:1662–1669.

Surgery Techniques: Transhiatal Esophagectomy without Thoracotomy

Paula Ugalde
Rodney J. Landreneau
Arjun Pennathur

In 1913, Denk (1) performed the first extrathoracic esophagectomy. With a vein stripper (metal ring), he avulsed the esophagus blindly from cadavers and experimental animals. Nevertheless, the first successful transhiatal esophagectomy (THE) was performed only in 1933. The patient had esophageal cancer and the procedure was carried out through combined abdominal and cervical incisions in 2 different stages; first for the resection and second to reestablish the alimentary tract (2).

Subsequently, the transthoracic technique with intrathoracic anastomosis achieved widespread use and acclaim (3). The blind mediastinal dissection and the fear that the stomach as a conduit would not reach the neck justified the abortion of the transhiatal technique. However, frequent postoperative complications associated with the necessary thoracotomy were high (4). As a result, in 1978 in the work of Orringer (5), THE emerged as an alternative operative approach that could be associated with less risk and morbidity (6).

In 1948, Sweet (10) and Garlock (11) both demonstrated that the stomach can be mobilized through the chest to allow a tension-less cervicogastric anastomosis. In the 1970s several case reports were published advocating THE for benign and malignant esophageal diseases (7–9). Orringer and Sloan (12) described the use of substernal gastric bypass in patients with surgically incurable esophageal cancer. Although this did not result in an effective palliative procedure due to major surgical complications (13), the rational for this surgery was to relieve dysphagia with a straightforward bypass (12). Orringer (14) showed that with proper mobilization, the stomach can easily reach the neck for the cervical anastomosis. In 1978, the first series of THE was published and the technique was popularized as an alternative approach for benign and malignant esophageal disease (5). Regardless of the level of esophageal pathology, the entire esophagus was removed and a high cervical gastroesophageal anastomosis was performed (5).

Orringer and colleagues have been instrumental in establishing the safety of THE and the techniques in this chapter are primarily derived from their work.

Esophageal reconstruction involves 3 important decisions: the necessity of removing the patient's esophagus, the route to re-establish the alimentary tract, and the organ to be used as conduit. The development of new modern anesthetic techniques, refinement of the operative techniques, and advances in critical care management have all allowed a significant decrease in the surgical morbidity and mortality rates of these patients (3). Nevertheless, the stage and biologic behavior of the tumor are important factors that will determine survival in patients with esophageal cancer (14).

At present, the 2 main approaches for an esophagectomy are transhiatal (THE) and transthoracic (TTE) (3).

Over the last years, technical advances have improved the effectiveness of both procedures in reestablishing continuity of the alimentary tract in a safe and efficient manner. However, there remains a controversy over the best method of treatment, which has been coupled with increasing efforts to reduce operative morbidity and mortality rates in a disease with somber prognosis. (15)

This chapter primarily focuses on open THE. Based upon Orringer's experience (5), a thoracotomy is seldom required to perform an esophagectomy in a benign esophageal disease Megaesophagus of achalasia and portal hypertension are exceptions due, respectively, to extensive pleural adhesions and the risk of bleeding. Some of the potential advantages of a transhiatal technique include a decrease in the incidence of respiratory complications (16), and the reduced risks of a cervical anastomotic leak in comparison to an intrathoracic anastomotic leak (17, 18).

PATIENT SELECTION

Patient selection is critical to optimizing surgical results. This includes risk assessment for this purpose and accurate staging.

Indications

All patients who are candidates for an esophagectomy, even after chemotherapy, radiotherapy, caustic injuries, achalasia, or previous surgery, can be considered for the transhiatal approach. The stomach is the preferred organ to use as conduit because of its rich blood supply, mobility, length to reach the neck, and the need for only one unique anastomosis. In case of esophageal cancer, a gastric conduit can be performed for tumors at all levels of the esophagus (19). This type of resection is safe and well tolerated (19–20).

Contraindications

Contraindications for THE include bronchoscopic evidence of tracheobronchial invasion, or distant metastasis, during preoperative assessment (21). In the absence of clinical contraindications, the most critical assessment is in the operating room, with the surgeon's palpation through the hiatus determining if the resection is feasible and safe. Firm adhesion of the esophagus to the aorta or the tracheobronchial tree, either from direct tumor transgression or dense adhesions, contraindicates a THE (22).

Preoperative Preparation

Ideally, at least 2 weeks before surgery, the patient should start pulmonary physiotherapy and smoking cessation. The nutritional status needs to be evaluated and optimized as soon as possible. If weight loss and nutritional depletion are severe, consideration should be given to supplemental feedings (20). In some instances, a feeding jejunostomy tube may be considered. Although colonic bowel preparation is not routinely required, patients with past history of gastric diseases or surgery should have their colon evaluated by a barium enema and prepared for surgery in case the stomach interposition is not feasible (21).

ANESTHESIA

Patients are typically monitored with continuous intra-arterial blood pressure monitoring, and 2 large-bore intravenous catheters should be placed in the patient for this purpose. This is important because the mediastinal blind blunt dissection compresses the heart and causes impaired diastolic filling, and because the estimated blood loses is between 0.5 L and 1 L (23).

An epidural catheter can be considered for better postoperative pain control and, consequently, better pulmonary function. A single-lumen endotracheal tube is normally used, except when the patient has a previous history of prior esophageal surgery or in upper or middle-third tumors, in which cases, a thoracotomy might be required.

Esophagoduodenoscopy is routinely performed at the beginning of the operative procedure under general anesthesia. This allows the surgeon to confirm the position of the tumor and review the surgical approach. Retroflexion is regularly performed to evaluate the gastroesophageal junction and cardia. It is prudent to avoid excessive air insufflation during the preoperative endoscopy.

OPERATIVE TECHNIQUE

The patient is positioned supine with the head in extension turned to the right on a shoulder roll. Prophylactic first-generation cephalosporin antibiotics are administered. The skin preparation includes the neck, anterior chest, and whole abdomen. The surgery is performed in a sequential fashion that starts in the abdomen, moves on to the neck and then combines both approaches.

Abdominal Phase: Laparotomy

The procedure begins with a midline incision starting from the xiphoid and extending to the umbilicus. In patients with cancer, it is important to first explore the abdomen to evaluate for metastasis in the peritoneum, liver, and periaortic and distant metastatic lymph nodes. The resection is aborted if distant metastases are encountered (21,23). If proceeding with the resection, carefully examine the stomach for scarring or any other evidence of prior disease.

Once the tumor is deemed to be resectable, start by dividing the triangular ligament for mobilization of the left hepatic lobe. A self-retaining retractor is placed to help with exposure. The mobilization of the stomach is started typically at the midpoint of the greater curvature. It is critical to handle the stomach gently, with care, and identify and preserve the gastroepliploic arcade. While the first assistant retracts the colon, dissection is started where the right gastroepiploic artery terminates through an avascular portion of the omentum toward the spleen. The transition between the short gastric vessels and the gastroepiploic arcade must be identified to avoid injuries to the right gastroepiploic artery. In addition, as the short gastric vessels are divided, care is taken to stay away from the spleen. Larger vessels should be ligated separately; the ultrasonic scalpel is useful for safely transecting the short gastric vessels. The remainder of the greater curve exposure is obtained by dividing the gastrocolic ligament on the anterior surface of the pancreas. The greater curve is, thus, mobilized from the left crus to the pylorus. The stomach is then retracted anteriorly and the posterior gastric attachments should then be divided.

The next step is to start dividing the gastrohepatic ligament with the electrocautery or an ultrasonic scalpel toward the right crus. Some prefer to preserve the right gastric artery. The left gastric vessels are identified. In view of unpredictable anatomic variations, it is important to recognize the celiac trunk and its branches and to identify any aberrant left hepatic artery, before dividing the left gastric vessels. The left gastric vessels can be divided with mechanical sutures or suture ligatures.

Once the stomach is completely mobilized, the duodenum is generously mobilized from its retroperitoneal location (Kocher maneuver) so the pylorus can be displaced from its usual position and the stomach gains maximal cephalad reach. A pyloromyotomy should be performed to avoid the possibility of delayed gastric emptying after vagotomy. Begin by placing a 4–0 silk stay suture at the most superior and inferior aspect of the pylorus. With traction on the stay sutures, the serosa and muscle across the pylorus are transversally scored with the electrocautery for a length of 1.5 cm. The dissection continues until the submucosa bulges out. The pyloromyotomy is covered with adjacent omentum. Alternatively, a pyloroplasty can be performed.

The phrenoesophageal ligament at the hiatus is divided as the crus of the diaphragm is opened anteriorly (23). The esophagogastric junction is encircled with a Penrose drain to use as a handle. With downward traction on the Penrose drain, the right hand enters the diaphragmatic hiatus to perform blunt finger dissection of the lower esophagus. At this point, it is important to ensure that the esophagus is free from pericardium, aorta, prevertebral fascia, and tracheobronchial tree. Fixation precludes resection or if deemed unsafe, do not hesitate to convert to a transthoracic resection (24).

Most of the esophagus can be released from the mediastinal attachments through the abdomen under direct vision, which allows the placement of clips in the blood vessels surrounding the esophagus. Placing the patient in reverse Trendelenburg position can aid the exposure. The major vagal trunks are divided as the esophagus is dissected from the pleura and pericardium. When the dissection is technically difficult, direct exposure of the esophagus is facilitated by small retractors in the diaphragmatic hiatus. The esophagus can be rotated in any direction and dissected routinely up to the level of the pulmonary veins and to the subcarinal area (25). No attempts should be made to include any surrounding soft tissue or lymph nodes in the specimen. In case of firm adhesions that cannot be separated from the mediastinal structures, the dissection should be abandoned and a right thoracotomy performed. The abdominal phase of the operation is concluded with the placement of a jejunostomy tube.

Cervical Phase

A 5 to 8 cm oblique incision, along the anterior border of the left sternocleidomastoid muscle, is made. The sternocleidomastoid muscle and carotid sheath are retracted laterally and the thyroid and larynx medially. During this phase, it is imperative that no retractor be placed against the tracheoesophageal groove to avoid injury to the recurrent laryngeal nerve. The middle thyroid vein is usually ligated and divided (21). Once the prevertebral fascia is reached, blunt dissection with an index finger is performed posterior to the esophagus as far caudal as possible.

Then, develop a plane between the trachea and the anterior surface of the esophagus; care must be taken not to injure the posterior membranous trachea. Start with sharp dissection, staying always posterior to the recurrent laryngeal nerve. Fingers must be kept closely applied to the wall of the esophagus. Once the anterior and posterior thoracic esophagus is mobilized, gently encircle it with a rubber drain and maintain an upward traction. With this maneuver, the esophagus can be liberated and mobilized from mediastinum down to the carina. When the upper third of the thoracic esophagus is firmly attached to the posterior membranous trachea, either because of tumor or inflammatory reaction, a partial median sternotomy might be necessary to provide good access and direct vision.

Transhiatal or Mediastinal Dissection

One hand is inserted through the diaphragmatic hiatus posterior to the esophagus while a half-sponge stick is placed through the cervical incision to dissect the esophagus off the prevertebral fascia and toward the abdomen (21). A gentle upward traction is applied in the encircling cervical rubber drain. Again, blunt dissection is carried out, keeping the fingers directly against the esophagus in the midline. This completes the liberation of the posterior esophagus.

The anterior mobilization is also performed from both abdominal and cervical incisions, with the fingers always directly against the anterior esophagus to avoid injury to the posterior membranous wall of the trachea. This part is usually more technically demanding. Through the hiatus the esophagus is held at the upper most level between the index and middle fingers and the remaining attachments are severed, with a downward motion from the superior mediastinum. At the subcarinal level, posterior pressure is exerted against the esophagus, thereby sweeping it away from the pericardium. The carina and left bronchus are vulnerable to injury if an inappropriate blunt dissection is performed. The vascular structure at risk is the azygos vein. Frequent assessment for blood pressure and constant communication with the anesthetist are essential in avoiding prolonged hypotension.

Once the esophagus is completely free, from the hiatus to the neck, divide it obliquely in its uppermost part distal to the cricopharyngeus muscle. Pull the surgical specimen through the abdomen. A careful inspection of the posterior mediastinum should be performed. Mediastinal packing for a couple of minutes is a prudent step and helps with hemostasis. In case of pleural entry, chest tubes should be inserted.

The stomach and esophagus are placed in the anterior abdominal wall to perform the partial proximal gastrectomy. To prepare the gastric tube, place traction in the highest point of the gastric fundus and another in the lowest point of the antrum so the stomach is stretched. An Endo GIA (gastrointestinal anastomosis) stapler (U.S. Surgical, Norwalk, Connecticut) is applied in the lesser curve toward the gastric fundus so the cardia and proximal stomach are resected. Allow 5 to 6 cm margins distal to the tumor. After each application of the stapler, the stomach is lengthened progressively cephalad, thereby maximizing the upward reach of the conduit. With most of the lesser curvature removed, the fundus can usually reach the neck without excessive tension and the stomach becomes a tubular structure instead of the usual reservoir (23). Even with gross 5 cm margin beyond the tumor, the gastric remnant is long enough to reach the cervical esophagus. In cases of benign disease or middle or upper esophageal cancer, more stomach can be preserved, saving the collateral circulation to the fundus. Some surgeons prefer to routinely oversew the staple line.

The entire forearm is passed through the diaphragmatic esophageal hiatus to ensure an adequate mediastinal tunnel for the new esophageal conduit. The stomach is gently pushed rather than pulled through the hiatus and delivered above the clavicles. It should pass through the original esophageal bed in the posterior mediastinum. This is a direct path, tension free, and does not require resection of the clavicle (23,25). The whole conduit should be palpated to assure proper positioning, without torsion ensuring proper orientation. When the gastric fundus appears in the cervical wound, it is gently grasped with a Babcock clamp and pulled upward as the other hand inserted from the abdomen gently pushes the stomach upward, making sure no twisting occurs. Every effort is made to minimize trauma to the mobilized stomach being used to replace the esophagus (26). The hiatus is re-approximated with non-absorbable sutures so that only 3 fingers pass alongside the stomach. Abdominal hemostasis and closure of the abdominal wound are completed prior to beginning the cervical esophagogastric anastomosis.

Cervical Esophagogastric Anastomosis

Several techniques have been described for the esophagogastric anastomosis, both manually or with mechanical sutures (12,23,25,27). In the 1990s, Dewar reported that the 2-layer interrupted anastomosis had the lowest leak rate (28).

If handmade, the traditional description of the Orringer technique is a single-layer, interrupted suture technique, constructing an end-to-side cervical esophagogastric anastomosis over a 46F bougie (6). A full-thickness of anterior gastric wall is excised 3 to 4 cm below the apex of the stomach to create an anterior gastric stoma. Interrupted 4–0 polyglycolic acid sutures are placed, and the anastomosis completed. A nasogastric (NG) tube is passed and placed above the pylorus. A muscle flap to protect the anastomosis has been suggested by some authors (23).

When performed with mechanical sutures, begin the anastomosis by placing the anvil of the circular Endo GIA stapler (U.S. Surgical, Norwalk, Connecticut) in the esophageal stump. Then, a 1.5 cm incision is made in the anterior gastric wall of the conduit distant from the gastric fundus, to allow the full insertion of the circular stapler. Once the esophagus and the stomach are aligned, the circular Endo GIA is closed into the anvil. The gastrotomy is closed with staplers.

Another option is to perform a side-to-side cervical anastomosis with a linear Endo GIA II 30–3.5 stapler (26). In this case, after performing the anterior gastrotomy, place 2 stay sutures to align the esophagus and the stomach. The stapler is inserted with the thinner anvil into the stomach and closed. Before firing, 2 suspension sutures are placed on either side of the anastomosis. Once fired, a NG tube is placed and the anastomosis can be completed in 2 layers. The gastric incision is closed with linear staplers and the cervical wound is closed over a drain.

POSTOPERATIVE CARE

The patients are usually extubated in the operating room, and the epidural catheter can be valuable in postoperative pain control. A chest X-ray is obtained in the recovery room to evaluate hemothorax, pneumothorax, and mediastinal widening. During the first 24 hours the patient must be under close observation and monitored. As soon as possible, respiratory physiotherapy is resumed and ambulation is encouraged. Early ambulation is a key factor in postoperative care.

The use of a feeding jejunostomy permits early postoperative discontinuation of intravenous feedings, and nutritional supplementation if necessary following the discharge from the hospital (18). Jejunostomy tube feeding is usually started in postoperative day 3, via slow infusion and, if well tolerated, can be progressively increased. Postoperative weight loss after esophagectomy is common, but it tends to stabilize within 1 to 3 months.

Postoperative protocols can vary. Some surgeons prefer to start oral intake after the barium swallow is done on or after postoperative day 7 and is confirmed to be normal; others remove the nasogastric (NG) tube by postoperative day 3 to 5. If the NG tube is removed by day 3 to 5, a liquid diet should begin 24 hours after removal and, on postoperative day 7, the barium swallow examination is obtained. Oral intake also is managed in different ways. Some prefer to leave the patients on a liquid diet while others advance in consistency. Patients may experience some degree of dysphagia independent of the type of anastomosis (18).

COMPLICATIONS

Hemorrhage

One of the greatest concerns with the use of THE has centered over the lack of direct visualization of the mediastinal dissection and, consequently, the risk of increased blood loss and the potential for catastrophic bleeding (22,29). This complication is rare and, when it occurs, is usually related to injury of larger vessels, such as the azygos and the aorta. Most of the arteries that nourish the esophagus originate directly from the aorta, divide into fine branches, and then penetrate the muscular wall to form an extensive interconnecting submucosal network. When these small vessels are torn, massive hemorrhage is rare and unusual (22). If the point of bleeding cannot be identified, the mediastinum should be packed and volume resuscitation started. If the bleeding continues, the procedure is converted to a thoracotomy.

The average bleeding for THE has been 500 mL to 1000 mL, but with experience, it has decreased (18). The key is to maintain the plane of dissection immediately on the muscular wall of the esophagus. Patients with tumors fixed to the aorta or periesophageal tissues should not undergo this procedure. In Orringer's series, less than 1% of patients required a thoracotomy for bleeding control (20).

Tracheal Tear

Tracheal tear is another major intraoperative complication with a lower rate of occurrence in experienced hands. Orringer reported an incidence of 1% in his series (20). Patients at risk include patients who have had preoperative radiation therapy, prior mediastinitis, or tumors with firm fixation to the posterior tracheal wall.

Upon identifying an airway laceration, the endotracheal tube should be guided under direct vision, distal to the tear to avoid loss of a large volume. Ideally, after the completion of the esophagectomy, the tear can be primarily repaired. The technique of the tracheal repair is dependent upon the site of the injury (22). When the tear is in the upper trachea, a partial sternotomy offers direct visualization. However, extensive tears involving carina or main bronchus should be approached by right thoracotomy.

Pleural Complications

Intraoperative pleural entry is a minor complication easily managed with immediate chest tube insertion. This occurs in 25% to 75% of all cases (22). In the Gurkan series, 44.6% of the patients submitted to an esophagectomy had pneumothorax (19).

Chylothorax has been reported in approximately 1% of cases (20). Chest tube drainage greater than 200 to 400 ml per shift for more than 48 hours should lead one to suspect of thoracic duct injury. The milky aspect of the fluid, the high levels of triglycerides, or the presence of chylomicrons in the pleural effusion confirm the diagnosis. Nonoperative treatment using tube thoracostomy and reduced-fat diet with administration of medium chain triglycerides or total parenteral nutrition may suffice; however, some surgeons advocate aggressive management by early surgical repair, via transthoracic ligation of the thoracic duct (30). Prolonged or massive drainage of chyle may perpetuate serious nutritional deficits and lymphocyte depletion, both of which may promote or magnify the effects of perioperative infective complications (30). When there is persistent high chylous drainage and no improvement with conservative management, surgical ligation of the thoracic duct should be performed.

Nerve Injury

Recurrent laryngeal nerve injury can be a devastating complication after esophagectomy, not only because of the hoarseness, impaired ability to cough, and secondary bronchial aspiration. Paresis of the recurrent nerve is usually related to the placement of retractors in the tracheoesophageal groove and usually resolves within weeks (31). Gurkan et al. (19) and Daniel (29) reported an incidence of 9%, while Orringer (31) reported a 1% incidence of recurrent laryngeal nerve injury in his series.

Anastomotic Leaks

The incidence of anastomotic leak reported in the literature vary from 13% to 20% (3,19,27,32). Although the relative merits of hand-sewn versus stapled approaches and single- versus multilayer closures have been debated, there is no definitive evidence that suggests that any anastomotic technique is associated with significantly superior results (22). In the Orringer series (20), cervical anastomosis leak occurred in 13% of cases, typically after retrosternal placement, radiation therapy, and prior operation at the gastroesophageal junction (20).

This complication of anastomotic leak in the neck is usually easy to manage (3,29,32). Mediastinitis in this context is rare, due to the cervical position of the anastomosis (19).

The clinical presentation can vary from a clinically silent fistula to a septic critically ill patient requiring immediate surgical intervention. In the first case, the diagnosis will probably be made during a routine contrast exam, and, in general, these leaks are small and contained (27). Early dilation has been suggested by some, not only to facilitate closure of the fistula but also to prevent a dense stricture from becoming established (33).

Symptomatic patients present with fever, cervical pain, erythema, and purulent discharge from the wound. The wound should be opened and drainage established. Spontaneous closure will often occur within 2 to 3 weeks, during which time adequate nutrition is maintained with enteral or parenteral nutrition. Some allow water ingestion to wash out the wound. To prevent anastomotic strictures and distal obstructions early esophageal dilatation has been advocated by some authors (33).

Some anastomotic leaks are characterized by significant gastric ischemia, which may be due to venous thrombosis or arterial insufficiency in the gastric fundus. Endoscopically, one can visualize necrosis that can compromise the whole circumference or part of the conduit. All these patients require urgent surgery to take down the stomach and perform a cervical esophagostomy and a tube gastrostomy. This type of complication carries a high mortality rate. Late anastomotic leaks are rare and usually occur with limited acute morbidity.

Splenectomy

Incidental spleenectomy, secondary to traction injury and bleeding, has been reported in about 3% of patients (20). A careful dissection around the greater curvature can prevent this type of injury.

RESULTS

The ability to perform a safe and efficient THE for both benign and malignant disease has been amply demonstrated (32,34), primarily through the work of Orringer (31). Many retrospective studies (16,29,35–40) have compared THE and TTE predominantly in cancer patients, resulting in conflicting arguments for one method over the other. Despite reports advocating one form of esophagectomy in preference to another, the optimal surgical approach that has the greatest survival with the lowest surgical morbidity and mortality has not been established (40–42).

The higher operative mortality previously reported (32,43) has been challenged by studies reporting a mortality of less than 8% for resection of esophageal carcinoma (4,16,19–20,29,44–46). Respiratory failure and sepsis are the most common causes of death (22). Although anastomotic leak, in general, is not associated with death, it is a major morbidity (19,45). Recent series have compared THE and TTE in regard to morbidity, mortality, and recurrence rates in esophageal cancer patients, and no statistical differences were found (32,39,41,44,47).

Although major debate still surrounds the use of THE as a cancer operation, several studies have not shown a significant difference when compared to TTE (3,35,41,42,44,48). Increasing experience with esophageal reconstruction techniques has resulted in lower operative morbidity and mortality rates and improved function of the esophageal substitutes (26). Yet, despite improvements, esophageal resection remains a formidable operation for patients whose nutritional and pulmonary status have been compromised by dysphagia. Differences in tumor extent, nutritional status, surgical technique, hospital volume, and surgeon experience are all important factors impacting the results of esophagectomies reported in the literature (49).

SUMMARY

The benefits of surgery in patients with resectable esophageal cancer are clearly established, offering patients a superior palliative or curative effect with acceptable morbidity and mortality (50). THE can be performed safely with low mortality and acceptable long-term function.

References

1. Denk W. Zur Radikaloperation des Osophaguskarzinoms. *Zentralbl Chir.* 1913;40:1065.
2. Turner GG. Excision of the thoracic esophagus for carcinoma with construction of extra-thoracic gullet. *Lancet.* 1933;2:1315–1316.
3. Boyle MJ, Franceschi D, Livingstone AS. Transhiatal versus transthoracic esophagectomy: complication and survival rates. *Am Surg.* 1999;65:1137–1142.
4. Katariya K, Harvey JC, Pina E, Beattie EJ. Complications of transhiatal esophagectomy. *J Surg Oncol.* 1994;57:157–163.
5. Orringer MB, Sloan H. Esophagectomy without thoracotomy. *J Thorac Cardiovasc Surg.* 1978;76:643–654.
6. Orringer MB. Transhiatal esophagectomy without thoracotomy. In: Pearson FG, Cooper JD, Deslauriers J, et al., eds. *Esophageal Surgery.* 2nd ed. New York: Churchill Livingstone; 2002:834–853.
7. Kirk RM. Palliative resection of oesophageal carcinoma without formal thoracotomy. *Br J Surg.* 1974;61:689–690.
8. Akiyama H, Sato Y, Takashashi F. Immediate pharyngogastrostomy following total esophagectomy by blunt dissection. *Jpn J Surg.* 1971;1:225–231.
9. Thomas AN, Dedo HH. Pharyngogastrostomy for treatment of severe caustic stricture of the pharynx and esophagus. *J Thorac Cardiovasc Surg.* 1977;73:817–824.
10. Sweet RH. The treatment of carcinoma of the esophagus and cardiac end of the stomach by surgical extirpation—203cases of resection. *Surgery.* 1948;23:952.
11. Garlock JH. Resection of thoracic esophagus for carcinoma located above arch of aorta: cervical esophagogastrostomy. *Surgery.* 1948;24:1.
12. Orringer MB, Sloan H. Substernal gastric bypass of the excluded thoracic esophagus for palliation of esophageal carcinoma. *J Thorac Cardiovasc Surg.* 1975;70:836–851.
13. Orringer MB. Substernal gastric bypass of the excluded esophagus-results of an ill-advised operation. *Surgery.* 1984;96:467–470
14. Orringer MB. Technical aids in performing transhiatal esophagectomy without thoracotomy. *Ann Thorac Surg.* 1984;38:128–132.
15. Vigneswaran WT, Trastek VF, Pairolero PC, Deschamps C, Daly RC, Allen MS. Transhiatal esophagectomy for carcinoma of the esophagus. *Ann Thorac Surg.* 1993;56:838–846.
16. Bolton JS, Sardi A, Bowen JC, Ellis JK. Transhiatal and transthoracic esophagectomy: a comparative study. *J Surg Oncol.* 1992;51:249–253.
17. Orringer MB, Orringer JS. Esophagectomy without thoracotomy: a dangerous operation? *J Thorac Cardiovasc Surg.* 1983;85:72–80.
18. Orringer MB. Transthoracic versus transhiatal esophagectomy: what difference does it make? *Ann Thorac Surg.* 1987;44:116.
19. Gurkan N, Terzioglu T, Tezelman S, Sasmaz O. Transhiatal oesophagectomy for oesophageal carcinoma. *Br J Surg.* 1991;78:1348–1351.
20. Orringer MB, Marshall B, Iannettoni MD. Transhiatal esophagectomy: clinical experience and refinements. *Ann Surg.* 1999;230:392–403.
21. Lin J, Iannettoni MD. Transhiatal esophagectomy. *Surg Clin North Am.* 2005; 85:593–610.
22. Gandhi SK, Naunheim KS. Complications of transhiatal esophagectomy. *Chest Surg Clin N Am.* 1997;7:601–612.
23. Zwischenberger JB, Sankar AB. Transhiatal esophagectomy. *Chest Surg Clin N Am.* 1995;5:527–542.
24. Orringer MB. Transhiatal esophagectomy without thoracotomy for carcinoma of the thoracic esophagus. *Ann Surg.* 1984;200:282–288.
25. Pinotti HW, Cecconello I, De Oliveira MA. Transhiatal esophagectomy for esophageal cancer. *Semin Surg Oncol.* 1997;13:253–258.
26. Orringer MB, Marshall B, Iannettoni MD. Transhiatal esophagectomy for treatment of benign and malignant esophageal disease. *World J Surg.* 2001;25:196–203.
27. Gelfand GA, Finley RJ, Nelems B, Inculet R, Evans KG, Fradet G. Transhiatal esophagectomy for carcinoma of the esophagus and cardia. Experience with 160 cases. *Arch Surg.* 1992;127:1164–1168.
28. Dewar L, Gelfand G, Finley RJ, Evans K, Inculet R, Nelems B. Factors affecting cervical anastomotic leak and stricture formation following esophagogastrectomy and gastric tube interposition. *Am J Surg.* 1992;163:484–489.
29. Daniel TM, Fleischer KJ, Flanagan TL, Tribble CG, Kron IL. Transhiatal esophagectomy: a safe alternative for selected patients. *Ann Thorac Surg.* 1992;54:686–690.
30. Orringer MB, Bluett M, Deeb GM. Aggressive treatment of chylothorax complicating transhiatal esophagectomy without thoracotomy. *Surgery.* 1988;104:720–726.
31. Orringer MB, Marshall B, Stirling MC. Transhiatal esophagectomy for benign and malignant disease. *J Thorac Cardiovasc Surg.* 1993;105:265–277.
32. Rao YG, Pal S, Pande GK, Sahni P, Chattopadhyay TK. Transhiatal esophagectomy for benign and malignant conditions. *Am J Surg.* 2002;184:136–142.
33. DiMusto PD, Orringer MB. Transhiatal esophagectomy for distal and cardia cancers: implications of a positive gastric margin. *Ann Thorac Surg.* 2007;83:1993–1999.
34. van Sandick JW, van Lanschot JJ, ten Kate FJ, Tijssen JG, Obertop H. Indicators of prognosis after transhiatal esophageal resection without thoracotomy for cancer. *J Am Coll Surg.* 2002;194:28–36.
35. Moon MR, Schulte WJ, Haasler GB, Condon RE. Transhiatal and transthoracic esophagectomy for adenocarcinoma of the esophagus. *Arch Surg.* 1992;127:951–955.
36. Siewert JR, Holscher AH. Current strategy in surgery for esophageal cancer. *Ann Ital Chir.* 1992;63:13–18.
37. Akiyama H, Tsurumaru M, Ono Y, Udagawa H, Kajiyama Y. Esophagectomy without thoracotomy with vagal preservation. *J Am Coll Surg.* 1994;178:83–85.
38. Bousamra M II, Haasler GB, Parviz M. A decade of experience with transthoracic and transhiatal esophagectomy. *Am J Surg.* 2002;183:162–167.
39. Rentz J, Bull D, Harpole D, et al. Transthoracic versus transhiatal esophagectomy: a prospective study of 945 patients. *J Thorac Cardiovasc Surg.* 2003; 125:1114–1120.
40. Johansson J, DeMeester TR, Hagen JA, et al. En bloc vs. transhiatal esophagectomy for stage T3 N1 adenocarcinoma of the distal esophagus. *Arch Surg.* 2004;139:627–633.
41. Hulscher JB, Tijssen JG, Obertop H, van Lanschot JJ. Transthoracic versus transhiatal resection for carcinoma of the esophagus: a meta-analysis. *Ann Thorac Surg.* 2001;72:306–313.
42. Hulscher JB, van Sandick JW, de Boer AG, et al. Extended transthoracic resection compared with limited transhiatal resection for adenocarcinoma of the esophagus. *N Engl J Med.* 2002;347:1662–1669.
43. Muller JM, Erasmi H, Stelzner M, Zieren U, Pichlmaier H. Surgical therapy of oesophageal carcinoma. *Br J Surg.* 1990;77:845–857.
44. Pac M, Basoglu A, Kocak H, et al. Transhiatal versus transthoracic esophagectomy for esophageal cancer. *J Thorac Cardiovasc Surg.* 1993;106:205–209.
45. Vigneswaran WT, Trastek VF, Pairolero PC, Deschamps C, Daly RC, Allen MS. Transhiatal esophagectomy for carcinoma of the esophagus. *Ann Thorac Surg.* 1993;56:838–846.
46. Gertsch P, Vauthey JN, Lustenberger AA, Friedlander-Klar H. Long-term results of transhiatal esophagectomy for esophageal carcinoma. A multivariate analysis of prognostic factors. *Cancer.* 1993;72:2312–2319.
47. Chu KM, Law SY, Fok M, Wong J. A prospective randomized comparison of transhiatal and transthoracic resection for lower-third esophageal carcinoma. *Am J Surg.* 1997;174:320–324.
48. Fok M, Siu KF, Wong J. A comparison of thanshiatal and transthoracic resection for carcinoma of the thoracic esophagus. *Am J Surg.* 1989;158:414–418.
49. Goldfaden D, Orringer MB, Appelman HD, Kalish R. Adenocarcinoma of the distal esophagus and gastric cardia. Comparison of results of transhiatal esophagectomy and thoracoabdominal esophagogastrectomy. *J Thorac Cardiovasc Surg.* 1986;91:242–247.
50. Linden PA, Sugarbaker DJ. Section V: techniques of esophageal resection. *Semin Thorac Cardiovasc Surg.* 2003;15:197–209.

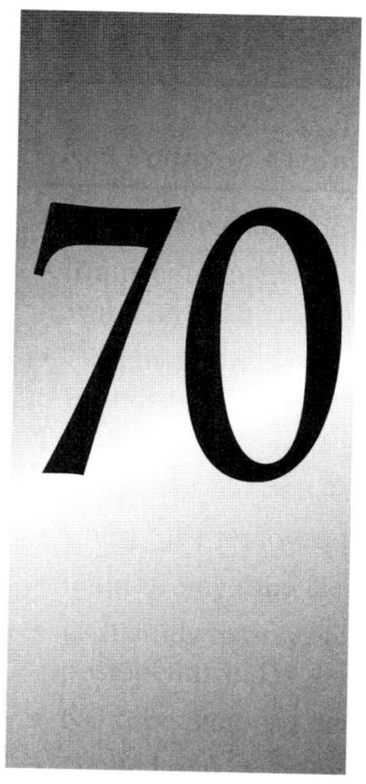

Surgery Techniques: Three-Field Esophagectomy

Inderpal S. Sarkaria
Nabil P. Rizk
Valerie W. Rusch

The extent of lymph node dissection required when surgically treating esophageal cancer is a source of considerable controversy. Much of this debate stems from different perspectives regarding the natural history of esophageal cancer and the role that surgery can play in treating this disease. For those who believe that esophageal cancer metastasizes early in its course, a more radical operation with an extended lymphadenectomy achieves little or no gain in most patients, at the cost of significantly increased morbidity (1). Within this paradigm, the goal of resection is simply to provide local control with the least possible morbidity in order to permit patients to receive systemic treatments. Transhiatal esophagectomy, championed by Orringer, is the traditional operation used in this type of resection, with the esophagus, stomach, and immediately adjacent lymph nodes removed through transabdominal mobilization of the esophagus with an anastomosis created in the neck. While a transhiatal esophagectomy strictly refers to the surgical approach and not the extent of lymphadenectomy, most believe that an aggressive lymphadenectomy would require some component of a transthoracic approach (2). The contrasting viewpoint regarding esophageal cancer considers that even in patients with locally advanced disease (including in the presence of nodal disease), there is the potential for a surgical cure. In these patients, an extended lymphadenectomy represents an extension of basic oncologic principles, with the possibility that a wider extent of resection clears nodal basins potentially harboring malignant cells and results in improved long-term survival (3–7). In the context of this viewpoint, the role of a more radical lymphadenectomy for esophageal cancer is especially relevant because the rich submucosal network of lymphatics allows for extensive longitudinal spread of tumor-bearing cells early in the disease process. Lymph node metastases can be found in up to 12% of superficial tumors with invasion into the (deep mucosa) submucosa and in up to 45% of those invading into the submucosa (8). Furthermore, the patterns of lymphatic spread also dictate the extent and location of the lymphadenectomy. Tumors of the upper and middle third of the esophagus usually follow patterns of lymphatic flow to the neck and upper mediastinum and those in the lower third to lymph node basins of the abdomen (9). The rationale for extended lymphadenectomies espoused by proponents of these approaches stems from this widespread pattern of lymphatic flow, in which tumor-bearing metastases of the thoracic esophagus may travel to lymph node basins from the neck to the abdomen.

DEFINITIONS

Fields of Lymph Node Dissection

The terminology regarding the extent of lymphadenectomy has come to revolve around the concept of different nodal "fields," of which 3 are described: abdominal, mediastinal, and high-mediastinal or cervical.

The first field describes nodal basins accessible through the abdominal dissection, including the lesser curve of the stomach; the left gastric, celiac, common hepatic, and splenic arteries; and tissues between the pancreas and diaphragmatic crus.

The second field describes nodal basins spanning the mediastinum proper, including the periesophageal nodes extending from the diaphragm up to at least the subcarinal region, with some also describing a dissection up to the thoracic inlet. Some surgeons also advocate clearance of the thoracic duct along with all periductal tissues within its mediastinal course as part of this portion of the dissection. A transthoracic approach to the surgery is felt by many to be necessary in order to accomplish the mediastinal component of the dissection, although isolated reports suggest that adequate 2-field dissection to the tracheal bifurcation may be accomplished through a radical transhiatal approach (10).

The third field includes nodal tissues within the superior and posterior mediastinum and neck, including the nodal chain along the course of the recurrent nerves bilaterally as well as the internal jugular and supraclavicular basins. Advocates of resection of this field cite significant rates of positive occult nodal disease in this area as well as significant rates of cervical nodal recurrence occurring in patients undergoing more limited lymphadenectomies (11,12).

It is important to note that there is no consensus of opinion regarding these definitions. Although an International Society of Diseases of the Esophagus consensus conference in the early 1990s sought to standardize definitions of these fields, there exists a small but significant difference in definitions of these dissections, particularly with respect to the third field. In the bulk of the Japanese literature, for instance, a superior mediastinal lymph node dissection along the bilateral recurrent nerves is often included within the scope of an "extended" or "total" second-field dissection. In this description, the third field strictly consists of those lymph node basins located exclusively within the supraclavicular fossae and along the cervical/jugular chains. The 2-field dissection described in the Western literature, on the other hand, refers to the standard infracarinal resection as described previously, with the third field describing superior mediastinal dissection along the bilateral recurrent laryngeal nerves as well as the cervical and supraclavicular basins. These differences in definition should be kept in mind when contrasting results of studies, particularly between Eastern and Western groups (13).

En Bloc Resection

The definitions of the different fields of lymphadenectomy become even more imprecise when the concept of an "en bloc" resection is introduced (2,14). This term derives from the principle of gaining wide radial margins of resection of tumor-bearing viscera. In terms of esophageal resection, it entails resection of the esophagus and tumor proper, along with extirpation of all periesophageal tissues laterally including the bilateral pleura, anteriorly to and including necessary portions of pericardium, and posteriorly together with all periaortic tissues and the thoracic duct. This term does not specifically refer to the extent of lymphadenectomy in terms of the fields described previously, but assumes at least a complete mediastinal and abdominal 2-field dissection from the tracheal bifurcation to the esophageal hiatus, including also described perigastric, left gastric, celiac, common hepatic, paracardial, and retroperitoneal nodal basins. First espoused by Logan and Skinner, proponents of the en bloc esophagectomy cite improved rates of survival and recurrence over lesser resections (2–4,14–25).

EVIDENCE

The evidence supporting a more extensive lymphadenectomy is primarily anecdotal. While there are many reported case series and retrospective comparisons of various surgical approaches in which there appears to be evidence supporting more aggressive surgical management, these data for the most part do not rise to the level of evidence needed to show a convincingly conclusive benefit of any 1 approach. In most retrospective series, a selection bias and stage migration likely explains improved outcomes after extensive lymphadenectomy. However, there are some tantalizing data that do provide a hint of the potential benefit of a more radical resection.

Two-Field versus a Lesser Lymphadenectomy

Transhiatal Esophagectomy Versus Transthoracic Esophagectomy

The primary source of evidence supporting the potential benefit of a more extensive lymphadenectomy comes from studies comparing transhiatal (THE) versus transthoracic (TTE) approaches to esophageal resection (9). Proponents of THE cite shorter operative times and improved rates of pulmonary and pain-related morbidity due to the lack of a thoracotomy. Conversely, proponents of TTE cite the benefits of direct and thorough anatomic mediastinal esophageal and nodal dissection, including decreased rates of intraoperative morbidity from injuries to tracheobronchial structures, the azygous vein, and thoracic duct. In addition to various series comparing the 2 approaches, 2 large meta-analyses by Hulscher et al. and Rindani et al. found no differences in long-term outcomes between patients undergoing THE versus TTE, with 5-year survival rates of approximately 20% to 25% (1,26–46). While Hulscher et al. reported increased rates of pulmonary-related morbidity and mortality in the immediate postoperative period in patients undergoing TTE, Rindani found no difference in cardiovascular- or pulmonary-related morbidity and cited increased rates of anastomotic and recurrent laryngeal nerve–related complications in patients undergoing THE.

Four randomized prospective studies compared THE to TTE (28,31,47,48). The long-term results of the largest trial were recently published and showed no differences in 5-year survival between the groups, with reported rates of approximately 35% (49). A subgroup analysis of patients with tumors involving the gastroesophageal junction found a 14% survival advantage for patients undergoing TTE versus THE (51% vs. 37%), although this was not statistically significant. In patients with N1 disease and fewer than 8 positive lymph nodes, 5-year locoregional disease-free survival was significantly greater for patients undergoing TTE compared to THE (64% vs. 23%).

Two large nonrandomized, multi-institutional studies utilizing prospectively maintained national databases investigated differences in morbidity and mortality between patients undergoing THE versus TTE (50,51). Rentz et al. utilized the Department of Veterans Affairs National Surgical Quality Improvement Program to compare 383 patients undergoing THE versus 562 undergoing TTE. There were no significant differences in the incidence of perioperative complications with the exception of an increased rate of wound dehiscence in patients undergoing THE versus THE (5% vs. 2%) (51). Connors et al. compared 11,914 patients undergoing THE versus 5,481 patients undergoing TTE drawn from the Nationwide Inpatient Sample database. There were no differences seen in morbidity or mortality between the groups. Low-volume centers (10 or fewer esophagectomies performed per year) had significantly higher rates of mortality for both procedures and higher rates of gastrointestinal and systemic complication in patients undergoing TTE (50).

En Bloc Resection

En bloc resections incorporate a more aggressive local resection that, by extension, results in a more complete lymphadenectomy, particularly in the first and second fields. Results from series evaluating this procedure are extrapolated by some as indirect evidence supporting a more aggressive lymphadenectomy. The concept of en bloc resection stems from basic oncologic theory that malignant tumors should be resected along with all surrounding potentially tumor-bearing tissues. In the case of esophageal cancers, this approach is concordant with surgeons who do not ascribe to the belief that all esophageal cancers necessarily represent disseminated disease beyond the scope of potential surgical cure at the time of diagnosis. Given the lack of a true serosa, the fibrous pericardial and subpleural origins and insertions of the lower esophageal longitudinal muscle may be considered a substitute for this layer. As originally described by Logan and then Skinner, en bloc resection entails complete removal of the primary tumor along with a surrounding fascial cylinder containing all related lymphatics, including pericardium, thoracic duct, azygous vein, intercostal vessels, bilateral pleurae, and a cuff of crura abutting the tumor bulk (2,14,15,52,53). An extensive lymphadenectomy of the midthoracic and abdominal fields is necessarily assumed as part of this dissection, although modifications of the technique may include sparing of the intercostal vessels, pericardium, thoracic duct, and azygous vein. Dissection of the cervical field is not explicitly addressed and not assumed within the scope of this dissection.

The concept of en bloc resection is more appropriate in the context of a Western patient population with a predominance of adenocarcinomas of the lower esophagus, allowing for extensive lateral peritumoral dissection below the level of the carina and tracheobronchial tree. Tumors of the mid- to upper esophagus are less amenable to en bloc resection, given the proximity of these vital structures.

Indications for en bloc resection in Western patients, as outlined by Skinner and Altorki, were initially limited to early stage I and II tumors of the mid- and lower esophagus and cardia of the stomach (53,19). During the past decade, these indications were expanded to include more advanced lesions with operative mortality rates of less than 5% (15,18,52,54,55). Despite morbidity rates as high as 40% to 50% and overall recurrence rates from 30% to 50%, proponents of this approach report local recurrence rates as low as 4.5%, with most nodal recurrences occurring outside the initial field of dissection (15,56–58). Reported 5-year survival rates for patients undergoing en bloc resections have been impressive, ranging from 37% to 50% (55). When compared to more limited transhiatal resections, significantly improved survival rates have been seen with en bloc resections in N1 patients with adenocarcinomas and fewer than 8 positive nodes in the surgical specimen (49,59). At least 1 single-institution experience by

Portale et al. reported en bloc resection to be an independent predictor of improved outcomes on multivariate analysis (60).

Three-Field versus a Lesser Lymphadenectomy

One of the most common rationales for extending the lymphadenectomy to a third field is to identify and remove unrecognized sites of nodal disease. In 1985, a Japanese study by Isono et al. analyzed cervical recurrences in patients after resection of squamous cell esophageal cancers and found such recurrences in more than one-third of cases (11). Lerut et al. reported a 75% rate of unforeseen cervical lymph node involvement in patients undergoing 3-field dissections (61). The frequency of cervical nodal metastases was similar between patients with adenocarcinomas or squamous carcinomas (23% vs. 25%, respectively) and resulted in pathological upstaging of 12% of patients in this series. The rates of cervical node metastasis are closely related to the location of the primary tumor, with up to 60% of proximal thoracic esophageal tumors having cervical lymph node metastases but only 20% and 12% for tumors of the middle and distal esophagus (61–63). A national Japanese initiative investigating the results of adding the third field of dissection to reduce this recurrence rate found improved survival rates over 2-field dissection, but also showed an increased morbidity, especially recurrent laryngeal nerve injuries (12). After resection, one-third of these patients were discovered to have cervical nodal metastases that would otherwise have gone unrecognized.

Akiyama et al. compared patients with N0 disease who had undergone 3-field dissection to those undergoing 2-field dissections (62). The authors found significantly improved survival in patients undergoing extended cervical dissections, with a 5-year survival of 84% versus 55% for those undergoing the more limited dissection. Although uniformly lower in both groups, this was also found for node-positive patients, with 5-year survival rates of 43% versus 28%, with a survival rate of 30% in patients with cervical metastases undergoing 3-field dissection.

Altorki et al. have reported the major experience with 3-field dissection in North America (63). This analysis includes mainly adenocarcinomas of the lower esophagus, reflecting the epidemiological patterns of esophageal carcinomas in the United States. The operative mortality in patients undergoing 3-field dissection was 5% with a morbidity of 47%, including a 6% rate of recurrent laryngeal nerve injury. The 5-year survival in patients with cervical metastases was 15% for adenocarcinomas versus 40% for squamous cell carcinomas.

In Europe, Lerut reported an overall 5-year survival of 42% in patients with either squamous cell carcinoma or adenocarcinoma undergoing 3-field resection (61). The rate of positive cervical nodes and adenocarcinomas was 26% versus 18% for those with squamous cancers. Five-year survival for patients with adenocarcinomas and positive cervical nodal metastases was 11%.

Kang et al. retrospectively compared 233 patients with squamous cell esophageal cancers undergoing resections using 1-, 2-, or 3-field lymphadenectomy (64). Positron-emission tomography and endoscopic ultrasound were not routinely used in preoperative staging. None of the patients received induction therapy. Group I included patients undergoing lymphadenectomy of peritumoral/paraesophageal nodes only, group II included patients undergoing peritumoral/paraesophageal and either upper thoracic or abdominal lymphadenectomy, and group III included patients undergoing resection of all 3 nodal fields. Overall mortality for the entire study was 2.1%, and overall morbidity was 39.9%. The 5-year survival was 21.2%, 36.3%, and 53.7% in groups I, II, and III respectively. Although 5-year survival rates trended toward improvement between the groups in patients with N1 disease, this was not statistically significant. Locoregional recurrence was significantly greater in group I versus groups II or III, but there was no significant difference in rates of distant recurrence.

Fujita et al. similarly found improved rates of survival for patients with upper or middle esophageal squamous cancers undergoing 3-field dissections (including cervical and supraclavicular basins) versus less extensive 2-field dissections (65). Although mortality rates were similar among the groups, morbidity involving the recurrent laryngeal nerve paresis, anastomotic leak, or tracheal ischemia was significantly higher with 3-field dissection. Patients with lower esophageal tumors did not experience advantage in short- or long-term outcomes from 3-field dissection.

CONFOUNDING ISSUES

Stage Migration

One of the main controversies regarding purported improved survival rates of patients undergoing extended lymphadenectomies revolves around the issue of staging. A common criticism of published studies is that they are not prospective randomized trials comparing 2 treatment modalities and that extended lymphadenectomies may simply stage patients more accurately. Studies of limited lymphadenectomy will necessarily include a significant percentage of patients with unrecognized additional nodal disease that would otherwise have been discovered with a more radical dissection (66). While more extensive lymphadenectomies certainly improve staging, the resultant stage migration introduces a considerable bias in the interpretation of comparisons made between these patients and those undergoing lesser resections with less adequate staging. It is difficult to assess whether performing 3-field lymphadenectomy for these professed gains are warranted in light of significant rates of serious perioperative morbidity, which also have consequences for long-term quality of life (67). At least 1 recent large observational study of more than 5,500 patients from the Surveillance, Epidemiology, and End-Results (SEER) database found that only total the number of lymph nodes removed (> 30) and the total number of negative lymph nodes (> 15) predicted improved survival in patients undergoing extended lymphadenectomies (68).

Isolated Cervical Recurrence Versus Multifocal Recurrence

Proponents of adding a third field of resection argue that a potential benefit of a more radical lymphadenectomy is to decrease disease recurrence at sites of unresected nodal disease. This argument would be legitimate if such recurrences developed in the absence of systemic disease. Although the incidence of cervical nodal recurrence in patients undergoing lesser dissections is significant, the incidence of isolated cervical recurrences in the absence of other systemic or locoregional recurrence is quite low (69–71). While Law et al. reported an 11% rate of cervical recurrence in a series of patients undergoing esophagectomy without cervical nodal dissection, only 4% of these recurrences were isolated to the neck alone (72). In comparison, the mediastinal and systemic recurrence rates were 25% and 26%, respectively. A similar study by Dresner et al. found an isolated cervical recurrence rate of only 1%, with mediastinal and systemic rates of recurrence of 21% and 18%, respectively (73). Yano et el. reported isolated cervical recurrences in 1.4% of patients even after 3-field dissection (74). Several small series and case reports anecdotally show long-term survival with additional resection in patients with recurrent isolated cervical node disease (74–76).

Completeness of Resection

A potential confounder in the data supporting more extensive lymphadenectomies is the likely importance of a complete gross and pathological (R0) surgical resection to long-term survival. The data from en bloc resections have consistently shown that a more extensive radical resection is associated with a higher likelihood of an R0 resection (22). As might be expected, however, a more "radical" operation for excision of the primary tumor will also be associated with a more extensive lymphadenectomy. Given this strong correlation, it is not possible from retrospective data to disassociate these 2 factors in analyses of survival.

Mucosal and Submucosal Lesions

Meticulous Japanese histologic classification studies of superficial squamous esophageal cancers have carefully defined rates of lymph node metastases based on precise levels of mucosal and submucosal tumor invasion (8). A national survey compared intraepithelial cancers contained within the basement membrane (m1) versus those contained within the muscularis mucosae (m2) versus those close to or infiltrating the muscularis mucosae (m3). Rates of metastatic lymph node disease between these groups was 0.0%, 3.3%, and 12.2%, respectively. Submucosal lesions were similarly divided into three histologic subgroups (sm1, sm2, sm3), with rates of lymph node metastases of 26.5%, 35.8%, and 45.9% seen among the three, respectively. This has led to the recommendation that endoscopic mucosal resections be limited to patients with m1 or m2 disease (77,78). The relatively high rates of nodal disease seen in patients with m3 or greater disease make esophagectomy with appropriate adenectomy a more suitable therapeutic choice (79). Newer endoscopic techniques incorporating high-frequency ultrasound combined with chromoendoscopy and magnification endoscopy are under investigation to help define these histologic subgroups and better assign appropriate therapy to patients with these cancers (80).

SUMMARY

The decision to perform en bloc resections and extended lymphadenectomies for esophageal cancer remains highly controversial, with no existing high prospective randomized trials to guide definitive recommendations regarding this issue. However, the preponderance of evidence suggests a true survival benefit and improved rates of locoregional control with en bloc infracarinal resections, especially for cancers of the middle and lower esophagus (81). Given these data, it is reasonable to recommend en bloc resections with 2-field lymphadenectomies in those patients with stages I to III esophageal carcinomas, good performance status, and no prohibitive comorbidities and at a center of excellence with experience performing these operations on a regular basis (82). The benefit of 3-field lymphadenectomy is still undefined. A decision to perform such an extended resection must consider substantial rates of significant perioperative morbidity with unclear improvements in survival or locoregional control.

SUGGESTED READINGS

Altorki NK. Lymph node dissection for carcinoma of the esophagus. In: Ferguson MK, editor. *Difficult decisions in thoracic surgery: an evidence-based approach*. 1st ed. London: Springer; 2007:225–233.

Law S, Wong J. Lymph node dissection in surgical treatment of esophageal neoplasms. *Surg Oncol Clin N Am*. 2007;16(1):115–131.

Vrouenraets BC, van Lanschot JJ. Extent of surgical resection for esophageal and gastroesophageal junction adenocarcinomas. *Surg Oncol Clin N Am*. 2006;15(4):781–791.

References

1. Orringer MB, Marshall B, Iannettoni MD. Transhiatal esophagectomy: clinical experience and refinements. *Ann Surg*. 1999;230:392–400.
2. Skinner DB. En bloc resection for neoplasms of the esophagus and cardia. *J Thorac Cardiovasc Surg*. 1983;85:59–71.
3. Altorki N. En-bloc esophagectomy—the three-field dissection. *Surg Clin North Am*. 2005;85:611–619.
4. Lerut T, Coosemans W, Decker G, et al. Extended surgery for cancer of the esophagus and gastroesophageal junction. *J Surg Res*. 2004;117:58–63.
5. Law S, Wong J. The current management of esophageal cancer. *Adv Surg*. 2007; 41:93–119.
6. Hulscher JB, van Sandick JW, Tijssen JG, et al. The recurrence pattern of esophageal carcinoma after transhiatal resection. *J Am Coll Surg*. 2000;191:143–148.
7. Korst RJ, Kansler AL, Port JL, et al. Downstaging of T or N predicts long-term survival after preoperative chemotherapy and radical resection for esophageal carcinoma. *Ann Thorac Surg*. 2006;82:480–484.
8. Kodama M, Kakegawa T. Treatment of superficial cancer of the esophagus: a summary of responses to a questionnaire on superficial cancer of the esophagus in Japan. *Surgery*. 1998;123:432–439.
9. Cense HA, van Eijck CH, Tilanus HW. New insights in the lymphatic spread of oesophageal cancer and its implications for the extent of surgical resection. *Best Pract Res Clin Gastroenterol*. 2006;20:893–906.
10. Rudiger Siewert J, Feith M, Werner M, et al. Adenocarcinoma of the esophagogastric junction: results of surgical therapy based on anatomical/topographic classification in 1,002 consecutive patients. *Ann Surg*. 2000;232:353–361.
11. Isono K, Onoda S, Okuyama K, et al. Recurrence of intrathoracic esophageal cancer. *Jpn J Clin Oncol*. 1985;15:49–60.
12. Isono K, Sato H, Nakayama K. Results of a nationwide study on the three-field lymph node dissection of esophageal cancer. *Oncology*. 1991;48:411–420.
13. Devesa SS, Blot WJ, Fraumeni JF Jr. Changing patterns in the incidence of esophageal and gastric carcinoma in the United States. *Cancer*. 1998;83:2049–2053.
14. Logan A. The surgical treatment of carcinoma of the esophagus and cardia. *J Thorac Cardiovasc Surg*. 1963;46:150–161.
15. Altorki N, Skinner D. Should en bloc esophagectomy be the standard of care for esophageal carcinoma? *Ann Surg*. 2001;234:581–587.
16. Altorki NK. Extended resections in the management of esophageal carcinoma. *Curr Opin Gen Surg*. 1994:113–116.
17. Altorki NK. The rationale for radical resection. *Surg Oncol Clin N Am*. 1999; 8:295–305.
18. Altorki NK, Girardi L, Skinner DB. En bloc esophagectomy improves survival for stage III esophageal cancer. *J Thorac Cardiovasc Surg*. 1997;114:948–955.
19. Altorki NK, Skinner DB. En bloc esophagectomy: the first 100 patients. *Hepatogastroenterology*. 1990;37:360–363.
20. Law S, Wong J. Two-field dissection is enough for esophageal cancer. *Dis Esophagus*. 2001;14:98–103.
21. Lerut T, Coosemans W, De Leyn P, et al. Is there a role for radical esophagectomy. *Eur J Cardiothorac Surg*. 1999;16(suppl 1):S44–S47.
22. Nigro JJ, DeMeester SR, Hagen JA, et al. Node status in transmural esophageal adenocarcinoma and outcome after en bloc esophagectomy. *J Thorac Cardiovasc Surg*. 1999;117:960–968.
23. Nigro JJ, Hagen JA, DeMeester TR, et al. Prevalence and location of nodal metastases in distal esophageal adenocarcinoma confined to the wall: implications for therapy. *J Thorac Cardiovasc Surg*. 1999;117:16–23.
24. Nigro JJ, Hagen JA, DeMeester TR, et al. Occult esophageal adenocarcinoma: extent of disease and implications for effective therapy. *Ann Surg*. 1999;230:433–438.
25. Williams VA, Peters JH. Adenocarcinoma of the gastroesophageal junction: benefits of an extended lymphadenectomy. *Surg Oncol Clin N Am*. 2006;15:765–780.
26. Hulscher JB, Tijssen JG, Obertop H, et al. Transthoracic versus transhiatal resection for carcinoma of the esophagus: a meta-analysis. *Ann Thorac Surg*. 2001;72:306–313.
27. Rindani R, Martin CJ, Cox MR. Transhiatal versus Ivor-Lewis oesophagectomy: is there a difference? *Aust N Z J Surg*. 1999;69:187–194.
28. Chu KM, Law SY, Fok M, et al. A prospective randomized comparison of transhiatal and transthoracic resection for lower-third esophageal carcinoma. *Am J Surg*. 1997; 174:320–324.
29. Gelfand GA, Finley RJ, Nelems B, et al. Transhiatal esophagectomy for carcinoma of the esophagus and cardia: experience with 160 cases. *Arch Surg*. 1992;127:1164–1167.
30. Gertsch P, Vauthey JN, Lustenberger AA, et al. Long-term results of transhiatal esophagectomy for esophageal carcinoma: a multivariate analysis of prognostic factors. *Cancer*. 1993;72:2312–2319.
31. Goldminc M, Maddern G, Le Prise E, et al. Oesophagectomy by a transhiatal approach or thoracotomy: a prospective randomized trial. *Br J Surg*. 1993;80:367–370.
32. Horstmann O, Verreet PR, Becker H, et al. Transhiatal oesophagectomy compared with transthoracic resection and systematic lymphadenectomy for the treatment of oesophageal cancer. *Eur J Surg*. 1995;161:557–567.
33. Putnam JB Jr, Suell DM, McMurtrey MJ, et al. Comparison of three techniques of esophagectomy within a residency training program. *Ann Thorac Surg*. 1994;57:319–325.
34. Vigneswaran WT, Trastek VF, Pairolero PC, et al. Transhiatal esophagectomy for carcinoma of the esophagus. *Ann Thorac Surg*. 1993;56:838–844.
35. Adam DJ, Craig SR, Sang CT, et al.. Oesophagogastrectomy for carcinoma in patients under 50 years of age. *J R Coll Surg Edinb*. 1996;41:371–373.
36. Ellis FH Jr. Standard resection for cancer of the esophagus and cardia. *Surg Oncol Clin N Am*. 1999;8:279–294.
37. Hofstetter W, Swisher SG, Correa AM, et al. Treatment outcomes of resected esophageal cancer. *Ann Surg*. 2002;236:376–384.
38. Karl RC, Schreiber R, Boulware D, et al. Factors affecting morbidity, mortality, and survival in patients undergoing Ivor Lewis esophagogastrectomy. *Ann Surg*. 2000; 231:635–643.
39. Kelsen DP, Ginsberg R, Pajak TF, et al. Chemotherapy followed by surgery compared with surgery alone for localized esophageal cancer. *N Engl J Med*. 1998;339: 1979–1984.
40. Lieberman MD, Shriver CD, Bleckner S, et al. Carcinoma of the esophagus: Prognostic significance of histologic type. *J Thorac Cardiovasc Surg*. 1995;109:130–138.
41. Sharpe DA, Moghissi K. Resectional surgery in carcinoma of the oesophagus and cardia: what influences long-term survival? *Eur J Cardiothorac Surg*. 1996;10:359–363.
42. Visbal AL, Allen MS, Miller DL, et al. Ivor Lewis esophagogastrectomy for esophageal cancer. *Ann Thorac Surg*. 2001;71:1803–1808.
43. Walsh TN, Noonan N, Hollywood D, et al. A comparison of multimodal therapy and surgery for esophageal adenocarcinoma. *N Engl J Med*. 1996;335:462–467.
44. Wright CD, Mathisen DJ, Wain JC, et al. Evolution of treatment strategies for adenocarcinoma of the esophagus and gastroesophageal junction. *Ann Thorac Surg*. 1994;58:1574–1578.
45. Morgan MA, Lewis WG, Hopper AN, et al. Prospective comparison of transthoracic versus transhiatal esophagectomy following neoadjuvant therapy for esophageal cancer. *Dis Esophagus*. 2007;20:225–231.
46. Bousamra M II, Haasler GB, Parviz M. A decade of experience with transthoracic and transhiatal esophagectomy. *Am J Surg*. 2002;183:162–167.
47. Hulscher JB, van Sandick JW, de Boer AG, et al. Extended transthoracic resection compared with limited transhiatal resection for adenocarcinoma of the esophagus. *N Engl J Med*. 2002;347:1662–1669.
48. Jacobi CA, Zieren HU, Muller JM, et al. Surgical therapy of esophageal carcinoma: the influence of surgical approach and esophageal resection on cardiopulmonary function. *Eur J Cardiothorac Surg*. 1997;11:32–37.
49. Omloo JM, Lagarde SM, Hulscher JB, et al. Extended transthoracic resection compared with limited transhiatal resection for adenocarcinoma of the mid/distal esophagus: five-year survival of a randomized clinical trial. *Ann Surg*. 2007;246:992–1001.
50. Connors RC, Reuben BC, Neumayer LA, et al. Comparing outcomes after transthoracic and transhiatal esophagectomy: a 5-year prospective cohort of 17,395 patients. *J Am Coll Surg*. 2007;205:735–740.
51. Rentz J, Bull D, Harpole D, et al. Transthoracic versus transhiatal esophagectomy: a prospective study of 945 patients. *J Thorac Cardiovasc Surg*. 2003;125:1114–1120.
52. Hagen JA, DeMeester SR, Peters JH, et al. Curative resection for esophageal adenocarcinoma: analysis of 100 en bloc esophagectomies. *Ann Surg*. 2001;234:520–530.
53. Skinner DB, Little AG, Ferguson MK, et al. Selection of operation for esophageal cancer based on staging. *Ann Surg*. 1986;204:391–401.
54. Collard JM, Otte JB, Fiasse R, et al. Skeletonizing en bloc esophagectomy for cancer. *Ann Surg*. 2001;234:25–32.
55. Tachibana M, Kinugasa S, Yoshimura H, et al. En-bloc esophagectomy for esophageal cancer. *Am J Surg*. 2004;188:254–260.
56. Peters JH, Hoeft SF, Heimbucher J, et al. Selection of patients for curative or palliative resection of esophageal cancer based on preoperative endoscopic ultrasonography. *Arch Surg*. 1994;129:534–539.
57. Hagen JA, Peters JH, DeMeester TR. Superiority of extended en bloc esophagogastrectomy for carcinoma of the lower esophagus and cardia. *J Thorac Cardiovasc Surg*. 1993;106:850–858.
58. Lerut T, Coosemans W, De Leyn P, et al. Reflections on three field lymphadenectomy in carcinoma of the esophagus and gastroesophageal junction. *Hepatogastroenterology*. 1999;46:717–725.

59. Johansson J, DeMeester TR, Hagen JA, et al. En bloc vs transhiatal esophagectomy for stage T3 N1 adenocarcinoma of the distal esophagus. *Arch Surg.* 2004;139:627–631.
60. Portale G, Hagen JA, Peters JH, et al. Modern 5-year survival of resectable esophageal adenocarcinoma: single institution experience with 263 patients. *J Am Coll Surg.* 2006; 202:588–596.
61. Lerut T, Nafteux P, Moons J, et al. Three-field lymphadenectomy for carcinoma of the esophagus and gastroesophageal junction in 174 R0 resections: impact on staging, disease-free survival, and outcome: a plea for adaptation of TNM classification in upper-half esophageal carcinoma. *Ann Surg.* 2004;240:962–972.
62. Akiyama H, Tsurumaru M, Udagawa H, et al. Radical lymph node dissection for cancer of the thoracic esophagus. *Ann Surg.* 1994;220:364–372.
63. Altorki N, Kent M, Ferrara C, et al. Three-field lymph node dissection for squamous cell and adenocarcinoma of the esophagus. *Ann Surg.* 2002;236:177–183.
64. Kang CH, Kim YT, Jeon SH, et al. Lymphadenectomy extent is closely related to long-term survival in esophageal cancer. *Eur J Cardiothorac Surg.* 2007;31:154–160.
65. Fujita H, Sueyoshi S, Tanaka T, et al. Optimal lymphadenectomy for squamous cell carcinoma in the thoracic esophagus: comparing the short- and long-term outcome among the four types of lymphadenectomy. *World J Surg.* 2003;27:571–579.
66. Hulscher JB, Van Sandick JW, Offerhaus GJ, et al. Prospective analysis of the diagnostic yield of extended en bloc resection for adenocarcinoma of the oesophagus or gastric cardia. *Br J Surg.* 2001;88:715–719.
67. Baba M, Aikou T, Natsugoe S, et al. Quality of life following esophagectomy with three-field lymphadenectomy for carcinoma, focusing on its relationship to vocal cord palsy. *Dis Esophagus.* 1998;11:28–34.
68. Schwarz RE, Smith DD. Clinical impact of lymphadenectomy extent in resectable esophageal cancer. *J Gastrointest Surg.* 2007;11:1384–1393.
69. Nakagawa S, Kanda T, Kosugi S, et al. Recurrence pattern of squamous cell carcinoma of the thoracic esophagus after extended radical esophagectomy with three-field lymphadenectomy. *J Am Coll Surg.* 2004;198:205–211.
70. Osugi H, Takemura M, Takada N, et al. Prognostic factors after oesophagectomy and extended lymphadenectomy for squamous oesophageal cancer. *Br J Surg.* 2002; 89:909–913.
71. Osugi H, Takemura M, Higashino M, et al. Causes of death and pattern of recurrence after esophagectomy and extended lymphadenectomy for squamous cell carcinoma of the thoracic esophagus. *Oncol Rep.* 2003;10:81–87.
72. Law SY, Fok M, Wong J. Pattern of recurrence after oesophageal resection for cancer: clinical implications. *Br J Surg.* 1996;83:107–111.
73. Dresner SM, Wayman J, Shenfine J, et al. Pattern of recurrence following subtotal oesophagectomy with two field lymphadenectomy. *Br J Surg.* 2000;87:362–373.
74. Yano M, Takachi K, Doki Y, et al. Prognosis of patients who develop cervical lymph node recurrence following curative resection for thoracic esophageal cancer. *Dis Esophagus.* 2006;19:73–77.
75. Motoyama S, Saito R, Okuyama M, et al. Long-term survival after salvage resection of recurrent esophageal cancer with anterior mediastinal lymph node involvement: report of a case. *Surg Today.* 2006;36:827–830.
76. Komatsu S, Shioaki Y, Ichikawa D, et al. Survival and clinical evaluation of salvage operation for cervical lymph node recurrence in esophageal cancer. *Hepatogastroenterology.* 2005;52:796–799.
77. Soetikno R, Kaltenbach T, Yeh R, et al. Endoscopic mucosal resection for early cancers of the upper gastrointestinal tract. *J Clin Oncol.* 2005;23:4490–4498.
78. Natsugoe S, Matsumoto M, Okumura H, et al. Prognostic factors in patients with submucosal esophageal cancer. *J Gastrointest Surg.* 2004;8:631–635.
79. Nozoe T, Kakeji Y, Baba H, et al. Two-field lymph-node dissection may be enough to treat patients with submucosal squamous cell carcinoma of the thoracic esophagus. *Dis Esophagus.* 2005;18:226–229.
80. Inoue H, Sasajima K, Kaga M, et al. Endoscopic in vivo evaluation of tissue atypia in the esophagus using a newly designed integrated endocytoscope: a pilot trial. *Endoscopy.* 2006;38:891–895.
81. Hulscher JB, van Lanschot JJ. Individualised surgical treatment of patients with an adenocarcinoma of the distal oesophagus or gastro-oesophageal junction. *Dig Surg.* 2005; 22:130–134.
82. Altorki NK. Lymph node dissection for carcinoma of the esophagus. In: Ferguson MK, editor. *Difficult decisions in thoracic surgery: an evidence-based approach.* 1st ed. London: Springer; 2007:225–233.

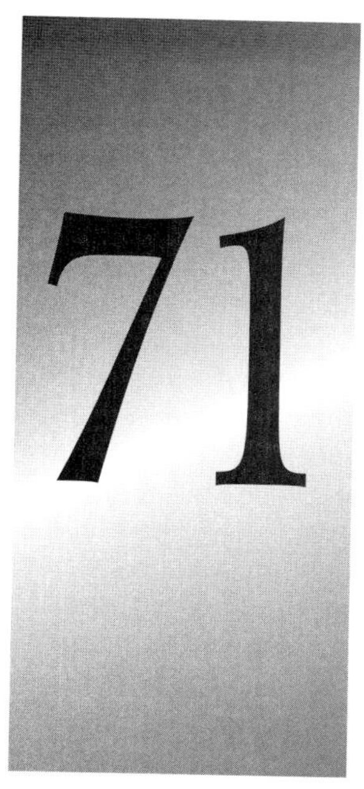

71 Surgery Techniques: En Bloc Esophagectomy

Paul C. Lee
Nasser K. Altorki

The prognosis of esophageal cancer remains dismal despite improvements in perioperative care, surgical techniques, chemotherapy, and radiotherapy over the last decade. More than 95% of patients will succumb to their disease following a diagnosis of esophageal cancer in the United States. Even with a curative resection (R0 resection), the 5-year survival of patients after transthoracic esophagectomy or transhiatal esophagectomy rarely exceeds 30% (1–4). The primary argument for the poor survival is the fact that the majority of patients develop metastatic disease following surgical resection, suggesting that the disease may already have disseminated at the time of diagnosis. While undoubtedly this is the case in most patients, a careful analysis of the patterns of failure following surgical resection also suggests inadequate locoregional control. After conventional surgical resection, the locoregional failure rates range from 30% to as high as 60% (5–8). Addition of preoperative chemotherapy and/or radiotherapy did not meaningfully reduce the high locoregional failure rate. Without adequate locoregional control, it is unlikely that a meaningful improvement in the survival of patients with esophageal cancer can be achieved.

Logan in 1963 first described en bloc resection for tumor of the lower esophagus and cardia (9). The reported 5-year survival was unparalleled at the time but at the cost of a high operative mortality. Skinner in 1979 revisited the en bloc approach and extended its use to tumors of the middle and proximal esophagus (10). A few years earlier, Orringer and Sloan had published their surgical technique on the transhiatal approach for esophagectomy without thoracotomy (11). The efficacy of radical en bloc esophagectomy remains controversial up to the present time, with the majority of surgeons favoring conventional techniques of esophageal resection through either a transthoracic or a transhiatal approach. However, we and others continue to advocate radical en bloc esophageal resection as the procedure of choice to maximize locoregional control and improve long-term survival in patients with esophageal carcinoma. At our institution, en bloc esophagectomy is offered to nearly all patients who have no evidence of distant metastases and no compelling medical contraindications.

The basic en bloc resection concept is removal of the tumor-bearing esophagus within a wide envelop of surrounding tissues. For tumors of the middle or lower thoracic esophagus, in addition to the tumor-bearing esophagus, the en bloc specimen would include both pleural surfaces laterally, the pericardium anteriorly, as well as the thoracic duct, and all lympho-areolar tissue wedged posteriorly between the esophagus and the spine. The associated lymphadenectomy includes en bloc resection of all nodal groups in the middle and lower mediastinum in addition to the upper abdomen. For selected patients, the lymphadenectomy is extended to include the superior mediastinal and cervical lymph nodes, also known as 3-field lymphadenectomy. Japanese surgeons first introduced the 3-field concept, prompted by the observation that up to 40% of patients resected by radical 2-field esophagectomy developed isolated recurrences in the cervical nodes (12). Isono and colleagues reported in 1991 the results of 3-field lymph node dissection and found that occult cervical node metastases occurred in one-third of patients (13). Even for lower-third tumors, 20% of patients harbored cervical metastases. Most Western surgeons have been reluctant to adopt the 3-field dissection technique. This is mostly due to skepticism that long-term survival can be achieved once nodal disease is present. A second reservation is the reported high morbidity associated with the operation, particularly injury to one or both recurrent laryngeal nerves reported in as many as 50% of patients (14,15).

PREOPERATIVE EVALUATION

Preoperative assessment is directed toward establishing the accurate clinical TNM stage of the disease, as well as assessing the patient's ability to tolerate the planned operation. Standard diagnostic and staging work-up includes an upper endoscopy with biopsy and a computed tomography (CT) of the chest and upper abdomen to evaluate the locoregional extent of the disease and exclude distant metastases. Most patients will also undergo endoscopic ultrasonography (EUS) as well as positron-emission tomography (PET). EUS is more accurate than CT in determining T and N factors, and is useful in selecting patients for clinical trials of preoperative induction therapy. PET is a generally more sensitive test for detection of distant visceral and skeletal metastases. Generally, patients are considered for surgical resection if preoperative evaluation revealed no evidence of distant metastases or clear evidence of direct tumor invasion of the airway or major vascular structures. The presence of extensive nodal disease is not considered a contraindication to resection unless it clearly extends beyond the proposed fields of dissection. Finally, all patients undergo detailed evaluation of pulmonary and cardiac function to determine their ability to withstand the planned procedure. Generally, patients with an FEV_1 less than 1.5 liters per second despite aggressive physiotherapy and optimal bronchodilator therapy are considered ineligible for en bloc resections. Cardiac disease, if suspected, is carefully assessed using either noninvasive stress testing or angiocardiography, if necessary.

OPERATIVE TECHNIQUE

The basic technical principle underlying the en bloc esophagectomy is resection of the tumor-bearing esophagus with a wide envelope of periesophageal tissue, which includes both pleural surfaces laterally, a patch of pericardium anteriorly, lymphovascular tissue and the thoracic duct posteriorly, along with the mediastinal lymph nodes from the tracheal bifurcation to the hiatus. An upper abdominal lymphadenectomy is performed that includes the common hepatic, celiac, left gastric, parahiatal, lesser curvature, and retroperitoneal lymph nodes (Figure 71.1). A third-field lymphadenectomy can be incorporated by extending the nodal dissection to include the superior mediastinal and cervical lymph nodes (Figure 71.2). En bloc esophagectomy is almost always carried out through 3 incisions: a right thoracotomy followed by a laparotomy and collar neck incision.

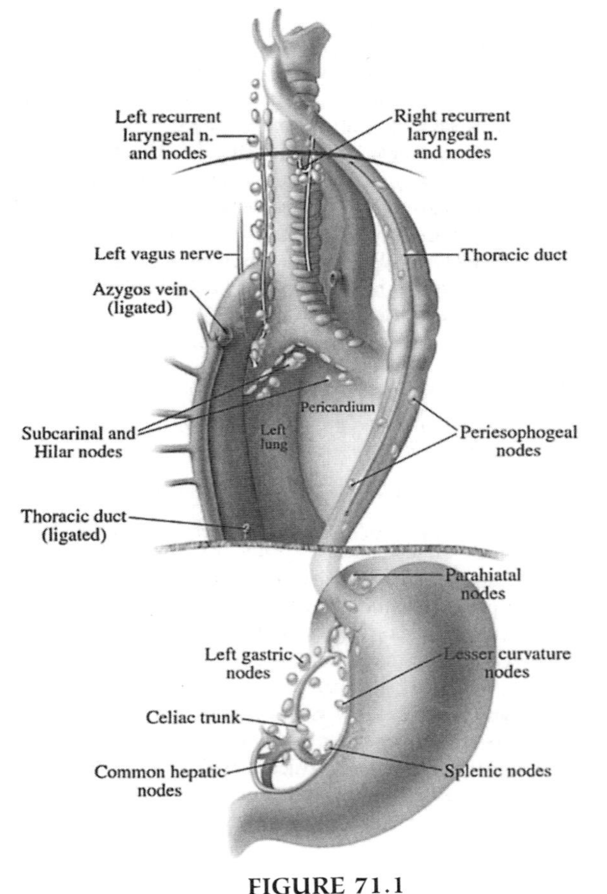

FIGURE 71.1

Mediastinal and upper abdominal lymph node fields in the en bloc resection. Shields et al. *General Thoracic Surgery* vol 2, Philadelphia: Lippincott Williams & Wilkins; 2005. Figure 131–21. With permission.

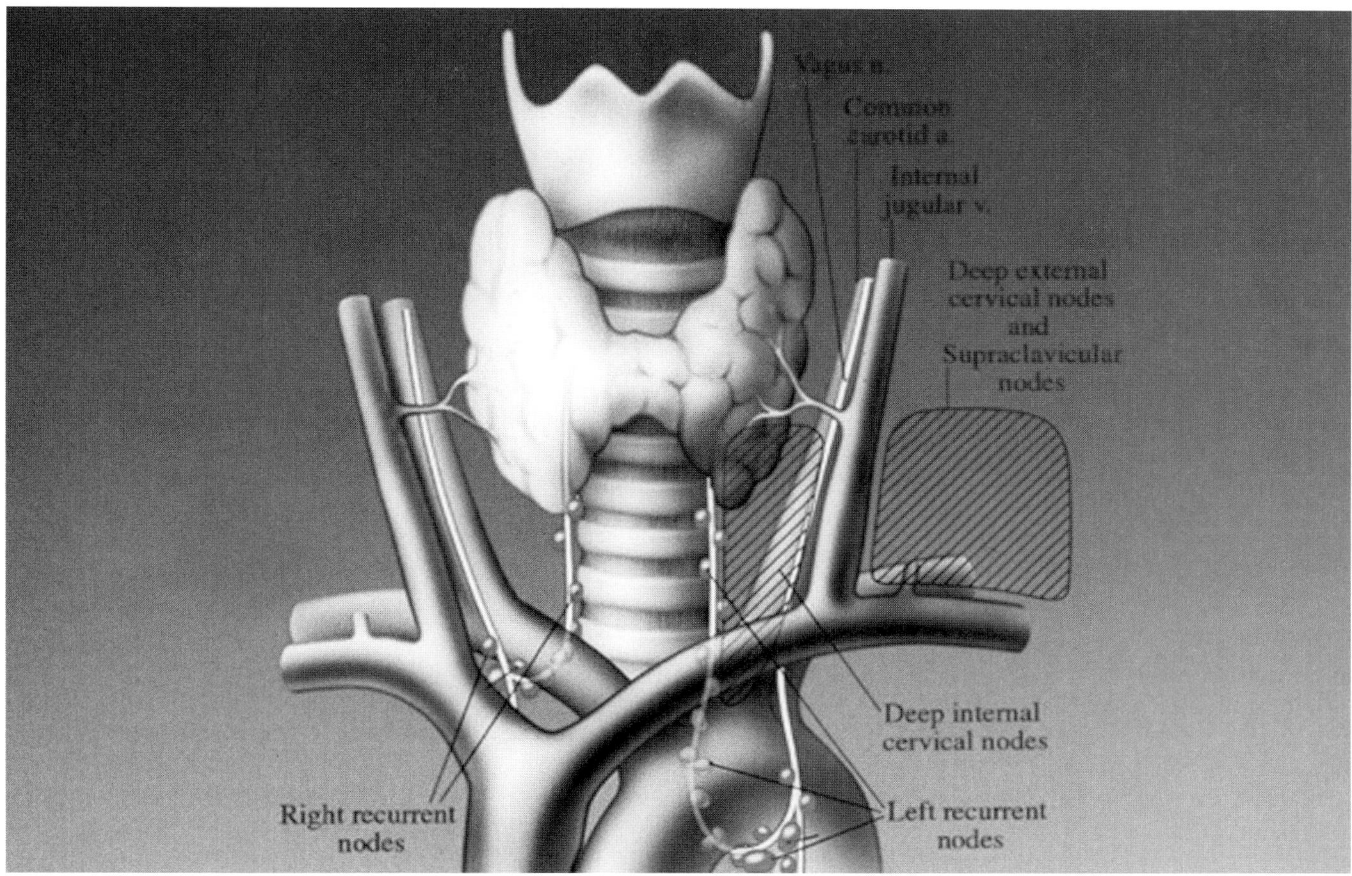

FIGURE 71.2

Recurrent and deep cervical nodal fields in the three-field lymphadenectomy. Shields et al. *General Thoracic Surgery* vol 2. Philadelphia: Lippincott Williams & Wilkins; 2005. Figure 131–20. With permission.

The Thorax

A right fifth interspace thoracotomy is performed regardless of the location of the tumor within the esophagus, removing a 1 cm segment of sixth rib posteriorly. The initial field of dissection comprises the middle and lower mediastinum and is bounded superiorly by the tracheal bifurcation, inferiorly by the esophageal hiatus, anteriorly by the hilum of the lung and pericardium, and posteriorly by the descending thoracic aorta and the spine. The en bloc resection begins by incising the mediastinal pleura over the anterior aspect of the azygous vein from the level of the azygous arch superiorly to the aortic hiatus inferiorly. The dissection proceeds medially anterior to the aorta and across the mediastinum to the opposite pleura, which is entered along the entire length of the incision. The thoracic duct is thus mobilized anteriorly toward the specimen (Figure 71.3). All lymphatic channels are clipped or ligated between the thoracic duct and the spine to minimize the occurrence of a chylothorax. At the caudal end of the dissection, the thoracic duct is ligated and divided as it enters the mediastinum through the aortic hiatus of the diaphragm. Superiorly, the thoracic duct is ligated and divided as it crosses to the left side of the mediastinum at the level of the aortic arch. In the superior mediastinum, the pleura is incised anteriorly along the tracheoesophageal groove. The esophagus is separated from the membranous trachea from the thoracic inlet to the carina. The arch of the azygous vein, but not its main trunk, is resected en bloc with the specimen. The anterior dissection is commenced by division of the azygous vein flushed with the superior vena cava. The dissection is carried along the right main bronchus and the posterior aspect of the hilum of the right lung. The hilar and subcarinal nodes are cleared en bloc with the specimen (Figure 71.4). A patch of pericardium is resected en bloc with the tumor-bearing esophagus for all but submucosal tumors (T_1) of the middle and lower thirds of the esophagus. Division of both left and right inferior pulmonary ligaments completes the esophageal

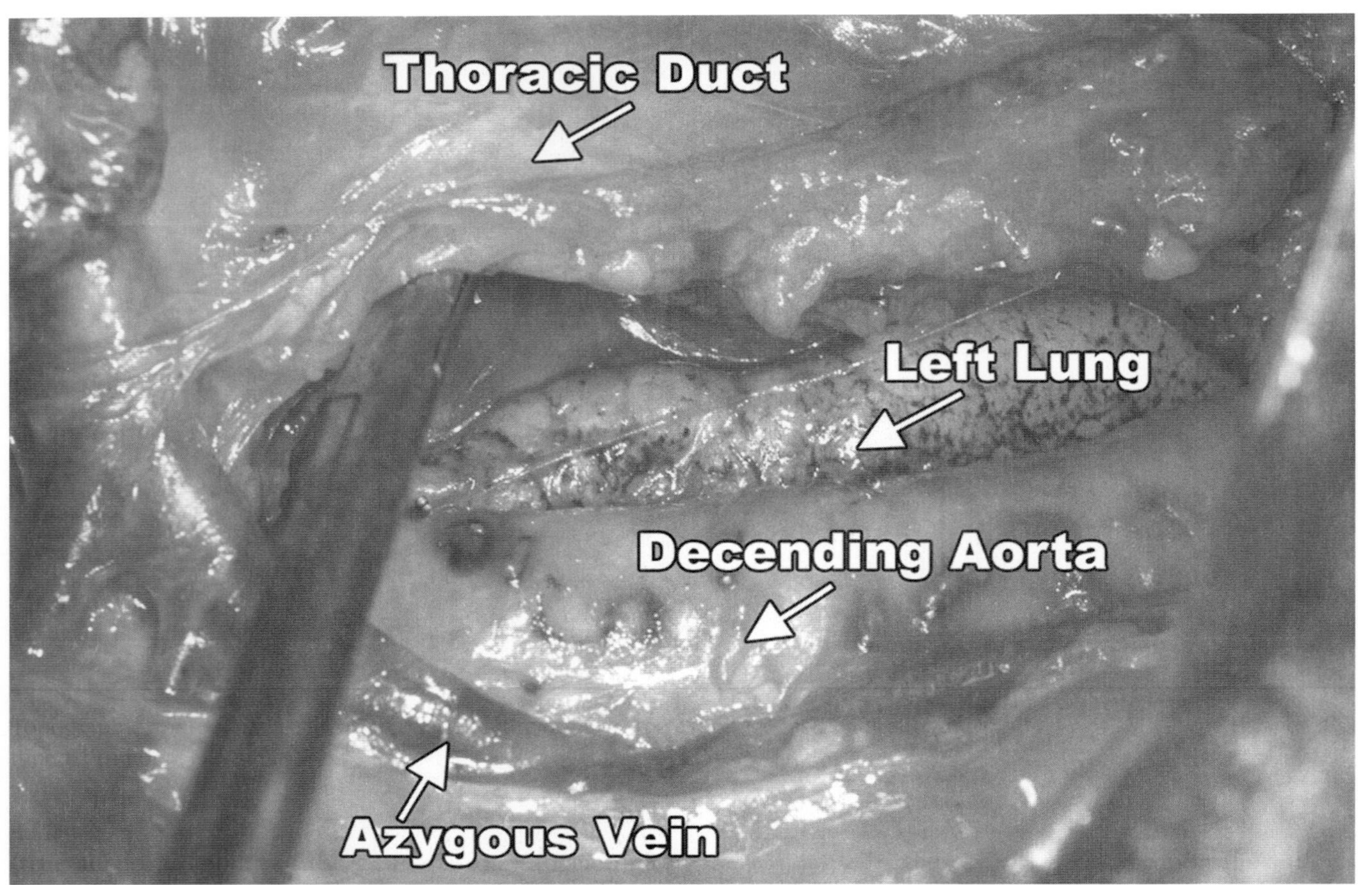

FIGURE 71.3

View from a right thoracotomy. The specimen including the thoracic duct is mobilized medially anterior to the aorta and across the mediastinum to the opposite pleura.

mobilization. For tumors traversing the hiatus, a 1-inch cuff of diaphragm is circumferentially excised en bloc with the specimen. The completed dissection clears all nodal tissue in the middle and lower mediastinum, which contains the right and left paraesophageal, para-hiatal, para-aortic, subcarinal, bilateral hilar, and aorto-pulmonary lymph nodes.

When a 3-field lymphadenectomy is incorporated with the en bloc esophagectomy, dissection of the "third-field" begins during the thoracic portion of the procedure and is later completed through a collar neck incision. Dissection of the superior mediastinal nodes includes the nodes along the right and left recurrent laryngeal nerves throughout their mediastinal course. The left recurrent nerve is exposed from the level of the aortic arch to the thoracic inlet, thereby allowing a left paratracheal node dissection. The nodes along the anterior aspect of the left recurrent nerve are carefully excised using a "no-touch" technique. The right recurrent nerve is carefully exposed near its origin at the base of the right subclavian artery. A good method for locating the right recurrent nerve is to follow the right vagus nerve from its divided end. The right recurrent nodal chain starts at that level and forms a continuous package extending through the thoracic inlet to the neck. Again, the right recurrent nerve is dissected using a strict no-touch technique. Through the cervical incision, the remainder of the recurrent nodes are dissected, as are the lower deep cervical nodes located posterior and lateral to the carotid sheath. Thus the third-field includes a continuous chain of nodes that extends from the superior mediastinum to the lower neck.

The Abdomen

The patient is repositioned supine for the next stage of the operation. The abdomen is entered through an upper mid-line incision. The omentum is separated from the colon in the avascular plane. The lesser sac is entered and the short gastric vessels are divided.

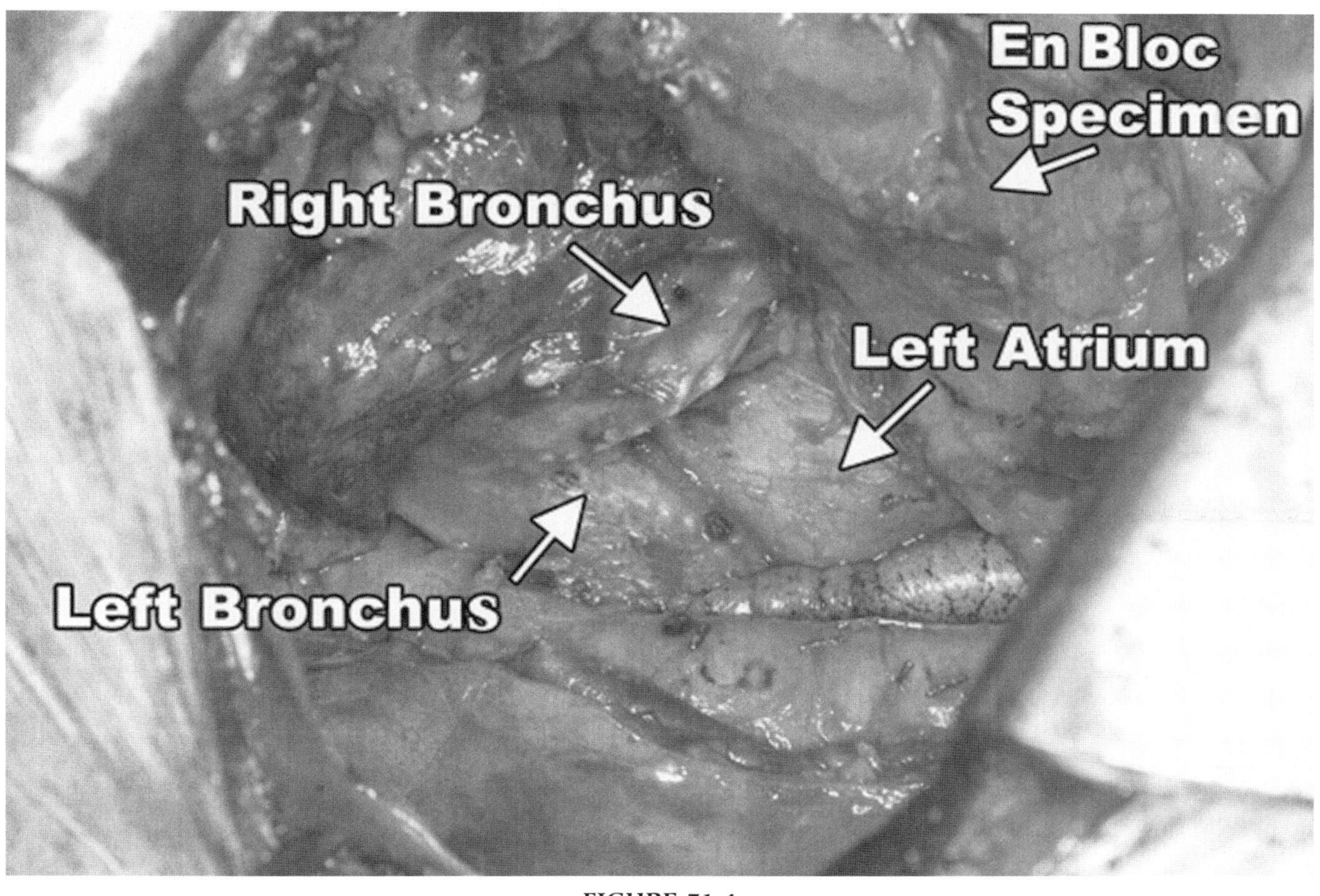

FIGURE 71.4

The en bloc specimen is completely mobilized, revealing the left lung, the carina, and the pericardium.

The retroperitoneum is incised along the superior border of the pancreas. The retroperitoneal lymphatic and areolar tissues are swept superiorly toward the esophageal hiatus and medially along the splenic artery to the celiac trifurcation. The nodes along the common hepatic artery are dissected toward the specimen and the left gastric artery is divided flush with its celiac origin. The boundaries of the retroperitoneal dissection are the dissected esophageal hiatus superiorly, the hilum of the spleen laterally, and the common hepatic artery and inferior vena cava medially (Figure 71.5). Finally, the lesser curvature of the stomach and left gastric nodes are included with the specimen as the gastric tube is fashioned. The omentum is resected as a separate specimen at least several centimeters outside the gastroepiploic arcade.

The Neck

A generous low-collar incision is performed and subplatysmal flaps are raised inferiorly and superiorly. The strap muscles are divided. The esophagus, which has been previously fully mobilized from the thorax, is retrieved from the prevertebral space. The esophagus is divided distally, and the specimen is delivered through the hiatus into the abdomen. The previously dissected recurrent nerves are easy to visualize and any residual nodal tissue is excised. When a 3-field lymphadenectomy is incorporated into the en bloc resection, the nodes posterior and lateral to the carotid sheath are removed along with the supraclavicular nodes, particularly for tumors of the middle and upper thirds of the esophagus. The dissection is bounded superiorly by the inferior belly of the omohyoid. Within the abdomen the specimen is transected distally to include the third or fourth branch of the left gastric artery. The gastric tube is prepared and the specimen is removed (Figure 71.6). The gastric tube is advanced through the posterior mediastinum to the neck. Gastrointestinal continuity is restored by a cervical esophagogastrostomy, which is performed as a single-layer running anastomosis with a monofilament

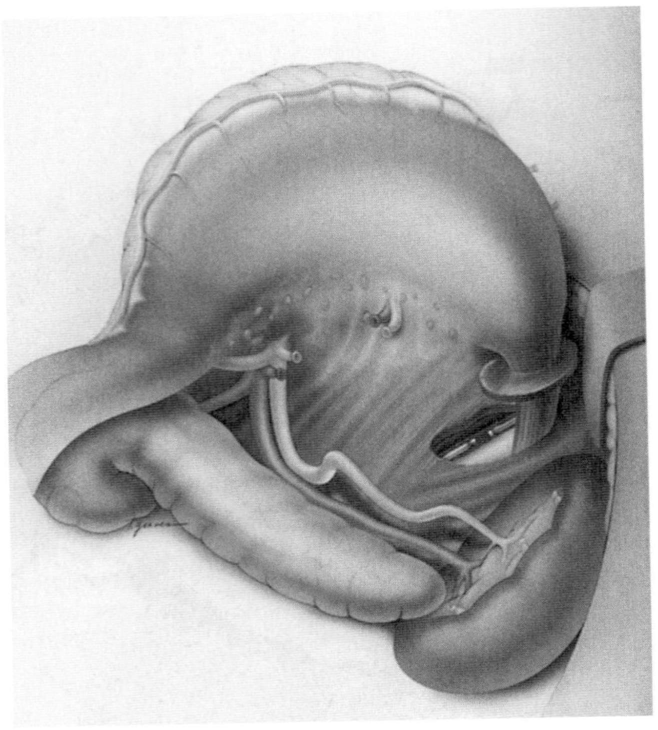

FIGURE 71.5

Illustration of en bloc dissection in the abdomen. Shields et al. *General Thoracic Surgery* vol 2. Philadelphia: Lippincott Williams & Wilkins; 2005. With permission.

absorbable suture or, more recently, employing a hybrid technique using a linear stapling device for the back wall and a continuous monofilament suture for the front wall. The gastric tube is secured to the hiatus and a feeding jejunostomy tube is placed for early postoperative enteral feeding.

Postoperative Care

In the past, all patients undergoing en bloc esophagectomy were cared for in an intensive care unit for 24 hours for fluid management and mechanical ventilation. Currently, with improved epidural pain control and aggressive pulmonary physiotherapy, patients who undergo a 2-field en bloc resection are extubated in the operating room. Patients who undergo a 3-field en bloc resection often require 24 hours of mechanical ventilation. Intense pulmonary hygiene is required, often with frequent bronchoscopies for the first 48 hours after extubation, since some patients have variable degrees of bronchorrhea. The bronchorrhea generally resolves on the third or fourth postoperative day. Patients often demonstrate significant sequestration of extracellular fluid and lymph postoperatively as a result of the removal of the thoracic duct and mediastinal lymphatics. Aggressive fluid replacement is necessary during the first 48 hours after surgery. Spontaneous diuresis usually occurs by the third postoperative day. Aggressive physical therapy is critical in getting patients out of bed and ambulating. Enteral jejunostomy feeding is commenced by the fourth or fifth postoperative days. Chest tubes are removed when drainage is less than 250 ml per day. Oral intake is begun once anastomotic integrity is confirmed by a barium study on the fifth postoperative day. Patients are discharged by the seventh or eighth postoperative day; they eat a regular diet but often require supplemental jejunostomy feeding at night. The jejunostomy tube is usually removed 4 weeks following hospital discharge if the usual postoperative anorexia resolves and oral intake is considered adequate.

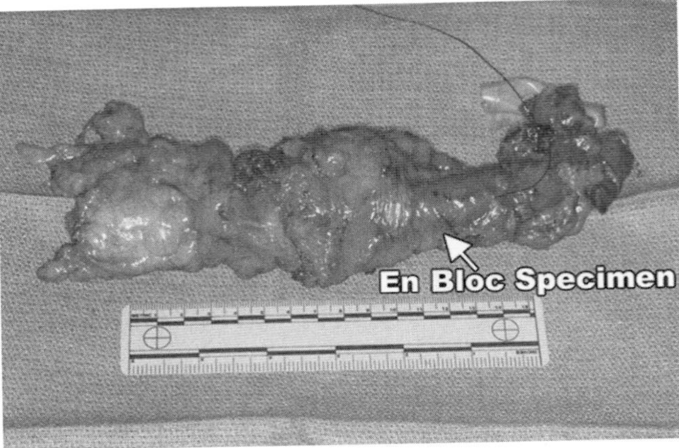

FIGURE 71.6

The en bloc specimen; note that the esophageal tumor is not seen, since it is resected within a wide envelope of adjacent tissues. Shields et al. *General Thoracic Surgery* vol 2. Philadelphia: Lippincott Williams & Wilkins; 2005. With permission.

RESULTS

In 2001, we reported a 10-year series of 111 patients who underwent en bloc esophagectomy with either a 2-field or 3-field dissection (16). The overall hospital mortality was 5.4%, which is similar to the mortality rates reported for conventional esophagectomy. Complications occurred in 54 patients and were considered minor in 11 and major in 43 (including 6 postoperative deaths) (38.7%) (Table 71.1).The most common morbidity was pulmonary related. Anastomotic leaks occurred in 13% of patients, and all healed with simple drainage. Since the introduction of the hybrid anastomotic technique, the anastomotic leak rate is about 5%.

TABLE 71.1
Surgical Complications

Leak	15 (13.5%)
Anastomotic	10 (9%)
Gastric tip necrosis	5 (4.5%)
Pulmonary	30 (27%)
Reintubation	17
Tracheostomy	10
Lobar collapse	9
Pneumonia	8
Cardiac	11 (11.7%)
Myocardial infarction	1
Supraventricular arrhythmia	10
Pericarditis	2
Infectious complications	11 (10%)
Wound	2
Abscess	1
Urinary tract infection	1
Empyema	8*
Chylothorax	2
Recurrent nerve injury (unilateral)	4
Other	11 (10%)
Splenectomy	1
Renal failure	1
Stroke	1
Pulmonary embolism	2
Delirium tremens	5
Peritonitis	1

*Including 6 patients with anastomotic leaks.
Altorki NK, Skinner D. Should en bloc esophagectomy be the standard of care for esophageal carcinoma? *Ann Surg.* 2001;234(5):581–587. With permission.

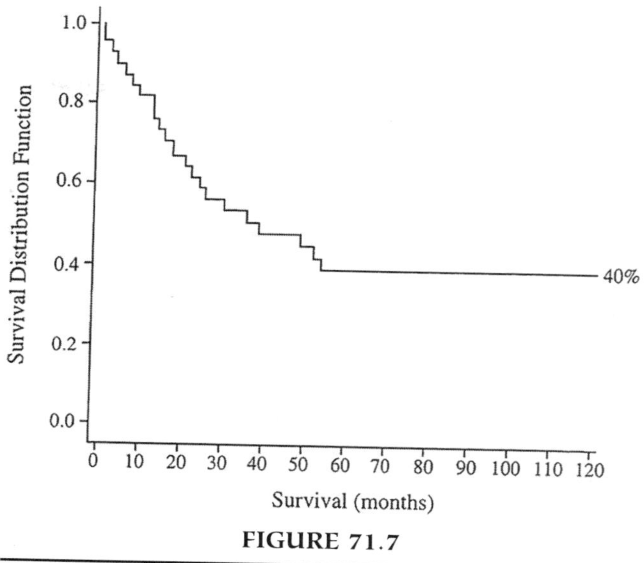

FIGURE 71.7

Overall survival for patients following en bloc esophagectomy. Altorki NK, Skinner D: Should en bloc esophagectomy be the standard of care for esophageal carcinoma? *Ann Surg.* 234:581–587, 2001. With permission.

Recurrent nerve injuries occurred in only 4 patients and were unilateral in all. None required tracheostomy as a result of recurrent nerve injury.

Overall 5-year survival for all patients was 40%, with a median survival of 38 months (Figure 71.7). Node-negative patients had a significantly improved 5-year survival of 75% compared to 26% in node-positive patients. More impressively, the 5-year survival for stage III patients was 39%, compared to 11% after conventional transthoracic esophagectomy as we and others have previously reported (17). This is especially important since most of the patients presenting with esophageal cancer already have stage III disease at presentation. An interesting observation is that for stage IV patients, 5-year survival was 27%. Survival was also significantly better in patients with locoregional N1 nodal metastases compared with distant M1a nodal metastases (31% vs. 21%, $P = 0.03$). Overall local recurrence rate was 8%, comparing favorably with the 31% to 45% of local recurrence reported after conventional esophagectomy.

More recently, Lerut et al. reported their results in a cohort of 174 patients with esophageal cancer treated by en bloc esophagectomy with 3-field lymphadenectomy (18). Hospital mortality was 1.2% and morbidity was 58%. Overall 3- and 5-year survival was 51% and 41.9%, with disease-free survival of 51.4% and 46.3%. The local recurrence rate was impressively low at 5.2%. The 5-year survival for node-negative patients was 80.2% compared to 24.5% for node-positive patients. The prevalence of metastatic disease to the cervical nodes was high, 23% for adenocarcinoma and 25% for squamous cell carcinoma. The 5-year survival in patients with positive cervical nodes in middle third carcinomas as 27.2%. This led the author to suggest that these nodes should be considered as regional (N1) rather than distant metastasis (M1b) in middle third carcinomas.

Finally, a randomized trial comparing transthoracic en bloc esophagectomy to transhiatal resection was published by Hulscher in 2002 (19). The difference in survival between the 2 groups was not statistically significant, but there was a trend toward a survival benefit with en bloc resection at 5 years. The overall and disease-free 5-year survival rates in the en bloc group were 39% and 39%, compared with 29% and 27% in the transhiatal group. Transthoracic en bloc esophagectomy was associated with higher morbidity than transhiatal esophagectomy, consistent with the increased complexity of the resection.

SUMMARY

En bloc esophagectomy can be performed with similar operative mortality compared to conventional transthoracic or transhiatal esophagectomy. It provides the widest surgical margins and the most thorough staging information through the incorporation of a 2- or 3-field lymphadenectomy. Locoregional recurrence rates are substantially lower compared to conventional esophagectomy. The superior 5-year survival rate reported suggests that en bloc resection with extended lymphadenectomy does appear to have a favorable impact on survival, especially in patients with nodal metastases.

References

1. Orringer MB, Marshall B, Iannettoni MD. Transhiatal esophagectomy: clinical experience and refinements. *Ann Surg.* 1999;230:392–403.
2. Ellis FH Jr, Heatly GJ, Krasna MJ, et al. Esophagogastrectomy for carcinoma of the esophagus and cardia: a comparison and results after standard resection in three consecutive eight-year intervals with staging criteria. *J Thorac Cardiovasc Surg.* 1997;113:836–846.
3. Lieberman MD, Shriver CD, Bleckner S, et al. Carcinoma of the esophagus. Prognostic significance of histologic type. *J Thorac Cardiovasc Surg.* 1995;109:130–138.
4. Putnam JB, Suell DM, McMurtrey MJ, et al. Comparison of three techniques of esophagectomy within a residency training program. *Ann Thorac Surg.* 1994;57:319–325.
5. Altorki NK. The rationale for radical resection. *Surg Oncol Clin North Am.* 1999;8:295–305.
6. Herskovic A, Martz K, Al-Sarraf M, et al. Combined chemotherapy and radiotherapy compared with radiotherapy alone in patients with cancer of the esophagus. *N Engl J Med.* 1992;326:1593–1598.
7. Kelsen DP, Ginsberg R, Pajak T. Chemotherapy followed by surgery compared with surgery alone for localized esophageal cancer. *N Engl J Med.* 1998;339:1979–1984.
8. Law S, Fok M, Chow S, et al. Preoperative chemotherapy versus surgical therapy alone for squamous cell carcinoma of the esophagus: a prospective randomized trial. *J Thorac Cardiovasc Surg.* 1997;114:210–217.
9. Logan A. The surgical treatment of carcinoma of the esophagus and cardia. *J Thorac Cardiovasc Surg.* 1963;46:150.
10. Skinner DB. En bloc resection for neoplasms of the esophagus and cardia. *J Thorac Cardiovasc Surg.* 1983;85:59–70.
11. Orringer MB, Sloan H. Esophagectomy without thoracotomy. *J Thorac Cardiovasc Surg.* 1978;76:643.
12. Isono K, Onoda S, Nakayama K, et al. Recurrence of intrathoracic esophageal cancer. *Jpn J Clinical Oncol.* 1985;15:49–60.
13. Isono K, Sato H, Nakayama K. Results of a nationwide study on three-field lymph node dissection of esophageal cancer. *Oncology.* 1991;48:411–420.
14. Fujita H, Kakegawa T, Yamana H, et al. Mortality and morbidity rates, postoperative course, quality of life, and prognosis after extended radical lymphadenectomy for esophageal cancer. Comparison of three-field lymphadenectomy with two-field lymphadenectomy. *Ann Surg.* 1995;222:654–662.
15. Nishihira T, Hirayama K, Mori S. A prospective randomized trial of extended cervical and superior mediastinal lymphadenectomy for carcinoma of the thoracic esophagus. *Am J Surg.* 1998;175:45–51.
16. Altorki NK, Skinner D. Should en-bloc esophagectomy be the standard of care for esophageal carcinoma? *Ann Surg.* 2001;234:581–587.
17. Altorki N, Girardi L, Skinner DB. En bloc esophagectomy improves survival for stage III esophageal cancer. *J Thorac Cardiovasc Surg.* 1997;114:948.
18. Lerut T, Nafteux P, Moons J RN MScN, et al. , Three-field lymphadenectomy for carcinoma of the esophagus and gastroesophageal junction in 174 R0 resection: impact on staging, disease-free survival, and outcome. *Ann Surg.* 2004;240:962–974.
19. Hulscher JB, Van Sandick JW, De Boer AGEM, et al. Extended transthoracic resection compared with limited transhiatal resection for adenocarcinoma of the esophagus. *N Engl J Med.* 2002;347:1662.

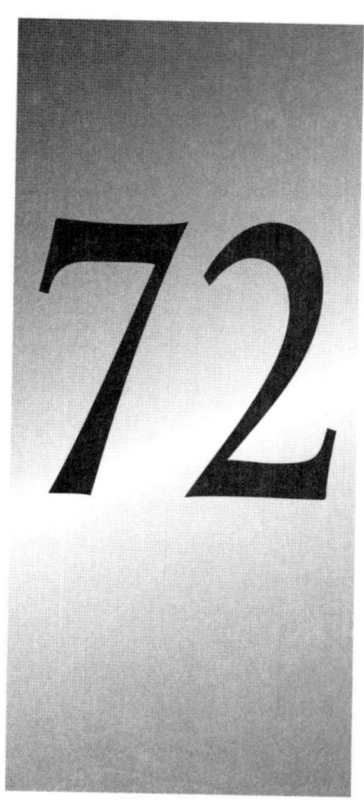

72 Surgery Techniques: Left Transthoracic and Thoracoabdominal Esophagectomy

Donald Edward Low
Matthew James Deeter

The presentation of esophageal cancer continues to evolve. Historically, it was most commonly a tumor of the upper to mid-esophagus of squamous cell origin. There has been a gradual epidemiologic shift associated with an increase of adenocarcinoma predominately involving the lower esophagus and gastroesophageal junction. Statistics from Surveillance, Epidemiology and End Results Program (SEER) note 54.0% adenocarcinoma, 38.8% squamous cell carcinoma, and 7.2% other histologic types among confirmed 2001–2004 cases (1). In spite of a continuing evolution in resective technique and multimodality therapy, the incidence and mortality rates of esophageal cancer in the United States remain remarkably similar, with an estimated 15,560 new cases and 13,940 deaths in 2007 (2).

The ultimate goal of therapy is the immediate relief of symptoms while providing the best opportunity to cure cancer and maintain the highest possible quality of life. Several treatment options are available. No one operative approach can be considered globally superior to the others in all situations. Selecting the right operation for the right patient involves many factors. The major variables that govern the selection of the best surgical approach include location of the tumor, extent of the disease, surgeon experience, and patient's physiologic status. Esophagogastrectomy by the left thoracoabdominal approach (LTA) offers many advantages (see summary below) and is the ideal approach for many patients, particularly those presenting with distal esophageal adenocarcinoma. It would not be considered an appropriate approach for some middle esophageal and most upper esophageal tumors, particularly those clinically staged at T3 or T4.

Some details of LTA's rich history have been obscured by time, but the broad pattern remains discernible. The initial report of the application of a left thoracoabdominal incision came from Tiegel and Wendel in Germany in 1909 (3). The first esophagectomy for cancer through the left chest was performed by Dr. Franz Tork in the United States in 1913 (4). Specific reports of LTA being applied for esophageal resection appear in the 1930s with Adams and Phemister (5) and in the 1940s from Sweet and Garlock (4). The operation was further popularized in North America for tumors of the esophagogastric junction by Dr. F. H. Ellis at the Lahey Clinic (3). More recently, LTA has been more frequently utilized in Europe, especially in the United Kingdom. There continues to be a misconception on the part of some surgeons that the approach limits the extent of the proximal resection and the surgeons' options for positioning the anastomosis high in the chest or neck due to the position of the aortic arch. The technical description in this chapter will demonstrate that these perceptions are incorrect.

ADVANTAGES OF LTA

Completeness of resection remains the main determinant of outcome. Extirpation of the entire thoracic esophagus is possible with LTA with the addition of a cervical incision. With appropriate technique, nearly the entire length of the esophagus can be mobilized and removed under direct vision. Additionally, LTA provides excellent exposure of the upper abdomen and is thus ideal for resection of adenocarcinoma or other tumors of the esophagogastric junction, cardia, or fundus. Some of the advantages of LTA are summarized below.

1. Unparalleled exposure is provided for resection of proximal gastric to distal thoracic esophageal lesions and for accomplishing a "complete" abdominal and thoracic lymph node dissection.
2. The thoracotomy is accomplished through the costal margin, which allows the chest to be opened like a book rather than spreading ribs against 2 fixed points, as with a standard thoracotomy. This results in less immediate and long-term postoperative pain.
3. The entire incision is located in 1 or 2 dermatomes, typically T7 or T8, making postoperative analgesia straightforward with a thoracic epidural.
4. Mobilization of the stomach (or other conduit) and the esophagus are performed synchronously through the same incision. The location of the anastomosis can easily be tailored in response to intraoperative findings, including resection margins to any level between the inferior pulmonary vein and the neck.
5. Conduit selection can be diversified easily to include the whole stomach, a narrow gastric tube, or a segment of colon or pedicled jejunum.
6. The entire abdominal and thoracic dissection is done under direct vision, which is particularly important when mobilizing a reoperative or scarred esophagus.
7. The mobilization of the cervical esophagus from the chest decreases the risk of recurrent nerve damage during a cervical anastomosis.
8. It provides excellent exposure of the thoracic esophagus and surrounding structures, including pericardium, aorta, left main bronchus, thoracic duct, and diaphragm. Dissection is accomplished under direct vision to minimize blood loss and to avoid inadvertent injury to surrounding structures. Direct vision also facilitates en bloc dissection in the case of T4 disease in the mid and lower thorax.

PERIOPERATIVE STANDARDIZED CLINICAL PATHWAYS

A program incorporating standardized clinical pathways designed around set goals significantly improves outcomes (6–8). A standardized clinical pathway organizes the approach to care and allows for continued improvement over time (see Table 72.1). Prior to surgery, it ensures information is collected or obtained, organized, and communicated within the medical team in an efficient manner. The pathway also provides clear expectations for the patient and their family. These expectations provide a framework around which they can better understand, plan, and organize for the time immediately around the operation, subsequent hospitalization, and recovery period. For many this reduces anxiety and improves cooperation. It provides milestones of recovery that may act as motivators. Specific improvements have previously been documented in the timing of initiation of early mobilization, nutrition, and discharge (8). Goals within the pathway can be updated over time as the management team gains experience and results improve.

LEFT THORACOABDOMINAL ESOPHAGECTOMY: TECHNICAL DESCRIPTION

Preoperative

Preoperative preparation includes a standard bowel preparation. Preoperative antibiotics are administered and a thoracic epidural is placed for pain control in the holding area or on entry into the operating room. Once in the operating room an arterial line and other appropriate monitoring are established. Below-the-knee sequential compression stockings are placed, and intubation with double lumen endotracheal tube is achieved.

Positioning/Setup

Setup includes standard thoracotomy and laparotomy trays, including a Balfour. Additionally, a reticulating arm retractor system such as Emdec Arm or Martin Arm (Gebrüder Martin GmbH & Co., Tuttlingen, Germany) facilitates exposure. An operative table capable of flexing with 2 rolled bolsters, an axillary roll, and an arm rest or sling facilitates positioning.

Positioning for the LTA is in a modified right lateral decubitus, as seen in Figures 72.1 and 72.2. The patient is positioned at approximately 70 degrees away from the vertical obliquely between the right lateral decubitus and supine position. The operative table is adjusted to provide for a mildly flexed position to open the rib spaces. The left arm is supported on a sling device. The patient is held in position by anterior and posterior rolled bolsters placed to center the left subcostal area for maximal exposure of the chest and abdomen. Positioning is aided by a combination of tape and a warming blanket placed across the hips, as seen in Figure 72.2.

TABLE 72.1
Esophageal Resection Standardized Clinic Pathway

- Initial contact (referral):
  - **Interview patient within 48 hours of referral**
  - Verbal review (telephone interview)
    - PMH
    - Current symptoms → e.g., swallowing/wt loss
    - Current investigations
    - Travel arrangements
    - Initial description of surgery/VM
  - Patient appointment made with respect to patient/ referring physician wishes, patient symptoms/status, patient availability
- Prior to VM appointment
  - Arrangements for previous notes, investigations, films, path sent or brought to VM
  - Arrange patient-tailored schedule, which is forwarded to patient
- Initial encounter (completes within 2–3 working days)
  - Consultations
    - Thoracic surgery
    - Medical oncology
    - Radiation oncology
    - Cardiology (>50 y.o. (risk factors))
  - Path review
  - Investigations
    - Contrast CT
    - PET/CT
    - EGD/EGD US – attended by surgeon
  - **Presentation at thoracic tumor board** (next conference following initial appointment)
  - Patient contacted with recommendations day following tumor board – reports sent to referring MD
- Pre-op arrangements
  - Initiate chemotherapy or chemoradiotherapy
  - Referral for neoadjuvant therapy
  - Reassessment following completion of neoadjuvant therapy
    - CT scan
    - EGD US
  - Reassessment done 2–4 weeks prior to operative date
  - **Individualized operative approach according to**
    - Tumor/Barrett's characteristics
    - Patient physiology
    - Previous surgery
- Surgery
  - Thoracic epidural placed preoperatively
  - Minimize blood loss/transfusions
  - **Conservative intraoperative fluid administration**
  - **Immediate extubation**
  - **Post-op anesthesia—PCEA**
  - Admit to ICU
- Post-op
  - Patient sits up and dangles evening of surgery
  - **Patient walks in hall morning POD #1**
  - Discharge from ICU 12–18 hours post-op
  - Walks the ward 3–4 × each day ± physical therapy consult
  - Chest tube 1 removed day 2
  - Chest tube 2 removed day 3, 4 or 5
  - Jejunostomy tube nutrition initiated day 3
  - Gastrografin/barium swallow day 4 or 5
  - NG tube removed day 5 or 6
  - Switch to oral/J-tube analgesics day 5 or 6
  - Dietary/home health consult day 5 or 6
  - Discharge day 7 or 8
  - Represent at next available tumor board following completion of path results
  - Review recommendations with patient within 24 hours
  - Forward recommendations to referring (outside MDs)

Additional padding is placed as needed to maintain positioning and for protection against pressure injury. The thoracic epidural catheter is protected by adhesive drape. A secure and safe position is assured by each member of the operating team prior to skin preparation.

Assessing Local Resectability in the Abdomen

The initial incision is made from the abdominal midline at midpoint between the umbilicus and xiphoid to the left costal margin (see Figure 72.3). The skin and subcutaneous tissues are opened to the level of the fascia. The anterior sheath of the rectus abdominus muscle and the external oblique are incised. The posterior sheath of the rectus is divided to provide access for evaluation for unresectable disease within the abdomen.

Inspection is performed for peritoneal implants, metastasis to the liver or omentum, and the extent of the abdominal component of the tumor (see Figure 72.4). The tumor is evaluated for locoregional invasion, which may preclude resection due to involvement of surrounding vital structures. Biopsies are taken as indicated.

Performing this initial evaluation allows the patient with unresectable disease to avoid a thoracotomy. If this occurs, a feeding gastrostomy or jejunostomy can be placed through this incision when appropriate.

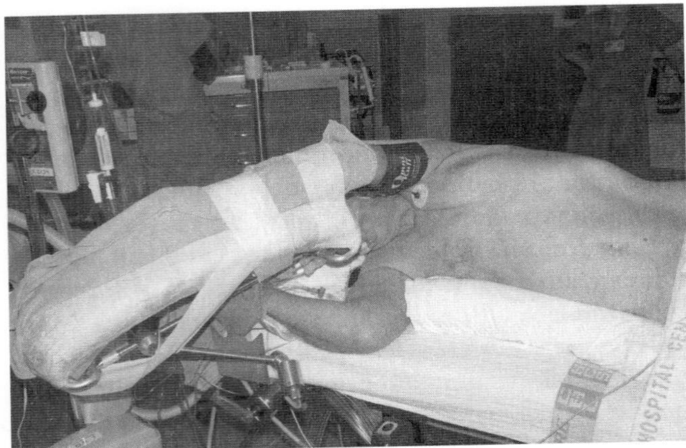

FIGURE 72.1

Anterior view of patient positioning.

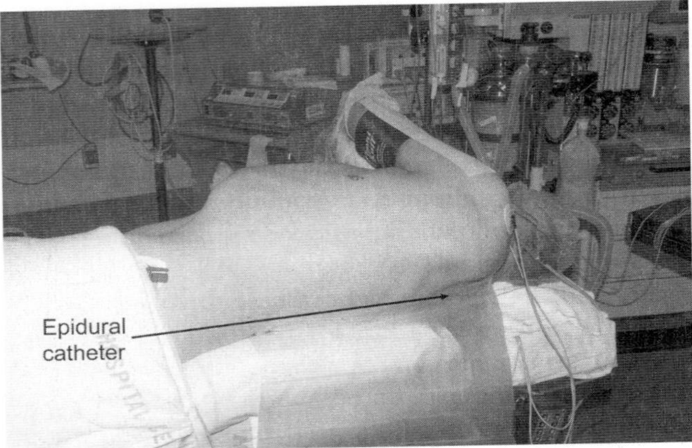

FIGURE 72.2

Posterior view of patient positioning.

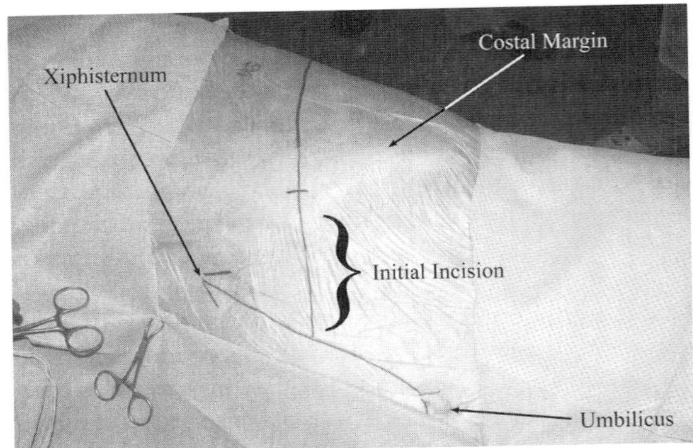

FIGURE 72.3

Initial abdominal incision.

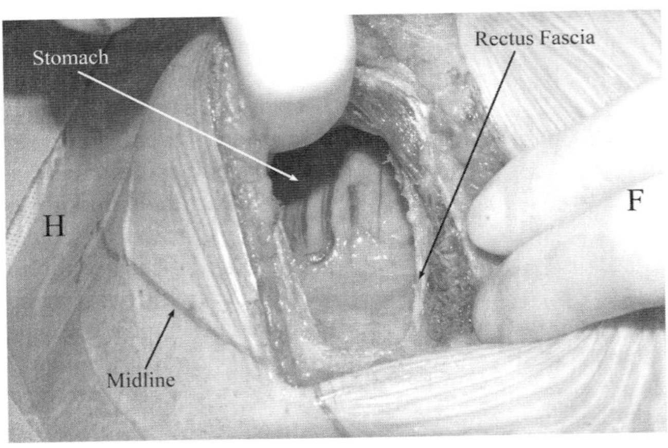

FIGURE 72.4

Initial abdominal access and assessment. Head (H) Feet (F).

Assessing Local Resectability in the Chest

If resectable disease is found, the incision is extended over the left chest. The incision should follow a generally straight line as a continuation of the initial incision to a point just posterior to the tip of the scapula. The skin and subcutaneous tissue are opened to the level of the fascia. The latissimus dorsi muscle is divided. The serratus anterior is divided posteriorly and detached from its rib insertions anteriorly (see Figure 72.5).

Entry into the chest is generally through the highest intercostal space where the costal margin remains narrow. The exact intercostal space that will provide the best exposure to thoracic esophagus as well as the upper abdomen is dependent on the particular patient's body habitus. This optimal space becomes apparent with palpation through the diaphragm from the abdomen. In most younger patients, the costal margin can be divided with scalpel, as seen in Figure 72.6. When it is calcified, rib cutting shears are required. This type of thoracotomy is much better tolerated as it opens the chest like a book rather than spreading the ribs against 2 fixed points. The diaphragm is opened radially for 8 to 12 cm dependent on the patient's body habitus, with care to avoid injury to the branches of the phrenic nerve in the area of the central tendon. See Figure 72.7.

With the diaphragm open, a Balfour retractor is placed with the blades on the chest wall and an upper hand retractor placed under the rib cage superiorly to provide better access to the upper chest. See Figure 72.8. The operative table can be rotated to the left or right to optimize exposure of the chest or abdomen.

The left lung is retracted anteriorly. The inferior pulmonary ligament is mobilized up to the level of the inferior pulmonary vein. The mediastinal pleura is divided

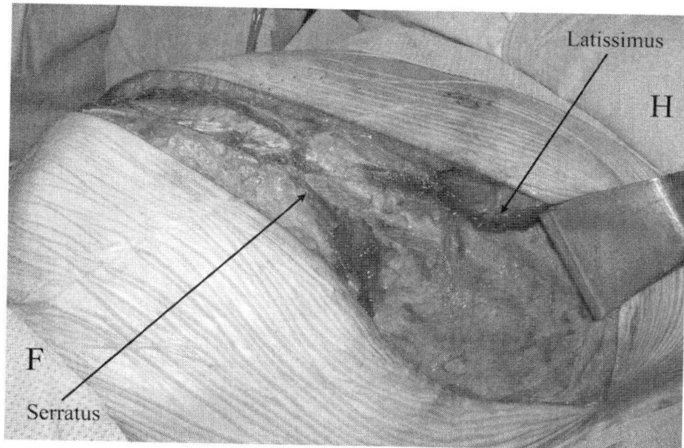

FIGURE 72.5

Initiation of chest incision.

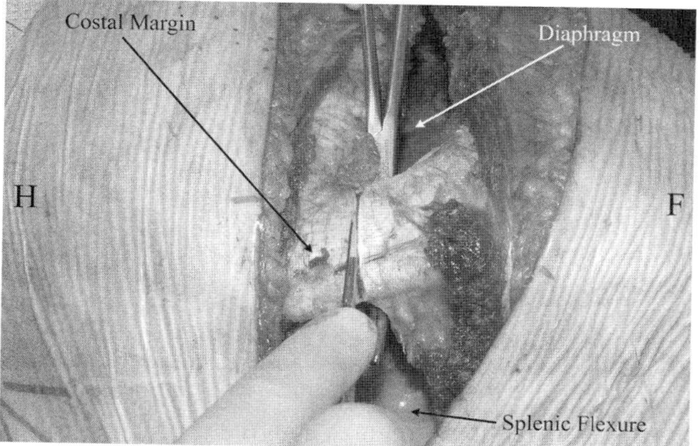

FIGURE 72.6

Costal margin is incised sharply.

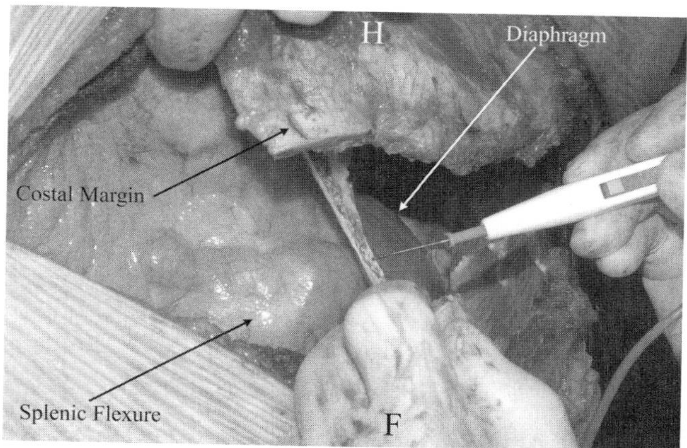

FIGURE 72.7

After opening the costal margin, the diaphragm is incised.

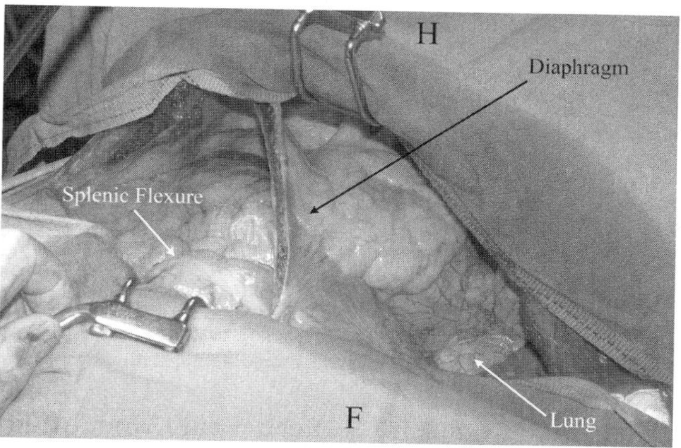

FIGURE 72.8

Placement of retractors to provide simultaneous access to the chest and abdomen.

laterally along the aorta and lateral to the esophagus. The periesophageal tissue, including all lymph nodes, is mobilized by careful dissection of the entire posterior aspect of the pericardium and inferior mediastinum. See Figure 72.9. This tissue is left attached to the esophagus, which is encircled initially manually, and then with a Penrose drain. Direct extension of the cancer into the pericardium, diaphragm, lung, or thoracic duct can be dealt with by en bloc resection where appropriate. The right pleura is resected if it comes into direct contact with the tumor.

Dissection is then continued superiorly, mobilizing the esophagus from attachments and taking all lymphatics and associated lymph nodes from the posterior mediastinal space. Feeding vessels from the aorta are identified individually and secured with cautery, clips, or a harmonic scalpel under direct vision. See Figure 72.10.

Great care is exercised to ensure continuity of the specimen. See Figure 72.11. Any nodes not encompassed in the specimen are removed and labeled as to origin at the time of removal to ensure proper tissue handling. The subcarinal lymph node packet can typically be taken en bloc. The anterior and posterior vagus nerves are identified and left intact at this stage. The esophagus is subsequently mobilized circumferentially from the hiatus. The specimen is thus mobilized from the peritoneal reflection to the inferior aspect of the aortic arch. See Figure 72.12.

Mobilizing the Stomach

Attention is then directed to the abdomen. During this period, the left lung can be re-expanded. Exposure is

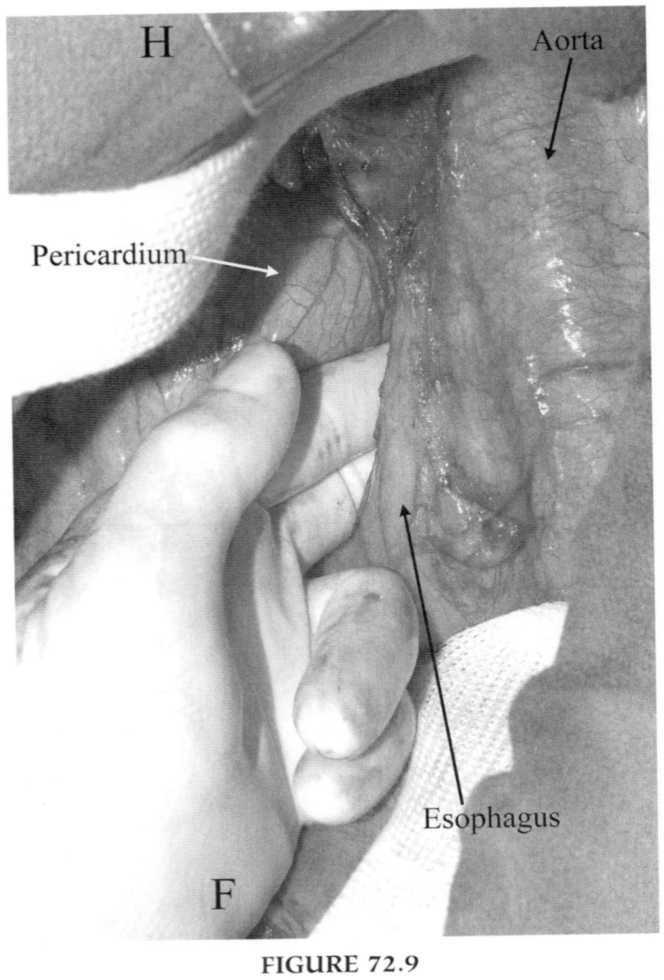

FIGURE 72.9

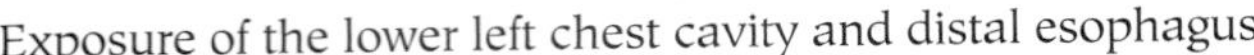

Exposure of the lower left chest cavity and distal esophagus.

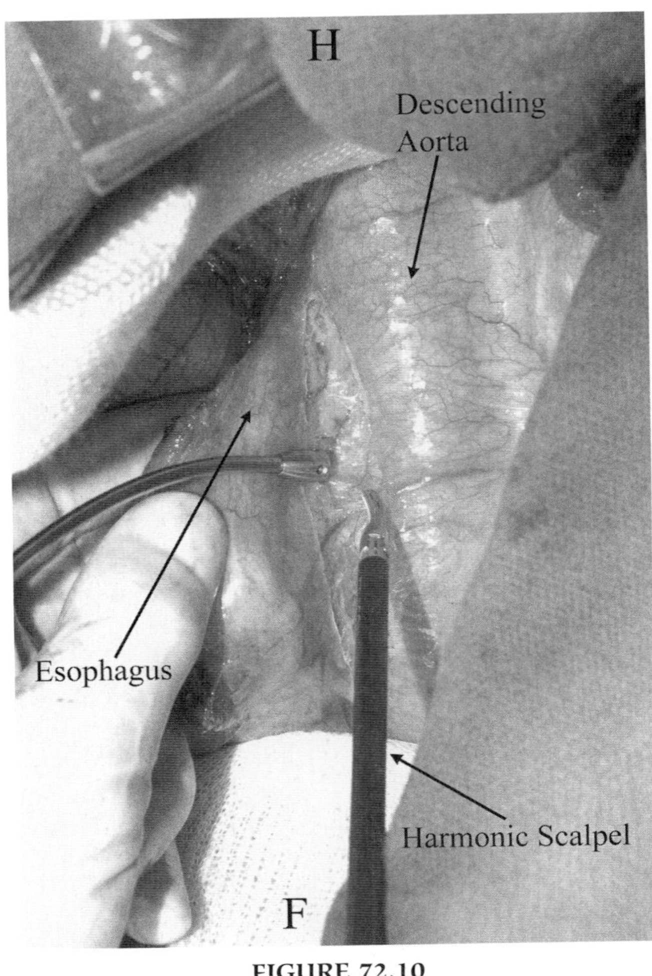

FIGURE 72.10

Exposure of the esophagus below the aortic arch.

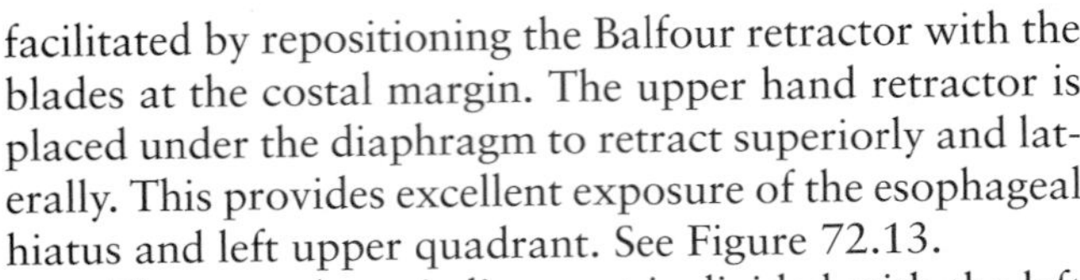

facilitated by repositioning the Balfour retractor with the blades at the costal margin. The upper hand retractor is placed under the diaphragm to retract superiorly and laterally. This provides excellent exposure of the esophageal hiatus and left upper quadrant. See Figure 72.13.

The gastrohepatic ligament is divided with the left lobe liver retracted separately. See Figure 72.14. Dissection is continued up over the anterior aspect of the hiatus. The right and left crus are dissected free. See Figure 72.15. The hiatus is mobilized circumferentially. Once the peritoneum is taken down, the dissection in the chest has usually facilitated easy encircling of the esophagus. The distal esophagus is encircled with a Penrose drain. See Figure 72.16. The left thoracoabdominal incision provides excellent exposure to the short gastric vessels. These vessels are taken down with a harmonic scalpel. See Figure 72.17.

The right gastroepiploic vessels are identified early and the course clearly determined. At all times dissection is carried out 1 to 2 cm away from the right gastroepiploic vessels. The watershed area of the right and left gastroepiploic vessels is carefully inspected for communicating vessels which are preserved if present. The greater curvature is mobilized down to the pylorus. See Figure 72.18.

A Kocher maneuver is carried out to mobilize the pylorus up to the level of the esophageal hiatus. The patency and quality of the pylorus is evaluated for the need for pyloroplasty. See Figure 72.19. In the absence of prior surgery or inflammatory change, this is seldom required in our experience.

With the greater curve mobilized and Kocher maneuver complete, the left gastric pedicle is approached posteriorly. The stomach is elevated, and any remaining retrogastric adhesions are taken down. The stomach is then drawn out of the abdominal cavity (see Figure 72.20), and the entire fatty and lymphatic mass around the lesser curve and upper pancreatic area and supraceliac region is dissected en bloc.

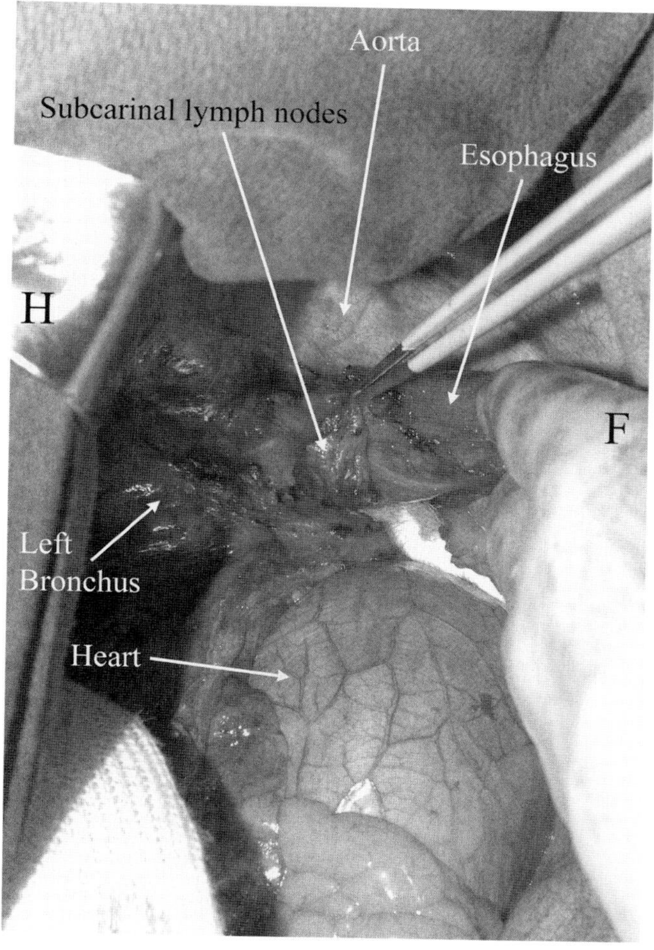

FIGURE 72.11

Mid-esophageal dissection including subcarinal nodes.

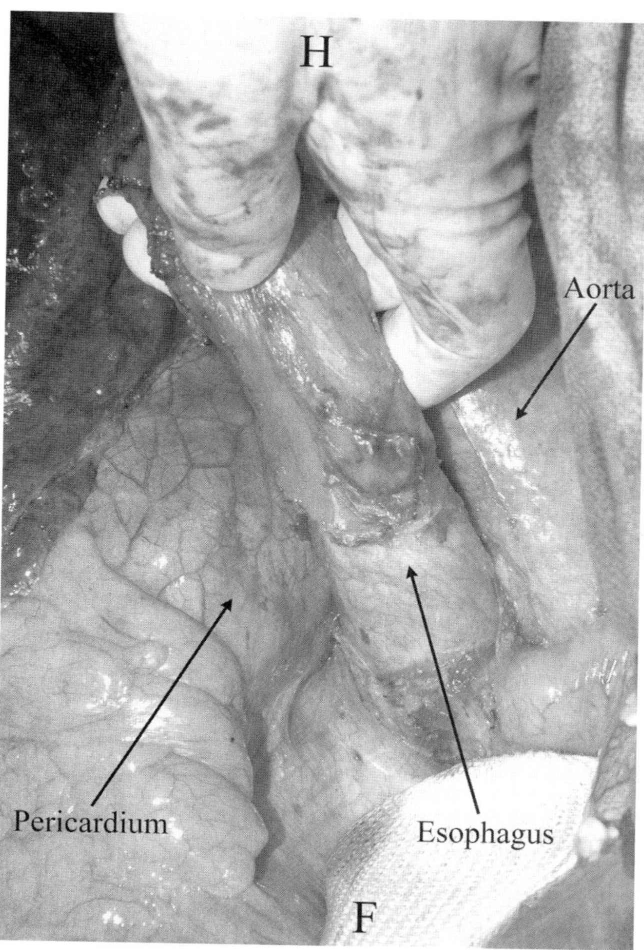

FIGURE 72.12

Mobilization of esophagus at the diaphragmatic hiatus.

Careful dissection is carried out to positively define the left gastric artery and vein. The left gastric artery is mobilized to its origin at the celiac axis. See Figure 72.21. All associated supra-celiac artery and suprapancreatic nodes are dissected free. The left gastric artery is suture ligated with 3–0 silk.

A feeding jejunostomy tube is then placed approximately 40 cm from the ligament of Trietz.

Return to the Chest

Attention then returns to the chest. Dissection in the periesophageal planes is carried up to a point just inferior to the aortic arch. Anterior and posterior vagus nerves are divided between clips. If the conduit's length is inadequate to reach the neck due to the planned extent of the gastric resection, an anastomosis can be done below the level of the aortic arch. See section on Intrathoracic Anastomosis. Dissection continues in the periesophageal plane underneath the aorta, mobilizing additional periesophageal lymph nodes. See Figure 72.22. This is the only part of the dissection that is done without direct visualization.

Once mobilization is completed under the arch, a window through the pleura over the esophagus is made above the aortic arch and to the left of the left subclavian artery. The window is initially opened with a small incision of the pleura on top of the dissecting finger then dilated with the surgeon's fingers. See Figure 72.23. Through this window, the dissection is continued in the periesophageal planes up into the base of the neck.

After dissection is completed, the esophagus can be brought out through this window above the aortic arch. See Figure 72.24.

Once circumferential mobilization of the esophagus is complete, the nasogastric tube is pulled back into the supra-aortic esophagus and secured with a transfixing

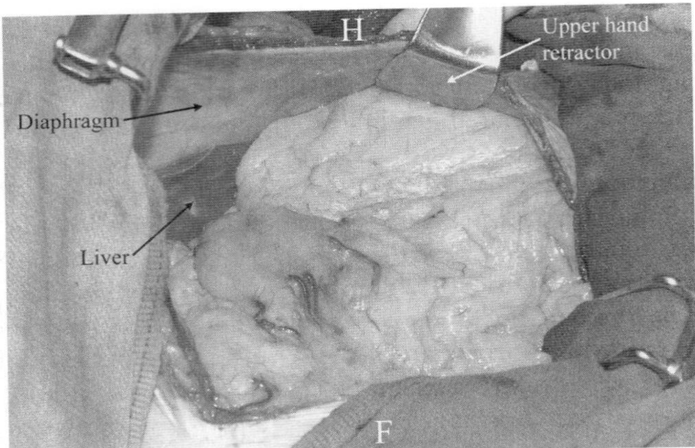

FIGURE 72.13

Initial upper abdominal exposure.

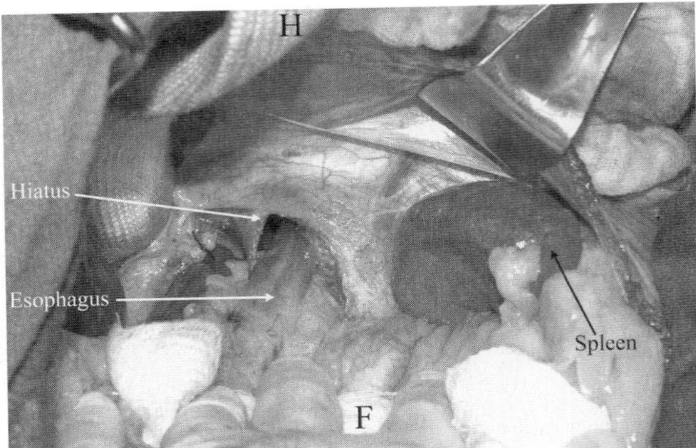

FIGURE 72.15

The hiatus is mobilized circumferentially.

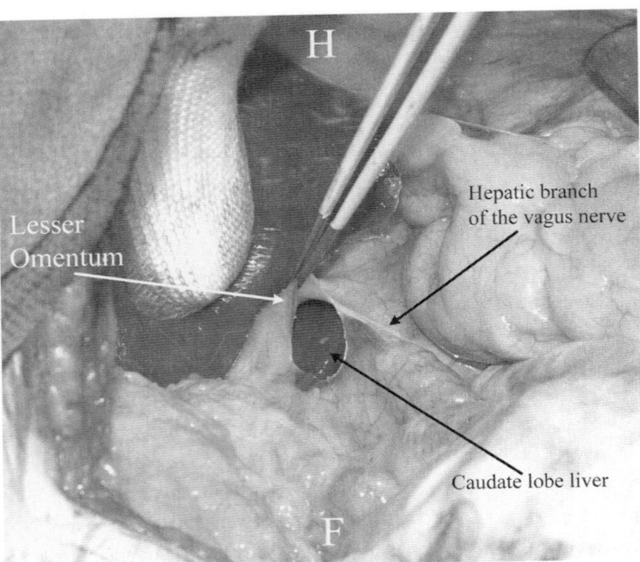

FIGURE 72.14

Initial mobilization of the stomach.

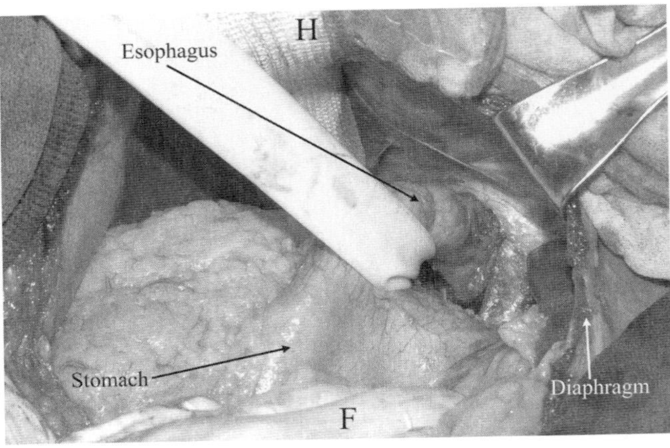

FIGURE 72.16

Completed mobilization of the esophagogastric junction.

suture. The esophagus is then divided sharply just distal to this point. See Figure 72.25. (Note: An additional length of esophagus is typically taken at the time of anastomosis in the neck.)

Conduit Construction

With dissection complete and the esophagus transected, the esophagus and attached tissues are delivered into the abdomen. See Figure 72.26. Fashioning the conduit is very easy and accurate through this exposure. The conduit is fashioned with the primary concern for adequate distal margin. Secondary considerations in conduit construction include retaining appropriate length while producing a relatively narrow conduit to promote emptying and reduce redundancy.

The lesser curve is prepared for division. Depending on the amount of gastric involvement the lesser curve can be cleaned for transection at any point between the third vein and the pylorus. See Figure 72.27.

Constructing the conduit is initiated in the fundus. See Figure 72.28. There should be a tendency for advancing in small controlled increments with each application of staples to allow for elongation of conduit and shaping to a consistent width and even resection margin of at least 4 to 5 cm. See Figure 72.29. The specimen is then taken to pathology by the surgeon to orient the specimen and obtain frozen section assessment of the proximal resection margin.

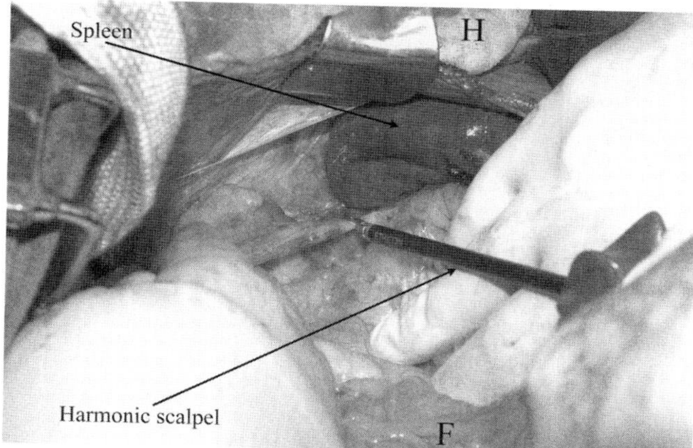

FIGURE 72.17

Taking down the short gastrics.

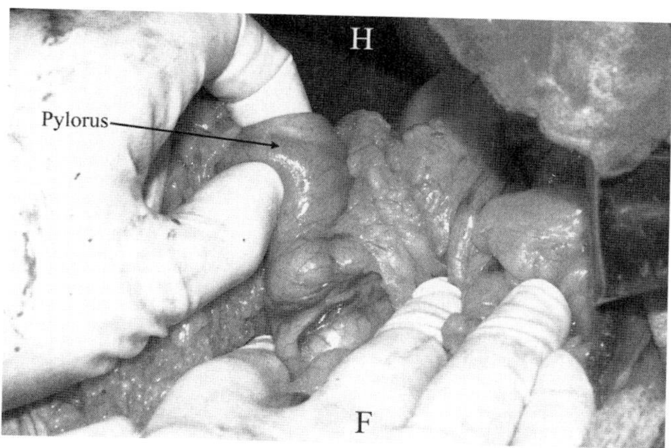

FIGURE 72.19

Following the Kocher maneuver, the pylorus is assessed.

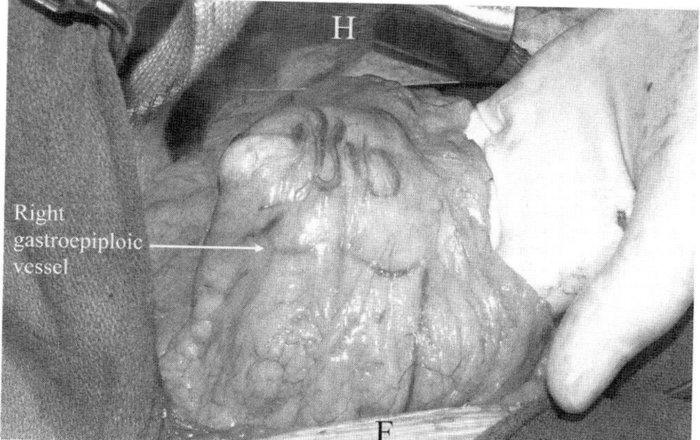

FIGURE 72.18

The entire greater curve is mobilized. The course of the right gastroepiploic artery is identified.

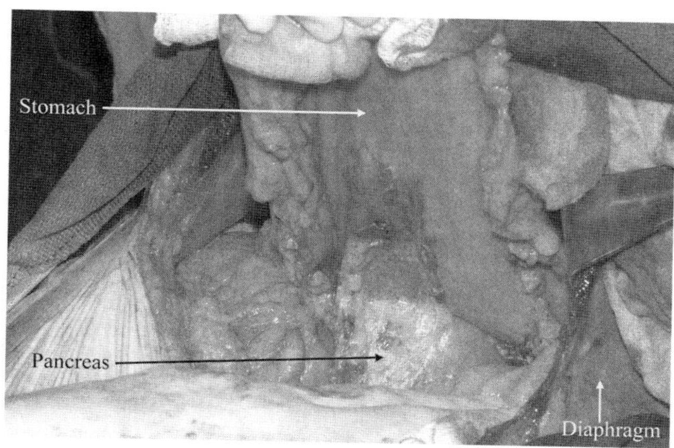

FIGURE 72.20

Exposure of the left gastric artery.

The extent of stomach available for esophageal replacement will depend on the amount of gastric involvement. Generally the stomach will be divided at the level of the fourth vein, as described above. With more extensive gastric involvement, however, the line of resection may be as far down as the incisura or even immediately above the pylorus if greater gastric resection margin is required or a particularly thin conduit would be considered advantageous for an individual patient.

The staple line along the tubularized stomach is oversewn in with 3–0 silk suture in a Lembert fashion. See Figure 72.30. The final 2 3–0 silk sutures at the apex of the conduit will subsequently be used to secure the apex of conduit to esophageal stump above the aortic arch.

The gastric conduit is passed through the hiatus, under the aortic arch and secured to the transected esophagus with the final 3–0 silk sutures, making sure to keep the conduit in the correct orientation. See Figure 72.31. This facilitates the gastric conduit being brought up into the neck during the cervical phase of the operation.

Great care is taken to ensure the correct orientation of the conduit, as any twisting or bending may compromise the vascular supply. See Figure 72.32. The neoesophagus is secured to the abdominal and thoracic aspects of the hiatus with 3–0 silk sutures to prevent herniation of abdominal contents.

Closure

The medial component of the diaphragm is closed with a running 2-O Vicryl. Individual interrupted Vicryl sutures are placed to approximate the remainder of diaphragm. See Figure 72.33. The interrupted sutures are tied from

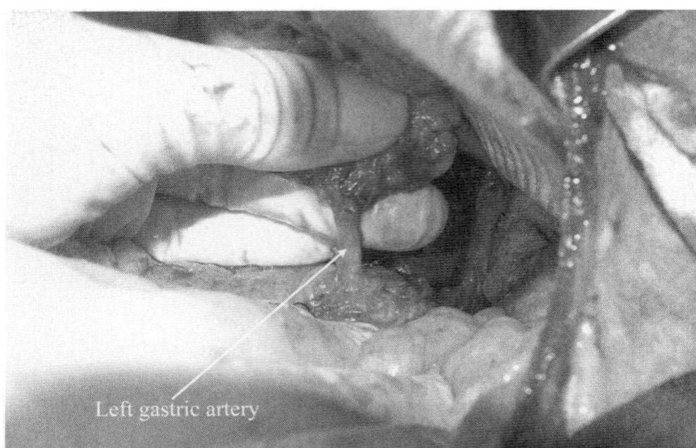

FIGURE 72.21

Left gastric artery.

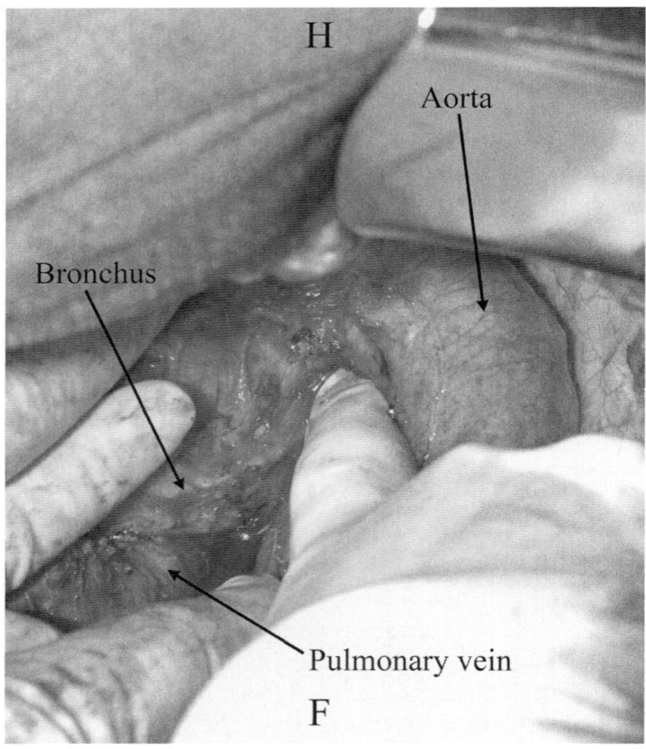

FIGURE 72.22

Dissection underneath the aortic arch.

within the abdomen once the costal margin has been brought together.

The costal margin is closed in an overlapping fashion to ensure stability, making no attempt to bring the costal margin together end to end. See Figure 72.34. This can be done with wire, but #1 Vicryl suture works extremely well. Anterior and posterior #24 chest tubes

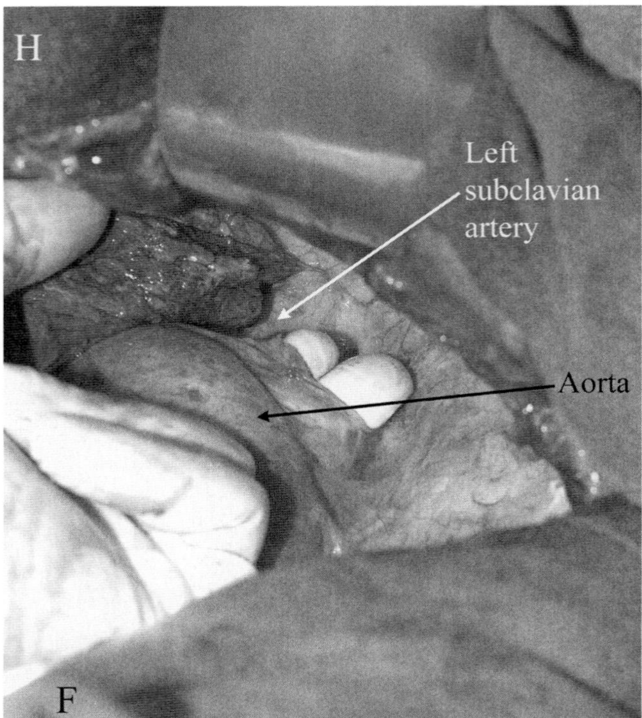

FIGURE 72.23

Surgeon's fingers underneath the aortic arch and through the window opened in the pleura just lateral to the left subclavian artery.

are placed in the left chest. The chest wall is closed with pericostal double strand #1 Vicryl suture. The layers of the chest wall and abdomen are closed in the standard fashion.

Cervical Phase

After completion of standard chest closure, the patient is repositioned supine. The neck is slightly extended. The heating blanket is brought up to cover majority of the torso and lower extremities. See Figure 72.35. A cervical incision is made along the anterior border of the left sternocleidomastoid muscle. See Figure 72.36. The skin, subcutaneous tissue, and platysma are divided.

The sternocleidomastoid and great vessels are retracted laterally as the dissection is carried down to the prevertebral space. See Figure 72.37. Exposure may be facilitated by division of the omohyoid muscle, middle thyroid vein, and the inferior thyroid artery. Typically, however, the esophagus is found to be completely mobilized from prior dissection in the chest. See Figure 72.38. This method of mobilization generally protects the recurrent nerve. The esophagus is encircled and brought up into the neck with the attached gastric conduit.

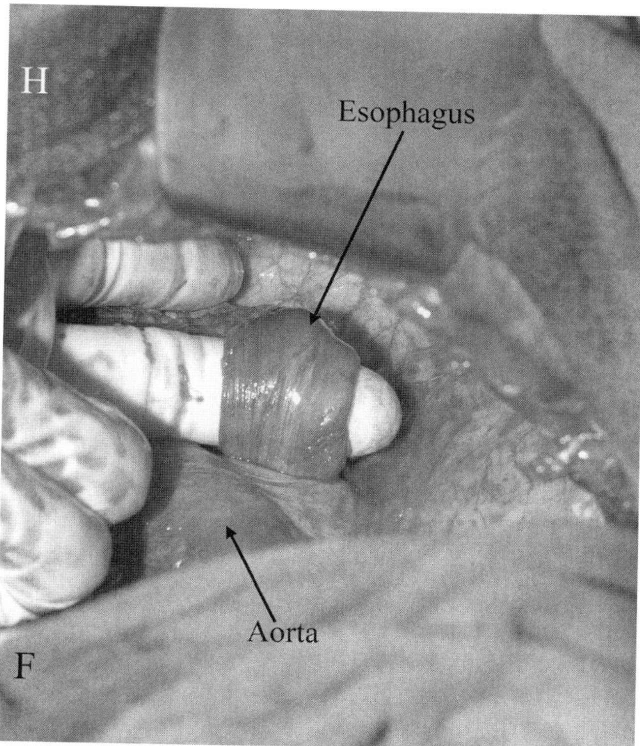

FIGURE 72.24

Mobilizing the esophagus above the aortic arch.

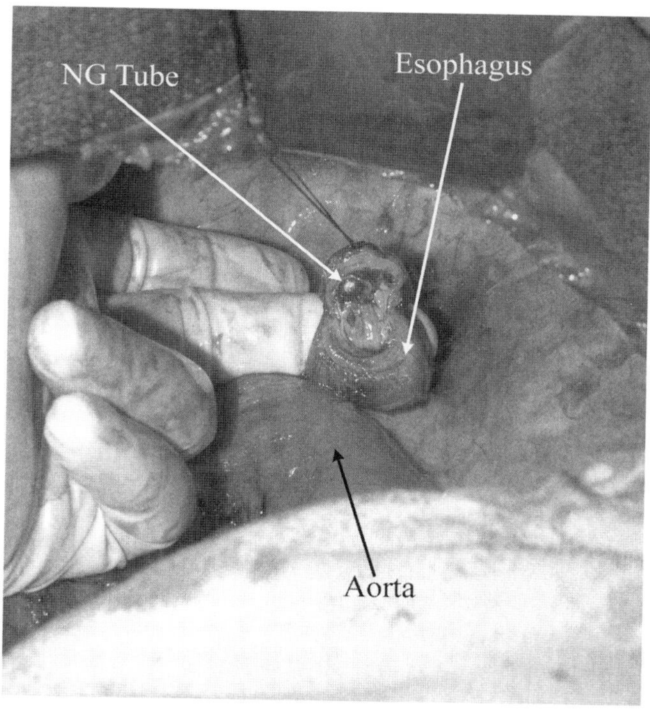

FIGURE 72.25

Partial transection of the esophagus above the aortic arch.

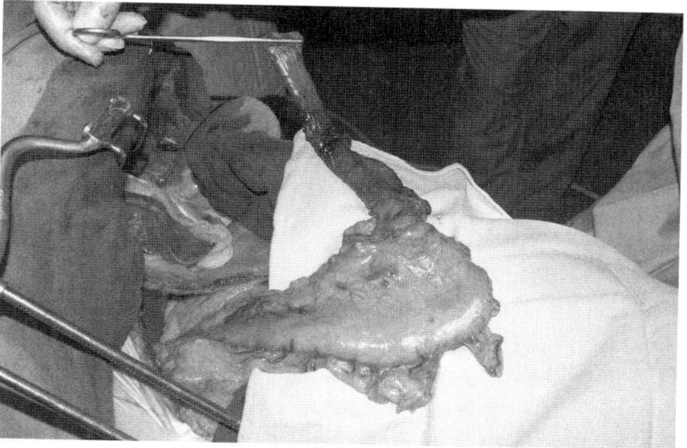

FIGURE 72.26

Esophagus and stomach reduced into the abdominal cavity.

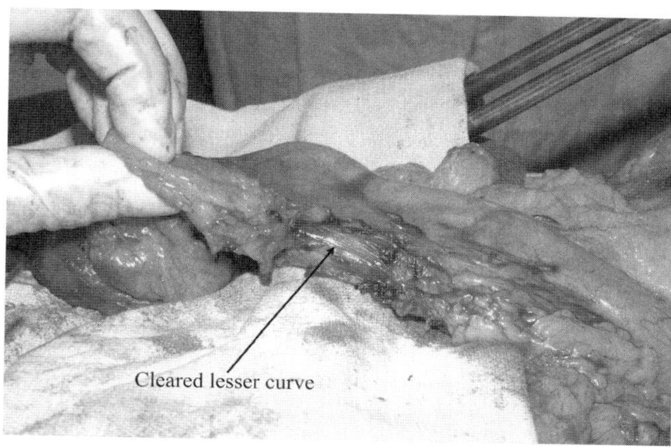

FIGURE 72.27

Preparing the stomach for fashioning the gastric conduit.

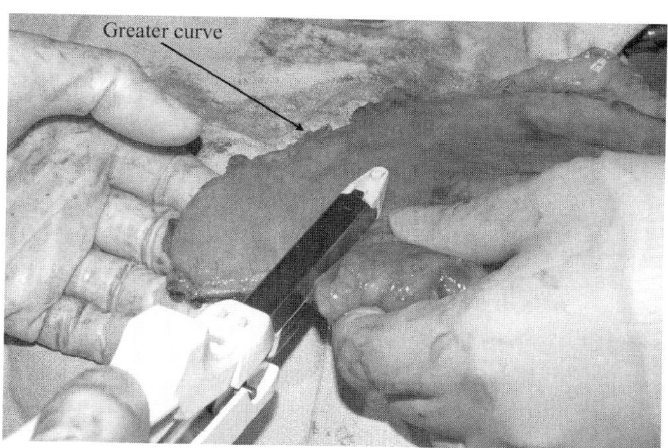

FIGURE 72.28

Constructing the gastric conduit.

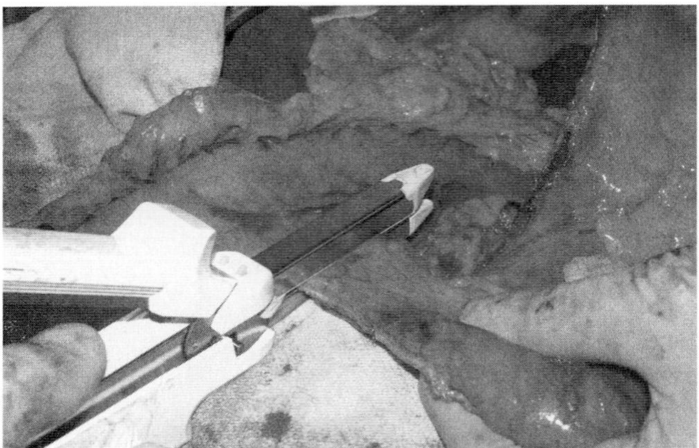

FIGURE 72.29

Completion of gastric resection and separating the specimen.

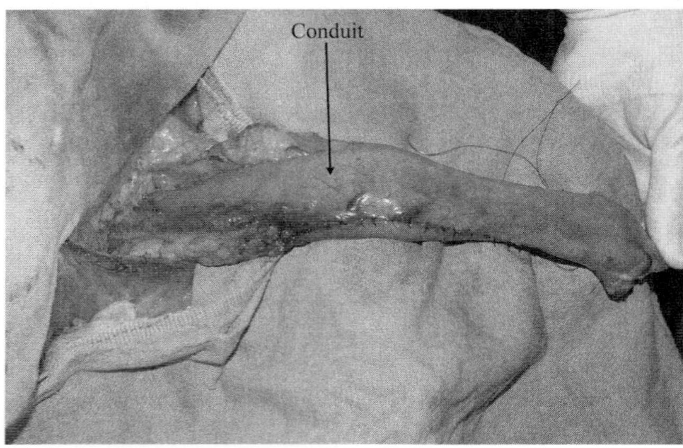

FIGURE 72.30

Completed gastric conduit.

The esophagus and attached stomach are brought up into the incision. See Figure 72.39. A hand-sewn or a longitudinal stapled anastomosis can be performed. The best method of gastroesophageal anastomosis remains debated. Orringer, Marshall, and Iannettoni have suggested that a stapled side-to-side gastroesophageal anastomosis reduces leaks and subsequent stricture (9). We believe the choice should be made by the individual surgeon, who ideally is aware of their personal leak and stenosis rate.

We typically utilize a 2-layer anastomosis, performed with inner layer of interrupted 3-O Vicryl and outer layer of 3-O silk. The nasogastric tube is advanced into the gastric conduit prior to completing the anterior wall of the anastomosis. An additional 2 to 4 cm of proximal esophagus is resected at the time of the anastomosis. See Figure 72.40. The anastomosis is returned

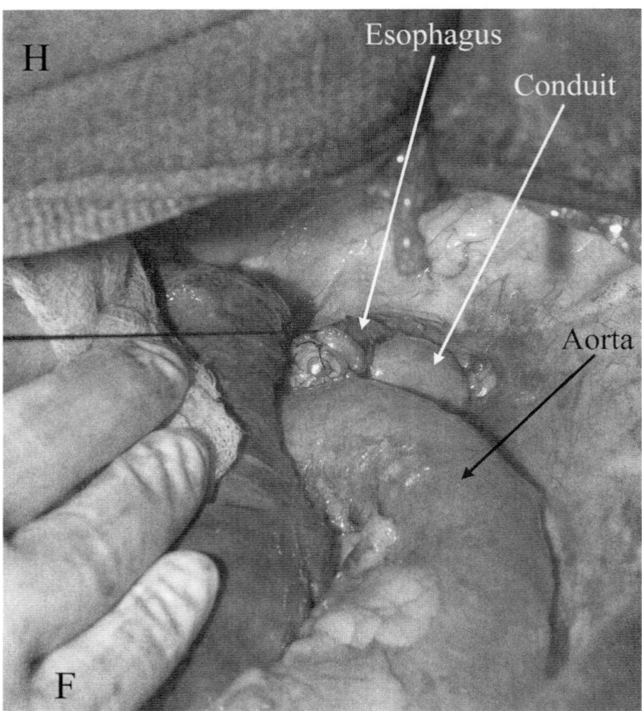

FIGURE 72.31

Gastric conduit is positioned in the bed of the esophagus and sutured to the proximal esophageal stump.

to the neck and will lie approximately 2 to 3 cm above thoracic inlet. See Figure 72.41.

A drain is passed posterior to the anterior head of the sternocleidomastoid to lie adjacent to the esophagus and cephalad to the anastomosis. See Figure 72.42. The wound is irrigated and aspirated. The fascia is closed with 3–0 Vicryl.

Intrathoracic Anastomosis

A cervical anastomosis will not be possible or desirable in all cases. The conduit may not be sufficient in length for a tension-free cervical anastomosis due to gastric involvement, prior surgery, or other factors. As noted above, an intrathoracic anastomosis can be achieved at any level between the inferior pulmonary ligament and the aortic arch. See Figures 72.43–72.46.

Esophageal dissection is carried just proximal to level of intended resection as seen in Figure 72.43. The anastomosis can be achieved in a hand-sewn or stapled fashion. A circular stapler can be utilized to construct an end-to-end anastomosis. A purse-string stapling device is placed to secure the anvil of the circular stapler in the proximal esophageal remnant as seen in Figure 72.44.

The esophagus is divided below the aortic arch. The anvil of the stapler is introduced into the esophagus and secured with the purse-string, as seen in Figure 72.45. The circular stapler is introduced into the conduit by way of a gastrotomy or, alternatively, through the site of a pyloroplasty. The center rod of the stapler is brought out of the fundus several centimeters from the staple line of the conduit.

The stapler is fired and the gastroesophageal anastomosis is completed as seen in Figure 72.46. The rings of esophagus and conduit resected around the center rod, "doughnuts" are removed from the staple cartridge and examined for completeness of anastomosis. The gastrotomy is closed. The abdomen and chest are closed in the standard fashion noted above.

ADDITIONAL POINTS

If the stomach is felt to be inappropriate for utilization as a replacement conduit, the abdominal component of the incision can be extended inferiorly along the abdominal midline to facilitate mobilizing the left or transverse colon or a Roux-en-Y segment of jejunum.

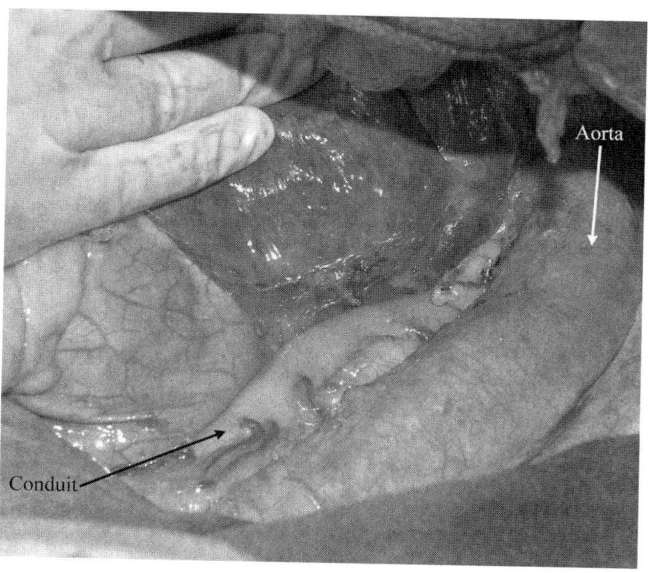

FIGURE 72.32

Gastric conduit in position in the posterior mediastinum.

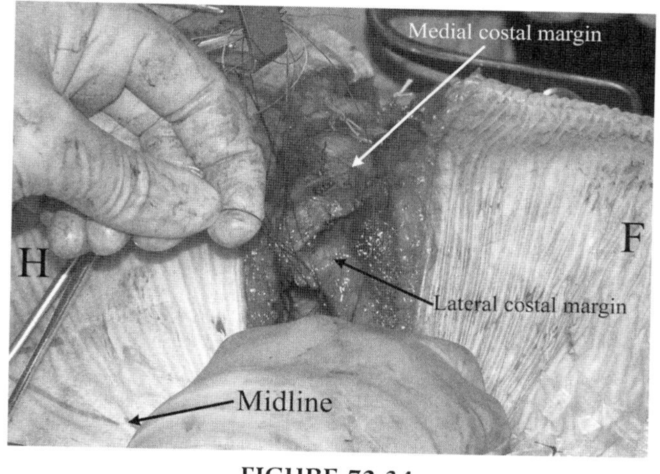

FIGURE 72.34

Final diaphragmatic sutures tied from the abdominal side once the costal margin is reapproximated.

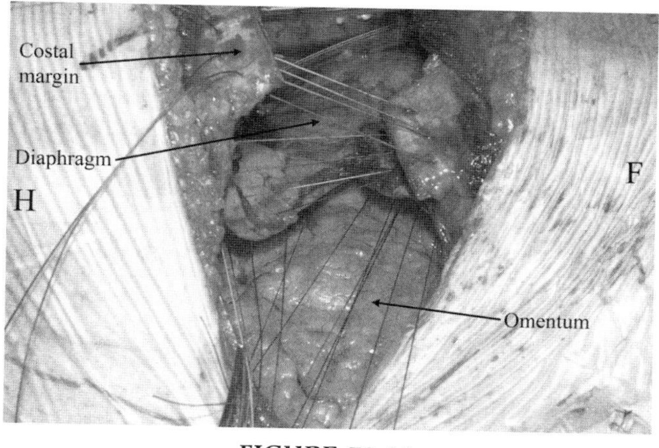

FIGURE 72.33

Closure of the diaphragm and costal margin.

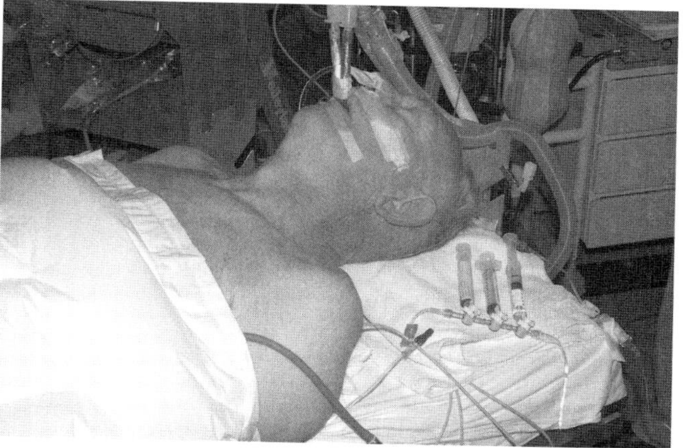

FIGURE 72.35

Patient is repositioned for cervical anastomosis.

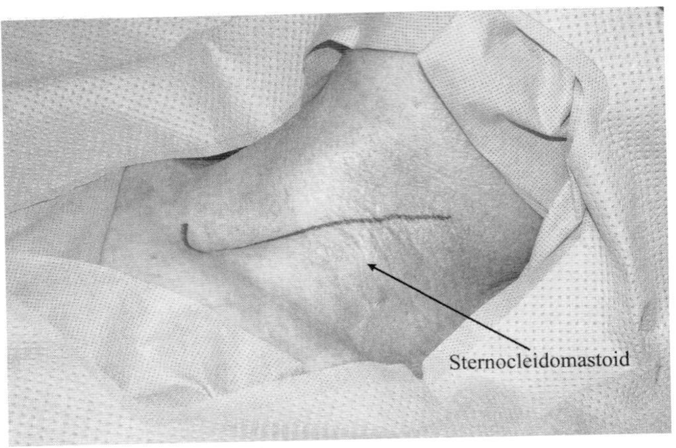

FIGURE 72.36

A fairly limited incision is required to gain access to cervical esophagus.

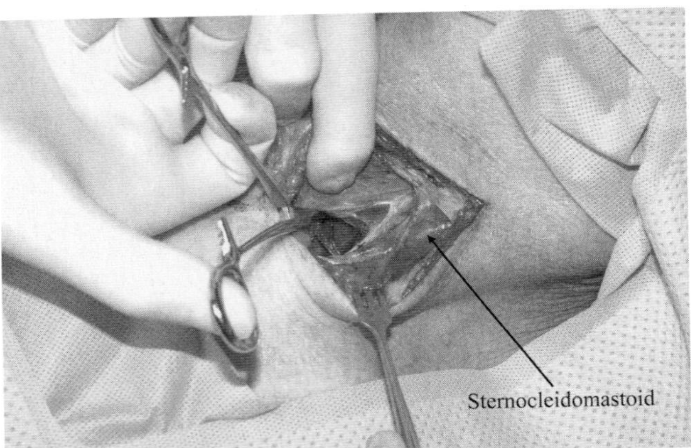

FIGURE 72.37

Access to the cervical esophagus.

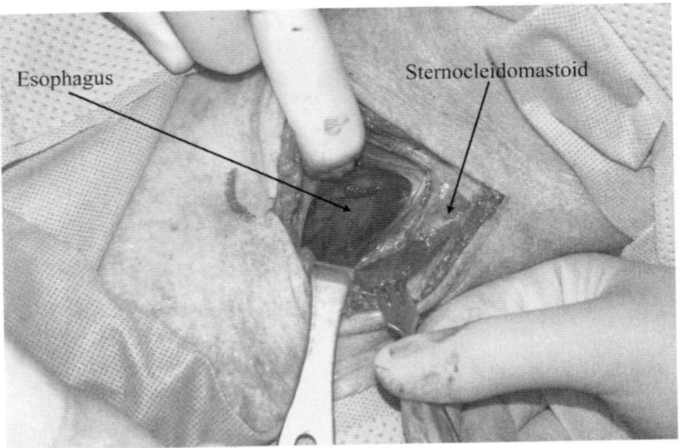

FIGURE 72.38

Dissection carries deep into the neck to the prevertebral space.

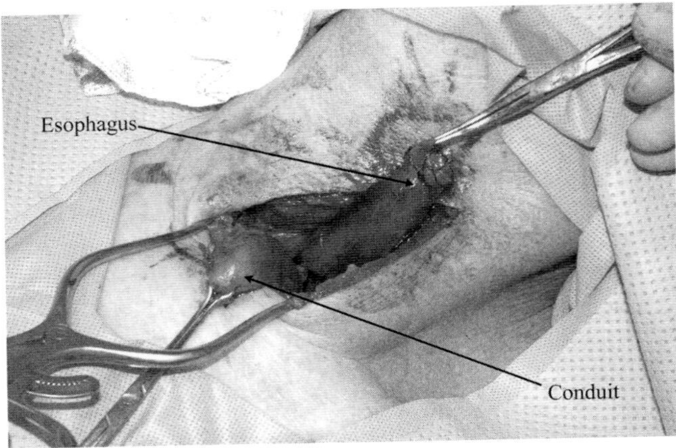

FIGURE 72.39

Initiating cervical anastomosis.

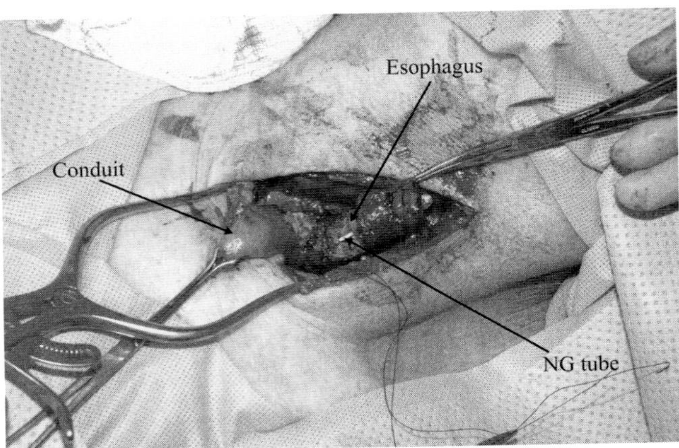

FIGURE 72.40

Cervical hand-sewn anastomosis.

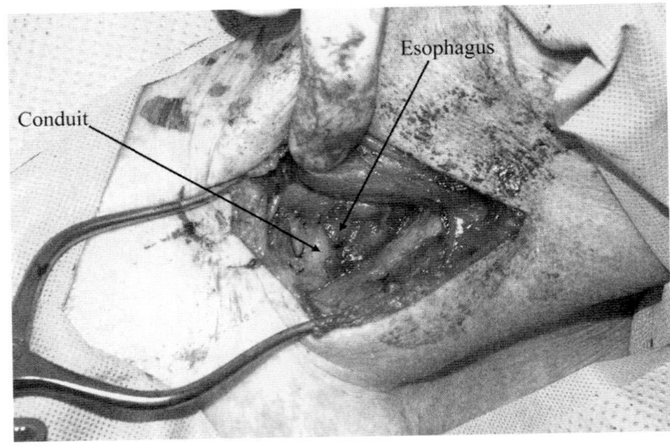

FIGURE 72.41

Completion of the cervical anastomosis.

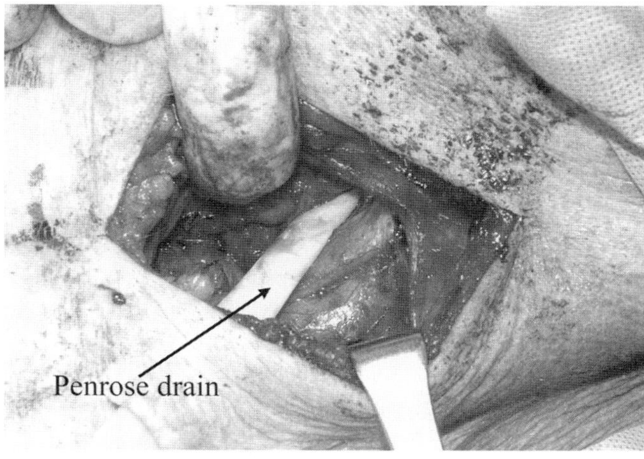

FIGURE 72.42

Placement of a cervical drain.

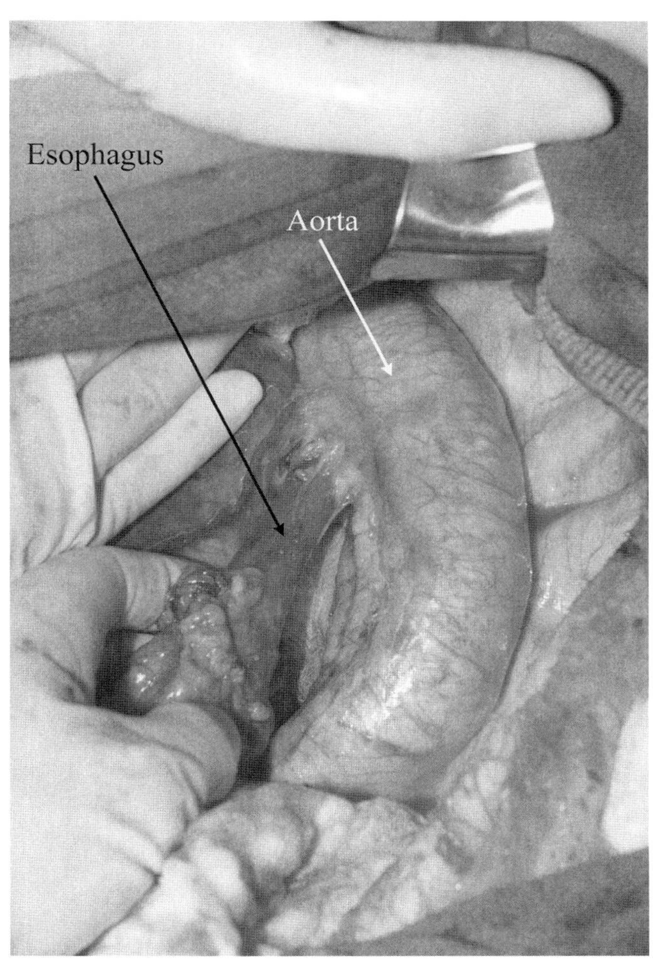

FIGURE 72.43

Esophagus prepared for transaction below aortic arch.

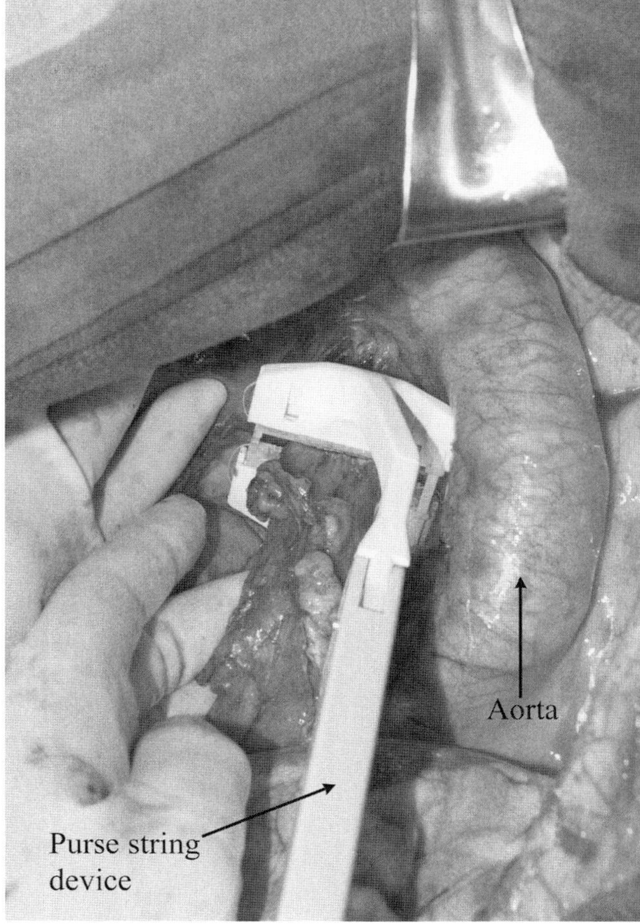

FIGURE 72.44

A purse string is placed in the esophagus below aortic arch.

As demonstrated in the technical description, the anastomosis can be placed below the aortic arch, as seen in Figure 72.46, or in the neck, as seen in Figure 72.41. Other surgeons have utilized an upper thoracic anastomosis by bringing the esophagus out through the supra-aortic window (see Figure 72.25) and placing the anastomosis over the aortic arch.

POST-OP CARE

The perioperative standardized clinical pathway can be seen in Figure 72.1. Key points in the immediate post-operative period are outlined in Table 72.2. In part, this process is facilitated by clear definition of steps and goals. The most important aspect is involving the entire care team, including all clinicians, supportive staff, the patient, and their families.

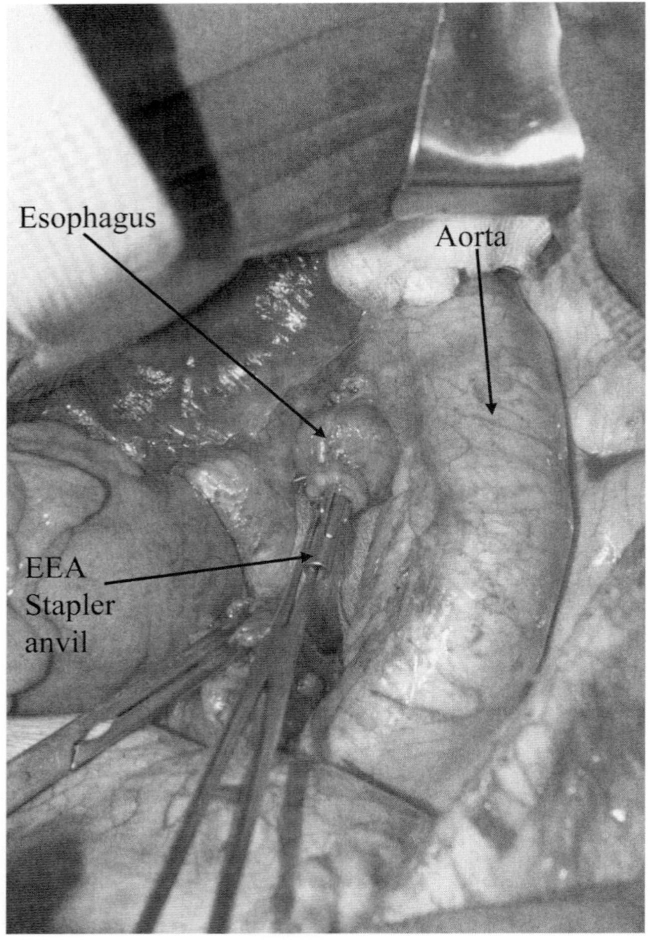

FIGURE 72.45

Anvil of circular stapler secured in the esophagus.

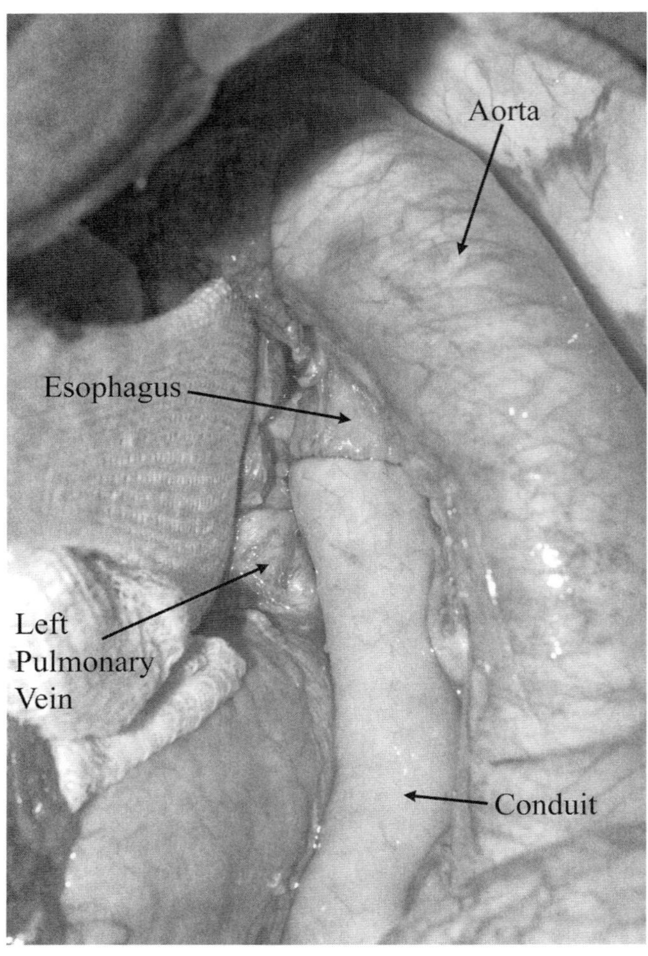

FIGURE 72.46

Completed intrathoracic gastroesophageal anastomosis.

OUTCOMES ASSOCIATED WITH LTA ESOPHAGECTOMY

We support the concept of a diversified approach to esophageal resection. However, the LTA is particularly well suited for management of distal esophageal and esophagogastric junction tumors, which currently comprise the most common presentation in the Western world.

Previous results have highlighted that the LTA esophagectomy is the most common operative approach used for esophageal cancer at our institution (8,10–12). An assessment of eating ability and dietary status between 1991 and 1998 (90% patients undergoing LTA) demonstrated that dietary intake was normal or only minimally limited in 85% of patients at a mean follow-up of 36 months (12). Similarly, a specific examination of long-term quality of life in patients undergoing esophageal resection for high-grade dysplasia or invasive cancer (60% of patients undergoing LTA) demonstrated that age- and sex-matched postoperative SF-36 scores were equal to the general population at a mean follow-up of 5 years (11).

A specific examination of benchmarks associated with outcomes between 1996 and 2002 in pancreaticoduodenectomy and esophageal resection (60% of patients undergoing LTA) showed significant advantages in multiple parameters compared to the medical literature published during the same period (10). Our results compared favorably with respect to several benchmarks including mortality 0% vs. 5.5%, operative blood loss 204 vs. 964 cc, anastomotic leak rate of 2.9% vs. 9.1% and hospital length of stay 11.1 vs. 16.6 days.

A major review of 340 consecutive patients (8) undergoing esophagectomy for cancer by a single surgeon at our institution between 1991 and 2006 (63% of

TABLE 72.2
Key Points in the Immediate Postoperative Period

- Immediate extubation in the operating room
- Transfer to intensive care unit with discharge to the ward 12 to 18 hours post-op
- Patient controlled epidural analgesia. Pain team rounds twice a day
- Patient mobilization out of bed morning pod #1 prior to transfer out of ICU
- Chest tube removed postoperative day 1 to 3
- Jejunostomy tube feeds begin day 3
- UGI study to assess anastomosis and gastric emptying postoperative day 4 to 5
- NG tube removed day 4 to 5
- Limited oral clear fluids begun day 5 to 6
- Shorten/remove the cervical Penrose day 6 to 7
- Dietary consultation day 5 to 6
- Hospital discharge day 7 to 8

patients undergoing LTA) has demonstrated that mortality levels can be extremely low in esophageal resection, contrary to national database reports in the literature (13). In our review, the mortality rate was 0.3% for the entire series. Just as importantly, significant improvements in the survival were demonstrated in the patients operated on between 1998 and 2004. Kaplan-Meyer 5-year survival of stage I, II, and III patients was 92.4%, 57.1%, and 34.5%, respectively. We credit these results to an organized team approach to management, guided by an evolving standardized clinical pathway. See Table 72.1. Although the majority of these patients had an LTA, we believe these results highlight the importance of flexibility in the management of esophageal cancer and demonstrate the safety and efficacy of a diversified approach to esophageal resection.

References

1. Ries LAG, Melbert D, Krapcho M, et al. (eds). *SEER Cancer Statistics Review, 1975–2004*. Bethesda, MD: National Cancer Institute. http://seer.cancer.gov/csr/1975_2004/, based on November 2006 SEER data submission, posted to the SEER website, 2007.
2. Jemal A, Siegel R, Ward E, et al. Cancer statistics, 2007. *CA Cancer J Clin*. 2007;57:43–66.
3. Forshaw MJ, Gossage JA, Ockrim J, et al. Left thoracoabdominal esophagogastrectomy: still a valid operation for carcinoma of the distal esophagus and esophagogastric junction. *Dis Esophagus*. 2006;19:340–345
4. Naef AP. The mid-century revolution in thoracic and cardiovascular surgery: part 3. *Interact Cardiovasc Thorac Surg*. 2004;3:3–10.
5. Lee RB, Miller JI. Esophagectomy for cancer. *Surg Clin North Am*. 1997;77(5):1169–1196.
6. Low DE. Evolution in perioperative management of patients undergoing oesophagectomy. *Br J Surg*. 2007;94:655–656.
7. Cerfolio RJ, Bryant AS, Bass CS, et al. Fast tracking after Ivor Lewis esophagogastrectomy. *Chest*. 2004;126:1187–1194.
8. Low DE, Kunz S, Schembre D, et al. Esophagectomy—It's not just about mortality anymore: standardized perioperative clinical pathways improve outcomes in patients with esophageal cancer. *J Gastrointest Surg*. 2007;11:1395–1402.
9. Orringer MB, Marshall B, Iannettoni MD. Eliminating the cervical esophagogastric anastomotic leak with a side-to-side stapled anastomosis. *J Thorac Cardiovasc Surg*. 2000;119:277–288.
10. Traverso LW, Shinchi H, Low DE. Useful benchmarks to evaluate outcomes after esophagectomy and pancreaticoduodenectomy. *Am J Surg*. 2004;187:604–608.
11. Moraca RJ, Low DE. Outcomes and health-related quality of life after esophagectomy for high-grade dysplasia and intramucosal cancer. *Arch Surg*. 2006;141:545–549.
12. Ludwig DJ, Thirlby RC, Low DE. A prospective evaluation of dietary status and symptoms after near-total esophagectomy without gastric emptying procedure. *Am J Surg*. 2001;181:454–458.
13. Birkmeyer JD, Siewers AE, Finlayson EV, et al. Hospital volume and surgical mortality in the United States. *N Engl J Med*. 2002;346:1128–1137.

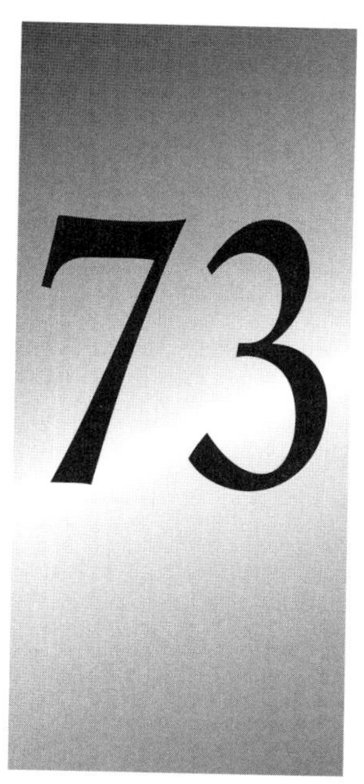

Surgery Techniques: Resection of Cancer Involving the Cervicothoracic Esophagus

Thomas K. Varghese, Jr.
Douglas E. Wood

Esophageal cancer is a deadly disease, accounting for 15,560 new cases in 2007 and 13,940 deaths (1). Less than 10% of all primary esophageal tumors involve the cervical esophagus, and they are invariably squamous cell carcinomas (2). These tumors usually present at an advanced stage and thus pose several challenges to the managing physician. A multidisciplinary team approach is ideal, with surgeons, radiation therapists, and medical oncologists working together to formulate a treatment plan. When a primary surgical-based intervention is planned, careful assessment of the extent of tumor is critical, as local invasion can significantly influence the planned resection. The surgeon must consider the reconstructive challenges of the surgical defect that impacts swallowing, speech, and respiration. If chemoradiation is used as initial modalities of treatment, patients should be closely followed to assess whether surgical salvage of treatment failures is feasible.

Surgical resection is a controversial therapy for cancers of the cervical esophagus. As these tumors are relatively uncommon, few surgeons have extensive experience with their management. Disappointing postoperative functional results, low rates of long-term survival, and improvements in locoregional therapy, including both radiotherapy and chemoradiotherapy, have generated considerable discussion regarding appropriate selection of treatment. However, resection remains a viable option in the management of patients with potentially curable cervical esophageal cancer (3). Malignant tumors of the larynx, hypopharynx, trachea, or thyroid can secondarily involve the cervical esophagus, and in these patients removal of the esophagus is only 1 component of the surgical intervention, as laryngectomy and resection of the proximal trachea may be required. Outcomes in these patients are not as good as those in whom only an esophagectomy and esophageal substitution are needed. However, with a meticulous systematic approach, success in terms of palliation and sometimes cure can be achieved.

ANATOMY

The cervical portion of the esophagus is approximately 5 cm long and descends between the vertebral column and trachea from the level of the sixth cervical vertebra to the level of the thoracic inlet (bounded by the suprasternal notch anteriorly and the interspace between the first and second thoracic vertebrae posteriorly). Important anatomical relations include the following (Figure 73.1):

- Anterior—posterior tracheal membrane.
- Posterior—prevertebral fascia.
- Recurrent laryngeal nerves lie in the right and left grooves between the trachea and esophagus.

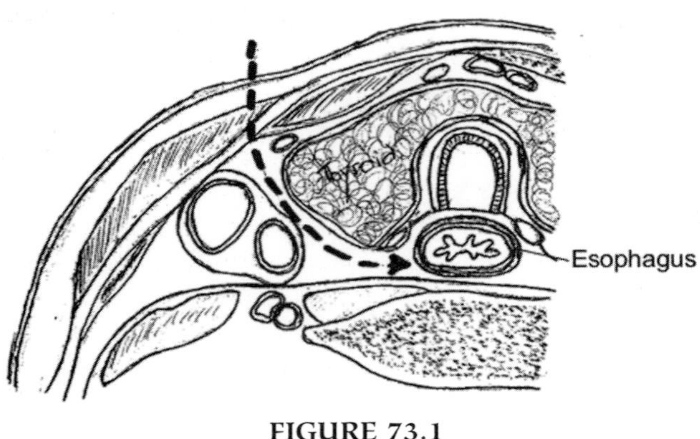

FIGURE 73.1

Horizontal section at the level of the sixth cervical vertebra showing the surgical approach to the cervical esophagus (dotted arrow).

- Laterally, the esophagus is bounded on each side by the carotid sheaths and the respective lobes of the thyroid gland.

The cricopharyngeus muscle represents the transition between the hypopharynx and cervical esophagus. The cervical esophagus is a muscular tube that has a squamous epithelial layer, a submucosa rich in lymphatics, a muscular layer, and an adventitial layer. The muscular layer is divided into an inner circular and outer longitudinal layer. The lymphatics of the cervical esophagus are almost coincident with the hypopharyngeal lymphatics and include drainage to the recurrent laryngeal, paratracheal, and jugular chain nodes. There is also some drainage of the cervical esophagus to the superior mediastinal lymph nodes. The vascular supply is derived from the inferior thyroid arteries with some contribution from the high thoracic vasculature. Finally, innervation to the cervical esophagus is provided by sympathetics, parasympathetics, and cranial nerves IX, X, and XI (the spinal accessory nerve).

CLINICAL PRESENTATION AND STAGING

Patients with cervical esophageal tumors usually present at an advanced stage and often have dysphagia. The overall appearance of these patients will likely reveal a malnourished individual. Respiratory symptoms may occur either from airway involvement or aspiration. Hoarseness can occur if the recurrent laryngeal nerve is involved. As the tumor increases in size, progressive dysphagia, severe dehydration, weight loss, chronic aspiration, and upper airway obstruction result.

Current staging of esophageal cancer is based on the tumor/node/metastasis classification developed by American Joint Committee on Cancer. Clearly, patient outcomes are worse with advanced stage of disease. Accurate staging depends on a thorough physical examination coupled with appropriate imaging studies. The extent of the tumor and lymph node involvement must be defined by clinical exam, operative endoscopy (fiberoptic laryngoscopy, bronchoscopy, and esophagoscopy), and imaging. A complete examination of the head and neck should be performed with a focus on the mucosa of the upper aerodigestive tract to evaluate the extent of the primary tumor and to assess for second primaries. Physical examination may reveal a neck mass, enlarged lymph nodes, or signs of metastatic disease. Speech and swallowing evaluation should also be performed.

In the treatment of cervical esophageal malignancies, the role of imaging involves the pretreatment evaluation of the extent of primary tumor and possible metastases, as well as the evaluation of the patient after treatment. The barium swallow (esophagram) can help in the diagnosis of malignancies in this region. It can also be used to image the distal extent of the disease in those patients where an endoscope cannot be passed distally. The primary imaging modality for pretreatment evaluation of the cervical esophagus is cross-sectional imaging with computed tomography (CT) of the neck, chest, and abdomen. In multiple studies examining the impact of cross-sectional imaging on the staging of hypopharyngeal or esophageal cancer, the clinical tumor stage was upstaged in up to 90% of patients (4). Accuracy of tumor staging, as compared to pathologic findings, is 58% for clinical examination and 80% for CT. Positron-emission tomography improves the ability to detect metastatic disease.

At operation, exploration is performed to determine whether there is involvement of the larynx or trachea. If such involvement is identified, laryngectomy and tracheal resection are necessary for a curative resection. Bilateral modified neck dissection is performed to remove all the regional lymph nodes. If a 5-cm margin of normal esophagus cannot be removed distal to the inferior extent of gross tumor, a total esophagectomy is performed. Some advocate total esophagectomy in all cases to accomplish a more complete excision and lymph node dissection. In selected patients, a segmental esophagectomy with or without laryngectomy can be performed, and reconstruction is achieved by means of a free jejunal graft with microvascular anastomosis.

SURGICAL CONSIDERATIONS

Preoperative Assessment

There are many factors to consider when anticipating surgical intervention (Table 73.1). The first decision entails appropriate patient selection. Staging studies are reviewed, and the medical fitness of the patient to undergo surgery is assessed. As respiratory complications are the most common after surgery, pulmonary function tests are obtained, and pulmonary physiotherapy measures are instituted. These include cessation of smoking, ambulation, and use of an incentive spirometer. The next decision centers on the extent of esophageal resection and approach. Location of the tumor, involvement of adjacent lymph nodes, and invasion of the adjacent trachea are influencing factors. The extent of resection is usually based on the preoperative staging. The reconstruction technique is then considered. Although there has been significant debate about the best method to replace the esophagus, in most situations the stomach remains the conduit of choice, whereas a colon or small bowel interposition is favored in instances where the stomach is inadequate or absent.

Operative Techniques

Communication between the surgeon and the anesthesiologist is needed to properly secure the airway. A tracheostomy or placement of an endotracheal tube under direct endoscopic vision may be needed in certain cases. The patient is positioned supine, with the arms tucked at the sides, and neck gently extended with a shoulder roll. The head is turned to the patient's right if a left lateral neck incision is planned or kept neutral for a collar incision. Absence of airway involvement can be determined by flexible bronchoscopy. Flexible esophagoscopy helps to confirm location of the tumor, extent of the tumor, as well as determination of whether the larynx can be preserved. In general, tumor involvement within 2 to 3 cm of the cricopharyngeus necessitates resection of the larynx. After removal of the flexible esophagoscope, a nasogastric tube is then carefully placed.

TABLE 73.1
Factors to Consider When Anticipating Surgical Intervention

1. Preoperative optimization
   a. Cessation of smoking
   b. Nutritional status assessment
   c. Cardiorespiratory assessment
   d. Epidural placement
2. Operative factors
   a. Airway status
   b. Extent of esophageal resection
   c. Decision whether to preserve the larynx
   d. Lymphadenectomy
   e. Exposure of the superior mediastinum
   f. Need for cervical exenteration
   g. Reconstruction method (gastric tube, jejunal free flap, colon interposition)
   h. Feeding tube
3. Postoperative management
   a. Care of airway
      i. Humidification of inspired air
      ii. Minimal trauma to the trachea
   b. Pulmonary physiotherapy measures
   c. Enteral feeding
   d. Nasogastric decompression
   e. Monitoring for hypoparathyroidism
   f. Postoperative contrast study

Resection

The cricoid cartilage is the anatomic landmark for the cricopharyngeus muscle and the origin of the cervical esophagus. The length between the cricoid cartilage and the upper sternal notch represents the approximate length of the cervical esophagus that is accessible through a cervical incision. Because of its natural deviation slightly to the left, the cervical esophagus is often approached through an oblique 5- to 6-cm incision parallel to the anterior border of the left sternocleidomastoid muscle (Figure 73.2). The left cervical incision is used in those tumors confined to the esophagus. The superior extent of the incision is just above the level of the cricoid cartilage. The platysma is divided, followed by identification and division of the omohyoid muscle. Ligation of the middle thyroid vein and inferior thyroid artery is often needed. The carotid sheath and its contents are retracted laterally, while the trachea and thyroid gland are retracted medially. Metal retractors are generally not used to retract in the tracheoesophageal groove to avoid injury to the recurrent laryngeal nerve. The dissection is continued to the prevertebral fascia posteriorly in a plane medial to the carotid sheath. The prevertebral space behind the esophagus is developed by blunt finger dissection, taking care to constantly keep the finger against the esophagus. Blunt finger dissection along the prevertebral fascia into the superior mediastinum mobilizes the high retrosternal esophagus away from the spine. The tracheoesophageal groove is located, and the plane between the cervical esophagus and trachea is developed. Exposure is done, taking care to avoid injury to the recurrent laryngeal nerve. A Penrose drain is used to encircle the esophagus. Superior retraction is done while bluntly dissecting the cervical esophagus from the superior mediastinum, taking care to keep the fingers against the esophagus. In such a manner, a 10-cm length of the esophagus can be mobilized down to the level of the carina.

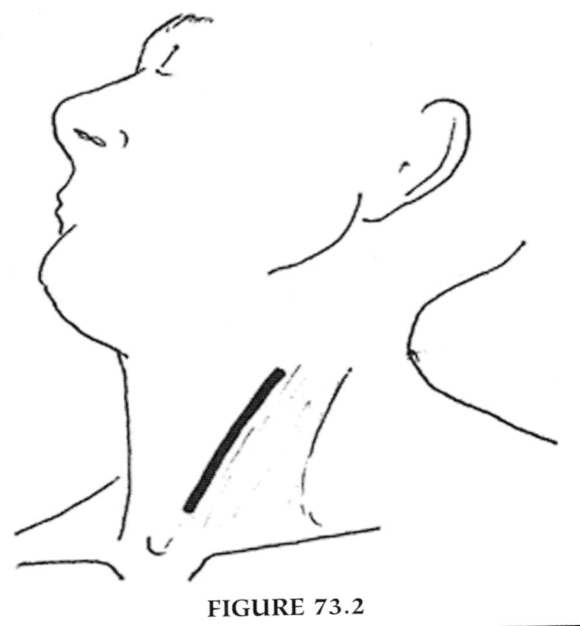

FIGURE 73.2

Left cervical incision for isolated cervical esophageal lesions.

However, tumors confined only to the cervical esophagus are rare. With more extensive tumors, the neck is explored initially through a collar incision (Figure 73.3). Esophageal mobilization is similar to that described previously, although the collar incision facilitates mobilization of more complex tumors by allowing the surgeon to approach the esophagus from both the right and the left. A clear proximal margin is often more difficult to attain than the distal. Care is taken to avoid injury to the adjacent structures, specifically the recurrent laryngeal nerves, larynx, and posterior tracheal membrane. In those patients with short necks or where further exposure of the low cervical or high thoracic esophagus is needed, an upper sternal split is used (5) (Figure 73.4). Although the cervicothoracic esophagus is encircled with a Penrose drain, the trachea is not encircled and instead is retracted with fingers along its anterolateral aspect, taking care not to injure the recurrent laryngeal nerves.

If the tumor extends to or below the thoracic inlet, the entire thoracic esophagus is resected using a transhiatal approach. Synchronous carcinomas in the esophagus have been cited in a number of reports to be as high as 6% to 15% (6–8). This has led many to advocate total esophagectomy in all patients. A transhiatal esophagectomy facilitates reconstruction with a gastric pull-up, avoids an intrathoracic anastomosis, and allows for removal of all esophageal squamous mucosa that may be at risk for recurrence or skip lesions.

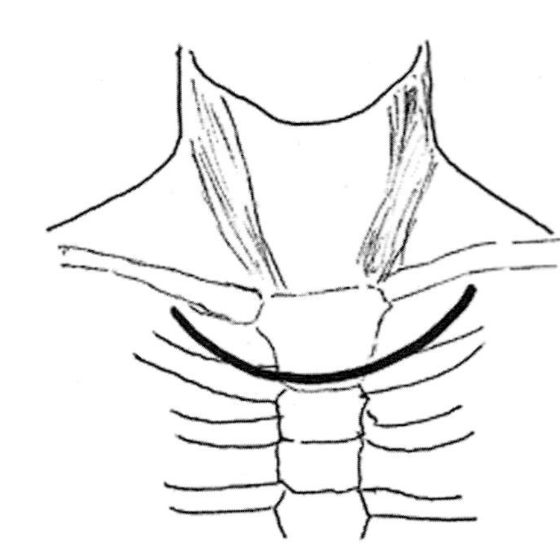

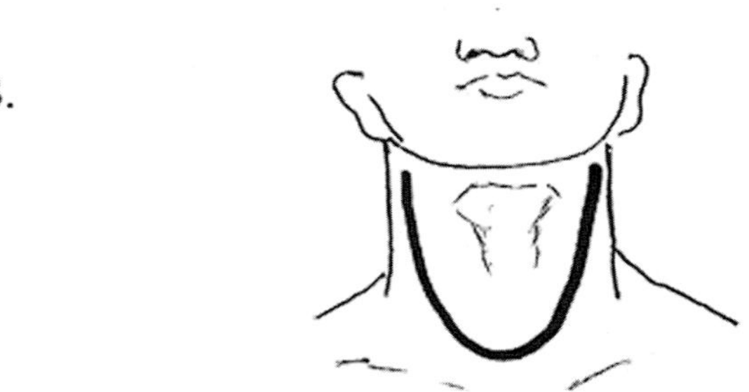

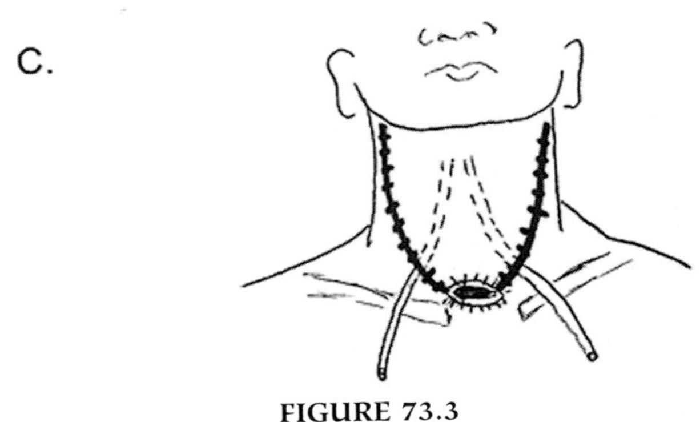

FIGURE 73.3

(A) Curved anterior thoracic incision with elevation of skin flaps as an alternative to the left cervical incision. (B) Low collar neck incision can be extended to form an apron incision with subsequent reflection of skin and subcutaneous flaps, including the superficial layer of the cervical fascia and the platysma. (C) Wound closure with bilateral drains and permanent tracheostomy brought out through the suprasternal notch. In those patients requiring extensive tracheal resection, a mediastinal tracheostomy is often needed.

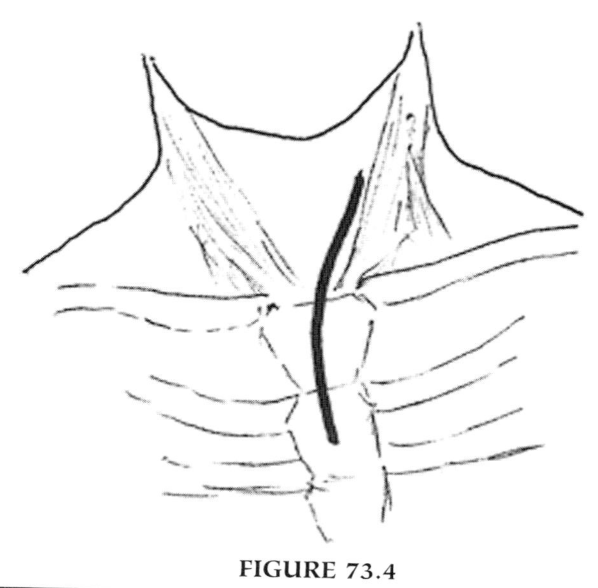

FIGURE 73.4

Extension of the left cervical incision onto the upper sternum.

Tumor involvement within 2 to 3 cm of the cricopharyngeus necessitates resection of the larynx. In these cases, the thyrohyoid membrane is entered just above the thyroid cartilage, the pharyngeal and pharyngeal mucosa is divided by carrying the incision laterally and posteriorly, and the hyoid bone is left behind. The epiglottis is grasped, retracted downward, and amputated. While achieving sufficient proximal margin, care is taken to ensure preservation of 1 or both thyroid lobes and its adjacent parathyroid glands. Hypoparathyroidism is one of the most significant morbidities associated with total laryngopharyngoesophagectomy with gastric transposition (9). Autotransplantation of the parathyroids may be required in those patients with contiguous involvement necessitating total thyroidectomy.

Cervical esophageal tumors involving the cervical trachea and secondary malignancies invading the upper aerodigestive system add complexity to the surgical resection. In these patients, cervical exenteration is needed. Cervical exenteration removes the larynx, a portion of the trachea, and the lower pharynx (10). Resecting a portion of the retrosternal trachea to achieve an adequate distal tracheal margin can make it difficult to elevate the remaining trachea out of the mediastinum for creation of the standard tracheostomy in the suprasternal notch. An anterior mediastinal tracheostomy is constructed in these patients (11). Removal of a plate of sternum, portions of the clavicles (at least 4 cm from its medial ends), and medial portions of the first and second ribs aids in the exposure. Bipedicled skin flaps allow the anterior chest wall soft tissue to reach the shortened trachea for a mediastinal tracheostomy, allowing a successful stoma with as little as 4 cm of trachea proximal to the carina. This usually requires division of the innominate artery and transposition of a muscle or omental flap to avoid the potential devastating consequence of a postoperative trachea-innominate artery fistula.

The control of regional metastasis is a core component of the management of cervical esophageal tumors. The regional lymph nodes must be assessed. Most squamous cell carcinomas requiring laryngopharyngoesophagectomy warrant bilateral neck dissections, as there may be up to 75% ipsilateral and 25% bilateral cervical nodal metastasis. Enlarged nodes mandate radical or modified radical neck dissections. En bloc resection of all tissues between the carotids, superior to the innominate artery and superficial to the prevertebral fascia, is performed.

Reconstruction

The extent of esophageal resection influences the choice for esophageal replacement. In all patients, feeding jejunostomy tubes should be placed. Most surgeons think that the gastric conduit is the best choice after total esophagectomy in terms of functional outcome. Sufficient length to the oropharynx is usually achieved (Figure 73.5). Advantages of the gastric pull-up after resection include a 1-stage procedure with 1 anastomosis and removal of the entire esophagus. Its disadvantage includes the morbidity of a combined abdominal and cervical dissection and frequent gastric reflux. In most series, hospital mortality had ranged from 8.6% to 13%, with anastomotic leak rates of 17% to 26% (6–8,12). The pharyngogastric anastomosis is performed with a single layer of interrupted 3–0 polyglycolic acid suture. The anastomosis may be marked with hemoclips for later radiographic localization and covered either with adjacent pharyngeal muscle or with omental fat attached to the high gastric fundus. A pyloromyotomy is performed as a drainage procedure. A 10-mm Jackson-Pratt drain is placed beside the anastomosis and brought out through a supraclavicular stab wound.

Reconstruction with colon is done when the stomach is not available as a conduit. There are some who advocate for the use of colon interposition to avoid disabling gastric reflux. The left colon is preferred because of sufficient length, a more reliable blood supply, similar diameter to the esophagus, and better functional results than the right. Results of large series comparing the use of stomach versus colon for esophageal replacement in a nonrandomized fashion have shown no significant difference in functional outcome (13). Large series, however, have shown a high morbidity and mortality rate when compared to gastric pull-up or free

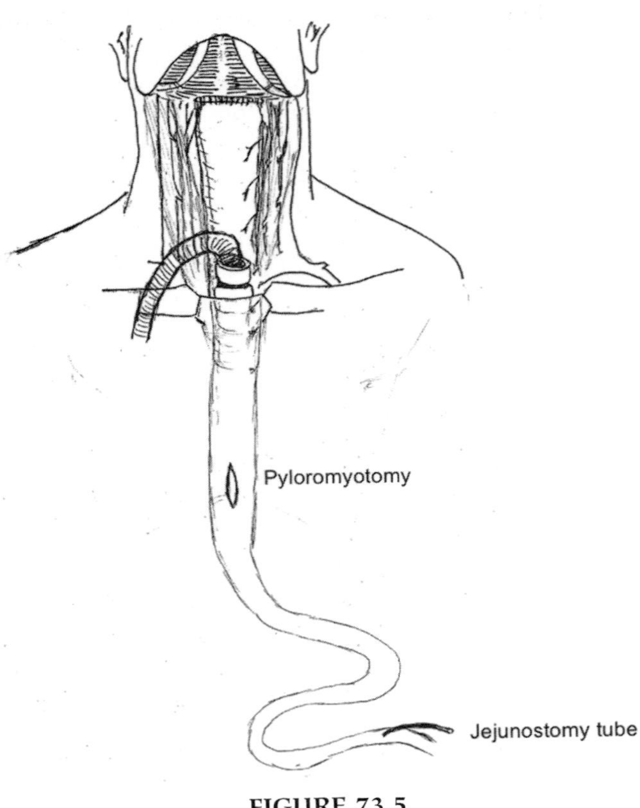

FIGURE 73.5

Gastric transposition after pharyngolaryngoesophagectomy. The advantage of the gastric pull-up is the single anastomosis in the neck. Pyloromyotomy is performed as a drainage procedure, while feeding jejunostomy tube assists in postoperative nutritional support.

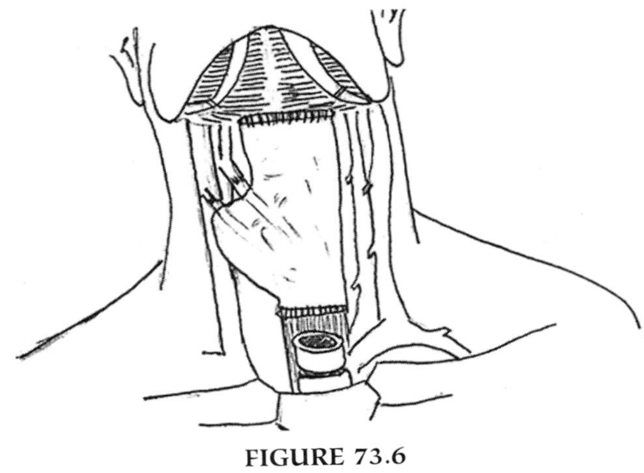

FIGURE 73.6

Free jejunal graft. The mesenteric artery is anastomosed to the superior thyroid or external carotid artery. The mesenteric vein is anastomosed to the superior thyroid vein or end to side to the jugular vein.

jejunal grafts. Disadvantages include the necessity for 2 abdominal and cervical anastomoses. Operative mortality has ranged from 11% to 18%, leak rates from 9% to 11%, and conduit necrosis rates from 5% to 31% (6–8,12).

In cases where segmental cervical esophageal resection is performed, free jejunal grafts have been utilized (Figure 73.6). Refinements in microvascular techniques have helped improve outcomes with free jejuna grafts. It is the procedure of choice in patients with segmental involvement of the cervical esophagus (less than 3 cm) with ability to obtain adequate distal esophageal margin in the neck, due to avoidance of mediastinal dissection, relatively low morbidity and mortality rates, and rapid return of function. The technique cannot be used in those tumors that extend below the level of the thoracic inlet. Disadvantages include the need for 3 intestinal and 2 microvascular anastomoses. Larger series of jejuna grafts have indicated an operative mortality of 6% to 7%, and fistula formation of 22% to 31% (6,14).

POSTOPERATIVE MANAGEMENT

With long operations, a period of ventilatory support is often needed in the postoperative period. As the majority of these patients will have a permanent tracheostoma, airway access is straightforward. Maintaining the position of the endotracheal tube above the tip of the carina is critical and can present challenges when only a short length of trachea remains (11). Trauma to the trachea is minimized, and humidified air is used to avoid concretion of secretions. A nasogastric tube facilitates decompression of the gastric conduit and minimizes reflux. Aggressive pulmonary physiotherapy measures are instituted, including chest physiotherapy, use of an incentive spirometer, and early ambulation. Enteral feeding through the feeding jejunostomy tube is started 48 to 72 hours postoperatively. On the seventh postoperative day, a barium contrast study is performed to assess the cervical anastomosis, assess transit through the conduit, and ensure that there is no obstruction at the jejunostomy tube site. If no anastomotic leak is detected, the nasogastric tube is discontinued after ensuring that the patient is ambulatory and can sit up while coughing and a clear liquid diet initiated. The diet is gradually advanced to a soft, solid diet. Depending on the adequacy of oral intake, patients may be discharged with supplemental tube feeds. Feeding tubes are kept in until the first postoperative visit and discontinued when adequate oral intake has been achieved. Serial calcium levels are measured to detect hypoparathyroidism.

RESULTS

Analysis of outcomes for cervical esophageal tumors is difficult because of the infrequency of procedures and the lack of prospective randomized reports comparing treatment modalities. Some authors group these tumors with hypopharyngeal carcinomas, while others report outcomes in conjunction with other esophageal cancers. Squamous cell carcinoma is the histology in more than 90% of patients, arising from the cervical esophagus, hypopharynx, or larynx. The remaining are usually secondary involvement of the esophagus from primary tumors of the thyroid and trachea. Cervical esophageal carcinomas are known to have a late onset and an unfavorable prognosis. Surgical resection is often not feasible in more than 40% of patients at the time of definitive diagnosis because of metastatic disease (15). The overall 5-year survival rates in various reports after complete resection have ranged from 13% to 26%. However, large-series data are limited because of the rarity of the lesions. A 1-year survival rate of 60% is much less than that seen with intrathoracic and distal esophageal tumors, usually because of recurrence of the primary tumor.

CONCLUSION

In many patients with cervical esophageal cancer, radiation or chemoradiation therapy is the preferred therapy. In the majority of patients with advanced disease, surgical resection should include pharyngoesophagectomy and total laryngectomy with definitive tracheostomy. The ideal reconstructive method should be a 1-stage procedure with low morbidity and mortality rate and with rapid restoration of swallowing function. In most cases reconstruction is performed with a gastric pull-up, with free jejunal grafts and colonic interposition used in those cases where the stomach is not available. In those that survive long term, general satisfaction is achieved with resolution of dysphagia and respiratory symptoms.

References

1. Jemal A, Siegel R, Ward E, et al. Cancer statistics 2007. *CA Cancer J Clin.* 2007;1:43.
2. Mendenhall W, Sombeck M, Parsons J, et al. Management of cervical esophageal carcinoma. *Semin Radiat Oncol.* 1994;4(3):179.
3. Chakkaphak S, Krishnasamy S, Walker SJ, et al. Treatment of carcinoma of the proximal esophagus. *Surg Gynecol Obstet.* 1989;168:307.
4. Schmalfuss IM. Imaging of the hypopharynx and cervical esophagus. *Magn Reson Imaging Clin N Am.* 2002;10:495.
5. Orringer M. Partial median sternotomy: anterior approach to the upper thoracic esophagus. *J Thorac Cardiovasc Surg.* 1984;87:124.
6. Perrachia A, Bardini R, Ruol A, et al. Surgical management of carcinoma of the hypopharynx and cervical esophagus. *Hepatogastroenterology.* 1990;37:371.
7. Pesko P, Sabljak P, Bjelovic M, et al. Surgical treatment and clinical course of patients with hypopharyngeal carcinoma. *Dis Esophagus.* 2006;19(4):248.
8. Akiyama H. Multifocal development in carcinoma of the esophagus. In: *Surgery for Cancer of the Esophagus.* Baltimore: Williams & Wilkins; 1990:239–258.
9. Krespi Y, Wurster C, Stone D, et al. Hypoparathyroidism following total laryngopharyngectomy and gastric pull-up. *Laryngoscope.* 1985;95:1184.
10. Grillo H, Mathisen D. Cervical exenteration. *Ann Thorac Surg.* 1990;49:401.
11. Orringer M. Anterior mediastinal tracheostomy with and without cervical exenteration. *Ann Thorac Surg.* 1992;54:628.
12. Carlson G, Schusterman M, Guillamondegui O. Total reconstruction of the hypopharynx and cervical esophagus: a 20-year experience. *Ann Plastic Surg.* 1992;29:408.
13. Deschamps C. Use of colon and jejunum as possible esophageal replacements. *Chest Surg Clin N Am.* 1995;5:555.
14. Triboulet J, Mariette C, Chevalier D, et al. Management of carcinoma of the hypopharynx and cervical esophagus. *Arch Surg.* 2001;136:1164.
15. Pingree T, Davis R, Reichman O, et al. Treatment of hypopharyngeal carcinoma: a 10 year review of 1362 cases. *Laryngoscope.* 1987;97:901.

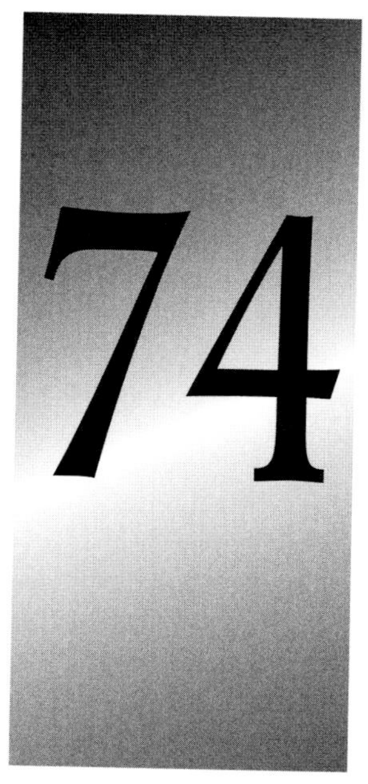

Surgery Techniques: Transhiatally Extended Total Gastrectomy

Hubert J. Stein

Because of its rising incidence, adenocarcinoma of the esophagogastric junction (AEG) has become an important clinical topic. The discussions surrounding the adequate management of such tumors and, in particular, the optimal surgical approach have in the past been overshadowed by confusion about the type of tumors that were included in various published reports. Some consider and treat all adenocarcinomas arising at or close to the esophagogastric junction as esophageal cancer, others as gastric cancer, and yet others as an entirely separate entity (1–3). Furthermore, individualized approaches, which increasingly also incorporate multimodal pre- and/or postoperative treatment strategies, have recently emerged (4–7). This has resulted in a variety of surgical procedures that are currently recommended for adenocarcinoma of the esophagogastric junction, ranging from simple local resection with esophagogastrostomy to a total ultraradical esophagogastrectomy with systematic 3-field (i.e., cervical, mediastinal, and abdominal) lymph node dissection and colon interposition. Obviously, these approaches vary widely in their invasiveness, the associated morbidity, postoperative mortality, and the functional sequelae in the long-term survivors.

Following a consensus conference of the International Society for Diseases of the Esophagus and the International Gastric Cancer Association, an agreement has been achieved for classification of adenocarcinoma arising in the vicinity of the esophagogastric junction (1) in order to provide a basis for comparison of treatment results with different approaches and between centers. This classification is based on topographic anatomic characteristics and the location of the tumor center above, at, or below the gastric cardia as suggested by Siewert in 1987 (8). The landmark that remains at the center of this anatomical classification is the endoscopic "cardia," defined as the oral end of the typical longitudinal gastric mucosa folds. In AEG type I, the tumor is located above this endoscopically defined cardia; in AEG type II, the tumor center or tumor mass is in the area of the endoscopic cardia; and in AEG type III, the tumor center or tumor mass is below this landmark (Figures 74.1 and 74.2).

The application of this classification system not only has shown marked differences between squamous cell esophageal cancer and adenocarcinoma of the distal esophagus in terms of etiology, tumor biology, type of affected patients, pattern of lymphatic spread, and prognosis, but also has revealed substantial differences between the various AEG subtypes (9–12). While type I tumors (adenocarcinoma of the distal esophagus) have emerged as a separate entity of esophageal carcinoma, which usually arise from metaplastic Barrett's esophagus as a consequence of chronic gastroesophageal reflux, the biology and morphology of type II tumors

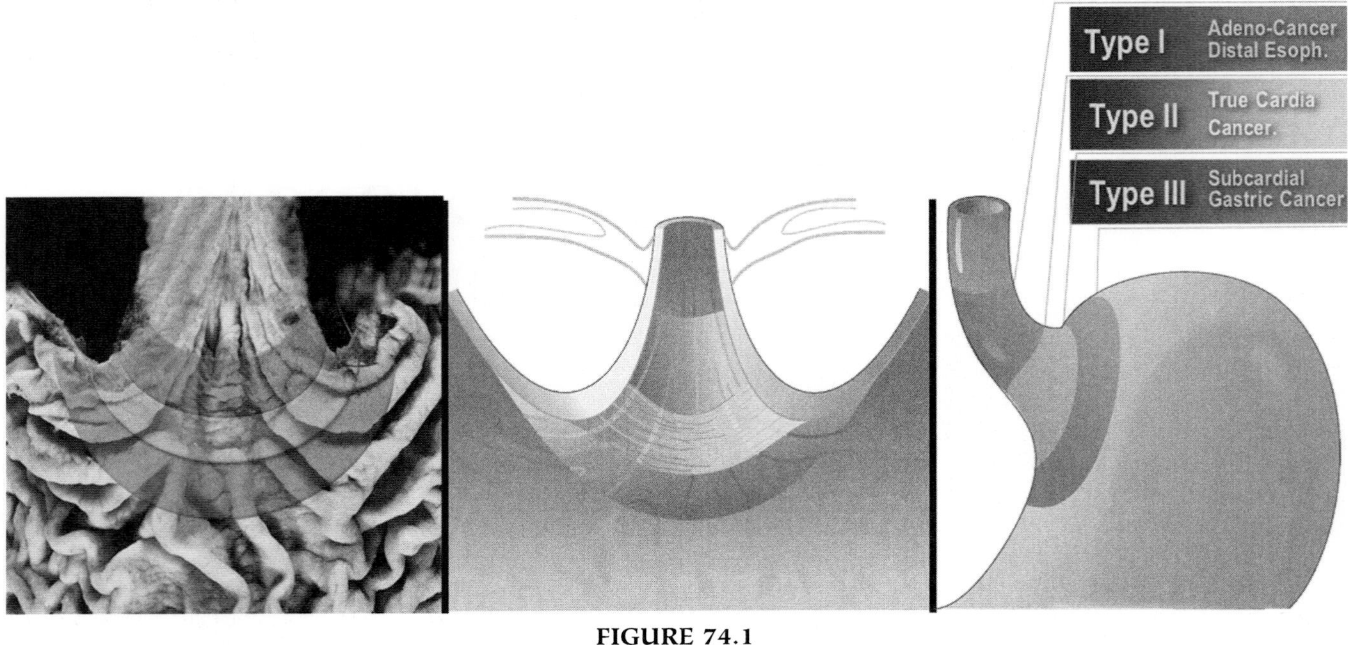

FIGURE 74.1

Topographic anatomic classification of adenocarcinoma of the esophagogastric junction into AEG type I, AEG type II, and AEG type III tumors (1).

(true adenocarcinoma of the gastric cardia) appears to be very similar to type III tumors (subcardiac gastric cancer). This is also reflected in the pattern of lymphatic and submucosal spread (Figure 74.3). The direction of lymphatic spread (i.e., the most likely location of lymph node metastases) in patients with type I tumors is the lower mediastinum and the upper abdomen (13,14). In contrast, lymphatic spread toward the mediastinum appears to be a late and less common event in patients with type II and type III tumors. The most common location of lymph nodes metastases in these patients is the left and right paracardiac region, along the left gastric artery, splenic artery, and, in later stages, toward the splenic hilum and left para-aortic region at the left renal hilum (Figure 74.4).

These observations should be taken into account when planning surgical treatment of such tumors. From the surgical oncology point of view, the extent of resection should be guided by the goals to achieve a complete tumor resection (a so-called R0 resection) and to perform an adequate lymphadenectomy with as little perioperative mortality, morbidity, and long-term side effects as possible. Surgical resection and lymphadenectomy for adenocarcinoma of the distal esophagus (type I tumors) should therefore be planned differently from that for squamous cell esophageal cancer and also differently from that for true adenocarcinoma of the gastric cardia (type II tumors) or carcinoma of the subcardiac region (type III tumors). The classification thus allows one to tailor the oncologic radicality required for complete tumor removal and lymph node clearance and to balance the perceived benefits of the surgical procedure against its risks (5,15,16).

Most agree that type I tumors require a subtotal esophagectomy and systematic mediastinal lymphadenectomy in addition to an upper abdominal lymph node dissection. Based on tumor biology and the pattern of lymphatic spread, subtotal esophagectomy and extensive mediastinal lymph node clearance, however, appear unnecessary in most patients with type II and type III tumors. In these patients, the focus should rather be directed toward clearance of the upper abdominal compartment and lower posterior mediastinum. This can be achieved in most instances without thoracotomy via a pure abdominal approach with wide splitting of the esophageal hiatus; that is, a total gastrectomy with transhiatal resection of the distal esophagus and systematic lymphadenectomy according to the rules of gastric cancer surgery and Roux-en-Y reconstruction. A clear oral margin obviously is mandatory. The required length of the clear proximal resection margin (i.e., the length of unaffected esophagus that needs to be resected to avoid local or anastomotic recurrences) has been a matter of debate but, as in rectal cancer, is overestimated in most publications. In any case, a clear oral resection should always be confirmed by intraoperative frozen sections.

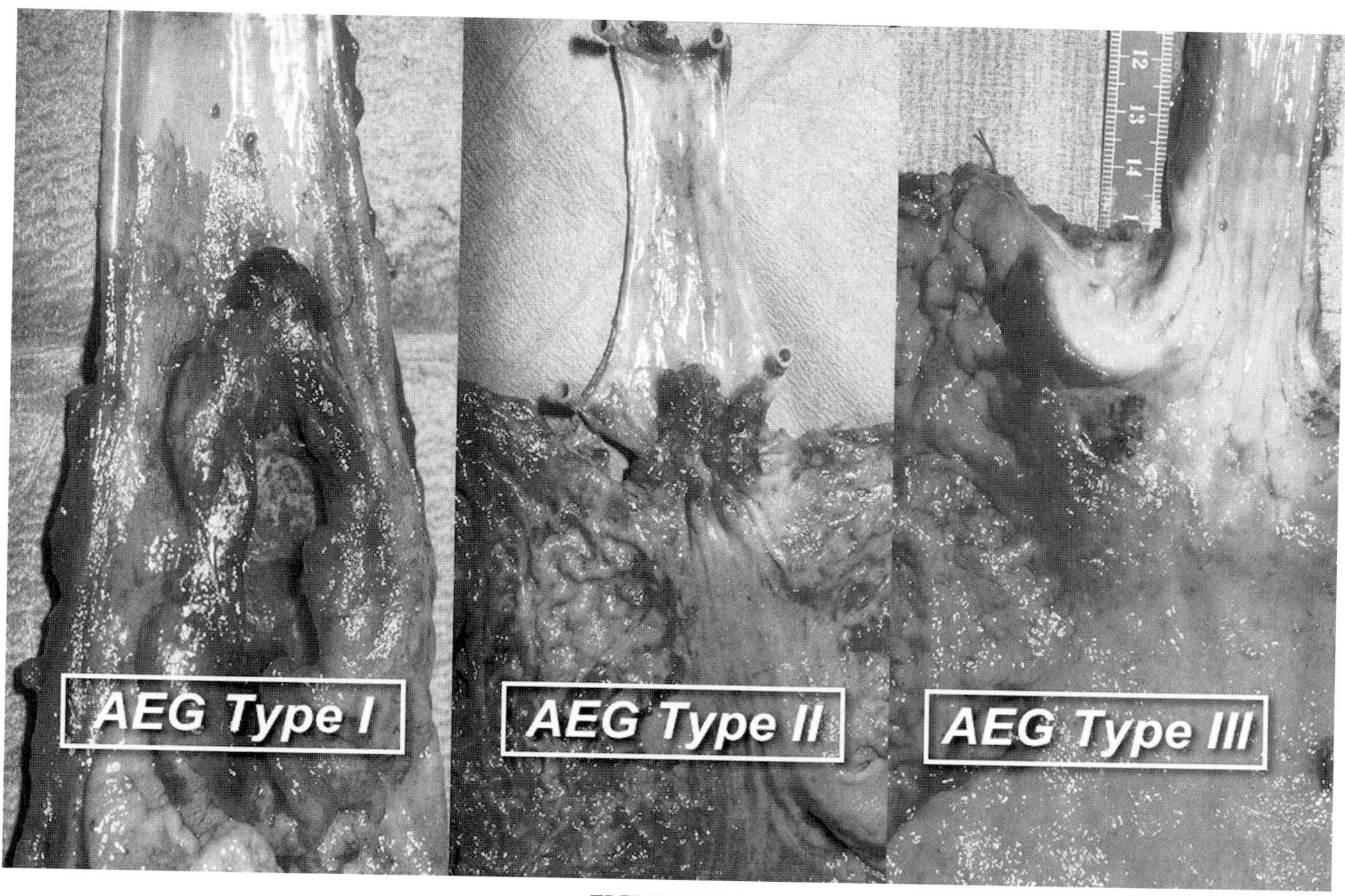

FIGURE 74.2

Typical specimen showing AEG type I, AEG type II, and AEG type III tumors.

In the author's experience, a subtotal esophagectomy has only rarely become necessary to achieve this goal in patients with type II or type III tumors. Based on the huge experience of Professor Siewert's Department of Surgery at TU Munich, a total gastrectomy with transhiatal resection of the distal esophagus, systematic upper abdominal and lower mediastinal lymphadenectomy, and Roux-en-Y reconstruction has become the procedure of choice for patients with type II and type III tumors of the esophagogastric junction (5,10,17).

TECHNICAL DETAILS OF TRANSHIATALLY EXTENDED TOTAL GASTRECTOMY FOR AEG TYPE II AND TYPE III TUMORS

Wide exposure is critical for good access to the esophagogastric junction and lower posterior mediastinum in oncologic surgery. This starts with placement of the patient on the operating table, as illustrated in Figure 74.5. A generous horizontal upper abdominal incision gives best exposure. In obese patients, an additional abdominal upper midline incision may occasionally be required. An overhead retractor placed as shown in Figure 74.6 elevates the sternum and "opens" the access to the esophagogastric junction and posterior mediastinum. In every patient with transmural tumor growth (pT2b or higher tumor category), a generous en bloc resection of the diaphragmatic crura and both pleural sheets should be performed, as shown in Figure 74.7. This will ensure clear circumferential resection margins. Access to the lower posterior mediastinum up to the level of the tracheal bifurcation can be achieved after a wide anterior or left lateral splitting of the diaphragm and insertion of specially designed over-long retractors, as shown in Figure 74.8. With this approach, the entire posterior mediastinum and retrucrural area can be cleared of lymphatic tissue under direct vision and up to 10 cm of the distal esophagus exposed. In most instances this suffices to place a purse-string clamp and divide the esophagus well above the tumor at the level of the tracheal bifurcation (Figure 74.9). Nevertheless, a clear proximal resection margin should always be confirmed by intraoperative frozen sections.

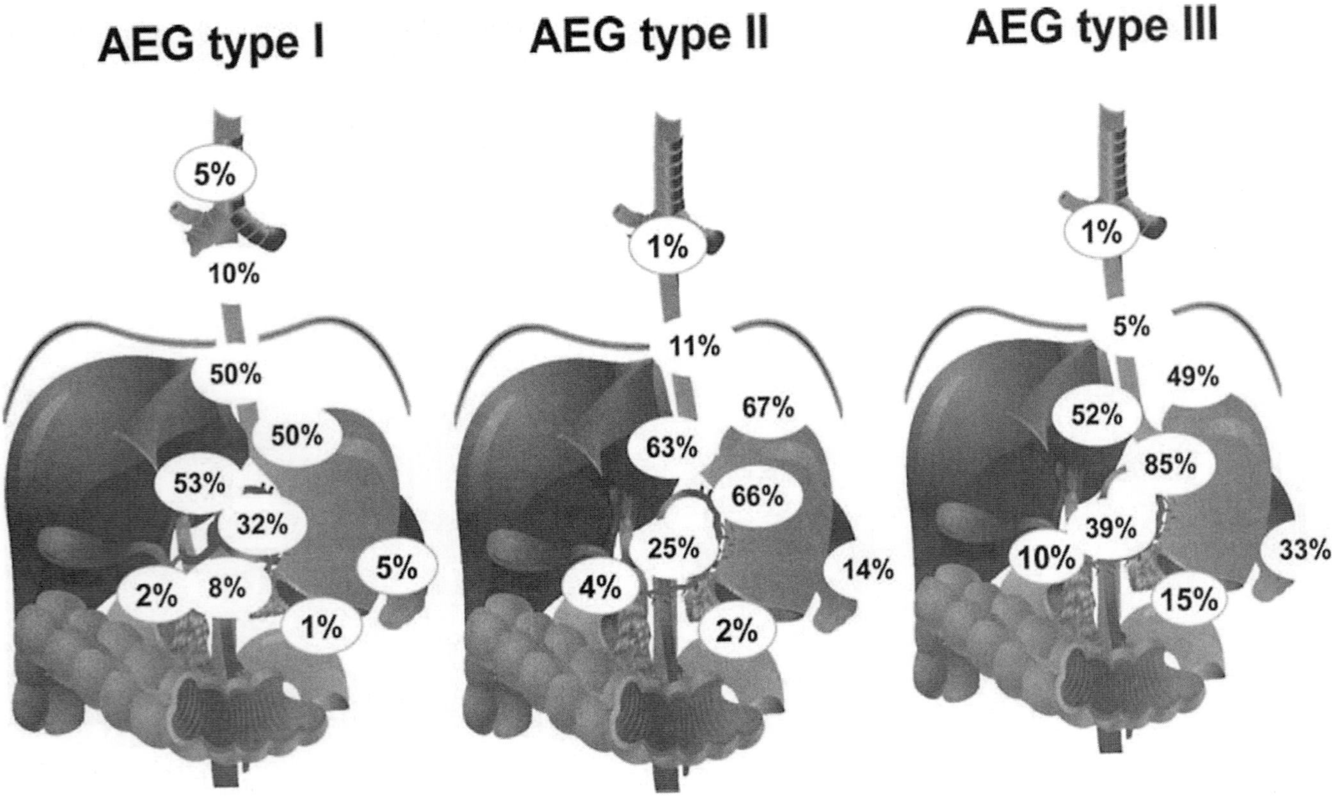

AEG type I

5%
10%
50%
50%
53%
32%
2%
8%
5%
1%

AEG type II

1%
11%
67%
63%
66%
25%
4%
14%
2%

AEG type III

1%
5%
49%
52%
85%
39%
10%
33%
15%

FIGURE 74.3

Pattern of lymphatic spread of type I, type II, and type III adenocarcinoma of the esophagogastric junction (AEG).

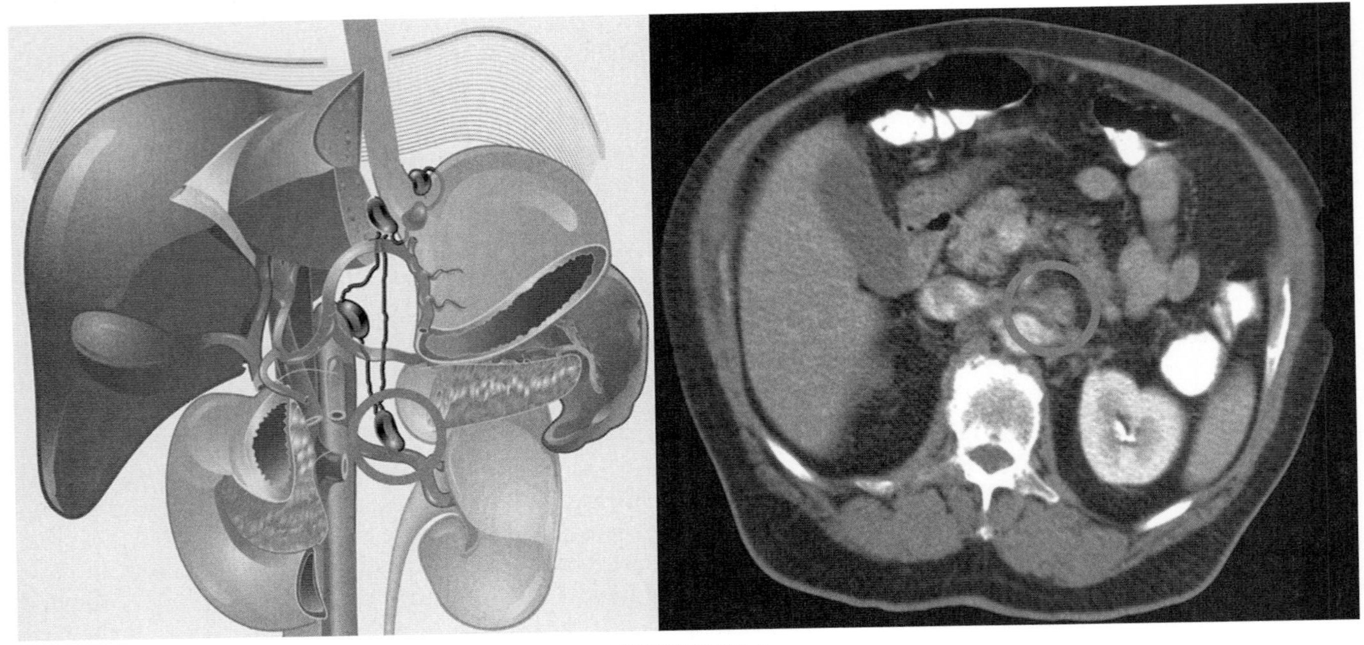

FIGURE 74.4

Lymphatic spread toward the left para-aortic region in adenocarcinoma of the gastric cardia due to direct lymphatic pathways.

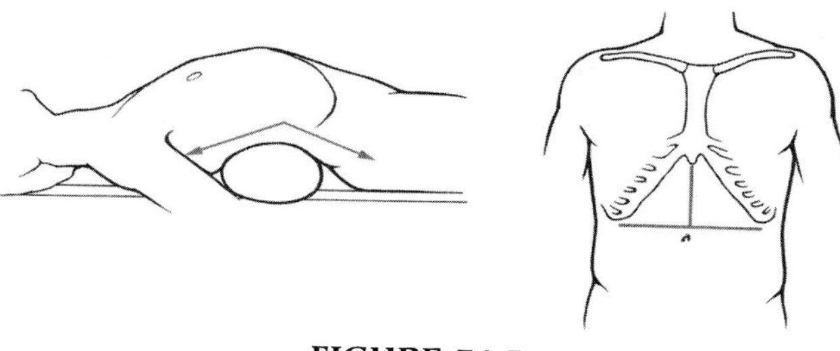

FIGURE 74.5

Transabdominal access to the esophagogastric junction and lower posterior mediastinum. Positioning of the patient and line of incision.

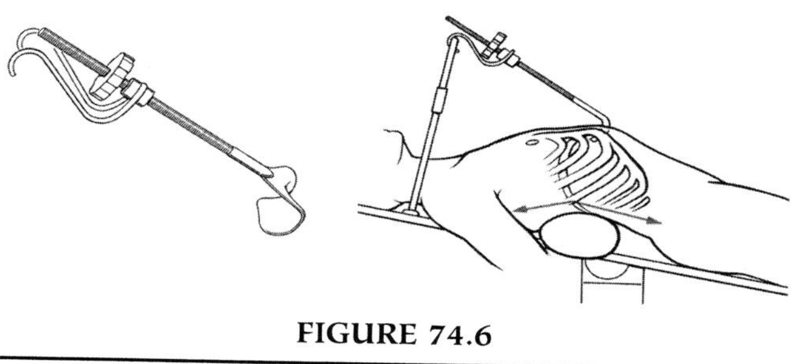

FIGURE 74.6

The use of an overhead retractor "opens" the access to the esophagogastric junction and lower posterior mediastinum.

The extent of upper abdominal lymphadenectomy is that of a formal D2 dissection performed en bloc with the total gastrectomy. Because of the frequent lymphatic spread toward the splenic hilum and retroperitoneum (Figure 74.2), a pancreas-preserving splenectomy and a retroperitoneal para-aortic lymphadenectomy toward the left adrenal gland and the hilus of the left kidney

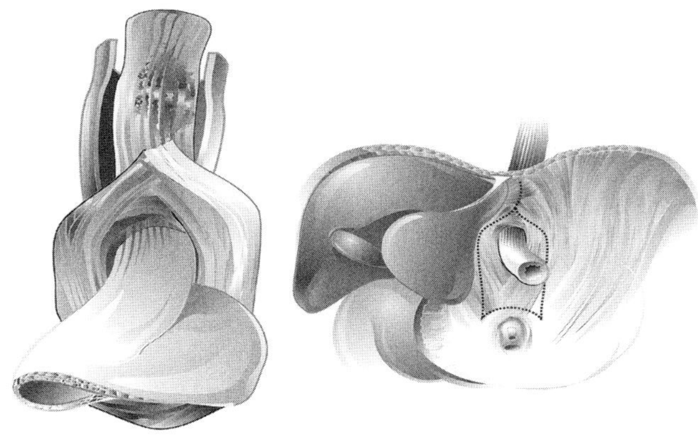

FIGURE 74.7

Wide local en bloc mobilization of the distal esophagus with surrounding structures (diaphragmatic crura and pleural sheet).

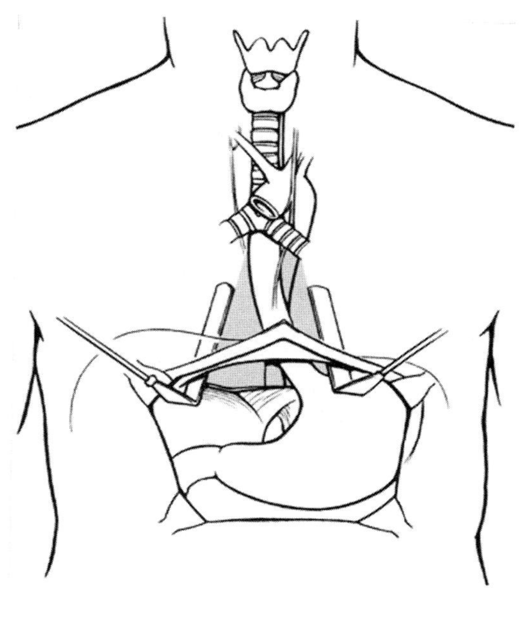

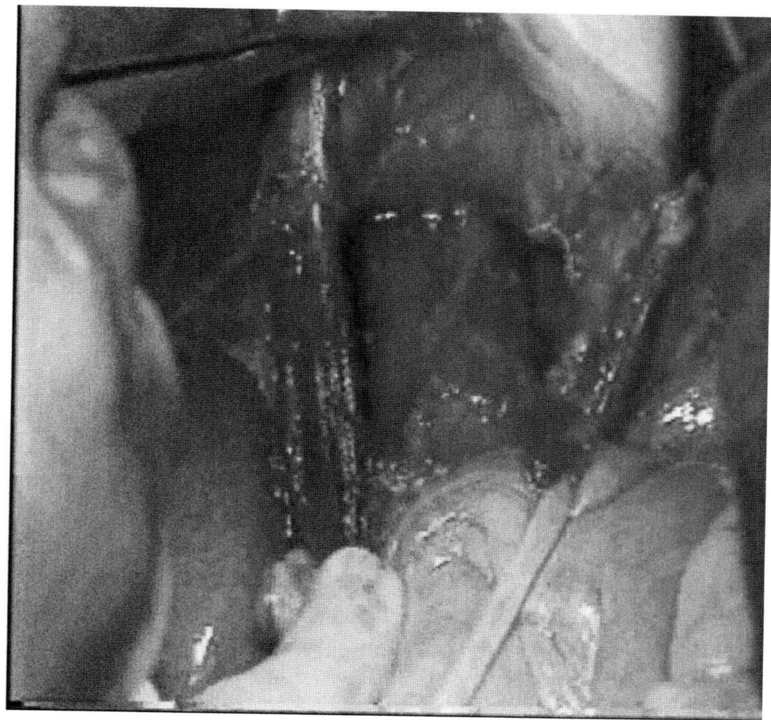

FIGURE 74.8

Wide exposure of the distal esophagus and lower posterior mediastinum after insertion of special retractors. Left: Graphic depiction. Right: Intraoperative view.

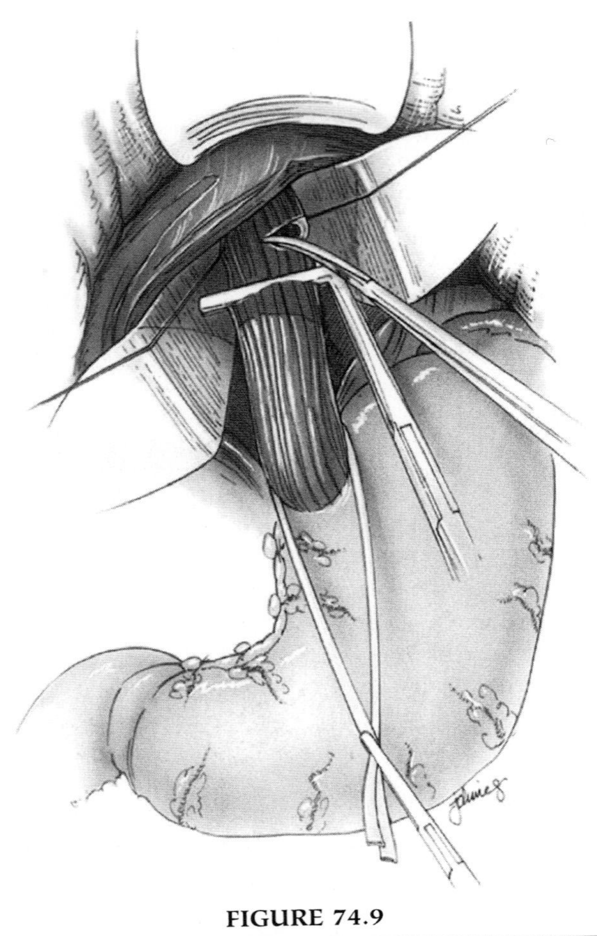

FIGURE 74.9

Transection of the esophagus well above the tumor.

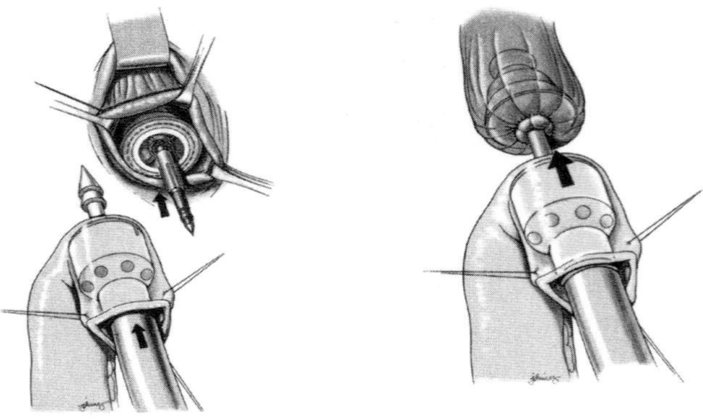

FIGURE 74.10

Esophagojejunal end-to-side anastomosis in the lower posterior mediastinum after transhiatally extended total gastrectomy and resection of the distal esophagus.

may be added (Figure 74.4). This extension of the procedure should, however, be considered only in patients with frank lymph node metastases in these areas because it may result in substantial morbidity. Whenever possible, a resection of the tail of the pancreas should be avoided because this is followed by septic complications in 20% to 25% of the patients (pancreatic fistulae and abscesses). The only indication for resection of the pancreatic tail is a direct tumor invasion into the pancreas.

From a technical and functional point of view, reconstruction with a pouch after total gastrectomy and a transhiatal resection of the distal esophagus does not make sense because the pouch would be located partially within the chest and cannot function as a reservoir. The fastest and easiest reconstruction is an end-to-side esophagojejunostomy in the Roux-en-Y technique (Figures 74.10 and 74.11). The distance between the esophagointestinal anastomosis and Roux loop should be at least 40 to 50 cm.

Modern circular stapler devices allow safe anastomosis high in the mediastinum without thoracotomy (Figure 74.10). A careful selection of a proximal jejunal loop with a good vascular arcade and a tension-free anastomosis are key to prevent leaks and stricture formation. Diaphanoscopy helps with identification and construction of the Roux loop.

OUTCOME OF TRANSHIATALLY EXTENDED TOTAL GASTRECTOMY WITH ROUX-EN-Y RECONSTRUCTION

The oncologic results and the long-term outcome of this approach are at least as good as those with more radical abdominothoracic procedures (Figure 74.12), while the surgical procedure is safer and the postoperative course smoother when thoracotomy is avoided (2,9,10,17). This experience was recently confirmed by a prospective randomized study from the National Cancer Center in Tokyo (18). In this study, the abdominothoracic approach for AEG type II and type III tumors was associated with a higher postoperative mortality rate and a significantly higher postoperative overall morbidity as compared to the transhiatal approach. There were no significant differences in long-term survival between the two procedures. Thus, a thoracotomy with subtotal esophagectomy and systematic mediastinal lymphadenectomy is not necessary for the vast majority of patients with adenocarcinoma of the gastric cardia or subcardiac region, even when distal esophageal invasion is present. The thoracotomy only adds morbidity without a survival benefit. Rather, a pure transabdominal/transhiatal approach is the access of choice whenever a clear oral resection margin can be achieved by this procedure (Table 74.1).

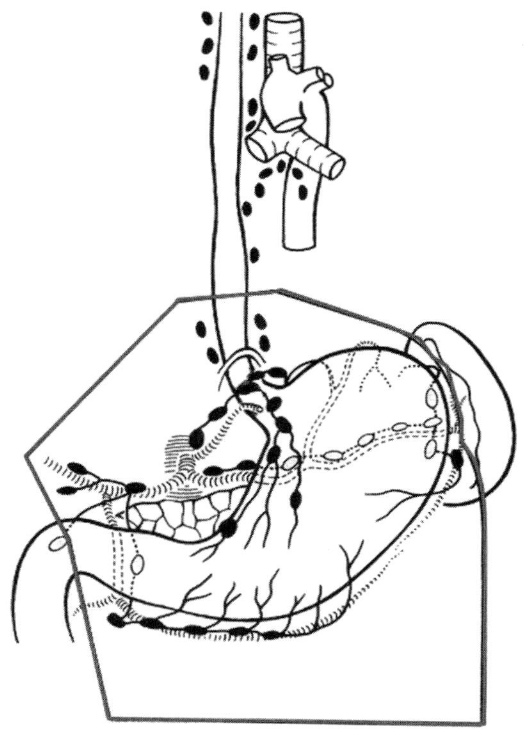

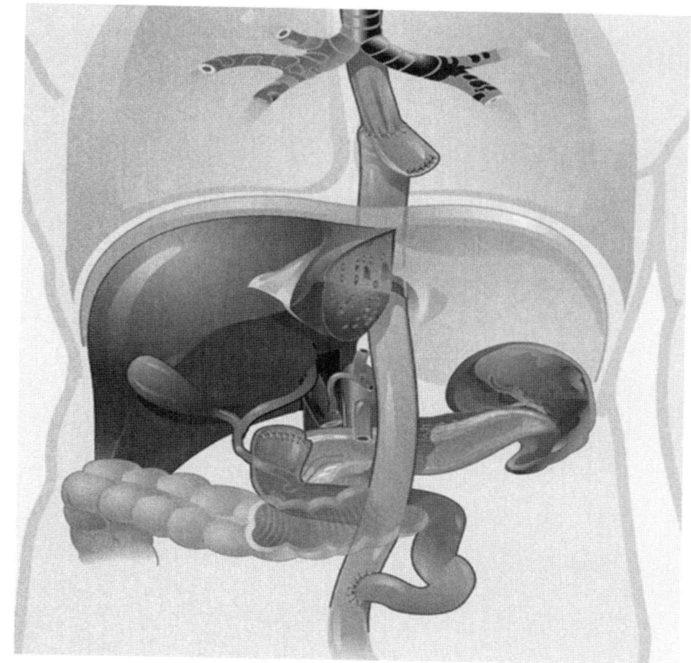

FIGURE 74.11

Left: Extent of resection. Right: Graphic depiction of a completed Roux-en-Y esophagojejunostomy immediately below the level of the tracheal bifurcation after total gastrectomy and transhiatal resection of the distal esophagus.

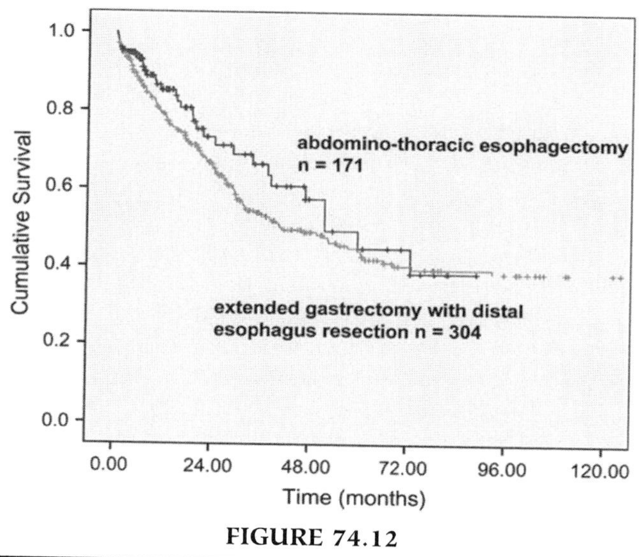

FIGURE 74.12

Long-term survival rates for AEG type II/III after abdominothoracic esophagectomy with proximal gastric resection versus transhiatally extended total gastrectomy (data from TU Munich series).

TABLE 74.1
Strengths and Weaknesses of Transhiatally Extended Total Gastrectomy for Adenocarcinoma of the Gastric Cardia (AEG Type II) and Subcardiac Gastric Cancer Infiltrating the Distal Esophagus (AEG Type III)

Strengths	Weaknesses
No thoracotomy required	Limited mediastinal exposure
Preservation of healthy esophagus	Narrow oral resection margin
Adequate abdominal lymphadenectomy	Limited mediastinal lymphadenectomy
Easy and safe reconstruction	Loss of potentially unaffected stomach

References

1. Siewert JR, Stein HJ. Classification of carcinoma of the oesophagogastric junction. *Br J Surg.* 1998;85:1457–1459.
2. Sauvanet A, Mariette C, Thomas P, et al. Mortality and morbidity after resection for adenocarcinoma of the gastroesophageal junction: predictive factors. *J Am Coll Surg.* 2005;201:253–262.
3. Papachristou DN, Fortner JG. Adenocarcinoma of the gastric cardia: the choice of gastrectomy. *Ann Surg.* 1980;192:58–64.
4. Stein HJ, Sendler A, Fink U, et al. Multidisciplinary approach to esophageal and gastric cancer. *Surg Clin N Am.* 2000;80:659–682.
5. Stein HJ, Feith M, Siewert JR. Individualized surgical strategies for cancer of the esophagogastric junction. *Ann Chir Gynaecol.* 2000;89:191–198.
6. Kitajima M, Kitagawa Y. Surgical treatment of esophageal cancer—the advent of the era of individualization. *New Engl J Med.* 2002;347:1705–1709.
7. Hulscher JB, van Landschot JJ. Individualised surgical treatment of patients with an adenocarcinoma of the distal esophagus or gastro-esophageal junction. *Dig Surg.* 2005;22:130–134.
8. Siewert JR, Hölscher AH, Becker K, et al. Versuch einer therapeutisch relevanten Klassifikation. *Chirurg.* 1987;58:25–34.
9. Siewert JR, Stein HJ. Adenocarcinoma of the gastroesophageal junction: classification, pathology and extent of resection. *Dis Esophagus.* 1996;9:173–182.
10. Siewert JR, Feith M, Werner M, et al. Adenocarcinoma of the esophagogastric junction: results of surgical therapy based on anatomical/topographic classification in 1,002 consecutive patients. *Ann Surg.* 2000;232:353–361.
11. Siewert JR, Stein HJ, Feith M, et al. Tumor cell type is an independent prognostic parameter in esophageal cancer: lessons learned from more than 1000 consecutive resections at a single institution in the Western world. *Ann Surg.* 2001;234:360–369.
12. Siewert JR, Feith M, Stein HJ. Biologic and clinical variations of adenocarcinoma at the esophago-gastric junction: relevance of a topographic-anatomic subclassification. *J Surg Oncol.* 2005;13:139–146.
13. Stein HJ, Feith M, Brücher BLDM, et al. Early esophageal cancer: pattern of lymphatic spread and prognostic factors for long term survival after surgical resection. *Ann Surg.* 2005;242:566–572.
14. Stein HJ, Feith M, Müller J, et al. Limited resection for early adenocarcinoma in Barrett's esophagus. *Ann Surg.* 2000;232:733–742.
15. Stein HJ, Sendler A, Siewert JR. Site dependent resection techniques for gastric cancer. *Surg Oncol Clin N. Am.* 2002;11:405–414.
16. Stein HJ, Siewert JR. Surgical approach to adenocarcinoma of the gastric cardia. *Operat Tech Gen Surg.* 2003;5:14–22.
17. Feith M, Stein HJ, Siewert JR. Adenocarcinoma of the esophagogastric junction: surgical therapy based on 1602 consecutive resected patients. *Surg Oncol Clin N Am.* 2006;15:751–764.
18. Sasako M, Sano T, Yamamoto S, et al. Left thoracoabdominal approach versus abdominal transhiatal approach for gastric cancer of the cardia or subcardia: a randomised controlled trial. *Lancet Oncol.* 2006;7:644–651.

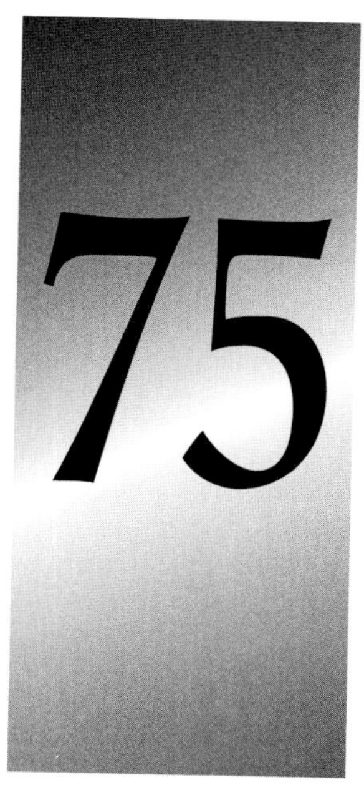

Surgery Techniques: Salvage Esophagectomy

Donn Spight

Esophageal cancer is an increasingly common malignancy associated with a dismal prognosis. More than 50% of patients present with dysphagia and are found to have locally advanced or disseminated malignancy at the time of diagnosis (1). Despite improvements in diagnostic tools, surgical instrumentation, and operative technique, the mortality of esophageal cancer remains unacceptably high. In a review of 122 reports on esophageal cancer surgery published between 1960 and 1979, the average rate of resection, mortality, and 5-year survival rates were 39%, 29%, and 4%, respectively (2,3). When reassessed for the period 1980–1988, Müller et al. reported the respective rates to be 56%, 13%, and 20%, respectively (4). Although the latter study identified favorable trends, the overall results for esophagectomy today remain similarly unsatisfactory leading many to look for other alternatives.

In large-volume centers, esophagectomy alone has proven effective in early stage cancers, while definitive chemoradiation therapy (CRT) is the treatment of choice for stage IV disease. The optimal treatment strategy for locoregionally advanced esophageal cancer has not been clearly defined (5). In Japan and Western countries, medical and radiation oncologists have reported improved survival of stage III patients treated with definitive CRT, thus blurring the boundaries of traditional treatment strategies (6). Fueled by unsatisfying surgical results and high mortality rates, the use of definitive CRT instead of surgery is increasing in frequency in the United States (30% vs. 34%) (7). The observation that 15% to 36% of surgical specimens show complete tumor eradication following neoadjuvant therapy has led some centers to offer definitive CRT to patients with potentially resectable tumors (8–12).

Persistent or recurrent local disease after definitive CRT treatment remains the greatest failure of this strategy. For a subset of carefully selected patients, salvage esophagectomy remains the only curative option. Operation after definitive CRT is infrequent even in experienced, high-volume tertiary referral centers. As experience with definitive CRT grows, the number of patients referred for salvage esophagectomy will increase.

THE CASE FOR DEFINITIVE CHEMORADIATION

Chemoradiation without surgery has not been compared with surgery alone in prospective clinical trials. Several studies have evaluated outcomes for chemoradiation followed by surgery versus definitive chemoradiation in potentially resectable esophageal tumors. Long-term follow-up studies from the Radiation Therapy Oncology Group trial (RTOG 85–01) reported a median survival of

14.1 months with a 5-year survival of 26% in a randomized cohort of T1–3, N0–1, M0 patients receiving chemoradiation therapy alone. Although designed to evaluate efficacy of CRT over radiation alone (0%, 5-year survival), the analysis of this multi-institutional trial revealed survival rates comparable to those reported in the surgical literature (8).

In the Federation Francaise de Cancerologie Digestive (FFCD 9102) trial, 445 patients with operable thoracic esophageal cancer, histologically squamous cell carcinoma (SCC), stage T3–4N0–1M0 were treated with 5-FU, super selective high-dose intraarterial cisplatin (CDDP) plus radiation (13). The 259 patients who had at least a partial response were randomized to receive additional chemorads or surgery. This study concluded that definitive CRT was an alternative to surgery in patients with locally advanced resectable esophageal cancer who respond to initial chemorads. The 2-year survival was 34% in the surgery group versus 40% in the definitive CRT group ($P = .56$). Median survival was 17.7 months versus 19.3 months respectively. The German Esophageal Cancer Study Group (GOCSG) concluded that CRT followed by surgery can no longer be recommended as a routine treatment in patients with good tumor response to induction chemoradiation therapy in a trial comparing preoperative CRT followed by surgery with definitive CRT alone (12). This trial randomized 172 patients with locally advanced SCC of the esophagus; stage T3–4N0–1M0 to 1 of the 2 groups. Although the local progression-free survival rate at 2 years (64% in surgery group vs. 40.7% in chemorads group) was significantly different ($P = .003$), overall survival was no different (39.9% and 35.5% at 2 years, 31.3% and 24.4% at 3 yrs.). Median survival of each group were not statistically different (14).

Despite flaws in these studies, proponents of definitive CRT postulate that patients who benefit most from esophagectomy are those who have had a complete pathologic response to induction therapy (15). They therefore contend that subsequent esophagectomy does not add true value but instead confirms a favorable prognosis at the cost of major surgery.

FAILURE OF DEFINITIVE CHEMORADIATION

Unfortunately, not all patients experience complete tumor eradication. Persistent or recurrent local disease after definitive CRT treatment remains the greatest drawback of this strategy: 11% to 26% of patients do not exhibit any morphologic tumor response leading to a dismal prognosis with a median survival of 9 months (13,16,17). The ability to predict who will respond remains a formidable challenge. Definitive CRT is now accepted as primary treatment of squamous cell cancer at many sites including head and neck, anus, and cervix (18). In esophageal cancer, squamous cell type is often more suitable for definitive CRT than adenocarcinoma due to tumor location (9). Adenocarcinomas are often located at or near the gastroesophageal junction (GEJ) where radiation doses must be limited due to fear of inclusion of abdominal viscera in the field.

Locoregional recurrence is defined as tumor detected more than 3 months after CRT. Persistence is defined by tumor detected within 3 months in the same site (6). Approximately 40% to 60% of patients do not achieve locoregional control after definitive chemoradiation therapy as evidenced by persistent or recurrent tumor at the primary site within 1 year (8,19). For many of these patients, salvage esophagectomy is not an option, as metastases are revealed upon restaging work-up or severe physiologic impairment precludes operative intervention. The reasons for treatment failure can be multifactorial. In the Trans Tasaman Radiation Oncology Group (TROG) study of definitive CRT, approximately 20% of patients failed to complete the prescribed protocol due to deterioration in performance status or toxicity (20). Local problems that prevented completion of therapy included esophageal fistualizaton and dysphagia (9). Patients treated with CRT alone often require dilatation or stents for palliation of strictures or local recurrence more often than those treated by surgery (12).

Esophageal surgery after definitive CRT is infrequent even in experienced high-volume tertiary referral centers. Although long-term survival is the primary goal, local control and freedom from dysphagia are important secondary endpoints for any treatment. Symptoms could be palliated with stent placement, but this approach would not be curative. Other treatments such as PDT and EMR have limited utility in this population. As experience with definitive CRT grows, the number of patients referred for salvage esophagectomy will increase.

MORBIDITY AND MORTALITY OF SALVAGE ESOPHAGECTOMY

Salvage esophagectomy is a high-risk operation that carries a mortality of over 10% even among specialized units (19). There is also increased morbidity as manifested by duration of ventilator dependence, ICU stay, overall hospital stay, and increased anastomotic leak rate. Therefore, physiologic fitness and functional status are extremely important considerations when evaluating patients for possible salvage esophagectomy. Zubrod performance status, FEV1, DLCO, and serum albumin are important preoperative predictors of complications after salvage esophagectomy (15,21–23).

In 2007, Gardner-Thorpe et al. performed a meta-analysis of 9 series containing a total of 105 patients (Table 75.1) (9). Operation after definitive CRT was infrequent even in tertiary referral centers. Approaches varied depending on the tumor site and institutional preference and included Ivor Lewis, transthoracic, and transhiatal. Performance of extended lymphadenectomy varied. The largest series was published by Nakamura et al., who reported 27 salvage procedures out of 660 (4.1%) esophagectomies between 1992 and 2002 (6). Looking across all of the published series, the overall anastomotic leak rate was 17.1% (range 6%–38%) (9). In-hospital mortality was 11.4%. This was compared to overall mortality rate of 2% reported over the same time period for all esophagectomies. Five-year survival rate was 25% to 35%. Median survival after salvage esophagectomy ranged from 7 to 32 months. Prognostic factors for increased survival were RO resection ($P = 0.006$) and longer interval between CRT and recurrence ($P = 0.002$). The median interval between completion of CRT and salvage esophagectomy was 4 to 18 months (6,19,24–26). The most common indications for salvage esophagectomy were persistent disease (52.4%) and locoregional recurrence (42.9%) (9).

Swisher et al. reported the MD Anderson experience from 1987 to 2000. Thirteen of 780 esophagectomies were performed after definitive CRT (5). Anastomotic leak rate was 38%. Pneumonia rate was 38%. Length of stay averaged 29.4 days and the in-hospital death rate was 15%. Salvage esophagectomy resulted in a 5-year survival of 25%. They noted improved survival after salvage procedure was associated with early path stage (T1NO, T2NO), prolonged time to relapse, and RO surgical resection.

TECHNICAL CHALLENGES OF SALVAGE ESOPHAGECTOMY

The challenges of the procedure are primarily due to the increased doses of radiation and the prolonged time interval to presentation after the completion of radiation. Neoadjuvant therapy for locally advanced esophageal cancer typically consists of cisplatin, 5-FU, and radiation. The average dose of radiation delivered to the esophagus is 41.4 Gy (range 30.0–60.0 Gy) in neoadjuvant groups, as compared to 57.7 Gy (range 30.9–90.0 Gy) in definitive CRT regimens (5). Treatment specifics of radiation therapy, such as total dose, treatment field, and fraction size, determine the extent of thoracic injury and, therefore, morbidity of subsequent salvage esophagectomy. The lungs are not usually affected by radiation < 45Gy for esophageal cancer because it is typically delivered via anterior and posterior opposed

TABLE 75.1
***a*Salvage Esophagectomy Series after Failure of Definitive Chemoradiation Therapy**

Reference	# of patients	Study interval	Country	Age	Sex ratio (M:F)	Radiation dose (Gy)	Chemotherapy
Leichman et al.	4	1983–1985	USA	60 (54–80)	2:2	50	Cisplatin and 5-FU or mitomycin C and 5-FU and bleomycin
Meunier et al	6	1991–1995	France	57 (40–65)	6:0	60	Cisplatin and 5-FU
Murakami et al.	4	1989–1996	Japan	60 (52–70)	2:2	60–66	Cisplatin and 5-FU
Wilson et al.	16	1993–1998	Canada	64	–	50	Cisplatin and 5-FU
Swisher et al.	13	1987–2000	USA	65 (45–83)	9:4	56–57	Cisplatin and 5-FU
Gotohda et al.	6	1998–2001	Japan	56 (46–66)	4:2	60	Cisplatin and 5-FU
Nakamura et al.	27	1992–2002	Japan	63 (36–79)	21:6	60	Cisplatin and 5-FU
Stahl et al.	5	1994–2002	Germany	–	–	65	Cisplatin and 5-FU and leucovorin and etoposide
Tomimaru et al.	24	1985–2004	Japan	63	22:2	62	Cisplatin and 5-FU and doxorubicin

[a]Adapted from Gardner-Thorpe et al. (9).

beams (6). However, radiation doses > 45 Gy require obliquely oriented beams to avoid spinal cord damage, which may lead to lung damage. Radiation damages mediastinal structures and causes inflammation early (weeks) and fibrosis later (months) (27). The resulting fibrosis becomes difficult to distinguish from residual or recurrent cancer. These indistinct planes between tumor and fibrotic masses within the irradiated mediastinal tissues increase the propensity for bleeding in the thoracic cavity and make the operation more difficult overall. In a series of 13 patients reported by Swisher et al., operations frequently took over 9 hours to complete with 2 intraoperative deaths (5). Salvage surgery took longer than other esophageal operations performed at MD Anderson (9 vs. 7 hrs. $P = .006$).

There have been numerous operative strategies to reduce the morbidity of the salvage esophagectomy; however, major complications such as respiratory failure, esophagogastric anastomotic leak, recurrent laryngeal nerve injury, chylothorax, pericardial effusion, airway necrosis, and fistulization persist regardless of the operative approach. Irradiation of the esophagus and stomach may affect their blood supply and this may be a contributing factor to leakage. All efforts should be made to avoid the use of irradiated esophagus for any anastomosis. Modifications to reduce the incidence of leaks include the use of a colonic interposition graft, jejeunal interposition with vascular anastomosis in neck (supercharged), or reinforcement of the anastomosis with viable tissue. Small caliber transnasal esophagoscopy can be a very useful tool to assess for ischemic changes. Subcutaneous or anterior mediastinal positioning of the conduit has been postulated to minimize the consequence of leakage (9). The liberal use of pericardial fenestration may decrease the postoperative morbidity from a pericardial effusion (1). Staged reconstruction can be utilized to decrease operative time and ensure conduit viability before anastomosis in sick patients. Placement of a feeding jejeunostomy tube is recommended, given the high rate of postoperative complication.

OUTCOMES

Numerous studies have shown that the prognosis of a patient with a non-curative salvage esophagectomy is extremely poor. Outcomes of salvage esophagectomy after definitive CRT has been shown to be comparable to elective neoadjuvant plus surgery when an RO resection is performed (6). Tomimaru et al. calculated that the odds ratio for improved long-term survival was 23.3 (95% CI 2.4–219.6) if an RO resection was achieved ($P = .006$) (25). Swisher et al. achieved median survival of 86 months and 5-year survival of 60% for those with RO resection (5). No patient with R1/R2 resection survived more than 13 months in any series (6,19,25). In a retrospective cohort evaluation of 24 salvage esophagectomy patients compared with historic controls treated with elective neoadjuvant followed by surgery, R1+R2 resection was more frequently performed in the salvage group (33% vs. 13%) (25). Multivariate analysis showed curability (RO vs. R1+R2) to be the strongest predictor of successful salvage surgery ($P = .0064$). The rate of noncurative surgery in patients diagnosed as T4 before CRT was 64% (7/11) in their study. None of these patients survived more than 10 months postop. Considering this high rate of failure, salvage surgery should be avoided in T4 stage patients. Instead palliative therapy such as intraluminal stenting, bypass, PDT, or EMR should be considered.

Prognostic factors for increased survival after salvage esophagectomy are RO resection ($P = .006$), and longer interval between CRT and recurrence ($P = .002$). Since salvage esophagectomy should be carried out only if RO resection is feasible, preoperative patient selection and re-staging become paramount to patient selection (9). In a study to individualize predictive factors of RO resection in patients with locally advanced disease, Piessen et al. performed a multivariate analysis of 98 patients deemed unresponsive to chemoradiation. They found that tumor height between 0 and 5 cm on barium swallow and aortic contact < 90 degrees on CT were predictive of RO resection (odds ratio 2.4, 95% CI 1.3–4.4, $P = .004$) (28).

Unfortunately, there is no highly sensitive and specific investigative modality to accurately re-stage patients after definitive CRT. In contrast to its well-established role in staging esophageal cancer before CRT, CT is inaccurate for restaging post treatment (29). Nodal disease is considered to be a relative contraindication to salvage esophagectomy, but standard PET alone cannot distinguish tumor from peritumoral lymph node disease (5). In a study of neoadjuvant CRT, the sensitivity of PET for response was 71% and specificity 82% compared with gold standard of histopathology after esophagectomy (30). Fusion PET/CT may prove more accurate in this respect. Endoscopy is important in detecting recurrence but may not be sufficient as a restaging diagnostic tool (31). Frequently, stenosis will preclude ability to perform a full exam. Even when completed, EUS cannot reliably distinguish postinflammatory changes from malignant nodes or direct spread of tumor. In a recent study, accuracy was 27% for T stage and 58% for N stage (31). Frozen section histology should be performed for any suspicious nodes with subsequent abortion of operation if they are positive. In addition, exclusion of patients with T4 disease on initial staging (before CRT) has been postulated to be the best strategy to avoid noncurative salvage operations (9).

CONCLUSION

Based on the results of prospective randomized controlled trials conducted by the Radiation Therapy Oncology Group (RTOG 85–01) and the Intergroup INT 0123 (RTOG 94–05), concurrent chemoradiotherapy has become the standard of care for patients with localized cancer of the thoracic esophagus selected for nonsurgical treatment (8,14,32). With its popularity supported by low morbidity and high postoperative quality of life, definitive chemotherapy is becoming more common as a viable treatment option for locoregionally advanced operable cancer (3,25). Unfortunately, not all patients will attain locoregional control after definitive chemoradiation therapy, and some will have persistent or recurrent tumor at the primary site within 1 year. The ability to predict who will respond remains at the forefront of esophageal cancer investigation.

As medical management strategies become more prevalent, salvage esophagectomy will be required more frequently to deal with treatment failures. The development of accurate re-staging methodologies is urgently needed for preoperative counseling. For a subset of carefully selected patients able to achieve an RO resection, salvage esophagectomy remains the only curative option. Given the technical difficulty and resultant morbidity and mortality, salvage esophagectomy's acceptability as a "back-up" for definitive chemoradiation must be evaluated carefully as a standard of care. For superficial tumors that remain persistent or recurrent at the local site, EMR may provide an alternate salvage technique (33). Invariably the best treatment strategy will arise from a multidisciplinary dialogue and, therefore, possible candidates should be referred to an esophageal cancer center of excellence, rich in experience, and capable of delivering high-quality team-based care.

References

1. Urschel JD, Ashiku S, Thurer R, et al. Salvage or planned esophagectomy after chemoradiation therapy for locally advanced esophageal cancer—a review. *Dis Esophagus.* 2003;16(2):60–65.
2. Earlam R, Cunha-Melo JR. Oesophageal squamous cell carcinoma: I. A critical review of surgery. *Br J Surg.* 1980;67(6):381–390.
3. Nishimaki T, Shimoji H, Sunagawa H. Recent changes and the future roles of esophageal cancer surgery. *Ann Thorac Cardiovasc Surg.* 2004;10(6):324–332.
4. Müller JM, Erasmi H, Stelzner M, et al. Surgical therapy of oesophageal carcinoma. *Br J Surg.* 1990;77(8):845–857.
5. Swisher SG, Wynn P, Putnam JB, et al. Salvage esophagectomy for recurrent tumors after definitive chemotherapy and radiotherapy. *J Thorac Cardiovasc Surg.* 2002;123(1):175–183.
6. Nakamura T, Hayashi K, Ota M, et al. Salvage esophagectomy after definitive chemotherapy and radiotherapy for advanced esophageal cancer. *Am J Surg.* 2004;188(3):261–266.
7. Daly JM, Karnell LH, Menck HR. National cancer data base report on esophageal carcinoma. *Cancer.* 1996;78(8):1820–1828.
8. Cooper JS, Guo MD, Herskovic A, et al. Chemoradiotherapy of locally advanced esophageal cancer: long-term follow-up of a prospective randomized trial (RTOG 85–01). radiation therapy oncology group. *JAMA.* 1999;281(17):1623–1627.
9. Gardner-Thorpe J, Hardwick RH, Dwerryhouse SJ. Salvage oesophagectomy after local failure of definitive chemoradiotherapy. *Br J Surg.* 2007;94(9):1059–1066.
10. Hironaka S, Ohtsu A, Boku N, et al. Nonrandomized comparison between definitive chemoradiotherapy and radical surgery in patients with T(2–3)N(any) M(0) squamous cell carcinoma of the esophagus. *Int J Radiat Oncol Biol Phys.* 2003;57(2):425–433.
11. MacFarlane SD, Hill LD, Jolly PC, et al. Improved results of surgical treatment for esophageal and gastroesophageal junction carcinomas after preoperative combined chemotherapy and radiation. *J Thorac Cardiovasc Surg.* 1988;95(3):415–422.
12. Stahl M, Stuschke M, Lehmann N, et al. Chemoradiation with and without surgery in patients with locally advanced squamous cell carcinoma of the esophagus. *J Clin Oncol.* 2005;23(10):2310–2317.
13. Bedenne L, Michel P, Bouche O, et al. Chemoradiation followed by surgery compared with chemoradiation alone in squamous cancer of the esophagus: FFCD 9102. *J Clin Oncol.* 2007;25(10):1160–1168.
14. Shinoda M, Hatooka S, Mori S, et al. Clinical aspects of multimodality therapy for resectable locoregional esophageal cancer. *Ann Thorac Cardiovasc Surg.* 2006;12(4):234–241.
15. Urschel JD, Sellke FW. Complications of salvage esophagectomy. *Med Sci Monit.* 2003;9(7):RA173–180.
16. Mariette C, Taillier G, Van Seuningen I, et al. Factors affecting postoperative course and survival after en bloc resection for esophageal carcinoma. *Ann Thorac Surg.* 2004;78(4):1177–1183.
17. Di Fiore F, Lecleire S, Rigal O, et al. Predictive factors of survival in patients treated with definitive chemoradiotherapy for squamous cell esophageal carcinoma. *World J Gastroenterol.* 2006;12(26):4185–4190.
18. Tobias JS, Ball D. Synchronous chemoradiation for squamous carcinomas. *BMJ.* 2001;322(7291):876–878.
19. Swisher SG, Wynn P, Putnam JB, et al. Salvage esophagectomy for recurrent tumors after definitive chemotherapy and radiotherapy. *J Thorac Cardiovasc Surg.* 2002;123(1):175–183.
20. Denham JW, Burmeister BH, Lamb DS, et al. Factors influencing outcome following radio-chemotherapy for oesophageal cancer: the Trans Tasman Radiation Oncology Group (TROG). *Radiother Oncol.* 1996;40(1):31–43.
21. Stein HJ, Brucher BL, Sendler A, et al. Esophageal cancer: patient evaluation and pretreatment staging. *Surg Oncol.* 2001;10(3):103–111.
22. Ferguson MK, Durkin AE. Preoperative prediction of the risk of pulmonary complications after esophagectomy for cancer. *J Thorac Cardiovasc Surg.* 2002;123(4):661–669.
23. Nagawa H, Kobori O, Muto T. Prediction of pulmonary complications after transthoracic oesophagectomy. *Br J Surg.* 1994;81(6):860–862.
24. Meunier B, Raoul J, Le Prise E, et al. Salvage esophagectomy after unsuccessful curative chemoradiotherapy for squamous cell cancer of the esophagus. *Dig Surg.* 1998;15(3):224–226.
25. Tomimaru Y, Yano M, Takachi K, et al. Factors affecting the prognosis of patients with esophageal cancer undergoing salvage surgery after definitive chemoradiotherapy. *J Surg Oncol.* 2006;93(5):422–428.
26. Gotohda N, Nishimura M, Yoshida J, et al. Salvage operation for esophageal cancer after radical chemoradiotherapy. *Kyobu Geka.* 2002;55(9):743–746; discussion 746–749.
27. Kato H, Fukuchi M, Miyazaki T, et al. Surgical treatment for esophageal cancer. current issues. *Dig Surg.* 2007;24(2):88–95.
28. Piessen G, Briez N, Triboulet JP, et al. Patients with locally advanced esophageal carcinoma nonresponder to radiochemotherapy: who will benefit from surgery? *Ann Surg Oncol.* 2007;14(7):2036–2044.
29. Jones DR, Parker LA Jr, Detterbeck FC, et al. Inadequacy of computed tomography in assessing patients with esophageal carcinoma after induction chemoradiotherapy. *Cancer.* 1999;85(5):1026–1032.
30. Munden RF, Macapinlac HA, Erasmus JJ. Esophageal cancer: The role of integrated CT-PET in initial staging and response assessment after preoperative therapy. *J Thorac Imaging.* 2006;21(2):137–145.
31. Beseth BD, Bedford R, Isacoff WH, et al. Endoscopic ultrasound does not accurately assess pathologic stage of esophageal cancer after neoadjuvant chemoradiotherapy. *Am Surg.* 2000;66(9):827–831.
32. Minsky BD, Pajak TF, Ginsberg RJ, et al. INT 0123 (Radiation Therapy Oncology Group 94–05) phase III trial of combined-modality therapy for esophageal cancer: high-dose versus standard-dose radiation therapy. *J Clin Oncol.* 2002;20(5):1167–1174.
33. Hattori S, Muto M, Ohtsu A, et al. EMR as salvage treatment for patients with locoregional failure of definitive chemoradiotherapy for esophageal cancer. *Gastrointest Endosc.* 2003;58(1):65–70.

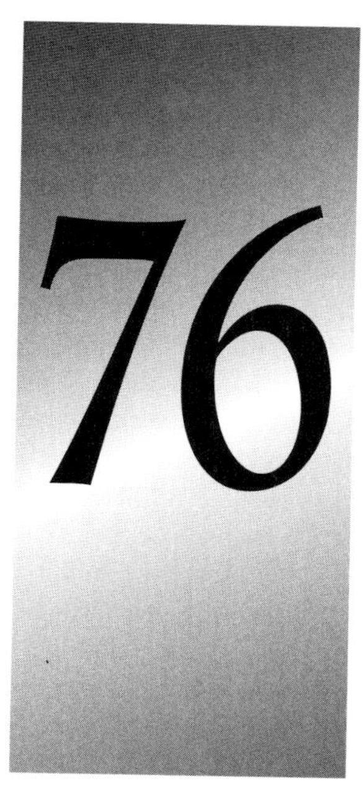

76 Surgery Techniques: Postoperative Care

Brant K. Oelschlager
Martin I. Montenovo

For the most part, fluid resuscitation after esophagectomy is like any other surgical procedure, with the amount and type of fluid dictated by the patient's clinical status (vital signs, urine output, hemodynamic monitoring, etc). However, because of the nature of the procedure and the common cardiopulmonary side effects and complications, many have suggested these patients have to be treated slightly different than other patients undergoing gastrointestinal resections. For example, Kita et al. (1) suggest that, in patients undergoing esophagectomy, a strict balance must be achieved, since excess fluid leads not only to pulmonary insufficiency but also to edema of the reconstructive organ, which may influence its oxygen partial pressures and, thus, its viability. This balance is accomplished by maintaining a fluid rate of 1.0 to 2.0 ml kg^{-1} h^{-1} and central venous pressure lower than 5 mm Hg during the operation. However, at the moment, there is not enough evidence that supports such restrictive fluid management in patients undergoing esophagectomy; therefore, most surgeons, including ourselves, base fluid resuscitation on the patient needs.

THE USE OF BLOOD TRANSFUSIONS

With the increasing use of neoadjuvant chemotherapy, many patients present with anemia and bone marrow suppression before esophagectomy. Moreover, resection carries with it substantial risk of bleeding; therefore, consideration of blood transfusion is relatively frequent. The hemoglobin level at which there is a benefit for circulation and oxygen delivery has been dropping over time. Also, there is evidence that blood transfusions may have a negative impact on the oncologic outcomes. The concept of packet red blood cells (PRBC) transfusions increasing recurrence of cancer was introduced by Gantt in 1981 (2). He hypothesized that if transfusions downregulated the host's immune surveillance against malignant cells, then transfusions could augment tumor growth. Since then, there have been many reports of cancer recurrence or cancer-related deaths secondary to transfusion, though all of these reports are retrospective and uncontrolled. Vamvakas and Blajchman (3) conducted a meta-analysis assessing the clinical relationship between transfusion and cancer-related death. Unfortunately, patients who received transfusions might have had larger, more advanced tumors, or more significant medical problems predisposing them to surgical complications and long hospital stays. As a result of these factors, a causal relationship between transfusion and cancer recurrence or death has not been definitively proven (4).

Some work has compared the effects of autologous and allogeneic blood transfusions on outcomes after surgical resection of malignancies. To date, there are

2 studies with level III evidence (5,6) by Motoyama et al. that indicate that the use of allogeneic blood transfusion rather than autologous blood during esophagectomy results in decreased 3-year survival and increased rates of cancer recurrence. Still, most patients should not require blood transfusion, making the role for autologous donation unclear.

In a related topic, there is considerable controversy regarding the ideal postoperative hemoglobin level. The age-old practice of keeping the hemoglobin above 10 g/dl has very little evidence-based support. Currently, in most patients, transfusion is started when hemoglobin levels are less than 7%. A multicenter, randomized, controlled clinical trial from Canada (7) demonstrated that a restrictive strategy of blood transfusion, in which patients were transfused only for a hemoglobin level of less than 7 g/dl, was at least as effective as and possibly was superior to a liberal transfusion strategy in critically ill patients. Herbert et al. suggest that hemodynamically stable, critically ill patients with cardiovascular disease (excluding patients with acute myocardial infarction and unstable angina) can be safely maintained at hemoglobin concentrations above 7% (8). Thus, surgeons and anesthesiologists should adopt a more stringent set of requirements for blood transfusion, and in doing so, even fewer patients will require transfusion.

ANALGESIA

Effective analgesia is a significant challenge after esophageal resection. These operations often require an upper abdominal incision and either a thoracotomy and/or neck incision as well. Severe postoperative pain can induce cardiovascular instability and impairs respiratory function (9). The introduction of thoracic epidural analgesia represents a key advance in perioperative pain control. Adequate pain management, particularly by epidural analgesia, can decrease perioperative stress and influence the postoperative immune response (10,11).

Thoracic epidural analgesia (TEA) blocks afferent nociceptive stimuli and inhibits efferent sympathetic outflow in response to painful stimuli. Starting with a bolus before the incision and giving a continuous infusion postoperatively minimizes the stress response. Myocardial oxygen demand and arrhythmias incidence can be reduced with the use of TEA, which also has the potential to improve supply by producing stenotic vessel dilation (12).

Some studies have also demonstrated that TEA improves the microcirculation of the distal gastric tube and increases the intestinal motility after a gastric pull-up. TEA reduces the activity of efferent sympathetic fibers innervating the mesenterial blood vessels resulting in venodilation and decreased vascular resistance. Sympaticolysis together with an improved venous return may explain the enhanced tissue perfusion in the anesthetized area (13). This effect may counteract the generally inadequate tissue perfusion at the anastomotic site, usually the main cause of anastomotic leakage, stricture, and ulceration; therefore, TEA may not only provide excellent pain relief but also represent an effective strategy to decrease the rate of anastomotic insufficiency.

In patients in whom TEA is contraindicated, there are several available alternatives. Intercostal nerve block is a valid alternative. The catheter is placed in a paravertebral space just below the level of the incision (for thoracic incisions). Effectiveness of this type of analgesia seems to be the most similar to epidural analgesia with the major advantage of the absence of related complications.

Continuous extrapleural analgesia in the postoperative period is another alternative that provides excellent results, especially when long-acting analgesics are used (14). Local anesthetics may be applied intraoperatively to incisions and as intercostal nerve blocks to limit immediate postoperative pain. Intravenous narcotics (until institution of oral analgesia) are generally always used either as the primary or supplementary analgesic. This can be administered by a nurse, but is more commonly provided via patient controlled analgesia (PCA) pumps, which provide more consistent pain control and patient satisfaction. Finally, non-steroidal analgesics can work synergistically with narcotics and can contribute to dramatically reducing the severity of postoperative pain (15); thus, unless there are contraindications to their use, they should be considered.

RESPIRATORY THERAPY

Respiratory problems remain a major cause of both morbidity and mortality after esophagectomy for cancer. The incidence of respiratory complications after esophagectomy has been estimated around 30%, and complications include pleural effusions, atelectasis, chylothorax, pneumonia, respiratory failure, and pulmonary embolism (16–18). The key to its management is prevention that encompasses a wide spectrum of efforts. The preoperative institution of pulmonary toilet exercises, ambulation, and smoking cessation are paramount for decreasing the risk of postoperative pulmonary complications (19).

Pneumonia and atelectasis are among the most common pulmonary complications after esophagectomy. Their risk can be minimized in the immediate postoperative period by providing adequate pain relief, early ambulation, pulmonary toilet exercises (such as coughing and deep breathing), incentive spirometric devices, and warming and humidification of inhaled gases (20–22). In patients with a history of chronic bronchitis, percussion and postural drainage can help clear secretions and may reduce the incidence of pulmonary infection (23).

Early extubation and epidural analgesia are the 2 postoperative factors that seem to make the biggest difference in reducing postoperative respiratory complications. It was demonstrated that there are far fewer respiratory complications (24,25) in patients who have adequate pain control and breathe spontaneously because there is more efficient pulmonary toilet when excreted through coughing and deep breathing maneuvers than if endotracheal suctioning is performed.

Results confirm this. For example, Nishi et al. (25) have shown that fatal respiratory complications after esophagectomy were reduced significantly by the introduction of epidural analgesia and aggressive postoperative physiotherapy and mobilization, avoiding whenever possible postoperative ventilation. Ballantyne et al. (26) assessed in a meta-analysis the postoperative pulmonary outcomes of epidural and systemic analgesia. Compared with systemic opioids, epidural analgesia decreased the incidence of atelectasis and had a tendency to reduce the incidence of pulmonary infections and pulmonary complications overall.

Supplemental Oxygen

The need for supplemental oxygen in patients who undergo an esophagectomy is nearly universal due to the nature of the operation. The causes of hypoxemia include low inspired-oxygen concentration, alveolar hypoventilation, ventilation/perfusion abnormalities, increased oxygen consumption, and decreased cardiac output. Furthermore, in the postoperative setting there are numerous factors that influence the patient's predisposition for the development of hypoxemia postoperatively, including factors unique to the patient (e.g., age, obesity, cardiopulmonary disease); intraoperatively related reasons (e.g., duration of anesthesia, operative site, one-lung ventilation) and events occurring postoperatively as a result of the surgery (e.g., atelectasis, reactive pleural effusions, abdominal distention, pain) (27).

The level of oxygen supplementation is an area of recent debate. In a prospective randomized trial, Shoemaker et al. (28) found that treatment aimed at achieving supranormal values of oxygen delivery was associated with improved survival in high-risk surgical patients. However, controversy surrounds these results because they were obtained in a heterogeneous population. In another report, Kusano et al. (29) investigated the impact of hemodynamic and oxygen transport variables on postoperative complications in patients undergoing esophagectomy for carcinoma. They demonstrated that low oxygen delivery during the first 12 hours after esophagectomy is associated with the risk of a complication and may lead to the earlier diagnosis of a potentially fatal complications, such as anastomotic leak and severe pneumonia. Therefore, oxygen delivery should be monitored carefully immediately after esophagectomy to predict severe postoperative complications.

At the very least, measurement of arterial oxygen saturation should be routine in the early postoperative period following esophagectomy, and arterial oxygen saturation levels should be used to titrate the amount given as a supplement either by face mask (5–10 l/min) or nasal cannula (1–6 l/min) with the main arterial oxygen saturation above 90% (30) The addition of supplemental oxygen after esophagectomy has many advantages, including the maintenance of an adequate cardiac and central nervous system function, since improving oxyhemoglobin saturation in patients with hypoxemia has been shown to reduce the incidence of cardiac arrhythmias, myocardial ischemia, and mental confusion; more rapid postoperative rewarming (31); a reduction in the incidence of nausea and vomiting (32); and lower wound infection rates (33–34).

Timing of Extubation

There is a considerable institutional variation in the duration of postoperative ventilation after esophagectomy, though the trend is toward early extubation in the operating room. Before the advent of thoracic epidural analgesia, the majority of the studies suggested that results after esophagectomy were better following a period of postoperative ventilation, some for up to 2 days (35). However, postoperative ventilation has not been shown to reduce respiratory complications after abdominal surgery in elective high-risk patients (36). Furthermore, there are potential problems associated with this approach including progressive deterioration in lung compliance, functional residual capacity, risk of aspiration, and sedation-related side effects. Weaning in the intensive care unit is often prolonged and difficult in mechanically ventilated patients, and is exacerbated by decreasing respiratory muscle strength in malnourished patients, with a tendency to develop muscle atrophy (37). As a result, mechanical ventilation after esophagectomy is associated with increased morbidity and mortality.

Over the last decade, with the advent of thoracic epidural analgesia, improved algorithms for fluid management and reduced operative time, early extubation has been advocated to reduce morbidity, mortality, and cost after esophagectomy (38–41). Early extubation after esophagectomy and reconstruction reduces intensive care unit stay and postoperative respiratory complications and does not lead to an increased risk of reintubation, especially when a thoracotomy is not performed (39–42).

Certainly there are specific conditions, such as cardiac instability, compromised myocardial function or perioperative infarction, acute lung injury, airway impairment due to edema or bleeding, severe neurologic impairment, or continued bleeding with high likelihood of returning to the operating theater, that could require continued ventilation support and intubation (38). Even after excluding these conditions, besides the normal criteria for extubation (being awake, adequate airway protection, and presence of cough reflex), these patients are at high risk for respiratory failure, and consideration for postoperative intubation should be given (43).

PREVENTION OF ARRHYTHMIAS

Supraventricular tachyarrhythmias, especially atrial fibrillation, have been described as occurring in 13% to 46% of all patients undergoing esophagectomy (44). While their development is associated with increase incidence of pulmonary complication, anastomotic leakage, surgical sepsis (43), many do not have other associated complications. Several factors have been identified as contributing to arrhythmias, such as age, history of chronic obstructive pulmonary disease (COPD) and cardiac disease, hypovolemia, fluid overload, electrolyte shift. Although the reasons for the increased risk of arrhythmias after esophagectomy are not well known, several hypotheses have been formulated, including loss of normal sinus node pacemaker cells with age, and irritation of the right side of the heart and pulmonary veins from surgery, injury, and/or inflammation of the vagal nerve (43). The inflammatory response to the sympaticovagal nerve fibers of the heart following surgical trauma may alter the autonomic modulation of atrial myocardial cells to endogenous cathecolamines. Thus, postoperatively the usual increased sympathetic tone can shorten the atrial refractory period and cause atrial reentry or trigger automaticity leading to arrhythmias. This explains why drugs that attenuate the adrenergic response to surgery, such as beta-blockers, are frequently used effectively to reduce arrhythmias after esophagectomy. Additionally, sympathetic blockade by thoracic epidural analgesia can reduce the occurrence of arrhythmias; in fact, in one study, atrial fibrillation was seen more frequently after the epidural catheter was removed (45).

The physiologic impact of a new-onset arrhythmia after esophagectomy depends upon ventricular response rate, duration of arrhythmia, and underlying cardiac function. Although most of the literature regarding management of postoperative arrhythmias is in the setting of cardiac surgery, it is reasonable to apply these findings in the non-cardiac setting.

Atrial fibrillation generally occurs 2 to 4 days after the operation (46–47), and episodes tend to be transient, frequent, and recurrent. Over 80% of patients with new-onset arrhythmias revert to sinus rhythm prior to discharge (47–51). In 20% to 30% of cases, no therapeutic intervention is required (48–50). Hemodynamic compromise is uncommon and few patients require urgent cardioversion (48–50).

Atrial fibrillation with a rapid ventricular response can worsen diastolic filling due to decreased filling time and loss of atrioventricular synchrony. For unstable patients who have hypotension, pulmonary edema, or unstable angina, urgent cardioversion is indicated. Intravenous ibutilide, a class III antiarrhythmic agent, is effective in stopping atrial fibrillation and flutter. It is an alternative for acute cardioversion in the hemodynamically stable patient (52).

For patients who do not have hemodynamic compromise and who have atrial fibrillation lasting for more than 15 minutes, initiation of therapy to control the ventricular rate is recommended. Intravenous beta blockers are a logical choice in postoperative patients with high sympathetic tone. In the AFFIRM study, beta-blockers were the most effective drug class for rate control, achieving the specified heart rate endpoints in 70% of patients compared with 54% with use of calcium channel blockers (53). Beta-blockers should be initiated cautiously in patients with atrial fibrillation and heart failure who have reduced ejection fraction (54).

Intravenous calcium channel blockers (verapamil and diltiazem) are also a good choice for the control of heart rate in atrial fibrillation and, furthermore, they are the only agents that have been associated with an improvement in quality of life and exercise tolerance. Due to their short duration of action, they should be administered in a continuous infusion. They are usually preferred for long-term use over beta-blockers in patients with bronchospasm or COPD (55). These agents should be avoided in patients with heart failure due to systolic dysfunction because of their negative inotropic effects (55).

Amiodarone is also effective for controlling the ventricular rate in patients with atrial fibrillation. It is usually considered a suitable alternative agent for heart rate control when conventional measures are ineffective (56). Digoxin has a delayed onset of action and works by increasing vagal tone. Thus, digoxin is typically ineffective for acute rate control in this setting because of its long onset of action; however, its one advantage is it does not drop the blood pressure (57).

Persistent atrial fibrillation is associated with increased risk of stroke or transient ischemic attack after 48 hours. Anticoagulation should be considered in this setting, weighing the potential benefits against the risk of postoperative bleeding (57).

Regarding the use of beta-blockers in the preoperative, the most recent guideline for management of atrial fibrillation states that unless contraindicated, treatment with a beta-blocker to prevent postoperative atrial fibrillation is recommended for patients undergoing cardiac surgery (Class I. Level of Evidence: A) (55).

Since the incidence of atrial fibrillation after noncardiac surgery is fairly low, prophylactic beta-blockers are indicated only for high-risk patients. However, when patients are on beta-blockers preoperatively, postoperative continuation is crucial (58).

DRAINAGE TUBES

Nasoenteral Tube

The use of nasoenteral tube for draining reconstructive organs after esophageal reconstruction is fairly standard practice for most surgeons. There is, however, little evidence to support its use. The theoretic benefits include: (a) decompression of the conduit to reduce the stress on staple lines and anastomosis, (b) providing an assessment of the degree of emptying of the reconstructive organ, (c) preventing accumulation of saliva, bile, and enteric secretions in the reconstructive organ, which can predispose to aspiration, and (d) possibility of use as a stent in a narrowed or inflamed anastomosis. However, nasoenteric tubes also have several potential drawbacks. They are uncomfortable and substantially interfere with the patient's quality of life while in place. A tube can cause erosion of the conduit if it is left for extended periods. Nasoenteral tubes also adversely affect pulmonary toilet exercises, leading to an increased risk of pneumonia. Finally, nasal alar pressure necrosis is a disfiguring and permanent complication of these tubes that is avoidable by properly securing the tube.

The timing of tube removal is variable, usually depending on surgeon's beliefs and personal preferences. Some surgeons prefer to leave the tube in until a contrast radiograph is performed, to rule out anastomotic leak and adequate emptying of the reconstructive organ. More surgeons, however, are removing the tube early based on the absence of abdominal distension, the presence of bowel sounds, evidence for bowel activity, and low outputs from the tube, which is often possible in the first 2 to 3 days. This algorithm is the author's preference. It is important to highlight that early removal of nasoenteric tubes promotes the return of normal bowel activity and facilitates early restoration of oral intake.

Local Drains

The use of local drains near a cervical anastomosis after esophagectomy and reconstruction is another nearly universal practice with little evidence to support its use. A randomized trial studying this issue showed that routine drainage conferred no benefit (59). Moreover, one report suggests that the risk of anastomotic leak is reduced if a drain is placed (60), while another showed that the presence of drain material in proximity to an esophagogastric anastomosis predisposes to anastomotic leakage (61). In case of an anastomotic leak, whether placement of a drain decreases the likelihood of catastrophic complications is unknown. However, it is true that some small leaks are controlled by these drains, thus requiring no further intervention.

Chest Tubes

Thoracostomy tubes are routinely placed when a thoracotomy is used as part of esophagectomy, and they are sometimes used when the pleura has been violated during transhiatal esophagectomy. The use of such tubes should be avoided whenever possible because of the risk of complications such as injury of the intercostal neurovascular bundle, associated pain that interferes with adequate pulmonary toilet postoperatively, and infectious risks from foreign bodies. Thoracostomy tubes should be used only to drain blood/fluid as well as air to allow complete lung expansion. Pleural effusions are common after esophagectomy; thus, consideration of thoracentesis or tube thoracostomy is often given. Our criteria used to removal of thoracostomy tubes are: the patient is not on positive pressure ventilation; there has been no air leak through the tube for at least 24 hours; and volume output is less than 250 ml/day.

It is uncommon for an intrathoracic or cervical anastomotic leak to be effectively drained by a standard thoracostomy tube placed at the time of esophageal reconstruction, since adhesions form quickly postoperatively and seal the tube tract from the region of the anastomosis. Therefore, leaving a thoracostomy tube in place for this purpose or until a contrast radiograph is performed should be discouraged. Moreover, placing the tube in close proximity to the anastomosis increases the risk of erosion and posterior leak.

NUTRITION

There is wide consensus that, after surgery, early oral/enteral feeding preserves gut integrity, maintains immunocompetence, reduces clinical infections, and accelerates wound healing (62–67). Because of the proximal anastomosis after esophagectomy, patients are usually restricted from taking anything by mouth for 4 to 7 days. This is very detrimental for all the aforementioned benefit mechanisms of enteral nutrition. Moreover, considering that a significant proportion of patients who undergo an esophagectomy and reconstruction present with significant weight loss and feeding problems as a result of an obstructing tumor (43), adequate nutrition is an even more important issue.

Beginning as early as the 1940s, several techniques for parenteral and enteral nutrition were devised that helped reverse negative nitrogen balance after major surgery. Nutritional repletion prior to major surgery has been shown to reduce postoperative complications and mortality; however, these benefits are only evident for the most seriously malnourished patients (68–69). As such, the use of postoperative nutritional therapy is generally recommended for several patients' settings: those who are severely malnourished (defined as > 15% weight loss accompanied by major organ dysfunction) prior to surgery, those who have severe complications, and those who are not expected to be able to eat adequately within 7 to 10 days after their operation (70).

Since a substantial number of patients will fit into one of these categories, a strategy is necessary to ensure nutritional supplementation if needed. The choice comes down to total parenteral nutrition (TPN) versus the routine placement of a feeding jejunostomy tube at the time of resection. The choice between TPN and enteral nutrition (EN) is debatable. The cost of TPN is at least 10 times that of EN and requires sophisticated nursing and biochemical monitoring. Furthermore, TPN is associated with several complications, including pneumothorax, vascular injury, air embolism, catheter embolization, venous thrombosis, catheter malposition, multiple and complex metabolic disturbances, line sepsis, infection at skin site, disruption of the intestinal microflora, intestinal bacterial translocation, impaired gut immune function. So too are there complications related to jejunostomy, including aspiration pneumonia, peritonitis, intestinal obstruction, jejunal necrosis, and pneumatosis intestinale (71–74). Several groups reported a jejunostomy-related mortality rate of between 4% and 10%, with a corresponding morbidity of between 45% and 82% (71–73). While these rates seem high and are not specifically for esophagectomy patients, neither course (TPN or EN) should be consider to be low risk. Our own practice is to place a small-caliber feeding jejunostomy that is used only if severe complications occur necessitating alternative nutritional support or for patients who are slow to resume adequate oral intake, which usually can be done in 7 to 8 days. Certainly, patient comorbid conditions will affect how aggressively to start jejunal feedings.

ANTIBIOTICS

Esophageal reconstructive surgery is classified as a clean contaminated procedure. However, patients who undergo an esophagectomy often have a compromised nutritional status, require invasive catheters in the early postoperative period, and have the usual risk of infection at the surgical sites. Thus, judicious use of antibiotics and adequate nutrition help prevent infection (43).

It has been demonstrated that patients who undergo this type of operation will benefit from perioperative systemic antibiotics (75). Use of an antibiotic dose just prior to beginning the operation and maintenance of adequate antibiotic levels throughout the operation (by appropriate redosing) reduces wound infection rates and may lessen the incidence of other infectious complications (76). There is no benefit in the use of extending antibiotic administration after the operation.

RADIOGRAPHIC IMAGING

Upper Gastrointestinal Images

Routine use of upper gastrointestinal images (UGI) after esophagectomy is common practice and is usually done 5 to 7 days after surgery. Postoperative contrast radiographs assess anatomic and functional components after esophageal reconstruction providing useful information regarding the anatomy of the reconstruction since they are able to show stricture of the anastomosis, redundancy of the reconstruction, and any narrowing where the reconstruction crosses the level of the diaphragm. Furthermore, they provide some information regarding the completeness of emptying (77). The other reason to do these X-rays is to assess for a subclinical leak, though its use for this purpose is clearly debatable, since many surgeons consider the absence of clinical signs of an anastomotic leak as a lack of need for any type of intervention.

When a contrast radiograph is done, a water-soluble contrast agent is generally used as the contrast medium of choice, since they have no known deleterious effects on the neck, mediastinum, pleural cavity, or peritoneal cavities, and are absorbed rapidly from these extraluminal spaces if a leak is present (78–81). However, water-soluble contrast agents are less radiopaque than barium and less adherent to sites of leakage, limiting their ability to depict perforations, particularly if the perforations are subtle (78–81). Some studies reported that when using water-soluble contrast agents, the false negative incidence was up to 40%, and moreover, such agents produce important pneumonitis if they are accidentally aspirated during the swallow (82–83).

The use of barium-sulfate, either full strength or diluted, improves the accuracy of leak detection and produces a much lower risk of pulmonary complications if accidentally ingested (84). Although more of the demonstrated leaks are clinically unimportant, some authors claimed that its discovery changes the patient's management. Swanson et al. (85) reported that in 53% of the patients with leaks detected only on images obtained with barium, the patient's management changed. Some surgeons have concerns that, if a leak is discovered, barium will be retained in the neck or mediastinum, which may interfere with healing or with subsequent radiographic evaluation of healing (86). However, some authors suggest that the presence of barium in a fistula tract encourages the development of granulation tissue and hastens closure of the fistula (77).

A different question revolves around the appropriate evaluation when an anastomotic leak is suspected clinically. An UGI is often quicker to do and does not require IV contrast with the inherent risks to kidneys. However, the false-negative rate of an UGI diminishes its utility as a single assessment. Besides the aforementioned potential problems with these studies, the use of barium and high ionic concentration contrast agents complicates the ability to get a CT scan. As a result, the differential diagnosis and index of suspicion for leak or other complications should be carefully considered when selecting a diagnostic study.

Chest X-Ray

In the immediate postoperative period, the gastric conduit is collapsed and projected as a soft tissue density adjacent to the cardiac border, either to the right, if access has been via the right chest or transhiatally, or to the left, if access has been via the left chest (87). For a certain period following surgery, there may be fluid within the pleural space, but delayed development of pneumothorax or hydropneumothorax may herald the presence of a leak.

Computed Tomography

The role of computed tomography (CT) is predominantly in assessing symptomatic postoperative complications. Imaging is performed post administration of intravenous contrast and, if possible, oral contrast medium. Imaging must include the chest and upper abdomen. In the immediate postoperative period, there are often locules of pleural air related to chest drains. Features of leak on CT are represented by signs of mediastinitis: mediastinal air, fluid collections, or a combination of these. Pleural effusions are common. Empyema may be indicated by pleural enhancement, loculations, and pleural adhesions (87). To date, there is not literature to support the use of CT scan over UGI in the detection of leaks.

ANTICOAGULATION

Venous thromboembolism (VTE) that manifests as deep vein thrombosis (DVT) or pulmonary embolism (PE) is a common complication of cancer (88–91) and is very important in the management of patients with esophageal cancer for several reasons. Patients with cancer have a 4-fold increased risk of developing VTE compared with individuals without cancer (92–93). Furthermore, cancer patients with VTE have a higher mortality rate than cancer patients without VTE, a consequence of both the thrombosis and the apparently more aggressive nature of cancer that is associated with VTE (94). The risk of VTE complications is further increased in patients who undergo cancer-related surgery (95–98) because cancer-related operations activate the body's clotting cascade and often involves venous trauma, and because patients tend to be immobilized for prolonged periods. Finally, cancer treatments (chemotherapy, radiation, etc) and the use of central venous catheters further heighten the VTE risk for cancer patients undergoing surgery (88).

For patients undergoing surgery for cancer, the incidence of venographically observed DVT may be as high as 20% to 40% in the absence of prophylaxis, rising to 40% to 60% in patients with additional risk factors (91).

The most commonly used thromboprophylaxis regimen consists of a single preoperative dose of unfractionated heparin (UFH) or low-molecular weight heparin (LMWH) continuing with subcutaneous doses every 8 to 24 hours postoperatively. Several studies have been performed to compare the effectiveness of UFH versus LMWH in patients with a malignancy. The prospective, randomized, double-blind multicenter Enoxaparin in Cancer (ENOXACAN) study (99) involved high-risk patients who were undergoing elective curative abdominal or pelvic surgery for cancer. A 40 mg once-daily dose of the LMWH, enoxaparin, initiated 2 hours before surgery, was found to be as effective and as safe as UFH given 3 times daily, initiated 2 hours before surgery, for the prevention of VTE.

The optimal duration of thromboprophylaxis in patients with cancer remains the subject of debate. Traditionally, thromboprophylaxis is given for the 7 to 10 days in the postoperative period, while the patient is in the hospital. However, there is evidence to suggest that late thrombotic events can occur up to 7 weeks after the procedure has been performed. The ENOXACAN II double-blind study (100) was set up to compare the efficacy and safety of extended prophylaxis with conventional 1-week prophylaxis in patients undergoing elective surgery for abdominal or pelvic cancer. The study demonstrated that high-risk patients with cancer experience a 60% reduction in the relative risk of venographically detected VTE after a 4-week period of prophylaxis with enoxaparin at 40 mg once-daily subcutaneous, compared with the 1-week regimen. There was no significant difference between both regimens in the incidences of bleeding at both 4 weeks and 3 months after surgery. As a result, many surgeons are treating patients with extended prophylaxis, as provided in this trial, for patients with esophageal cancer.

Mechanical prophylaxis is recommended for patients who have a contraindication to anticoagulant prophylaxis or a high risk of bleeding (91). It includes early and frequent ambulation, graduated compression stockings, and intermittent pneumatic compression devices. Although no mechanical prophylaxis measure has been shown to reduce the risk of death or PE, there is evidence that efficacy may be improved when mechanical prophylaxis is used in combination with anticoagulant prophylaxis (91). For those at highest risk, such as patients with prior history of thromboembolic disease or risk of bleeding, temporary/removable vena caval filters can be placed.

References

1. Kita T, Tadanori M, Kishi Y. Fluid management and postoperative respiratory disturbances in patients with transthoracic esophagectomy for carcinoma. *J Clin Anesth.* 2002;14:252–256.
2. Gantt CL. Red blood cells for cancer patients. *Lancet.* 1981;2:363.
3. Vamvakas EC, Blajchman MA. Deleterious clinical effects of transfusion-associated immunomodulation: fact or fiction? *Blood.* 2001;97:1180–1195.
4. Englesbe MJ, Pelletier SJ, Diehl KM, et al. Transfusions in surgical patients. *J Am Coll Surg.* 2005;200:249–254.
5. Motoyama S, Saito R, Kamata S, et al. Survival advantage of using autologous blood transfusion during surgery for esophageal cancer. *Surg Today.* 2002;32:951–958.
6. Motoyama S, Okuyama M, Kitamura M, et al. Use of autologous instead of allogeneic blood transfusion during esophagectomy prolongs disease-free survival among patients with recurrent esophageal cancer. *J Surg Oncol.* 2004;87:26–31.
7. Herbert PC, Wells G, Blajchman MA, et al. A multicenter, randomized, controlled clinical trial of transfusion requirements in critical care. Transfusion Requirements in Critical Care Investigators, Canadian Critical Care Trials Group. *N Engl J Med.* 1999;340:409–417.
8. Herbert PC, Wells G, Blajchman MA, et al. A multicenter, randomized, controlled clinical trial of transfusion requirements in critical care. *N Engl J Med.* 1999;340:340–409.
9. Tsue SL, Low S, Fok M. Postoperative analgesia reduces mortality and morbidity after oesophagectomy. *Am J Surg.* 1997;173:472–478.
10. Volk T, Schenk M, Voigt K, et al. Postoperative epidural anesthesia preserves lymphocyte, but not monocyte, immune function after major spine surgery. *Anesth Analg.* 2004;98:1086–1092.
11. Yokoyama M, Itano Y, Katayama H, et al. The effects of continuous epidural anesthesia and analgesia on stress response and immune function in patients undergoing radical esophagectomy. *Anesth Analg.* 2005;101:1521–1027.
12. Groban L, Dolinski SY, Zvara DA, et al. Thoracic epidural analgesia: its role in post-thoracotomy atrial arrhythmias. *J Cardiothorac Vasc Anesth.* 2000;14:662–65.
13. Lazar G, Kaszaki J, Abraham S, et al. Thoracic epidural anesthesia improves the gastric microcirculation during experimental gastric tube formation. *Surgery.* 2003;134:799–805.
14. Francois T, Blanloeil Y, Pillet F, et al. Effect of intrapleural administration of bupivacaine or lidocaine on pain and morphine requirement after esophagectomy with thoracotomy: A randomized, double-blind and controlled study. *Anesth Analg.* 1995;80:718–723.
15. Joris J. Efficacy of nonsteroidal anti-inflammatory drugs in postoperative pain. *Acta Anaesthesiol Belg.* 1996;47:115–123.
16. Tsutsui S, Moriguchi S, Morita M, et al. Multivariate analysis of postoperative complications after esophageal resection. *Ann Thorac Surg.* 1992;53:1052–1056.
17. Nagawa H, Kobori O, Muto T. Prediction of pulmonary complications after transthoracic oesophagectomy. *Br J Surg.* 1994;81:860–862.
18. Millikan K, Silverstein J, Hart V, et al. A 15-year review of esophagectomy for carcinoma of the esophagus, and cardia. *Arc Surg.* 1995;130:617–624.
19. Moores LK. Smoking and postoperative pulmonary complications. An evidence-based review of the recent literature. *Clin Chest Med.* 2000;21:139–46.
20. Hall JC, Tarala RA, Tapper J, et al. Prevention of respiratory complications after abdominal surgery: a randomized clinical trial. *Br Med J.* 1996;312:148–153.
21. Chumillas S, Ponce JL, Delgado F, et al. Prevention of postoperative pulmonary complications through respiratory rehabilitation: a controlled clinical study. *Arch Phys Med Rehabil.* 1998;79:5–9.
22. Hall JC, Tarala R, Harris J, et al. Incentive spirometry versus routine chest physiotherapy for prevention of pulmonary complications after abdominal surgery. *Lancet.* 1991;337:953–956.
23. Stiller KR, Munday RM. Chest physiotherapy for the surgical patient. *Br J Surg.* 1992;79:745–749.
24. Watson A, Allen PR. Influence of thoracic epidural analgesia on outcome after resection for oesophageal cancer. *Surgery.* 1994;115:429–432.
25. Nishi M, Hiramatsu Y, Hioki K, et al. Pulmonary complications after subtotal oesophagectomy. *Br J Surg.* 1988;75:527–530.
26. Ballantyne JC, Carr D, deFerranti S, et al. The comparative effects of postoperative analgesic therapies on pulmonary outcome: cumulative meta-analyses of randomized, controlled trials. *Anesth Analg.* 1998;86:598–612.
27. Marley RA. Postoperative oxygen therapy. *J Perianesth Nurs.* 1998;13:394–412.
28. Shoemaker WC, Appel PL, Kram HB, et al. Prospective trial of supranormal values of survivors as therapeutic goals in high risk surgical patients. *Chest.* 1988;94:1176–1186.
29. Kusano C, Baba M, Takao S, et al. Oxygen delivery as a factor in the development of fatal postoperative complications after oesophagectomy. *Br J Surg.* 1997;84:252–257.
30. Powell C, Menon DK, Jones JG. The effects of hypoxemia and recommendations for postoperative oxygen therapy. *Anaesthesia.* 1996;51:769:72.
31. Frank SM, Hesel TW, El-Rahmany HK, et al. Warmed humidified inspired oxygen accelerates postoperative rewarming. *J Clin Anesth.* 2000;12:283–287.
32. Greif R, Laciny S, Rapf B, et al. Supplemental oxygen reduces the incidence of postoperative nausea and vomiting. *Anesthesiology.* 1999;91:1246–1252.
33. Knighton DR, Halliday B, Hunt TL. Oxygen as an antibiotic. The effect of inspired oxygen on infection. *Arch Surg.* 1984;119:199–204.
34. Greif R, Akca O, Horn EP, et al. Supplemental perioperative oxygen to reduce the incidence of surgical-wound infection. *N Engl J Med.* 2000;342:161–167.
35. Patti MG, Wiener-Kronish JP, Way LW, et al. Impact of transhiatal esophagectomy on cardiac and respiratory function. *Am J Surg.* 1991;162:563–567.
36. Shackford SR, Virgilio RW, Peters RM. Early extubation versus prophylactic ventilation in the high risk patient: a comparison of postoperative management in the prevention of respiratory complications. *Anesth Analg.* 1981;60:76–80.
37. Demling RH, Read T, Lind LJ, et al. Incidence and morbidity of extubation failure in surgical intensive care patients. *Crit Care Med.* 1988;16:573–577.
38. Caldwell MT, Murphy PG, Page R, et al. Timing of extubation after oesophagectomy. *Br J Surg.* 1993;80:1537–1539.
39. Yap FH, Lau JY, Jount GM, et al. Early extubation after transthoracic oesophagectomy. *Hong Kong Med J.* 2003;9:98–102.
40. Chandrashekar MV, Irving M, Wayman J, et al. Immediate extubation and epidural analgesia allow safe management in a high-dependency unit after two-stage oesophagectomy: results of eight years of experience in a specialized upper gastrointestinal unit in a district general hospital. *Br J Anaesth.* 2003;90:474–449.
41. Watson A, Allen PR. Influence of thoracic epidural analgesia on outcome after resection for esophageal cancer. *Surgery.* 1994;115:429–432.
42. Robertson SA, Skipworth RJE, Clarke DL, et al. Ventilatory and intensive care requirements following oesophageal resection. *Ann R Coll Surg Engl.* 2006;88:354–357.
43. Aceto P, Congedo E, Cardone A, et al. Postoperative management of elective esophagectomy for cancer. *Rays.* 2005;30:289–294.
44. Amar D, Burt ME, Bains MS, et al. Symptomatic tachydysrhythmias after esophagectomy : incidence and outcome measures. *Ann Thorac Surg.* 1996;61:1506–1509.
45. Murthy SC, Law S, Whooley BP, et al. Atrial fibrillation after esophagectomy is a marker for postoperative morbidity and mortality. *J Thorac Cardiovasc Surg.* 2003;126:1162–1167.
46. Polancyk CA, Goldman L, Marcantonio ER, et al. Supraventricular arrhythmia in patients having noncardiac surgery: clinical correlates and effect on length of stay. *Ann Intern Med.* 1998;129:279–285.
47. Goldman L. Supraventricular tachyarrhythmias in hospitalized adults after surgery. Clinical correlates in patients over 40 years of age after major noncardiac surgery. *Chest.* 1978;73:450–454.
48. Batra GS, Molyneux J, Scott NA. Colorectal patients and cardiac arrhythmias detected on the surgical high dependency unit. *Ann R Coll Surg Engl.* 2001;83:174–176.
49. Walsh SR, Oates JE, Anderson JA, et al. Postoperative arrhythmias in colorectal surgical patients : incidence and clinical correlates. *Colorect Dis.* 2006;8:212–216.
50. Brathwaite D, Weissman C. The new onset of atrial arrhythmias following major noncardiothoracic surgery is associated with increased mortality. *Chest.* 1998;114:462–468.
51. Valentine RJ, Rosen SF, Cigarroa JE, et al. The clinical course of new-onset atrial fibrillation after elective aortic operations. *J Am Coll Surg.* 2001;193:499–504.
52. Ellenbogen KA, Stambler BS, Wood MA, et al. Efficacy of intravenous ibutilide for rapid termination of atrial fibrillation and atrial flutter: a dose-response study. *J Am Coll Cardiol.* 1996;28:130–136.
53. Olshansky B, Rosenfeld LE, Warmer AL, et al. The Atrial Fibrillation Follow-up Investigation of Rhythm Management (AFFIRM) study: approaches to control rate in atrial fibrillation. *J Am Coll Cardiol.* 2004;43:1201–1208.
54. Hunt SA. ACC/AHA 2005 guideline update for the diagnosis and management of chronic heart failure in the adult: a report of the American College of Cardiology/American Heart Association Task Force on Practice Guidelines. *J Am Coll Cardiol.* 2006;47:1503–1505.
55. Fuster V, Rydén LE, Cannom DS, et al. ACC/AHA/ESC 2006 Guidelines for the management of patients with atrial fibrillation. *J Am Coll Cardiol.* 2006;48:149–246.
56. Clemo HF, Wood MA, Gilligan DM, et al. Intravenous amiodarone for acute heart rate control in the critically ill patient with atrial tachyarrhythmias. *Am J Cardiol.* 1998;81:594–598.
57. Heintz KH, Hollenberg SM. Perioperative cardiac issues: postoperative arrhythmias. *Surg Clin N Am.* 2005;85:1103–1114.

58. Stippel DL, Taylan C, Schröder W, et al. Supraventricular tachyarrhythmia as early indicator of a complicated course after esophagectomy. *Dis Esoph.* 2005;18:267–273.
59. Choi HK, Law S, Chu KM, et al. The value of neck drain in esophageal surgery: a randomized trial. *Dis Esoph.* 1998;11:40–42.
60. Horstmann O, Becker H, Verreet PR, et al. Insufficiency of cervical esophagogastrostomy: results of a prospective randomized trial. In: Peracchia A, Rosati R, Bonavina L, et al. editors. *Recent Advances in Diseases of the Esophagus.* Bologna: Monduzzi Editore: 1996:1023–1027.
61. Cui Y, Urschel JD. Latex rubber (Penrose drain) is detrimental to esophagogastric anastomotic healing in rats. *J Cardiovasc Surg (Torino).* 2000;41:479–481.
62. Page CP. The surgeon and gut maintenance. *Am J Surg.* 1989;158:485–494.
63. Moore EE, Jones TN. Benefits of immediate jejunostomy feeding after major abdominal trauma—a prospective, randomized study. *J Trauma.* 1986;26:874–881.
64. Alverdy JC, Aoys E, Moss GS. Total parenteral nutrition promotes bacterial translocation from the gut. *Surgery.* 1988;104:185–189.
65. Moore FA, Feliciano DW, Andreassy RJ, et al. Early enteral feeding, compared with parenteral, reduces post-operative septic complications. *Ann Surg.* 1992;216:172–183.
66. Willmore DW, Smith RJ, O'Dwyer ST, et al. The gut: a central organ after surgical stress. *Surgery.* 1987;104:917–923.
67. Adams S, Dellinger EP, Wertz MJ, et al. Enteral versus parenteral nutritional support following laparotomy for trauma: a randomized prospective trial. *J Trauma.* 1986;26:882–891.
68. Veterans Affairs Total Parenteral Nutrition Cooperative Study Group. Perioperative total parenteral nutrition in surgical patients. *N Engl J Med.* 1991;22:525–532.
69. Torosian MH. Perioperative nutrition support for patients undergoing gastrointestinal surgery: critical analysis and recommendations. *World J Surg.* 1999;23:565–559.
70. Waizberg DL, Plopper C, Terra RM. Postoperative total parenteral nutrition. *World J Surg.* 1999;23:560–564.
71. Smith RC, Hartemink RJ, Hollinshead JW, et al. Fine bore jejunostomy feeding following major abdominal surgery: a controlled randomized clinical trial. *Br J Surg.* 1985;72:459–461.
72. Smith-Choban P, Max MH. Feeding jejunostomy: small bowel stress test? *Am J Surg.* 1988;155:112–117.
73. Maki DG. Maximal barrier precautions during insertion reduce the risk of central venous catheter-related bacteremia. *Infect Control Hosp Epidemiol.* 1994;15:227–230.
74. Brotman S, Marshall WJ. Complications from needle catheter jejunostomy in posttraumatic surgery. *Contemp Surg.* 1985;27:52–56.
75. Page CP, Bohnen JM, Fletcher JR, et al. Antimicrobial prophylaxis for surgical wounds. Guidelines for clinical care. *Arch Surg.* 1993;128:79–88.
76. Classen DC, Evans RS, Pestotnik SL, et al. The timing of prophylactic administration of antibiotics and the risk of surgical wound infection. *N Engl J Med.* 1992;30:281–286.
77. Ferguson MK. Postoperative management. In: Ferguson MK. *Reconstructive Surgery of the Esophagus.* Armonk, NY: Futura Publishing Company; 2002:285–305.
78. Foley MJ, Ghahremani GG, Rogers LF. Reappraisal of contrast media used to detect upper gastrointestinal perforations. *Radiology.* 1982;144:231–237.
79. Dodds WJ, Stewart ET, Vlymen WJ. Appropriate contrast media for evaluation of esophageal disruption. *Radiology.* 1982;144:439–441.
80. Phillips LG, Cunningham J. Esophageal perforation. *Radiol Clin N Am.* 1984; 22:607–613.
81. Levine MS. What is the best oral contrast agent to use for the fluoroscopic diagnosis of esophageal rupture? *AJR.* 1994;162:1243.
82. Fan ST, Lau WY, Yip WC, et al. Limitations and dangers of gastrografin swallow after esophageal and upper gastric operations. *Am J Surg.* 1988;155:495–497.
83. Goel AKK, Sinha S, Chattopadhyay TK. Role of gastrografin study in the assessment of anastomotic leaks from cervical oesophagogastric anastomosis. *Aust NZ J Surg.* 1995;65:8–10.
84. Tanomkiat W, Galassi W. Barium sulfate as contrast medium for evaluation of postoperative anastomotic leaks. *Acta Radiol.* 2000;41:482–485.
85. Swanson J, Levine M, Redfern R, et al. Usefulness of high-density barium for detection of leaks after esophagogastrectomy, total gastrectomy, and total laryngectomy. *AJR.* 2003;181:415–420.
86. Gollub MJ, Bains MS. Barium sulfate: a new (old) contrast agent for diagnosis of postoperative esophageal leaks. *Radiology.* 1997;202:360–362.
87. Upponi S, Ganeshan A, Slater A, et al. Imaging following surgery for oesophageal cancer. *Clin Radiol.* 2007;62:724–731.
88. Lee AY, Levine MN. Venous thromboembolism and cancer: risks and outcomes. *Circulation.* 2003;107:117–121.
89. Thodiyil PA, Walsh DC, Kakkar AK. Thromboprophylaxis in the cancer patient. *Acta Haematol.* 2001;106:73–80.
90. Svendsen E, Karwinski B. Prevalence of pulmonary embolism at necropsy in patients with cancer. *J Clin Pathol.* 1989;42:805–809.
91. Geerts WH, Pineo GF, Heit JA, et al. Prevention of venous thomboembolism: The Seventh ACCP Conference on Antithrombotic and Thrombolytic Therapy. *Chest.* 2004;126:338S–400S.
92. Baron JA, Gridley G, Weiderpass E, et al. Venous thromboembolism and cancer. *Lancet.* 1998;351:1077–1080.
93. Nordstrom M, Lindblad B, Anderson H, et al. Deep venous thrombosis and occult malignancy: an epidemiological study. *BMK.* 1994;308:891–894.
94. Sorensen HT, Mellemkjaer L, Olsen JH, et al. Prognosis of cancers associated with venous thromboembolism. *N Engl J Med.* 2000;343:1846–1850.
95. Ricles FR, Levine MN. Epidemiology of thrombosis in cancer. *Acta Haematol.* 2001;106:6–12.
96. Gallus AS. Prevention of postoperative deep leg vein thrombosis in patients with cancer. *Thromb Haemost.* 1997;78:126–132.
97. Bergqvist D. Venous thromboembolism and cancer: prevention of VTE. *Throm Res.* 2001;102:V209–V13.
98. Kakkar AK, Williamson RC. Prevention of venous thromboembolism in cancer patients. *Semin Thromb Hemost.* 1999;25:239–243.
99. ENOXACAN Study Group: Efficacy and safety of enoxaparin versus unfractionated heparin for prevention of deep vein thrombosis in elective cancer surgery: a double-blind randomized multicenter trial with venographic assessment. *Br J Surg.* 1997;84:1099–1103.
100. Bergqvist D, Agnelly G, Cohen AT, et al. Duration of prophylaxis against venous thromboembolism with enoxaparin after surgery for cancer. *N Engl J Med.* 2002;346:975–980.

77 Managing the Complications of Multimodality Therapy

Robert C. Miller
Andrew Y. Kee
David A. Schomas
Matthew J. Iott
Sumita Bhatia
Aminah Jatoi

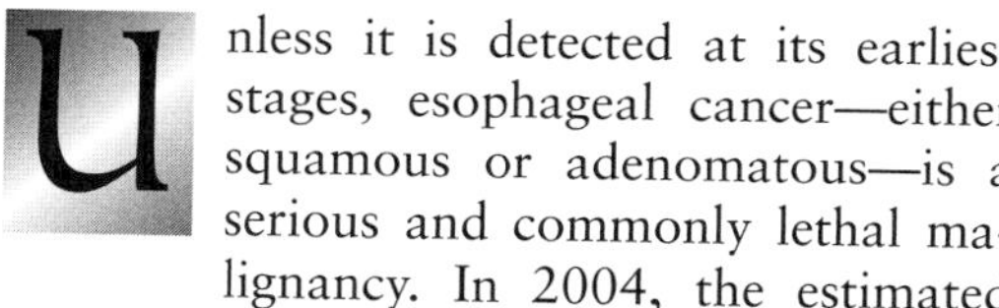

Unless it is detected at its earliest stages, esophageal cancer—either squamous or adenomatous—is a serious and commonly lethal malignancy. In 2004, the estimated incidence in the United States was 14,250 and the estimated mortality was 13,300. It is the seventh leading cause of cancer death among men in the United States, accounting for 4% of total male cancer deaths. In the 30 years after the early 1970s, 5-year overall survival for all stages of esophageal cancer improved, increasing from 5% to 8% ($P < .05$), but, with the high death rate, better treatment modalities are greatly needed (1).

Progress in the treatment of esophageal cancer with radiotherapy, chemotherapy, and surgery has been slow since the early 1980s. Regrettably, the majority of patients with esophageal cancer present with locally advanced disease involving tumors that either extend through the wall of the esophagus or involve regional lymph nodes or distant metastases. For patients without metastatic disease at diagnosis, trimodality therapy (radiotherapy, chemotherapy, and surgery) has gained increasing acceptance since the publication of the results of a randomized control trial in Dublin by Walsh et al. (2). The results showed a significant improvement in survival among patients receiving neoadjuvant radiotherapy and chemotherapy before resection compared with those who underwent only surgery. Previously, the Radiation Therapy Oncology Group (RTOG) had shown that radiotherapy in combination with chemotherapy had greater efficacy than radiotherapy alone in the treatment of locally advanced esophageal carcinoma (3). Although these studies did show improvement with greater intensity of therapy, the majority of the patients still succumbed to metastatic disease, often within a short period. However, a subset of long-term survivors after trimodality therapy or radiotherapy in combination with chemotherapy does demonstrate the utility of such treatment despite potential toxicity. The optimal sequencing of modalities, as well as the necessity of combining radiotherapy, chemotherapy, and surgery, remains to be determined. The majority of clinical trials reported to date have not had sufficient statistical power to convincingly answer this question (4). However, the early advances shown with the use of multiple modalities in the treatment of this malignant disease suggest that the use of intense treatment regimens will continue in the foreseeable future.

Although a greater intensity of therapy has improved long-term outcomes, it has been accompanied by considerable toxicity and, at times, higher mortality. The combination of radiotherapy, chemotherapy, and surgery can exacerbate the negative aspects of each modality. Patients undergoing trimodality therapy typically experience some measure of esophagitis, nausea, vomiting, decreased blood cell counts, and susceptibility to neutropenic infection, anorexia, weight loss, or other acute effects. In the long term, radiotherapy carries the risk of injury to the lungs, heart, spinal cord, vertebral bodies, small bowel, or other organs within the radiation field. Surgical excision of the tumor is a significant undertaking with its own associated morbidity and potential mortality, which may be exacerbated by other treatment modalities and patient comorbidities. This is well documented in reports from large randomized clinical trials.

The RTOG 85–01 trial compared a regimen of external beam radiotherapy (5,000 cGy) along with 5-fluorouracil (5-FU) (1,000 mg/m^2 of body surface area daily for 4 days) and cisplatin (75 mg/m^2 on the first day) with a regimen of radiotherapy alone (to a total dose of 6,400 cGy) in patients with squamous cell carcinoma or adenocarcinoma of the thoracic esophagus. More patients in the combined-modality group (33% vs. 18% of the patients who received only radiotherapy) experienced severe or life-threatening (grade 3 or 4) complications involving the upper aerodigestive tract in the acute phase of treatment and its aftermath. Grade 3 or 4 hematologic toxicity affected 48% in the combined-modality group and 3% in the radiotherapy-alone group. Overall, grade 4 toxicity was reported for 20% of the patients in the combined-modality group and for only 3% in the radiotherapy-alone group. Grade 3 toxicity was reported for 44% of the patients in the combined-modality group and for 25% in the radiotherapy-alone group. However, this increased toxicity in the combined-modality group was accompanied by an increase in survival at 2 years of 38% (vs. 10% for the radiotherapy-alone group) (5). In the long term, among patients receiving combined-modality therapy, 20% had grade 3 esophageal complications and 2% had grade 4 complications, and 4% had grade 3 hematologic toxicity and 2% had grade 4 toxicity. Long-term toxicity was similar, however, for esophageal injury in the radiotherapy-alone group, with 19% of the patients experiencing grade 3 or 4 toxicity (6).

The addition of combined-modality therapy before surgery clearly increases short-term patient morbidity, but whether this affects surgical morbidity and mortality is unclear. The results from the Medical Research Council esophageal cancer trial, as well as others, have not shown an increase in postoperative complications or postoperative deaths. The Medical Research Council study reported no statistically significant difference in nonfatal postoperative complications (overall rate, 41% in the combined-modality therapy group and 42% in the surgery-alone group). The rate of postoperative deaths was similar in both groups (10%), but 3% of the patients in the combined-modality therapy group did die before surgery could be undertaken. Reported toxicities in this trial are similar to those of the RTOG trial, with patients receiving combined-modality therapy experiencing neutropenia, mucositis, stomatitis or mouth ulcers, nausea, and vomiting (7).

The study by Walsh et al. (2) demonstrated similar, although less toxic, results. In that study, patients received 40 Gy of preoperative external beam radiotherapy along with 5-FU (15 mg/kg daily for 5 days) and cisplatin (75 mg/m^2 of body surface area on day 7 of weeks 1 and 6). Preoperatively, 10% of the patients in the multimodality regimen had grade 3 toxicity, as defined by the World Health Organization criteria, and 2 patients had grade 4 toxic reactions: one cardiac and the other involving the digestive tract. One patient had fatal bleeding due to tumor hemorrhage during combined-modality therapy. Postoperatively, the rates of respiratory complications and cardiac complications were similar between patients who received radiotherapy and chemotherapy preoperatively and those who did not. This study reported 5 deaths during hospitalization among the patients receiving combined-modality therapy and 2 postoperative deaths among patients undergoing surgery alone (2).

Less well documented are issues relating to patient quality of life, fatigue, depression, or financial concerns associated with the increase in intensity of therapy.

ESOPHAGITIS

Esophagitis is a common complication among esophageal cancer patients undergoing radiotherapy. With standard fractionation, the symptoms usually begin 2 to 4 weeks after the start of therapy; they can be very challenging to manage near the end of treatment. Patients with esophagitis initially present with dysphagia that requires dietary modifications. Malnutrition, dehydration, and the eventual need for a feeding tube occur in up to 74% of the patients during treatment (8). The degree of radiation-induced esophagitis is dependent on fractionation, total dose, volume of esophagus treated, and choice of chemotherapy.

Dysphagia and odynophagia are common initial symptoms in patients undergoing radiotherapy. Obtaining a thorough history is critical before attributing symptoms to esophagitis. Because the mean age of patients at diagnosis is 69 years, life-threatening causes such as cardiac ischemia need to be considered in the differential diagnosis (9). If dysphagia is attributed to radiation-induced esophagitis, the history and physical examination, including vital signs, are important for assessing the patient's nutritional and hydration status.

Patients with mild esophagitis are encouraged to consume adequate fluids and a relatively soft diet. Mild forms of pain medications may be necessary initially for dysphagia. Medications commonly used include Haddad's solution (mixture of equal parts of liquid simethicone, diphenhydramine, and lidocaine) and Capital's solution (acetaminophen, 120 mg, and codeine, 12 mg in 5 mL).

With higher doses of radiation, the esophageal mucosa continues to break down, creating areas of ulceration or pseudomembrane formation. Patients frequently report worsening dysphagia and pain, resulting in reduced oral intake of fluids and poorer nutrition. An average adult needs to consume 2 L of fluid per day to maintain adequate kidney function (10). Increased water intake is required in patients who are undergoing chemotherapy. A decrease in blood pressure with standing, reduced skin turgor, thirst, dizziness, and fatigue are common signs and symptoms of moderate to severe dehydration. Mild to moderate dehydration can be managed with better control of pain to improve oral intake. Stronger pain medications such as liquid oxycodone are commonly prescribed during this phase of esophagitis.

Patients with more severe dehydration often have orthostatic hypotension or dizziness (or both). Oral intake is further compromised by nausea and vomiting related to decreased profusion of vital organs. Intravenous fluid supplements must be provided on either an outpatient basis or an inpatient basis, depending on the severity and other comorbid health problems.

Patients' nutritional reserves are greater than their fluid reserves. A well-nourished adult can use nutritional reserves for up to 2 weeks before needing medical intervention. Nutrition is monitored and assessed weekly during radiotherapy. Patients who initially report solid food dysphagia due to their esophageal cancer commonly report improvement in their swallowing ability during the first half of their radiotherapy. As the absorbed radiation dose increases, the mucosal damage eventually leads to pain, gradual onset of dysphagia and odynophagia, and a resultant decrease in nutritional intake. Consultation with a dietitian and intake of a softer diet is the most common approach in initial management. Continued monitoring of the patient's weight throughout treatment is important in assessing the patient's nutritional status.

Placement of a percutaneous endoscopic jejunostomy (PEJ) or percutaneous endoscopic gastrostomy (PEG) tube should be considered for patients who frequently need intravenous hydration or who lose weight despite conservative intervention. Feeding tubes pose an increased risk of cellulitis, nausea and vomiting, and formula-associated diarrhea or constipation. Regular visits with a dietitian are necessary while using a feeding tube to ensure an adequate nutritional level. Patients continue to have treatment-related discomfort requiring pain medications. Some medications, such as oxycodone, are available as a liquid; medications that do not have a liquid form can be flushed with water. Long-acting pain medications, such as the fentanyl transdermal system, can be used for extended relief.

Parenteral nutrition is not recommended for patients with esophagitis alone. In a meta-analysis of 82 randomized controlled trials, the American Gastroenterological Association released a technical review of the clinical efficacy of parenteral nutrition (11). Subjects in 19 of the trials were oncology patients, with 3 trials involving radiotherapy. The meta-analysis discouraged parenteral nutrition since it does not alter the survival of patients receiving radiotherapy or chemotherapy and there appears to be a clinically significant risk of infectious complications.

The side effects of radiotherapy on nutrition and hydration continue for many weeks, with the most severe effects peaking between the last weeks of radiotherapy and 2 weeks after treatment. Patients should be counseled on the effects of esophagitis, with the expectation that adverse effects may continue for many weeks. Information on dehydration and malnutrition should be reviewed with symptoms that warrant medical attention. Esophageal cancer patients are prone to have many complications, so that a cooperative, integrated, multispecialty evaluation and management are needed to ensure that the patients receive the highest quality of care.

NAUSEA, VOMITING, AND DIARRHEA

Gastrointestinal tract toxicity manifesting as nausea, vomiting, or diarrhea affects most patients during treatment of esophageal cancer. Nausea, vomiting, or diarrhea of grade 2 or less are reported to occur in 56% to 94%, 56% to 93%, and 23% to 97% of patients, respectively. Nausea, vomiting, or diarrhea of grade 3 or 4 (severe toxicity) occur in 5% to 12%, 5% to 10%, and 1% to 4% of patients, respectively (2,5,12–15). Management of these side effects is crucial to the timely completion of therapy without treatment interruptions or deterioration in performance status.

Cisplatin has been classified as a high-risk (> 90%) emetogenic agent, and 5-FU has been classified as a low-risk (10%–30%) agent (16). Chemotherapy-induced nausea and vomiting has been classified as delayed, anticipatory, breakthrough, or acute (between 24 and 120 hours) (17). Initial nonpharmacologic procedures include avoidance of aggravating foods and use of oral rehydration. However, the following discussion focuses on pharmacologic treatments of acute nausea and vomiting.

There are 5 classes of pharmacologic agents used for the treatment of chemotherapy-induced nausea and vomiting: dopamine antagonists, corticosteroids, serotonin antagonists, neurokinin antagonists, and cannabinoids (Table 77.1). The current routine usually involves a combination of a serotonin antagonist, corticosteroids, and a neurokinin antagonist. The serotonin receptor antagonists such as ondansetron, granisetron, and dolasetron have equivalent efficacy and safety profiles and can be substituted for one another (17). The neurokinin antagonists are a new class of antiemetics. Aprepitant is the first member of this class to gain regulatory approval. This drug acts in the brainstem emetic center and in the gastrointestinal tract. Corticosteroids (dexamethasone and methylprednisolone) are also highly effective, especially in the prevention of chemotherapy-induced

TABLE 77.1
Summary of Antiemetic Regimens in Oncology

Recommendation category	Current recommendations
Specific emetic risk category	
High (>90%) emetic risk	The 3-drug combination of a 5-HT3 serotonin receptor antagonist, dexamethasone, and aprepitant is recommended before chemotherapy. For all patients receiving cisplatin and all other agents of high emetic risk, the 2-drug combination of dexamethasone and aprepitant is recommended. The Update Committee no longer recommends the combination of a 5-HT3 serotonin receptor antagonist and dexamethasone on days 2 and 3.
Moderate (>30%–90%) emetic risk	The 3-drug combination of a 5-HT3 serotonin receptor antagonist, dexamethasone, and aprepitant is recommended for patients receiving AC. For patients receiving chemotherapy of moderate emetic risk other than AC, the 2-drug combination of a 5-HT3 receptor serotonin antagonist and dexamethasone is recommended. For patients receiving AC, aprepitant as a single agent is recommended on days 2 and 3. For all other chemotherapies of moderate emetic risk, single-agent dexamethasone or a 5-HT3 serotonin receptor antagonist is suggested for the prevention of emesis on days 2 and 3.
Low (10%–30%) emetic risk	Dexamethasone, 8 mg, is suggested. No routine preventive use of antiemetics for delayed emesis is suggested.
Minimal (<10%) emetic risk	No change from the original guideline. No antiemetic should be administered routinely before or after chemotherapy.
Chemotherapy	
Combination chemotherapy	No change from the original guideline. Patients should receive antiemetics appropriate for the chemotherapeutic agent of greatest emetic risk.
Multiple consecutive days of chemotherapy	No change from the original guideline. It is suggested that antiemetics appropriate for the risk class of the chemotherapy, as outlined above, be administered for each day of the chemotherapy and for 2 days after, if appropriate.
Antiemetic agents	
Lower therapeutic index	For persons receiving chemotherapy of high emetic risk, there is no group of patients for whom agents of lower therapeutic index are appropriate first-choice antiemetics. These agents should be reserved for patients intolerant of or refractory to 5-HT3 serotonin receptor antagonists, NK1 receptor antagonists, and dexamethasone.
Adjunctive drugs	Lorazepam and diphenhydramine are useful adjuncts to antiemetic drugs but are not recommended as single agents.
Combinations of antiemetics	It is recommended that 5-HT3 serotonin receptor antagonists be administered with dexamethasone and aprepitant in patients receiving chemotherapy of high emetic risk and in patients receiving AC. A 5-HT3 serotonin receptor antagonist combined with dexamethasone should be used in patients receiving agents of moderate emetic risk other than AC.

Abbreviations: AC = anthracycline and cyclophosphamide; 5-HT3 = 5-hydroxytryptamine-3; NK1 = neurokin 1. From Kris et al (17). Used with permission.

emesis. Dexamethasone is valuable when administered in combination with a serotonin receptor antagonist and aprepitant when cisplatin is being administered. Other drugs such as benzodiazepines (lorazepam and alprazolam) and antihistamines (diphenhydramine) are useful adjuncts.

Current recommendations for patients receiving cisplatin are to administer serotonin receptor antagonists with dexamethasone and aprepitant (17). The American Society of Clinical Oncology recommendations recently changed for patients at least 24 hours after chemotherapy treatment from administering a combination of serotonin receptor antagonist and dexamethasone to administering the 2-drug combination of dexamethasone and aprepitant (17).

Complicating matters is the fact that nausea and vomiting are not only the result of chemotherapy but also the result of radiotherapy to the upper abdomen and esophagus. For radiation-induced nausea, serotonin receptor antagonists are the mainstay of treatment, and daily administration is recommended during radiotherapy (17).

The highest frequency of diarrhea occurs with bolus rather than infusional administration of 5-FU. Treatment should be tailored to the severity of the signs and symptoms. As appropriate, management should include hemodynamic support, parenteral nutrition, and antibiotics (Figure 77.1). Management should include nonpharmacologic and pharmacologic interventions to diminish diarrhea and clinical evaluations to assess fluid volume status. Initial nonpharmacologic procedures include avoidance of aggravating foods and oral rehydration.

Common pharmacologic interventions include the use of loperamide and diphenoxylate. Although both have a rapid onset of action, loperamide has been recommended in treatment guidelines for its superior effectiveness (18). Other second-line treatments are also available. Anticholinergic drugs can be effective but are not commonly used because of the unpleasant side-effect profile. They can, however, be useful to relieve cramping associated with diarrhea. Deodorized tincture of opium and paregoric (camphorated tincture of opium) are both effective antidiarrheals as well.

NUTRITIONAL SUPPORT

During the course of combined-modality treatment for esophagus cancer, it is necessary to monitor the patients' ability to maintain adequate hydration. As treatment-related side effects such as nausea, vomiting, diarrhea, esophagitis, and anorexia persist, patients are at increased risk of dehydration and poor nutrition. Nutritional status can affect patients' electrolyte balance, with the sequelae of symptoms associated with potentiating fluid volume depletion. Proper fluid intake, including water from food, is estimated at 1,600 mL per day. This is essential to preserving patients' hydration and subsequent quality of life during treatment. Therefore, fluid volume status should be closely observed.

Providers should obtain a detailed history along with a physical examination when assessing patients for dehydration and malnutrition. Typical noninvasive parameters for assessing and monitoring hydration status include mucous membrane moisture, skin turgor, capillary refill, orthostatic blood pressure, the amount and quality of urine output, thirst, and weight loss. Clinical manifestations of orthostatic hypotension may include symptoms such as dizziness, light-headedness or vertigo, fatigue, weakness, muscle spasms, quavering, headache, impaired cognition, blurred vision, nausea, and palpitations. The more severe symptoms of abdominal pain, chest pain, confusion, and lethargy can also occur. It is important to remember that elderly patients' signs and symptoms of dehydration may be nonspecific. As signs and symptoms of dehydration develop, fluid volume deficits should be replaced in a timely manner. The best avenue for rehydration in patients who have treatment-related side effects is intravenous infusion (19).

The type of intravenous fluid used for fluid replacement depends on the provider's preference in addition to the likely electrolyte deficiencies. Patients who are hypernatremic may need dextrose in water or hypotonic saline solutions depending on the suspected source of water loss. Isotonic or hypertonic saline fluid may be necessary for patients who are hyponatremic. Along with fluid replacement, potassium supplementation may be necessary. The amount and rapidity of intravenous fluid replacement depend on the patients' cardiac status as well as overall health status (20).

The decision to place a feeding tube before or during the initiation of combined-modality therapy can be problematic. Most patients have some degree of dysphagia or odynophagia at the time of consultation. They will experience relief of dysphagia during radiotherapy and chemotherapy, with an increased ability to take in solids and liquids midway through the course of radiotherapy. However, this is accompanied by treatment-related esophagitis, anorexia, and other adverse effects that may make intake of adequate calories problematic.

Our current practice is to seek a multispecialty consultation with gastroenterology, medical oncology, radiation oncology, thoracic surgery, and possibly nutritional support professionals before the initiation of external beam radiotherapy and chemotherapy. At that time, the decision is made on whether to place an enteral feeding tube before treatment. Typically, the decision is based on an assessment of the patient's performance status, daily caloric intake, and degree of weight loss. Patients

Cancer treatment–induced diarrhea

Uncomplicated
CTC grade 1 or 2 diarrhea with no complicating signs or symptoms

Nonspecific management
- Stop intake of all lactose-containing products, alcohol, and high-osmolar supplements
- Drink 8-10 large glasses of clear liquids a day (eg, sports drinks, broth)
- Eat frequent small meals (eg, bananas, rice, applesauce, toast, plain pasta)
- Record the number of stools and report symptoms of life-threatening sequelae (eg, fever or dizziness on standing)
- For grade 2 diarrhea, hold cytotoxic chemotherapy until symptoms resolve and consider dose reduction

Specific treatment
- Administer standard dosage of loperamide: initial dose, 4 mg; then 2 mg every 4 h or after every unformed stool
- Consider clinical trial participation

Reassess in 12-24 h

Diarrhea unresolved

Diarrhea resolving
- Continue to follow instructions for dietary modification
- Gradually add solid foods to diet
- Discontinue use of loperamide after 12-h diarrhea-free interval

RT-induced: continue use of loperamide

Persistent diarrhea (CTC grade 1 or 2)
- Administer loperamide, 2 mg every 2 h
- Administer oral antibiotics
- Observe patient for response

RT-induced: oral antibiotics not generally recommended

Reassess in 12-24 h

Diarrhea unresolved

Diarrhea resolved
- Continue to follow instructions for dietary modification
- Gradually add solid foods to diet
- Discontinue use of loperamide after 12-h diarrhea-free interval

RT-induced: continue use of loperamide

Persistent diarrhea (CTC grade 1 or 2) (no fever, dehydration, neutropenia, or blood in stool)

Evaluate in office or outpatient center
- Check stool work-up (blood, fecal leukocytes, *Clostridium difficile, Salmonella, Escherichia coli, Campylobacter*, infectious colitis)
- Check CBC and electrolytes
- Perform abdominal examination
- Replace fluids and electrolytes as appropriate
- Discontinue use of loperamide and begin second-line agent
  - Octreotide (100-150 mcg SC TID, with dose escalation up to 500 mcg TID)
  - Other second-line agent (eg, tincture of opium)

RT-induced: continue use of loperamide or other oral agent; no work-up required

Complicated
CTC grade 3 or 4 diarrhea or grade 1 or 2 with ≥1 of the following signs or symptoms:
- Cramping
- Nausea/vomiting (≥grade 2)
- Decreased performance status
- Fever
- Sepsis
- Neutropenia
- Frank bleeding
- Dehydration

Progression to severe diarrhea (CTC grade 3 or 4 with or without fever, dehydration, neutropenia, or blood in stool)

Admit to hospital*
- Administer octreotide (100-150 mcg SC TID, or 25-50 mcg/h IV if dehydration is severe, with dose escalation up to 500 mcg TID)
- Administer IV fluids and antibiotics as needed (eg, fluoroquinolone)
- Stool work-up, CBC, and electrolyte profile
- Discontinue cytotoxic chemotherapy until all symptoms resolve; resume chemotherapy at reduced dose

who have lost more than 10% to 15% of their weight because of the tumor and who have evidence of malnutrition should be particularly evaluated for intervention. Any decision to place a feeding tube should be made in conjunction with the patient's thoracic surgeon to avoid compromising the planned resection and future anastomosis. Initially, radiographically assisted placement of a PEJ feeding tube is considered; if this is unsuccessful or not feasible, surgical placement is an option. If necessary, a PEG tube can be considered, but the exact placement of the tube must be carefully considered to avoid future difficulty with surgery. For patients who experience nausea and vomiting that is not manageable with medications, consideration should be given to placement of a feeding tube if these symptoms cannot be controlled with oral or intravenous antiemetics and if the patient cannot be adequately rehydrated with intravenous fluids. Additionally, refractory esophagitis, odynophagia, or dysphagia should also lead to consideration of a feeding tube if the patient has significant weight loss (> 10%) and other conservative measures fail. The majority of patients should be able to tolerate treatment with a combination of aggressive oral antiemetics as outlined above.

CHRONIC TOXICITY ISSUES

Cardiac complications after radiotherapy are well documented for various diseases such as breast cancer and Hodgkin's disease. The correlation between chronic radiation injury and heart complications in patients with esophageal cancer is complicated by the overall poor prognosis, making this a less critical issue when compared with treating young patients with curable diseases. However, this is still an issue of concern in combined-modality therapy for patients with esophageal cancer (either with primary therapy or with neoadjuvant or adjuvant therapy). This can be particularly difficult in lower esophageal and gastroesophageal junction tumors in which the tumor itself lies directly behind the cardiac ventricles. In these situations, conformal or intensity-modulated radiotherapy can decrease the dose delivered to the myocardium but make it impossible to completely avoid irradiation of the heart itself. Once again, although there is not a great deal of prospective evidence showing cardiac injury with esophageal irradiation, extrapolation from other studies does point out this risk. A study by Jagsi et al. (21) from the University of Michigan included 828 patients who received radiotherapy for breast cancer over a 16-year period. The 10-year cumulative myocardial infarction rates were 2.7% for left-sided irradiation in which the heart was potentially treated and 1.2% for right-sided breast cancer. The overall incidence reported was low compared with more closely followed populations because of the methodology of this study, but it does illustrate the increased risk of cardiotoxicity with cardiac irradiation. Additional findings of increased risk are well documented with Hodgkin's lymphoma irradiation as demonstrated by Hancock et al. (22) and others (23,24). A prospective study by Marks et al. (25) has demonstrated the use of myocardial scintigraphy and echocardiograms to identify left ventricular abnormalities after irradiation.

A more pressing concern in both the short term and the long term is pneumonitis. Radiation pneumonitis typically occurs between several weeks and 6 months after the conclusion of thoracic radiotherapy. It probably occurs in 5% to 15% of patients treated definitively for lung cancer with life-threatening pneumonitis developing in a minority of those patients. It is characterized by a dry cough, dyspnea, and a characteristic infiltrate on computed tomography or chest radiography conforming to but not limited to the radiation portal. Occasionally, the reaction can be severe and proceed to acute respiratory distress syndrome. An increased white blood cell count and sedimentation rate may be noted. These findings can often make differentiation from infectious pneumonia difficult, although both entities can coexist at the same time. The development of the inflammatory response associated with a lung infection may contribute to the cytokine cascade accompanying and propagating radiation pneumonitis. Lung cancer patients are at risk of recurrent lung infections even without lung radiotherapy, so the differential diagnosis is broad for a patient with dyspnea and radiographic abnormalities that develop after lung radiotherapy. Patients should be adequately treated for pneumonia when presenting with "radiation pneumonitis" and a complete pulmonary work-up is in order.

FIGURE 77.1

(See facing page) American Society of Clinical Oncology anti-diarrheal guidelines. Asterisk indicates that intensive outpatient management should be considered for radiation-induced diarrhea and for select patients with chemotherapy-induced diarrhea unless the patient has sepsis, fever, or neutropenia. CBC = complete blood cell count; CTC = common toxicity criteria; IV = intravenous; mcg = micrograms; RT = radiotherapy; SC = subcutaneous; TID = 3 times per day. (Modified from Kornblau S, Benson AB III, Catalano R, et al. Management of cancer treatment–related diarrhea: issues and therapeutic strategies. *J Pain Symptom Manage*. 2000;19:118–129. Used with permission.)

Bronchoscopy with bronchoalveolar lavage, bacterial and fungal cultures, and biopsies should be considered before committing the patient to long-term treatment for a presumed diagnosis of pneumonitis due to radiotherapy. Treatment for mild cases consists simply of observation. Pulmonary symptoms typically resolve over 1 to 3 months. For more severe cases, long-term treatment with prednisone may be indicated. Prednisone should be given initially at 60 to 100 mg per day and continued until the symptoms improve. A very slow taper should be considered: decrease the daily dosage by 10 mg per week, to 20 to 40 mg; then decrease the daily dosage by 10 mg every other week; then decrease it to 5 mg per day for 2 weeks; then decrease it to 5 mg every other day for 2 weeks; and then stop the use of prednisone. If the dosage is tapered too quickly, patients may have a recurrence of symptoms. Consideration should be given to pneumocystis pneumonia prophylaxis with trimethoprim-sulfamethoxazole during long-term treatment with corticosteroids.

With the widespread use of 3-dimensional treatment planning, dose-volume histograms for estimating the risk of symptomatic pneumonitis have become an integral part of the field design. Graham et al. (26) reviewed pneumonitis incidence in relation to various dosimetric parameters in 99 patients. They concluded that the percentage of lung volume that received a dose greater than 20 Gy (V20) best reflected the risk of radiation pneumonitis. A strong correlation was noted between the severity of pneumonitis and higher V20 values. No fatal pneumonitic events were noted with a V20 less than 32%. The incidence of events rated grade 3 to 5 increased to 23% with a V20 greater than 40% (Table 77.2). The authors concluded that plans with V20 values of 35% to 40% should not be used. Tsujino et al. (27), from Hyogo Hospital in Japan, reported similar results. The only predictive factor for pneumonitis of grade 2 or greater in that study was V20. However, most recent reports have emphasized the importance of the volume of lung receiving doses in the range of 10 to 13 Gy having a greater importance in predicting pneumonitis, which may have a greater influence on radiotherapy delivery in esophageal cancer (28–30).

TABLE 77.2
Incidence of Radiation Pneumonitis as a Function of Lung V20

	Incidence of pneumonitis, %	
V20, %	**Grade 2**	**Grades 3–5**
<22	0	0
22–31	8	8
32–40	13	5 (1 was grade 5)
>40	19	23 (3 were grade 5)

V20 = lung volume that received a dose >20 Gy. From Graham et al (26). Used with permission.

CHEMOTHERAPY COMPLICATIONS

Since complications relating to chemotherapy administration are varied, reflecting the choice of agents used during multimodality therapy, a comprehensive review of potential toxicities is not possible in this chapter. However, in practice, the combination of 5-FU and cisplatin is often used in this setting, since it perhaps carries the longest track record of use with irradiation. As a result of receiving these chemotherapy agents, patients can experience some degree of fatigue, nausea and vomiting, mucositis, esophagitis, diarrhea, myelosuppression with attendant risk of neutropenia and fevers, and, occasionally, hearing loss and peripheral neuropathy. It should be noted that rates of hospitalization vary among medical centers, but a large subset of patients—approximately 40%—appear to require hospitalization during such concomittant therapy (31–33).

SURGICAL COMPLICATIONS AFTER MULTIMODALITY THERAPY

An increase in surgical complications soon after neoadjuvant radiotherapy and chemotherapy has not been demonstrated in the limited data available from large-scale clinical trials and other studies (34). Later, pulmonary fibrosis and other chronic radiotherapy changes can lead to an increased risk of injury with attempts at resection. In addition, fibrotic responses at sites of tumors responding to neoadjuvant therapy can make dissection difficult when this fibrosis involves critical mediastinal structures. Anastamotic leaks, bleeding, chylothorax, tracheobronchial injury, and other intrathoracic injuries are risks for patients after multimodality therapy or after surgery alone, with anastamotic leaks being the most common technical injury. Medical complications of surgery include bleeding, arrhythmias, pneumonia, and alcohol withdrawal. Patients who undergo resection of proximal tumors may be at higher risk of surgical morbidity than those with distal tumors. Patients receiving a higher dose of radiotherapy to normal lung tissues during neoadjuvant therapy can have a higher risk of postoperative injury. Careful preoperative planning and evaluation can identify patients at risk of postoperative cardiac and pulmonary risk factors because of preexisting medical conditions and smoking habits (30,35–37).

QUALITY OF LIFE AFTER MULTIMODALITY THERAPY

Quality-of-life research in esophageal cancer has been modest despite the negative effect that esophageal cancer can have from dysphagia and esophageal obstruction due to local progression and from other symptoms due to regional and metastatic progression (38–40).

Therapy for esophageal carcinomas, whether surgery, chemotherapy, or radiotherapy (or a combination), is characterized by somatic discomfort and loss of function, both acutely and chronically. Patients reported significant negative changes in quality of life in the 1-year period after treatment but typically showed improvement with time in the absence of tumor progression (41). Although various reports have been published describing the effect of surgical intervention on quality of life, few reports correlate quality of life with outcomes and survival (42,43). A report from Taiwan of 110 patients with squamous cell carcinoma correlated dysphagia scores with overall survival but did not correlate survival with other quality-of-life measures (44). Absent from these reports are multidimensional analyses correlating quality-of-life measures with patient demographics, tumor characteristics, and multiple treatment interventions. In particular, further research in assessing the effect of neoadjuvant chemotherapy or radiotherapy on quality of life would be of clinical utility for practitioners because of the potential toxicity of such treatments in conjunction with their disputed clinical benefits (45,46).

References

1. Jemal A, Tiwari RC, Murray T, et al, American Cancer Society. Cancer statistics, 2004. *CA Cancer J Clin*. 2004;54:8–29.
2. Walsh TN, Noonan N, Hollywood D, et al. A comparison of multimodal therapy and surgery for esophageal adenocarcinoma. *N Engl J Med*. 1996;335:462–467. Erratum in: *N Engl J Med*. 1999;341:384.
3. Cooper JS, Guo MD, Herskovic A, et al., Radiation Therapy Oncology Group. Chemoradiotherapy of locally advanced esophageal cancer: long-term follow-up of a prospective randomized trial (RTOG 85–01). *JAMA*. 1999;281:1623–1627.
4. Enzinger PC, Mayer RJ. Esophageal cancer. *N Engl J Med*. 2003;349:2241–2252.
5. Herskovic A, Martz K, al-Sarraf M, et al. Combined chemotherapy and radiotherapy compared with radiotherapy alone in patients with cancer of the esophagus. *N Engl J Med*. 1992;326:1593–1598.
6. al-Sarraf M, Martz K, Herskovic A, et al. Progress report of combined chemoradiotherapy versus radiotherapy alone in patients with esophageal cancer: an intergroup study. *J Clin Oncol*. 1997;15:277–284. Erratum in: *J Clin Oncol*. 1997;15:866.
7. Medical Research Council Oesophageal Cancer Working Group. Surgical resection with or without preoperative chemotherapy in oesophageal cancer: a randomised controlled trial. *Lancet*. 2002;359:1727–1733.
8. Heath EI, Burtness BA, Heitmiller RF, et al. Phase II evaluation of preoperative chemoradiation and postoperative adjuvant chemotherapy for squamous cell and adenocarcinoma of the esophagus. *J Clin Oncol*. 2000;18:868–876.
9. Ries LAG, Melbert D, Krapcho M, et al. *SEER Cancer Statistics Review, 1975–2004*. Bethesda, M.D.: National Cancer Institute. (Accessed August 27, 2007, at http://seer.cancer.gov/csr/1975_2004/.)
10. Rose B, Post TW, eds. *Clinical Physiology of Acid-Base and Electrolyte Disorders*. 5th ed. New York: McGraw-Hill, 2001:285–287.
11. Koretz RL, Lipman TO, Klein S, et al. American Gastroenterological Association [AGA] technical review on parenteral nutrition. *Gastroenterology*. 2001;121:970–1001.
12. Minsky BD, Pajak TF, Ginsberg RJ, et al. INT 0123 (Radiation Therapy Oncology Group 94–05) phase III trial of combined-modality therapy for esophageal cancer: high-dose versus standard-dose radiation therapy. *J Clin Oncol*. 2002;20:1167–1174.
13. Bedenne L, Michel P, Bouché O, et al. Chemoradiation followed by surgery compared with chemoradiation alone in squamous cancer of the esophagus: FFCD 9102. *J Clin Oncol*. 2007;25:1160–1168.
14. Burmeister BH, Smithers BM, Gebski V, et al., Trans-Tasman Radiation Oncology Group, Australasian Gastro-Intestinal Trials Group. Surgery alone versus chemoradiotherapy followed by surgery for resectable cancer of the oesophagus: a randomised controlled phase III trial. *Lancet Oncol*. 2005;6:659–668.
15. Cunningham D, Allum WH, Stenning SP, et al, MAGIC Trial Participants. Perioperative chemotherapy versus surgery alone for resectable gastroesophageal cancer. *N Engl J Med*. 2006;355:11–20.
16. Grunberg SM, Osoba D, Hesketh PJ, et al. Evaluation of new antiemetic agents and definition of antineoplastic agent emetogenicity: an update. *Support Care Cancer*. 2005 Feb;13:80–84. Epub December 14, 2004.
17. Kris MG, Hesketh PJ, Somerfield MR, et al, American Society of Clinical Oncology. American Society of Clinical Oncology guideline for antiemetics in oncology: update 2006. *J Clin Oncol*. 2006;24:2932–2947. Epub May 22, 2006. Erratum in: *J Clin Oncol*. 2006;24:5341–5342.
18. Benson AB III, Ajani JA, Catalano RB, et al. Recommended guidelines for the treatment of cancer treatment-induced diarrhea. *J Clin Oncol*. 2004;22:2918–2926.
19. Post TW, Rose BD. Clinical manifestations and diagnosis of volume depletion in adults. Waltham, MA: UpToDate. (Accessed August 31, 2007, at http://uptodateonline.com/utd/content/topic.do?topicKey=fldlytes/13927&selectedTitle=1~465&source=search_result.)
20. Rose BD. Maintenance and replacement fluid therapy in adults. Waltham, MA: UpToDate. (Accessed August 31, 2007, at http://uptodateonline.com/utd/content/topic.do?topicKey=fldlytes/13345&selectedTitle=1~4920&source=search_result.)
21. Jagsi R, Griffith KA, Koelling T, et al. Rates of myocardial infarction and coronary artery disease and risk factors in patients treated with radiation therapy for early-stage breast cancer. *Cancer*. 2007;109:650–657.
22. Hancock SL, Donaldson SS, Hoppe RT. Cardiac disease following treatment of Hodgkin's disease in children and adolescents. *J Clin Oncol*. 1993;11:1208–1215.
23. Aleman BM, van den Belt-Dusebout AW, De Bruin ML, et al. Late cardiotoxicity after treatment for Hodgkin lymphoma. *Blood*. 2007;109:1878–1886. Epub November 21, 2006.
24. Mauch PM, Kalish LA, Marcus KC, et al. Long-term survival in Hodgkin's disease relative impact of mortality, second tumors, infection, and cardiovascular disease. *Cancer J Sci Am*. 1995;1:33–42.
25. Marks LB, Yu X, Prosnitz RG, et al. The incidence and functional consequences of RT-associated cardiac perfusion defects. *Int J Radiat Oncol Biol Phys*. 2005;63:214–223.
26. Graham MV, Purdy JA, Emami B, et al. Clinical dose-volume histogram analysis for pneumonitis after 3D treatment for non-small cell lung cancer (NSCLC). *Int J Radiat Oncol Biol Phys*. 1999;45:323–329.
27. Tsujino K, Hirota S, Endo M, et al. Predictive value of dose-volume histogram parameters for predicting radiation pneumonitis after concurrent chemoradiation for lung cancer. *Int J Radiat Oncol Biol Phys*. 2003;55:110–115.
28. Seppenwoolde Y, Lebesque JV, de Jaeger K, et al. Comparing different NTCP models that predict the incidence of radiation pneumonitis: normal tissue complication probability. *Int J Radiat Oncol Biol Phys*. 2003;55:724–735.
29. Schallenkamp JM, Miller RC, Brinkmann DH, et al. Incidence of radiation pneumonitis after thoracic irradiation: dose-volume correlates. *Int J Radiat Oncol Biol Phys*. 2007;67:410–416.
30. Lee HK, Vaporciyan AA, Cox JD, et al. Postoperative pulmonary complications after preoperative chemoradiation for esophageal carcinoma: correlation with pulmonary dose-volume histogram parameters. *Int J Radiat Oncol Biol Phys*. 2003;57:1317–1322.
31. Pizzo PA. Management of fever in patients with cancer and treatment-induced neutropenia. *N Engl J Med*. 1993;328:1323–1332.
32. Hughes WT, Armstrong D, Bodey GP, et al. 2002 guidelines for the use of antimicrobial agents in neutropenic patients with cancer. *Clin Infect Dis*. 2002;34:730–751. Epub February 13, 2002.
33. Smith TJ, Khatcheressian J, Lyman GH, et al. 2006 update of recommendations for the use of white blood cell growth factors: an evidence-based clinical practice guideline. *J Clin Oncol*. 2006;24:3187–3205. Epub May 8, 2006.
34. Rice DC, Correa AM, Vaporciyan AA, et al. Preoperative chemoradiotherapy prior to esophagectomy in elderly patients is not associated with increased morbidity. *Ann Thorac Surg*. 2005;79:391–397.
35. Putnam JB Jr. Complications of multimodality therapy. *Chest Surg Clin N Am*. 1998;8:663–680.
36. Doty JR, Salazar JD, Forastiere AA, et al. Postesophagectomy morbidity, mortality, and length of hospital stay after preoperative chemoradiation therapy. *Ann Thorac Surg*. 2002;74:227–231.
37. Hölscher AH, Vallböhmer D, Brabender J. The prevention and management of perioperative complications. *Best Pract Res Clin Gastroenterol*. 2006;20:907–923.
38. Headrick JR, Nichols FC III, Miller DL, et al. High-grade esophageal dysplasia: long-term survival and quality of life after esophagectomy. *Ann Thorac Surg*. 2002;73:1697–1702.

39. McDougall NI, Johnston BT, Kee F, et al. Natural history of reflux oesophagitis: a 10 year follow up of its effect on patient symptomatology and quality of life. *Gut.* 1996;38:481–486.
40. Kuster GG, Foroozan P. Early diagnosis of adenocarcinoma developing in Barrett's esophagus. *Arch Surg.* 1989;124:925–927.
41. Blazeby JM, Sanford E, Falk SJ, et al. Health-related quality of life during neoadjuvant treatment and surgery for localized esophageal carcinoma. *Cancer.* 2005;103:1791–1799.
42. Deschamps C, Nichols FC III, Cassivi SD, et al. Long-term function and quality of life after esophageal resection for cancer and Barrett's. *Surg Clin North Am.* 2005;85:649–656, xi.
43. Blazeby JM, Kavadas V, Vickery CW, et al. A prospective comparison of quality of life measures for patients with esophageal cancer. *Qual Life Res.* 2005;14:387–393.
44. Fang FM, Tsai WL, Chiu HC, et al. Quality of life as a survival predictor for esophageal squamous cell carcinoma treated with radiotherapy. *Int J Radiat Oncol Biol Phys.* 2004;58:1394–1404.
45. Miller RC, Atherton PJ, Kabat B, et al. Assessment of quality of life in patients with esophageal cancer after combined modality therapy [abstract]. Presented at the 14th annual meeting of the Federation of European Cancer Societies, Barcelona, Spain, September 2007 *Eur J Cancer.* 2007.
46. Miller RC, Atherton PJ, Kabat B, et al. Assessment of quality of life in patients with esophageal cancer after combined modality therapy [abstract]. *Int J Radiat Oncol Biol Phys.* 2007;69 Suppl:S584.

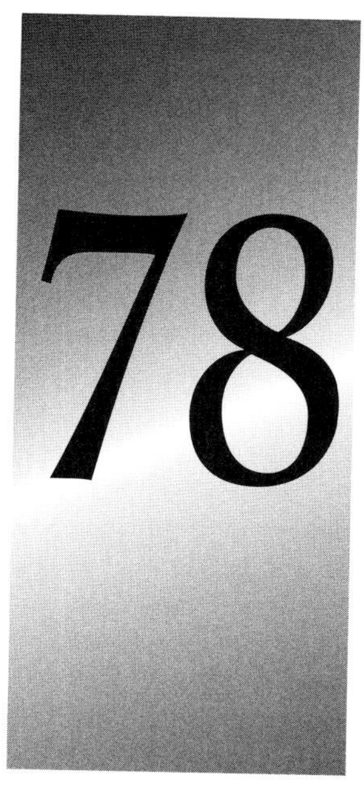

Postoperative Care and Management of the Complications of Surgical Therapy

Kai Engstad
Paul Henry Schipper

The first esophagectomy was performed by Franz Torek on March 14, 1913. However, widespread success with esophagectomy did not occur until the 1940s. Most reported operative series during the 1950s and 1960s focus on technique but do not systematically report mortality or morbidity, which were high. Contemporary mortalities range from 0.5% to 10% (1–8). These mortalities are strikingly lower than those achieved during the early history of esophageal surgery. The evolution of esophageal surgery has in large part been the development of techniques to avoid complications and to reduce the severity of complications when they do occur.

In 1,700 esophagectomies performed at multiple Veterans Administration hospitals between 1991 and 2001 and reported in the National Surgical Quality Improvement Program (NSQIP) database, there was a 10% mortality rate and a 50% morbidity rate. The most common postoperative complications in this series were pneumonia in 21%, ventilator dependence > 48 hours in 22%, and unplanned reintubation in 16% (9). In 2006, 1,665 esophagectomies were submitted to the Society of Thoracic Surgery General Thoracic Database, spanning a time period from January 2002 to June 2006. In this database, the most common postoperative complication was "atrial arrhythmia requiring therapy" in 15.7%. Second was anastamotic leak in 9.7%, followed by reintubation 7.6%, pneumonia 6.6%, wound infection 4.2%, and tracheostomy 3.5%. Less common complications were myocardial infarction, pulmonary embolism, deep venous thrombosis, renal failure, chylothorax, recurrent laryngeal nerve palsy, gastric outlet obstruction, and urinary tract infection. It is clear from these lists that the most common complications of esophageal surgery are the most common complications of thoracic surgery in general, namely atrial arrhythmia and pulmonary. This chapter will discuss the management of these complications.

PULMONARY

The most common complications post esophagectomy in the VA NSQIP study were pneumonia and pulmonary related (unplanned re-intubation and ventilator dependence > 48 hours) (9). In the STS database re-intubation and pneumonia were the second and third most common morbidity.

Ferguson et al. showed that post esophagectomy, pneumonia, prolonged ventilation, and respiratory failure were significant predictors of mortality (10). D'Amico et al. have shown that developing pneumonia post esophagectomy resulted in a 20% mortality, quadruple the rate of those not developing pneumonia (11). In a review of the literature examining the relation of pneumonia to mortality, 50% to 100% of reported mortalities post esophagectomy involved pulmonary complications (11). Pulmonary complications not only affect survival in the perioperative period but long-term survival. Kinugasa found a 27% 5-year survival in patients experiencing pneumonia post esophagectomy versus 53% in those who did not (12).

As with many complications, treatment begins with prevention and the appropriate and tailored selection of operative approach. The rate of pulmonary complications post transhiatal esophagectomy is less than the rate post transthoracic esophagectomy. Orringer et al. reported a 3% rate of pneumonia after transhiatal esophagectomy (13). The Mayo Clinic experience with Ivor-Lewis esophagectomy reported a 12.3% rate of pneumonia (14). A meta-analysis performed by Hulscher et al. looked at 24 papers comparing the transhiatal to the transthoracic esophagectomy. He found a 50% increased risk of pulmonary complications in the transthoracic approach (15,16).

Preoperatively, patients should be evaluated for their risk of pulmonary complications. A history probing for exercise tolerance, cigarette smoking, and respiratory symptoms is taken. Preoperative chest radiographs and computed tomography (CT) scans are examined not only for the esophagus and lymph nodes with an eye toward staging but also for the character of the lung parenchyma for emphysema or other pathology. If there is any question of respiratory insufficiency, pulmonary function testing is obtained. Accompanying a patient on a stair-climbing exercise can give invaluable information. A patient who ascends 4 flights of stairs with ease is unlikely to be at increased risk of pulmonary complications. Patients who are current smokers should be counseled to quit and offered the pharmacologic and follow-up assistance necessary to successfully quit. The risk of complications post thoracic surgery in non-smokers is less than the risk of complications in smokers. It is not well established how long someone has to be a non-smoker to obtain this risk reduction and the risk of pulmonary complications may increase in the first 2 weeks after quitting. Stopping cigarettes for at least 4 weeks prior to surgery is advised (17,18).

Preoperative counseling on incentive spirometry (including giving the patient an inspirometer on which to practice), early ambulation, and the importance of good pain control and coughing post esophagectomy can recruit the patient and their family as an ally against pneumonia and pulmonary complications. A preoperative program of pulmonary rehabilitation may reduce postoperative pulmonary complications, especially in high-risk patients (19,20).

Postoperatively, esophagectomy patients require extra attention to their pulmonary status. Pain should be controlled via either epidural or IV PCA (21,22). Patients should be up to a chair the evening of or the morning after the procedure with ambulation shortly thereafter. The average hospital length of stay ranges from 10 to 15 days. Patients should ambulate 4 times a day every one of these days. Pulmonary protocols can be developed utilizing available resources, such as respiratory therapy, pulmonary rehabilitation, specialized nursing, and physical therapy. An observant and involved physician and surgeon, however, are required to "keep the wheels on the wagon."

Because of the risk of aspiration and the subsequent pneumonia, attention to laryngeal-pharyngeal function as detailed below is important in preventing pneumonia.

LARYNGOPHARYNGEAL DYSFUNCTION AFTER ESOPHAGECTOMY

There are multiple factors that lead to postoperative respiratory complications, most of which are common to many thoracic procedures: bleeding, pain, pulmonary toilet, preoperative pulmonary function, and so on. The most common specific cause of pulmonary morbidity after esophagectomy, however, is laryngotracheal dysfunction. This refers to a broad range of disorders including those of swallowing, airway protection, and speech. Commonly, these problems are attributed to recurrent laryngeal nerve injury.

The recurrent laryngeal nerve provides sensory innervation to the pharynx and motor innervation to the cricopharyngeous. Denervation results in insufficient glottic closure during swallowing with resultant aspiration and dysphagia. Vocal cord immobility associated with these injuries also predisposes patients to frank aspiration, decreased cough strength, and pulmonary complications. Superior laryngeal nerve injuries, particularly after intervention on the cervical esophagus, are often underestimated. The superior laryngeal nerve is responsible for tension of the vocal cord and sensory innervation of the upper larynx, and injury to the nerve classically results in voice fatigue but also has been shown to result in pharyngeal fatigue during repetitive swallowing. This dysfunction is often hard to demonstrate clinically or on routine testing.

Examination of the literature to determine the true incidence of injury after esophageal resection is difficult. Most studies include patients who have clinical signs of injury; however, it is estimated that 30% to 50% of patients sustaining injury may be asymptomatic. Studies using direct laryngoscopy have demonstrated rates of 15% to 30% of postoperative vocal cord paralysis. Most of these were associated with a cervical anastomosis. In the same series, 50% of patients with nerve injury went on to develop respiratory complications. Of those without evidence of nerve injury, the pulmonary complication rate was still 30%. High levels of aspiration (47%) and swallowing difficulties (67%) have been demonstrated in patients after transhiatal esophagectomy, and failure of symptom improvement in patients having had medialization procedures for vocal cord paralysis suggest a more complex pathophysiology than simply nerve injury.

Based on the subtlety of presentation, high incidence, and potential for significant morbidity, a high index of suspicion should be had for these injuries. Clinical evaluation also appears unreliable. If one considers that dysfunction is a result of both motor and sensory denervation, then tests that directly evaluate these 2 factors should be most accurate in the detection of abnormalities in swallowing. One such test is fiberoptic endoscopic evaluation of swallowing with sensory testing (FEESST). Both videofluoroscopic swallow study (VFSS) and modified barium swallow with fiberoptic endoscopic evaluation of swallowing (FEES) are considered equivalent in evaluation of the motor mechanics of swallowing but only indirectly assess sensory function. Routine contrast esophagography as used to evaluate the patient for postoperative anastomotic leak is probably insufficiently sensitive to adequately evaluate for aspiration.

As many patients presenting for esophageal resection may have swallowing dysfunction, some authors have recommended preoperative evaluation to identify patients at high risk and to apply speech therapy preoperatively to help prevent postoperative complications.

In the operating room, prevention of these injuries is key to avoid postoperative problems. Avoiding retractor placement in the tracheoesophageal groove, meticulous dissection of the cervical esophagus, and identification of the recurrent laryngeal nerve should serve to minimize injuries.

In the early postoperative period, early assessment of swallowing is advised. The morbidity of pneumonia after esophagectomy is significant and rivals that of anastomotic leak. Evaluation by VFSS, FEES, or FEEST will help guide clinicians as to when and if oral intake may be safely instituted. When new or persistent abnormalities of swallowing are detected, specific measures to improve swallowing and airway control may be instituted. These include speech therapy and interventions such as using a chin tuck maneuver, shown to decrease aspiration in over 80% of patients with aspiration.

When vocal cord paralysis is diagnosed, then vocal cord medialization should be performed, especially in the presence of aspiration. Studies have shown that this is associated with improved outcome with high success rates. When comparing early to delayed medialization, those with early medialization had lower rates of pneumonia and shorter hospitalization, making early medialization the preferred option.

ATRIAL FIBRILLATION

Atrial fibrillation is one of the most common complications after esophageal surgery, and after thoracic surgery in general. Murthy and colleagues, examining 921 esophagectomies performed between 1982 and 2000, found postoperative atrial fibrillation occurred in 22% of patients. The STS Database reported 15.7% of esophagectomies experienced atrial fibrillation that required therapy. The NSQIP database did not collect atrial fibrillation as a complication. In non-cardiac thoracic surgery, preoperative factors that may increase a patient's risk of postoperative atrial fibrillation include increasing age, male gender, preexisting atrial fibrillation, and preexisting cardiac conditions such as congestive hear failure (CHF) or valvular disease (23). Murthy and colleagues confirm increasing age and cardiac disease as risk factors, and add 2 others: increasing degree of thoracic dissection and increasing intraoperative blood loss. Several medications have been examined as preoperative atrial fibrillation prophylaxis. None of these studies were done in esophagectomy patients exclusively. The closest approximations are series involving non-cardiac thoracic surgery, the bulk of which are pulmonary resections. Of the medications examined, beta-blockers are the most intensely examined. Beta-blockers reduce the frequency of postoperative atrial fibrillation but have not been shown to reduce secondary measures such as hospital length of stay or stroke rate. Amar evaluated postoperative prophylactic diltiazem after pulmonary resection and found a reduction in the rate of atrial fibrillation from 25% to 15%. This reduction, however, did not reduce hospital length of stay or cost of hospitalization (24). Amiodarone has been found to reduce the rate of atrial fibrillation post cardiac surgery by up to 50% (23). Lanza et al. found it could reduce the rate of atrial fibrillation, stroke, and length of stay post non-cardiac thoracic surgery (25). In Lanza's study, amiodarone was delivered postoperatively 200 mg 3 times a day orally. Esophagectomy patients are not immediately able to take oral medications. Amiodarone can be crushed and delivered through a feeding tube; however, the bioavailability of amiodarone delivered to the jejunum is variable and enhanced by the presence of food, especially lipids. The effect of an ileus on the absorption of amiodarone is not known. Prophylactic IV amiodarone, while an attractive option, has not been studied in esophagectomy patients to date.

In summary, atrial fibrillation occurs commonly after esophagectomy. Prophylactic beta-blockers, amiodarone, and diltiazem have been used to decrease the incidence of this arrhythmia in thoracic surgery but have not been well studied in esophagectomy patients.

MYOCARDIAL INFARCTION AND PULMONARY EMBOLISM

The management of myocardial infarction and pulmonary embolism post esophageal resection does not differ from standard postoperative considerations. However, because the blood supply to the conduit is sometimes tenuous, care must be taken to maintain systemic pressure and cardiac output. If the patient's extremities are cool and mottled from a low-flow state, it is likely the conduit is mottled as well. If a patient has sustained a myocardial infarction, pulmonary embolism, or atrial fibrillation, the surgical team should be vigilant for evidence of conduit ischemia and anastamotic leak.

CHYLOTHORAX AFTER ESOPHAGECTOMY

Chylothorax is a pleural collection of lymphatic fluid composed of lymphocytes, immunoglobulins, triglycerides, fat soluble vitamins, and proteins. A postoperative chylothorax after esophagectomy is a potentially morbid though fortunately uncommon complication. Reported incidence after esophagectomy is 1% to 3.4% and depends on operative approach, with a higher incidence noted for thoracic approaches (26–28).

Chylothorax is generally heralded by the appearance of a large volume of chest tube output or a new pleural effusion. If the patient is not eating by mouth or receiving tube feedings, the fluid will be straw colored. The diagnosis can be confirmed by the finding of a triglyceride level greater than 100 mg/dl in pleural fluid. The clinical diagnosis can be confirmed by the finding of milky drainage on institution of feeds containing fat either orally or by enteral feeding tube access. Neither the characteristic milky appearance of chyle nor the elevated triglycerides will be present until fat-containing foods are delivered to the small intestines. Some patients receiving preoperative radiation treatment to the mediastinum can have significant inflammation in the operative bed and high-volume serous chest tube output post esophagectomy without having a chylothorax or an injury to the thoracic duct. Patients with this type of chest tube output do not have a chylothorax and will not respond to the maneuvers used to treat chylothorax. Given time and good nutrition, this type of leakage almost always heals and seals.

The thoracic duct is prone to injury during esophagectomy secondary to its structure and anatomic position in the chest. A fragile, 1 to 2 mm, tubular structure, it generally enters the chest through the aortic hiatus and passes to the right side of the mediastinum before crossing towards the left at the level of T5 and draining into the jugulosubclavian junction in the neck. Damage and resultant leakage can be the result of either damage to the duct itself or injury to one of its branches. The duct can potentially be damaged anywhere along its course, and the clinical appearance of the leak will change depending on the level of the leak. Injury of the duct above the level of the arch may drain chyle into a neck drain; injury in the midportion may drain chyle into a chest tube; injury near the hiatus may result in chylous ascites or chylothorax.

Unlike blood, chyle is devoid of clotting factors and will not seal or clot on its own. Continued loss results in caloric and lymphocyte depletion, with resultant malnutrition and immunocompromise—a highly morbid combination in a group of patients often already malnourished and immunocompromised both as a result of underlying disease and therapy. Delaying treatment of chylothorax has resulted in reported mortalities approaching 50% (29).

Indications for surgical therapy are persistently high output unresponsive to conservative therapy. Conservative therapy usually consists of complete restriction of enteral intake and the institution of total parenteral nutrition (TPN). Some authors have used enteral feeds containing only medium chain fatty acids, which are directly absorbed by small bowel enterocytes without passage through the lymphatic system. The success of this approach is variable and the use of TPN without any enteral feeding is more reliable. Steps should be taken to ensure complete drainage of the chest and accurate measurement of chest tube output. Drainage of greater than 1 L per day or 400 cc per 8-hour period, despite maximal medical therapy, are indications for surgery. Because of the nutritional and immunologic consequences of a chylothorax, conservative management should not be used for more than 1 week in patients with high-level drainage. If drainage is noted to decrease dramatically in response to conservative measures, then continued nonoperative management is reasonable. Nutritional markers and electrolytes should be followed. Once output falls to less than 200 to 300 ml per day, feeding can be instituted. In general, a fat-containing diet either orally or enterally is used. If output remains low and nonchylous then drains may be removed.

Care taken in dealing with the thoracic duct at the original operation can prevent this complication. If visualized, the duct should be avoided or ligated. Various techniques have been proposed, including vascular clips, pledgeted sutures, simple ligation, or sealing with alternative energy sources. In the abdomen, the cisterna chylae is vulnerable during the lymphatic dissection around the celiac axis and left gastric artery. The lymphatic tissue around these arteries should be ligated. Low in the chest, the thoracic duct is generally located just medial to the ascending portion of the azygous vein in the fatty tissue between the aorta, esophagus, and right pleura. In a transthoracic esophagectomy, a wide lymphatic dissection can include the thoracic duct, in which case identifying it and ligating it at the level of the diaphragm and at the level of the arch of the aorta can avoid future leak.

In a sick, debilitated patient, the decision to operate may not be easy but the mortality of persisting with nonoperative approaches in the face of failing conservative management is associated with substantial mortality compared with invasive approaches.

Prior to returning to the operating room, careful planning is needed. In general, the intraoperative tenets include identification and control of the leak, possible obliteration of the pleural space, and establishing or maintaining good drainage of the pleural space.

Contrast lymphangiography can help identify the precise location of the leak but is a technically involved radiologic procedure not available at many institutions. A nuclear medicine lymphoscintogram does not localize the leak any further than simply observing what tube or body cavity from which the chyle is draining. Just prior to reoperation, fat in the form of cream or oil should be given to the patient enterally in order to help identify the area of leakage. Parekh et al. recommends 60 to 90 ml of cream given enterally starting 6 hours before the procedure and continuing during the procedure (30). At our institution, we use 250 ml of half-and-half given over 1 hour, followed by 2 to 3 hours of 100 ml/hour including during the procedure.

Either minimally invasive or open approaches to the thorax can be used and in general should be on the side of the chylothorax. After entry into the chest, the conduit should be mobilized and the site of leakage identified. When identified, the area of leakage should be controlled with clips or sutures. If generalized oozing is seen, then systematic clipping of all branches and application of fibrin glue may be effective. In addition, the thoracic duct should be identified as low in the chest as possible and mass ligated just above the diaphragm. The addition of mechanic pleurodesis may be helpful. If the duct was partially resected during the periesophageal lymphadenectomy, both ends may be leaking, one end low in the chest bringing chyle from the abdomen, the second high near the arch of the aorta, leaking chyle retrograde from the upper thorax. Both ends should be identified and ligated.

Injury to the cisternae chylae can result in chylothorax or chylous ascites. On thoracoscopy, chyle seen arising from the aortic or esophageal hiatus represents a leak originating below the level of the diaphragm, possibly from the cisternae chylae. This leak can be approached through laparotomy or laparoscopy, again identifying the site of the leak and ligating it with pledgeted sutures.

An alternative intervention with percutaneous access to the cisterna chyle and embolization of the thoracic duct has also been reported. While apparently effective, this approach requires expertise in interventional radiology, which may not be available in many centers.

FUNCTIONAL CONDUIT DISORDERS

Digestive tract reconstruction after esophageal reconstruction results in substantial alteration in foregut function, which falls under the general categorization of functional conduit disorders. The most common method of recreating gastrointestinal continuity after esophageal resection involves use of gastric conduit, though both colonic and small bowel may be used under select circumstances. While surgeons are often focused on the life-threatening complications early in the postoperative period, more insidious long-term issues with digestive function substantially affect patients' quality of life (31,32).

These issues should not be taken lightly as they affect a majority of patients to some degree. In fact, normal digestive function is found in a minority of patients (33,34).

The most common functional issues are dumping, delayed gastric emptying, and reflux.

DUMPING

Up to 50% of patients may suffer from dumping syndrome, which in a minority may be disabling (33–36). Dumping is categorized into early and late varieties based on temporal association with food ingestion. After esophagectomy, the majority of patients suffer from the early variety, with a lesser percentage suffering from the late variety or, even more uncommonly, both. Mechanisms of dumping are poorly understood and are felt to reflect alterations in gastrointestinal hormone secretion as well as anatomic factors related to surgery and subsequent reconstruction. Symptoms are manifested by gastrointestinal symptoms such as cramping, bloating, nausea, and diarrhea, as well as vasomotor symptoms such as flushing, diaphoresis, syncope, and palpitation.

Early dumping, 10 to 30 minutes after eating, is felt to result from rapid transit of hyperosmolar gastric contents into the small bowel. After esophagectomy, decreased reservoir capacity and alteration in pyloric anatomy contribute to this process.

Late dumping, 1 to 3 hours after eating, is manifested by systemic vascular symptoms. Rapid emptying of carbohydrates into the small bowel triggers insulin release in an exaggerated fashion with resultant hypoglycemia and symptoms (37).

Diagnosis is usually clinical but can be confirmed by noting symptoms after glucose challenge or finding of hypoglycemia in the hours after eating. Studies showing rapid gastric emptying may be noted but do not appear to correlate well with symptoms.

Treatment is generally with diet modification. Avoidance of high carbohydrate loads can be accomplished by advising patients to avoid simple sugars, eating more frequent small meals, and restricting fluid intake with meals. The majority of patients respond to these simple measures. In the small majority of patients with refractory symptoms, pharmacologic measures may be useful. Propanolol, prednisolone, verapamil, and methysergide maleate have been used to alleviate vasomotor symptoms associated with dumping. Literature support for these, however, is primarily case series and case reports (38–40).

Octreotide has been found to be effective in the treatment of dumping syndrome. It acts by both delaying gastric emptying and small bowel motility as well as inhibiting secretion of gastrointestinal hormones and insulin. Doses of 25 to 100 micrograms subcutaneously administered 30 minutes prior to eating have been found to be effective. Use is limited by diarrhea and inconvenience.

Acarbose is an inhibitor of the conversion of carbohydrates to monosaccharides. This results in lowering of postprandial glucose and subsequent insulin secretion. It may be useful in the treatment of delayed dumping but its side effects of diarrhea and flatulence may limit its use.

Surgical techniques may have an effect on the development of dumping, and sparing of vagal nerves under selected circumstances may preserve gastric motility.

DELAYED GASTRIC EMPTYING

Following esophageal resection, delayed gastric emptying is commonly seen. This is felt to result from denervation of the gastric conduit and disruption of pyloric function secondary to vagotomy. How to deal with the pylorus is also an area of controversy, experience with vagal denervation and need for pyloroplasty or pyloromyotomy comes from surgery for the treatment of ulcer disease. The patient with a normal stomach formed into a gastric conduit appears different, however. Studies looking at the addition of a pyloric drainage procedure—whether pyloroplasty, pyloromyotomy, or more recently injection of Botox—do not demonstrate clear benefit.

Formation of the gastric conduit itself may play a role in postoperative function. Narrow conduits appear to empty more rapidly, removal of the majority of the distal lesser curvature decreases contractile force. Placement of the conduit in an extra anatomic position as opposed to the more common posterior mediastinum also seems to increase the incidence of delayed gastric emptying. Clearly, torsion of the conduit will affect its function and should be avoided.

Pharmacologic therapy is the mainstay of treatment. Various prokinetic agents, metaclopramide, cisapride, and erythromycin, have been used with varying degrees of success. Of these, erythromycin appears most effective. An agonist against the motilin receptor, it has been shown to promote gastric emptying. In some patients, postoperative balloon dilation or injection of Botox into the pylorus may be attempted.

REFLUX

Esophagectomy and subsequent reconstruction causes disruption of normal anti-reflux mechanisms, such as the distal esophageal sphincter and the diaphragmatic hiatus. Positive abdominal pressure and negative thoracic pressure promote reflux as well. It is therefore not surprising that reflux is extremely common after esophageal resection. Symptoms are generally pain and may include aspiration and cough. Bile reflux may be promoted by the addition of a pyloric drainage procedure. Other surgical factors implicated in the finding of reflux include the height of the anastomosis in the chest with a higher level anastomosis and complete intrathoracic placement of the stomach being less prone to reflux. However, even patients with cervical anastomosis demonstrate reflux when studied. Symptomatic patients should be treated with H2 blockers or proton pump inhibitors. Surgical strategies to prevent reflux such as creating valve-like anastomoses or intercostal muscle wraps are described but are uncommonly performed.

ANASTAMOTIC STRICTURE

Improved results in the therapy of both patients with benign and malignant esophageal disease undergoing esophagectomy have led to the realization that not only is survival important but quality of life is a key component of successful treatment. Postoperative dysphagia, often a result of esophageal stricture, is a factor that may have a substantial effect on quality of life.

The definition of what constitutes a stricture is not clear. In general, however, the combination of dysphagia along with either endoscopic or radiographic finding of esophageal narrowing is used. It has been shown that up to a third of patients with dysphagia will not have an anatomic stricture (41). Without a clear definition, the incidence of stricture is hard to establish with reported rates of 10% to 50%.

Etiology is multifactorial. Key components in the pathogenesis of postoperative strictures include anastomotic technique, anastomotic leak, conduit ischemia. Late strictures are generally benign and result from chronic reflux or malignant and result from recurrence.

Anastomotic technique has been identified as a factor in stricture formation. In terms of anastomotic size, it has been observed that using larger diameter circular staplers substantially decreases the incidence of stricture. When hand-sewn anastomosis is looked at, a 2-layer technique appears to increase the incidence of stricture. Side-to-side stapled anastomosis, as popularized by Orringer, has shown to result in lower rates of stricture formation.

Anastomotic leak and stricture formation are closely tied together with a substantial portion of patients with leaks developing strictures. Institution of early dilation in these patients has been shown to result in decreased stricture formation (42).

Ischemia of the conduit also plays a role in the development of stricture. Studies evaluating gastric blood flow, or endoscopic evidence of mucosal ischemia, demonstrate a clear association with stricture formation. Care taken during conduit preparation, avoidance of injury to the right gastroepiploic artery, gentle transposition of the conduit into the neck or chest, and avoiding anastomosis adjacent to staple lines should help minimize stricture formation.

Stricture after esophagectomy generally presents in the first 2 to 6 months after surgery. Presentation of dysphagia in the immediate postoperative period should make one suspicious for either a technical error such a narrow anastomosis or a nerve injury as previously discussed. Late presentation should prompt one to think of local or mediastinal tumor recurrence or of reflux.

Dilation has been demonstrated to be an effective treatment for stricture (41,42). This can be performed either with balloon or bougienage. In the largest reported series of patients undergoing cervical esophagogastric anastomoses, any patient with symptoms underwent early dilation. This resulted in over 50% of patients undergoing at least one dilation. Long-term follow-up showed that less than 20% of patients had the need for long-term dilations (28). Treatment with balloon dilation showed similar results. Multiple dilations may be needed. Reoperation is rarely needed.

CONDUIT NECROSIS

Reconstruction of the foregut after esophagectomy is complex and complications may result in substantial morbidity and mortality. Preparation and preservation of the conduit is essential to good short- and long-term results. Conduit choice is limited and generally consists of either stomach or, less commonly, colon or jejunum. In all cases, preservation of conduit blood supply is key.

Conduit ischemia is a rare complication. A recent review of the literature found it occurred on average in 3.2% of gastric (0.5%–10.4%), 5.1% of colonic (0%– 13%), and 4.2% of jejunal (0%–11.3%) conduits (43).

Factors contributing to conduit necrosis are generally felt to be technical and involve injury or twisting of their vascular pedicles. It is theorized that intraoperative and perioperative hypotension may contribute to ischemia.

A high index of suspicion is needed to make the diagnosis. Regardless of the conduit used, persistent tachycardia, fevers, leukocytosis, hypotension, or anastomotic leak should trigger an evaluation of the conduit. Flexible esophagoscopy can be used to directly examine the mucosa for signs of ischemia. Small-caliber esophagoscopy can be performed at bedside with topical anesthetic and offers an excellent view of the anastamosis and mucosal integrity. Endoscopy, however, cannot confirm full thickness necrosis. Contrast esophagography may indirectly suggest ischemia and may show anastomotic disruption. In patients with cervical anastomosis, direct examination of the conduit may be possible. Occasionally, operative re-exploration may be needed.

Once the diagnosis is made, prompt reoperative exploration should follow. Basic tenets regardless of conduit type include resection of necrotic bowel, drainage of the mediastinum, cervical esophageal diversion, and distal enteral feeding access, if not previously placed.

Rarely is regaining immediate esophagointestinal continuity prudent. Generally, delayed reconstruction with an alternative conduit in 3 to 6 months is recommended. Various nonoperative strategies such as anticoagulation, steroids, vasodilators have been proposed. None are recommended.

As mentioned previously, the best way to prevent ischemic complications is careful conduit construction, preservation of blood supply, careful transposition through the mediastinum, and meticulous handling of the conduit. Various techniques have been proposed to decrease the incidence of conduit ischemia. "Super charging" the conduit near the proximal anastomosis by microvascular augmentation has been described for all 3 types of conduit (44–46). Ischemic conditioning of the gastric conduit by staged conduit construction followed by resection has shown promise as a mechanism to prevent ischemia but superior results have not yet been clearly demonstrated (47,48).

LEAK

Esophageal leak remains a major cause of morbidity and mortality after esophageal resection in spite of improvements in operative and perioperative care. Associated with conduit ischemia and often resulting in stricture, leaks result in both acute and chronic complications.

Incidence of leak varies widely in the literature. Differences in anastomotic technique, both hand-sewn versus stapled, as well as variation in anastomotic location, appear to affect leak rate.

Orringer, in a recent publication detailing 2,000 transhiatal esophagectomies with cervical anastamosis, reports an overall leak rate of 12% with a leak rate of 9% in the last 944 patients. No such single institution series have been published for transthoracic approaches, but met-analysis showed a leak rate of 7% in a total of over 2,500 patients (16). Location of the leak also has a substantial effect on morbidity and mortality. Mediastinitis is rare after cervical anastomotic leak; however, after a thoracic leak, it is more common.

Martin et al. reported 621 transthoracic esophagectomies with intrathoracic anastamosis performed between 1970 and 2004. They found no difference in the leak rate of 4.8% during the period 1970 to 1986 and 6.3% between 1987 and 2004. They did, however, find a significant decrease in the leak associated mortality between these 2 eras from 43% to 3.3%. This decrease in mortality was attributed to more frequent reoperation, use of tissue flaps to reinforce repairs on reoperation, and possibly quicker use of enteral nutrition in the later era (49).

Nutrition in many patients presenting for esophageal resection may be compromised, both as a result of mechanic complications of their esophageal disease or as a result of underlying malignancy and subsequent therapy. Nutritional markers have been found to correlate with an increased rate of anastomotic leak and efforts should be made to maximize nutrition in the preoperative period.

As part of the multimodality treatment of esophageal malignancy, many patients receive neoadjuvant chemoradiation. This does not appear to be a substantial risk factor for esophageal leak despite concerns expressed by surgeons.

As mentioned, ischemia of the conduit is intimately associated with the development of anastomotic disruption. Conduit ischemia should be prevented by preservation of the vascular supply, gentle handling, and positioning of the conduit to ensure a tension-free anastomosis. The proximal esophagus should also be gently handled and extensive dissection should be avoided.

Excellent results have been reported for both single- and double-layer hand-sewn anastomoses as well as by both circular stapled and side-to-side stapled anastomosis. It is felt that a hand-sewn anastomosis may be more versatile, in particular when using jejunal or colonic conduits. Stapled anastomosis, on the other hand, is probably faster, more reproducible, easier to teach, and may be useful in areas where exposure is difficult, such as high in the chest. Surgeon experience and consistent refinement and application of a technique are probably the most important factors.

Colon and jejunal conduits can be "super-charged" by creating proximal arterial and venous anastamosis between the conduit and vessels of the neck and superior mediastinum. Alternatively, the stomach can be "prepared" as a conduit by performing a laparoscopy or laparotomy 1 to 2 weeks prior to the planned esophagectomy. At this procedure, the small gastric vessels and left gastric artery are divided, partially devascularizing the stomach. This promotes expansion of the capillary beds of the stomach and compensatory hypertrophy of the right gastroepiploic artery (50).

Postoperative decompression of the conduit may decrease the mechanic stress of the anastomosis.

The diagnosis of anastomotic disruption depends both on timing and location. Early leaks in the first hours or days after surgery present with signs of sepsis, chest tube output, which is bilious in nature, or undrained collection in the thoracic cavity. These require no formal diagnostic testing and are the result of conduit necrosis or serious error in the construction of the anastomosis.

Most leaks present in more subtle fashion. In a series of 621 transthoracic esophagectomies and intrathoracic anastamosis, Martin et al. reported a median of 9 days until detection of a leak. Most authors report median hospital stays of 10 to 18 days after esophagectomy, making an anastamotic leak a complication appearing later in the hospital course. Their presentation depends primarily on their location. Cervical leaks generally manifest with fever, drainage from the wound, and signs of local infection in the first postoperative week. Thoracic leaks can be more insidious. Systemic signs of infection such as fever, tachycardia, tachypnea, leukocytosis are generally the first signs. Increasing fluid collections on thoracic imaging or a new air leak from the chest tube may be seen. Atrial fibrillation is not uncommon. A high clinical index of suspicion and prompt diagnosis is needed to prevent deterioration.

Most surgeons obtain a contrast esophagram 5 to 10 days after surgery to exclude leak. Any clinical suspicion of an anastomotic problem should lead to prompt evaluation. There is some controversy over contrast agent of choice. Barium is a more sensitive agent and avoids the risk of chemical pneumonitis resulting from aspiration of water soluble agents.

Concerns about mediastinal extravasation of barium with resultant morbidity are unfounded. However, the argument is moot as contrast materials (Omnipaque, Visipaque), which provide good resolution on radiography but are inert if aspirated or leak into an extravisceral space, are available.

Endoscopy can be used to evaluate the conduit for ischemic changes, though it is not sensitive for diagnosis of leak. A pink mucosa is reassuring, however, the finding of necrotic mucosa does not tell one whether the necrosis is full thickness. We have found the small caliber endoscope to be a very useful tool for this purpose. The conduit can be inspected at the bedside, transnasally, unsedated, with topical anesthetic only. The scope is small and easily traverses the anastamosis. CT scanning may show pleural cavity collections and air, which may suggest leak.

Management of a leak is dependent on the patient's clinical condition, the location of the leak, and the severity of the leak. Intrathoracic and cervical leaks are discussed separately. If a long segment of native esophagus is left between the cricopharyngeus and the anastamosis, it is possible for a "cervical" anastamosis to fall back into the thoracic cavity, such that a leak from this anastamosis behaves more like a thoracic anastamosis.

INTRATHORACIC LEAK

Asymptomatic, contained intrathoracic leaks can be observed. A swallow study is repeated in 1 to 3 weeks and oral nutrition instituted when the leak has resolved. Management of a contained but symptomatic intrathoracic leak is initially IV antibiotics, resuscitation, and percutaneous drainage but may require operative intervention. Patients who continue to show signs of active infection require operation. Uncontained leaks of intrathoracic anastamosis almost always require operative intervention. Intravenous antibiotics and resuscitation can be initiated during the planned return to the operating room. If conduit necrosis is found, the necrotic areas are resected, the remaining conduit returned to the abdomen, the mediastinum debrided and drained, the proximal esophagus diverted, and distal enteral access ensured. If the conduit is found viable and the patient is hemodynamically stable, the anastamosis can be repaired but should be buttressed with a pedicled tissue flap such as serratus, latissimus, or intercostal muscle. Martin et al. found that with early aggressive management of uncontained intrathoracic leaks and more conservative management of contained leaks, in the modern era, mortality in patients with a leak was 3% and no different than in those without (49).

CERVICAL LEAK

Anastamotic leaks from a cervical anastamosis are considered to be more frequent but less dangerous. Reported leak rates range from 8% to 15% (16,26,51–55). Some leaks are small, contained, asymptomatic, and found on routine esophagram. These can be observed and will generally heal. The patient is kept nothing by the mouth or on clear liquids until the leak heals. This can be checked with esophagram in 1 to 2 weeks, or, alternatively, not checked and the patient's diet advanced and followed clinically. Larger leaks or leaks that do not drain well or are accompanied by cellulitis or systemic signs of infection require drainage. This can be accomplished at the bedside or in the operative suite. The neck incision is opened and all loculations drained. Patients are then maintained nothing by the mouth with enteral nutrition through a jejunostomy. Some authors will have patients drink several glasses of water a day to flush out the wound. Most leaks treated in this manner will close in 2 to 3 weeks. As with any anastamotic leak, the viability of the conduit should be confirmed either by operative inspection or endoscopy.

In more than 50% of cases, a healed anastamotic leak will develop a stricture (56). Because of this high rate, some authors recommend early and prophylactic dilatation (42). Please see the above discussion on treatment of esophageal stricture.

ACKNOWLEDGMENT

The authors thank Jill Rose for her help in preparing this manuscript.

RECOMMENDED READING

Complications of Esophageal Surgery ed. Cameron D. Wright, MD. Thoracic Surgery Clinics, Volume 16(1), February 2006.

Challenges in Esophageal Reconstruction ed. Mark Orringer, MD. Seminars in Thoracic and Cardiovascular Surgery, Volume 19(1), Spring 2007.

References

1. Sauvanet A, Baltar J, Le Mee J, et al. Diagnosis and conservative management of intrathoracic leakage after oesophagectomy. *Br J Surg.* 1998;85:1446–1449.
2. Whooley B, Law S, Alexandrou A, et al. Critical appraisal of the significance of intrathoracic anastomotic leakage after esophagectomy for cancer. *Am J Surg.* 2001;181:198–203.
3. Patil P, Patel S, Mistry R, et al. Cancer of the esophagus: esophagogastric anastomotic leak—a retrospective study of predisposing factors. *J Surg Oncol.* 1992;49:163–167.
4. Crestanello J, Deschamps C, Cassivi S, et al. Selective management of intrathoracic anastomotic leak after esophagectomy. *J Thorac Cardiovasc Surg.* 2005;129:254–260.
5. Huang G, Wang L, Liu J, et al. Surgery of esophageal carcinoma. *Sem Surg Oncol.* 1985;1:74–83.
6. Pickleman J, Watson W, Cunningham J, et al. The failed gastrointestinal anastomosis: an inevitable catastrophe? *J Am Coll Surg.* 1999;188:473–482.
7. Karl R, Schreiber R, Boulware D, et al. Factors affecting morbidity, mortality, and survival in patients undergoing Ivor Lewis esophagogastrectomy. *Ann Surg.* 2000;231:635–643.
8. Griffin S, Shaw I, Dresner S. Early complications after Ivor Lewis subtotal esophagectomy with two-field lymphadenectomy: risk factors and management. *J Am Coll Surg.* 2002;194:285–297.
9. Bailey S, Bull D, Harpole D, et al. Outcomes after esophagectomy: A ten-year prospective cohort. *Ann Thorac Surg.* 2003;75:217–222.
10. Ferguson M, Martin T, Reeder L, et al. Mortality after esophagectomy: risk factor analysis. *World J Surg.* 1997;21:599–603.
11. Atkins B, Shah A, Hutcheson K, et al. Reducing hospital morbidity and mortality following esophagectomy. *Ann Thorac Surg.* 2004;78:1170–1176.
12. Kinugasa S, Tachibana M, Yoshimura H. Postoperative pulmonary complications are associated with worse short- and long-term outcomes after extended esophagectomy. *J Surg Oncol.* 2004;88.
13. Orringer M, Marshall B, Iannettoni M. Transhiatal esophagectomy: Clinical experience and refinements. *Ann Surg.* 1999;230:392–403.
14. Visbal A, Allen M, Miller D, et al. Ivor Lewis esophagogastrectomy for esophageal cancer. *Ann Thorac Surg.* 2001;71:1803–1808.
15. Hulscher J, van Sandwick J, De Boer A, et al. Extended transthoracic resection compared with limited transhiatal resection for adenocarcinoma of the esophagus. *N Engl J Med.* 2002;347:1662–1669.
16. Hulscher J, Tijssen J, Obertop H, et al. Transthoracic versus transhiatal resection for carcinoma of the esophagus: a meta-analysis. *Ann Thorac Surg.* 2001;72:306–313.

17. Barrera R, Shi W, Amar D, et al. Smoking and timing of cessation: impact on pulmonary complications after thoracotomy. *Chest*. 2005;127:1977–1983.
18. Nakagawa M, Tanaka H, Tsukuma H. Relationship between the duration of the preoperative smoke-free period and the incidence of postoperative pulmonary complications after pulmonary surgery. *Chest*. 2001;120:705–710.
19. Chumillas S, Ponce J, Delgado F. Prevention of postoperative pulmonary complications through respiratory rehabilitation: a controlled clinical study. *Arch of Phys Med Rehab*. 1998;79:5–9.
20. Ferguson M, Durkin A. Preoperative prediction of the risk for pulmonary complications after esophagectomy for cancer. *J Thorac Cardiovasc Surg*. 2002;123:661–669.
21. Watson A, Allen P. Influence of thoracic epidural analgesia on outcome after resection for esophageal cancer. *Surgery*. 1994;115:429–432.
22. Whooley B, Law S, Murthy S. Analysis of reduced death and complication rates after esophageal resection. *Ann Surg*. 2001;233:338–344.
23. Mayson S, Greenspon A, Adams S, et al. The changing face of postoperative atrial fibrillation prevention. A review of current medical therapy. *Cardiol Rev*. 2007;15:231–241.
24. Amar D, Roistacher N, Rusch V, et al. Effects of diltiazem prophylaxis on the incidence and clinical outcome of atrial arrhythmias after thoracic surgery. *J Thorac Cardiovasc Surg*. 2000;120:790–798.
25. Lanza L, Visbal A, DeValeria P, et al. Low-dose oral amiodarone prophylaxis reduces atrial fibrillation after pulmonary resection. *Ann Thorac Surg*. 2003;75:223–230.
26. Rindani R, Martin C, Cox M. Transhiatal versus Ivor-Lewis oesophagectomy: is there a difference? *Aust N Z J Surg*. 1999;69:187–194.
27. Dugue L, Sauvanet A, Farges O, et al. Output of chyle as an indicator of treatment for chylothorax complicating oesophagectomy. *Br J Surg*. 1998;85:1147–1149.
28. Orringer M, Marshall B, Chang A, et al. Two thousand transhiatal esophagectomies. Changing trends, lessons learned. *Ann Surg*. 2007;246:363–374.
29. Patel H, Tan B, Yee J, et al. A 25-year experience with open primary transthoracic repair of paraesophageal hiatal hernia. *J Thorac Cardiovasc Surg*. 2004;127:843–849.
30. Parekh K, Iannettoni M. Complications of esophageal resection and reconstruction. *Sem Thorac Cardiovasc Surg*. 2007;19:79–88.
31. Langenhoff B, Krabbe P, Wobbes T. Quality of life as an outcome measure in surgical oncology. *Br J Surg*. 2001;88:643–652.
32. Kredder H, Wright J, McLeod R. Outcome studies in surgical research. *Surgery*. 1997;121:223–225.
33. McLarty A, Deschamps C, Trastek V. Esophageal resection for cancer of the esophagus: long-term function and quality of life. *Ann Thorac Surg*. 1997;63:1568–1572.
34. Headrick J, Nichols F, Miller D. High-grade esophageal dysplasia: long-term survival and quality of life after esophagectomy. *Ann Thorac Surg*. 2002;73:1697–1702.
35. Orringer M, Stirling M. Esophageal resection for achalasia: indications and results. *Ann Thorac Surg*. 1989;47:340–345.
36. Wang L, Huang M, Huang B. Gastric substitution for resectable carcinoma of the esophagus: an analysis of 368 cases. *Ann Thorac Surg*. 1992;53:289–294.
37. Donington J. Functional conduit disorders after esophagectomy. *Thorac Surg Clin*. 2006;16:53–62.
38. Chandos B. Dumping syndrome and the regulation of peptide YY with varapamil. *Am J Gastroenterol*. 1992;87:1530–1531.
39. Shibata C, Funayama Y, Fukushima K. Effect of steroid therapy for late dumping syndrome after total gastrectomy: report of a case. *Dig Dis Sci*. 2004;49:802–804.
40. Christoffersson E, Wallensten S. Drug therapy in the dumping syndrome. *Nord Med*. 1971;86:1589–1590.
41. Rice T. Anastomotic stricture complicating esophagectomy. *Thorac Surg Clin*. 2006;16:63–73.
42. Chang A, Orringer M. Management of the cervical esophagogastric anastomotic stricture. *Thorac Cardiovasc Surg*. 2007;19:66–71.
43. Wormuth J, Heitmiller R. Esophageal conduit necrosis. *Thorac Surg Clin*. 2006;16:11–22.
44. Sekido M, Yamamoto Y, Minakawa H. Use of the "supercharge" technique in esophageal and pharyngeal reconstruction to augment microvascular blood flow. *Surgery*. 2003;134:420–424.
45. O'Rourke I, Threlfall G. Colonic interposition for oesophageal reconstruction with special reference to microvascular reinforcement to microvascular reinforcement of graft circulation. *Aust N Z J Surg*. 1986;56:767–777.
46. Heitmiller R, Gruber P, Swier P. Long-segment substernal esophageal replacement with internal mammary vascular augmentation. *Dis Esophagus*. 2000;13:240–242.
47. Urschel J. Ischemic conditioning of the stomach may reduce the incidence of esophagogastric anastomotic leaks complicating esophagectomy: a hypothesis. *Dis Esophagus*. 1997;10:217–219.
48. Urschel J, Takita H, Antkowiak J. The effect of ischemic conditioning on gastric wound healing in the rat: implications for esophageal replacement with stomach. *J Cardiovasc Surg*. 1997;38:535–538.
49. Martin L, Swisher S, Hofstetter W, et al. Intrathoracic leaks following esophagectomy are no longer associated with increased mortality. *Ann Surg*. 2005;242:392–402.
50. Jobe B, Kim C, Minjarez R, et al. Simplifying minimally invasive transhiatal esophagectomy with the inversion approach. *Arch Surg*. 2006;141:857–866.
51. Swanson S, Batirel H, Bueno R, et al. Transthoracic esophagectomy with radical mediastinal and abdominal lymph node dissection and cervical esophagogastrostomy for esophageal carcinoma. *Ann Thorac Surg*. 2001;72:1918–1924.
52. Goldminc M, Maddern G, Le Prise E, et al. Oesophagectomy by a transhiatal approach or thoracotomy: a prospective randomized trial. *Br J Surg*. 1993;80:367–370.
53. Urschel J. Esophagogastrostomy anastomotic leaks complicating esophagectomy: a review. *Am J Surg*. 1995;169:634–640.
54. Katariya K, Harvey J, Pina E, et al. Complications of transhiatal esophagectomy. *J Surg Oncol*. 1994;57:157–163.
55. Gurkan N, Terzioglu T, Tezelman S, et al. Transhiatal oesophagectomy for oesophageal carcinoma. *Br J Surg*. 1991;78:1348–1351.
56. Mitchell J. Anastomotic leak after esophagectomy. *Thorac Surg Clin*. 2006;16:1–9.

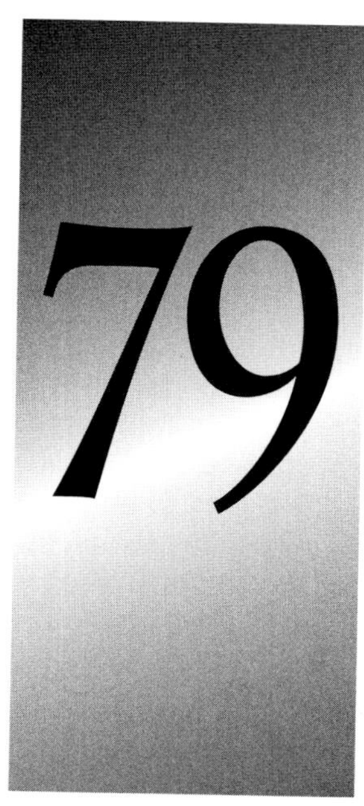

79 Quality of Life after Esophagectomy

Jonathan Ford Finks

Patient reported outcomes, such as health-related quality of life (QOL), have become increasingly recognized as important outcome measures in evaluating therapies for esophageal and other cancers. The focus among investigators and regulatory agencies has widened to include not only traditional outcome measures, such as mortality, morbidity, and complications, but patient-based measures as well, such as symptom assessment, performance status, and QOL. Indeed, the Oncologic Drugs Advisory Committee of the FDA has recommended that approval for new anticancer drugs be based on their beneficial effects on QOL and/or survival (1). Moreover, improving QOL in cancer patients is now a key goal of the American Cancer Society (2), and the Working Group of the American Society of Clinical Oncology has emphasized the importance of patient outcomes, such as survival and quality of life, rather than tumor response rates in assessing the success of cancer treatment (3).

Incorporating QOL measures is especially important when evaluating therapy for a disease such as esophageal cancer, for which prognosis is poor and treatment is particularly harsh. Even with definitive therapy, long-term prognosis is poor. Two-year survival following esophagectomy for esophageal cancer ranges between 20% and 60%, while 5-year survival is between 10% and 40% (4–6). Furthermore, esophagectomy, the only curative treatment, is an extensive procedure with associated major morbidity rates of 44% to 50% and mortality rates between 4% and 11% (7–10). Given these therapeutic limitations, the impact of surgery on symptoms, function, and overall QOL takes on greater importance and must be taken into consideration when balancing the risks and benefits of treatment.

Moreover, in cases where esophagectomy may not offer a significant survival advantage over chemoradiation alone, as with some locally advanced tumors (11,12), differential treatment effects on QOL may be the deciding factor in determining the course of therapy. The same holds true when comparing palliative therapies as well. Finally, symptom control and QOL outcomes may also help determine the optimal surgical approach and reconstruction technique (e.g., cervical vs. intrathoracic anastomosis), since the approach to esophagectomy may not significantly affect overall survival (5,13).

DEFINING AND MEASURING QUALITY OF LIFE

While it is easy to appreciate the importance of QOL outcomes, defining and measuring health-related QOL is more complex. The World Health Organization has defined health as not merely the "absence of infirmity or disease" but also a state of "physical, mental and social well-being" (14). While there is no standard definition for heath-related QOL, it is generally thought to encompass aspects of physical, social, and psychologic (including emotional and cognitive) function that are affected by health conditions and interventions (15,16). Following esophagectomy, QOL incorporates not only physiologic outcomes, such as degree of dysphagia and reflux and ability to eat, but also psychological and social outcomes, such as the ability to work and perform activities of daily living, social interaction, energy level, and emotional state (17). In fact, the degree of disease-specific symptoms (e.g., dysphagia, reflux) has been shown to correlate poorly with overall and other aspects of QOL in patients with esophageal cancer, suggesting that other domains of QOL need to be evaluated separately (18–20).

Given its subjective, complex, and multidimensional nature, measurement of QOL is a significant challenge. The ideal instrument for measuring QOL should be reliable, responsive, interpretable, and valid (21,22). Validity refers to the degree to which an instrument measures what it was intended to measure. Reliability refers to the extent to which an instrument is free from measurement error and reproducible, or consistent, across multiple measurements (23). In addition to being valid and reliable, a QOL instrument must be responsive, allowing for detection of clinically important changes in QOL over time, even if those changes are small. Finally, QOL measures must be interpretable, such that differences in scores correspond to very small, small, moderate, and large differences in clinical outcome (22).

Experimental evidence suggests that QOL questionnaires should also be designed to be completed by the patients themselves. In a study of patients with esophageal cancer, Blazeby and colleagues compared results when 1 doctor, 52 patients, and 39 caregivers independently completed a well-validated QOL survey (24). They showed that agreement was poor to moderate in most QOL scales and items between healthcare providers and patients. In another study, QOL following resection of esophageal cancer was assessed by both patients and a psychologist, using separate validated instruments. While both the self and external evaluations showed significant correlation, QOL was consistently rated as being higher by the external observer (20). Clearly the patient is best able to evaluate their own QOL and should be the one who answers the questionnaire.

There are a variety of different tools available for evaluating QOL. Generic instruments, such as the Medical Outcomes Study SF-36, are designed to provide a broad summary of QOL measures and apply to a wide range of patient populations, regardless of the underlying condition. They are often unresponsive, however, to changes in clinically important aspects of a patient's condition. This drawback has led to the use of disease-specific questionnaires that focus on aspects of health status relevant to a particular subset of patients, such as cancer patients (22). Several such instruments have been developed and validated and are currently in use.

One of the most widely used and extensively validated instruments to evaluate QOL in patients with esophageal cancer was developed by the European Organization for Research and Treatment of Cancer (EORTC). The instrument includes a core cancer-specific scale, the QLQ-30, as well as a supplemental esophageal-specific module, the OES-18, designed to improve the sensitivity and specificity of the core instrument. The QLQ-30 is a 30-item scale, which incorporates 5 functional scales (physical, role, social, emotional, and cognitive), a global health scale, and 3 symptom scales (pain, nausea/emesis, and fatigue). Six single items assess 5 additional symptoms common to patients with cancer (loss of appetite, insomnia, dyspnea, constipation, and diarrhea), as well as the perceived financial impact of the disease and its treatment. The OES-18 includes 4 symptom scales (dysphagia, eating, reflux, and odynophagia) and 6 single items (dry mouth, taste, speech, coughing, choking, and difficulty swallowing saliva). In the function and global QOL scales, a higher score is equivalent to better function. In the symptoms scales and items, a higher score indicates worse symptoms. In general, a mean score difference of 10 points is considered clinically significant. In validation studies, both the core and esophageal-specific modules were able to distinguish between esophageal cancer patients undergoing palliative versus curative treatment and demonstrated treatment-induced changes over time (15,18,25).

QUALITY OF LIFE AFTER ESOPHAGECTOMY FOR CANCER

Using the EORTC instrument and other similar scales, several investigators have examined functional status, symptoms, and overall QOL following esophagectomy for esophageal cancer. Not surprisingly, nearly all studies have found that esophagectomy has a substantial negative impact on quality of life, affecting nearly all functional domains. Esophagectomy also results in significant, debilitating, and, often, long-lasting symptoms. While QOL often recovers to preoperative levels within 1 to 2 years after surgery, a significant subset of patients experience an irreversible decline in functional status and global QOL following esophagectomy.

Cross-Sectional Studies

In the only population-based study, Viklund et al. evaluated QOL indicators in 282 esophageal cancer patients

6 months following esophagectomy from the Swedish Esophageal and Cardia Cancer Register (26). Their scores were compared to a random reference sample from the general population as well as from a group of patients with a diagnosis of cancer. Compared to the reference group, study patients had significantly diminished global QOL, functional scores, and general symptoms. The most affected functional scales were role and social function. Fatigue, appetite loss, diarrhea, and dyspnea were the predominant general symptoms in the study group. While difficulty eating was the dominant esophageal-specific symptom, study patients also had difficulty with cough, reflux, odynophagia, dysphagia, and taste. This study was somewhat limited, however, by the short follow-up period and lack of preoperative QOL data.

In another large cross-sectional study with long-term follow-up, Deschamps et al. evaluated symptoms and QOL measures in 107 patients with stage I or II esophageal cancer who had survived longer than 5 years after esophagectomy (27). Assessed using the SF-36, a generic survey instrument, QOL outcomes were compared to national norms. The authors found that physical function scores were significantly below the national norm and energy level was somewhat decreased. Conversely, ability to work, social interaction, daily activities, emotional function, and health perception were all similar to the reference population, while study patients scored higher than the national norm in the area of mental health. Despite fairly good QOL scores, however, only 16% of the patients were asymptomatic at the time of the survey. Dysphagia remained a problem in 25% of patients, and 43% had required at least 1 dilation. Reflux symptoms were present in 60% of patients, half of whom required antacids. Half of the patients experienced postprandial dumping symptoms and 49% never regained the weight lost following surgery.

In a similar study, De Boer et al. evaluated 35 patients 2 to 5 years following transhiatal esophagectomy for esophageal cancer, using a modified symptom scale and the SF-36 QOL instrument (28). As with the previous study, the authors found that most QOL indices were similar to the reference population, while emotional function was higher. Yet over 50% of patients still suffered significant symptoms. In particular, patients complained of early satiety, fatigue, dysphagia, and heartburn. The authors also found that emotional issues, such as worry and psychological irritability, had a greater correlation with overall QOL than did disease-specific symptoms. In both of these studies, the apparently low QOL impact of surgery may in part reflect the generic nature of the instrument used to measure QOL. The SF-36 may be somewhat less sensitive to the specific QOL issues of patients with esophageal cancer than other disease-specific scales (29).

Longitudinal Studies

Other investigators have examined longitudinal effects on global QOL, function outcomes, and symptoms following esophagectomy for esophageal cancer. Lagergren et al. evaluated QOL with the EORTC instruments in 47 patients who had survived 3 years after esophagectomy (30). They found that all functional scores, except emotional function, had deteriorated significantly after surgery (Figure 79.1). By 12 months, however, scores for role, cognitive, and social function had returned to baseline, whereas scores for global QOL and physical function never recovered to baseline levels. By contrast, emotional function improved steadily after surgery and was better at 3 years than at baseline.

The authors also assessed general and esophageal symptoms in these patients. Fatigue, pain, sleeplessness, and loss of appetite were the dominant general symptoms prior to surgery. All symptom scores deteriorated after surgery, particularly those for appetite loss and dyspnea (Figure 79.2). Within 6 to 12 months, most symptom scores had recovered to baseline levels. Dyspnea and diarrhea, however, remained significant problems at 3 years, affecting 50% and 40% of patients, respectively. Significant esophageal-specific symptoms at baseline included dysphagia, eating restrictions, reflux, odynophagia, dry mouth, taste, and coughing. All of these symptom scores worsened postoperatively (Figure 79.3). Nearly all of these symptom scales had returned to baseline by 12 months, and dysphagia scores were better at 3 years than at baseline. Reflux symptoms, conversely, were significantly worse after surgery and never returned to preoperative levels, affecting nearly 75% of patients at 3 years.

Using a mood scale and a QOL tool with somewhat different subscales than those of the EORTC instrument, Brooks et al. evaluated mood states and QOL over 12 months in 38 patients who had undergone esophagectomy (31). They found deterioration in global QOL, as well as in the physical and functional subscales, after surgery, with a gradual return to baseline scores within 9 months. Similarly, scales for esophageal symptoms worsened after therapy and returned to baseline within 9 months. Emotional and social subscales were relatively unaffected by the operation. Overall mood dysfunction was highest at baseline and 1 month postoperatively, with a gradual improvement over 9 months. Depression scores, however, remained relatively stable throughout the study period. Fatigue was a significant problem at 1 month post-op but steadily improved over the next several months.

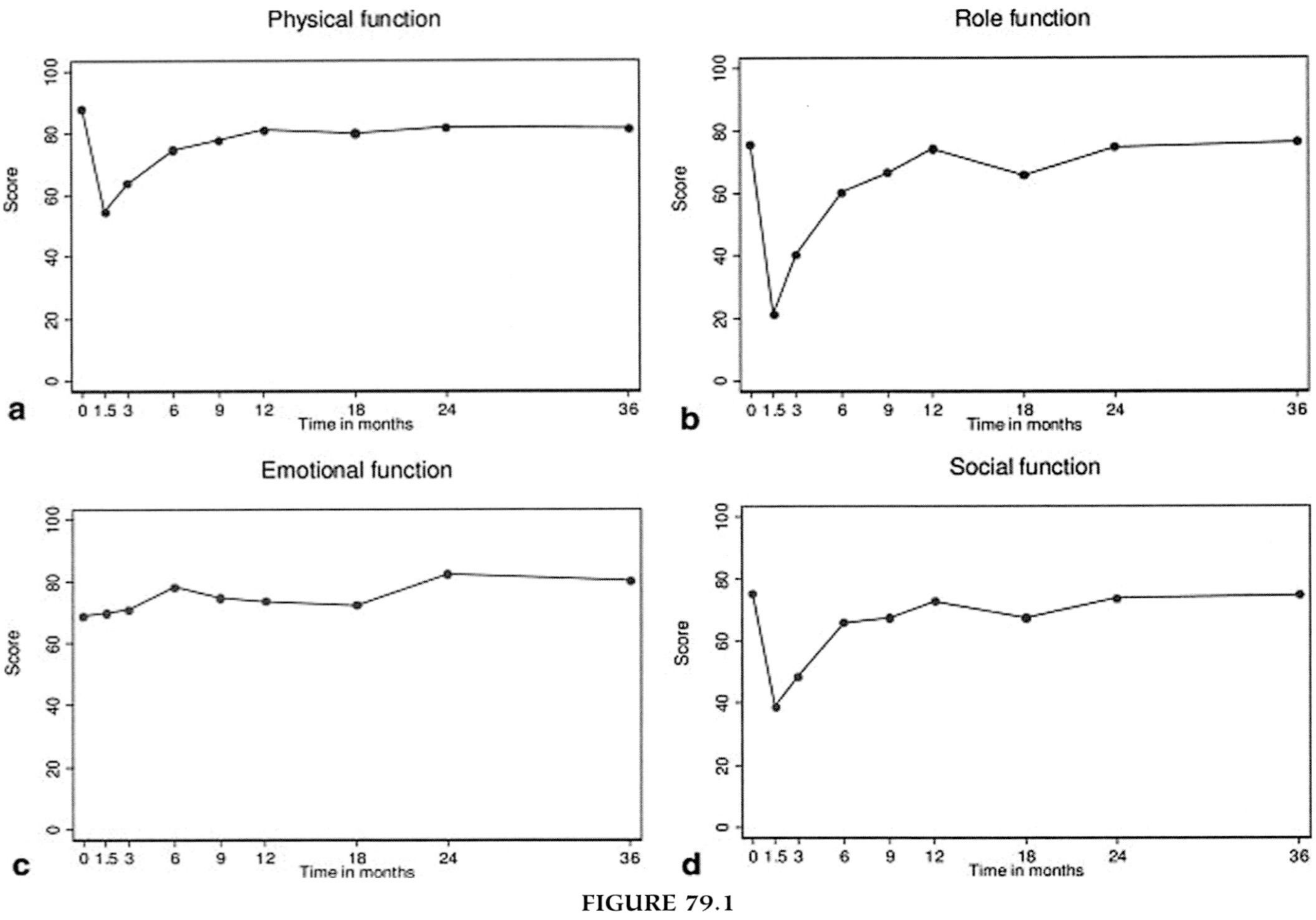

FIGURE 79.1

Health-related quality of life function scores among 47 long-term survivors after esophagectomy for esophageal cancer (higher scores indicate better function) (30).

Employing the EORTC scales, Zieren and colleagues assessed QOL over 1 year in 30 patients who had undergone esophagectomy (20). Their study excluded those who died or had recurrent disease diagnosed within the year. Role and physical function deteriorated significantly following surgery but recovered to baseline levels within 6 to 9 months. Global QOL also deteriorated postoperatively but returned to baseline levels within 3 to 6 months and exceeded preoperative levels by 12 months. Emotional and social dysfunction was less common, although 33% had some degree of emotional problem, particularly depression and anxiety. When present, emotional and social dysfunction had a significant impact on the evaluation of overall QOL. Regarding symptoms, dysphagia was the dominant symptom before surgery but had improved by hospital discharge. Postoperatively, fatigue, weight loss, and pain were the most significant symptoms. They all returned to baseline by 3 months, however, and were better than preoperative levels by 12 months.

FACTORS PREDICTING DIMINISHED QUALITY OF LIFE

Several studies have evaluated factors associated with diminished QOL following esophagectomy. Viklund and colleagues examined factors affecting quality of life at 6 months postoperatively in 100 patients who had undergone esophagectomy for esophageal cancer (32). They found that the occurrence of surgical complications was the main predictor of reduced scores of global QOL, physical and role functioning (Table 79.1). In particular, complications affecting QOL included anastomotic leak, infection, respiratory insufficiency, cardiac complications, and the need for reoperation. QOL was not affected by the choice of surgical approach or the occurrence of anastomotic stricture. These findings were supported in the study by Deschamps et al. of 107 patients who were over 5 years out from esophagectomy (27). These authors found that anastomotic leak was associated with decreased physical functioning and health

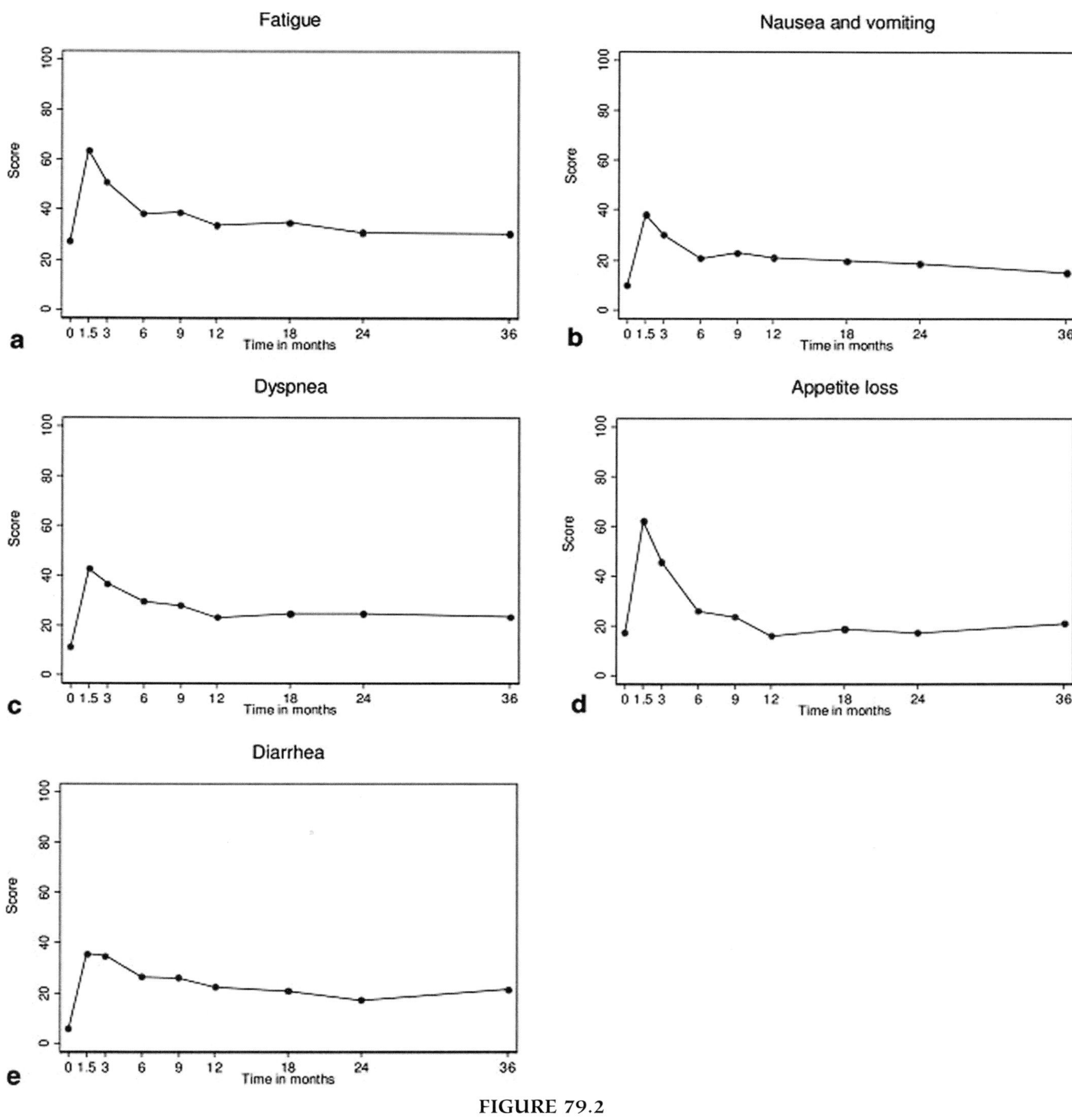

FIGURE 79.2

General symptom scores among 47 long-term survivors after esophagectomy for esophageal cancer (higher scores indicate worse symptoms) (30).

perception, while the need for dilation adversely affected social functioning.

In a study with 12 month follow-up, Zieren et al. found that tumor recurrence and anastomotic stricture were the only factors that significantly correlated with lowered quality of life (20). In this study, patients with symptomatic recurrent disease had significantly lower scores on the global QOL, physical, role, and emotional function scales and experienced worse disease symptoms than patients who were disease-free at the time of

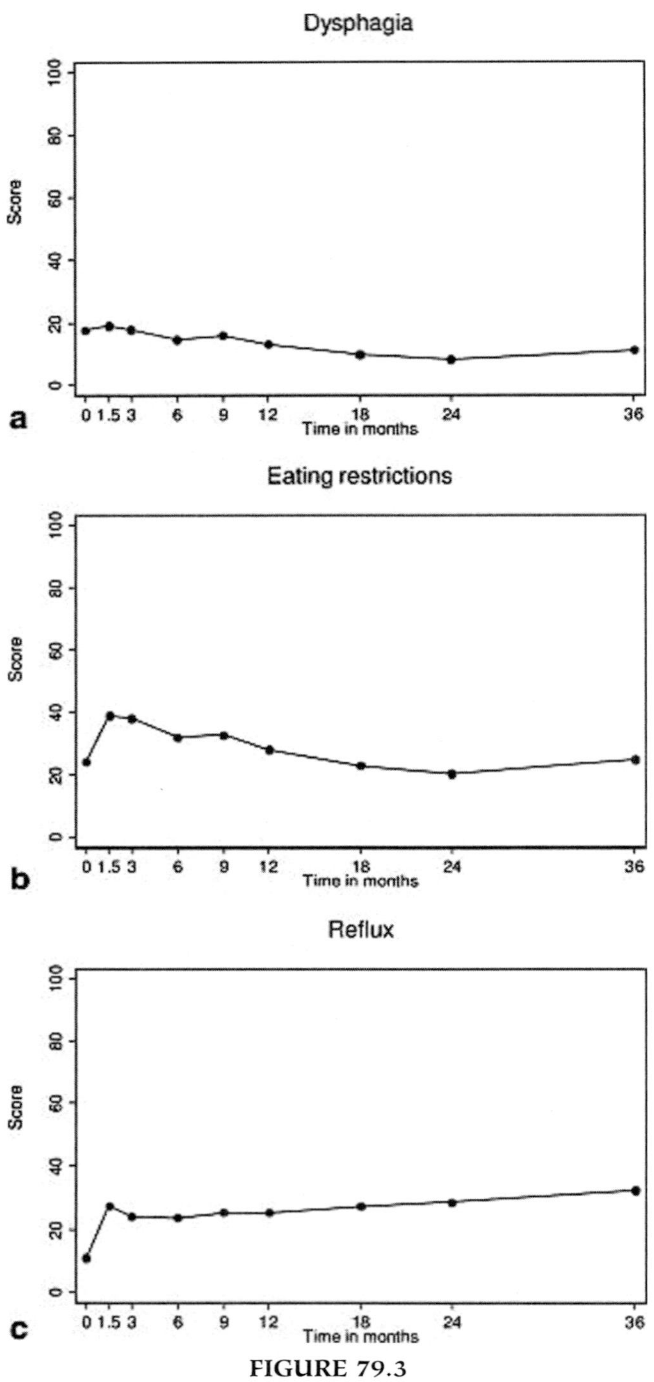

FIGURE 79.3

Esophageal-specific symptom scores among 47 long-term survivors after esophagectomy for esophageal cancer (higher scores indicate worse symptoms) (30).

the study. Even patients with asymptomatic recurrent disease showed lower scores on global QOL and emotional function. Similarly, in a study with 3-year follow-up, Blazeby et al. found that patients who survive for at least 2 years after esophagectomy recover most aspects of QOL within 6 to 9 months from surgery (33). Patients who die within 2 years, however, suffer an irreversible and progressive decline in QOL, with scores similar to patients initially selected for palliative only treatment. These 2 studies point to the importance of accurate preoperative staging to identify those patients who are unlikely to be cured by surgery and who may benefit more, from the QOL standpoint, from less aggressive therapies.

EFFECT OF ANASTOMOTIC SITE ON QUALITY OF LIFE

Several studies have suggested that the site of anastomosis following esophagectomy may affect postoperative symptoms. For example, reflux symptoms appear to be more common after intrathoracic than cervical anastomosis (34–36). This potential disparity in postoperative symptoms, combined with the lack of a clear survival advantage for either approach, makes the effects of operative approach on QOL a more compelling outcome to evaluate when comparing surgical strategies.

Egberts and colleagues studied 105 patients for 2 years after esophagectomy using the EORTC QOL instrument (4). A third of patients had a cervical anastomosis (25 with concomitant thoracotomy; 8 without), and the remainder had an intrathoracic anastomosis. In both groups, all QOL functional scores, particularly role function, dropped from baseline in the early postoperative period and never fully recovered to preoperative levels (Figure 79.4). Global QOL also dropped after surgery but recovered by 12 months to near-baseline levels. There was no significant difference in any of the QOL scales between the cervical and intrathoracic groups. Overall, symptom scales were also similar between groups (Figure 79.5). Specifically, dysphagia and reflux scores improved over time and were not significantly different between groups. Pain and nausea/vomiting, however, were significantly worse in patients with intrathoracic anastomoses.

In a similar study, de Boer and colleagues compared QOL outcomes for 3 years following esophagectomy in 199 patients who had undergone a transhiatal (THE) or extended transthoracic (TTE) resection (37). They employed a modified symptom scale, the Rotterdam Symptom Checklist, and a generic QOL instrument, the SF-20. Results from the symptom surveys revealed that physical symptoms and activity level diminished after surgery but returned to baseline levels within 1 year. Psychologic symptoms continued to improve after surgery and stabilized within the first year above baseline levels. Global QOL, despite an initial drop postoperatively, gradually recovered to higher than preoperative levels.

TABLE 79.1
Surgery-Related Factors and Variables Representing Global, Physical and Role Measures of Quality of Life Among 100 Patients after Esophagectomy for Cancer of the Esophagus or Gastric Cardia (Higher Score Indicates Better Quality of Life) (32)

		Measures of quality of life in mean scores (score) with standard deviations (SD) and P-values (P)		
Variable	**Patients (number)**	**Global score (SD)**	**Physical score (SD)**	**Role score (SD)**
No complication (reference)	56	65 (21)	82 (19)	74 (30)
Reoperation	9	56 (26) $P = 0.42$	63 (23) $P = 0.014$*	37 (31) $P = 0.002$*
Anastomotic leakage	8	53 (16) $P = 0.10$	65 (19) $P = 0.024$*	38 (32) $P = 0.008$*
Infections	9	48 (23) $P = 0.05$*	62 (25) $P = 0.024$*	43 (32) $P = 0.01$*
Respiratory insufficiency	14	51 (26) $P = 0.08$	68 (22) $P = 0.03$*	48 (31) $P = 0.007$*
Cardiac complications	10	49 (22) $P = 0.04$*	71 (25) $P = 0.13$	53 (29) $P = 0.05$
Technical complications	7	61 (22) $P = 0.67$	73 (19) $P = 0.16$	50 (36) $P = 0.08$
Anastomotic strictures	4	60 (30) $P = 0.90$	87 (22) $P = 0.51$	71 (39) $P = 1.00$

With kind permission from Springer Science+Business Media: World Journal of Surgery, Influence of Surgery-related Factors on Quality of Life after Esophageal or Cardia Cancer Resection, Pernilla Viklund, July 1, 2005; 29(7), 841–848.
*Statistically significant difference.

The only significant differences between the groups occurred at 3 and 6 months after operation, where patients who had undergone THE reported significantly fewer physical symptoms than those in the TTE group. At 3 months postoperatively, the THE patients also had better activity levels than TTE patients. By 1 year, however, these differences between the 2 surgical groups had disappeared.

Analysis of the generic QOL surveys in this study revealed a similar pattern. Following surgery, QOL declined sharply, particularly for physical, role, and social functioning. All of these indices returned to baseline levels within 6 to 9 months. At 3 months postoperatively, QOL was better for THE than TTE patients. Although there were no statistically significant differences beyond that point, there was an overall trend toward improved QOL scores for patients in the THE group.

EFFECTS OF CHEMORADIATION THERAPY ON QUALITY OF LIFE

The last decade has seen a rise in the use of adjuvant and neoadjuvant chemoradiothearapy in the treatment of locally advanced esophageal cancer. Because survival advantages over surgery alone are still modest, the impact that different therapies have on QOL outcomes should play a role in determining optimal treatment strategies. Comparative studies to date have evaluated QOL measures in multimodal therapy versus surgery alone, as well as with definitive chemoradiation versus surgery.

Multimodal Therapy vs. Surgery Alone

Blazeby et al. used the EORTC scales to compare QOL outcomes over 12 months between patients who had received neoadjuvant chemotherapy or chemoradiotherapy prior to esophagectomy and those undergoing surgery alone (38). During neoadjuvant therapy, most aspects of QOL deteriorated, and patients experienced a rise in general symptoms associated with treatment toxicity. After esophagectomy, patients in all groups experienced a sharp decline in physical, role, and social function but recovered most aspects of QOL by 6 to 9 months. Overall, postoperative QOL scores were similar between all 3 groups of patients, except that those who had undergone multimodal therapy reported earlier recovery with regard to dysphagia and nausea/vomiting than those who had undergone surgery alone. Despite having a temporary negative effect on QOL, neoadjuvant therapy did not delay postoperative recovery of QOL measures.

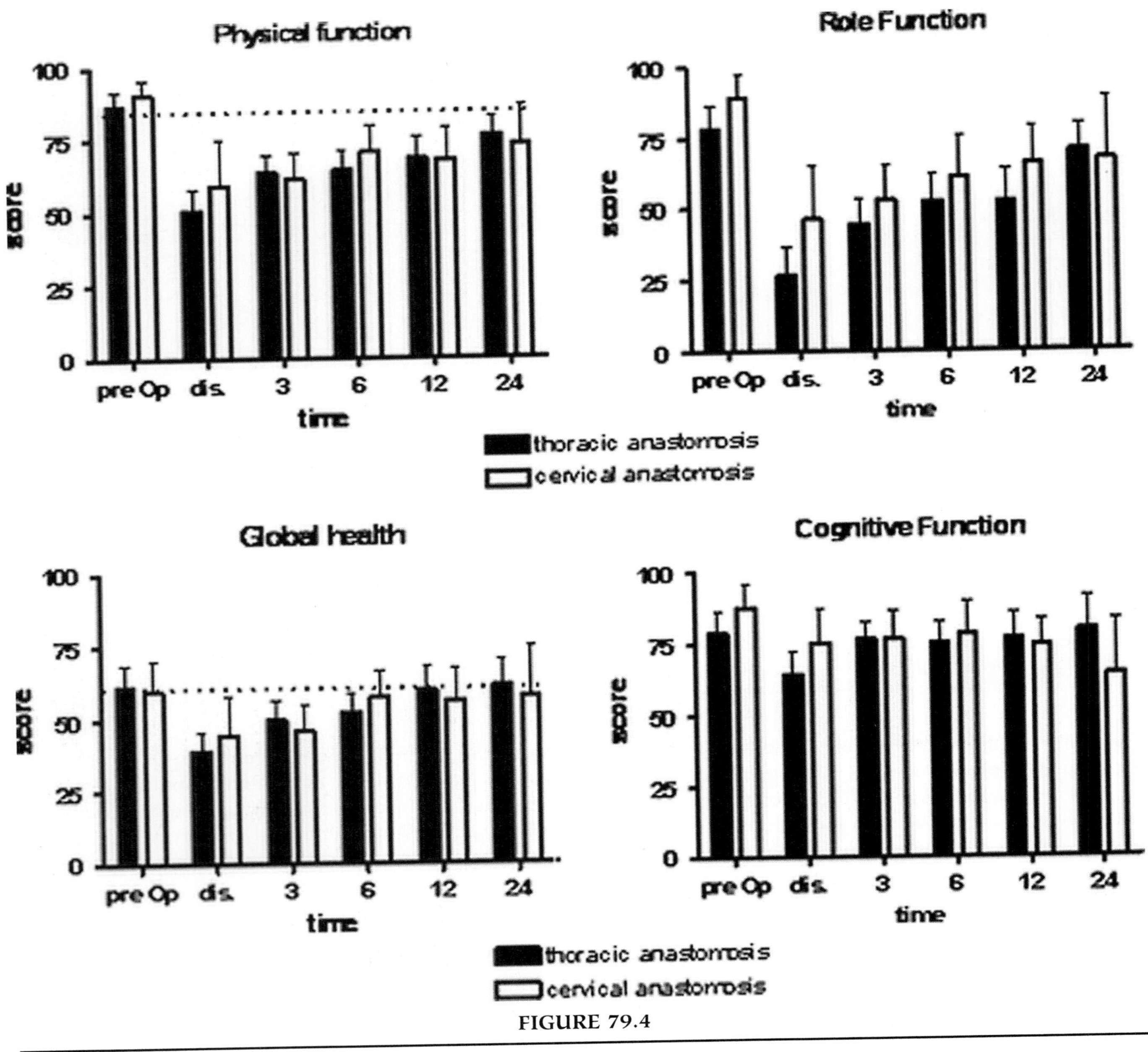

FIGURE 79.4

Comparison of functional scores in patients after esophagectomy with either a cervical or intrathoracic anastomosis. Mean values of corresponding items are displayed and 95% confidence interval is indicated as error bars. Functional scores of an age-matched healthy population is shown in dotted lines (4). With kind permission from Springer Science+Business Media: World Journal of Surgery, Influence of Surgery-related Factors on Quality of Life after Esophageal or Cardia Cancer Resection, Pernilla Viklund, July 1, 2005; 29(7), 841–848.

These findings were echoed in a similar study by Reynolds and colleagues (39). These authors also used the EORTC instruments to compare QOL over 1 year in 202 patients who had undergone esophagectomy with or without neoadjuvant chemoradiotherapy. Physical and role function scores were reduced preoperatively in the multimodal treatment group, although dysphagia scores had improved. In both groups, most QOL measures had recovered to baseline levels by 6 months. In the surgery-alone group, however, physical and role function remained impaired at 12 months, while social functioning and financial concerns were problematic for the multimodal treatment group. Finally, global QOL scores were better in those who had undergone multimodal therapy than those who had surgery alone.

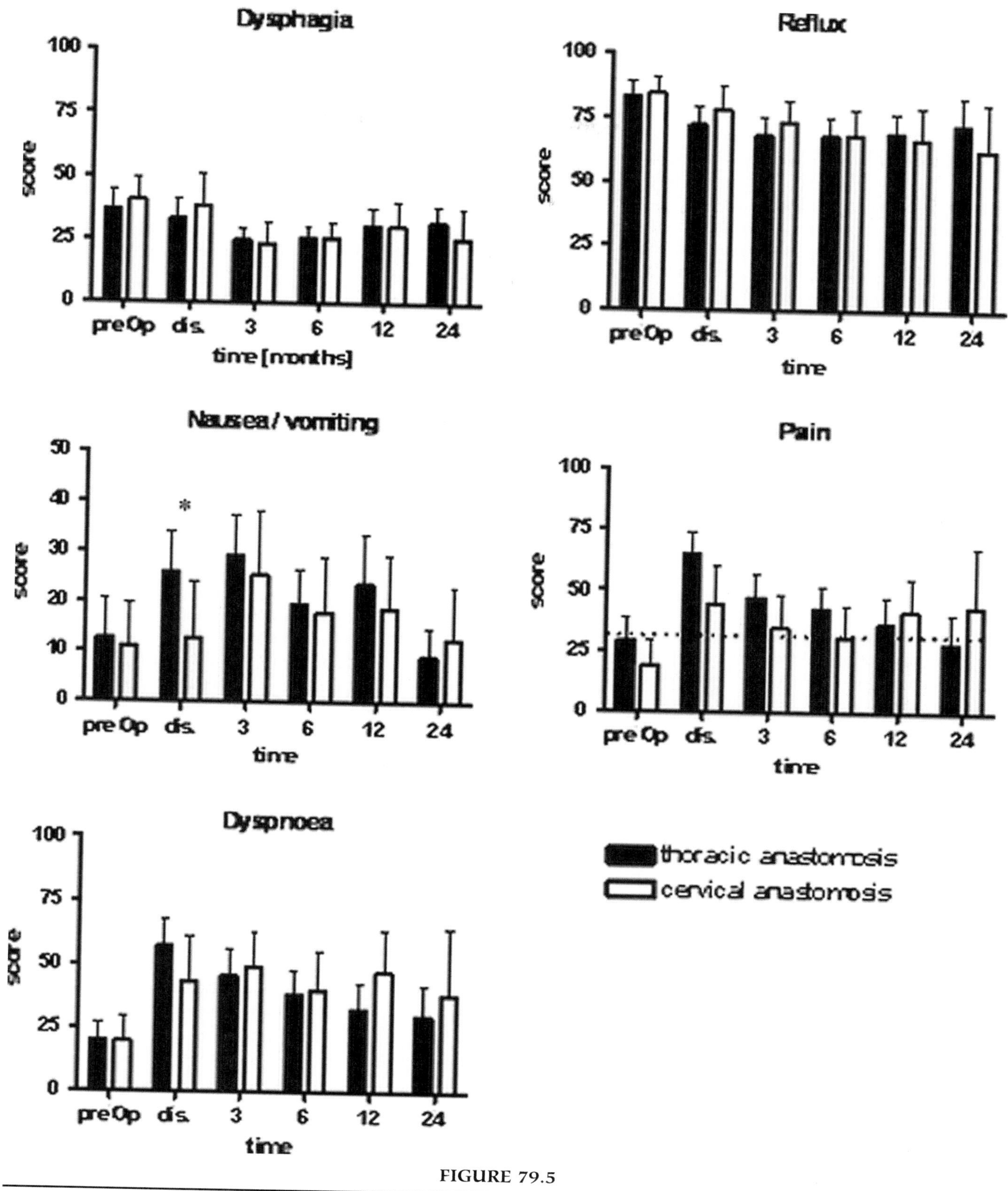

FIGURE 79.5

Comparison of symptom scores in patients after esophagectomy with either a cervical or intrathoracic anastomosis. Mean values of corresponding items are displayed and 95% confidence interval is indicated as error bars (P = 0.025) (4). With kind permission from Springer Science+Business Media: World Journal of Surgery, Influence of Surgery-related Factors on Quality of Life after Esophageal or Cardia Cancer Resection, Pernilla Viklund, July 1, 2005; 29(7), 841–848.

Definitive Chemoradiation vs. Surgery

Avery et al. compared short-term QOL outcomes between definitive chemoradiation therapy and surgery in patients with locally advanced esophageal cancer (29). At the expected worst time (12 weeks after starting chemoradiotherapy and 6 weeks after esophagectomy), patients in the surgery group showed a greater decline in physical, role, and social function and reported more problems with fatigue, dyspnea, nausea/vomiting, and diarrhea than patients treated with chemoradiotherapy. At the expected recovery time (9 months after chemoradiotherapy and 6 months after esophagectomy), QOL scores had returned to baseline levels in the chemoradiotherapy group. In the surgery group, however, scores for role function, dyspnea, diarrhea, and cough remained well below baseline levels. Furthermore, reflux symptoms were significantly worse for patients who had undergone surgery. This study was somewhat limited by the fact that some patients in the surgery group had undergone multimodal therapy, which may have had an impact on QOL scores for these patients.

As part of a multicenter, randomized trial comparing chemoradiation plus surgery to chemoradiation alone for locally advanced esophageal cancer, Bonnetain and colleagues evaluated QOL measures over 2 years after treatment (40). They used the Spitzer Index, a cancer-specific questionnaire that is completed by the provider and not the patient. The authors found that the QOL Index was significantly worse in the surgery arm at the first follow-up after treatment. However, there were no significant differences in QOL over time and longitudinal QOL among 2-year survivors did not differ between treatment groups. As with other studies discussed, the lack of a disease-specific QOL instrument may have limited the ability of this study to detect differences in esophageal-specific treatment effects.

CONCLUSION

Esophagectomy has a significant negative impact on most aspects of health-related QOL. While QOL typically improves over the first 1 to 2 years, many aspects may not return to baseline levels. This appears especially true in patients who develop recurrent disease or suffer major complications from surgery. While esophagectomy is generally successful at relieving dysphagia, patients are often left with long-lasting and sometimes debilitating symptoms, particularly reflux, dyspnea, and diarrhea. These detrimental treatment effects, combined with the overall poor prognosis, underline the value of including QOL outcomes when comparing different therapies or making treatment decisions. From the patient perspective, these outcomes may prove to be the most important.

References

1. Beitz J, Gnecco C, Justice R. Quality-of-life end points in cancer clinical trials: the U.S. Food and Drug Administration perspective. *J Natl Cancer Inst Monogr.* 1996;(20):7–9.
2. Gondek K, Sagnier PP, Gilchrist K, et al. Current status of patient-reported outcomes in industry-sponsored oncology clinical trials and product labels. *J Clin Oncol.* 2007;25(32):5087–5093.
3. American Society of Clinical Oncology. Outcomes of cancer treatment for technology assessment and cancer treatment guidelines. *J Clin Oncol.* 1996;14(2):671–679.
4. Egberts JH, Schniewind B, Bestmann B, Schafmayer C, Egberts F, Faendrich F, Kuechler T, Tepel J. Impact of the site of anastomosis after oncologic esophagectomy on quality of life—a prospective, longitudinal outcome study. *Ann Surg Oncol.* 2007.
5. Hulscher JB, van Sandick JW, de Boer AG, et al. Extended transthoracic resection compared with limited transhiatal resection for adenocarcinoma of the esophagus. *N Engl J Med.* 2002;347(21):1662–1669.
6. Wijnhoven BP, Tran KT, Esterman A, et al. An evaluation of prognostic factors and tumor staging of resected carcinoma of the esophagus. *Ann Surg.* 2007;245(5): 717–725.
7. Connors RC, Reuben BC, Neumayer LA, et al. Comparing outcomes after transthoracic and transhiatal esophagectomy: a 5-year prospective cohort of 17,395 patients. *J Am Coll Surg.* 2007;205(6):735–40.
8. Lagarde SM, Reitsma JB, de Castro SM, et al. Prognostic nomogram for patients undergoing oesophagectomy for adenocarcinoma of the oesophagus or gastro-oesophageal junction. *Br J Surg.* 2007;94(11):1361–1368.
9. Rodgers M, Jobe BA, O'Rourke RW, et al. Case volume as a predictor of inpatient mortality after esophagectomy. *Arch Surg.* 2007;142(9):829–839.
10. Viklund P, Lindblad M, Lu M, et al. Risk factors for complications after esophageal cancer resection: a prospective population-based study in Sweden. *Ann Surg.* 2006;243(2):204–211.
11. Chiu PW, Chan AC, Leung SF, et al. Multicenter prospective randomized trial comparing standard esophagectomy with chemoradiotherapy for treatment of squamous esophageal cancer: early results from the Chinese University Research Group for Esophageal Cancer (CURE). *J Gastrointest Surg.* 2005;9(6):794–802.
12. Stahl M, Stuschke M, Lehmann N, et al. Chemoradiation with and without surgery in patients with locally advanced squamous cell carcinoma of the esophagus. *J Clin Oncol.* 2005;23(10):2310–2317.
13. Walther B, Johansson J, Johnsson F, et al. Cervical or thoracic anastomosis after esophageal resection and gastric tube reconstruction: a prospective randomized trial comparing sutured neck anastomosis with stapled intrathoracic anastomosis. *Ann Surg.* 2003;238(6):803–812; discussion 812–814.
14. Breslow L. A quantitative approach to the World Health Organization definition of health: physical, mental and social well-being. *Int J Epidemiol.* 1972;1(4):347–355.
15. Blazeby JM, Conroy T, Hammerlid E, et al. Clinical and psychometric validation of an EORTC questionnaire module, the EORTC QLQ-OES18, to assess quality of life in patients with oesophageal cancer. *Eur J Cancer.* 2003;39(10):1384–1394.
16. Rock EP, Scott JA, Kennedy DL, et al. Challenges to use of health-related quality of life for Food and Drug Administration approval of anticancer products. *J Natl Cancer Inst Monogr.* 2007;(37):27–30.
17. Stein HJ, von Rahden BH, Siewert JR. Survival after oesophagectomy for cancer of the oesophagus. *Langenbecks Arch Surg.* 2005;390(4):280–285.
18. Blazeby JM, Williams MH, Brookes ST, et al. Quality of life measurement in patients with oesophageal cancer. *Gut.* 1995;37(4):505–508.
19. van Knippenberg FC, Out JJ, Tilanus HW, et al. Quality of Life in patients with resected oesophageal cancer. *Soc Sci Med.* 1992;35(2):139–145.
20. Zieren HU, Jacobi CA, Zieren J, Muller JM. Quality of life following resection of oesophageal carcinoma. *Br J Surg.* 1996;83(12):1772–1775.
21. Blazeby JM, Vickery CW. Quality of life in patients with cancers of the upper gastrointestinal tract. *Expert Rev Anticancer Ther.* 2001;1(2):269–276.
22. Guyatt GH, Feeny DH, Patrick DL. Measuring health-related quality of life. *Ann Intern Med.* 1993;118(8):622–629.
23. Switzer GE, Wisniewski SR, Belle SH, et al. Selecting, developing, and evaluating research instruments. *Soc Psychiatry Psychiatr Epidemiol.* 1999;34(8):399–409.
24. Blazeby JM, Williams MH, Alderson D, et al. Observer variation in assessment of quality of life in patients with oesophageal cancer. *Br J Surg.* 1995;82(9):1200–1203.
25. Osoba D, Rodrigues G, Myles J, et al. Interpreting the significance of changes in health-related quality-of-life scores. *J Clin Oncol.* 1998;16(1):139–144.
26. Viklund P, Wengstrom Y, Rouvelas I, et al. Quality of life and persisting symptoms after oesophageal cancer surgery. *Eur J Cancer.* 2006;42(10):1407–1414.
27. Deschamps C, Nichols FC III, Cassivi SD, et al. Long-term function and quality of life after esophageal resection for cancer and Barrett's. *Surg Clin North Am.* 2005;85(3):649–656, xi.

28. De Boer AG, Genovesi PI, Sprangers MA, et al. Quality of life in long-term survivors after curative transhiatal oesophagectomy for oesophageal carcinoma. *Br J Surg.* 2000;87(12):1716–1721.
29. Avery KN, Metcalfe C, Barham CP, et al. Quality of life during potentially curative treatment for locally advanced oesophageal cancer. *Br J Surg.* 2007;94(11):1369–1376.
30. Lagergren P, Avery KN, Hughes R, et al. Health-related quality of life among patients cured by surgery for esophageal cancer. *Cancer.* 2007;110(3):686–693.
31. Brooks JA, Kesler KA, Johnson CS, et al. Prospective analysis of quality of life after surgical resection for esophageal cancer: preliminary results. *J Surg Oncol.* 2002;81(4):185–194.
32. Viklund P, Lindblad M, Lagergren J. Influence of surgery-related factors on quality of life after esophageal or cardia cancer resection. *World J Surg.* 2005;29(7):841–848.
33. Blazeby JM, Farndon JR, Donovan J, et al. A prospective longitudinal study examining the quality of life of patients with esophageal carcinoma. *Cancer.* 2000;88(8):1781–1787.
34. Chen J, Wei G, Shao L. A comparative study of cervical and thoracic anastomoses after esophagectomy for esophageal carcinoma [in Chinese]. *Zhonghua Zhong Liu Za Zhi.* 1996;18(2):131–133.
35. McLarty AJ, Deschamps C, Trastek VF, et al. Esophageal resection for cancer of the esophagus: long-term function and quality of life. *Ann Thorac Surg.* 1997;63(6):1568–1572.
36. Schmidt CE, Bestmann B, Kuchler T, et al. Quality of life associated with surgery for esophageal cancer: differences between collar and intrathoracic anastomoses. *World J Surg.* 2004;28(4):355–360.
37. de Boer AG, van Lanschot JJ, van Sandick JW, et al. Quality of life after transhiatal compared with extended transthoracic resection for adenocarcinoma of the esophagus. *J Clin Oncol.* 2004;22(20):4202–4208.
38. Blazeby JM, Sanford E, Falk SJ, et al. Health-related quality of life during neoadjuvant treatment and surgery for localized esophageal carcinoma. *Cancer.* 2005;103(9):1791–1799.
39. Reynolds JV, McLaughlin R, Moore J, et al. Prospective evaluation of quality of life in patients with localized oesophageal cancer treated by multimodality therapy or surgery alone. *Br J Surg.* 2006;93(9):1084–1090.
40. Bonnetain F, Bouche O, Michel P, et al. A comparative longitudinal quality of life study using the Spitzer quality of life index in a randomized multicenter phase III trial (FFCD 9102): chemoradiation followed by surgery compared with chemoradiation alone in locally advanced squamous resectable thoracic esophageal cancer. *Ann Oncol.* 2006;17(5):827–834.

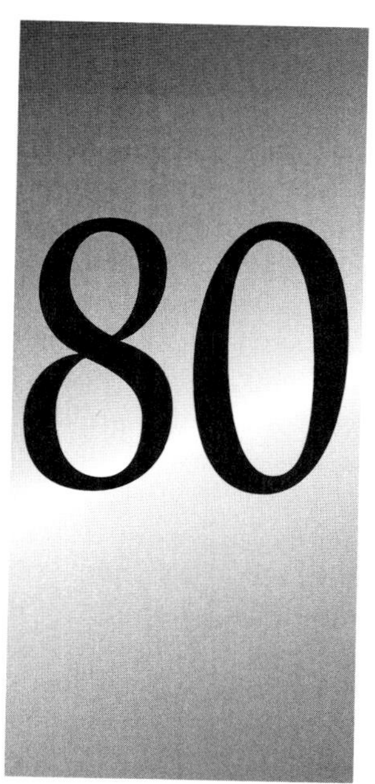

80 Proper Follow-Up after Definitive Therapy

Marek Polomsky
Jeffrey H. Peters

The epidemiology of esophageal cancer has dramatically changed over the past few decades, with increasing numbers of people being diagnosed with adenocarcinoma, and especially patients younger than 50 years old (1,2). Several developments have resulted in increasing numbers of patients surviving long term. Improvements in preoperative staging, such as detection of occult esophageal cancer at an earlier stage when the disease is confined to the mucosa or submucosa, have contributed to this prolonged survival (3). The link between Barrett's esophagus and esophageal adenocarcinoma has been established, resulting in increasing surveillance programs through liberal use of flexible endoscopy to investigate foregut symptoms, which has also increased patients having surgical resection and improvement in long-term survival (4). New surgical techniques, including the en bloc esophagectomy for control of locoregional disease, and new neoadjuvant and adjuvant therapies have also resulted in increasing numbers of patients surviving long term (5). Yet the risk of developing locoregional or systemic recurrence remains all too common. As such, clinical follow-up of patients post resection and the potential benefit of diagnostic strategies aimed toward the early identification of recurrent disease have gained increasing importance.

There is no current consensus on either the methodologies for, or the benefits of postoperative surveillance in patients with resected esophageal cancer. No prospective randomized control trials exist, and few other studies are available to guide recommendations. Thus, most clinicians follow individual follow-up routines that range from nothing to quarterly clinical, biochemical, and radiographic assessment. The ideal radiologic, laboratory, and endoscopic modalities are unknown, as is the optimal frequency of evaluation. The ultimate goal of a surveillance strategy is to increase survival and improve quality of life. Whether early detection and treatment of recurrent disease accomplishes this is also unknown.

RECURRENCE PATTERNS FOLLOWING ESOPHAGECTOMY AND THE BENEFIT OF TREATMENT

Knowledge of the timing and patterns of recurrence following esophagectomy for cancer is fundamental to any surveillance strategy. Esophageal cancer may recur locally, within the field of previous resection, within distant nodes outside the field of dissection, or systemically. These patterns have been studied in a variety of settings over the past several decades. The vast majority (75%–80%) of recurrences occur in the first 2 years post resection (Figure 80.1) (6). The probability of recurrence is highly associated with T and N stage, with both the presence of and number of metastatic lymph nodes being the most significant predictors of both local and systemic recurrence.

Several studies have shown the local recurrence rates after transhiatal esophagectomy to be in the range of 23% to 47% (Table 80.1) (7–10). Hulscher et al. examined recurrence patterns in 149 patients following transhiatal resection alone (7). The median interval between operation and recurrence was 11 months, ranging from 1.4 to 62.5 months. At a median follow-up of 2 years, slightly over half of the patients (52.6%) developed recurrent disease. Half of these were locoregional only, one-fourth systemic, and one-fourth both (Table 80.2).

In contrast, local recurrence rates after en bloc esophagectomy have been reported to be as low as 1% to 10% (Table 80.1) (11–15). Hagen et al. reported recurrence patterns in 100 patients following 2-field en bloc esophagogastrectomy (13). Only 1 of the 100 patients developed recurrence within the resection field (Table 80.3). Nodal recurrence outside of the surgical field occurred in 9 patients at a median of 35 months post resection. Systemic recurrence developed in 31 patients (31%) at a median of 10 months post resection. The risk of systemic recurrence increased with transmural invasion, more than 4 lymph nodes, and ratio of involved to uninvolved nodes greater than 10%. The evidence strongly suggests that transthoracic en bloc resection results in better control of local-regional disease. This is in contrast to the widespread practice of relying on adjuvant radiochemotherapy to improve local

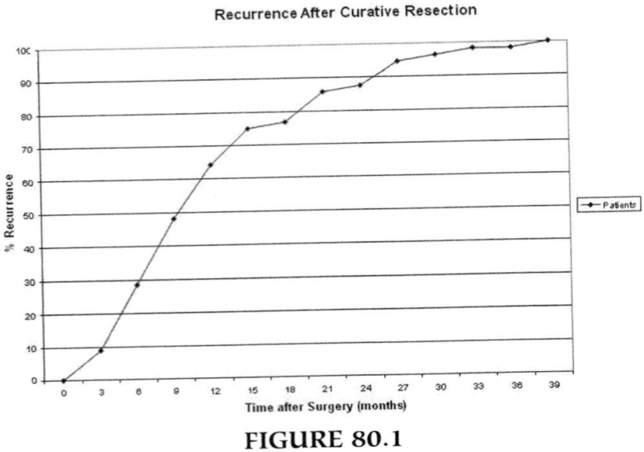

FIGURE 80.1

In examining 108 patients that had recurrence after esophagectomy for SCC, the majority of recurrences occurred in the first 2 years following resection. (Law et al. 1996)

TABLE 80.1
Reported Ability of Transthoracic EBE and THE to Control Locoregional Disease

Author	Year	No. of subjects	Local recurrence (%)
EBE			
Matsubara et al. (11)	1994	171	10%
Altorki & Skinner (12)	2001	111	8%
Hagen et al. (13)	2001	100	1%
Collard et al. (14)	2001	324	4%
Swanson et al. (15)	2001	250	5.6%
Range			1%–10%
THE			
Hulscher et al. (7)	2000	137	23%
Becker et al. (8)	1987	35	31%
Gignoux et al. (9)	1987	56	47%
Nygaard et al. (10)	1992	186	35%
Range			23%–47%

Modified from Johansson J, DeMeester TR, Hagen JA, et al. En bloc vs. transhiatal esophagectomy for stage T3 N1 adenocarcinoma of the distal esophagus. *Arch Surg*. 2004;139:627–631.

TABLE 80.2
Recurrence Pattern of Esophageal Carcinoma after Transhiatal Resection

Recurrence	N	% of patients	% of recurrences
Local only	32/72	21%	45%
Systemic only	21/72	14%	29%
Both	19/72	12%	26%

Modified from Hulscher, van Sandick JW, Tijssen JG, et al. The recurrence pattern of esophageal carcinoma after transhiatal resection. *J Am Coll Surg*. 2000;191:143–148.

TABLE 80.3
One Hundred En Bloc Resections for Esophageal Adenocarcinoma

Patterns of recurrent disease

Within the operative field: 1 patient

Systemic metastases: 31 patients

Latent nodal metastates: 9 patients

Modified from Hagen JA, DeMeester SR, Peters JH, et al. Curative resection for esophageal adenocarcinoma: analysis of 100 en bloc esophagectomies. *Ann Surg*. 2001;234:520–530.

control, which has not seen great success (Table 80.4). Nigro et al. reported that virtually all tumor recurrences in patients after en bloc resection were either distant (nodes outside the field of dissection) or systemic (3).

The impact of adjuvant therapy on both local and systemic recurrence has been reported in several studies. Shimada et al. analyzed 258 patients undergoing radical esophagectomy with extended lymphadenectomy with various adjuvant therapies for esophageal SCC between 1990 and 1998 to determine treatment response and prognostic factors in patients with recurrent esophageal cancer (16). Ninety-five (37%) patients had a recurrence with mean follow-up of 22 months. Recurrence occurred in lymph nodes in 45 (47%) patients and in distant metastases in 35 (37%) patients. Overall clinical response was seen in 26 of 76 (34%) patients who had recurrence treated nonsurgically with chemotherapy or radiotherapy. One-year survival after recurrence was higher in treatment group versus non-treated group (31% vs. 0%, $P < .001$) (Figure 80.2). One-year survival after recurrence was higher in the responder group versus the

TABLE 80.4
Local Recurrence after Varied RO Surgical Resections

Surgical resection	n	Local recurrence within operative field
En bloc (13)	94	1%
Ivor-Lewis (47)	100	14%
Transhiatal (7)	144	35%
Chemo & surgery (17)	124	32%
Chemo & RT & surgery (48)	50	19%

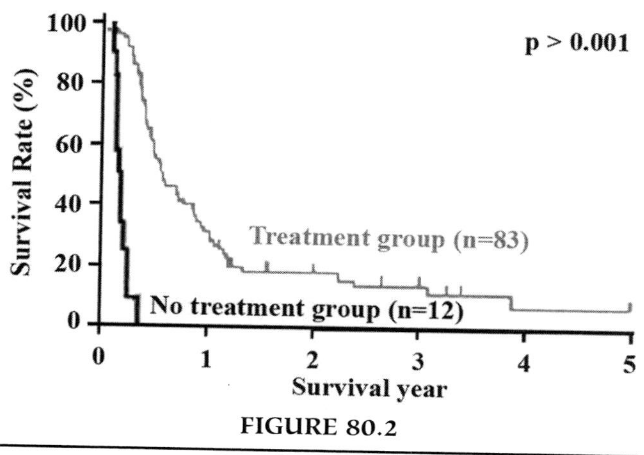

FIGURE 80.2

Treatment response and prognosis of patients after recurrence of esophageal cancer. (Shimada et al. 2003)

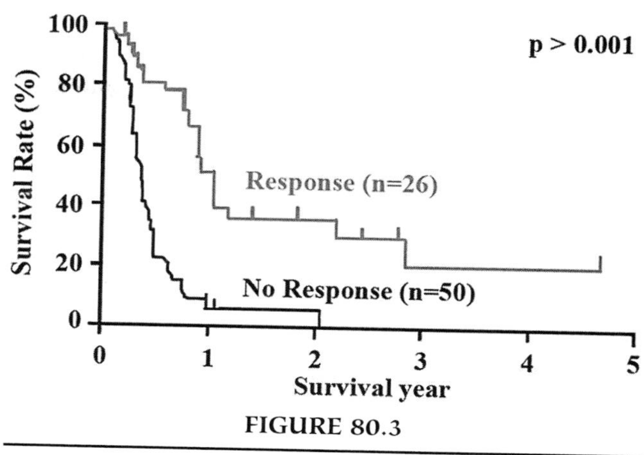

FIGURE 80.3

Treatment response and prognosis of patients after recurrence of esophageal cancer. (Shimada et al. 2003)

nonresponder group (60% vs. 17%, $P < .001$) (Figure 80.3). Treatment response was significantly associated with type of recurrence, history of perioperative adjuvant therapy, time of recurrence, number of recurrent tumors, albumin concentration, S-CRP, and S-p53-Abs. Since S-CRP and S-p53-Abs were independent prognostic factors after multivariate analysis, the authors point out the markers as potential promising predictive factors. Patients who do not respond to treatment can be spared significant side effects and toxicities of the various chemoradiotherapy treatments.

In a multi-institutional randomized trial comparing preoperative chemotherapy followed by surgery with surgery alone for patients with local and esophageal cancer, Kelsen et al. demonstrated that preoperative chemotherapy (combination of cisplatin and fluorouracil) did not improve overall survival (17). Preoperative chemotherapy also did not affect the rate of overall recurrence at locoregional or distant sites. However, when assessing patients whose resection was curative, the patients with surgery alone had higher frequency of first failures of therapy at a distant site of disease than the patients who received preoperative chemotherapy (50% vs. 41%), whereas locoregional failure was equal between the 2 groups (Table 80.5). In the United Kingdom, the Medical Research Council Adjuvant Gastric Infusional Chemotherapy (MAGIC) trial that assessed patients with resectable adenocarcinoma of the stomach, esophagogastric junction, or lower esophagus randomly assigned to either perioperative chemotherapy and surgery (250 patients) or surgery alone (253 patients), local recurrence occurred in 14.4% of perioperative chemotherapy group vs. 20.6% of surgery-alone group, as compared to distant metastases occurring in 24.4% of perioperative chemotherapy group vs. 36.8% of surgery-alone group (18). Similarly pointed out, preoperative chemotherapy decreases systemic but not locoregional recurrence.

TABLE 80.5
Patterns of First Failure Following Resection for Esophageal Carcinoma

Outcome	Surgery	Chemotherapy & surgery
Resection RO (curative)	129	124
Failure pattern	**No. (%)**	**No. (%)**
Locoregional	24 (19)	31 (25)
Local plus distant	15 (12)	9 (7)
Distant only	49 (38)	42 (34)
Any local	39 (31)	40 (32)
Any distant	64 (50)	51 (41)

Modfied from Kelsen DP, Ginsberg R, Pajak TF, et al. Chemotherapy followed by surgery compared with surgery alone for localized esophageal cancer. *N Engl J Med.* 1998;339:1979–1984.

TABLE 80.6
Combined-Modality Therapy for Esophageal Cancer: Patterns of Failure

	High dose (64.8 Gy) (*n* = 109)		Standard dose (50.4 Gy) (*n* = 109)	
	No.	**%**	**No.**	**%**
Alive/no failure	21	19	27	25
Any failure	88	81	82	75
Persistent local disease	36	33	37	34
Local failure	10	9	13	12
Regional failure	8	7	8	7
Distant failure	10	9	17	16
Regional and distant failure	0	0	2	2
Total local/regional persistence/failure	54	50	60	55
Treatment-related death	11	10	2	2
Second primary cancer	4	4	1	1
Cancer death/or not specified	3	3	0	0
Dead of intercurrent disease	6	6	2	2

Modified from Kelsen DP, Ginsberg R, Pajak TF, et al. Chemotherapy followed by surgery compared with surgery alone for localized esophageal cancer. *N Engl J Med.* 1998;339:1979–1984.

The ability of radiation therapy to control local disease has not been shown conclusively (Table 80.6) (19). Hofstetter reported the outcomes of 994 patients who underwent esophageal resection from 1970 to 2001 (20). The overall recurrence rate was 43%. Of 216 patients that received neoadjuvant chemoradiation, locoregional recurrence was significantly less (17% vs. 25%, $P = .01$), and there was a tendency toward less distant recurrence (31% vs. 35%, $P = .12$). A meta-analysis of randomized controlled trials of neoadjuvant chemoradiation versus surgery alone revealed lower locoregional recurrences with an odds ratio of 0.38 when compared to those not receiving neoadjuvant treatments (21).

CLINICAL AND DIAGNOSTIC FOLLOW-UP METHODOLOGIES

The clinical intensity and diagnostic modalities employed during postoperative follow-up for esophageal and other solid tumors vary greatly. That being said, the basis of every follow-up routine is a detailed history and thorough physical examination. The questions asked in the interview should focus on the symptoms that may relate to recurrence; in esophageal cancer, for example, this would include evidence of weight loss, anorexia, fatigue, pain, and recurrent dysphagia.

Regular follow-up visits have been recommended for colorectal follow-up, even in the most simple surveillance strategies. It seems appropriate that office visits every 3 months, at least for the first 2 years, should form the basis for esophageal cancer follow-up. Since the median time to systemic recurrence is less than 1 year, laboratory studies including liver function tests should be also obtained, preferably concomitantly with each office visit.

Patients who present with signs or symptoms of recurrence, pertinent evaluation should be obtained, possibly including chest X-ray, laboratory studies, endoscopy, barium esophagram, CT and/or PET scanning. Although barium esophagram is useful in the preoperative evaluation of esophageal cancer, no studies demonstrate its utility in postoperative surveillance.

Endoscopic Evaluation

The utility of endoscopy and endoscopic ultrasound prior to esophageal resection has been established (22). Few studies, however, assess the utility of upper endoscopy and endoscopic ultrasound (EUS) after resection. Conventional endoscopy with liberal biopsy will miss extramural recurrence. Although EUS may aid as a diagnostic tool in the detection of anastomotic recurrence and locoregional recurrence, it is unclear if it improves detection over conventional studies such as CT and is unlikely to alter survival, particularly in patients that are asymptomatic.

Catalano et al. reported a review on EUS in 30 asymptomatic and 10 symptomatic patients 1 to 2 years after resection (23). Ten percent (3/30) of asymptomatic patients were found to have unsuspected recurrence at the anastomosis. Of these, 1 patient had a positive endoscopic biopsy, and none were detected on CT scan. Forty percent (4/10) of symptomatic patients had recurrence on EUS, all of which were seen on standard endoscopy with biopsy. One patient in the asymptomatic group underwent resection. In both groups, patients with recurrence had either transumural (T3, T4) or lymph node involvement (N1) at initial surgery. The authors recommend surveillance EGD-EUS at 6-month intervals for 2 years in patients with transmural and/or lymph node involvement.

Fockens et al. studied 43 asymptomatic patients after localized resection of cancer of esophagus or gastric cardia that were followed at 6-month intervals for 2 years by EUS (24). Sixteen out of 66 examinations were abnormal, demonstrating 100% sensitivity, 96% specificity, and PPV of 92%, when focusing on suspicious lymph nodes or focal wall thickening. Sixty-seven percent of patients were without symptoms when recurrence was discovered. Authors concluded that EUS should be used as an adjunctive modality to conventional endoscopy for postoperative surveillance.

Muller et al. reported a retrospective analysis of 27 patients with EUS after gastric resection, 10 patients after esophageal resection, and 49 patients after transanal or anterior resection of rectal or sigmoid carcinoma (25). Endoscopic ultrasound had sensitivity of 92% and specificity of 84% for examination after esophageal resection and partial or total gastrectomy, and sensitivity of 98% and specificity of 66% after sigmoid or rectal resection, prompting authors to conclude that endoscopic ultrasound is an accurate means of detecting tumor recurrence.

CT, PET, and PET/CT

Computed tomography (CT) and/or FDG-PET scanning are routinely used in the preoperative staging of esophageal carcinoma. FDG-PET may be useful for re-staging following neoadjuvant chemotherapy and/or chemoradiation (26). There is considerably less data assessing the benefit of CT scan, PET scan, or combined PET/CT surveillance on survival following esophageal cancer resection. Few studies have tried to ascertain the detection rates of esophageal cancer recurrence following surgical resection. PET scan has shown to be sensitive for whole body assessment of systemic disease and recurrence (27).

BENEFITS OF POSTOPERATIVE FOLLOW-UP STRATEGIES IN NON-ESOPHAGEAL SOLID TUMORS

Given the paucity of data regarding the ideal follow-up strategy for esophageal cancer, a review of studies focused upon other GI solid tumors is useful. The most widely studied solid tumor is colorectal cancer. Follow-up strategies in colorectal cancer vary from relatively simple, including history and physical examinations and CEA laboratory monitoring, to considerably more intensive, including regular CT scans, chest X-rays, abdominal ultrasound, and colonoscopy. In general, the more resource-intense programs focus on later stage II and III patients, since stage I patients are cured by resection alone having 93% 5-year survival (28).

The American Society of Clinical Oncology (ASCO) published updated colorectal surveillance guidelines in 2005 based on 3 meta-analyses of 6 randomized trials comparing various surveillance programs (Table 80.7) (29). Four trials compared intensive to minimal follow-up, and 2 trials compared intensive to conventional follow-up (30–35). Testing strategies and follow-up specifics varied slightly among the studies. Postoperative CEA levels and liver imaging were used in 4 of the trials. Five of the 6 individual trials failed to demonstrate a survival benefit of the more intensive follow-up program. Significant methodologic criticisms have been made, however. Some of the studies lacked power to detect significant differences. The method of randomization was not fully described in each study. Four of the 6 studies included stage

TABLE 80.7
Randomized Trials of Follow-Up in Colorectal Cancer after Resection

Author	Year	5-Year survival rate (%)	
		Less intense	More intense
Makela et al. (30)	1995	54	59
Ohlsson et al. (31)	1995	67	75
Kjedsen et al. (32)	1997	68	70
Schoemaker et al. (33)	1998	70	76
Pietra et al. (34)	1998	58	73 ($P < .05$)
Secco et al. (35)	2002	48	63

Modified from Desch CE, Benson AB III, Somerfield MR, et al. Colorectal cancer surveillance: 2005 update of an American Society of Clinical Oncology practice guideline. *J Clin Oncol.* 2005;23:8512–8519.

I patients, and, given their favorable outcome, may have limited the ability to detect differences between surveillance groups. Very little data on the complications and consequences of follow-up testing or quality of life in follow-up programs were provided.

In contrast to the individual studies, several meta-analyses have demonstrated increased survival following an intensive follow-up program therapy (Table 80.8) (36–38). This includes a 7% absolute risk reduction of intervention compared to control for pooled 5-year mortality rate, with a RR of 0.80–0.81. Of note, the number of recurrences was similar in both groups (intensive vs. control). However, patients with more intensive surveillance had earlier documentation of recurrence and the incidence of asymptomatic recurrence was significantly more common in the intensive follow-up group as opposed to the less intensive group. Patients with more intensive surveillance were more likely to have surgery for metastatic or recurrent disease, with a higher reoperation rate. In addition, the use of CEA screening and liver imaging during follow-up demonstrated a survival benefit in the pooled analysis. Thus, earlier detection leading to reoperation when possible, particularly in asymptomatic patients, and the use of CEA levels and liver CT scans may explain improved survival of more intensive surveillance in colorectal cancer. This occurs at the expense of increased cost, potential complications, and perhaps lessened quality of life of a more intensive surveillance program.

Current guidelines for surveillance following resection for colorectal cancer include:

1. Office visits with full history and physical every 3 to 6 months for first 3 years, every 6 months during years 4 and 5, and yearly thereafter.
2. CEA every 3 months for first 3 years.
3. Annual CT scan for first 3years.
4. Preoperative or perioperative colonoscopy or within 6 months of surgery, then after 3 years, and if normal every 5 years.

Surveillance methods not recommended following resection for colorectal cancer include fecal occult blood test, CXR, LFTs, CBC, and PET scan.

Tjandra et al. recently performed a meta-analysis that included 2 further randomized trials in addition to the previous 6 trials reviewed above (39). Consistent with the previous meta-analyses, the results confirmed a reduction in mortality given a more intensive surveillance protocol. Overall mortality was 21.8% in the intensive follow-up group compared to 25.7% in the minimal follow-up group (OR = .74, P = .01). Cancer-related mortality was not significantly different between the 2 groups, however (11.5% vs. 12.5%, OR = .91, P = .52). Mortality was significantly lower in patients followed with CEA, colonoscopy, CXR, and liver USG compared to control patients that did not use those modalities. Similar to previous reports, there was no difference between all-site recurrence, although the incidence of asymptomatic recurrence and the curative reoperation rate was higher in the more intensive follow-up group. As mentioned, the survival benefit from intensive follow-up was not related to improvement in cancer-related mortality. Detecting an earlier phase of disseminated disease, coupled with the morbidity and mortality of subsequent therapy for recurrent disease, may balance the benefit of earlier intervention. Thus other factors, such as psychologic and behavioral changes as well as dietary and lifestyle modifications, may be attributed for the overall survival benefit. Further studies are needed to optimize the surveillance strategies.

As in esophageal cancer, surveillance strategies for gastric cancer have been less well defined. Most (95%) of patients with gastric cancer will recur within 4 years

TABLE 80.8

Meta-Analyses of Colorectal Cancer Post-Treatment Surveillance Randomized Control Trials

Author	Year	No. of articles analyzed	5-Year mortality across trials		Absolute risk difference		Effect on 5-year mortality	
			Control	Intervention	%	95% CI	RR	95% CI
Figueredo et al. (36)	2003	6	37%	30%	7	3 to 12	0.8	.7 to .91
Renehan et al. (37)	2002	5	37%	30%	7	2 to 12	0.81	.7 to .94
Jeffery et al. (38)	2002	5	37%	30%	7	2 to 12	0.81	.53 to .84

Modified from Desch CE, Benson AB III, Somerfield MR, et al. Colorectal cancer surveillance: 2005 update of an American Society of Clinical Oncology practice guideline. *J Clin Oncol.* 2005;23:8512–8519.

of curative resection (40). Kodera et al. reviewed 197 patients with recurrence enrolled in a follow-up program following curative resection from 1985 to 1996 (41). Half (50%) of the recurrences were diagnosed within 1 year and 75% within 2 years after surgery. Eighty-eight patients (45%) were asymptomatic when the recurrence was first diagnosed. Detection of early asymptomatic recurrences allowed more patients to be treated with chemotherapy and undergo resection of metastatic lesions. Overall survival after curative resection was not different between the symptomatic and asymptomatic recurrence, however. This was due to the detection and diagnosis of symptomatic recurrence later after surgery than the asymptomatic recurrence. Even though survival after detection was longer, the disease-free survival was shorter, resulting in no effect on overall survival (Figure 80.4). The authors concluded that surveillance strategies that pick up earlier asymptomatic recurrence may not be worth the cost and effort because they do not increase overall post-resection survival.

In a larger study from a tertiary referral center where a high volume of curative gastric surgery is performed, Bennett et al. examined 561 gastric cancer patients with recurrence following curative resection from 1985 to 2000 (42). The aim of the study was to elucidate outcomes following detection of recurrence and to look at variables that may be prognostic and predictive of postrecurrence survival. Median survival was 13.5 months for asymptomatic patients and 4.8 months for symptomatic patients, a significant difference ($P < .001$). Median disease-specific survival was 29.4 months for asymptomatic patients and 21.6 months for symptomatic patients ($P < .05$). Disease-free survival

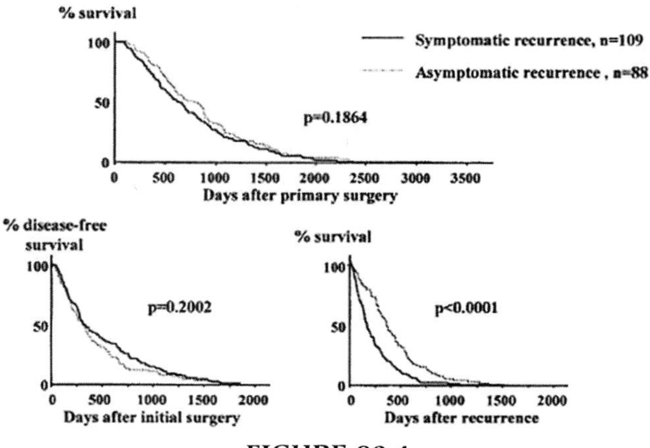

FIGURE 80.4

Overall survival, disease-free survival, and survival after detection of recurrence in 197 patients with gastric carcinoma who had recurrent disease after curative resection. (Kodera et al. 2003)

(or recurrence-free survival) was similar in symptomatic and asymptomatic patients (12.4 vs. 10.8 months, P = ns). Thus the difference in overall and postrecurrence survival is not due to lead time bias of the disease-free survival as was seen in previous studies. Improved overall survival likely resulted from earlier detection of asymptomatic recurrence (Figure 80.5). Variables associated with poor postrecurrence survival included symptomatic recurrence, advanced stage, poor differentiation, short disease-free interval, and multiple sites of recurrence. This study points out that following detection of recurrence, survival patterns in asymptomatic patients are more favorable than with symptomatic patients.

These data taken together suggest that for colorectal and gastric cancer, a more intensive surveillance strategy may improve postrecurrence and overall survival.

FOLLOW-UP STRATEGIES IN ESOPHAGEAL CANCER

The current NCCN oncology practice guidelines for follow-up of esophageal cancer include:

1. History and physical examinations every 4 months for 1 year, every 6 months for 2 years, and then annually.
2. Blood chemistry profile and CBC as clinically indicated.
3. Chest X-ray and other radiologic modalities as clinically indicated.
4. Endoscopy as clinically indicated, although not mandatory on scheduled visits. (43)

These guidelines are, of course, relatively vague, leaving considerable room for individual variability.

Kato et al. studied 55 patients with thoracic esophageal squamous cell carcinoma who underwent radical esophagectomy and were followed by PET twice per year, CT 3 times per year, and endoscopy once during first 2 years if asymptomatic (44). Symptomatic patients had earlier and additional evaluations. There were a total of 27 (49%) recurrences in the 55 patients, 19/55 (35%) locoregional, and 15/55 (27%) distant, with 8/55 (15%) being symptomatic. In patients with locoregional recurrences, FDG-PET had 100% sensitivity, 75% specificity, and 84% accuracy, which compared to 84%, 86%, and 85% for CT. There was a high false-positive rate leading to low specificity due to increased physiologic uptake in the gastric tube. In patients with distant recurrence, FDG-PET had an 87% sensitivity, 95% specificity, and 93% accuracy, which compared to 87%, 98%, and 95% for CT. FDG-PET was better diagnostically in locoregional recurrence, whereas it and CT were equal with distant mets. In addition to the low specificity due to FDG uptake in gastric graft, further limitations of PET

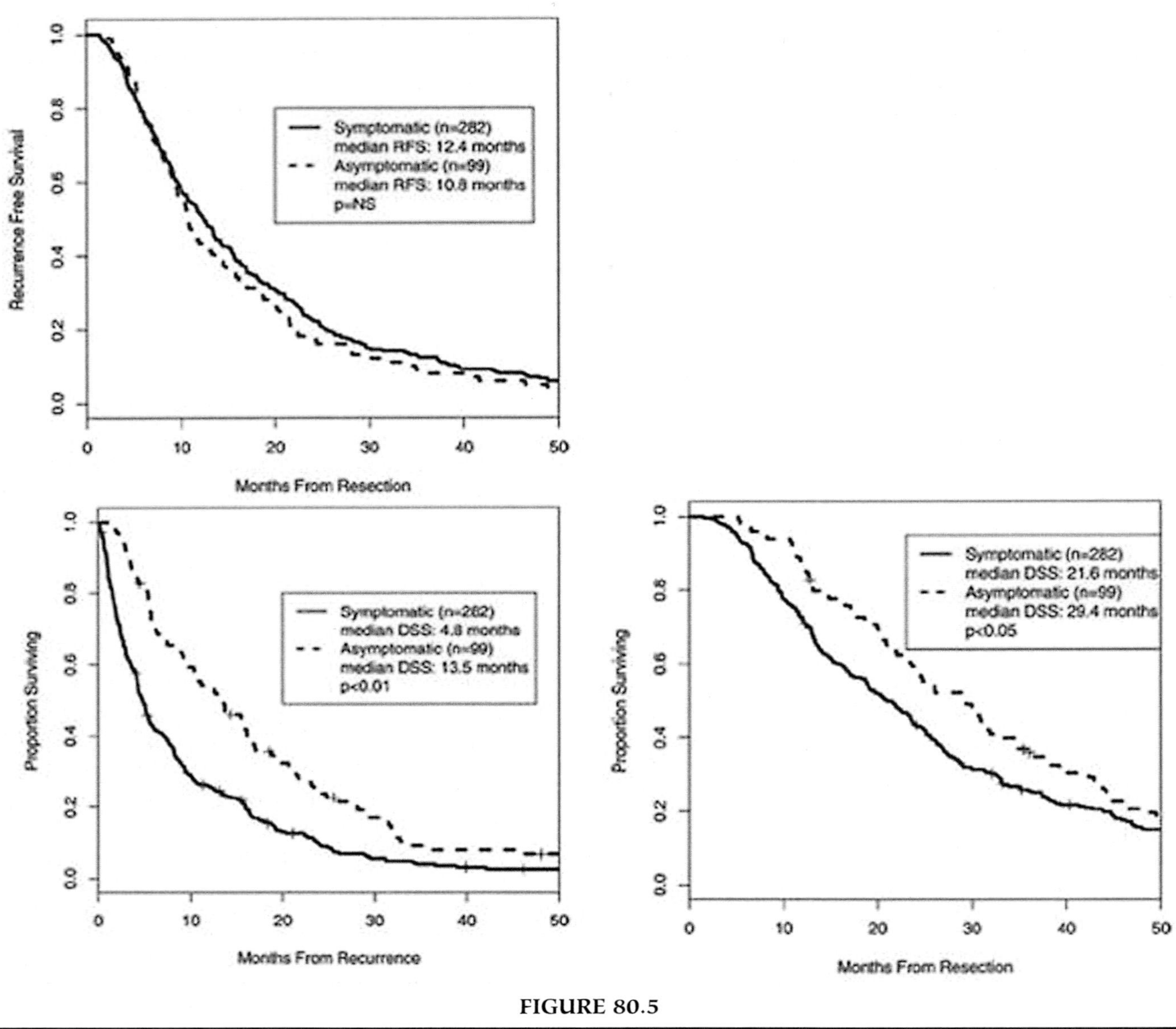

FIGURE 80.5

Recurrence-free survival, disease-free survival, and overall disease-specific survival of 282 symptomatic and 99 asymptomatic patients who had gastric cancer recurrence after resection. (Bennet et al. 2005)

scan include poorer spatial resolution than CT scan and partial volume effects leading to missing small tumors. CT scan has difficulty in distinguishing the esophagus and its surroundings and thus its limited use in picking up locoregional recurrences. The authors conclude that combined PET-CT is likely to be most useful for detecting asymptomatic recurrences in patients following curative resection.

There are remarkably few studies of the benefit of treatment once recurrence is identified. A few small series or case reports of surgical resection of isolated metastases have been reported. Yamashita and colleagues in Tokyo compared 16 patients with supraclavicular or mediastinal nodal recurrence treated with salvage radiotherapy (56.6 Gy) with or without chemotherapy to 39 patients with mediastinal or distant recurrence treated with palliative radiotherapy and 27 patients receiving planned postoperative radiotherapy (45). The median survival was 13.8 months in the salvage treatment group, 3.5 months in the palliative therapy group, and 19.1 months in patients receiving planned postoperative treatment. Fifty-six percent of the salvage group survived 1 year, and 19% of the salvage group survived 2 years. The authors concluded that symptomatic relief occurred in a substantial percentage of patients and that long-term survival was possible. Although this study is far from perfect and is concerned with a different treatment group, it does suggest that treating postoperative recurrence may be beneficial.

The authors' practice includes an office visit, symptom assessment, and weight, along with CBC, liver functions tests, and CT scan every 3 months for the first 2 years, every 6 months for next 3 years, and annually after 5 years. More recently, a combined PET/CT is included annually in place of a CT scan. Given a median time to recurrence of less than 1 year, and the majority of recurrences occurring within 2 years, surveillance is frequent for first 2 years postoperatively. Following 2 years, the frequency may be decreased in asymptomatic individuals without signs of recurrence. While evidence-based data specific to esophageal cancer are lacking, early recognition of recurrent disease is likely beneficial. Unlike the routine use of colonoscopy for CRC surveillance, upper endoscopy is uncommonly fruitful, as anastomotic and intraluminal recurrence is uncommon. Prospective trials and retrospective studies with cost analysis are needed to further clarify post-operative surveillance strategies following curative resection.

References

1. American Cancer Society. *Cancer Facts and Figures 2006*. Atlanta: American Cancer Society; 2006.
2. Devesa SS, Blot WJ, Fraumeni JF Jr. Changing patterns in the incidence of esophageal and gastric carcinoma in the United States. *Cancer*. 1998;83:2049–2053.
3. Nigro JJ, Hagen JA, DeMeester TR, et al. Occult esophageal adenocarcinoma: extent of disease and implications for effective therapy. *Ann Surg*. 1999;230:433–438; discussion 438–440.
4. van Sandick JW, van Lanschot JJ, Kuiken BW, et al. Impact of endoscopic biopsy surveillance of Barrett's oesophagus on pathological stage and clinical outcome of Barrett's carcinoma. *Gut*. 1998;43:216–222.
5. Ohga T, Kimura Y, Futatsugi M, et al. Surgical and oncological advances in the treatment of esophageal cancer. *Surgery*. 2002;131:S28–S34.
6. Law SY, Fok M, Wong J. Pattern of recurrence after oesophageal resection for cancer: clinical implications. *Br J Surg*. 1996;83:107–111.
7. Hulscher JB, van Sandick JW, Tijssen JG, et al. The recurrence pattern of esophageal carcinoma after transhiatal resection. *J Am Coll Surg*. 2000;191:143–148.
8. Becker CD, Barbier PA, Terrier F, et al. Patterns of recurrence of esophageal carcinoma after transhiatal esophagectomy and gastric interposition. *AJR Am J Roentgenol*. 1987;148:273–277.
9. Gignoux M, Roussel A, Paillot B, et al. The value of preoperative radiotherapy in esophageal cancer: results of a study of the E.O.R.T.C. *World J Surg*. 1987;11:426–432.
10. Nygaard K, Hagen S, Hansen HS, et al. Pre-operative radiotherapy prolongs survival in operable esophageal carcinoma: a randomized, multicenter study of pre-operative radiotherapy and chemotherapy. The second Scandinavian trial in esophageal cancer. *World J Surg*. 1992;16:1104–1109; discussion 1110.
11. Matsubara T, Ueda M, Yanagida O, et al. How extensive should lymph node dissection be for cancer of the thoracic esophagus? *J Thorac Cardiovasc Surg*. 1994;107:1073–1078.
12. Altorki N, Skinner D. Should en bloc esophagectomy be the standard of care for esophageal carcinoma? *Ann Surg*. 2001;234:581–587.
13. Hagen JA, DeMeester SR, Peters JH, et al. Curative resection for esophageal adenocarcinoma: analysis of 100 en bloc esophagectomies. *Ann Surg*. 2001;234:520–530; discussion 530–531.
14. Collard JM, Otte JB, Fiasse R, et al. Skeletonizing en bloc esophagectomy for cancer. *Ann Surg*. 2001;234:25–32.
15. Swanson SJ, Batirel HF, Bueno R, et al. Transthoracic esophagectomy with radical mediastinal and abdominal lymph node dissection and cervical esophagogastrostomy for esophageal carcinoma. *Ann Thorac Surg*. 2001;72:1918–1924; discussion 1924–1925.
16. Shimada H, Kitabayashi H, Nabeya Y, et al. Treatment response and prognosis of patients after recurrence of esophageal cancer. *Surgery*. 2003;133:24–31.
17. Kelsen DP, Ginsberg R, Pajak TF, et al. Chemotherapy followed by surgery compared with surgery alone for localized esophageal cancer. *N Engl J Med*. 1998;339:1979–1984.
18. Cunningham D, Allum WH, Stenning SP, et al. Perioperative chemotherapy versus surgery alone for resectable gastroesophageal cancer. *N Engl J Med*. 2006;355:11–20.
19. Minsky BD, Pajak TF, Ginsberg RJ, et al. INT 0123 (Radiation Therapy Oncology Group 94–05) phase III trial of combined-modality therapy for esophageal cancer: high-dose versus standard-dose radiation therapy. *J Clin Oncol*. 2002;20:1167–1174.
20. Hofstetter W, Swisher SG, Correa AM, et al. Treatment outcomes of resected esophageal cancer. *Ann Surg*. 2002;236:376–384; discussion 384–385.
21. Urschel JD, Vasan H. A meta-analysis of randomized controlled trials that compared neoadjuvant chemoradiation and surgery to surgery alone for resectable esophageal cancer. *Am J Surg*. 2003;185:538–543.
22. Rosch T. Endosonographic staging of esophageal cancer: a review of literature results. *Gastrointest Endosc Clin N Am*. 1995;5:537–547.
23. Catalano MF, Sivak MV Jr, Rice TW, et al. Postoperative screening for anastomotic recurrence of esophageal carcinoma by endoscopic ultrasonography. *Gastrointest Endosc*. 1995;42:540–544.
24. Fockens P, Manshanden CG, van Lanschot JJ, et al. Prospective study on the value of endosonographic follow-up after surgery for esophageal carcinoma. *Gastrointest Endosc*. 1997;46:487–491.
25. Muller C, Kahler G, Scheele J. Endosonographic examination of gastrointestinal anastomoses with suspected locoregional tumor recurrence. *Surg Endosc*. 2000;14:45–50.
26. Levine EA, Farmer MR, Clark P, et al. Predictive value of 18-fluoro-deoxy-glucose-positron emission tomography (18F-FDG-PET) in the identification of responders to chemoradiation therapy for the treatment of locally advanced esophageal cancer. *Ann Surg*. 2006;243:472–478.
27. Skehan SJ, Brown AL, Thompson M, et al. Imaging features of primary and recurrent esophageal cancer at FDG PET. *Radiographics*. 2000;20:713–723.
28. O'Connell JB, Maggard MA, Ko CY. Colon cancer survival rates with the new American Joint Committee on Cancer sixth edition staging. *J Natl Cancer Inst*. 2004;96:1420–1425.
29. Desch CE, Benson AB III, Somerfield MR, et al. Colorectal cancer surveillance: 2005 update of an American Society of Clinical Oncology practice guideline. *J Clin Oncol*. 2005;23:8512–8519.
30. Makela JT, Laitinen SO, Kairaluoma MI. Five-year follow-up after radical surgery for colorectal cancer. Results of a prospective randomized trial. *Arch Surg*. 1995;130:1062–1067.
31. Ohlsson B, Breland U, Ekberg H, et al. Follow-up after curative surgery for colorectal carcinoma. Randomized comparison with no follow-up. *Dis Colon Rectum*. 1995;38:619–626.
32. Kjeldsen BJ, Kronborg O, Fenger C, et al. A prospective randomized study of follow-up after radical surgery for colorectal cancer. *Br J Surg*. 1997;84:666–669.
33. Schoemaker D, Black R, Giles L, et al. Yearly colonoscopy, liver CT, and chest radiography do not influence 5-year survival of colorectal cancer patients. *Gastroenterology*. 1998;114:7–14.
34. Pietra N, Sarli L, Costi R, et al. Role of follow-up in management of local recurrences of colorectal cancer: a prospective, randomized study. *Dis Colon Rectum*. 1998;41:1127–1133.
35. Secco GB, Fardelli R, Gianquinto D, et al. Efficacy and cost of risk-adapted follow-up in patients after colorectal cancer surgery: a prospective, randomized and controlled trial. *Eur J Surg Oncol*. 2002;28:418–423.
36. Figueredo A, Rumble RB, Maroun J, et al. Follow-up of patients with curatively resected colorectal cancer: a practice guideline. *BMC Cancer*. 2003;3:26.
37. Renehan AG, Egger M, Saunders MP, et al. Impact on survival of intensive follow up after curative resection for colorectal cancer: systematic review and meta-analysis of randomised trials. *BMJ*. 2002;324:813.
38. Jeffery GM, Hickey BE, Hider P. Follow-up strategies for patients treated for non-metastatic colorectal cancer. *Cochrane Database Syst Rev*. 2002;(1):CD002200.
39. Tjandra JJ, Chan MK. Follow-up after curative resection of colorectal cancer: a meta-analysis. *Dis Colon Rectum*. 2007;*50*(11):1783–1799.
40. D'Angelica M, Gonen M, Brennan MF, et al. Patterns of initial recurrence in completely resected gastric adenocarcinoma. *Ann Surg*. 2004;240:808–816.
41. Kodera Y, Ito S, Yamamura Y, et al. Follow-up surveillance for recurrence after curative gastric cancer surgery lacks survival benefit. *Ann Surg Oncol*. 2003;10:898–902.
42. Bennett JJ, Gonen M, D'Angelica M, et al. Is detection of asymptomatic recurrence after curative resection associated with improved survival in patients with gastric cancer? *J Am Coll Surg*. 2005;201:503–510.
43. National Comprehensive Cancer Network. *The NCCN Esophageal Cancer Clinical Practice Guidelines in Oncology (Version 2.2007)*; 2006. http://www.nccn.org. Accessed November 5, 2008.
44. Kato H, Miyazaki T, Nakajima M, et al. Value of positron emission tomography in the diagnosis of recurrent oesophageal carcinoma. *Br J Surg*. 2004;91:1004–1009.
45. Yamashita H, Nakagawa K, Tago M, et al. Salvage radiotherapy for postoperative loco-regional recurrence of esophageal cancer. *Dis Esophagus*. 2005;18:215–220.
46. Johansson J, DeMeester TR, Hagen JA, et al. En bloc vs. transhiatal esophagectomy for stage T3 N1 adenocarcinoma of the distal esophagus. *Arch Surg*. 2004;139:627–631; discussion 631–633.
47. King RM, Pairolero PC, Trastek VF, et al. Ivor Lewis esophagogastrectomy for carcinoma of the esophagus: early and late functional results. *Ann Thorac Surg*. 1987;44:119–122.
48. Urba SG, Orringer MB, Turrisi A, et al. Randomized trial of preoperative chemoradiation versus surgery alone in patients with locoregional esophageal carcinoma. *J Clin Oncol*. 2001;19:305–313.

VI

PALLIATION

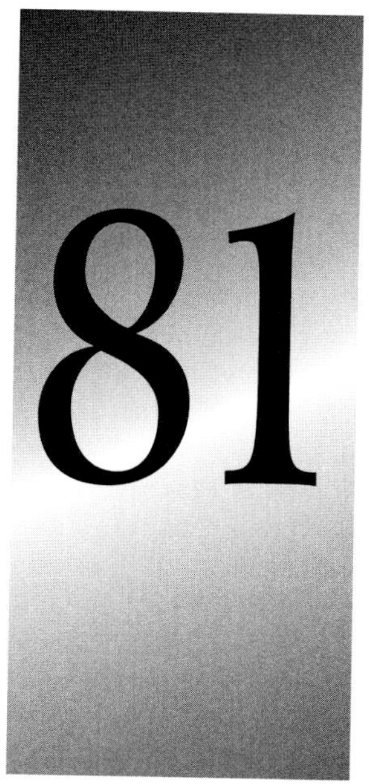

Guidelines for Palliative Care: Hospital and Hospice

Rachelle E. Bernacki
Steven Z. Pantilat

Patients with esophageal cancer have a high burden of symptoms including pain, dysphagia, nausea, and dyspnea (1,2). These symptoms can arise from the disease itself as well as from the therapies used to treat it. They can arise at any point in the course of illness and can significantly diminish quality of life. Palliative care is the field of medicine focused on symptom management and improving quality of life for patients living with a life-threatening illness such as esophageal cancer. Palliative care expertise includes the assessment and treatment of pain and other symptoms, and the relief of suffering caused by physical, psychosocial, and spiritual aspects of disease. Unlike hospice, which requires that a physician endorse a 6-month prognosis in order for a patient to qualify for service, palliative care, sometimes also referred to as supportive care, is provided in conjunction with curative treatment at any point in the disease trajectory from the time of diagnosis (Figure 81.1). As a patient becomes sicker, palliative care may become a greater focus of care either because curative treatments are no longer available or because the patient no longer desires them. Palliative care is provided by an interdisciplinary team including physicians, nurses, social workers, pharmacists, psychologists, and chaplains (3,4). Palliative care teams not only treat the patient but also attend to the needs of the family, understanding that family can include any person the patient identifies as part of their support network. Palliative care is best started early in the course of illness and across multiple-care settings; therefore, communication among the varied settings and continuity of care is essential to achieving quality care for patients (Table 81.1).

While *palliative care* refers to an approach to care focused on symptom management and improving quality of life, *palliative medicine* is used to describe the medical specialty focused on providing palliative care. Despite the emergence of palliative medicine as a recognized medical specialty, all physicians who care for patients with life-limiting illness need to be able to provide appropriate pain and symptom management and identify and treat other sources of suffering in their patients. In order to achieve this goal, all physicians need training in palliative care. Even with such training, physicians will identify some patients who have such complex needs that referral to a specialized palliative medicine team will be appropriate.

Palliative care can be provided in any setting, including hospitals, clinics, nursing homes, emergency facilities, prisons, and home (Table 81.2). Hospice is the most common way for people in the United States to receive palliative care at the end of life (5). To qualify for hospice benefits, a patient must have a life expectancy of 6 months or less. Hospice is covered by Medicare as well as most health insurance. In the United States, the

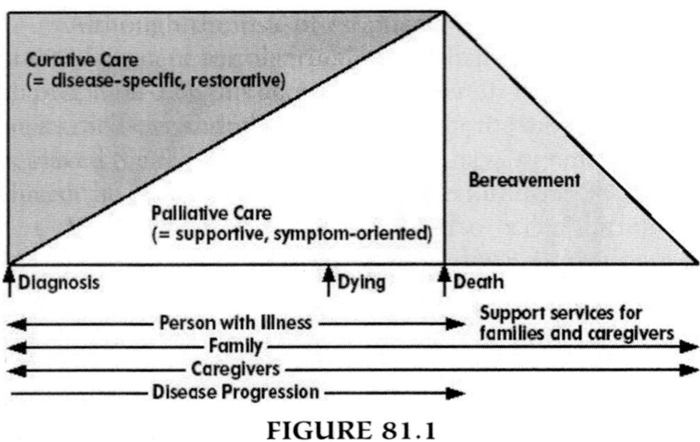

FIGURE 81.1

Palliative care model. From http://hab.hrsa.gov/tools/primarycareguide/images/PCG fig15_1b.gif

vast majority of patients receiving hospice services do so at home. Patients enrolled in home hospice generally have a primary caregiver, who is guided by a hospice nurse who visits on an as-needed basis, typically ranging from 1 to 3 times per week depending on the patient's status. A nursing aide might visit the home and bathe the patient twice a week. The hospice agency can help the family arrange for other custodial care as needed by the patient. Durable medical equipment (hospital bed, wheelchair, commode, etc.) and medications related to symptom management are provided at no charge to the patient under the hospice benefit. While hospice providers can manage most symptoms at home, if a crisis occurs, the patient can be admitted to an acute care facility until symptoms are under control.

STRUCTURE AND PROCESSES OF CARE

Care should be provided in the setting the patient chooses. If it is not possible to provide care in the patient's preferred location, the alternate setting should provide flexible visiting hours, adequate space for visitors, and sufficient respite for care providers. When the patient cannot be in their preferred setting, creative measures are taken to make the alternate care setting as comfortable and familiar as possible.

A key element of palliative care is effective communication in order to elicit a patient's preferences and goals of care. Understanding the needs and goals of the patient and family is essential for providing high quality palliative care. Palliative care teams also provide coordination of care and create plans to deal with potential crises, thereby allowing the patient to remain in their setting of choice. Palliative care providers also need good prognostication skills in order to help patients and families define goals of care and make appropriate decisions and plans. For example, when a family calls and states that a patient is eating poorly, it is important to know whether this represents a potentially reversible esophageal obstruction that could be relieved with a stent or is a sign that the patient is approaching the final days to weeks of life (6–8). Prognostic information is important in helping patients make treatment decisions. For example, one patient may want a stent placed in order to be able to eat and drink and survive to attend a granddaughter's marriage, while a different patient in a similar clinical situation may decide that he does not want to undergo yet another procedure. When the disease progresses, communication becomes even more important to ensure that all involved have the same understanding

TABLE 81.1
Palliative Care Services

- provides relief from pain and other distressing symptoms
- affirms life and regards dying as a normal process
- intends neither to hasten or postpone death
- integrates the psychological and spiritual aspects of patient care
- offers a support system to help patients live as actively as possible until death
- offers a support system to help the family cope during the patients illness and in their own bereavement
- uses a team approach to address the needs of patients and their families, including bereavement counseling, if indicated
- will enhance quality of life, and may also positively influence the course of illness
- is applicable early in the course of illness, in conjunction with other therapies that are intended to prolong life, such as chemotherapy or radiation therapy
- includes those investigations needed to better understand and manage distressing clinical complications

Information from World Health Organization's Definition of Palliative Care. Accessed online December 14, 2007 at: http://www.who.int/cancer/palliative/definition/en/

TABLE 81.2
Palliative Care Models

Model	*Care setting*
Consultation team	Usually in a hospital or nursing home; often includes social work evaluations
Combined hospice program and palliative care program	Hospital, nursing home, freestanding hospice inpatient facilities
Dedicated inpatient unit	Acute hospitals, nursing homes
Hospice-based palliative care in the home	Home
Outpatient palliative care practice or clinic	Hospital or private practice

Information from National Consensus Project for Quality Palliative Care. Clinical practice guidelines for quality palliative care. Accessed online November 28, 2007, at: http://www.nationalconsensusproject.org/Guidelines_Download.asp.

of the prognosis and plan of care. Finally, when possible, recognizing the signs and symptoms of the final stages of illness is helpful for coordinating care and logistics in the time near death. Although it is impossible to know exactly what will happen to any particular patient, experienced palliative care providers can use data, scores such as Karnofsky or Eastern Cooperative Oncology Group (ECOG), and clinical experience to offer patients and families estimates such as hours to days, days to weeks, weeks to months, and months to a year that communicate prognosis while recognizing the inherent uncertainty of such predictions.

Palliative medicine teams formulate and document care plans based on patient wishes, then convey them to patient, family, and other providers. Care plans change according to the needs of the patient and family, and should involve additional input from other specialists (radiation oncologists, anesthesiologists, complementary medicine providers) (9–14). Functional and cognitive status, disease trajectory, cultural and spiritual preferences, and home support must be considered in formulating care plans. For example, a patient with esophageal cancer may want to remain at home during the final days and weeks of life, but his wife, who is the primary caregiver, has trouble managing his medications due to mild cognitive impairment. In this situation, home nursing services or hospice can provide a weekly mediset and provide daily phone call reminders to administer the medicines. As death nears, the team may address the possibility of pursuing an inpatient hospice given the wife's limitations.

PALLIATIVE CARE DOMAINS

The key aspects of palliative care can be divided into 5 domains, including physical; psychological and psychiatric; social; spiritual, religious, and existential; and cultural aspects of care (15). Specific components of four domains are outlined in Table 81.3.

TABLE 81.3
Palliative Care Domains

Area	*Examples*
Physical	Pain, shortness of breath, nausea, fatigue, weakness, anorexia, insomnia, confusion, constipation, treatment side effects, functional capacities, treatment efficacy and alternatives (and patient and family preferences)
Psychological/psychiatric	Anxiety, depression, care-giving needs or capacity of family; stress; grief and bereavement risks for the patient and family (i.e., depression and co-morbid complications); coping strategies
Social	Family structure and geographic location; cultural concerns and needs; finances; sexuality; living arrangements; caregiver availability; access to transportation; access to prescription and over-the-counter medicines
Spiritual/religious/existential	Spiritual background, beliefs, and practices of the patient and family; hopes and fears; life completion tasks; wishes regarding care setting for death

Information from National Consensus Project for Quality Palliative Care. Clinical practice guidelines for quality palliative care. Accessed online November 28, 2007, at: http://www.nationalconsensusproject.org/Guidelines_Down/oad.asp.

Physical Aspects of Care

Physical symptoms associated with esophageal cancer include pain, dyspnea, dysphagia, nausea, vomiting, fatigue, weakness, anorexia, insomnia, anxiety, depression, confusion, and constipation. Pharmacologic, nonpharmacologic, and complementary therapies can help alleviate these symptoms. In esophageal cancer, feeding and nutrition issues are often addressed early in the course of the disease in anticipation of the need to make decisions in the future.

The goal of pain and symptom management is reduction of the symptoms to a level the patient defines as satisfactory (16, 17). Providers should be careful not to state that all symptoms will be completely alleviated, because while that is sometimes possible, more often, symptoms such as pain and nausea are attenuated to an acceptable level. Pain from esophageal cancer often requires the use of opioids, and physicians must be willing to prescribe opioids and in sufficient doses to relieve pain. Physicians should also reassure patients that addiction is rare, somnolence transitory at stable doses, and side effects manageable.

Psychological and Psychiatric Aspects of Care

In addition to addressing physical aspects of care, palliative care should address psychological issues and psychiatric needs and support emotional growth. Physicians should acknowledge the stress involved in caring for patients with life-threatening illness and address caregiver needs. Physicians must recognize the importance of maintaining a relationship with the patient even after referral to hospice and understand that patients and families are particularly vulnerable to feeling abandoned at this time by their physicians. Making follow-up appointments for patients and calling on the telephone can help reassure patients that a referral to hospice is not abandonment by the physician. Physicians must also be aware of normal and complicated grief and address those appropriately. Hospice programs provide bereavement services and follow-up for 12 months after the death of the patient. Finally, all providers can discuss and offer coping strategies to determine the most constructive approach to dealing with loss based on individual family needs and temperament.

Social and Practical Aspects of Care

A palliative care social worker can promote access to care by providing referral to services that meet identified needs as well as to community resources and volunteers that can help in the home or with transportation. Collaboration with pharmacists can ensure that patients have access to necessary medications; home nursing agencies can ensure proper equipment is available. Family structure and living arrangements, geographic location, finances, and caregiver availability are considered and reflected in the care plan. For example, an older patient with esophageal cancer may have a partner who is ill and unable to provide care. In such a situation, where the support system is already at its limit, the palliative care team must develop a plan to insure appropriate care and safety for the patient and his partner. Sending a patient home without adequate support can often lead to readmission; addressing needs early and activating community support can allow patients to remain at home as long as possible. Different teams may provide these services in differing ways. Some teams have dedicated social workers to address these issues, whereas other teams may use case managers or nurses to focus on these matters. It is important to realize the care coordination involved is more than a physician or nurse can do alone; the interdisciplinary nature of palliative care draws upon the strengths of each field.

Spiritual, Religious, and Existential Aspects of Care

Beliefs surrounding illness and death are profoundly influenced by a patient's and family's religious and spiritual values. The salient spiritual needs of patients at the end of life encompass questions of meaning, value, and relationship. Physicians may not recognize these spiritual needs, may not believe they have a duty to address these issues, and may not understand how best to respond to them; however, physicians can play a key role in helping patients express these needs by routinely asking patients about their religious and spiritual beliefs and practices (18) and how these impact on the patient's view of illness. Chaplains and other members of the spiritual care service can address such issues in a non-threatening and supportive way and even help facilitate religious or spiritual rituals as well as contact spiritual communities identified by the patient and family. Sometimes religious beliefs can be seen as a barrier to providing good end-of-life care, but if addressed sensitively and appropriately, they can be navigated and enrich the experience for the patient and the medical team. For example, one patient and his family had a strong religious belief in a miraculous cure of metastatic esophageal cancer. The palliative care team chaplain explored this belief more explicitly and was able to negotiate a treatment plan that was respectful of the families' belief but also practical. The chaplain directly addressed that forgoing additional chemotherapy would not change whether a miracle was possible. The patient was then referred to hospice care, where he benefited from continued support.

Cultural Aspects of Care

End-of-life concerns are also deeply affected by a patient's and family's cultural values. Culture often defines how patients and families understand illness, suffering, and dying. Encounters between physicians and patients of different backgrounds are common given the diversity in the United States and, therefore, there are many opportunities for cross-cultural misunderstandings (19). Desire for life-prolonging therapies and technology, the locus of decision-making, and disclosure of information are all influenced by cultural norms. While autonomy may prevail in the United States, some cultures prefer that families make medical decisions as a unit (20). One common scenario encountered is when an adult child does not want to reveal to their sick parent that they have cancer. Palliative medicine providers may address this issue by asking the patient, "I have information regarding your condition. Some patients prefer to hear the information directly from me and make their own decisions, and others prefer to have me talk to someone else and let them make the decisions. What do you think?" Such communication can demonstrate respect for the patient's culture without assuming that the patient will conform to their cultural norms. Skilled communication, genuine curiosity, and openness to differences can increase the likelihood that patients and families are satisfied with the process and outcomes of care.

CARE OF THE IMMINENTLY DYING PATIENT

When possible, the transition to the actively dying phase should be recognized and communicated to the patient, family, and care providers. If the patient is at home, hospice nurses can be a key resource to families at this time. Many families worry about whether they will know when the person is actively dying. They are often concerned it will be a painful process and that their loved one will suffer a great deal. By understanding the signs and symptoms of impending death and knowing how to address the symptoms that do arise, physicians can explain to family members what to expect and reassure them that their loved one will receive good care.

While each person experiences the final stages differently, common symptoms exist. These terminal symptoms include loss of appetite, dehydration, and drowsiness. Many patients become anorexic and lose their appetite in the last weeks of life. Family members often want to feed patients who are unable to eat. Although physicians may recognize that feeding will not help the patient and may even harm by leading to aspiration, they must also recognize that feeding is a primary means of nurturing. Physicians can redirect this desire by promoting other important factors such as good oral and skin care. Most patients are unable to drink in their final days, and many families will ask about intravenous fluids. At this time of life, artificial hydration can lead to pulmonary edema and dyspnea, ascites, peripheral edema, and infections at intravenous catheter sites and should be discouraged. Symptoms such as dry mouth and thirst can be addressed by attentive oral care. Because patients may become unable to take medications orally, the rectal and subcutaneous routes may be used, which some patients with esophageal cancer may be already familiar with. If the patient is incontinent of urine, diapers and heavy towels may be used to avoid catheterization, but catheterization can be done based on patient and family preference.

Changes in respiratory status are common in imminently dying patients. Breathing usually becomes shallow as death nears and periods of apnea are common. Secretions that accumulate in the pharynx due to the patient being too weak or unresponsive to swallow or cough can produce a rattling sound that can be distressing to the family. Deep suctioning should be avoided as it can lead to gagging and may be uncomfortable. Glycopyrrolate, atropine, or scopolamine can be effective in reducing rattle by decreasing the amount of mucus and saliva produced. Rooms should be cool and well ventilated, and a fan can aid in reducing the sensation of dyspnea. It may be appropriate to stop taking blood pressure and monitor only respiratory rate and pulse in order to avoid disturbing the patient. The pulse rate typically increases and is weak and irregular in the final hours to days of life.

Drowsiness and decreased responsiveness is common; rarely, patients become confused or agitated. When possible, confusion or agitation should be treated according to the cause. If the patient is experiencing agitation due to increased pain, pain should be treated with opioids as appropriate, or if thought due to dyspnea, treated with oxygen and opioids. Behavioral interventions such as brushing a patient's hair or providing music can be highly effective in treating agitation. When these measures do not work and the cause is uncertain, agitation can be treated with low doses of neuroleptics such as haloperidol.

ETHICAL AND LEGAL CONSIDERATIONS

Ethical and legal issues commonly arise in palliative care. Advance care planning can help communicate patient preferences across different health care settings and should be discussed early. In such discussions, physicians should encourage patients to appoint surrogate decision makers and educate them on how to make decisions and discuss choices with their loved one. All physicians should follow accepted ethical principles, including respect for autonomy, acting in the patient's best interest, avoiding harm, treating patients equally, and maintaining confidentiality. At the point when the patient is no longer able to express his wishes, the team should turn to the patient's previously expressed wishes to help guide care. Palliative care teams also discuss with patients and families the need for wills, guardianship agreements, and financial documentation prior to the loss of decision-making capacity.

Some patients may make requests for their physician to assist them to die. Such requests for aid in dying are often triggered by pain, depression, or other distress. Physicians must address these issues whenever a patient raises the issue of assisted suicide because treating pain and depression and making referrals to hospice reduces these requests. Physician aid in dying is only legal in the states of Oregon and Washington and there only with specific safeguards.

Palliative care aims for the relief of suffering caused by physical, psychosocial, and spiritual aspects of disease and utilizes an interdisciplinary team to provide care. With focused symptom management and clear goals of care, patients living with esophageal cancer can improve their quality of life and maximize valuable time with friends, family, and loved ones.

References

1. Boyce HW. Esophageal malignancies and premalignant conditions. In: Kirsner J, ed. *The Growth of Gastroenterologic Knowledge During the Twentieth Century.* Malvern, PA: Lea & Febiger; 1994:11–34.
2. Boyce HW. Tumors of the esophagus. In: Sleisinger MH, Fordtran JS, eds. *Gastrointestinal Disease.* Philadelphia, PA: WB Saunders; 1993:401–418.
3. Bruera E, Portenoy R, eds. *Topics in Palliative Care, Volume 5.* New York: Oxford University Press; 2001.
4. Brescia, FJ. Specialized care of the terminally ill. In: DeVita VT, Hellman S, Rosenberg SA, eds. *Cancer: Principles & Practice of Oncology,* Philadelphia: J.B. Lippincott; 2004:3077–3012.
5. Teno JM, Clarridge BR. Family perspectives on end-of-life care at the last place of care. *JAMA.* 2004; 291(1):88–93.
6. Boyce HW. Stents for palliation of esophageal cancer. *N Engl J Med.* 1993;329(18): 1345–1346.
7. Heit HA, Johnson LF, Siegel SR, et al. Palliative dilation for dysphagia in esophageal carcinoma. *Ann Intern Med.* 1978;89:629–631.
8. Knyrim K, Wagner HJ, Bethge N. A controlled trial of an expansile metal stent for palliation of esophageal obstruction due to inoperable cancer. *N Engl J Med.* 1993;329 (18):1302–1307.
9. Iyer R, Wilkinson N, Demmy T, et al. Controversies in the multimodality management of locally advanced esophageal cancer: evidence-based review of surgery alone and combined-modality therapy. *Ann Surg Oncol.* 2004;11:665–673.
10. Javle M, Ailawadhi S, Yang GY, et al. Palliation of malignant dysphagia in esophageal cancer: a literature-based review. *J Support Oncol.* 2006;4:365–373,379.
11. Lightdale CJ, Kulkarni KG. Role of endoscopic ultrasonography in the staging and follow-up of esophageal cancer. *J Clin Oncol.* 2005;23:4483–4489.
12. Loizou LA, Grigg D, Atkinson M, et al. A prospective comparison of laser therapy and intubation in endoscopic palliation for malignant dysphagia. *Gastroenterology.* 1991;100:1303–1310.
13. Macdonald JS, Smalley SR, Benedetti J, et al. Chemoradiotherapy after surgery compared with surgery alone for adenocarcinoma of the stomach or gastroesophageal junction. *N Engl J Med.* 2001;345:725–730.
14. Urba S. Combined modality therapy of esophageal cancer—standard of care? *Surg Oncol Clin N Am.* 2002;11:377–386.
15. Singer P, Martin DK. Domains of quality end-of-life care from the patient's perspective. *JAMA.* 1999;281:163–168.
16. American Pain Society Quality of Care Committee. Quality improvement guidelines for the treatment of acute pain and cancer pain. *JAMA.* 1995;274(23):1874–1880.
17. Benedetti C, Brock C, et al. NCCN practice guidelines for cancer pain. *Oncology Huntington.* 2000:14(11A):135–150.
18. Sulmasy DP. Spiritual issues in the care of dying patients ". . . It's okay between me and God" *JAMA.* 2006;296:1385–1392.
19. Kagawa-Singer M, Blackhall LJ. Negotiating cross-cultural issues at the end of life: "you got to go where he lives." *JAMA.* 2001;286:2993–3001.
20. Crawley LM, Marshall PA, et al. Strategies for culturally effective end-of-life care. *Ann Intern Med.* 2002;136(9):673–679.

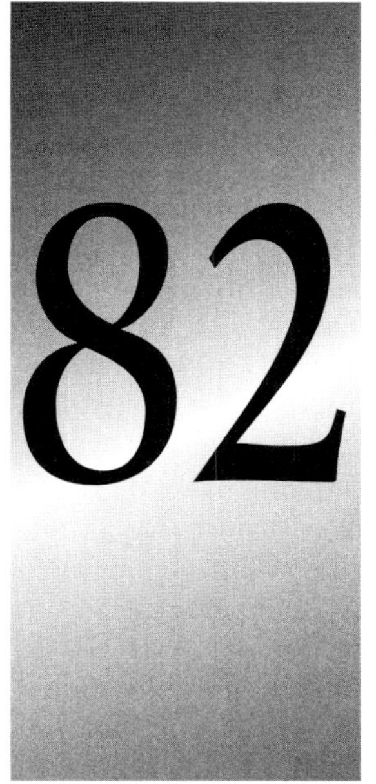

82 Care of the Psychosocial Needs of the Patient and Family

Mindy Hartgers
Jessica Mitchell
Aminah Jatoi

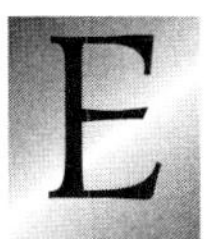

Esophageal cancer is an aggressive malignancy, and it requires aggressive therapy. For example, patients with locally advanced disease often receive aggressive combination therapy that includes concomitant chemotherapy and radiation followed by surgery (1). However, prescribing such therapy entails more than adhering to protocol standards that fall under the rubrics of 3 foregoing treatment modalities. One critical component of health care for patients with esophageal cancer falls outside the realm of chemotherapy or radiation or surgery and comprises its own separate therapeutic modality: psychosocial support.

To our knowledge, the literature provides little guidance for health care providers on how best to provide psychosocial support to esophageal cancer patients and their families. Typing in the search terms *esophageal cancer* and *psychosocial* yields only 14 hits, most of which refer to articles that bear little relevance to the subject at hand. This chapter therefore attempts to pull from a diverse medical literature in an effort to construct a practical tool on how best to recognize and address the psychosocial needs of esophageal cancer patients and their families.

THE IMPORTANCE OF CONSISTENT INFORMATION

The psychosocial needs of patients and their families cannot be met within an environment of confusion that arises when oncologists and non-oncologists are incongruent in their discussions of prognosis and therapeutic options. Such inconsistencies can lead to increased anxiety and distress on the part of patients and their families.

Thus, a major requirement for compassionately discussing treatment options with patients and their family members focuses on imparting accurate information. Girgis and others surveyed 84 cancer patients, 64 oncologists, and 140 oncology nurses on how best to break bad news (2). The one point that all respondents agreed upon is that "patients have a legal and moral right to accurate and reliable information and that patients should be given the diagnosis and prognosis honestly."

The importance of providing honest and accurate information on prognosis poses a significant challenge for patients with esophageal cancer for one major reason: despite multiple clinical trials, there is no established standard of care that dictates how best to provide cancer therapy. As one example, for locally advanced esophageal cancer, not all studies have been consistent in outlining a clear role for trimodality therapy (1). Some oncology health care providers proceed with concomitant chemotherapy and radiation, followed by surgery; others recommend only the former and include surgery only in the event of residual cancer. Similarly, recent data suggest that neoadjuvant chemotherapy without radiation followed by surgery and then more chemotherapy offers a reasonable therapeutic approach for patients with locally advanced esophageal cancer. As a second example, there appears to be no consensus on how best to prescribe chemotherapy for patients with metastatic disease (3). Despite the fact that previous studies suggest a survival advantage with the use of chemotherapy, medical oncologists continue to prescribe a variety of first-line regimens, noting that even with the most promising of regimens, the median survival remains under 1 year—too short to enable any such regimen to be deemed a standard. Hence, in the absence of well-established therapeutic approaches, the risk of health care providers, particularly non-oncologists, to impart inconsistent patient education information is high.

As a result of this risk, several points on prognosis may be inconsistently stated by members of the health care provider team, particularly primary care providers, who face the challenging task and responsibility of imparting up front or corroborative cancer-related information to patients and their families as treatment decisions are shifting and evolving in a rapid manner. Again, when oncology health care providers and non-oncology health care providers are not providing identical information about the goals of cancer therapy and prognosis, the psychosocial needs of the patient are clearly not being attended to, and any incongruent recommendations often provide tremendous anxiety for the patient and his/her family members.

To our knowledge, there have been no studies that outline gaps in the accuracy of esophageal cancer information and treatment options among primary health care providers, but the existence of such gaps are suggested by 2 recent studies. First, Sigouin and Jadad surveyed 1998 cancer patients, 871 family physicians, and 30 oncologists about their familiarity with peer reviewed internet information (4). Survey response rates were 72%, 44%, and 97%, respectively, for each of the above groups. Among patients, only 1% were aware of the Cochrane Collaboration, and only 13% were aware of Medline. More surprisingly, although most oncologists knew about these resources, 33% of family physicians were not aware of the existence of the Cochrane Collaboration and its role and as many as 8% were not aware of Medline. This lack of awareness of these major sources of information among primary care physicians suggests that the dissemination of important health care information, including cancer-related information, may not be as widespread as hoped. Such knowledge deficits are compounded even further in esophageal cancer patients for whom a lack of clear-cut treatment standards, as discussed above, is also lacking.

Studies have not assessed whether health care providers know about the benefits of chemotherapy in patients with metastatic esophageal cancer, but in non-small cell lung cancer—a far more common malignancy—40% of surveyed physicians did not think that chemotherapy provided a survival advantage over best supportive care, despite numerous robust and randomized trials that indicate otherwise (5). In view of the fact that esophageal cancer is a far less common malignancy, it appears that the benefits of chemotherapy may not be known among all health care providers, particularly non-oncologists, who see patients with metastatic esophageal cancer.

Thus, in an effort to practice in accordance with the statement that "patients have a legal and moral right to accurate and reliable information and that patients should be given the diagnosis and prognosis honestly" and in an effort to sidestep the possibility of providing patients with inaccurate information, 2 major points on the treatment of esophageal cancer are discussed below.

First, patients with locally advanced esophageal cancer do sustain some chance for cure, even in the setting of local lymph node involvement. It is important to realize that a subgroup of patients, even those with dysphagia and weight loss, can ultimately be cured of their cancer. Various surgical series show that in general 20% of patients who undergo an esophagectomy with complete extirpation of their cancer can go on to live 5 years without cancer recurrence (1). Although controversial, the use of multimodality therapy that includes chemotherapy and radiation up front followed by surgery or, alternatively, the use of chemotherapy before and after surgery may improve cure rates. It is important for non-oncologists to recognize the curative goals of such approaches and to convey such information accurately when discussing options with a newly diagnosed esophageal cancer patient.

On a separate but related note, a commonly encountered, emotionally challenging scenario deals with trimodality therapy. Locally advanced esophageal cancer patients are sometimes hospitalized while receiving concomitant chemotherapy and radiation, and their inpatient care on occasion is managed by non-oncologists. Although the expectation is that these patients will go on to surgery, some become reluctant or are too ill to complete the entire planned treatment package and instead opt out of surgery. Non-oncologists may forget that chemotherapy and radiation alone—in the absence of surgery—can cure patients with locally advanced esophageal cancer, particularly those with squamous cell carcinoma, and that, in effect, some of these patients face the prospect of living a long life after having received only chemotherapy and radiation. In a seminal study, Cooper and others observed that at 5 years, as many as 26% of patients remained alive (6). Thus, in the spirit of conveying "prognosis honestly" to patients, it is important for health care providers to engage in ongoing conversations with esophageal cancer patients and to provide them with accurate information, particularly during times when the original treatment plan needs to be altered.

A second important point on prognosis in esophageal cancer focuses on the treatment of metastatic disease. Despite the poor prognosis associated with metastatic esophageal cancer, chemotherapy does play a pivotal role in providing a survival advantage to otherwise healthy cancer patients with a good performance status, and this point must be duly noted when discussing prognosis with patients with this malignancy. Four published trials, primarily in gastric cancer patients, have investigated chemotherapy versus best supportive care (3). Given the proximity of the esophagus to the stomach, the similar adenocarcinoma histology, and the general trend of similar clinical behavior, these studies are often invoked to suggest the efficacy of chemotherapy in adenocarcinoma of the esophagus as well. Although these trials are fraught with controversial study designs, the fact remains that 3 of 4 showed a survival advantage of a few months with chemotherapy. Admittedly, benefits are modest. All 4 of the chemotherapy trials referenced above tested multidrug regimens, but the median survival with chemotherapy was consistently less than 1 year, despite the fact that chemotherapy gained patients a statistically significant improvement in survival. In fact, in perhaps the most favorable median survival reported to date, Cunningham and others observed that the combination of oxaliplatin, capecitabine, and epirubicin provided a 11.2 month median survival (7).

FURTHER EVIDENCE OF THE IMPORTANCE OF HONESTY

Once the clinical facts about prognosis are well established among members of the health care team, how should prognosis be discussed with an esophageal patient and his/her family? Several studies indicate that the best way to proceed is to be up front in asking patients what they want to know about, to be honest in responding, and to allow time for the patient and family members to ask follow-up questions. Parker and others surveyed 351 patients with a variety of malignancies, 31% of which included gastrointestinal malignancies, to probe into what factors relevant to patient–health care provider communication were most valued by patients (8). These factors that earned the highest, most valued ratings include the following: "doctor being up to date on research on my type of cancer"; "doctor telling me best treatment option"; "having doctor take time to answer all my questions completely"; "doctor is honest about the severity of my illness"; "feeling confident about my doctor's skill"; and "being given enough time to ask all of my questions." (Table 82.1)

In contrast, factors that earned the lowest, or least valued, ratings included the following: "doctor holding my hand/touching my arm when giving news"; "doctor helps me figure out how to tell others about my cancer"; "doctor warning me there will be unfavorable news"; "having another health care provider present to offer support"; and "comforting me if I become emotional." (Table 82.1)

Interestingly, the above comments suggest once again that what patients value the most is honesty. But honesty can be difficult. As part of the Schwartz Center Rounds, Dias and others recently provided a provocative, patient-reported account of the consequences of honest discussions with patients and the consequences of a lack of such discussions (9). In this report, a patient described her experience with "13 abdominal surgeries, 4 months of chemotherapy, and 6 weeks of radiation therapy" for a malignancy that had never been able to be completely eradicated. Ironically, in reflecting on her own care, the patient focused and contrasted many of her own cancer experiences with those of her 86-year-old,

TABLE 82.1
What Do Patients Value When Given Bad News

Highly ranked by patients	Not so highly ranked
"doctor being up to date on research on my type of cancer"	"doctor holding my hand/touching my arm when giving news"
"doctor telling me best treatment option"	"doctor warning me there will be unfavorable news"
"having doctor take time to answer all my questions completely"	"having another health care provider present to offer support"
"doctor is honest about the severity of my illness"	"comforting me if I become emotional"
"feeling confident about my doctor's skill"	
"being given enough time to ask all of my questions"	

previously healthy father, who had been overheard to comment to the patient, "I will never suffer like that. I think what you're going through is just torture."

Subsequently, the patient's father developed rectal bleeding, which eventually prompted a barium enema that revealed an "irregularity." Never making contact with his doctor other than via a quick phone conversation, the patient's father ultimately went to a gastroenterologist for a colonoscopy after which he was told, "I don't know why you're here. You clearly have a blockage. You should have gone to a surgeon 3 weeks ago." After this devastating news was provided to the patient, multiple telephone conversations occurred between the patient's father and the patient and various doctors, but none of these conversations took place in person. Later in the day, as the patient completed a phone conversation with her father and described her father's reaction, she related how, "I could hear the distress in his voice. Evidently, he got off the phone, didn't say a word to my mother, walked right by her, walked into another room where he had a gun, which nobody knew about, walked out of the house, and shot himself in the head." Yes, being honest about bad news can be difficult, but not taking the time to be honest can be even worse.

The above tragic episode is a rare occurrence, but it nonetheless underscores the importance of providing information when patients appear to be seeking it. Moreover, although several studies have clearly demonstrated how health care providers encounter stress and a variety of other negative emotions when breaking bad news, the above scenario convincingly demonstrates how a lack of information can cause patients and their families to experience severe emotional distress.

HOW TO DISCUSS PROGNOSIS EFFECTIVELY

From a practical standpoint, how can health care providers strike such a balance of "being honest but at the same time encouraging, hopeful, and supportive," as recently discussed in a review by Fallowfield and Jenkins (10)? Stay away from ambiguous or technical terms in imparting information and instead rely on simple, straightforward wording. (See Table 82.2.) For example, when an esophageal cancer patient learns that his lymph nodes were "positive," such wording might suggest to a lay person that this finding is in fact "positive," when in fact such is not the case. A less equivocal statement is: "Your lymph nodes also have cancer cells within them."

As another example, upon looking at unfavorable radiographs, health care providers often offer to patients the comment, "Your cancer is progressing." The term *progressing* can carry positive connotations for some patients, when in fact the intention on the part of the health care provider is to inform the patient of evidence of a malignancy that has become refractory to cancer treatment. A less ambiguous statement is: "Your cancer is growing and getting worse, despite the chemotherapy." A greater sensitivity to daily jargon employed by health care providers might lead to better word choices and more honest and straightforward conversations.

A third such example is derived from anecdotes taken from the authors of this chapter. Often esophageal patients are told that they have a "30% chance that their cancer will respond to therapy." In effect, the health care provider is saying that 30% of esophageal patients will demonstrate some evidence of tumor shrinkage. However, patients can sometimes interpret the above statement to suggest that they hold a 30% chance of cure. Thus, clarifying goals of therapy with meticulous accuracy and precision allows for easier, less troubling conversations at a later date. This approach also allows the patient and family members more time for processing grave prognostic information.

In addition, the need to spend time with patients and families when giving bad news is important. Fallowfield and Jenkins commented upon the fact that time constraints often curtail necessary, sometimes exhaustive conversations (10). At the same time, however, these authors offer the observation, "Too much emphasis is perhaps placed on the communication of bad news by one individual." In fact, communication needs can sometimes be met by means of conversations that

TABLE 82.2
Word Choices in Explaining Cancer Facts

Problematic wording	Somewhat preferable wording
"Your lymph nodes were 'positive'."	"Your lymph nodes also had cancer cells present."
"Your cancer is progressing."	"Your cancer is growing and getting worse, despite the chemotherapy."
"There's a 30% chance your cancer will respond to chemotherapy."	"There's a 30% chance your cancer will shrink in the short term with chemotherapy."

occur with several health care providers or the same health care provider during multiple visits and conversations. Patients with esophageal cancer are likely to benefit from this approach of imparting information during multiple visits, as information on diagnosis and therapy is often directed and implemented by multiple health care providers, including the primary care provider, the gastroenterologist, the medical oncologist, the radiation oncologist, and the surgeon. Hence, despite the complexity of issues esophageal cancer patients must contend with, a multidimensional team can—and should—provide a major advantage for patients as they cope with the psychosocial issues associated with their malignancy.

Another practical point deals with an issue as seemingly minor as physician posture. Bruera and others studied 168 cancer patients, providing them with a video sequence of either a sitting or standing health care provider who was breaking bad news (11). Health care providers who were sitting were viewed as more compassionate and as spending more time with the patient. Women patients responded more favorably to physicians who sat. A subtle bedside maneuver, this simple gesture of sitting when conveying bad news can help demonstrate to patients that the health care provider does truly desire to spend time and answer questions in a forthcoming manner.

Several recent studies suggest that health care providers can learn many of the skills required for breaking bad news effectively, and several recent publications on the topic highlight the important of skills training. Although a survey from 1998 observed that only 6% of medical oncologists had ever received formal training in breaking bad news, the emergence of a variety of medical school–based and electronic tutorials are likely changing this statistic and making such instruction more accessible to health care providers (10).

TALKING ABOUT SIDE EFFECTS

Talking about prognosis outlines only a small segment of important information for patients with esophageal cancer. The complexity of cancer care among patients with this malignancy gives rise to a host of challenging issues that require ongoing candid discussions between the health care provider and the patient and his/her family. The following discussions vary based on whether patients have (a) metastatic disease, (b) locally advanced disease, or (c) advanced disease of any stage with limited antineoplastic options.

For patients with metastatic esophageal cancer with either an adenocarcinoma or squamous cell carcinoma histology, median survival remains under 1 year. However, the oncology community is demonstrating increasing interest in treating patients with triplet (3-drug) chemotherapy regimens in an effort to maximize survival, if only by a few more weeks. The trade-off of this modest prolongation of life is more frequent and more severe treatment-related toxicities.

One example of this approach involves recent phase III data with the agent docetaxel and provided some of the justification for the Food and Drug Administration's approval of this drug in this setting (12). Van Cutsem and others reported on 445 patients with metastatic esophageal and gastric cancer (13). Patients had been randomly assigned to receive either doxetaxel, cisplatin, 5-fluorouracil versus cisplatin, 5-fluorouracil. Time to cancer progression was the primary endpoint of this study and improved with the addition of docetaxel. Patients who received all 3 drugs had a time to cancer progression of 5.6 months in contrast to 3.7 months among patients who received only 2 drugs. Additionally, overall survival was also improved with the median survival being 9.2 months and 8.6 months among patients who received 3 and 2 drugs, respectively. Adverse events included febrile neutropenia, which required hospital admission in 63% and 27% of patients who received 3 drugs and 2 drugs, respectively. Severe diarrhea occurred in 19% and 8% of patients, respectively, and severe neurosensory changes occurred in 8% and 3% of patients, respectively. Finally, death within 30 days after the last infusion of chemotherapy occurred in 23 patients (10%) and 19 patients (8%), respectively.

Is it worth it? Does an 18-day median survival advantage justify higher rates of hospitalization for febrile neutropenia, severe diarrhea, neurosensory changes, and a somewhat shorter interval between chemotherapy administration and death? The answer to these questions is impossible for a health care provider to address alone and require that the patient and his/her family participate in such decision-making if this patient is deemed a potential candidate for such a more aggressive treatment approach. Although it might be difficult for patients to fully understand the real meaning of side effects such as myelosuppression and infection, diarrhea, and neuropathy in the absence of having received the treatment and having withstood its toxicity, the answers to such questions nonetheless require a team approach with patient input. Thus, the task of providing honest information on side effects is imperative for patients in order that they might play a role in deciding the best treatment to receive based on their own personal values.

Along similar lines, patients with locally advanced esophageal cancer have the option of receiving either chemotherapy and radiation versus chemotherapy and radiation followed by surgery. Both approaches can be offered with curative intent. A recent study from Bedenne and others suggested that both approaches are equivalent, but the relatively small sample and other factors relevant to the study design allow proponents of either approach ample justification for continuing with either approach (14), and at many medical centers within the United States, surgery continues to be accepted as a mainstay treatment modality.

However, Blazeby and others examined serial quality of life scores among 55 cancer patients who had undergone an esophagectomy (15). Scores did not return to their preoperative level until 9 months after surgery. Among esophageal cancer patients who have already experienced other surgeries such as an appendectomy, hernia repair, or cholecystectomy, the prospect of a 9-month recovery period might be close to mind-boggling and initially incomprehensible. Therefore, it should be clearly explained to patients in order that they know and can better cope with what is ahead of them in a postoperative setting. The question "Is it worth it?" recurs in many aspects of treating esophageal cancer, and inviting input from patients with full disclosure of such postoperative issues allows for an answer that is in alignment with the patient's values.

IMPACT OF PSYCHOSOCIAL SUPPORT

Despite all the challenges faced by patients with esophageal cancer, few studies have examined what sorts of interventions might truly help patients who find themselves having to contend with a diagnosis of esophageal cancer. Kuchler and others performed a randomized controlled trial to evaluate the effect of psychosocial support on survival among patients with a variety of gastrointestinal malignancies, including cancer of the esophageal, stomach, liver, gallbladder, pancreas, colon, or rectum (16). A total of 271 surgical patients participated.

Psychosocial support consisted of a therapist providing "individualized care based on findings from the psychotherapeutic intake interview." As per Kuchler and others, "Therapists provided ongoing emotional and cognitive support to foster 'fighting spirit' and to diminish 'hopelessness and helplessness'." This intervention occurred in both the preoperative and postoperative setting over a period of several months.

Results were surprising. A multivariate analysis that considered tumor stage, residual tumor burden, and site of malignancy suggested that such psychotherapeutic support appeared to enhance survival. (Figure 82.1). In fact, at 10 years, 21.3% of patients who had been randomized to the experimental group, which received psychotherapeutic counseling, were alive compared to 9.6% who had been randomized to the control group. The authors concluded, "The results of this study indicate that patients with gastrointestinal cancer, who undergo surgery for stomach, pancreatic, primary liver, or colorectal cancer, benefit from a formal program of psychotherapeutic support during the inpatient hospital stay in terms of long-term survival."

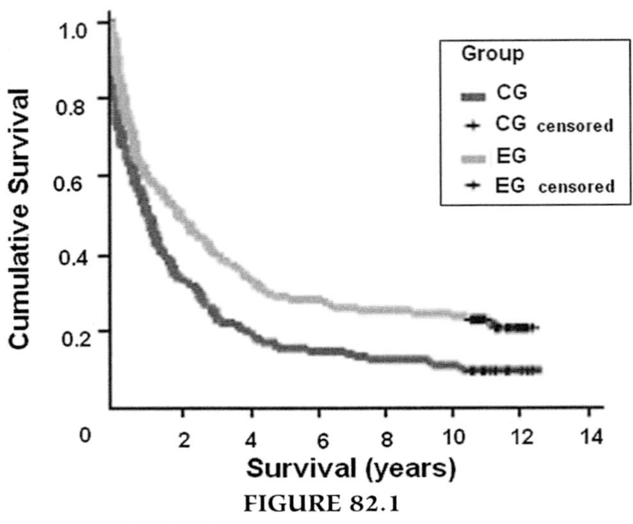

FIGURE 82.1

At 10 years, 21.3% of patients who had been randomized to the experimental group (EG) that received psychotherapeutic counseling were alive compared to 9.6% who had been randomized to the control group (CG). (Reproduced from Kuchler T, Bestmann B, Rappat S, et al. Impact of psychotherapeutic support for patients with gastrointestinal cancer undergoing surgery: 10-year survival results of a randomized trial. *The Journal of Clinical Oncology.* 2007;25(19):2702–2708. Reprinted with permission. © 2008 American Society of Clinical Oncology. All Rights Reserved.)

The foregoing findings are indeed provocative. At the beginning of this chapter, the term *psychosocial support* was described as a separate therapeutic modality that should be utilized in the treatment of patients with esophageal cancer. Psychosocial support appears to help patients as they receive their cancer treatment, but the foregoing survival advantage described by Kuchler suggests that psychosocial support may also offer more tangible benefits and directly improve cancer outcomes. Clearly, further research is warranted on improving the psychosocial aspects of therapy among patients with esophageal cancer.

References

1. McKian KP, Miller RC, Cassivi SD, et al. Curing patients with locally advanced esophageal cancer. *Dis Esophagus.* 2006;19:448–453.

2. Girgis A, Sanson-Fisher RW, Schofield MJ. Is there a consensus between breast cancer patients and providers on guidelines for breaking bad news? *Behav Med.* 1999;25:69–77.

3. Grunberger B, Raderer M, Schidinger M, et al. Palliative chemotherapy for recurrent and metastatic esophageal cancer. *Anticancer Res.* 2007;27:2705–2714.
4. Sigouin C, Jadad AR. Awareness of sources of peer-reviewed research evidence on the internet. *JAMA.* 2002;287:2867–2869.
5. Stinchcombe TE, Detterbeck FC, Lin L, et al. Beliefs among physicians in the diagnostic and therapeutic approach to non-small cell lung cancer. *J Thoracic Oncol.* 2007;2:819–826.
6. Cooper JS, Guo MD, Herskovic A, et al. Chemoradiotherapy of locally advanced esophageal cancer: long-term follow-up of a prospective randomized trial (RTOC 85–01). *JAMA.* 1999;281:1623–1627.
7. Cunningham D, Starling N, Rao S, et al. Capecitabine and oxaliplatin for advanced esophagogastric cancer. *N Engl J Med.* 2008;358:36–46.
8. Parker PA, Baile WF, de Moor C, et al. Breaking bad news about cancer: patients' preferences for communication. *J Clin Oncol.* 2001;19:2049–2056.
9. Dias L, Chabner BA, Lynch TJ, et al. Breaking bad news: a patient's perspective. *Oncologist.* 2003;8:587–596.
10. Fallowfield L, Jenkins V. Communicating sad, bad, and difficult news in medicine. *Lancet.* 2004;363:312–319.
11. Bruera E, Palmer JL, Pace E, et al. A randomized, controlled trial of physician postures when breaking bad news to cancer patients. *Palliat Med.* 2007;21:501–505.
12. Thuss-Patience PC, Kretzschmar A, Reichardt P. Docetaxel in the treatment of gastric cancer. *Future Oncol.* 2006;2:603–620.
13. Van Cutsem E, Moiseyenko VM, Tjulandin S, et al. Phase III study of docetaxel plus fluorouracil compared with cisplatin and fluorouracil as first-line therapy for advanced gastric cancer: a report of the V325 Study Group. *J Clin Oncol.* 2006;24:4991–4997.
14. Bedenne L, Michel P, Bouche O, et al. Chemoradiation followed by surgery compared with chemoradiation alone in squamous cancer of the esophagus: FFCD 9102. *J Clin Oncol.* 2007;25:1160–1168.
15. Blazeby JM, Farndon JR, Donovan J, et al. A prospective longitudinal study examining the quality of life of patients with esophageal carcinoma. *Cancer.* 2000;88:1781–1787.
16. Kuchler T, Bestmann B, Rappat S, et al. Impact of psychotherapeutic support for patients with gastrointestinal cancer undergoing surgery: 10-year survival results of a randomized trial. *J Clin Oncol.* 2007;25:2702–2708.

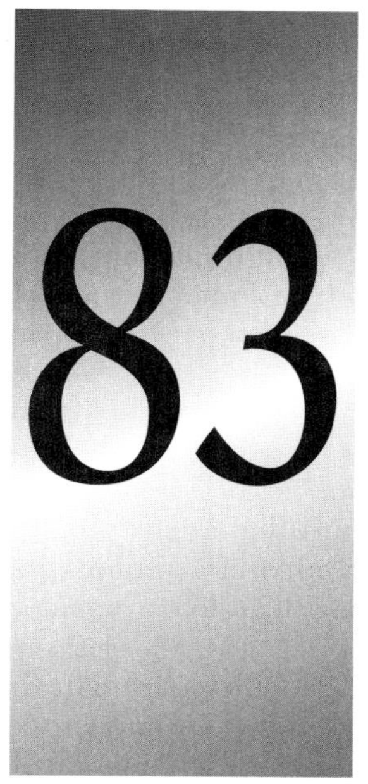

Objective Scoring Systems in the Palliative Setting

Marvin Omar Delgado-Guay
Sriram Yennurajalingam

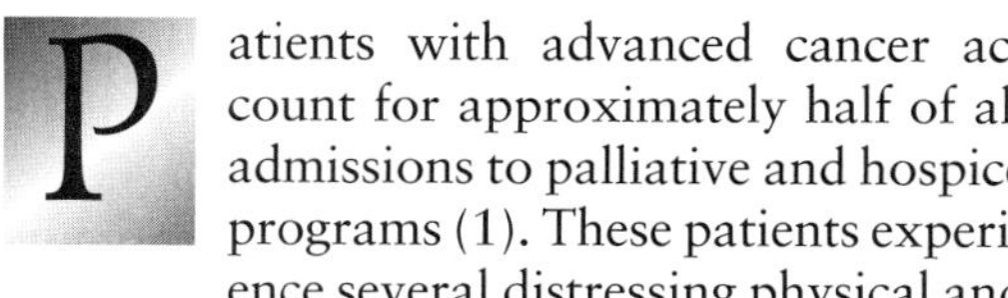

Patients with advanced cancer account for approximately half of all admissions to palliative and hospice programs (1). These patients experience several distressing physical and psychosocial symptoms before they die. The frequency of these symptoms has been studied and varies significantly from one study to another (1–6). Our primary goal as health care providers is to identify and treat these symptoms, which present both diagnostic and therapeutic challenges.

For the patient, these symptoms and the distress they cause are linked to the disease experience. In clinical practice, patients present with multiple symptoms requiring simultaneous assessment and management. It is very important to have an effective strategy that requires a multidimensional assessment of and a specific plan for each patient, respecting the treatment goals and the patient's wishes. This chapter describes instruments for assessing symptoms and some specific conditions, such as delirium, in patients with advanced cancer requiring palliative care (Figure 83.1).

SYMPTOM ASSESSMENT INSTRUMENTS

Good symptom assessment precedes effective symptom treatment. Symptom assessment is very important because symptoms directly affect patient distress, quality of life (QOL), and survival (7). Symptoms can be related to disease, treatment, concurrent comorbid illnesses, or a combination of all 3 (7,8). The early stages of cancer are associated with considerable symptomatology, and the symptom burden (symptoms and their interference with life) increases with cancer stage, possibly reflecting tumor burden (9–11). One important point to consider is that symptom burden decreases patient QOL (7,12). QOL is a multidimensional construct with specific emotional, physical, and social aspects (12–14). The presence of symptoms affects, but does not necessarily determine, QOL (7).

At present, there is no gold standard for symptom assessment in palliative care (1,7). Assessment tools allow for the identification of many more symptoms than do simple unstructured evaluations (15,16). Efficient symptom-assessment instruments include the Edmonton Symptom Assessment Scale, the Memorial Symptom Assessment Scale, and the Symptom Distress Scale.

The Edmonton Symptom Assessment Scale (ESAS) is used to assess 10 common symptoms (pain, fatigue, nausea, depression, anxiety, drowsiness, shortness of breath, appetite, sleep problems, and feeling of well-being) experienced by patients with cancer or chronic illness (17–20). In this scale, the patient rates the intensity of symptoms on a 0 to 10 numerical scale, with 0 representing "no symptom" and 10 representing the "worst possible symptom."

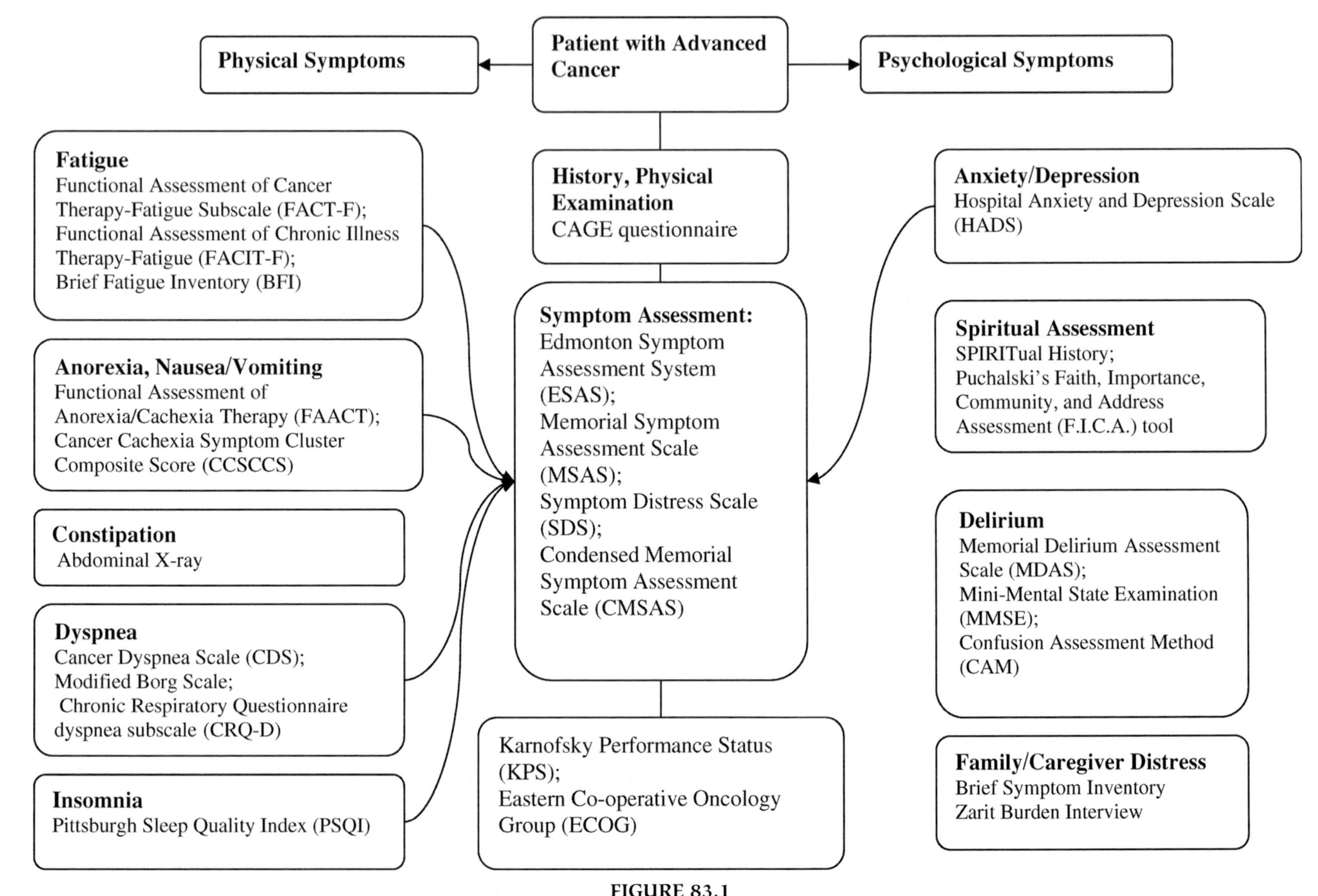

FIGURE 83.1

Some assessment tools used to evaluate physical, psychosocial, and spiritual symptoms of patients with advanced cancer in the palliative care setting.

The ESAS, which is available in Spanish, has been found to be reliable in cancer patients and to have internal consistency, criterion validity, and concurrent validity (21). It is widely used in palliative care research (22). Its ease of use and visual representation make it an effective and practical bedside tool (1,16,23,24) that allows the health care provider to track symptoms over time with regard to intensity, duration, and responsiveness to therapy. The ESAS was recently validated against a widely used scale, the Hospital Anxiety and Depression Scale (HADS), for assessing the presence of depression and anxiety in advanced cancer patients (25). The appropriate period for intermittent assessment is 1 week, and about 5 minutes is needed to complete the questionnaire.

The Memorial Symptom Assessment Scale (MSAS), a lengthier assessment tool, is mostly used for research purposes. With the MSAS, patients rate the frequency, severity, and distress associated with 32 physical and psychological symptoms (26). There is a short-form MSAS (MSAS-SF) that captures the patient-rated distress associated with 26 physical symptoms and the frequency of 4 psychological symptoms (27). Another tool that can be completed in 2 to 4 minutes and contains both QOL and survival information is the condensed MSAS (CMSAS), which provides equivalent information that approximates to the original 32 items (28). The Symptom Distress Scale (SDS) is a patient-rated instrument that assesses the intensity, frequency, and distress level associated with 9 physical and 2 psychological symptoms (29, 30). It is important to recognize that research instruments may differ from those used for clinical practice (28).

INSTRUMENTS FOR ASSESSMENT OF PROGNOSIS AND FUNCTION

Functional status is important for planning the setting of care, which can be at hospice, hospital, or home (31), and is considered an independent predictor of survival (32). The most frequently used performance status assessment scales in oncology practice for treatment planning and research are the Karnofsky Performance Status score and the Eastern Co-operative Oncology Group score. These tools have been shown to have reliable prognostic value (1,33–36).

The Karnofsky Performance Status score allows patients to be classified according to their functional impairment. This can be used to compare the effectiveness of different therapies and to assess the prognosis in individual patients. The lower the Karnofsky score, the worse the survival in most serious illnesses (35,37). However, Glare et al., in a systematic review of physicians' clinical predictions of survival, reported that performance status, anorexia, and dyspnea added limited information to these predictions (38). We found it interesting that physicians typically tended to overestimate survival.

The Eastern Co-operative Oncology Group score the ECOG Performance Status Rating measures how cancer affects the daily living abilities of the patient (39). The scale ranges from 0 (fully active, no restrictions) to 5 (dead), where lower scores represent better mobility. The Edmonton Functional Assessment Tool is used by physiotherapists and trained nurses to determine the functional performance of patients with advanced cancer and to evaluate other factors that contribute to functional impairment such as communication, mental status, pain, and dyspnea (40, 41).

The Functional Independence Measure can be used in the research setting to assess the functional status of advanced cancer patients (42,43). This tool includes 18 items that are used to evaluate independence in sphincter control, self-care, mobility, locomotion, communication, and social cognition.

Activities of Daily Living scales are very important for evaluating the level of physical impairment in our patients. Specifically, the Katz index of Activities of Daily Living (ADL) assesses activities such as eating, bathing, dressing, toileting, transferring, and continence (1). The Instrumental Activities of Daily Living (IADL) assesses more complex life activities, such as light housework, laundry, meal preparation, transportation, grocery shopping, using the telephone, medication management, and money management (1). The inability to perform 1 or more IADL helps us identify persons with cognitive impairment. These tools help us to identify physical limitations, distressing symptoms, and other related clinical problems seen in advanced stages of illness.

ASSESSMENT OF OTHER CLINICAL PROBLEMS

Assessment of Dyspnea

Dyspnea is a subjective experience of difficult, labored, and uncomfortable breathing (44–49). Patients with high dyspnea scores present with lower QOL (50).

Despite the fact that dyspnea is a distressful symptom, physicians consistently underrate it (44,51); in contrast, caregivers consistently appear to overrate symptom scores for dyspnea as well as those for pain and constipation in cancer patients newly admitted to palliative care and hospice (44).

Dyspnea can be assessed using numerical, verbal analog, or visual analog scales (52). Tools that assess the intensity of dyspnea include the Support Team Assessment Schedule (53) and the Edmonton Symptoms Assessment Scale (17,54). No one scale, however, can accurately reflect the far-reaching effects of breathlessness on the patient with advanced disease and on the patient's family. Thus, a combination of tools to assess dyspnea in advanced disease has been suggested, which includes a unidimensional scale (such as the visual analog scale), a disease-specific or multidimensional scale (such as the Cancer Dyspnea Scale) (55) and other methods to gauge psychosocial and caregiver distress (51). In a recent systematic review, Dorman et al. (56) concluded that the Numeric Rating Scale (57), the Modified Borg Scale (58,59), and the Chronic Respiratory Questionnaire dyspnea subscale (60) appeared to be the most suitable for use in palliative care, but further evaluation is required before adopting any scale as standard.

Assessment of Delirium

In patients with advanced cancer, delirium causes significant distress. Delirium, defined as a transient and potentially reversible disorder of cognition and attention, frequently complicates care at the end of life. In general, the etiology of delirium is multifactorial, especially in patients with advanced cancer and in elderly patients (61–71). Delirium is frequently misdiagnosed as depression or dementia (71). This confusion might be secondary to unfamiliarity with terminology, fluctuation of symptom intensity, and failure to objectively assess cognition (71–74). Delirium impedes communication with family members and caregivers at a time when it is often most desired (64,65). It is important to recognize delirium because it can make the reliable reporting of symptoms difficult for patients, who frequently present with disinhibition (64,65,74), are unable to participate in decisions about therapeutic interventions, and benefit from supportive psychotherapy (64).

Another important consideration is that if delirium is not recognized, not only family members but also health care providers can misinterpret the agitation as a sign of pain, resulting in escalated doses of opioids that can produce toxicity and complicate the delirium. To facilitate the diagnosis of delirium and impose relatively little burden on patients, instruments with adequate psychometric properties have been created, such as the Memorial Delirium Assessment Scale (MDAS) (61–63,67), the Mini-Mental State Examination (MMSE) (75), and the Confusion Assessment Method (CAM) (76).

The MDAS, a validated tool used in our palliative care practice, was designed to measure the severity of delirium and therefore captures behavioral manifestations as well as cognitive deficits (62). This instrument measures relative impairment in awareness, orientation, short-term memory, digit span, attention capacity, organizational thinking, perceptual disturbance, delusions, psychomotor activity, and sleep-wake cycle. Items are rated from 0 (none) to 3 (severe), depending on the level of impairment, with a maximum possible score of 30. The higher the score, the more severe the delirium. A total MDAS score of 7 out of 30 yields the highest sensitivity (98%) and specificity (96%) for delirium diagnosis (61).

Because cognitive impairment is not specific to delirium, the MMSE should be limited to screening for cognitive failure. The MMSE is the most used cognitive screening tool (75,77) and has been shown to have adequate interrater (0.82) and test-retest (0.89) reliability (75). The MMSE has been used for detecting delirium or combined delirium and dementia (78–80). The MMSE has not been used for evaluating other components of delirium such as psychomotor agitation, hallucinations, or delusions and may not detect mild cognitive failure. One of the advantages of the MMSE is that it can be administered by nurses, assistants, or volunteers (44). A strategy of assessing at regular intervals encourages early recognition of either cognitive failure or delirium.

Delirium also can be detected using the CAM (76). The CAM can be administered by a trained clinician as a 9-item scale or simplified algorithm. The algorithm indicates the presence of an acute-onset fluctuating course, inattention, disorganized thinking, and altered levels of consciousness. CAM for the intensive care unit (CAM-ICU) can be administered by a trained nurse and takes 2 minutes to complete (81). This tool has a high sensitivity (93%–100%) and specificity (98%–100%). When a patient in the ICU is verbal and nonintubated, the standard CAM can be used to detect subtle delirium (82).

Assessment of Fatigue

Fatigue is a multidimensional syndrome, often with multiple contributing causes (83–85), and is defined as a "decrement in performance of either physical or psychological tasks" (86). The National Comprehensive Cancer Network (87) defines cancer-related fatigue as "a distressing persistent, subjective sense of tiredness or exhaustion related to cancer or cancer treatment that is not proportional to recent activity and interferes with usual functioning."

Fatigue is a major problem for patients with advanced cancer (84) and is one of the most common symptoms encountered in palliative care patients (88–90), for whom the prevalence of fatigue ranges from 48% to 78% (91). Fatigue can be assessed by characterizing its severity and temporal features (onset, course, duration, and daily pattern) and by evaluating exacerbating, contributing, and relieving factors, its impact on daily life, and associated distress (88,92). In palliative care practice, patients present with multiple symptoms, which can be assessed using

ESAS. The presence of physical and/or psychological symptoms such as pain, sleep problems, depression, and anxiety significantly correlate with fatigue (88).

Fatigue also can be evaluated, for research purposes, with the Functional Assessment of Cancer Therapy-Fatigue (FACT-F) subscale (93), the Functional Assessment of Chronic Illness Therapy-Fatigue (FACIT-F) subscale (94), and the Brief Fatigue Inventory, which also has been validated as a measure of fatigue in patients with cancer (95). The FACIT-F subscale, used primarily in cancer patients to measure fatigue, consists of 13 items. Patients rate the intensity of fatigue and its related symptoms on a scale of 0 ("not at all") to 4 ("very much"). Test-retest reliability coefficients for the fatigue subscale have ranged from 0.84 to 0.90. This scale has demonstrated strong internal consistency (alpha = 0.93–0.95).

Other multidimensional tools include the multidimensional assessment of Fatigue Inventory, Multidimensional Fatigue Symptom Inventory, and revised Piper Fatigue Scale.

Assessment of Anorexia/Cachexia

The clinical assessment should include a careful history focused on nutritional issues and a physical examination. The subjective loss of appetite expressed by the patient can be assessed with a numerical rating scale such as the ESAS or other symptom-evaluation tools, as previously described (17–20,27,88). It is important to evaluate body weight, an assessment commonly used in the clinical practice. Measurement of the mid-upper arm circumference may also have prognostic value (96).

In the research setting, the 12-item Functional Assessment of Anorexia/Cachexia Therapy (FAACT) symptom-specific subscale, in addition to FACIT-G, is used to measure patients' concerns about their anorexia/cachexia during the past 7 days. The FAACT has internal consistency and a reliability coefficient (Cronbach's alpha) of 0.88 for its 12 components (94). Patients rate the intensity of anorexia/cachexia and its related symptoms on a scale of 0 ("not at all") to 4 ("very much").

Assessment of Nausea and Constipation

Nausea is a subjective symptom, frequently secondary to multiple causes. Nausea is commonly accompanied by other symptoms, such as pain, insomnia, anorexia, fatigue, anxiety, and depression; it is important to assess for these other symptoms at the same time because they can contribute to or worsen nausea, increasing patient and family distress. To record the intensity and frequency of this distressing symptom, a validated multidimensional tool such as the ESAS should be used, not only for the initial evaluation but also at regular intervals to evaluate the response to treatment (1).

Constipation is a difficult condition to assess and treat because of the wide variety of presenting symptoms (1). Patients with advanced disease present with higher risk factors for severe constipation; thus, it is important to carefully obtain a complete clinical history of bowel habits, including bowel pattern and the stool characteristics. The "Rome criteria" (romecriteria.org) helps in the assessment of constipation but does not consider QOL (1).

Abdominal X-ray films are helpful in assessing bowel gas pattern and in ruling out ileus or bowel obstruction. By dividing the film into 4 quadrants by drawing a large X, a "constipation score" can be obtained. Each quadrant is assigned a score of 0 to 3, with 0 indicating no stool in the lumen, 1 indicating stool occupancy of less than 50%, 2 indicating a greater than 50% occupancy, and 3 indicating complete occupancy of stool in the lumen. Overall scores for all 4 quadrants may range from 0 to 12, with a score of 7 or more indicating severe constipation (1).

Assessment of Sleep Disturbances

Sleep disturbance negatively affects QOL (97–100). Sleep deprivation heightens physical, psychological, social, and existential suffering, diminishes the coping capacity, and exacerbates symptoms such as pain and discomfort by increasing the perceived level of illness severity (100–101). Insomnia is underreported; Engstrom et al. (101) showed that only 16% of cancer patients with sleep disturbances reported their problem to health care providers.

It is important to assess sleep disturbances and to identify and treat associated symptoms. Several tools are used to evaluate sleep disturbances, one of which is the ESAS. Another effective tool used in the research setting is the Pittsburgh Sleep Quality Index (PSQI) (102), which measures sleep quality and patterns. It differentiates "poor" from "good" sleep by measuring 7 areas: subjective sleep quality, sleep latency, sleep duration, habitual sleep efficiency, sleep disturbances, use of sleeping medication, and daytime dysfunction over the past month. The subject self-rates each of these 7 areas. Scoring of answers is based on a 0 to 3 scale. A global score of 5 or greater (with 21 being the maximum global score) indicates a "poor" sleeper (a diagnosis of sleep disturbance). The PSQI can be used for both an initial assessment and ongoing comparative measurements across all health care settings. The PSQI has internal consistency and a reliability coefficient (Cronbach's alpha) of 0.83 for its 7 components. Numerous studies using the PSQI have supported its high validity and reliability. The screening performance of the ESAS for sleep disturbances is being studied, using the PSQI as a gold standard (102,103).

Assessment of Anxiety and Depression

Mood disorders are among the most prevalent and important of the psychiatric illnesses (104,105). Depression coexists with a number of physical symptoms in patients with advanced cancer. Its frequency varies widely, but it is considered to be present in approximately 25% of these patients (17,105–110). Mood disorders in medically ill patients are underdiagnosed and are therefore undertreated (108–111). To improve the accuracy of screening for depression, several self-reporting tools have been created that are easy to administer without extensive training (25,112). Lloyd-Williams et al. (112) showed the association between depression and physical symptoms in patients with advanced cancer using a 7-item verbal rating scale.

The ESAS has been widely used in the clinical setting for multiple symptoms and has been validated for use in patients with advanced cancer (17–20). Vignaroli et al. evaluated the screening performance of ESAS for depression and anxiety compared with that measured by the Hospital Anxiety and Depression Scale (HADS) and concluded that the ideal cutoff point of ESAS of 2 out of 10, is sensitive for the presence of depression and anxiety in patients in the palliative care setting (25).

HADS (113,114) is a brief, self-administered, widely used screening tool to measure psychological distress in patients. It is sensitive to change, both during the course of disease and in response to medical and psychological interventions. HADS consists of 14 items on 2 subscales (7 for anxiety and 7 for depression). Ratings are made on 4-point scales representing the degree of distress during the previous week. The 2 scales are then scored separately. A score of 7 or less indicates non-cases, 8 to 10 doubtful cases, and 11+ definite cases for anxiety and/or depression (with ranges of 0–21 for each subscale). Also, a one-third cut-off of the range (a score of 14–15) has been proposed as the indicator for severe disorder. In different studies, HADS showed good reliability and validity in assessing symptom severity, anxiety disorders, and depression in somatic, psychiatric, and primary care patients and even in the general population (113,114).

Assessment of Spirituality and Religiosity

Spirituality and religiosity are important considerations when evaluating patients with terminal illness and can influence coping strategies and QOL. The presence of spiritual pain can be important in patients with chronic or acute pain and other physical and psychological symptoms. The line between assessment and intervention is blurred, and simply inquiring about an area such as religious or spiritual coping may be experienced by the patient as an opening for further exploration and validation of the importance of this experience.

There is no widely accepted measure of spirituality. Research that purports to measure spirituality usually measures religiousness. Available tools examine spiritual history and have the advantage of engaging the patient in dialogue, identifying possible areas of concern, and indicating the need for providing resources such as referral to a chaplain or support group. One tool is called SPIRITual History (115), with SPIRIT an acronym for the 6 domains explored: S, spiritual belief system; P, personal spirituality; I, integration with a spiritual community; R, ritualized practices and restrictions; I, implications for medical care; and T, terminal events planning. The 6 domains include 22 items that may be covered in as little as 10 or 15 minutes or integrated into general interviewing over several appointments.

Another way to assess spirituality and religiosity is with Puchalski's and Romer's (115) Faith, Importance/Influence, Community, and Address (F.I.C.A.) assessment tool. F.I.C.A. includes questions to explore each of these areas (e.g., What is your faith? How important is it? Are you part of a religious community? How would you like me as your provider to address these issues in your care?). Although developed as a spiritual history tool for use in primary care settings, F.I.C.A. lends itself to any patient population. The relative simplicity of the approach has led to its adoption by many medical schools.

Assessment of Chemical Coping

The CAGE questionnaire (116–118) is used to screen for alcohol abuse at any period of life (have you ever felt that you should Cut down on your drinking? Have you been Annoyed by people criticizing your drinking? Have you ever felt bad or Guilty about your drinking? Have you ever had a drink to get rid of a hangover, i.e., an *E*ye-opener?) An abnormal score, defined as 2 positive answers to the 4 questions, has been shown to have prognostic value in opioid management in patients with cancer who experience pain (116–118).

Assessment of Family Distress and Caregiver Burden

The Brief Symptom Inventory and its short form (119) provide an overview of a caregiver's symptoms and their intensity at a specific point in time. The BSI is an 18-item self-reported symptom inventory designed to reflect the psychological symptom patterns of psychiatric and medical patients and nonpatients. This inventory reports profiles of 9 primary symptom dimensions and 3 global indices of distress. Each item is rated on a 5-point scale of distress ranging from 0 ("not at all") to 4 ("extremely"). The depression and anxiety subscales of the BSI are well established. The approximate completion time for these items is 5 minutes. The internal consistency estimates of these 2 subscales are 0.85 (depression) and 0.81 (anxiety). Estimates of the construct validity of these subscales also are satisfactory.

In the Zarit Burden Interview, "caregiver burden" is an all-encompassing term to describe the physical, emotional, and financial toll of providing care. It is the most widely referenced scale in studies of caregiver burden and has been demonstrated to have high internal consistency (Cronbach's $\alpha = 0.94$) (120).

CONCLUSION

Most patients receiving palliative care experience multiple symptoms that significantly affect QOL. Recognition of these symptoms as multidimensional complexes and the use of appropriate and validated assessment tools would provide optimal objective measures for managing these distressing symptoms and thereby improve patient QOL.

References

1. Dalal S, Del Fabbro E, Bruera E. Symptom control in palliative care–part 1: oncology as a paradigmatic example. *J Palliat Med.* 2006;9:391–408.
2. Reuben D, Mor V, Hiris J. Clinical symptoms and length of survival in patients with terminal cancer. *Arch Intern Med.* 1988;148:1586–1591.
3. Hopwood P, Stephens R. Symptoms at presentation for treatment in patients with lung cancer. Implications for the evaluation of palliative treatment. The Medical Research Council (MRC) Lung Cancer Working Party. *Br J Cancer.* 1995;71:633–636.
4. Talmi Y, Bercovici M, Waller A, et al. Home and in-patient hospice care of terminal head and neck cancer. *J Palliat Care.* 1997;13:9–14.
5. Conill C, Verger E, Henriquez I, et al. Symptom prevalence in the last week of life. *J Pain Symptom Manage.* 1997;14:328–331.
6. Addington-Hall J, McCarthy M. Dying from cancer: results of a national population based investigation. *Palliat Met.* 1995;9:295–305.
7. Kirkova J, Davis M, Walsh D, et al. Cancer symptom assessment instruments: a systematic review. *J Clin Oncol.* 2006;24:1459–1473.
8. Coyle N, Adelhardt J, Foley K, et al. Character of terminal illness in the advanced cancer patient: pain and other symptoms during the last four weeks of life. *J Pain Symptom Manage.* 1990;5:83–93.
9. Corner J, Hopkinson J, Fitzsimmons D, et al. Is late diagnosis of lung cancer inevitable? Interview study of patients' recollections of symptoms before diagnosis. *Thorax.* 2005;60:314–319.
10. Cleeland C, Reyes-Gibby C. When is it justified to treat symptoms? Measuring symptom burden. *Oncology.* 2002;16:64–70.
11. Cleeland C, Mendoza T, Wang X, et al. Assessing symptom distress in cancer patients: The M. D. Anderson Symptom Inventory. *Cancer.* 2000;89:1634–1646.
12. Portenoy R, Thaler H, Kornblith A, et al. Symptom prevalence, characteristics and distress in a cancer population. *Qual Life Res.* 1994;3:183–189.
13. Bruley D. Beyond reliability and validity: analysis of selected quality of life instruments for use in palliative care. *J Palliat Med.* 1999;2:299–390.
14. Veikova G, Stark D, Selby P. Quality of life instruments in oncology. *Eur J Cancer.* 1999;35:1571–1580.
15. Stromgren A, Goldschmidt D, Groenvold M, et al. Self-assessment in cancer patients referred to palliative care: A study of feasibility and symptom epidemiology. *Cancer.* 2002;94:512–520.
16. Stromgren A, Groenvold M, Pedersen L, et al. Does the medical record cover the symptoms experienced by cancer patients receiving palliative care? A comparison of the record and patient self-rating. *J Pain Symptom Manage.* 2001;21:89–96.
17. Bruera E, Kuehn N, Miller M.J, et al. The Edmonton Symptom Assessment System (ESAS): a simple method for the assessment of palliative care patients. *J Palliat Care.* 1991;7:6–9.
18. Porzio G, Ricevuto E, Aielli F, et al. The Supportive Care Task Force at the University of L'Aquila: 2-years experience. *Support Care Cancer.* 2005;13:351–355.
19. Rees E, Hardy J, Ling J, et al. The use of Edmonton Symptom Scale (ESAS) within a palliative care unit in the UK. *Palliat Med.* 1998;15:213–214.
20. Stromgren AS, Groenvold M, Peterson M.A, et al. Pain characteristics and treatment outcome for advanced cancer patients during the first week of specialized palliative care. *J Pain Symptom Manage.* 2004;27:104–113.
21. Chang V, Hwang S, Feuerman M. Validation of the Edmonton Symptom Assessment Scale. Cancer 2000;88:2164–2171.
22. Chochinov H, Tataryn D, Clinch J, et al. Will to live in the terminally ill. *Lancet.* 1999;354:816–819.
23. Philip J, Smith W, Craft P, et al. Concurrent validity of the modified Edmonton Symptom Assessment System with the Rotterdam Symptom checklist and the Brief Pain Inventory. *Support Care Cancer.* 1998;6:539–541.
24. Walke L, Gallo W, Tinetti M, et al. The burden of symptoms among community-dwelling older persons with advanced chronic disease. *Arch Intern Med.* 2004;164:2321–2324.
25. Vignaroli E, Pace E, Willey J, et al. The Edmonton Symptom Assessment System as a screening tool for depression and anxiety. *J Palliat Med.* 2006;9:296–303.
26. Portenoy R, Thaler H, Kornblith A, et al. The Memorial Symptom Assessment Scale: an instrument for the evaluation of symptom prevalence, characteristics and distress. *Eur J Cancer.* 1994;30A:1326–1336.
27. Chang V, Hwang S, Feuerman M, et al. The Memorial Symptom Assessment Scale Short Form (MSAS-SF). Validity and reliability. *Cancer.* 2000;89:1163–1171.
28. Chang V, Hwang S, Kasimis B, et al. Shorter symptom assessment instruments: The Condensed Memorial Symptom Assessment Scale (CMSAS). *Cancer Invest.* 2004;22:526–536.
29. McCorkle R, Young K. Development of a symptom distress scale. *Cancer Nurs.* 1978;1:373–378.
30. McCorkle R, Quint-Benoliel J. Symptom distress, current concerns and mood disturbance after diagnosis of life-threatening disease. *Soc Sci Med.* 1983;17:431–438.
31. Fortinsky R, Granger C, Sletzer G. The use of the functional assessment in understanding home care needs. *Med Care.* 1981;19:489–497.
32. Vigano A, Dorgan M, Buckingham J, et al. Survival prediction in terminal cancer patients: a systematic review of the medical literature. *Palliat Med.* 2000;14:363–374.
33. Coates A, Gebski V, Signorini D, et al. Prognostic values of quality of life scores during chemotherapy for advanced breast cancer. *J Clin Oncol.* 1992;10:1833–1838.
34. Miller F. Predicting survival in the advanced cancer patient. *Henry Ford Hosp Med.* 1991;391:81–84.
35. Schag C, Heinrich R, Ganz P. Karnofsky performance status revisited: reliability validity and guidelines. *J Clin Oncol.* 1984;2:187–193.
36. Yates J, Chalmer B, Mc Kegner F. Evaluation of patients with advanced cancer using the Karnofsky performance status. *Cancer.* 1980;45:2220–2224.
37. Mor V, Laliberte L, Morris JN, et al. The Karnofsky Performance Status Scale. An examination of its reliability and validity in a research setting. *Cancer.* 1984;53(9):2002–2007.
38. Glare P, Virik K, Jones M, et al. A systematic review of physician's survival predictions in terminally ill cancer patients. *Br Med J.* 2003;327:195.
39. Oken MM, Creech RH, Tormey DC, et al. Toxicity and response criteria of the Eastern Cooperative Oncology Group. *Am J Clin Oncol.* 1982;5:649–655.
40. Kaasa T, Wessel J. The Edmonton Functional Assessment Tool: further development and validation for use in palliative care. *J Palliat Care.* 2001;17:5–11.
41. Kaasa T, Wessel J, Darrah J, et al. Inter-rater reliability of formally trained and self-trained raters using the Edmonton Functional Assessment Tool. *Palliat Med.* 2000;14:509–517.
42. Marcianiak C, Sliwa J, Spill G, et al. Functional outcome following rehabilitation of the cancer patient. *Arch Phys Med Rehabil.* 2004;77:54–57.
43. Garrard P, Farnham C, Thompson A, et al. Rehabilitation of the cancer patient: experience in a neurological unit. *Neurorehabil Neural Repair.* 2004;18:76–79.
44. Del Fabro E, Dalal S, Bruera E. Symptom control in palliative care–part III. Dyspnea and delirium. *J Palliat Med.* 2006;9:422–436.
45. Doyle D, Hanks G, Cherny N, et al. *Oxford Textbook of Palliative Medicine.* 3rd edition. New York: Oxford University Press; 587–610.
46. Hardy JR, Turner R, Saunders M, et al. Prediction of Survival in a hospital-based continuing care unit. *Eur J Cancer.* 1994;30:284–288.
47. Kvale P, Simoff M, Prakash U. Palliative care. *Chest.* 2003;123:284–311.
48. Sutton L, Demark-Wahnefried W, Clipp E. Management of terminal cancer in elderly patients. *Lancet Oncol.* 2003; 4: 149–151.

49. Silvestri G, Sherman C, Williams T, et al. Caring for the dying patient with lung cancer. *Chest*. 2002;122:1028–1036.
50. Smith EL, Hann DM, Ahles TA, et al. Dyspnea, Anxiety, body consciousness, and quality of life in patients with lung cancer. *J Pain Symptom Manage*. 2001;21:323–329.
51. Nekolaichuk CL, Bruera E, Spachynski K, et al. A comparison of patient and proxy symptom assessment in advanced cancer patients. *Palliat Med*. 1999;13:311–323.
52. Bausewein C, Farquahar M, Booth S, et al. Measurement of breathlessness in advanced disease: a systematic review. *Resp Med*. 2007;101:399–410.
53. Ripamonti C. Management of dyspnea in advanced cancer patients. *Support Care Cancer*. 1999;7:233–243.
54. Chang VT, Hwang SS, Feuerman M. Validation of the Edmonton Symptom Assessment Scale. *Cancer*. 2000;88:2164–2171.
55. Henoch I, Bergman B. Validation of a Swedish version of a cancer dyspnea scale. *J Pain Symptom Manage*. 2006;31:353–361.
56. Dorman S, Byrne A, Edwards A. Which measurement scales should we use to measure breathlessness in palliative care? A systematic review. *Palliat Med*. 2007;21:177–191.
57. Gift A, Narsavage G. Validity of the numeric rating scale as a measure of dyspnea. *Am J Crit Care*. 1998;7:200–204.
58. Borg G. Perceived exertion as an indicator of somatic stress. *Scand J Rehab Med*. 1970;2:92–98.
59. Borg G. A category scale with ration properties for intermodal and interindividual comparisons. In: Geissler H, Petzoldt T, eds. *Psychophysical Judgements and the Process of Perception*. Berlin: Deutscher Verlag; 1982:25–34.
60. Guyatt G, Berman L, Townsend M, et al. A measure of quality of life for clinical trials in chronic lung disease. *Thorax*. 1987;42:773–778.
61. Lawlor P, Nekolaichuk C, Gagnon B, et al. Clinical utility, factor analysis, and further validation of the Memorial Delirium Assessment Scale in patients with advanced cancer. *Cancer*. 2000;88:2859–2867.
62. Centeno C, Sanz A, Bruera E. Delirium in advanced cancer patients. *Palliat Med*. 2004;18:184–194.
63. Rooij SE, Schuurmans MJ, van dal Mast RC, et al. Clinical subtypes of delirium and their relevance for daily clinical practice: a systematic review. *Int J Geriatr Psychiatry*. 2005;20:609–615.
64. Lawlor P, Fainsinger R, Bruera E. Delirium at the end of life. Critical issues in clinical practice and research. *JAMA*. 2000;284:2427–2429.
65. Lawlor P, Gagnon B, Mancini I, et al. Occurrence, causes, and outcome of delirium in advanced cancer patients: a prospective study. *Arch Intern Med*. 2000;160: 786–794.
66. Lipowski Z. Delirium. *JAMA*. 1987;258:1789–1792.
67. Yennurajalingam S, Braiteh F, Bruera E. Pain and terminal delirium research in the elderly. *Clin Geriatr Med*. 2005;21:93–119.
68. Liptzin B, Levkoff S. An empirical study of delirium subtypes. *Br J Psychiatry*. 1992;161:843–845.
69. Minagawa H, Uchitomi Y, Yamawaki S, et al. Psychiatric morbidity in terminally ill cancer patients: a prospective study. *Cancer*. 1996;78:1131–1137.
70. Massie M, Holland J, Glass E. Delirium in terminally ill cancer patients. *Am J Psychiatry*. 1983;140:1048–1050.
71. Inouye S. Delirium in older persons. *N Engl J Med*. 2006;354:1157–1165.
72. Bruera E, Miller L, McCallion J, et al. Cognitive failure in patients with terminal cancer: a prospective study. *J Pain Symptom Manage*. 1992;7:192–195.
73. Inouye S. The dilemma of delirium: clinical and research controversies regarding diagnosis and evaluation of delirium in hospitalized elderly medical patients. *Am J Med*. 1994;97:278–288.
74. Bruera E, Fainsinger R, Miller M, et al. The assessment of pain intensity of pain intensity in patients with cognitive failure: a preliminary report. *J Pain Symptom Manage*. 1992;7:267–270.
75. Folstein M, Folstein S, McHugh P. Mini-mental state: a practical method for grading the cognitive state of patients for the clinician. *J Psychiatry Res*. 1975;12:189–198.
76. Inouye S, van Dyck C, Alessi C, et al. Clarifying confusion: the confusion assessment method: a new method for detection of delirium. *Ann Intern Med*. 1990;113:941–948.
77. Malloy P, Cummings J, Duffy J. Cognitive screening instruments in neuropsychiatry: A report of the committee of research of the American Neuropsychiatric Association. *J Neuropsychiatr Clin Neurosci*. 1997;9:189–197.
78. Tombaugh T, McIntyre N. The mini-mental state examination: a comprehensive review. *J Am Geriatr Soc*. 1992;40:992–935.
79. O'Neill D, O'Shea B, Walsh J. Screening for dementia and delirium using an adapted Folstein Mini-Mental State Examination. *Ir Med J*. 1989;82:24–25.
80. Bruera E, Schoeller T, Wenk R, et al. A prospective multicenter assessment of the Edmonton staging system for cancer pain. *J Pain Symptom Manage*. 1995;10:348–355.
81. Ely E, Inouye S, Bernard g, et al. Delirium in mechanically ventilated patients: validity and reliability of the confusion assessment method for the intensive care unit (CAM-ICU). *JAMA*. 2001;286:2703–2710.
82. McNicoll L, Pisani M, Ely E, et al. Detection of delirium in the intensive care unit: comparison of the confusion assessment method for the intensive care unit with confusion assessment ratings. *J Am Geriatr Soc*. 2005;53:495–500.
83. Yennurajalingam S, Bruera E. Palliative management of fatigue at the close of life "It feels like my body is just worn out." *JAMA*. 2007;297:295–304.
84. Glaus A, Crow R, Hammond S. A qualitative study to explore the concept to fatigue/tiredness in cancer patients and in healthy individuals. *Support Care Cancer*. 1996;4:82–96.
85. Liao S, Ferrel BA. Fatigue in older population. *J Am Geriatr Soc*. 2000;48:426–430.
86. Sharpe MC, Archnard LC, Banatvala JE. A report-chronic fatigue syndrome, guidelines for research. *J R Soc Med*. 1991;84:118–121.
87. National Comprehensive Cancer Network Practice Guidelines. Cancer-related fatigue panel 2006 guidelines. Rockledge, PA: National Comprehensive Cancer Network; March 2006. http://www.nccn.org.
88. Del Fabbro E, Dalal S, Bruera E. Symptom control in palliative care—part II: cachexia/anorexia and fatigue. *J Palliat Med*. 2006;9:409–421.
89. Jenkins C, Schulz M, Hanson J, et al. Demographic, symptom, and medication profiles of cancer patients seen by a palliative care consult team in a tertiary referral hospital. *J Pain Symptom Manage*. 2000;19:174–184.
90. Portenoy R. Cancer-related fatigue: an immense problem. *Oncologist*. 2000;5:350–352.
91. Smets EM, Garssen B, Schuster-Uitterhoeve AL, et al. Fatigue in cancer patients. *Br J Cancer*. 1993;68:220–224.
92. Portenoy R, Itri L. Cancer-related fatigue. Guidelines for evaluation and management. *Oncologist*. 1999;4:1–10.
93. Cella DF, Tulsky DS, Gray G, et al. The Functional Assessment of Cancer Therapy scale: development and validation of the general measure. *J Clin Oncol*. 1993;11:570–579.
94. Cella D. *Manual of the Functional Assessment of Chronic Illness Therapy (FACIT) Measurement System*. Center on Outcomes, Research and Education (CORE). Evanston, Northwestern Healthcare and Northwestern Education. Version 4, 1997.
95. Mendoza T, Wang X, Cleeland C, et al. The rapid assessment of fatigue severity in cancer patients. *Cancer*. 1999;85:1186–1196.
96. Ferrigno D, Buccheri G. Anthropometric measurements in non-small cell lung cancer. *Supp Care Cancer*. 2001;9:522–527.
97. Fortner B, Stepanski E, Wang S, et al. Sleep and quality of life in breast cancer patients. *J Pain Symptom Manage*. 2002;24:471–480.
98. Zammit G, Weiner J, Damanto N, et al. Quality of life in people with insomnia. *Sleep*. 1999;22(Suppl 2):S379–385.
99. Redeker N, Lev E, Ruggiero J. Insomnia, fatigue, anxiety, depression, and quality of life of cancer patients undergoing chemotherapy. *Sch Inq Nurs Pract*. 2000;14:275–290; discussion 291–298.
100. Katz D, McHorney C. The relationship between insomnia and health-related quality of life in patients with chronic illness. *J Fam Pract*. 2002;51:229–235.
101. Engstrom C, Strohl R, Rose L, et al. Sleep alterations in cancer patients. *Cancer Nurs*. 1999;22:143–148.
102. Beck-Little R. Weinrich SP. Assessment and management of sleep disorder in the elderly. *J Gerontologic Nursing*. 1998; 24(4): 21–29.
103. Buysse DJ, Reynolds CF, Monk TH, et al. Pittsburgh Sleep Quality Index: a new instrument for psychiatric practice and research. *Psychiatr Res*. 1989;28(2):192–213.
104. Massie MJ. Prevalence of depression in patients with cancer. *J Natl Cancer Inst Monogr*. 2004;32:57–71.
105. Block S. Assessing and managing depression in the terminally ill patient. *Ann Intern Med*. 2000;32:209–218.
106. Hotopf M, Chidgey J, Addington-Hall J, et al. Depression in advanced disease: a systematic review. Part 1: Prevalence and case finding. *Palliat Med*. 2002;16:81–97.
107. Massie MJ, Gagnon P, Holland JC. Depression and suicide in patients with cancer. *J Pain Symptom Manage*. 1994;9:325–340.
108. Radbruch L, Nauck F, Ostgathe C, et al. What are the problems in palliative care? Results from a representative survey. *Support Care Cancer*. 2003;11:442–445.
109. Ng K, von Guten C. Symptoms and attitudes of 100 consecutive patients admitted to an acute hospice/palliative care unit. *J Pain Symptom Manage*. 1998;16:307–316.
110. Reuben D, Mor V, Hiris J. Clinical symptoms and length of survival in patients with terminal cancer. *Arch Intern Med*. 1998;148:1586–1591.
111. Kurtz M, Kurtz J, Stommel M, et al. Physical functioning and depression among older persons with cancer. *Cancer Practice*. 2001;9:11–18.
112. Lloyd-Williams M, Dennis M, Taylor F. A prospective study to determine the association between physical symptoms and depression in patients with advanced cancer. *Palliat Med*. 2004;18:558–563.
113. Johnston M, Pollard B, Hennessey P. Construct validation of the hospital anxiety and depression scale with clinical populations. *J Psychosomatic Res*. 2000;48:579–584.
114. Bjelland I, Dahl AA, Haug TT, et al. The validity of the Hospital Anxiety and Depression Scale: an updated literature review. *J Psychosom Res*. 2002;52:69–77.
115. Puchalski C, Romer A. Taking a spiritual history allows clinicians to understand patients more fully. *J Palliat Med*. 2000;3:129–137.
116. Bruera E, Moyano J, Seifert L, et al. The frequency of alcoholism among patients with pain due to terminal cancer. *J Pain Symptom Manage*. 1995;10:599–603.
117. Bruera E, Watanabe S. New developments in the assessment of pain in cancer patients. *Support Care Cancer*. 1994;2:312–318.
118. Bruera E, Schoeller T, Wenk R, et al. A prospective multicenter assessment of the Edmonton Staging System for cancer pain. *J Pain Symptom Manage*. 1995;10:348–355.
119. Derogatis LR, Melisaratos N. The Brief Symptom Inventory: an introductory report. *Psychol Med*. 1983,13:595–605.
120. Zarit S, Reever K, Bach-Peterson J. Relatives of the impaired elderly: correlates of feelings of burden. *Gerontologist*. 1980;20:649–655.

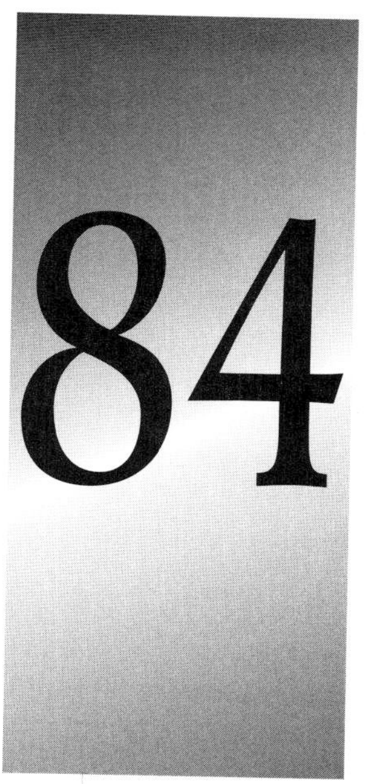

Guidelines for Pain Control in the Esophageal Cancer Patient

Kimberly Marie Kaplan

When we talk of esophageal pain, we can focus on either acute or chronic pain. In most standard terms, chronic pain refers to pain that has persisted for at least 6 months. This chapter will focus on chronic esophageal cancer pain, starting with a brief introduction of chronic pain itself. The chapter centers on palliative care but also will discuss treatments that are appropriate for non-malignant esophageal pain in order to emphasize the differences in treatment between malignant and non-malignant pain. We will then move into the pathophysiologic aspects of chronic pain and then discuss medication as well as interventional therapies. Medication management will include anticonvulsants, antidepressants, and a brief history of the opioid therapies. We will conclude with a discussion of sympathetic blockade for chronic esophageal pain and intrathecal therapies, the latter of which is a treatment used mainly for malignant esophageal pain.

Chronic pain is a debilitating disorder with an estimated cost to society totaling billions of dollars (1). The treatment of chronic pain represents a challenging problem to modern medicine. This is in part due to its poorly understood pathophysiology, its intractability to surgery, and impact on the psychosocial aspect of the patient.

The goal of pain management is not just control of pain but the ability of a patient to regain control of his or her psyche and maintain quality of life.

All methods of pain management attempt to either control the cause of the pain or alter the perception of the pain. Most therapeutic approaches as labeled as pharmacologic or non-pharmacologic. Nonpharmacologic approaches include behavioral techniques, radiation therapy, and surgery. Pharmacologic approaches obviously include the medication management that often relies upon chronic opioid therapies in the cancer patient.

PAIN PATHOPHYSIOLOGY

The transmission of pain from peripheral pain receptors to the brain is mediated by spinothalamic, spinomesencephalic, spinoreticular, spinolimbic, spinocervical, and dorsal column pathways. Neurons in the spinal cord transmit information to a number of regions of the brain stem, including the thalamus, periaqueductal gray, and bulbar reticular formation, as well as to limbic structures, hypothalamus, and amygdala of the limbic system and cortical centers via the thalamus. Much of the nociceptive processing involving the cognitive and affective components of pain is mediated by higher centers, such as the limbic system and thalamus. In addition, there is a descending analgesic system that incorporates many of the same components as the higher centers.

The approaches to acute esophageal pain, cancer esophageal pain, and chronic esophageal pain differ somewhat. Some pathologies are believed to heal and with healing will come pain resolution. Acute postoperative and posttraumatic esophageal pain fall into these categories. Thus, these 2 pathologies are generally treated with non-steroidal analgesics as a first-line approach.

The treatment of esophageal cancer pain, however, is considered to require aggressive analgesic therapy, and thus is considered safe to treat aggressively because the duration of treatment will be time-limited secondary to the disease process.

However, the use of potent analgesics in chronic noncancer pain has been subject to much more rigorous debate. Chronic pain does not share the same time course, and the cultural and social factors that envelop chronic pain sufferers suggest a much more complicated moral dilemma when applying concepts of palliation to potentially productive members of society. Although the moral imperative clearly is to treat the suffering of chronic noncancer pain patients in a palliative manner, the clinical data would suggest that the best outcome and quality of life actually are achieved with interdisciplinary approaches to chronic pain.

The World Health Organization analgesic ladder, delineated 15 years ago, is the appropriate path to follow in the treatment of cancer pain. It starts with using a non-opioid for the management of mild pain; step 2 is represented by weak opioids (e.g., codeine, hydrocodone); and step 3 uses opioids without a ceiling effect and is typically recommended for moderate to severe pain. There are some pain physicians who recommend skipping step 2, as pain in most patients is well managed using just steps 1 and 3. It is often the case that when a cancer patient arrives in one's office, he or she suffers from pain beyond the scope of agents listed in step 2, and step 3 becomes the next logical succession. Acetaminophen and nonsteroidal anti-inflammatory drugs can be used as adjuvants at any step.

How does one choose which agent to use as one's move upwards on the prescribing ladder? The choice of medication that is best for a specific patient is influenced by multiple factors such as medical history, drug allergy or intolerance, preferred route of administration, half-life, and availability. For the majority of cancer patients at the end of life, good pain relief while maximizing function is achievable.

NEUROPATHIC PAIN

Neuropathic therapy often involves multi-drug therapy. The basis for using multi-drug therapy for neuropathic pain is the recognition that there may be more than one underlying mechanism of the identified disorder.

Neuropathic pain includes diverse chronic pain disorders, such as postherpetic neuralgia, post-stroke central pain, painful diabetic neuropathy, and post-traumatic neuralgia, among others. Cancer pain often incorporates an element of neuropathic pain. The main defining characteristic of neuropathic pain is that the pain develops from disease of or injury to the somatic sensory systems. Among those mechanisms are peripheral sensitization, which implicates Substance P among others. Many other pathophysiologic pathways have been proposed to explain the phenomenon which is neuropathic pain; however, many are beyond the scope of this chapter.

Opioids are becoming a more accepted treatment for neuropathic pain but suffice it to say that many pain medicine physicians would still start antidepressant and anticonvulsant therapies prior to initiating any chronic opioid therapy. In cancer patients, the rules get broken and opioids tend to be given earlier in the disease process. Two first-line accepted treatments for esophageal cancer pain are the antidepressant and anticonvulsant or antineuropathic agents that are detailed below.

ANTIDEPRESSANTS

Antidepressant medications are among the most commonly prescribed psychotropic drugs used as single or adjuvant agents in the treatment of pain syndromes. We will discuss the tricyclic antidepressants (TCAs) and the selective serotonin reuptake inhibitors (SSRIs).

The TCAs or "tricyclics" are referred to as such because of their characteristic 3-ring structure. They are further categorized as either secondary or tertiary amine agents, depending on the amine group at the end of the carbon side chain.

The mechanism responsible for the antidepressant effects of TCAs is unknown. They act in the central nervous system to block the reuptake of the monoamine neurotransmitters norepinephrine and, serotonin from the synaptic cleft.

For the patient who can tolerate the side effects, a trial of a TCA probably offers the best likelihood of response for neuropathic pain. These medications are not often beneficial until one reaches approximately 80–100 mg daily. These medications can be increased safely every week; however, the wide variability in response rates and side effects dictates waiting several weeks before titrating upward.

For patients who are unable to tolerate a medication from the tertiary-amine class, a secondary-amine TCA may be administered in the same manner as described above. Nortriptyline is considered more potent than the other TCAs. Desipramine is less predictably sedating than the other TCAs, and some patients find it mildly stimulating (2).

Selective Serotonin Reuptake Inhibitor Antidepressants

Fluoxetine in 1987 for use in depression started the popularity of selective serotonin reuptake inhibitor antidepressants. However, the addition of venlafaxine added something new to the armamentarium of pain physicians.

These agents prolong the presence of serotonin in the synaptic cleft by blocking its reuptake into presynaptic neurons. Since being introduced, these medications have earned approval of many pain management practitioners. Duloxetine is the newest member of the family and widely prescribed, with therapeutic doses ranging from 60 mg to 120 mg daily. Duloxetine is classified as an SNRI (serotonin and norepinephrine reuptake inhibitor) (2).

KETAMINE

Ketamine was developed as an anesthetic. It has weak primary analgesic properties when used by itself in small doses. In other circumstances and uses, however, it exerts strong adjuvant analgesic properties by inhibiting the binding of glutamate to the NMDA-R, which is probably its most critical mechanism of action. There is growing evidence that NMDA-R antagonists, such as ketamine, palliate spontaneous, neuropathic pain. However, there may be other mechanisms to ketamine's action. There is no agreement on a single, uniform best ketamine protocol or dose. Often, however, reduction of opioid doses in cancer patients is achieved within the first few hours of a ketamine intravenous infusion or oral ketamine therapies. One should strongly consider the routine use of a small dose of benzodiazepine or neuroleptic while initiating treatment to minimize the psychotomimetic side effects.

OPIOIDS

Opioids are drugs that have been used for decades to treat pain in patients. Effects from opioids depend on the dose taken at one time, how the drug is delivered, a patient's history with the drug, the patient's psychological and emotional stability, and the simultaneous use of alcohol or other drugs. Opiates are drugs derived from opium and include well-known derivatives such as morphine and codeine. Opioids refer to drugs with morphine-like activity and can be naturally occurring, semisynthetic, or synthetically derived.

The proper use of opioids involves selecting a particular drug and route of administration and determining the suitable initial dose, the frequency of administration, and the incidence and severity of side effects; whether the analgesic will be given in an inpatient or ambulatory setting must also be determined.

The Short-Acting Opioid Analgesics

Without the brain, there is no experience known as pain. Opioid therapies combat that pain, not only at the central nervous system level but also at the spinal level. The short-acting opioid analgesics are often used for breakthrough pain. The short-acting medication discussed in this chapter will be tramadol.

Tramadol is a synthetic analog of codeine. IV Tramadol at dose of 50 to150 mg is equivalent to IV morphine at does of 5 to 15 mg. Tramadol is a useful agent for treating mild to moderate pain. However, tramadol may induce seizures, especially when used in conjunction with proconvulsive drugs and in epileptic patients.

The Long-Acting Opioid Analgesics

Morphine is the prototypical opioid to which all other analgesics are compared in determining their relative analgesia potency. It is the standard of comparison for parenteral and oral opioid analgesics. The opioids, including morphine, provide analgesia at both a spinal cord and at a cerebral cortex level. Opioids produce analgesia by binding to opioid receptors both within and outside of the central nervous system. Relative potency of intramuscular morphine to oral morphine on repeated administration is 1:2 or 1:3. Slow-release formulations of morphine can be administered on an 8-hour basis, 12-hour basis, or 24-hour basis. These formulations use either hydrophobic or hydrophilic matrices to allow a graded release of the drug as the pill passes through the gastrointestinal tract.

In addition to possessing pain-relieving properties, the opiates possess other effects. These include sedation, nausea, decreased pain perception, and feelings of euphoria.

Methadone is another long-acting opioid derivative with unusual pharmacodynamic and pharmacokinetic properties. Methadone's NMDA antagonist properties set it aside from the other analgesic therapies and perhaps make it a better opioid analgesic when neuropathic as well as nociceptive pain must be considered.

It is a popular choice for cancer pain, probably due to several factors, among which is its relatively long terminal half-life, which allows for less repeated dosing. Studies of methadone in opioid-dependent patients suggest that its terminal half-life ranges from 25 to 52 hours. Recently, an increased number of deaths have been associated with the use of methadone, and the FDA has alerted physicians about methadone-induced cardiorespiratory adverse effects.

Oral oxycodone is approximately 7 to 9.5 times more potent than oral codeine and 1.5 times more potent than oral morphine. Unlike morphine, oxycodone is currently marketed for pain management in only 1 controlled-release formulation.

Fentanyl is available in parenteral, transdermal, and transmucosal formulations. It is 80 to 100 times more potent than morphine when given by the IV route. The oral transmucosal formulation of fentanyl (Actiq, Cephalon) is indicated for the treatment of breakthrough pain in cancer patients already tolerant to opioid analgesics.

Fentanyl administered via a transdermal delivery system (i.e., the patch) attains variable plasma concentrations and is associated with a risk for respiratory depression (as are all opioid analgesics).

As the understanding of the pharmacologic aspects and clinical experience of opioids become more widespread in the medical communities, medical professionals have become more accepting of the use of opioids for the treatment of pain in both acute and chronic settings. The variety of opium derivatives, from naturally occurring to synthetic, from partial agonist to antagonist, allows the medical professional the flexibility to cater a treatment regimen that takes into account the myriad of medical complexity, types of pain, and potential side effects affecting their patients. Ongoing and future research and advances in the clinical use of opioid drugs together with parallel growth in the understanding of opioid mechanisms hopefully will counteract under treatment of pain and fear of opioid therapy.

SYMPATHETIC BLOCKS

Many pain clinics perform blockade of the sympathetic pathways. Sympathetic blockade is used diagnostically to determine if a patient's particular pain complaint involves components of the sympathetic nervous system. There are many different approaches to sympathetic blockade of the esophagus.

Blockade of sympathetic transmission can be accomplished by a variety of approaches, including epidural, intrathecal, or stellate ganglion blockade. A neuroaxial block which includes epidural or intrathecal will very likely result in blockade of all neuronal fibers: autonomic, sensory, and motor.

The indications for sympathetic blocks are very broad, representing the wide range of clinical symptoms the sympathetic nervous system can affect. Usually, pain physicians use sympathetic blocks for disorders of the upper-thoracic area (which includes the esophagus) and pain disorders of the upper extremities. This includes disorders such as complex regional pain syndrome type 1 and complex regional pain syndrome type II.

There are some signs to watch for to help determine if one has a successful diagnostic block. Horner's syndrome, which involves the triad of ptosis, miosis, and facial anhydrosis, is often the constellation of symptoms and signs that accompany a successful stellate ganglion block of the upper extremity. However, one does not need to achieve a Horner's syndrome to confirm a properly placed stellate ganglion block. In addition to a Horner's syndrome, there is often an increase in skin temperature.

A positive result to a diagnostic sympathetic block can be followed by a therapeutic block that often incorporates alcohol or phenol. These blocks are beneficial in that they let the patient scale back on their opioid consumption. Most pain practitioners reserve neurolysis procedures for those patients with malignant pain (2).

INTRATHECAL DRUG DELIVERY

Despite significant, positive advances in opioid formulations ranging from long-acting tablets to lollipops, the most potent way to administer opioids is by the intrathecal route.

Chronic infusion of a wide array of intrathecal medications for severe chronic pain or spasticity has become an accepted medical practice and offers an alternative therapy for patients unresponsive to conventional modalities. An array of distinct pharmacologic classes of analgesics are in use as single agents and in combination. Continued research into new drugs such as ketorolac, gabapentin, octreotide, neurotrophin-3 antisense oligonucleotide, glial-derived neurotrophic factor, and others may show promise. Restraint must be shown until preclinical and clinical trials demonstrate the safety of these drugs, and appropriate patient selection must be integral to the process to permit the best chance of success. An in-depth, systematic review of combination spinal analgesic chemotherapy by Walker et al. has provided evidence to support various single and combination drug therapies, and a treatment algorithm devised by the Polyanalgesic Consensus Conference of 2003 details much needed guidelines for their use. A wide range of opioid have been studied intraspinally. Fentanyl, sufentanil, and meperidine have been studied intraspinally and are routinely used. Other opioids that have been studied are buprenorphine, diamorphine, sufentanil, alfentanil, lofentanil, butorphanol, hydromorphone, nalbuphine, methadone, nicomorphine, pentazocine, phenoperidine, meptazinol, and tramadol. At this time, there is a general lack of comparative data for these drugs. The major difference between the various opioids intraspinally is latency of onset, duration of analgesia, and adverse effects. The quality of analgesia appears to be similar for all drugs (3).

In conclusion, there is no specific plan or spreadsheet that will dictate a patient's pain management needs or requests. Pain management must be catered to the individual, and the discussions above are only an outline. Combining drug therapies with psychologic support, and other alternative modalities, such as acupuncture and physical therapy techniques, give one the equation most likely to lead to success.

THE TEAM APPROACH

History and examination of the patient by appropriate health care professionals in multidisciplinary pain centers allow triage that guide management. Drugs, physical, and psychological measures are, most of the time, sufficient to relieve pain and improve quality of life. This however, takes time. Perhaps the most important role of the pain practitioner is to educate and assure patients that their quality of life and function can improve despite unchanging Visual Analog Scale (VAS) scores.

References

1. Kaplan KM, Brose WG. Intrathecal methods. *Neurosurg Clin North Am.* 2004;15:289–296.
2. Warfield CA, Fausett HJ. *Manual of Pain Management.* 2nd ed. Philadelphia: Lippincott, Williams, & Wilkens; 2001.
3. Farrow-Gillespie A, Kaplan KM. Intrathecal analgesic drug therapy. *Curr Pain Headache Rep.* 2006;10(1):.
4. Arantes S, Ferreira C, Baptista C, Moutinho R, Marcos A, Carvalho CJ. Low back pain: our multidisciplinary pain clinic reality [in Portuguese]. *Centro Hospitalar De Villa Nova De Gaia.*
5. Buvanendran A, Rueben S. Opioid analgesics for the management of postoperative pain. *Anesthesiol News.* 2007.

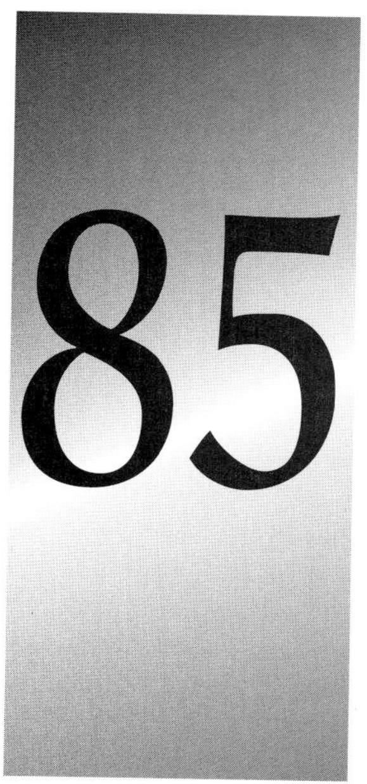

Endoscopic Palliation of Dysphagia: Photodynamic Therapy

Paula Ugalde
James D. Luketich

Von Tappeiner (1) originally described *photodynamic action* at the beginning of the 20th century. This reaction was based on the ability of acridine, in the presence of oxygen, to produce cytotoxicity to living organisms after light stimulation. However, it was not until 1942 that Auler and Banzer discovered the tumor cell selectivity of porphyrins when they noted in vivo fluorescence of tumor tissue after systemic application of a porphyrin (2). Then, in 1955, Samuel Schwartz (3) developed a hematoporphyrin derivative (HPD) by acetylation and reduction of hematoporphyrin, which was found to be twice as phototoxic as hematoporphyrin.

By the 1970s, photodynamic therapy had finally gained popularity, and several groups in North America and Europe expanded their investigations using photodynamic treatment for several cancers, including skin, bladder, lung, gynecologic, breast, brain, and esophageal cancer (4–10). In the 1990s, the U.S. Food and Drug Administration approved the purified HPD Photofrin (porfimer sodium; Quadra Logic Technologies Phototherapeutics, Inc., Vancouver, Canada) for the treatment of obstructive esophageal cancer (11).

The incidence of esophageal carcinoma has increased over the past 2 decades (12), and it is now the eighth most common cancer around the world (13). At diagnosis, nearly 60% of patients are either extremely poor operative candidates or have unresectable cancer that extends beyond the locoregional confines, leaving only a small percentage eligible for potentially curative resection (14). Thus, clinicians are often dealing with an advanced-stage, incurable carcinoma in newly diagnosed patients.

In patients with unresectable or incurable carcinoma who present with dysphagia, an important goal is to provide symptomatic relief, which may improve nutritional status, the sensation of well-being, and, ultimately, the overall quality of life (15). Malignant dysphagia results from a partially or completely obstructed esophageal lumen leading to malnutrition, aspiration, and sialorrhea. The return to oral intake through the least invasive procedure and shortest hospital stay is the ideal palliation. This type of management is far superior and more cost effective than feeding tubes or parenteral nutrition.

The primary nonsurgical method for palliation of dysphagia is endoscopic therapy (16–22). Ideally, the surgeon dealing with esophageal cancer patients should be well-versed in all endoscopic interventions. Currently available modalities include thermocoagulation (laser), bipolar electrocautery, balloon dilatation, expandable metal stent insertion, endoesophageal brachytherapy, and, more recently, photodynamic therapy (PDT) (23–28). One modality often is chosen over another based on the availability of instrumentation, physician expertise, and patient preference.

The ideal palliative method should be safe, effective, durable, have low cost and be associated with minimal morbidity and mortality. Some patients will require more than one palliative method to sustain lumen patency during the course of their disease. In this chapter, we review the use of PDT as an endoscopic palliation procedure for malignant dysphagia.

PRINCIPLES OF PHOTODYNAMIC THERAPY

In the palliative setting of advanced esophageal cancer, PDT is an easy, safe, and effective treatment modality. However, the cost of PDT is significant (29). Ideal candidates for this procedure have locally advanced esophageal cancer with primarily endoluminal disease and minimal stricture or extrinsic compression.

MECHANISM OF ACTION

A photosensitizer that can accumulate in tumor tissue marked for destruction is required for PDT. Porfimer sodium is the most widely used photosensitizer and achieves an exited state after exposure to light (30). The activated drug generates oxygen-free radicals that selectively kill the tumor cells (14). This cytotoxic effect leads to tumor ablation and ultimately endoluminal patency (31). In addition to directly killing cancer cells, PDT appears to shrink or destroy tumors in 2 other ways: it can damage blood vessels in the tumor and also activate the immune system to attack the tumor cells (11).

PROCEDURE

A simple 2-stage process, PDT can be performed in the outpatient setting and may be repeated and/or be used along with other therapies, such as surgery, radiation, or chemotherapy. Photofrin is injected into the bloodstream 24 to 48 hours prior to the procedure (2 mg/kg). This agent is absorbed by cells all over the body but there is some selectivity to malignant cells. Under general anesthesia, flexible endoscopy is performed to visualize the tumor. Then, with an optical fiber passed through the endoscope, a 630 nm wavelength of laser light is delivered onto the tumor. The photosensitizer absorbs the light energy, achieves an exited state, and through a photochemical reaction produces tumoricidal oxygen free radicals (32).

Patients are discharged home 2 to 3 hours post-procedure with instructions to maintain a liquid diet for 24 to 48 hours and then to progressively advance the consistency of the diet. Patients also need to be advised to avoid sunlight and other sources of ultraviolet light. We prefer to repeat the endoscopy 2 days after the PDT to assess tumor response, debride any necrotic tumor, and perform a second light application to remaining viable areas of tumor (33). Also, during this second endoscopy, esophageal dilation can be performed in attempt to avoid secondary strictures (34).

The non-thermal laser light activates the drug, allowing it to destroy the esophageal tumor while sparing nearby healthy tissue. This way, the risk to the integrity of the underlying structures is minor compared to thermal laser techniques (30). Since the light cannot pass through more than about 1 cm of tissue depth (35), PDT is not effective for large, bulky tumors unless several treatments are administered. Also, there is a strong correlation between the dose of light delivered per square centimeter of tissue and the depth of tissue necrosis (25). The length of ablation can be managed by using various length laser light probes (1 to 5 cm) (36). Finally, the tumor cytotoxicity continues for days after the application (33). Photosensitivity continues for 4 to 6 weeks and patients need to be well-educated on assessing their own photosensitivity and a careful return to sun exposure. We generally recommend complete avoidance of direct sunlight for 4 to 6 weeks. After this period, we recommend patients test for remaining sun sensitivity by exposing a forearm to sun for 10 minutes. The patient should then wait several hours and assess the response. If redness is present, we recommend additional avoidance of sunlight and a retrial at a later date.

RESULTS

Several studies have shown that PDT is effective as the primary modality in management of most patients with malignant dysphagia from obstructing esophageal cancer (25,34,37–38). This method delivers rapid relief of dysphagia and allows oral intake of a soft to regular diet 5 to 7 days after the procedure (25). Some patients may have temporary worsening of the dysphagia secondary to edema and some limitations in oral diet will still be required, but the large majority will be able to avoid the need for enteral nutrition. Within days of treatment the patient will note improvement of the malignant dysphagia, have minimal pain, and, in some cases of gastroesophageal junction tumors, have less reflux (33). The durability of the relief of dysphagia is variable, mostly depending on the rate of progression of the cancer (38). The benefits of this procedure are listed in Table 85.1.

The main drawback of PDT is the formation of esophageal strictures requiring dilations (31). Further, the combination of radiation therapy, chemotherapy, and PDT

TABLE 85.1
Benefits of Photodynamic Therapy

- Performed on an outpatient basis
- Relatively pain free
- Requires minimal sedation
- Involves less risk than other esophageal cancer treatments, such as surgery

TABLE 85.2
Complications (29)

- Esophageal stricture
- Esophageal perforation
- Photosensitivity for approximately 30 to 45 days
- Local swelling/inflammation
- Substernal chest pain
- Nausea
- Fever
- Cough and shortness of breath
- Odynophagia
- Pleural effusion
- Leukocytosis

increases the risk of stricture formation. In our series of 215 patients, this complication occurred in only 1.6% of patients (34), which is very low compared with that seen when PDT is used as curative treatment (as high as 50%) (35). As part of this protocol, most of the patients underwent dilation with debridement of necrotic tumor on day 2 after PDT treatment (34). In this experience, more than 90% of patients experienced improvement of dysphagia 4 weeks after PDT and sustained a symptom-free interval for 11 weeks. The mean survival of this series was 5.9 months (37). It is important to note that patients with marked extrinsic compression generally underwent placement of expandable metal stents and did not receive PDT as the primary therapy.

Two prospective randomized clinical trials (25,39) have compared the palliation of PDT with porfimer sodium versus Nd:YAG thermal ablation in advanced esophageal cancer patients. Both trials concluded that PDT has equal efficacy to Nd:YAG but with longer duration of response and that PDT can be accomplished with greater ease and fewer complications than Nd:YAG (25,39).

McCaughan and colleagues (40) used PDT to treat 77 patients with esophageal carcinoma over a 12-year period. Median survival for all patients was 6.3 months. The only significant variable affecting survival after PDT treatment was the clinical stage. Researchers are working to improve PDT by developing new photosensitizing drugs and evaluating new ways of delivering the proper amount of light to the cancer.

COMPLICATIONS

The main disadvantage of PDT is the skin photosensitivity in patients who have a limited life expectancy. Porfimer sodium makes the skin and eyes sensitive to light for approximately 6 weeks after treatment (14,41). Thus, patients are advised to avoid direct sunlight and bright indoor light for at least this period. Though the activating light is focused on the tumor, PDT can cause burns, swelling, pain, and scarring in nearby healthy tissue. This issue is carefully explained to the patient and family. It may not be the best choice for patients with a limited life span whose demographics and lifestyle include significant sun exposure.

Other known complications of PDT are esophageal stricture, perforation, Candida esophagitis, pleural effusion, fever, and chest pain (25,37–38). Typical complications are listed in Table 85.2. The costs of specialized equipment and the photosensitizing agent are significant. For example, a vial of 75 mg of photofrin can cost up to $2,000.00 or more and patients generally receive 2 mg/kg, thus 2 vials are frequently needed. The cost of the laser delivery device has decreased in recent years but can be $40,000 to $200,000 depending on the laser delivery device chosen. Less expensive delivery devices are becoming more available today.

CONTRAINDICATIONS

PDT should not be performed in patients with acute porphyria, poor kidney or liver function, thrombosis of main blood vessels, leukopenia, thrombocytopenia, and terminal tumor stage (11). Disadvantages of PDT include the need for expensive equipment that is not universally available, and the life style changes required to avoid sunlight exposure.

CONCLUSION

Despite various treatment options for palliation of malignant dysphagia, the optimal strategy remains unknown. For palliation, PDT is a simple, safe, and effective technique that can be performed in the outpatient setting. However, it has a high cost. It may become more efficient and more widely used if more effective sensitizers become available and if the light source for PDT can be simplified and made more affordable.

References

1. von Tappeiner H. Ueber die Wirkung fluorescierenden Stoffe auf Infusiorien nach Versuche von O. Raab. *Munch Med Wochenschr*. 1900;47:5.
2. Auler H, Banzer G. Untersuchungen uber die Rolle der Porphyrine bei geschwulstkranken Menschen und Tieren. *Z Krebsforsch*. 1942;53:65–68.
3. Schwartz SK, Abolon K, Vermund H. Some relationship of porphyrins, X-rays and tumors. *Univ Minn Med Bull*. 1955;27:1–37.
4. Dougherty TJ, Grindey GB, Fiel R, et al. Photoradiation therapy. II. Cure of animal tumors with hematoporphyrin and light. *J Natl Cancer Inst*. 1975;55:115–121.
5. Kelly JF, Snell ME, Berenbaum MC. Photodynamic destruction of human bladder carcinoma. *Br J Cancer*. 1975;31:237–244.
6. Dougherty TJ, Lawrence G, Kaufman JH, et al. Photoradiation in the treatment of recurrent breast carcinoma. *J Natl Cancer Inst*. 1979;62:231–237.
7. Hayata Y, Kato H, Konaka C, et al. Hematoporphyrin derivative and laser photoradiation in the treatment of lung cancer. *Chest*. 1982;81:269–277
8. Ward BG, Forbes IJ, Cowled PA, et al. The treatment of vaginal recurrences of gynecologic malignancy with phototherapy following hematoporphyrin derivative pretreatment. *Am J Obstet Gynecol*. 1982;142:356–357.
9. McCaughan JS Jr, Hicks W, Laufman L, et al. Palliation of esophageal malignancy with photoradiation therapy. *Cancer*. 1984;54:2905–2910
10. Friesen SA, Hjortland GO, Madsen SJ, et al. 5-Aminolevulinic acid-based photodynamic detection and therapy of brain tumors (review). *Int J Oncol*. 2002;21:577–582.
11. Wiedmann MW, Caca K. General principles of photodynamic therapy (PDT) and gastrointestinal applications. *Curr Pharm Biotechnol*. 2004;5:397–408.
12. Maier A, Anegg U, Fell B, et al. Effect of photodynamic therapy in a multimodal approach for advanced carcinoma of the gastro-esophageal junction. *Lasers Surg Med*. 2000;26:461–466.
13. Kamangar F, Dores GM, Anderson WF. Patterns of cancer incidence, mortality, and prevalence across five continents: defining priorities to reduce cancer disparities in different geographic regions of the world. *J Clin Oncol*. 2006;24:2137–2150.
14. Warren WH. Palliation of dysphagia. *Chest Surg Clin N Am*. 2000;10:605–623.
15. Maier A, Tomaselli F, Gebhard F, et al. Palliation of advanced esophageal carcinoma by photodynamic therapy and irradiation. *Ann Thorac Surg*. 2000;69:1006–1009.
16. Fleischer D, Kessler F. Endoscopic Nd:YAG laser therapy for carcinoma of the esophagus: a new form of palliation treatment. *Gastroenterology*. 1983;85:600–606.
17. Jensen DM, Machicado G, Randall G, et al. Comparison of low-power YAG laser and BICAP tumor probe for palliation of esophageal cancer strictures. *Gastroenterology*. 1988;94:1263–1270.
18. Song HY, Choi KC, Cho BH, et al. Esophagogastric neoplasm: palliation with a modified Gianturco stent. *Radiology*. 1991;180:349–354.
19. Bown SG. Palliation of malignant dysphagia: surgery, radiotherapy, laser, intubation alone or in combination? *Gut*. 1991;32:841–844.
20. Grund KE, Storek D, Farin G. Endoscopic argon plasma coagulation (APC): first clinical experiences in flexible endoscopy. *Endosc Surg Allied Tech*. 1994;2:42–46.
21. Nguyen NT, Luketich JD. Photodynamic therapy for obstructing esophagus cancer. *Can J Gastroenterol*. 1998;12:147B.
22. Nguyen NT, Luketich JD. The terminal patient: palliation of dysphagia in advanced esophageal cancer. In: Carrau RL, Murry T, eds. *Comprehensive Management of Swallowing Disorders*. San Diego: Singular Publishing Group; 1999:377–381.
23. Payne-James JJ, Spiller RC, Misiewicz JJ, et al. Use of ethanol-induced tumor necrosis to palliate dysphagia in patients with esophagogastric cancer. *Gastrointest Endosc*. 1990;36:43–46.
24. Loizou LA, Grigg D, Atkinson M, et al. A prospective comparison of laser therapy and intubation in endoscopic palliation for malignant dysphagia. *Gastroenterology*. 1991;100:1303–1310.
25. Heier SK, Rothman KA, Heier LM, et al. Photodynamic therapy for obstructing esophageal cancer: light dosimetry and randomized comparison with Nd:YAG laser therapy. *Gastroenterology*. 1995;109:63–72.
26. De Palma GD, di Matteo E, Romano G, et al Plastic prosthesis versus expandable metal stents for palliation of inoperable esophageal thoracic carcinoma: a controlled prospective study. *Gastrointest Endosc*. 1996;43:478–482.
27. Kozarek RA, Raltz S, Brugge WR, et al. Prospective multicenter trial of esophageal Z-stent placement for malignant dysphagia and tracheoesophageal fistula. *Gastrointest Endosc*. 1996;44:562–567.
28. Mitty RD, Cave DR, Birkett DH. One-stage retrograde approach to Nd:YAG laser palliation of esophageal carcinoma. *Endoscopy*. 1996;28:350–355.
29. Adler DG, Baron TH. Endoscopic palliation of malignant dysphagia. *Mayo Clin Proc*. 2001;76:731–738.
30. Hopper C. Photodynamic therapy: a clinical reality in the treatment of cancer. *Lancet Oncol*. 2000;1:212–219.
31. Moghissi K, Dixon K, Thorpe JA, et al. The role of photodynamic therapy (PDT) in inoperable oesophageal cancer. *Eur J Cardiothorac Surg*. 2000;17:95–100.
32. Chen M, Pennathur A, Luketich JD. Role of photodynamic therapy in unresectable esophageal and lung cancer. *Lasers Surg Med*. 2006;38:396–402.
33. Christie NA, Patel AN, Landreneau RJ. Esophageal palliation—photodynamic therapy/stents/brachytherapy. *Surg Clin North Am*. 2005;85:569–582.
34. Litle VR, Luketich JD, Christie NA, et al. Photodynamic therapy as palliation for esophageal cancer: experience in 215 patients. *Ann Thorac Surg*. 2003;76:1687–1693.
35. Sibille A, Lambert R, Souquet JC, et al. Long-term survival after photodynamic therapy for esophageal cancer. *Gastroenterology*. 1995;108:337–344.
36. Narayan S, Sivak MV Jr. Palliation of esophageal carcinoma. Laser and photodynamic therapy. *Chest Surg Clin N Am*. 1994;4:347–367.
37. Luketich JD, Christie NA, Buenaventura PO, et al. Endoscopic photodynamic therapy for obstructing esophageal cancer: 77 cases over a 2-year period. *Surg Endosc*. 2000;14:653–657.
38. McCaughan JS Jr, Williams TE Jr, Bethel BH. Palliation of esophageal malignancy with photodynamic therapy. *Ann Thorac Surg*. 1985;40:113–120.
39. Lightdale CJ, Heier SK, Marcon NE, et al. Photodynamic therapy with porfimer sodium versus thermal ablation therapy with Nd:YAG laser for palliation of esophageal cancer: a multicenter randomized trial. *Gastrointest Endosc*. 1995;42:507–512.
40. McCaughan JS Jr, Ellison EC, Guy JT, et al. Photodynamic therapy for esophageal malignancy: a prospective twelve-year study. *Ann Thorac Surg*. 1996;62:1005–1010.
41. Greenwald BD. Photodynamic therapy for esophageal cancer. Update. *Chest Surg Clin N Am*. 2000;10:625–637.

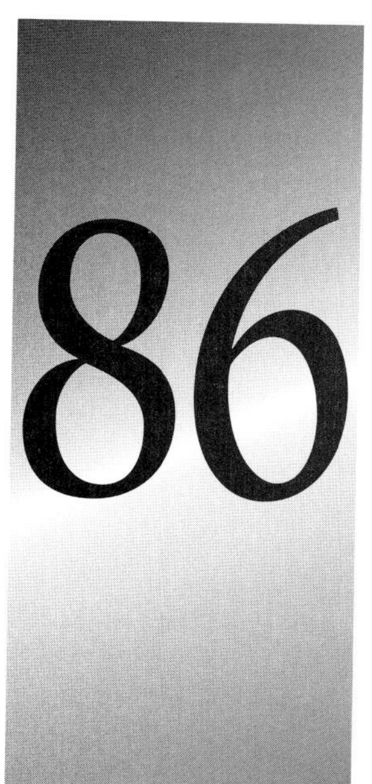

Endoscopic Palliation of Dysphagia: Stenting

Todd Huntley Baron

The initial stents used for palliation of malignant dysphagia were rigid stents, which continued to be used in some countries. However, the use of self-expandable metal stents (SEMS) has essentially replaced these rigid stents for palliation of malignant dysphagia (1). The first Food and Drug Administration (FDA) approved expandable esophageal stent was introduced in 1994. Recently, self-expandable plastic stents (SEPS) have been increasingly used for palliation of malignant dysphagia. This chapter will review the use of stents for palliation of malignant dysphagia.

MALIGNANT DYSPHAGIA

Esophageal cancer is the primary cause of malignant dysphagia, a major cause of morbidity and mortality. Cancer of the esophagus and gastroesophageal junction (GEJ) is increasingly diagnosed in more than 400,000 patients per year worldwide. Esophageal cancer is the eighth most common malignancy and sixth leading cause of cancer-related death (2). Esophageal cancer carries a dismal prognosis, with an overall 5-year survival rate of less than 20% (2). More than 50% of patients have unresectable disease at the time of diagnosis, due to either metastases or poor medical condition. Most of these patients live less than 6 months, and palliation is the major goal to relieve dysphagia. Malignant dysphagia, defined as difficulty with swallowing due to cancer, typically results from a partially or completely obstructed esophageal lumen. Obstruction can occur not only as a result of intrinsic lesions (esophageal cancer) but from extrinsic compression due to lung cancer or other mediastinal malignancies. Patients with malignant dysphagia often lose their ability to eat safely and comfortably, which leads to malnutrition, aspiration, and sialorrhea.

A wide variety of recently developed palliative treatments are currently available for relief of inoperable malignant dysphagia. The main options include endoscopic stent placement, radiation therapy (external-beam or brachytherapy), chemotherapy, photodynamic therapy, and nutritional support.

Rigid Plastic Stents

Rigid plastic esophageal prostheses were first placed surgically and later, endoscopically. These devices have fixed internal and external diameters (Figure 86.1). The largest diameter that can be achieved is still smaller than what is achieved with self-expandable stents. Because the stent diameters are fixed and relatively large in comparison to the stricture, large-bore dilation is required. In one series of 91 patients undergoing rigid plastic stent

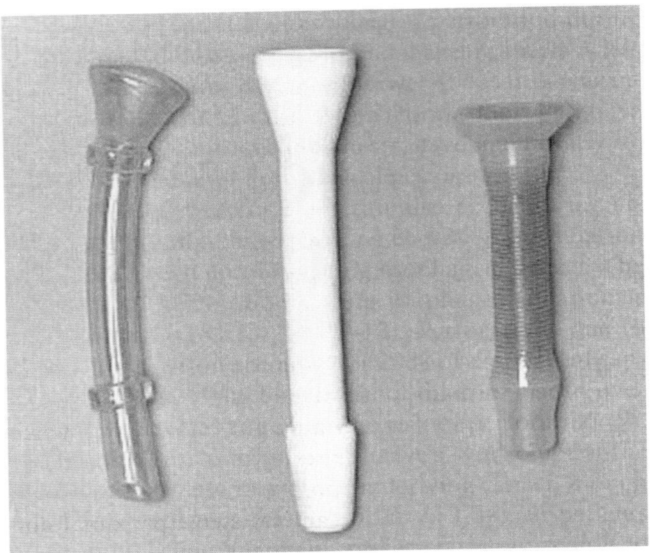

FIGURE 86.1

Representative rigid esophageal stents.

placement using Celestin and Atkinson tubes, the prosthesis was successfully placed in only 77 patients (3). Minor complications related to prosthesis placement (pain, obstruction, and migration) occurred in 40% of patients, and severe complications (perforation, fistulae, bleeding, and death) occurred in 20%. In another study of 71 patients, modified Tygon plastic stents with diameters of 9 to 14 mm were placed after stepwise dilation was performed over several sessions (4). After a median of 2 (range 1–5) dilation sessions, stent insertion was technically successful in all patients. Three patients had to undergo endoscopy within 24 hours because of pain or stent migration. No procedure-related perforation, hemorrhage, or respiratory complications occurred. Improvement or stabilization of dysphagia with oral intake could be achieved in 89%. Migration occurred in 8 patients, food obstruction in 5, and tumor overgrowth in 4. Nonetheless, rigid stents have been shown to palliate malignant dysphagia and seal esophago–respiratory fistulae. They continued to be used in countries where resources are limited, especially where the patient must pay for the device.

Self-Expandable Metal Stents

During the past 15 years, SEMS composed of wire mesh have become available for the treatment of malignant dysphagia and are now used almost exclusively as compared to rigid plastic stents; SEMS have a number of advantages over the previously used conventional plastic prosthetic tubes (5). They are supplied in a tightly bound form on a delivery catheter, greatly reducing the predeployment diameter of the delivery system to only 5 to 10 mm, requiring little or no dilation before placement. After its placement, the stent gradually expands, decreasing the risk of stent-related placement complications compared with plastic stents. Moreover, the luminal diameter achieved ranges between 16 and 24 mm and due to its flexibility there is significant improvement in the quality of swallowing when compared to plastic prosthetic tubes (6). Despite the reduction of complications related to stent insert, delayed complications may be as frequent following SEMS placement (7,8).

The currently available SEMS from various manufacturers differ in design and expanded luminal diameter (Figure 86.2). In addition, the radial expansile forces and degree of shortening also differ. The first-generation SEMS were uncovered. Tumor ingrowth through the wire mesh of the stent occurred in 20% to 30% of cases that led to recurrent dysphagia. The second-generation SEMS have an external or internal covering to prevent tumor ingrowth. In a randomized study of 62 patients with malignant inoperable esophageal obstruction at the GEJ, obstructing tumor ingrowth was significantly more likely in the uncovered stent group (9/30) than in the covered group (1/32) ($P = 0.005$) (9). However, covered SEMS are more likely to migrate than uncovered SEMS, especially when deployed in the region of the distal esophagus and cardia. In one study, the migration rate was nearly twice for covered than for uncovered stents (12% vs. 7%) (9). In a retrospective study of 152 patients, stent migration occurred in 0% of uncovered stents and 10% of covered stents (10).

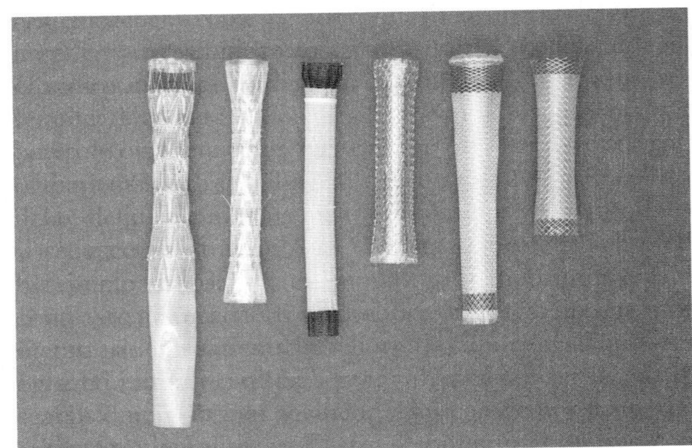

FIGURE 86.2

Representative covered expandable metal esophageal stents. From left to right: Dual anti-reflux modification of the esophageal Z-stent (Cook Endoscopy), Covered Z-stent with anti-migration hooks (Cook Endoscopy), Ultraflex (Boston Scientific), Ali-Maxx (Alveolus), Flamingo esophageal stent (Boston Scientific), and Wallstent II esophageal stent (Boston Scientific).

Most SEMS have large internal diameter, flexibility, relatively atraumatic ends, and in some cases can be repositioned (11). At present, there are 4 expandable metal esophageal stents available in the United States (Table 86.1) (12).

The Ultraflex stent (Boston Scientific, Natick, MA, USA) (Figure 86.2) consists of a knitted nitinol wire tube. The covered version has a polyurethane layer extending up to 1.5 cm of either end. The stent has a proximal flare with 2 sizes: 28 mm (distal diameter 23 mm) and 23 mm (distal diameter 17 mm) with midsection diameters of 22 mm and 18 mm, respectively. The delivery system is available in a proximal or distal release version. The degree of shortening after deployment is 30% to 40%. The radial force of the Ultraflex stent is the lowest amongst the currently available SEMS (1). The delivery system works by pulling a handle that leads to unraveling of a constraining string with subsequent stent expansion.

The Wallstent (Boston Scientific) is made from a stainless steel, cobalt-based alloy and is formed into a tubular mesh. It is available in 2 designs: the Wallstent II and the Flamingo Wallstent (available only in Europe) (Figure 86.2). The Wallstent II is covered with a silicone polymer layer, with 2 cm left exposed at the proximal and distal ends. It flares to 28 mm at both ends, with a diameter of 20 mm at its midsection. The degree of shortening after placement is about 20% to 30%. The delivery system is similar to the biliary Wallstent, in which a handle is withdrawn that then withdraws a covering constraining sheath. Wallstent can be re-constrained up to 50% of deployment. The Flamingo Wallstent has a much wider proximal flange intended to reduce the higher stent migration rate after placement across the GEJ. The conical shape of the stent is designed to apply a variable radial force throughout the length of the stent to address anatomic differences in the distal esophagus and gastric cardia. The stent is covered by a polyurethane layer, which is applied from the inside, extending up to 2 cm of either end. A large-diameter (proximal and distal diameters 30 and 20 mm) and a small-diameter stent (proximal and distal diameters 24 and 16 mm) are available. The Wallstent II and the Flamingo Wallstent have strong radial force and are both very pliable, with the diameter of the stent being unaffected even when angulated.

The Z-stent (Cook Endoscopy, Winston-Salem, NC, USA) consists of a wide Z-mesh of stainless steel

TABLE 86.1
Available Types of Covered Metal Stents

	Ultraflex	Wallstent II	Z-Stent	Alimaxx	Flamingo Wallstent	Choo Stent
Stent material	Nickel titanium (nitinol)	Cobalt-based alloy	Stainless steel	Nitinol	Cobalt-based alloy	Nitinol
Delivery system diameter (F)	16	18	28	21	18	28
Covering	Partial	Partial	Partial	Full	Full	Full
Design	Mesh	Mesh	Zig-zag		Mesh	Zig-zag
Radial force	+	+++	++		+++	++
Length (cm)	10, 12, 15	10, 15	6, 8, 10, 12, 14	7, 12, 15	12, 14	8, 11, 14, 17
Lumen diameter—flanges	23, 28	28	21, 25	27, 23 proximal 25, 21 distal	24, 30	
Lumen diameter—shaft	18, 23	20	18, 22	18, 22	16, 20	18
Release System	Proximal/Distal	Distal	Distal	Distal	Distal	Distal
Flexibility	+++	++	+	++	++	+
Degree of shortening	30%–40%	20%–30%	0%–10%	0%	20%–30%	0%–10%
FDA approved	Yes	Yes	Yes	Yes	No	No
Manufacturer	Boston Scientific, Natick, MA, USA	Boston Scientific, Natick, MA, USA	Cook Medical, Winston-Salem, NC, USA	Alveolus, Charlotte, NC, USA	Boston Scientific, Natick, MA, USA	MI Tech, Seoul, Korea

available in partially covered or fully covered by a polyethylene layer (Figure 86.2). It flares to 25 mm at both ends with a diameter at its midsection of either 18 mm or 22 mm. The stent requires assembly onto a delivery catheter. The Z-stent does not shorten on release and is the least flexible of the currently available SEMS. It is available with or without fixation barbs in the central segment (Figure 86.2). The Z-stent is also available with an antireflux valve (Dua modification) to prevent gastroesophageal reflux when placed across the gastroesophageal junction (GEJ) (Figure 86.2).

The Alimaxx stent (Alveolus, Charlotte, NC, USA) (Figure 86.2) is composed of nitinol and fully covered internally (lined). The delivery system is shorter than the other stents to allow the physician to deploy the stent with one hand. There are no clinical studies regarding the outcome for this stent for palliation of malignant dysphagia.

Stents from outside the United States

M.I.Tech Co., Ltd., Seoul, Korea, manufactures a variety of esophageal SEMS. These include the Choostent™, the Dostent™, and the Hanarostent™. The Choostent (Table 86.1) is completely covered with large flanges at each end. A retrieval lasso is present. The Dostent is designed specifically for obstruction at the lower esophagus and GEJ. It has a tricuspid antireflux valve. The Hanarostent has an *S*-shaped antireflux valve situated within the distal end of the stent.

Taewoong-Medical Co., Ltd, Seoul, Korea, manufactures the Niti-S stent, which is available in 3 varieties. One is completely covered and designed for removability. Another combines flared ends of 26 mm and a double-layer configuration consisting of an inner polyurethane layer to prevent tumor ingrowth and an outer uncovered nitinol wire tube. The latter allows the mesh of the stent to embed itself in the esophageal wall and prevent migration. A modification of this stent is available with an antireflux valve (Figure 86.3).

ELLA-CS, s.r.o., Czech Republic, manufactures the FerX-ELLA (stainless steel) and SX-ELLA (nitinol) esophageal stents. Each is available with and without and without an antireflux valve.

Comparison of Different Types of Covered Stents for Palliation of Malignant Disease

Several studies have been published that directly compare the outcome of different types of covered SEMS. A retrospective study, including 96 patients, compared the uncovered Ultraflex, covered and uncovered versions of the Wallstent, and the covered Z-stent. No differences were found in outcome and complication rate between the different stent types (13). Covered versions of the Wallstent and the Ultraflex stent were compared in another retrospective study, which showed a higher early complication rate with the Wallstent, but a higher reintervention rate with the Ultraflex stent (14).

In a prospective trial, 100 patients were randomized to receive the covered Ultraflex stent, the Flamingo Wallstent, or the Z-stent. There were no significant differences in the improvement of dysphagia, the occurrence of complications, or the recurrence of dysphagia, although there was a trend toward a higher complication rate with the Z-stent (Ultraflex stent: 24%, Flamingo Wallstent: 18%, and Z stent: 36%) (15). In another prospective trial, the Ultraflex stent and the Flamingo Wallstent were compared in patients with distal esophageal cancer. The 2 stent types were equally effective in the palliation of dysphagia in this patient group and the complication rate associated with their use was also comparable (23% in both) (16).

Though not a comparative study, data about the Niti-S stent come from a prospective study of 42 patients with malignant esophageal obstruction. Stent migration occurred in 7% of patients and stent occlusion from either tumor or hyperplastic tissue overgrowth was observed in 5% of patients after a mean follow-up of 6 months (17).

From the above data, it can be concluded that there are only minor differences in efficacy and complication rates between the most commonly used expandable metal esophageal stents. Some practical tips for the endoscopist when choosing a stent include: careful attention to results of trials, realizing that a single-center study is unlikely to address all possible scenarios; and individually meeting with stent manufacturer's representatives and have them display their products (predeployed and fully deployed) to decide which delivery system and stent the endoscopist feels most comfortable with. For endoscopists who are inexperienced with different SEMS, deployment of one type of stent in several patients allows for a comfort level to be reached in which to decide on the stent design. They should also talk with colleagues and experts in the field about the advantages and disadvantages of each stent for specific clinical scenarios. Since the differences in cost among stent types are relatively small in comparison to the overall cost in caring for these patients, it is unlikely to play a large role in determining which stent type to use (18).

ENDOSCOPIC PLACEMENT OF SELF-EXPANDABLE STENTS

Placement of SEMS for malignant dysphagia is usually performed as an outpatient procedure and in experienced hands can usually be performed in 15 to 30 minutes. Using moderate sedation, the patient is placed in

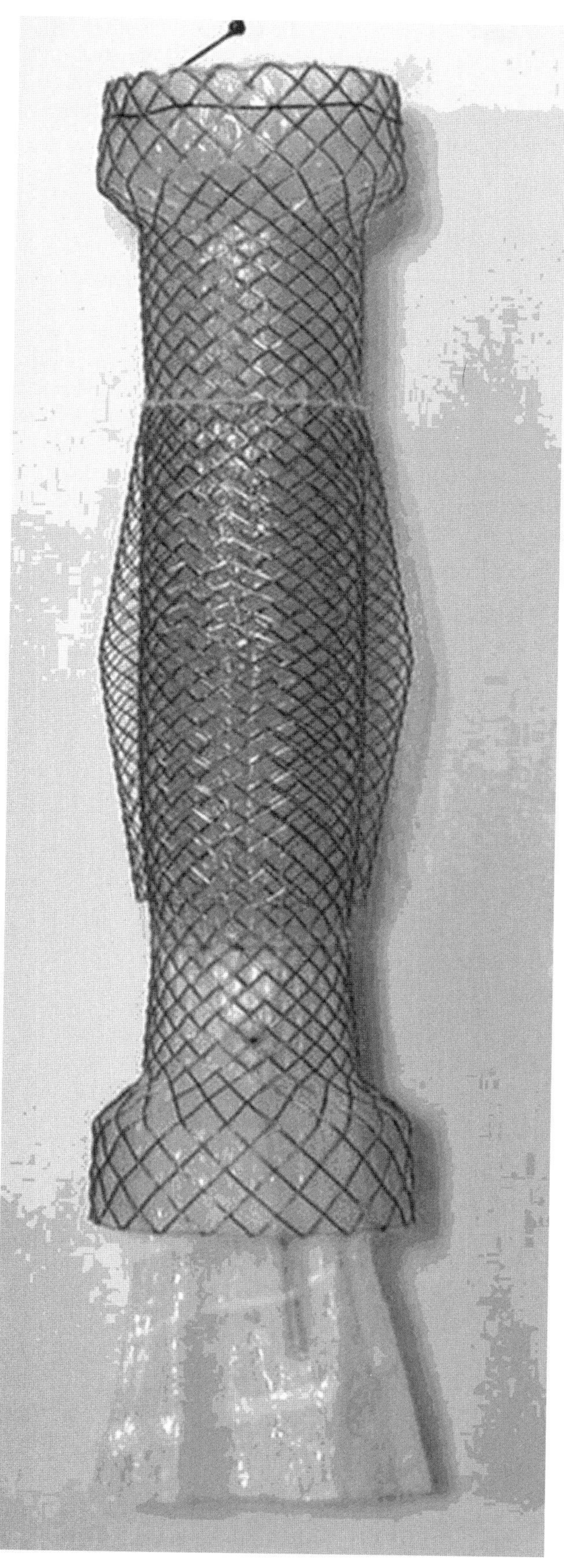

the left lateral decubitus or prone position. Placement is frequently done using fluoroscopic assistance, though placement under endoscopic visualization alone by passing the endoscope alongside the predeployed stent is also possible (19,20) Application of an endoscopically visible marker at the level of the proximal portion of the stent has been described to facilitate endoscopic visualization (21), though this is usually not necessary to visualize the proximal end of the stent. SEMS can also be placed under fluoroscopy alone without the use of endoscopy. In addition to the fluoroscopic markers on the stent, other fluoroscopic "markers" can be used to mark the location of the stricture to assist in placement. Usually the proximal and distal margins of the stricture are identified endoscopically and correlative radiopaque markers are used. These markers can be external skin markers or internal markers such as tissue clips or intramucosal injection of a radiopaque contrast agent. Unfortunately, external markers may become inaccurate with patient rotation (22).

Predilation of the stricture may be required up to a diameter of 10 to 12 mm to facilitate complete assessment of the stricture length and location. Alternatively, a small caliber endoscope may be used to assess the stricture and obviate the need for dilation. It should be noted that aggressive stricture dilation increases the risk of perforation. The next step is to place a guidewire (preferentially a stiff guidewire; i.e., a 0.038 inch Savary wire, Cook Endoscopy) across the stricture into the stomach or duodenum and withdraw the endoscope. The preloaded stent is then advanced over the wire. Endoscopic visualization during deployment can be achieved by reintroducing the endoscope alongside the predeployed stent (Figure 86.4). The stent is deployed as previously mentioned.

When the stent is placed across the GEJ, the proximal covered portion should lie at least 2 cm above the tumor margin and one must be careful not to place an excessive amount of distal stent into the stomach. This is to prevent impaction against—and subsequent ulceration of—the posterior wall of the stomach by the distal end (1). After deployment, the placement of the upper end of the stent in regard to the upper tumor margin can be assessed endoscopically. However, one should avoid passing the endoscope through the stent, especially if there is resistance at the level of the waist, because of the risk of dislodging the stent due to friction with the endoscope. Repositioning the stent after deployment from distal to proximal is much easier than proximal to distal

FIGURE 86.3

Niti-S Esophageal Covered Stent (Double Anti-Reflux Type) (Taewoong-Medical Co).

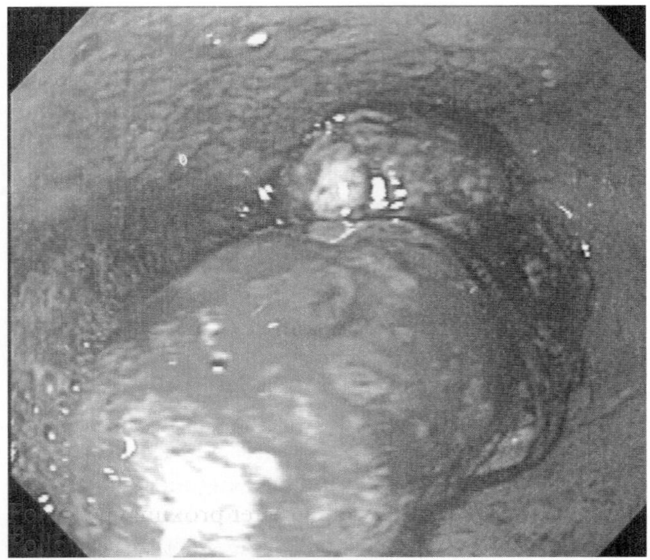

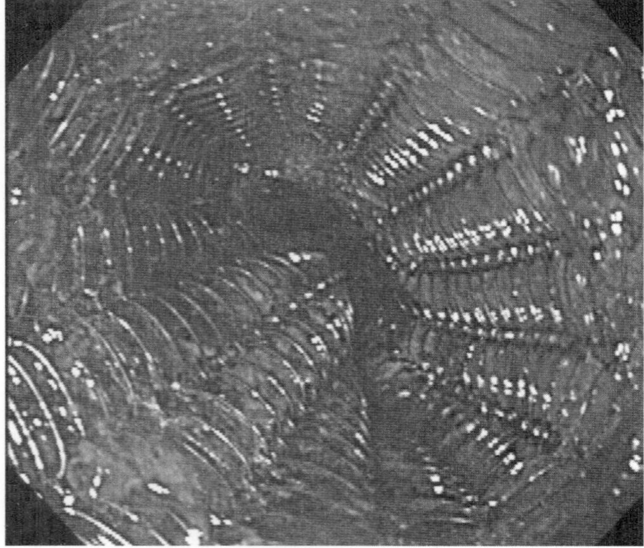

FIGURE 86.4

Endoscopic placement of expandable stent. (A) Endoscopic view of obstructing mass. (B) Endoscopic view immediately after deployment.

and can be achieved by pulling at the upper rim of the stent or at the string attached to the inside of the proximal flange (Ultraflex and Alimaxx), causing the radial diameter to decrease (2). The Z-stent can be withdrawn using a string that is attached to the end of the stent and attached to the delivery system. After correct position is confirmed, the string is cut at the end of the procedure just before removal of the delivery system.

In many centers, SEMS are placed by interventional radiologists. Interventional radiologists place esophageal stents with great accuracy and low complication rates. The results of radiologic placement are similar to endoscopic stent insertion. The advantages of radiologic stent insertion are the ability to traverse very small strictures that cannot be crossed endoscopically and the ability to visualize and treat small fistulae and perforations at the time of stenting (24).

EFFICACY AND COMPLICATIONS

The technical success rate for placement of esophageal SEMS is close to 100%. Failure may occur if the lumen cannot be traversed with a guidewire. The complications of stent placement and methods to avoid and treat them are described in detail elsewhere (22). Complications may be classified as intraprocedural and postprocedural (immediate and delayed) (Table 86.2).

Almost all patients experience improvement of dysphagia, which can be sustained until a specific complication arises. The dysphagia grade usually improves from a mean of 3 (able to eat liquids only) to a mean of 1 (able to eat most solid foods), with no difference in effectiveness between the Ultraflex stent, the Wallstent, and the Z-stent (12). Some patients with advanced cancer of the distal esophagus may fail to experience relief of symptoms following technically successful stent placement

TABLE 86.2
Complications of Esophageal SEMS

- Immediate
  - Aspiration
  - Airway compromise
  - Malposition
  - Delivery system entrapment
  - Stent dislodgement
  - Perforation
- Early
  - Bleeding
  - Chest pain
  - Nausea
- Late
  - GERD/aspiration
  - Re-obstruction
    - Tumor
    - Food impaction
  - Migration
  - Tracheoesophageal fistula
  - Bleeding

because of gastroparesis due to neural involvement by the tumor, peritoneal carcinomatosis, or other yet unidentified sites of intestinal obstruction. These patients can be managed by enteral tube placement, which may include nasoduodenal, percutaneous endoscopic gastrostomy (PEG), or percutaneous endoscopic jejunostomy tube (PEJ) placement. If PEG or PEJ tube placement is required, one should be careful not to dislodge the stent as the tube is withdrawn through the stent lumen (22).

Procedure-related complications after SEMS placement have remained fairly stable over the years and mainly consist of perforation, aspiration pneumonia, hemorrhage and severe pain, occurring in approximately 10% of patients (22).

Delayed complications following stent placement include bleeding, fistula formation, GE reflux, stent migration, food bolus obstruction and tumor overgrowth at either end of the stent, which occur in up to 35% to 45% of patients (12,22). Tumor overgrowth can be treated with either ablative therapies (i.e., argon plasma coagulation) or placement of subsequent stents (so-called stent-within-stent deployment). Repositioning or removal of a migrated metal stent can be achieved using a retrieval forceps, an inflated balloon catheter, or a polypectomy snare. Alternatively, if the stent has migrated completely out of the stricture and into the stomach, it may be reasonable to leave it there and place another stent for palliation of symptoms (25). The decision to retrieve the stent depends on the patient's performance status. If left in place, there is a small risk of distal stent migration out of the stomach and into the small bowel with resultant obstruction or perforation. If an additional stent is placed, one should consider using a different stent type and/or larger diameter. In some cases, placement of an uncovered stent can be entertained, though there are no data on this approach. Finally, although there is no proof that endoclip placement on the proximal end of the stent prevents migration, it can be used in an attempt to secure the position of the stent (22).

Another potential cause of recurrent dysphagia is the development of hyperplastic inflammatory tissue, over and through the uncovered meshes at the ends of partially covered stents (26). This complication occurs more frequently in those patients who live longer than 2 to 4 months (26).

Stents Placed across the GEJ

SEMS placed across the GEJ provide inferior palliation and have higher complication rates when compared to stents placed in the mid-esophagus (23,27). Specific problems include higher stent migration rates (since the distal part of the stent projects freely into the gastric fundus and does not contribute to anchoring), increased frequency of hemorrhage from erosion to the posterior gastric wall, decreased quality of swallowing from stent angulation between the esophagus and the cardia, and increased frequency of GE reflux symptoms.

The design of the stent may play a role in reducing stent migration. The Flamingo Wallstent, which is specially designed for tumors of the distal esophagus/cardia, has a shift in the braiding angle between its proximal and distal part, which allows the distal part to stretch in response to peristalsis. The Ultraflex stent and the Wallstent have proximal and distal uncovered segments that allow the normal mucosa above and below the tumor to project into the stent lumen. The Z-stent is available with metal barbs on the outside so as to anchor into the tumor.

Perhaps the most important way to prevent migration is the use of stents with a greater proximal flange diameter (i.e., 28 mm for the Wallstent II and the Ultraflex stents and 30 mm for the Flamingo Wallstent) and with increased diameter at their mid-portion (i.e., 22 mm for the Z-stent). A prospective randomized trial testing covered versions of the Ultraflex stent, the Flamingo, and the Z-stent demonstrated that 12 of 13 migrations occurred with small-diameter stents. In contrast, only one migration occurred with large-diameter stents placed for distal esophagus/cardia tumors. No differences in complications were noted between small and large-diameter stents (15). In a large study of 338 patients with dysphagia from obstructing esophageal or gastric cardia cancer who were treated with different types of SEMS of either small or large diameter, improvement in dysphagia was similar between the 2 groups (28). The occurrence of major complications, such as hemorrhage, perforation, fistula, and fever, was increased in patients with a large-diameter Z-stent compared with those treated with a small-diameter stent (40% vs. 20%; adjusted hazard ratio 5), but not in patients with large-diameter Ultraflex or Flamingo Wallstent. Dysphagia from stent migration, tissue overgrowth, and food bolus obstruction occurred more frequently in patients with a small-diameter stent than in those with a large-diameter stent. The authors concluded that large-diameter stents reduce the risk of recurrent dysphagia from stent migration, tissue overgrowth, or food obstruction. Increasing the diameter in some stent types may, however, increase the risk of stent-related local esophageal complications.

Many experts advocate the use of proton-pump inhibitors (PPIs) for patients in whom the stent crosses the lower esophageal sphincter to prevent reflux symptoms. PPIs improve reflux symptoms, but not the risk of aspiration. Recently, stents with an antireflux mechanism have been developed. In one type of anti-reflux stent, the distal cover is extended beyond the lower metal cage so as to form a "windsock-type" valve (Figure 86.2). Several studies have been published using anti-reflux stents (29–33). A randomized study comparing the anti-reflux Z-stent (25 patients) with a standard open Flamingo Wallstent (25 patients) showed that GE reflux symptoms occurred in 3/25 (12%) patients in the anti-reflux stent group versus 24/25 (96%) patients in the open stent group ($P<0.001$). No differences were found in the degree of dysphagia improvement or complications (30). However, similar superior results with the placement of anti-reflux stents were not reproduced in a subsequent randomized trial (33). Additionally, in a prospective single-arm study of anti-reflux Z-stent placement in 17 consecutive patients, 4 patients (22%) experienced permanent reflux symptoms and an additional 9 (50%) continued to take PPIs on a regular basis (34).

Two studies have reported 24-h pH-monitoring after anti-reflux stent placement (31,32). In a randomized study comparing the FerX-Ella stent with and without a "windsock-type" anti-reflux valve, 24-h pH monitoring showed increased esophageal acid exposure with the anti-reflux stent, suggesting that the anti-reflux valve failed to prevent GE reflux (32). A different type of anti-reflux stent with a reflux valve consisting of 3 leaflets, similar to the tricuspid valve of the heart, has also been also introduced. An initial study suggested that this stent is effective in preventing GE reflux (31).

More recently, 36 patients were randomized to receive the Hanarostent with S-shaped anti-reflux valve, the DoStent with tricuspid anti-reflux valve, or an open stent. Twenty-four-hour pH monitoring showed that the DeMeester score was significantly lower in the group with S-shaped anti-reflux stent than in the other groups. The fraction of the total recording time during which esophageal pH was below 4 was approximately 3% when using the S-shaped anti-reflux stent compared to 29% in the Dostent group and 15% in the standard open stent group ($P < 0.001$) (35). Further research is needed to establish the optimal design of an anti-reflux valve attached to the stent. Moreover, additional studies are needed to assess the efficacy of the anti-reflux stents, particularly in comparison to an open stent in conjunction with PPI use.

In summary, the currently available evidence suggests that it is probably best to deploy the largest available stent diameter of the individual manufacturer when placing stents across the GEJ in order to reduce the risk of stent migration. However, further studies are needed to establish the balance between the advantage of preventing stent migration and the potential increased risk of complications associated with the use of large-diameter stents. Placement of a stent with an anti-reflux valve may prevent GE reflux in patients in whom the stent extends across the GEJ. PPI therapy should be given indefinitely in patients in whom anti-reflux stents do not control symptoms and to those patients without anti-reflux stents.

ROLE OF CHEMOTHERAPY, RADIATION, AND STENT PLACEMENT FOR PALLIATION OF MALIGNANT DYSPHAGIA

The safety of placing SEMS in patients with incurable cancer of the esophagus after previous administration of radiation and/or chemotherapy is controversial (36–38). A large study with 200 prospectively followed patients concluded that the incidence of complications and the outcome after metal stent placement were not affected by prior radiation and/or chemotherapy. Only retrosternal pain occurred more frequently in patients who had undergone prior treatment (39). However, in a retrospective study of 116 patients, prior chemoradiotherapy was the only independent predictive factor of postprocedure major complications with an odds ratio of 5.6 (40).

In contrast, very little has been written about the effect of concomitant radiation and stent placement for palliation of dysphagia. In one study, patients receiving concurrent radiation and chemotherapy ($n = 12$) had prolonged survival (median 318 days after diagnosis, 225 days after stent) compared with patients of equal tumor staging, but without additional therapy ($n = 17$; median 157 days after diagnosis, $P<0.001$; 138 days after stent, $P<0.05$) (41). This has not been confirmed in prospective studies.

Patients with incurable esophageal cancer due to metastasis, but who are in relatively good general condition, are increasingly considered candidates for palliative chemotherapy. A disadvantage of stent placement and concomitant chemotherapy is the potential risk of stent migration into the stomach if the tumor responds to chemotherapy.

Unfortunately, despite the initial improvement in dysphagia following SEMS placement, recurrent dysphagia occurs in almost one-third of patients and requires repeat intervention (11). Therefore, some groups have proposed alternative methods of palliation using single-dose brachytherapy. A randomized trial comparing single-dose brachytherapy vs. metal stent placement for palliation of dysphagia in 209 patients with inoperable esophageal cancer showed that dysphagia improved more rapidly after stent placement, but long-term relief of dysphagia was better in the brachytherapy group (42). Complications occurred less frequently after single brachytherapy. There was no difference in median survival; however, patients assigned to brachytherapy had more days with almost no dysphagia during follow-up than those assigned to stent placement (115 days vs. 82 days, $P = 0.015$).

Subsequently, a prognostic model for identification of patients with esophageal cancer in whom stent placement would be preferable to brachytherapy was developed based upon predicted survival (43). For the poor prognosis group, the difference in dysphagia-adjusted survival was 23 days in favor of stent placement compared with brachytherapy (77 vs. 54 days, $P = 0.16$). For the other prognostic groups (intermediate or relatively good prognosis), brachytherapy resulted in a better dysphagia-adjusted survival.

PALLIATION OF DYSPHAGIA FROM EXTRINSIC COMPRESSION

Most outcome data following stent placement come from palliation of intrinsic lesions as a result of esophageal cancer. In one study, of 46 patients efficacy of palliation of dysphagia after SEMS placement was compared in 22 patients who had intrinsic and 24 patients with extrinsic malignant stenoses (44). Almost all of the patients in the extrinsic group received Wallstents. Significant improvement in dysphagia was seen in both groups, but the improvement was significantly greater in the intrinsic group than the extrinsic group ($P = 0.01$). The reason for this is probably multifactorial, but one likely factor is the greater force required to overcome extrinsic compression.

PALLIATION OF DYSPHAGIA FROM HIGH CERVICAL STRICTURES

Almost all prospective studies of expandable stents exclude patients with cervical strictures. Frequently, a distance of 2 cm below the upper esophageal sphincter is mentioned as being needed before one should consider placing a stent. This is not based upon scientific data, however, and there are several retrospective series that have been published showing that it is feasible to place stents very proximally in the esophagus and still achieve effective palliation (45,46). In the senior authors' experience, the outcome following stent placement in this group of patients is less predictable in terms of relief of dysphagia and development of foreign body sensation. It is recommended that because of the size of the esophageal lumen in the proximal esophagus, smaller diameter stents and those with a shorter length proximal flange (if available) should be used when placing stents in this area so as to potentially minimize foreign body sensation (47).

SELF-EXPANDABLE PLASTIC STENTS

The Polyflex stent (initially developed by Rüsch AG, Kernen, Germany, and distributed by Boston Scientific Corporation, now owned by Boston Scientific) was developed in order to overcome overgrowth and ingrowth of non-tumoral, inflammatory tissue when placed for malignant disease. The Polyflex stent can easily be removed, since no embedding occurs.

The Polyflex stent, the only available non-metallic expandable stent, is composed of polyester mesh embedded in silicone and is completely covered (Figure 86.5). The stent flares to 25 mm at the proximal end for the largest diameter. The expanded mid-body diameter ranges from between 16 and 21 mm. The stent needs to be loaded onto the delivery device before stent placement, which takes approximately 5 to 10 minutes. In addition, the diameter of the relatively inflexible delivery device is between 12 to 14 mm, which is larger than that of the most commonly used SEMS (12).

The Polyflex stent has been shown to be safe and effective for the palliation of malignant dysphagia. In one study Polyflex stents were placed in 33 patients with malignant dysphagia; no tissue hyperplasia was observed after a mean follow-up of 150 days. Stent occlusion was caused by tumor overgrowth in 10% of patients. The

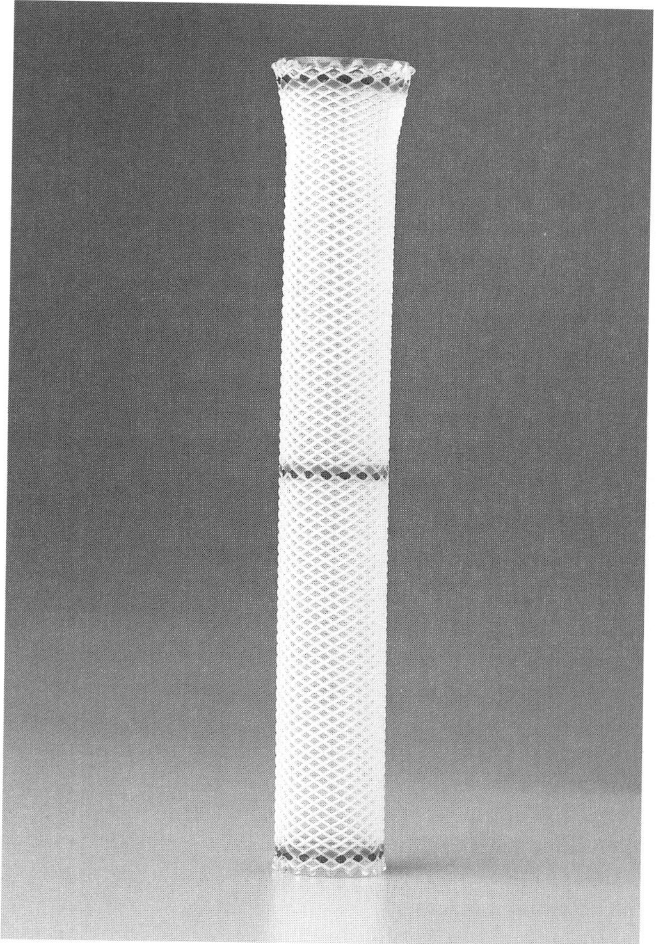

FIGURE 86.5

Polylfex esophageal stent (Boston Scientific).

migration rate was 6% (48). In another study of 16 patients, one episode of tumor overgrowth was reported; however, stent migration in this study occurred in 25% (49). In one study of 66 patients in whom the Polyflex stent was placed for palliation of malignant dysphagia, migration was seen in only 4.5% (50). No tumor ingrowth occurred. However, a landmark randomized trial of 101 patients in which the Polyflex stent was compared to the Ultraflex stent for the palliation of malignant dysphagia showed similar efficacy but a significantly higher migration rate in the Polyflex group (51).

TREATMENT OF MALIGNANT ESOPHAGEAL FISTULA

Progressive esophageal carcinoma can infiltrate into surrounding tissue with subsequent development of a fistula, most commonly between the esophagus and the respiratory tract (i.e., the trachea or bronchi). Primary lung cancer and some other mediastinal malignancies may produce tracheoesophageal fistulae as well (52). In addition, fistulae may develop as a result of radiation therapy. Finally, pressure necrosis caused by the proximal edge of a previously placed metal stent can also result in the development of a fistula. Treatment of fistulae should be immediate, as fistula formation is a potential life-threatening complication; in the case of a tracheoesophageal fistula, it may result in serious pulmonary infections from aspiration pneumonia.

Palliative surgery is associated with a mortality rate of up to 50% (12). Therefore, endoscopic placement of a covered stent is considered the palliative treatment of choice (Figure 86.6). Several retrospective and prospective series have been published reporting the outcome of endoscopic placement of a covered stent for this indication (53–59). In the majority of these publications, complete sealing of the fistula was established in more than 90% of patients. The complication rate varied between 10% and 30%.

In some patients with esophageal cancers that infiltrate into the trachea, dysphagia and dyspnea may develop simultaneously. Moreover, in some cases placement of a stent in the esophagus to seal a fistula can result in obstruction of the trachea and result in acute dyspnea. In these circumstances the placement of a stent into the trachea and/or bronchi in conjunction with or after esophageal stent placement can be performed (parallel stent placement). Stents placed in the trachea are usually uncovered and embed themselves in the mucosa of the respiratory tract (60). Complications occur more commonly with parallel stent placement. Fatal complications have been described, such as perforation and bleeding caused by tissue necrosis due to the high radial force exerted by both stents (61).

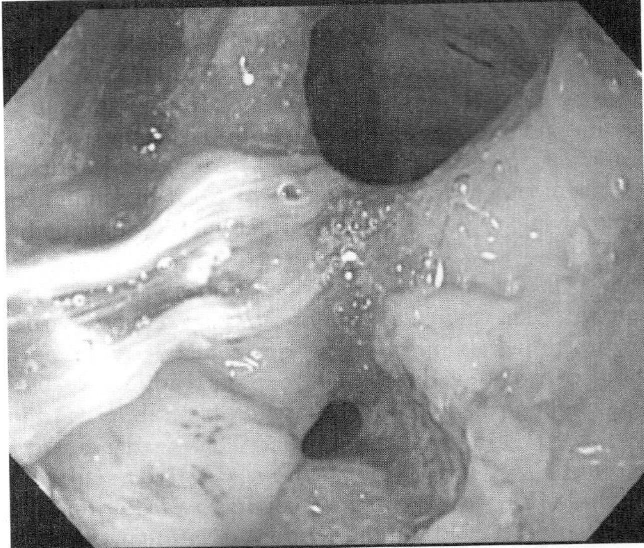

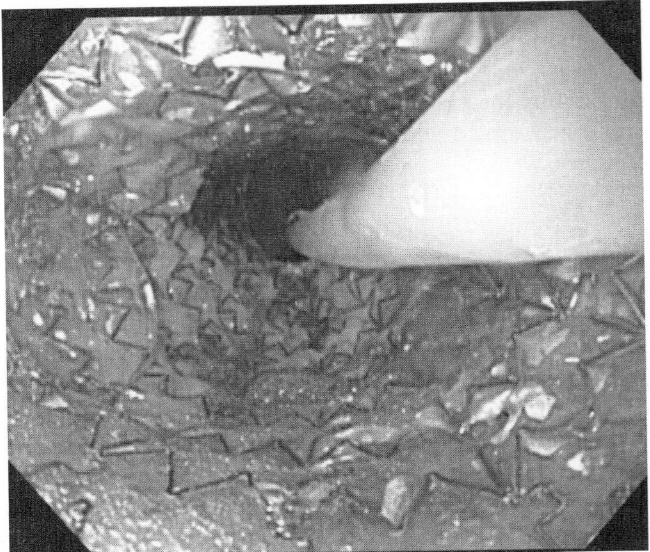

FIGURE 86.6

Endoscopic placement of covered stent for treatment of malignant tracheoesophageal fistula (TEF). (A) Endoscopic view of large TEF. (B) Endoscopic view immediately after deployment of covered stent.

CONCLUSION

The currently available endoscopic treatment modalities for the palliation of malignant dysphagia outside of self-expandable stent placement are, as yet, not optimal for achieving rapid and sustained dysphagia relief with minimal morbidity and mortality. Self-expanding stents are effective in improving dysphagia; however, the number of re-interventions needed for management of recurrent dysphagia remains higher than initially anticipated. The introduction of newer generation stents may reduce stent migration and non-tumoral tissue overgrowth and result in a decrease in the need for re-intervention.

Future developments in stent design include biodegradable stents, stents with a radioactive coating, and drug-eluting stents. Biodegradable stents have been developed for benign stenoses (62,63), but a possible application could also be the treatment of dysphagia in patients undergoing palliative chemotherapy. The incorporation of β-emitting agents and cytotoxic agents in esophageal stents may increase their efficacy, particularly in the prevention of tumor overgrowth at both ends of the stent. In healthy dogs, placement of radioactive stents caused fibrosis with radiation damage to the esophageal wall. However, serious complications such as perforation or fistula formation were not observed (64). The safety and efficacy of radioactive and drug-eluting stents in malignant esophageal strictures need to be further evaluated in clinical trials.

References

1. Siersema PD, Marcon N, Vakil N. Metal stents for tumors of the distal esophagus and gastric cardia. *Endoscopy.* 2003;35:79–85.
2. Parkin DM, Bray F, Ferlay J, et al. Global cancer statistics, 2002. *CA Cancer J Clin.* 2005;55:74–108.
3. Chavy AL, Rougier M, Pieddeloup C, et al. Esophageal prothesis for neoplastic stenosis. A prognostic study of 77 cases. *Cancer.* 1986;57:1426–1431.
4. Bohnacker S, Thonke F, Hinner M, et al. Improved endoscopic stenting for malignant dysphagia using Tygon plastic prostheses. *Endoscopy.* 1998;30:524–531.
5. Knyrim K, Wagner HJ, Bethge N, et al. A controlled trial of an expansile metal stent for palliation of esophageal obstruction due to inoperable cancer. *N Engl J Med.* 1993;329:1302–1307.
6. Roseveare CD, Patel P, Simmonds N, et al. Metal stents improve dysphagia, nutrition and survival in malignant oesophageal stenosis: a randomized controlled trial comparing modified Gianturco Z-stents with plastic Atkinson tubes. *Eur J Gastroenterol Hepatol.* 1998;10:653–657.
7. Kozarek RA, Ball TJ, Brandabur JJ, et al. Expandable versus conventional esophageal prostheses: easier insertion may not preclude subsequent stent-related problems. *Gastrointest Endosc.* 1996;43:204–208.
8. Eickhoff A, Knoll M, Jakobs R, et al. Self-expanding metal stents versus plastic prostheses in the palliation of malignant dysphagia: long-term outcome of 153 consecutive patients. *J Clin Gastroenterol..* 2005;39:877–885.
9. Vakil N, Morris AI, Marcon N, et al. A prospective, randomized, controlled trial of covered expandable metal stents in the palliation of malignant esophageal obstruction at the gastroesophageal junction. *Am J Gastroenterol.* 2001;96:1791–1796.
10. Saranovic DJ, Djuric-Stefanovic A, Ivanovic A, et al. Fluoroscopically guided insertion of self-expandable metal esophageal stents for palliative treatment of patients with malignant stenosis of esophagus and cardia: comparison of uncovered and covered stent types. *Dis Esophagus.* 2005;18:230–238.
11. Ross WA, Alkassab F, Lynch PM, et al. Evolving role of self-expanding metal stents in the treatment of malignant dysphagia and fistulas. *Gastrointest Endosc.* 2007;65:70–76.
12. Siersema PD. New developments in palliative therapy. *Best Pract Res Clin Gastroenterol.* 2006;20:959–978.
13. May A, Hahn EG, Ell C. Self-expanding metal stents for palliation of malignant obstruction in the upper gastrointestinal tract. Comparative assessment of three stent types implemented in 96 implantations, *J Clin Gastroenterol.* 1996;22:261–266.
14. Schmassmann A, Meyenberger C, Knuchel J, et al. Self-expanding metal stents in malignant esophageal obstruction: a comparison between two stent types. *Am J Gastroenterol.* 1997;92:400–406.
15. Siersema PD, Hop WC, van Blankenstein M, et al. A comparison of 3 types of covered metal stents for the palliation of patients with dysphagia caused by esophagogastric carcinoma: a prospective, randomized study. *Gastrointest Endosc.* 2001;54:145–153.
16. Sabharwal T, Hamady MS, Chui S, et al. A randomized prospective comparison of the Flamingo Wallstent and Ultraflex stent for palliation of dysphagia associated with lower third oesophageal carcinoma. *Gut.* 2003;52:922–926.
17. Verschuur EM, Homs MY, Steyerberg EW, et al. A new esophageal stent design (Niti-S stent) for the prevention of migration: a prospective study in 42 patients. *Gastrointest Endosc.* 2006;63:134–140.
18. Baron TH. A practical guide for choosing an expandable metal stent for GI malignancies: is a stent by any other name still a stent? *Gastrointest Endosc.* 2001;54:269–272.
19. Rathore OI, Coss A, Patchett SE, et al. Direct-vision stenting: the way forward for malignant oesophageal obstruction. *Endoscopy.* 2006;38:382–384.
20. Martin DF. Endoscopy is superfluous during insertion of expandable metal stents in esophageal tumors. *Gastrointest Endosc.* 1997;46:98–99.
21. Austin A, Khan Z, Cole AT, et al. Placement of self-expanding metallic stents without fluoroscopy. *Gastrointest Endosc.* 2001;54:157–159.
22. Baron TH. Minimizing endoscopic complications: endoluminal stents. *Gastrointest Endosc Clin N Am.* 2007;17:83–104.
23. Baron TH. Expandable metal stents for the treatment of cancerous obstruction of the gastrointestinal tract. *N Engl J Med.* 2001;344:1681–1687.
24. Morgan R, Adam A. The radiologist's view of expandable metallic stents for malignant esophageal obstruction. *Gastrointest Endosc Clin N Am.* 1999;9:431–435.
25. Rollhauser C, Fleischer DE. Late migration of a self-expanding metal stent and successful endoscopic management. *Gastrointest Endosc.* 1999;49:541–544.
26. Mayoral W, Fleischer D, Calcedo J, et al. Nonmalignant obstruction is a common problem with metal stents in the treatment of esophageal cancer, *Gastrointest Endosc.* 2000;51:556–559.
27. Spinelli P, Cerrai FG, Ciuffi M, et al. Endoscopic stent placement for cancer of the lower esophagus and gastric cardia. *Gastrointest Endosc.* 1994;40:455–457.
28. Verschuur EM, Steyerberg EW, Kuipers EJ, et al. Effect of stent size on complications and recurrent dysphagia in patients with esophageal or gastric cardia cancer. *Gastrointest Endosc.* 2007;65:592–601.
29. Dua KS, Kozarek R, Kim J, et al. Self-expanding metal esophageal stent with antireflux mechanism. *Gastrointest Endosc.* 2001:53;603–613.
30. Laasch HU, Marriott A, Wilbraham L, et al. Effectiveness of open versus antireflux stents for palliation of distal esophageal carcinoma and prevention of symptomatic gastroesophageal reflux. *Radiology.* 2002;225:359–365.
31. Do YS, Choo SW, Suh SW, et al. Malignant esophagogastric junction obstruction: palliative treatment with an antireflux valve stent. *J Vasc Interv Radiol.* 2001;12:647–651.
32. Homs MY, Wahab PJ, Kuipers EJ, et al. Esophageal stents with antireflux valve for tumors of the distal esophagus and gastric cardia: a randomized trial. *Gastrointest Endosc.* 2004;60:695–702.
33. Wenger U, Johnsson E, Arnelo U, et al. An antireflux stent versus conventional stents for palliation of distal esophageal or cardia cancer: a randomized clinical study. *Surg Endosc.* 2006;20:1675–1680.
34. Schoppmeyer K, Golsong J, Schiefke I, et al. Antireflux stents for palliation of malignant esophagocardial stenosis. *Dis Esophagus.* 2007;20:89–93.
35. Shim CS, Jung IS, Cheon YK, et al. Management of malignant stricture of the esophagogastric junction with a newly designed self-expanding metal stent with an antireflux mechanism. *Endoscopy.* 2005;37:335–339.
36. Kinsman KJ, DeGregorio BT, Katon RM, et al. Prior radiation and chemotherapy increase the risk of life-threatening complications after insertion of metallic stents for esophagogastric malignancy, *Gastrointest Endosc.* 1996;43:196–203.
37. Siersema PD, Hop WC, Dees J, et al. Coated self-expanding metal stents versus latex prostheses for esophagogastric cancer with special reference to prior radiation and chemotherapy: a controlled, prospective study, *Gastrointest Endosc.* 1998:47:113–120.
38. Bartelsman JF, Bruno MJ, Jensema AJ, et al. Palliation of patients with esophagogastric neoplasms by insertion of a covered expandable modified Gianturco-Z endoprosthesis: experiences in 153 patients. *Gastrointest Endosc.* 2000;51:134–138.
39. Homs MY, Hansen BE, van Blankenstein M, et al. Prior radiation and/or chemotherapy has no effect on the outcome of metal stent placement for esophagogastric carcinoma. *Eur J Gastroenterol Hepatol.* 2004;16:163–170.
40. Lecleire S, Di Fiore F, Ben-Soussan E, et al. Prior chemoradiotherapy is associated with a higher life-threatening complication rate after palliative insertion of metal stents in patients with oesophageal cancer. *Aliment Pharmacol Ther.* 2006;23:1693–1702.
41. Ludwig D, Dehne A, Burmester E, et al. Treatment of unresectable carcinoma of the esophagus or the gastroesophageal junction by mesh stents with or without radiochemotherapy. *Int J Oncol.* 1998;13:583–588.
42. Homs MYV, Steyerberg EW, Eijkenboom WMH, et al. Single-dose brachytherapy versus metal stent placement for the palliation of dysphagia from oesophageal cancer; multicenter, randomised trial. *Lancet.* 2004;364:1497–1504.
43. Steyerberg EW, Homs MYV, Stokvis A, et al. Stent placement or brachytherapy for palliation of dysphagia from esophageal cancer: a prognostic model to guide treatment selection. *Gastrointest Endosc.* 2005;62:333–340.
44. Bethge N, Sommer A, Vakil N. Palliation of malignant esophageal obstruction due to intrinsic and extrinsic lesions with expandable metal stents. *Am J Gastroenterol.* 1998;93:1829–1832.
45. Eleftheriadis E, Kotzampassi K. Endoprosthesis implantation at the pharyngo-esophageal level: problems, limitations and challenges. *World J Gastroenterol.* 2006;12:2103–2108.
46. Macdonald S, Edwards RD, Moss JG. Patient tolerance of cervical esophageal metallic stents. *J Vasc Interv Radiol.* 2000;11:891–898.
47. Shim CS, Jung IS, Bhandari S, et al. Management of malignant strictures of the cervical esophagus with a newly-designed self-expanding metal stent. *Endoscopy.* 2004;36:554–557.
48. Dormann AJ, Eisendrath P, Wigginghaus B, et al. Palliation of esophageal carcinoma with a new self-expanding plastic stent. *Endoscopy.* 2003;35:207–211.

49. Costamagna G, Shah SK, Tringali A, et al. Prospective evaluation of a new self-expanding plastic stent for inoperable esophageal strictures. *Surg Endosc.* 2003;17:891–895.
50. Szegedi L, Gal I, Kosa I, et al. Palliative treatment of esophageal carcinoma with self-expanding plastic stents: a report on 69 cases. *Eur J Gastroenterol Hepatol.* 2006;18:1197–1201.
51. Conio M, Repici A, Battaglia G, et al. A randomized prospective comparison of self-expandable plastic stent and partially covered self-expandable metal stent in the palliation of malignant esophageal dysphagia. *Am J Gastroenterol.* 2007;102(12):2667–2677.
52. Yoruk Y. Esophageal stent placement for the palliation of Dysphagia in lung cancer. *Thorac Cardiovasc Surg.* 2007;55:196–198.
53. Do YS, Song HY, Lee BH, et al. Esophagorespiratory fistula associated with esophageal cancer: treatment with a Gianturco stent tube. *Radiology.* 1993;187:673–677.
54. Bethge N, Sommer A, Vakil N. Treatment of esophageal fistulas with a new polyurethane-covered, self-expanding mesh stent: a prospective study. *Am J Gastroenterol.* 1995;90:2143–2146.
55. Kozarek RA, Raltz S, Brugge WR, et al. Prospective multicenter trial of esophageal Z-stent placement for malignant dysphagia and tracheoesophageal fistula, *Gastrointest Endosc.* 1996;44:562–567.
56. Low DE, Kozarek RA. Comparison of conventional and wire mesh expandable prostheses and surgical bypass in patients with malignant esophagorespiratory fistulas. *Ann Thorac Surg.* 1998;65:919–923.
57. May A, Ell C. Palliative treatment of malignant esophagorespiratory fistulas with Gianturco-Z stents. A prospective clinical trial and review of the literature on covered metal stents. *Am J Gastroenterol.* 1998;93:532–535.
58. Raijman I, Siddique I, Ajani J, et al. Palliation of malignant dysphagia and fistulae with coated expandable metal stents: experience with 101 patients *Gastrointest Endosc.* 1998;48:172–179.
59. Dumonceau JM, Cremer M, Lalmand B, et al. Esophageal fistula sealing: choice of stent, practical management, and cost. *Gastrointest Endosc.* 1999;49 70–78.
60. van den Bongard HJ, Boot H, Baas P, et al. The role of parallel stent insertion in patients with esophagorespiratory fistulas. *Gastrointest Endosc.* 2002;55:110–115.
61. Binkert CA, Petersen BD. Two fatal complications after parallel tracheal-esophageal stenting. *Cardiovasc Interv Radiol.* 2002;25:144–147.
62. Fry SW, Fleischer DE. Management of a refractory benign esophageal stricture with a new biodegradable stent. *Gastrointest Endosc.* 1997;45:179–182.
63. Sandha GS, Marcon NE. Expandable metal stents for benign esophageal obstruction. *Gastrointest Endosc Clin N Am.* 1999;9:437–446.
64. Won JH, Lee JD, Wang HJ, et al. Self-expandable covered metallic esophageal stent impregnated with beta-emitting radionuclide: an experimental study in canine esophagus. *Int J Radiat Oncol Biol Phys.* 2002;53:1005–1013.

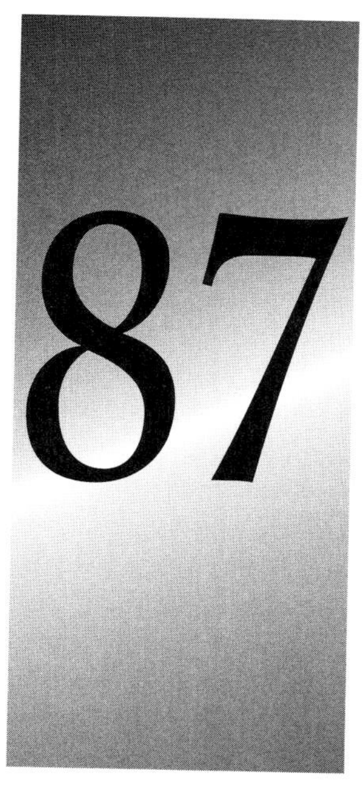

Endoscopic Palliation of Dysphagia: Laser

Jon P. Walker
Robert H. Hawes
Brenda J. Hoffman

The advent of thermal therapy for malignant dysphagia emerged in the early 1980s when Fleischer and Kessler reported the successful use of a neodymium: yttrium-aluminum-garnet (Nd:YAG) laser system to debulk obstructing esophageal tumors, resulting in the complete palliation of 5 patients with non-operable malignant dysphagia (1). Up to that point, therapeutic modalities for palliation of dysphagia were limited. The historic procedure of choice for palliation was surgery, which carried significant procedure-related morbidity and mortality, and subsequent detrimental effects on quality of life. Prosthetic tube intubation for palliation was theoretically safe and efficacious. In fact, intubation was often successful in providing some improvement in malignant dysphagia; however, despite the benefit of providing palliation with a single procedure, there were a number of drawbacks associated with this modality. Morbidity rates as high as 25% were reported with complications such as perforation, hemorrhage, ulcers, and severe chest pain. In addition, recurrent dysphagia was reported frequently due to tumor over- and undergrowth. Prosthetic stents cannot be used for patients with lesions in the cervical esophagus due to bolus sensation and subsequent inability of patients to tolerate. Finally, patients were rarely able to tolerate a completely normal diet, and diets were often limited to soft foods and thick liquids. Dilation therapy had been a known modality for decades and provided safe and near immediate dysphagia relief. However, dilation often lasted no more than several days to weeks and required multiple repeated procedures, which had a negative impact on quality of life.

External beam radiation demonstrated some promise in providing adequate tumor regression to provide relief of dysphagia in a low morbidity and mortality setting. However, radiation therapy did carry some morbidity, which was usually delayed and related to radiation-induced fibrotic stenosis, fistulas, or severe esophagitis. In addition, radiation therapy–induced improvement occurred over a longer period of time, which was a significant issue in patients with a limited lifespan. Brachytherapy could be provided in a setting to allow for less radiation and more rapid relief time. However, few studies have adequately explored the utility of brachytherapy alone, as other modalities that show greater promise have arisen.

Since that first report by Fleischer, a number of studies have explored the use of the Nd:YAG laser system. Laser therapy has been evaluated for safety, efficacy, survival, cost-effectiveness, and quality of life benefits. Laser therapy has been compared to a number of other therapeutic modalities, both as separate procedures and in combination. Numerous reports have demonstrated safety, efficacy, and a positive impact on patient quality of life. Despite the proven benefits of laser therapy, there has been a trend back to prosthetic devices, as self-expandible metal stents have been developed and improved to allow for a perceived single-step palliation protocol. However, the innovation of thermal therapy has also continued, with the replacement of the Nd:YAG laser system by argon plasma beam coagulation. This simple, easier, and less expensive thermal modality continues to have a role in palliation of lesions not amenable to stent therapies, such as treatment of tumor undergrowth, ingrowth, or overgrowth after stenting (2–5).

FUNDAMENTALS OF ND:YAG LASER

Nd:YAG laser therapy is indicated for the palliation of dysphagia induced by malignancies anywhere from the cervical esophagus to the gastric cardia. The lesions that have been treated have reflected the evolution of esophageal cancer; initially, lesions treated were primarily squamous cell but in time have shifted to adenocarcinoma. The lesions range from exophytic, mucosal lesions to submucosal lesions or non-esophageal lesions that are causing external compression. Patients undergoing treatment are deemed non-operable for a number of reasons ranging from distal metastatic disease to poor medical condition.

Nd:YAG works by emission of an invisible light beam (wavelength 1064 nm) delivered via a quartz fiber housed within a Teflon sheath and passed through the working channel of a standard or therapeutic endoscope. The laser is directed by a separate Xenon aiming light. A separate stream of nitrogen or carbon dioxide gas is passed down a coaxial sheath to keep the laser fiber free of debris and blood, as well as keeping the fiber cool during the treatment process. The laser is absorbed by tissue and results in molecular agitation and heating, which results in a degree of tissue injury that is dependent on the amount of light absorbed (6). The typical treatment involves an 80 to 100 watt application of 0.5 to 1 second pulse on a focused spot of malignant tissue from a distance of 5 to 10 mm from the lesion. However, several reports have demonstrated the use of a lower energy level, with only 40 to 50 watt. These studies have demonstrated similar efficacy, with the same to lower major complications (7–8). The short duration pulse, which is induced by a foot pedal, allows for a controlled amount of energy delivery. This limits the risk of overtreatment and subsequent perforation or fistula formation. The tissue appearance is reflective of the tissue response to treatment (9–10). White tissue, which occurs at temperatures of 60°C, is demonstrative of protein denaturation and coagulation, the goal of flat infiltrating lesions (6,9). As temperatures reach 100°C, tissue boils and vaporization begins, resulting in the appearance of a "divot" (6,9). Black tissue, which occurs as temperatures exceed 100°C, is demonstrative of carbonization and vaporization, the goal of bulky, exophytic lesions (6,9). The typical depth of penetration has been reported to be 3 to 6 mm. The goal is 2-fold: first, to effect necrosis and sloughing of obstructing tumor tissue and second, to cause fibrosis, which limits tumor regrowth at that particular focus.

Initially, treatments began at the proximal end of the tumor and proceeded distally. However, because treatment results in bleeding and edema, visualization was impaired and it can become difficult to follow the lumen. As a result, most reports after 1985 describe a distal to proximal treatment progression. This ensures that the lumen is kept in view and reduced the perforation rate. In some cases, this treatment technique required dilation before the endoscope could be passed into the stomach.

The primary goal of initial therapy was to attain an adequate degree of luminal patency, to allow easy passage of either a standard or therapeutic upper endoscope. This theoretically correlates with dysphagia improvement. Treatment protocols typically scheduled treatment every other to every fourth day, until the desired goal is achieved. Most reports found it required 2 to 4 treatment sessions to achieve the desired goal. However, using a retrograde approach, Pietrafitta and Mitty have reported achievement of luminal patency in 1.6 and 1 session, respectively (11–12). Follow-up protocols involved either a scheduled or on-demand re-treatment (10). This is due to the frequency of tumor recurrence and fibrotic occlusion, both of which are easiest treated in their earliest stages (10).

The initial reports of Nd:YAG treatment involved an inpatient stay with every other day treatment protocols until dysphagia improved. However, given the short life expectancy of patients with advanced esophageal cancer, cost and quality of life issues lead to a trend toward shortened hospital stays and outpatient therapy. In fact, Lightdale and colleagues demonstrated that outpatient treatment protocols had a significant cost benefit with no difference in efficacy or complication rate (13).

LASER THERAPY EFFICACY AND SAFETY

Over the 10 years in which Nd:YAG laser therapy became the dominant treatment choice for palliation of malignant dysphagia, a number of studies examined the efficacy and safety of the procedure. Efficacy can be assessed in terms of luminal patency achieved or by functional success (i.e., the degree of dysphagia relief). Success in achieving luminal patency has been reported to be greater than 90% (14–16). From a functional standpoint, studies typically used a dysphagia scale from 0 to 4 (0: no dysphagia; 4: unable to tolerate any oral intake). Most studies reported dysphagia improvement rates ranging from 70% to 100% (8–10,13–14,16–19). However, complete resolution of dysphagia was rare and if achieved, was short lasting (9,13,17,19). Few studies reported on global physiologic effects of tumor debulking, but one study, while failing to demonstrate improvement in patient weight or albumin, did identify a notable reduction in the decline of both factors (9,20). The initial dysphagia relief interval was generally found to last for about 4 weeks (15–17). In fact, some protocols called for scheduled re-evaluation every 4 weeks (9–10). Most studies demonstrated that retreated lesions required only 1 to 2 treatment sessions to maximize effect, as opposed to the 2 to 4 sessions required with initial treatment (9,15). Average survival times after initial treatment were generally reported to be 4 to 6 months (9,17,19). One important point from a quality of life perspective was that the Nd:YAG laser regimen was noted in multiple studies to result in some degree of dysphagia relief at death. Krasner and Bourke reported at least partial relief of dysphagia in 85% and 73% of patients at death, respectively (9,17). Another long-term study by Naveau was less optimistic, reporting only 39% improvement maintained at 3 months and 22% improvement maintained at 6 months (14). Rutgeerts noted that 63% of patients were able to maintain some degree of dysphagia relief until death (16).

The numerous studies on use of the Nd:YAG laser therapy have consistently demonstrated a high degree of safety. The quality control measures of short pulses of controlled energy to the malignant tissues from a specified distance are effective in limiting the depth and extent of thermal injury. However, as with any thermal therapy, there are reported major complications, and for Nd:YAG laser treatment, these consisted of hemorrhage, perforation, tracheoesophageal fistula, aspiration, and stenosis. Rutgeerts also reported a fairly substantial rate of sepsis after laser treatment. But this was not the experience of most endoscopists during Nd:YAG therapy (16). A review of the early documented studies find the complication rate tended to vary from 1% to 20% (8–10,14,16–19). However, the complication rates may be somewhat skewed, since some patients underwent other therapeutic modalities in addition to laser therapy. In one study in which 7 perforations were reported in 76 patients, only 2 perforations were in patients treated with laser therapy only. Two others underwent dilation performed prior to therapy and 3 others had plastic esophageal stents placed post laser therapy (9).

During laser therapy, there can also be adverse effects of the carbon dioxide being insufflated through a coaxial channel. High CO_2 flow rates combined with the technique of distal to proximal treatment of the tumor traps the CO_2 in the downstream gut. One can quickly distend the gut and overwhelm the absorption rate of CO_2 if the endoscopist is not constantly cognizant to aspirate air and smoke via the endoscope. Overdistension of the gut can trigger a vasovagal response, and cecal perforation has been reported. Bown and colleagues suggested the utility of nasogastric tube during the procedure for continuous decompression (10). Another potential problem is the presence of free air in the peritoneum or mediastinum from dissection of air through the tumor tissue (3,15). This was postulated in two studies in which a pneumomediastinum or pneumoperitoneum was present post-procedure and the work-up revealed no clear source of perforation.

The procedure-related mortality rate is difficult to truly assess. Most studies tend to report mortality rates in the range of 0% to 5% (8–10,18,20). However, one has to take into account the wide variability in the general medical condition of patients from study to study. Most patients undergoing Nd:YAG laser palliation were very advanced in their disease process with limited reserve to withstand a major complication. In addition, these mortality rates are similar to those of other therapeutic and palliative modalities (21).

FACTORS EFFECTING Nd:YAG SUCCESS

Patient and tumor characteristics have played a significant role in determining the success of Nd:YAG laser therapy. Tumor factors amenable to Nd:YAG laser therapy were clarified by David Fleischer: (a) tumor length less than 5 centimeters, (b) tumor location in the straightest portion of the middle third of the esophagus, and (c) exophytic mucosal tumors (22). In another study, Fleischer expanded on these characteristics to note that cervical esophageal lesions are least conducive to successful therapy, and lesions in the gastroesophageal junction are near equally difficult to achieve successful relief of dysphagia due to the angulation (3). In the same study, it was noted that recurrent cancers at an anastomotic site are very amenable to laser treatment (3). Submucosal spread presents a unique challenge due to the inability to delineate clear margins and the need to simultaneously treat normal tissue to reach malignant tissue (10). Not only are submucosal lesions more difficult to treat, but they also resulted in more frequent post-procedure chest pain, and theoretically are at higher risk for adverse outcomes such as perforation, fistula, and stricture (3).

Other groups have demonstrated similar findings with only slight variations. Lightdale and colleagues recognized the least success with (a) cervical esophageal lesions, (b) tumor length greater than 8 centimeters, and (c) infiltrating or extraluminal tumors (13).

While Mellow and Pinkas were in general agreement with Fleischer and Lightdale regarding the difficulty in treating cervical esophageal lesions, they found that the most important predictive factors were more functional than anatomic (15). They demonstrated that the most important factors effecting success included anorexia, pharyngeal dysphagia, and pretreatment performance status with performance status being the most important (15). This appraisal was echoed by Alexander et al. (23). Naveau added that benefits after the initial treatment session may also be a positive predictive factor of future treatment success (14).

The interaction between tumor histology and laser sensitivity has been debated. Naveau and colleagues, examining long-term outcomes after laser therapy, compared adenocarcinoma and squamous cell carcinoma. They found no significant difference in outcome after 3 months. However, after 6 months, adenocarcinoma was associated with less benefit than squamous cell carcinoma (14). Bourke and colleagues examined this same issue and found no difference in long-term effects of laser therapy (17). Other studies examining both short- and long-term effects have also failed to demonstrate histology as a predictive factor in laser success.

COMBINATION THERAPY

The combination of laser and radiotherapy was first reported by Bader and colleagues when administering several brachytherapy sessions, following laser recanalization with promising results (24). However, subsequent studies, despite demonstrating relative safety, have failed to demonstrate a clear benefit to combination therapy (25–28). Sander and colleagues, using iridium afterloading combined with laser versus laser alone, noted a prolonged dysphagia-free first interval with combination therapy in the squamous cell group but not the adenocarcinoma group (26). Again, there was no survival benefit, and despite longer dysphagia-free intervals, more procedures were required for the patients undergoing combined therapy.

Using combination external beam radiation and laser therapy, Sargeant demonstrated a significant improvement in initial dysphagia control and between procedure intervals of 5 vs. 9 weeks compared to laser alone (27). However, there was no survival benefit, and this improvement translated to one saved procedure over the short lifespan of the study patients. In a small study of 19 patients with laser therapy and onetime brachytherapy, there was a small prolongation of time to next laser treatment (28). However, this study was uncontrolled and compared to results of historic controls.

Combination of laser therapy and chemotherapy has been much more limited but appears to show some promise. Highley, comparing patients treated with laser therapy alone or laser therapy as an adjunct to 5-flourouracil, cisplatin, and epirubicin, demonstrated not only that fewer laser treatments were needed to maintain improvement in dysphagia scores, but there was also a significant survival benefit of 9.7 vs. 5.5 weeks (29). Although the study was small, it does suggest the potential for further studies evaluating combined chemotherapy/laser therapy palliative protocols.

LASER THERAPY VERSUS OTHER PALLIATIVE MODALITIES

Metal Wall Stents

Since laser therapy was shown to palliate dysphagia as well or better than plastic stents but with a slightly better complication profile, it rapidly became the modality of choice for palliation of malignant dysphagia (30–32). However, with the advent of expandable metal stents, they quickly replaced plastic stents for the treatment of malignant dysphagia (33–35). This resulted in the resurgence of the use of stents to palliate dysphagia, and despite their high cost, due to the ease of placement, almost immediate relief of dysphagia, and need for only one procedure, SEMS have become the primary modality used for palliation of malignant dysphagia.

A number of groups have compared SEMS to laser therapy on a variety of factors, including efficacy, safety, cost-effectiveness, survival, and quality of life benefits (37–40). Adam and colleagues reported a significantly better early improvement in dysphagia scores with the SEMS group compared to laser therapy group (36). However, other groups using similar dysphagia scoring systems failed to identify a similar benefit and have seen no significant difference between the two modalities (37–40). Dallal and Xinopoulos have both documented that there are increased cost associated with laser therapy (37,40). However, Xinopoulos noted that this benefit was slight and Sihvo documented no cost-effective benefit (39). One possible reason could be the high morbidity associated with stent placement that was reported by several groups (37–39). Chest pain and stent migration were the 2 most common complications. Because of the additional cost associated with treatment of pain and stent migration, the initial cost-benefit of SEMS is quickly ameliorated. Another cost-effective drawback would be the need for additional procedures to address tumor growth into or around the stent, including repeat stent or laser therapy.

Recent studies have failed to demonstrate a consistent quality of life benefit of SEMS over laser therapy.

While Xinopoulos demonstrated only a mild benefit in quality of life, Dallal demonstrated a significantly worse health-related quality of life assessed at 1 month post treatment with SEMS (37,40). In addition to the role that procedural morbidity can play in quality of life, it has also been suggested that increased patient interaction with the medical team associated with the more frequent laser therapy sessions may have a beneficial psychologic effect on the patient and may improve their sense of overall quality of life (39).

Finally, while Dallal has demonstrated a significant survival benefit of laser therapy over SEMS placement, no other comparison study has demonstrated a significant difference in survival time between the 2 modalities (37–40). However, with the continued innovation of stents along with the increasing experience of clinicians placing these devices, the complications are likely to decrease and the cost-effective benefit will likely continue to improve. In fact, the most recent comparison by Xinopolous and colleagues in 2004 did show both a slight cost-effective and quality of life benefit of SEMS over laser therapy (40).

Despite the slight differences between the 2 modalities, it is clear that both are efficacious in providing some degree of dysphagia relief. While the present-day modality of choice appears to be SEMS placement, there *are* clinical situations that may support the use of one modality over the other. SEMS is clearly the modality of choice for lesions associated with tracheoesophageal fistula and when dysphagia is caused by external compression. In addition, SEMS have a clear advantage in lesions greater than 6 cm in length, tumors with a tortuous lumen, and tumors that are predominantly submucosal. For gastroesophageal junction (GEJ) lesions, both procedures have potential advantages and disadvantages. Though they are easy to place, SEMS bridging the GEJ have a greater tendency to migrate and results in a greater degree of acid reflux and GERD-related complications. Therefore, some clinicians may prefer to treat GEJ lesions with laser therapy. However, this location presents challenges for the Nd:YAG laser due to the difficult angulation of the lumen and lesion. Finally, lesions in the cervical esophagus are difficult to address with both modalities. The foreign body sensation and discomfort associated with stent placement is very problematic. Alternatively, laser treatment is technically difficult and associated with less therapeutic benefit. The improvement in chemotherapy alone or in combination with external beam radiotherapy has resulted in most cervical tumors being treated by the oncologist and radiation therapist.

Finally, the complementary benefits of the 2 modalities cannot be overlooked. One of the most significant drawbacks to SEMS is tumor in-, over-, or undergrowth. While covered stents prevent ingrowth, tumor overgrowth and undergrowth continues to be a problem. The use of laser therapy for treatment of this over- or undergrowth has been reported to be both safe and efficacious (3–4). Alternatively, in patients with unsuccessful laser therapy, development of a tracheoesophageal fistula, or a laser treatment resulting in a perforation, placement of a covered stent can provide a useful adjunct for palliation and treatment.

Photodynamic Therapy

The past 2 decades have witnessed the emergence of photodynamic therapy (PDT). By using light-sensitizing, chemotherapeutic agents, tumors can theoretically be ablated by direct exposure to light. This modality has been used extensively for the treatment and palliation of a wide range of precancerous and cancerous processes from bladder transitional cell carcinoma to Barrett's esophagus with high-grade dysplasia. PDT has also been used with some success in the palliation of malignant dysphagia and is described further in Chapter 85.

When compared to thermal therapies, PDT has a number of advantages and disadvantages. With PDT there is no smoke production and no gaseous distention, and it is technically very simple. Disadvantages include a waiting period between administrations of light sensitizing agent (approximately 1–2 days with dihematoporphyrin ethers), shallow depth of penetration, high expense, stricture formation, and finally, the lifestyle modifications that are required to prevent sunburn (avoidance of sun exposure for approximately 1 month).

Studies by Lightdale, using porfimer sodium, and Heier, using dihematoporphyrin ethers, have compared PDT and laser therapy (41,42). Both studies demonstrated a similar initial improvement in dysphagia, with a similar number of initial treatment session required to achieve this benefit. However, PDT appeared superior to laser therapy after 1 month. Lightdale demonstrated that after 1 month, 32% of PDT patients maintained some degree of tumor response versus only 20% in the laser group (41). Heier demonstrated that 1 month after initial treatment, the PDT group had a statistically higher Karnovsky scores than the laser group, along with trends toward better dysphagia grade and dietary response (42). In addition, Heier demonstrated a longer duration of initial response in the PDT group (84 days vs. 57 days) (42). The exact reason for this difference is not quite clear. Explanations include a possible immunological response to PDT therapy (41).

Both procedures had an acceptable safety profile. The PDT group in both studies reported sunburn (41–42). Heier reported a tracheoesophageal fistula and 2 strictures in the PDT group (42). There were no complications in the laser group. However, Lightdale found a significantly higher complication rate in the laser group, with perforations noted in 1% in the PDT group vs. 7% in the laser group (41). In addition, Lightdale noted a significantly higher rate of procedure termination due to adverse effects in the laser group than the PDT group (42).

Overall these findings demonstrate that while initial benefits are similar, PDT might be a more efficacious long-term modality. PDT may have an even greater benefit in tumors more difficult to treat with laser therapy. These include long lesions (greater than 6 cm) and tumors in the most distal and proximal aspects of the esophagus. Safety comparisons are not consistent and further studies would need to be performed to clearly demonstrate the superiority of either modality.

INTRATUMORAL CHEMOTHERAPEUTIC INJECTION

Comparisons between laser therapy and direct chemotherapeutic injection into an obstructing lesion have failed to demonstrate a consistent superiority of one modality over the other (43–44). In a study by Carazzone, 47 patients were randomized to laser therapy or intratumoral injection of ethanol (44). Both groups were found to have similar initial dysphagia improvement, as well as similar initial dysphagia-free times. Pain was reported in 18 ethanol-treated patients and only 1 in the laser group. One perforation occurred in the ethanol group; no major complications occurred in the laser group. In another study by Angelini, 34 patients were randomized to either laser therapy or intratumoral injection of polidocanol (43). There was a similar initial improvement in dysphagia, and no significant difference was reported in initial dysphagia-free time. One perforation occurred in the polidocanol group and no major complications were reported in the laser group. Overall, these studies demonstrate a fairly similar efficacy profile. While they both seem to be similar in terms of major complication rate, the increased incidence of chest pain in patients receiving intratumoral ethanol injections may have effects on quality of life, making this a potentially suboptimal modality compared to laser therapy.

ALTERNATIVE THERMAL MODALITIES

Argon plasma beam coagulation (APC) had been an established modality in the operating room theater for years, before its introduction to the field of endoscopy. By ionizing a rapid flow of argon gas, a monopolar electrical current is created and a focus of thermal energy is delivered to a specific point. The use of APC offers a number of technical advantages over Nd:YAG laser therapy. It is a smaller system, and it is cheaper and easier to use. The complex and cumbersome safety features associated with laser use do not apply to APC. Tissue temperatures are much lower with APC therapy than laser, resulting in less tissue vaporization and more coagulation, a theoretic advantage in terms of tissue injury (45). In addition, depth of thermal injury from APC has been demonstrated to be 1 to 3 mm, compared to a depth of 3 to 6 mm, associated with laser therapy (45–46). In a study of 42 post-resection esophageal specimens treated with varying degrees of APC energy, only one was noted to have thermal injury of the muscularis propria (46). This slightly more shallow depth in addition to the lower focal treatment temperatures would provide a theoretical advantage over laser therapy, in terms of risk factors for perforation, fistula formation, and pain.

Several studies have been reported examining the use of APC for malignant dysphagia palliation (2,4,5,45–48). When using YAG laser reports as historic controls, APC appears comparable to laser therapy in terms of overall relief of dysphagia, complications, treatment-related mortality, and survival time. In the largest study to date, Heindorff and colleagues reported the use of APC in the palliation of 83 patients with esophageal or gastric cardia cancers. Complete improvement of dysphagia allowing for a normal diet occurred in 58% of patients after only 1 treatment. Another 26% were able to tolerate a normal diet after more than 1 treatment. Although 16% of patients were never able to tolerate a normal diet, all patients in this group noted some improvement in dysphagia. Complications, the majority of which were perforations, were reported in 10% of patients. A 1% treatment-related mortality rate was reported. The exact initial dysphagia free time was difficult to assess since patients were followed up every 4 weeks for repeat procedure and treatment.

Others studies evaluating APC as a palliative modality have been smaller but slightly less optimistic in their findings. A retrospective study by Erikson did not report specific figures in terms of dysphagia relief, but noted a majority of patient who presented with dysphagia grades of 3 or greater improved to 2 or less after initial APC therapy (47). It was noted that repeat APC was required about 4 weeks after initial improvement. A 13% complication rate was noted, primarily perforation, with 1 tracheoesophageal fistula and a 6.5% procedure-related mortality rate. Robertson reported the use of APC in 9 patients (5). All patients were rendered completely asymptomatic for a median of 6 weeks prior to need for pretreatment, with no procedure-related complications reported. In one small aspect of a larger study, Akhtar reported on APC use in 3 patients with malignant dysphagia secondary to esophageal cancer (2). Only 1 patient benefited from APC treatment. The other 2 required stent placement. Survival times appear to be in the range of 3 to 6 months (2,4,5,47). APC was also demonstrated by Akhtar and Robertson to be highly beneficial for treatment of growth in and around a previously placed stent (2,5).

At approximately the same time that the successful use of laser therapy was being reported, a separate thermal modality was also being developed, which utilized bipolar electrocoagulation. Until the early 1980s, this modality was used primarily to treat gastrointestinal bleeding. Bipolar electrocoagulation produces a focused heat source generated when 2 oppositely charged probes are applied to a specific site of tissue and the circuit is completed. The physics of this technology limits the depth of penetration of heat. In 1985, Johnston and colleagues reported the use of a specially designed BICAP probe, consisting of a bipolar electrocoagulation device incorporated into an olive-shaped dilator; similar to an Eder-Puestow dilator (49). BICAP probe diameters are 6 mm, 9 mm, 12 mm, and 15 mm (6,49). After an initial endoscopic examination to assess the length, location, and degree of stenosis, a guidewire is passed into the stomach. The BICAP device is then passed down the guidewire to either the distal or proximal end of the lesion. The BICAP probe diameter utilized depends on the lumen size. In some cases of very stenotic tumors, limited dilation was required prior to application of the BICAP probe. When in position, the probe is activated producing a 360-degree thermal tissue injury. As the tissue continues to heat, it dries and there is an increased resistance and subsequent decrease in current, thus theoretically limiting depth of penetration (6). The reported theoretic depth of the BICAP probe ranges from 2 to 4mm, but this may be deeper in tissue that is compressed by the probe. Nonetheless, this calculates to a theoretic increase in lumen size of 4 to 8mm (50). The probe is passed in either a distal or proximal direction. Some have reported slowly pushing through the lesion, then withdrawing while the probe is applying heat. Others report passing the probe to the distal end, and then activating the coagulation, and slowly withdrawing the probe through the lesion. While the BICAP probe was originally designed for 360-degree thermal therapy, probes have been developed with the capability of 180-degree therapy.

While few centers presently use BICAP thermal therapy, the studies evaluating its safety and efficacy were quite promising. In Johnston and colleagues' original study, 20 patients were treated with BICAP probe (51). In a mean of 1.7 initial treatment sessions, there was a significant improvement in overall dysphagia grade, with a mean interval to the need for repeat treatment of 7.6 weeks. Overall survival was not different from historic reports of other modalities. There was, however, a 20% rate of major complications with 2 patients developing hemorrhage and 2 patients developing fistulas. Other minor complications noted were self-limited chest pain and low-grade fevers. McIntyre found similar results in a comparison of 17 patients treated with BICAP to 13 patients treated with prosthetic tube (52). He noted an 88% improvement rate after BICAP therapy. Thirteen of 17 patients required only 1 treatment with an average duration of initial benefit of 4 weeks. Only 1 complication, a tracheoesophageal fistula, was noted. These findings were statistically similar to the prosthetic tube group. While the initial benefit lasted a shorter period of time than Johnston reported, there was also a lower complication rate. Johnston notes that the major drawbacks included the number of instruments required and the lack of clear visualization of all tumors being treated (51). The noted advantages included ease of application, speed of treatment, simplicity, and low cost of equipment. There was no necrotic debris to clear. It was effective for submucosal and cervical lesions, as well as long lesions. As with all thermal therapy, there does not appear to be a difference in response to BICAP based on histology (7,49). However, 1 study has reported a slightly higher failure rate in adenocarcinomas, as compared to squamous cell carcinoma (8). Potential complications are similar to other thermal modalities. Two studies have demonstrated a significant rate of delayed strictures after BICAP therapy (8,53). This was not seen consistently in other studies and may be secondary to probe application to normal tissue.

The benefits associated with BICAP therapy would appear to suggest superiority over laser therapy. However, this has not been demonstrated in the literature, and it appears as though each modality has its specific indications. Jensen and colleagues compared 14 patients treated with laser therapy to 14 patients treated with BICAP tumor probe therapy (7). Each group received only 1 initial treatment session. No statistical significance was demonstrated in dysphagia improvement at follow-up. Both groups reported an 86% improvement in dysphagia, allowing for a soft or semi-solid diet. Pain or edema requiring dilation was more common in the laser group, as was the incidence of delayed stricturing. Survival time was also similar. One tracheoesophageal fistula was reported in the BICAP group, in a patient with a non-circumferential lesion. No major complications were reported in the laser group. This study highlighted the differences in tumor characteristics that may be amenable to treatment by 1 modality or the other. Long, circumferential, submucosal, or cervical lesions may be more amenable to BICAP therapy. Shorter, non-circumferential, exophytic lesions in the middle and lower third of the esophagus would be more amenable to laser therapy. It has also been suggested that BICAP may be slightly less effective for cardia and lower third lesions, as well as anastomotic lesions (8). Non-circumferential lesions should never be treated with BICAP probe therapy. While an 180-degree probe is available, it is still not recommended in these circumstances.

In the present day, only APC is used as a thermal modality for the palliation of malignant dysphagia. Unfortunately, despite the early reports of safety and efficacy, BICAP therapy has failed to be maintained as a major modality for palliation. While it is possible to pass a small caliber endoscope to visualize the treatment of the most proximal aspects of the lesion, the inability to visualize the entire thermal delivery has likely been a key component in the demise of BICAP probe palliation. And while numerous studies have demonstrated the efficacy and safety of laser therapy, APC is similar to or slightly superior in virtually all aspects. In addition, APC is cheaper, more mobile, and easier to learn and manage.

SUMMARY

Thermal therapy utilizing the Nd:YAG laser has proven to be a safe and efficacious modality for the palliation of malignant dysphagia. A number of studies in the early 1980s demonstrated the superior efficacy, morbidity, and mortality profile compared to both palliative surgery and esophageal plastic tube intubation, and Nd:YAG laser rapidly became the procedure of choice for palliation of malignant dysphagia.

While laser therapy can be applied with some degree of effectiveness to any lesion in any region of the esophagus, lesions deemed most conducive to successful treatment tend to be shorter lesions, usually less than 6 cm or on a surgical anastomosis, in the straight part of the middle third of the esophagus, and exophytic, mucosal lesions. Submucosal extrinsic compression tumors, lesions in the cervical esophagus, and lesions on the gastroesophageal junction tend to be more difficult to treat with laser therapy. Limited studies have shown promise in the added benefit of the combination of laser with radiation or chemotherapy. Any lesion associated with mucosal disruption or tracheoesophageal fistulae are best addressed with SEMS placement.

After an initial course of approximately 2 to 4 sessions, Nd:YAG produces a variable success rate of about 70% to 90%, and improvement tends to last for about 4 weeks before repeat treatment is required. Major complications include perforation, tracheoesophageal fistula, bleeding, and delayed strictures and tend to occur in 0% to 10% of patients treated.

Since the 1990s, placement of covered and uncovered SEMS has become the modality of choice secondary to the perception of a one-time procedure providing adequate long-term palliation and a subsequent cost-effective and quality of life benefit. Early studies comparing the 2 modalities failed to consistently demonstrate this clear benefit. This was primarily due to the low but significant complication rate related to bleeding, stent migration, and chest pain. However, the most recent studies are suggestive that this risk is becoming less frequent and the cost-effective benefits are becoming clearer.

Despite the relatively universal use of SEMS as the primary modality of choice for palliation, there continues to be a role for thermal therapy. Argon plasma coagulation, which has generally replaced the Nd:YAG laser for thermal therapy, can provide treatment to areas of the esophagus, such as the cervical esophagus, that are not amenable to stenting due to poor patient tolerance. In addition, APC can still have a benefit in the treatment of tumor over- or undergrowth. Thus, the outlook for thermal therapy as a palliative modality in esophageal cancer continues to show promise.

References

1. Fleischer D, Kessler F. Endoscopic NdYAG laser therapy for carcinoma of the oesophagus: a new form of palliative treatment. *Gastroenterology*. 1983;85:600–606.
2. Akhtar K, Byrne JP, Bancewicz J, et al. Argon beam plasma coagulation in the management of cancers of the esophagus and stomach. *Surg Endosc*. 2000;14:1127–1130.
3. Fleischer D, Sivak MV. Endoscopic Nd-YAG laser therapy as palliation for esophageal cancer. *Gastroenterology*. 1985;89:827–831.
4. Heindorff H, Wojdemann M, Bisgaard T, et al. Endoscopic palliation of inoperable cancer of the oesophagus or cardia by argon electrocoagulation. *Scand J Gastroerol*. 1998;33:21–23.
5. Robertson GSM, Thomas M, Jamieson J, et al. Palliation of oesophageal carcinoma using the argon beam coagulator. *Br J Surg*. 1996; 83:1769–1771.
6. Reilly HF, Fleischer DE. Palliative treatment of esophageal carcinoma using laser and tumor probe therapy. *Gastrointest Clin North Am*. 1991;20:731–742.
7. Jensen DM, Machicado G, Randall G, et al. Comparison of low-power YAG laser and BICAP tumor probe for palliation of esophageal cancer strictures. *Gastroenterology*. 1988;94:1263–1270.
8. Maunoury V, Brunetand JM, Cochelard D, et al. Endoscopic palliation for inoperable malignant dysphagia: long-term follow up. *Gut*. 1992;33:1602–1607.
9. Krasner N, Barr H, Skidmore C, et al. Palliative laser therapy for malignant dysphagia. *Gut*. 1987;28:792–798.
10. Bown SG, Hawes R, Matthewson K, et al. Endoscopic laser palliation for advanced malignant dysphagia. *Gut*. 1987;28:799–807.
11. Pietrafitta JJ, Bowers GJ, Dwyer RM. Prograde versus retrograde endoscopic laser therapy for the treatment of malignant esophageal obstruction: a comparison of techniques. *Lasers Surg Med*. 1988;8:288–293.
12. Mitty RD, Cave DR, Birkett DH. One-stage retrograde approach to Nd:YAG laser palliation of esophageal carcinoma. *Endoscopy*. 1996;28:350–355.
13. Lightdale CJ, Zimbalist E, Winawer SJ. Outpatient management of esophageal cancer with endoscopic Nd-YAG laser. *Am J Gastro*. 1987;82:46–50.
14. Naveau S, Chiesa A, Poymard T, et al. Endoscopic Nd-YAG laser therapy as palliative treatment for esophageal and cardia cancer. *Dig Dis Sci*. 1990;35:294–301.
15. Mellow MH, Pinkas H. Endoscopic laser therapy for malignancies affecting the esophagus and gastroesophageal junction. *Arch Int Med*. 1985;145:1443–1446.
16. Rutgeerts P, Vantrappen G, Broeckaert L, et al. Palliative Nd:YAG laser therapy for cancer of the esophagus and gastroesophageal junction: impact on the quality of remaining life. *Gastrointest Endosc*. 1988;34:87–90.
17. Bourke MJ, Hope RL, Chu G, et al. Laser palliation of inoperable malignant dysphagia: initial and at death. *Gastrointest Endosc*. 1996;43: 29–32.
18. Buset M, des Marez B, Baize M, et al. Palliative endoscopic management of obstructive esophagogastric cancer: laser or prosthesis? *Gastrointest Endosc*. 1987;33:357–361.

19. Schulze S, Fischerman K. Palliation of oesophagogastric neoplasms with Nd:YAG laser treatment. *Scand J Gastroenterol.* 1990;25:1024–1027.
20. Abdel-Wahab M, Gad-Elhak N, Denewer A, et al. Endoscopic laser treatment of progressive dysphagia in patients with advanced esophageal carcinoma. *Hepatogastroenterol.* 1998;45:1509–1515.
21. Siersema PD, Dees J, van Blankenstein M. Palliation of malignant dysphagia from oesophageal cancer. *Scan J Gastroenterol.* 1998;33:75–88.
22. Fleischer D. Washington symposium on endoscopic laser therapy. *Gastrointest Endosc.* 1985;31:397–400.
23. Alexander GL, Wank KK, Ahlquist DA, et al. Does performance status influence the outcome of Nd:YAG laser therapy of proximal esophageal tumors? *Gastrointest Endosc.* 1994;20:451–454.
24. Bader M, Dittler HJ, Ultsch B, et al. Palliative treatment of malignant stenosis of the upper gastrointestinal tract using a combination of laser and afterloading radiotherapy. *Endoscopy.* 1986;18:27–31.
25. Renwick P, Whitton V, Moghissi K. Combined endoscopic laser therapy and brachytherapy for palliation of oesophageal carcinoma: a pilot study. *Gut.* 1992;33:435–438.
26. Sander R, Hagenmueller F, Sander C, et al. Laser versus laser plus afterloading with iridium 192 in the palliative treatment of malignant stenosis of the oesophagus: a prospective, randomized, and controlled study. *Gastrointest Endosc.* 1991;37:433–440.
27. Sargeant IR, Tobias JS, Blackman G, et al. Radiotherapy enhances laser palliation of malignant dysphagia: a randomized study. *Gut.* 1997;40:362–369.
28. Spencer GM, Thorpe SM, Sargeant IR, et al. Laser and brachytherapy in the palliation of adenocarcinoma of the oesophagus and cardia. *Gut.* 1996;39:726–731.
29. Highley MS, Parnis GA, Trotter GA, et al. Combination chemotherapy with epirubicin, cisplatin, and 5-fluorouracil for the palliation of advanced gastric and oesophageal adenocarcinoma. *Br J Surg.* 1994;81:1763–1765.
30. Alderson D, Wright PD. Laser recanalization versus endoscopic intubation in the palliation of malignant dysphagia. *Br J Surg.* 1990;77:1151–1153.
31. Carter R, Smith JS, Anderson JR. Laser recanalization versus endoscopic intubation in the palliation of malignant dysphagia: a randomized prospective study. *Br J Surg.* 1992;79:1167–1170.
32. Loizou LA, Grigg D, Atkinson M, et al. A prospective comparison of laser therapy and intubation in endoscopic palliation for malignant dysphagia. *Gastroenterology.* 1991;100:1303–1310.
33. DePalma GD, diMatteo E, Romano G, et al. Plastic prosthesis versus expandable metal stents for palliation of inoperable esophageal thoracic carcinoma: a controlled prospective study. *Gastrointest Endosc.* 1996;43:478–482.
34. Knyrim K, Wagner HJ, Bethge N, et al. A controlled trial of an expansile metal stent for palliation of esophageal obstruction due to inoperable cancer. *N Engl J Med.* 1993;329:1302–1307.
35. Siersema PD, Dees J, van Blankenstein M. Coated self-expanding metal stents versus latex prostheses for esophagogastric cancer with special reference to prior radiation and chemotherapy: a controlled, prospective study. *Gastrointest Endosc.* 1998;47:113–120.
36. Adam A, Ellul J, Watkinson AF, et al. Palliation of inoperable esophageal carcinoma: a prospective randomized trial of laser therapy and stent placement. *Radiology.* 1997;202:344–348.
37. Dallal HJ, Smith GD, Grieve DC, et al. A randomized trial of thermal ablative therapy versus expandable metal stents in the palliative treatment of patients with esophageal carcinoma. *Gastrointest Endosc.* 2001;54:549–557.
38. Gevers AM, Macken E, Hiele M, et al. A comparison of laser therapy, plastic stents, and expandable metal stents for palliation of malignant dysphagia in patients without a fistula. *Gastrointest Endosc.* 1998;48:383–388.
39. Sihvo EIT, Pentikainen T, Luostarinen ME, et al. Inoperable adenocarcinoma of the oesophagogastric junction: a comparative clinical study of laser coagulation versus self-expanding metallic stents with special reference to cost-analysis. *Eur J Surg Onc.* 2002;28:711–715.
40. Xinopoulos D, Dimitroulopoulos D, Moschandrea I, et al. Natural course of inoperable esophageal cancer treated with metallic expandible stents: quality of life and cost-effective analysis. *J Gastroenterol Hepatol.* 2004;19:1397–1402.
41. Lightdale CJ, Heier SK, Marcon NE, et al. Photodynamic therapy with porfimer sodium versus thermal ablation therapy with Nd:YAG laser for palliation of esophageal cancer: a multicenter randomized trial. *Gastrointest Endosc.* 1995; 42:507–512.
42. Heier SK, Rothman KA, Heier LM, et al. Photodynamic therapy for obstructing esophageal cancer: light dosimetry and randomized comparison with Nd:YAG laser therapy. *Gastroenterology.* 1995;109:63–72.
43. Angelini G, Pasini AF, Ederle A, et al. Nd:YAG laser versus polidocanol injection for palliation of esophageal malignancy: a prospective, randomized study. *Gastrointest Endosc.* 1991;37:607–610.
44. Carazzone A, Bonavina L, Segalin A, et al. Endoscopic palliation oesophageal cancer: results of a prospective comparison of Nd:YAG laser and ethanol injection. *Eur J Surg.* 1999;165:351–356.
45. Grund KE, Storek D, Farin G. Endoscopic argon plasma coagulation (APC). *Endosc Surg Allied Technol.* 1994;2:42–46.
46. Watson JP, Bennett MK, Griffin SM, et al. The tissue effect of argon plasma coagulation on esophageal and gastric mucosa. *Gastrointest Endosc.* 2000;52:342–345.
47. Eriksen JR. Palliation of non-resectable carcinoma of the cardia and oesophagus by argon beam coagulation. *Dan Med Bull.* 2002;49:346–349.
48. Manner H, May A, Faerber M, et al. Safety and Efficacy of a new high power argon plasma coagulation system in lesions of the upper GI tract. *Digest Liver Dis.* 38;2006:471–478.
49. Johnston J, Quint R, Petruzzi C, et al. Development and experimental testing of a large BICAP probe for palliative treatment of obstructing esophageal and rectal malignancy [abstract]. *Gastrointest Endosc.* 1985;31:156.
50. Jensen DM. Palliation of esophagogastric cancer via endoscopy. *Gastroenterol Clin Biol.* 1987;11:361–363.
51. Johnston JH, Fleischer D, Petrini J, et al. Palliative bipolar electrocoagulation therapy of obstructing esophageal cancer. *Gastrointest Endosc.* 1987;33:349–353.
52. McIntyre AS, Morris DL, Sloan RL, et al. Palliative therapy of malignant esophageal stricture with the bipolar tumor probe and prosthetic tube. *Gastrointest Endosc.* 1989;35:531–535.
53. Fleischer D, et al. Stricture formation following BICAP tumor probe therapy for esophageal cancer [Abstract]. *Gastrointest Endosc.* 1987;33:83.

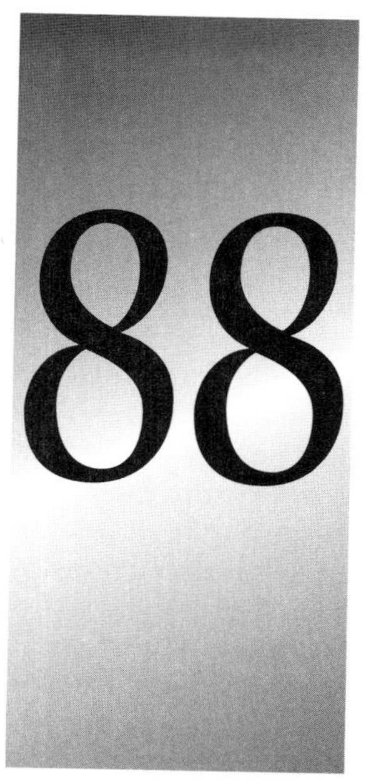

Endoscopic Palliation of Dysphagia: Brachytherapy

Atif J. Khan
Phillip M. Devlin

The incidence of esophageal carcinoma is rising at a substantial rate in the United States, due mainly to the increasing frequency of adenocarcinomas (1,2). In 2007, there were an estimated 15,560 new cases of esophageal cancer resulting in an estimated 13,940 deaths (3). Approximately 30% of diagnosed patients will have disease that is metastatic (4), and over 50% of patients with esophageal cancer are diagnosed with disease that is inoperable. Non-operative combined modality therapy can achieve local control in only approximately a half of treated patients (5–7). Median survival for patients with progressive disease is 3 to 5 months. Given these grim realities, the need for effective palliation in these patients cannot be overemphasized, in whom the ability to swallow without obstruction or pain for the duration of their remaining life is a vital parameter of overall quality of life.

Surgical methods for palliation can include limited resection with reconstruction and surgical bypass/feeding tubes. The more common treatment options for palliation of dysphagia include endoluminal therapies such as self-expanding metal stents, laser therapy, and photodynamic therapy (PDT), as well as endoluminal brachytherapy with or without external beam radiation therapy (EBRT). Laser therapy often requires multiple sessions to achieve durable palliation. A course of EBRT is often not practical for patients with advanced, metastatic, or recurrent disease, and those with poor performance status. Stents and endoluminal brachytherapy can offer durable palliation with fewer interventions and fewer trips to the physician's office. This chapter will focus on the use of brachytherapy for palliation of esophageal cancer.

DATA

Either alone or with chemotherapy, EBRT has been shown to be highly efficacious for the palliation of dysphagia in numerous reports (8–12). These studies, and others, convincingly demonstrate palliation of dysphagia in 70% to 80% of patients treated with EBRT. Approximately one-half of these patients will have durable palliation lasting until the time of death.

The study by Coia and colleagues is notable for its relatively large numbers and careful analysis of dysphagia as an endpoint (12). Using a previously described swallowing score, the authors analyzed 102 patients treated with EBRT and concurrent mitomycin C and continuous infusion 5-FU for esophageal cancer on prospective non-randomized trials at the Fox Chase Cancer Center: of the 102 patients, 49 were treated with palliative intent; 95% of patients had dysphagia at the outset; and after the 6-week course of treatment, 83% of patients experienced improvement. The median time to maximum improvement was 4 weeks, with a range of 1 to 21 weeks. Benign strictures occurred in 12% of patients. In the group treated for palliation, 91% of patients had improvement of their dysphagia and 67% of patients experienced palliation until death.

EBRT has the advantage that, unlike endoluminal modalities, it can treat the deep aspect of the obstructing tumor mass in addition to the visible endoluminal component. It suffers from the inconvenience of (typically) 2 weeks of daily treatments, after which it takes approximately 2 weeks to achieve palliation.

Brachytherapy has been employed for palliation of esophageal cancer for several years and several reports have documented its efficacy. It is difficult to compare the data reported for EBRT with those reported for brachytherapy due to uncontrolled selection biases inherent in patients referred for brachytherapy, who often have failed EBRT or are unable to travel for daily EBRT fractions.

The efficacy of brachytherapy was shown by Jager and colleagues, who reported their series of 88 patients treated with a single fraction of intraluminal brachytherapy (13). Patients with preexisting fistulas, gastroesophageal junction/cardia tumors, and complete obstruction were not included. Seven patients had received prior EBRT. Dose was prescribed at a depth of 1 cm from the central axis with a 1 cm superior-inferior margin on the visualized lesion. The first 51 patients were treated with medium-dose rate (MDR)^{137}Cs with treatment times ranging between 2.5 to 5 hours, while the remaining 37 patients were treated with HDR. Dysphagia improved in 67% of evaluable patients. Thirteen percent of patients reported no change in dysphagia and 20% had progression. Non-fatal bleeding occurred in 1 patient, and fistulae developed in 5 patients (6%). Two of the 7 patients who received prior EBRT developed severe dysphagia due to ulceration.

Sharma et al. treated 58 patients with advanced/metastatic or recurrent esophageal carcinoma with HDR intraluminal brachytherapy at the Tata Memorial Hospital in Mumbai (14). Fifteen patients had received prior palliative EBRT to doses of 20 to 30 Gy in 3 to 4 Gy fractions. A 6 mm catheter was used to deliver 12 Gy in 2 weekly fractions of 6 Gy at a depth of 1 cm. Overall improvement in dysphagia was reported in 48% of patients, while 15% of patients developed strictures, 10% ulceration, and 5% fistulas. The median time to stricture development was 4.2 months.

Sur and associates attempted to identify optimal fractionation for HDR intraluminal brachytherapy in their report on 172 patients randomized to either 12 Gy in weekly 6 Gy fractions, 16 Gy in weekly 8 Gy fractions, or 18 Gy in weekly 6 Gy fractions (15). Patients with lesions greater than 6 cm in the thoracic esophagus and with the ability to swallow at least liquids were included. A 0.6 cm catheter was used and dose was prescribed to a depth of 1 cm. A margin of 2 cm above and below the tumor was treated. After preliminary analysis, the 12 Gy arm was closed due to higher rates of persistent disease compared to the other 2 groups. In the final analysis, there was no statistical difference in dysphagia-free survival, although the rates of persistence/recurrent tumor were higher in the 12 Gy arm. The dysphagia-free survival for the entire group at 12 months was 29%. Benign fibrotic strictures were highest in the 18 Gy arm (42% vs. 14%–25%). The mean to stricture formation was 128 days. When comparing other palliative modalities, the authors concluded that 16 Gy in 2 fractions or 18 Gy in 3 fractions using HDR brachytherapy was the most effective palliative modality for these patients.

In the multi-national follow-up trial, Sur et al. conducted a randomized comparison of 18 Gy in 3 fractions versus 16 Gy in 2 fractions in a study that was sponsored by the International Atomic Energy Agency (16); 232 patients with squamous cell carcinomas greater than 5 cm in the thorax and performance status greater than 50 were randomized. Fractions were delivered on alternate days and dose was prescribed at a depth of 1 cm. Proximal and distal margins of 2 cm on the visualized tumor were included in the treatment volume. No differences were seen in outcome between the 2 randomized groups. Approximately 80% of patients had no dysphagia at 3 months and 60% had no dysphagia at 12 months. The median duration of dysphagia-free survival was 7.1 months. The medial survival of the whole group was 7.9 months. The incidence of strictures (11%) and fistulas (10%) was equal in the 2 groups. The study demonstrated the efficacy of palliation by means of endoluminal brachytherapy for these patients.

Two studies have directly compared metal stent placement with brachytherapy for palliation of dysphagia in esophageal cancer patients. In the study by Homs et al., 9 hospitals in the Netherlands randomized a total of 209 patients to either placement of a self-expanding metal stent or to single-dose brachytherapy (17). All patients had inoperable or metastatic esophageal cancer and preexistent dysphagia. Tumors greater than 12 cm and tumors with fistulas were excluded, as were patients with any prior radiation. For patients randomized to stent, the partly covered Ultraflex stent (Boston Scientific, Natick, MA) was introduced and deployed under fluoroscopy, and placement was verified endoscopically and radiographically. Stent length was chosen to give at least a 1.5 cm margin on the target lesion in both proximal and distal directions.

For patients randomized to the brachytherapy arm, a 10 mm catheter was positioned to cover the target lesion. The target volume included 2 cm proximal and distal margins on the tumor, and a single dose of 12 Gy was delivered at a depth of 1 cm from the source axis.

All patients received sucralfate for 4 weeks after brachytherapy. Patients in whom the distal end of the stent or the active length of the brachytherapy was below the GEJ received lifelong omeprazole.

Dysphagia improved more rapidly after stent placement, but by 30 days after treatment, dysphagia score improvement was equal in the 2 groups. At 30 days, dysphagia score improved by at least 1 grade in 73% of patients who had brachytherapy and in 76% of patients who had stent placement. Beyond 30 days, brachytherapy produced better dysphagia scores until about 350 days when the 2 treatments equalized again. Patients in the brachytherapy group had more days with no dysphagia (grade 0–1) during follow-up than those assigned to stent placement (115 vs. 82, $P = 0.015$). The stent group had significantly more complications ($P = 0.02$), most prominent of which was a significantly higher incidence of late hemorrhage (13% vs. 5%). Median survival was not different, and the number of patients eventually treated for recurrent or persistent dysphagia was not different. Fistulas were uncommon at 3% in each group. Total medical costs for the 2 methods were comparable. The authors concluded that single-dose brachytherapy gave better long-term relief of dysphagia and was better tolerated.

The second randomized trial comparing stent insertion to brachytherapy was conducted in Sweden by Bergquist et al. (18). A total of 65 patients with preexistent dysphagia were randomized to Ultraflex stent insertion or endoluminal brachytherapy delivered in 3 fractions of 7 Gy (HDR) at 1 to 2 week intervals. A 10 mm or 17 mm applicator was used to deliver dose to the target lesion with a 1 cm margin, and dose was prescribed to a depth of 1 cm. Clinical assessments were coupled to health-related quality of life questionnaires at regular intervals. Similar to the Dutch study, stenting was more effective in the first month, but that in patients with longer survival (beyond 3 months), brachytherapy offers better palliation and better quality of life.

Another option for palliation in patients with esophageal tumors is coagulation/vaporization with the neodymium yttrium aluminum garnet (Nd:YAG) laser. The tumor is treated under direct visualization and this method can achieve recanalization in 90% of appropriately selected patients. However, the response to laser therapy is not durable. Typically, repeat interventions are required every 4 to 6 weeks.

A randomized trial of laser recanalization alone or with EBRT (30 Gy in 10 fractions) showed that adding RT increased the interval between laser treatments (19). In addition, a randomized trial comparing laser recanalization with or without endoluminal brachytherapy has been reported by Spencer et al. (20). In this study, 22 patients referred to the Middlesex Hospital in London for palliation of dysphagia due to previously untreated, inoperable, exophytic adenocarcinoma of the esophagus were randomized to either additional brachytherapy or observation after laser recanalization. A dose of 10 Gy was delivered at 1 cm from the source using an HDR afterloader. The median time to dysphagia recurrence was longer in the brachytherapy group (19 weeks) than in the observation group (5 weeks), and this difference was statistically significant ($P < 0.001$). Furthermore, the patients treated with brachytherapy required less than half the number of treatments per month alive than those treated with laser alone ($P = 0.04$). This study clearly demonstrated the efficacy of a single fraction of endoluminal brachytherapy when added to laser recanalization.

Concerns regarding the toxicity of esophageal brachytherapy have been accentuated by the results of RTOG 9207 (21). In that study, 49 patients with inoperable esophageal cancer received 50 Gy EBRT with concurrent chemotherapy (cisplatin/5-FU), followed by a 2-week break, and then an endoluminal brachytherapy "boost." Brachytherapy consisted of 15 Gy as weekly 5 Gy fractions using HDR or 20 Gy with LDR and was delivered through a 4 to 6 mm catheter. Significantly, patients received chemotherapy during the brachytherapy portion of the treatment. The dose in the HDR group was reduced to 10 Gy in 2 fractions due to a high number of observed fistulas (6 patients). The LDR arm was closed due to poor accrual. In the final report, the median survival for all patients was 11 months and the local persistence/recurrence rate was 63%. A total of 6 patients developed fistulas (14.6%), resulting in the deaths of 3 of these patients. The 1-year actuarial fistula development rate was 17.5%.

As described by the authors of the study, factors contributing to the high rate of fistula formation probably include the use of more cycles of chemotherapy, the use of chemotherapy concurrent with brachytherapy, smaller diameter catheters leading to higher surface mucosal doses, and higher total brachytherapy doses. Notably, no fistulas occurred after the dose was reduced to 10 Gy in 2 fractions. In contrast, other authors have reported fewer esophageal complications in patients receiving a brachytherapy boost after concurrent chemotherapy and EBRT. In the palliative setting, without chemotherapy and with appropriately large applicators, fistula rates less than 10% are to be expected, as was demonstrated in the previously discussed randomized Dutch study.

TECHNIQUE

The goal of applicator placement is to pass the applicator beyond the target lesion so that a minimum 1.5 to 2 cm margin on tumor is covered both in the proximal and distal directions. The most widely available and commonly used applicator is a flexible single channel catheter. For application in the esophagus, a longer (100–150 cm) catheter is needed. As discussed above, narrow-bore catheters lead to higher mucosal doses so catheters with a diameter of 0.6 to 1 cm are preferred.

Applicator placement should occur in a controlled setting with the patient under moderate sedation or general anesthesia. Experienced endoscopists are necessary collaborators for the procedure. Commonly, the applicator can be placed transnasally after locally active anesthetic agents have been applied to the nasal mucosa. Placement of the applicator beyond the target lesion should be verified by endoscopy.

In situations where an obstructive lesion does not allow passage of the catheter, the gastrostomy tube can be used to help in applicator placement (2). First, the catheter can be passed through the nose and led out of the mouth. Next, the endoscope is passed through the mouth and advanced down the esophagus, past the target lesion, until the gastrostomy tube is visualized. A long suture or snare is inserted into the gastrostomy tube and grasped by the endoscope. The endoscope can then be withdrawn, thus bringing the suture out through the patient's mouth. The distal end of the suture, still at the level of the gastrostomy tube, requires attention so as to not be pulled up into the esophagus. The weighted end of the catheter can now be secured to the suture or snare and can together be pulled back through the esophagus by gently pulling the suture at the gastrostomy end and advancing the catheter at the nasal end.

If the endoscope cannot pass the obstruction, a thin biopsy catheter may be advanced beyond the lesion. As before, this catheter can now "catch" one end of a snare at the level of the gastrostomy tube and then be pulled back to the level of the mouth. The applicator can then be carefully advanced past the lesion as described above.

Neoplastic erosion and invasion of the esophagus can significantly weaken its ability to withstand instrumentation and intervention. Care must be taken to avoid the creation of a false lumen by the surgical instruments. Highly skilled and experienced endoscopists are required to minimize the potential risks of mucosal injuries, bleeding, perforation, and mediastinitis.

DOSE AND FRACTIONATION

The goal of palliative brachytherapy in this setting is to control the luminal component of the disease. Brachytherapy should not be expected to control deep esophageal wall disease or peri-esophageal disease. The American Brachytherapy Society has published guidelines for the use of brachytherapy both in the curative and palliative settings (22). The guidelines for palliation with brachytherapy have been reproduced in Table 88.1. Dose is prescribed at a depth of 1 cm from the source position. As described on Table 88.1, both low- and

TABLE 88.1
American Brachytherapy Society Recommendations for the Palliative Treatment of Esophageal Cancer

Recurrent after EBRT and short life expectancy

Brachytherapy:

HDR—total dose of 10–14 Gy, 1 or 2 fractions

LDR—total dose of 20–40 Gy, 1 or 2 fractions, 0.4–1.0 Gy/hr

No previous EBRT

EBRT:

30–40 Gy in 2–3 Gy fractions

Brachytherapy:

HDR—total dose of 10–14 Gy, 1 or 2 fractions

LDR—total dose of 20–25 Gy, single course, 0.4–1.0 Gy/hr

No previous EBRT, life expectancy > 6 months

EBRT:

45–50 Gy in 1.8–2.0 Gy fractions, 5 fractions/week, week 1–5

Brachytherapy:

HDR—total dose of 10, 5 Gy per fraction, 1 fraction/week, starting 2–3 weeks after EBRT

LDR—total dose of 20 Gy, single course, 0.4–1.0 Gy/hr, starting 2–3 weeks after EBRT

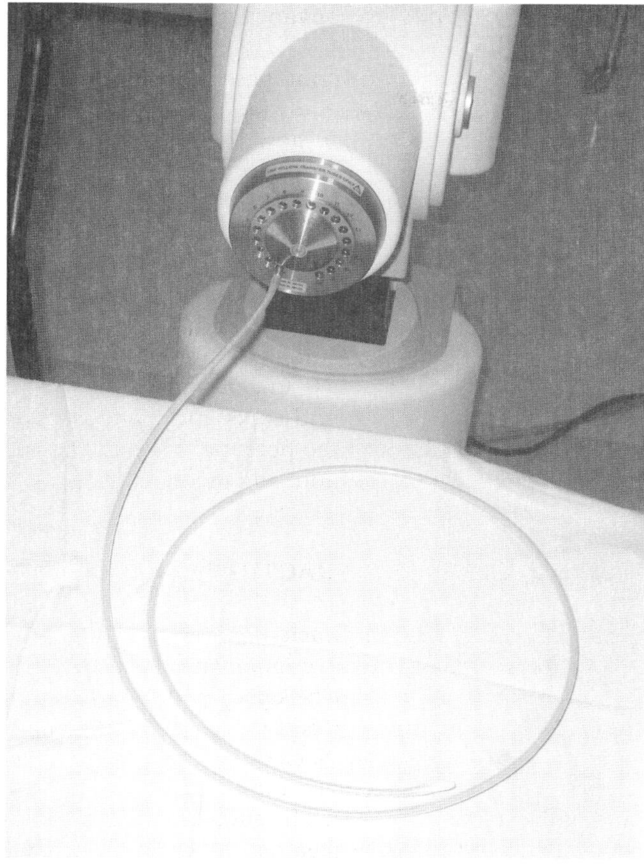

FIGURE 88.1

An HDR remote afterloading unit (Microselectron, Nucletron, Netherlands) with an attached intraluminal esophageal applicator (Nucletron, Netherlands).

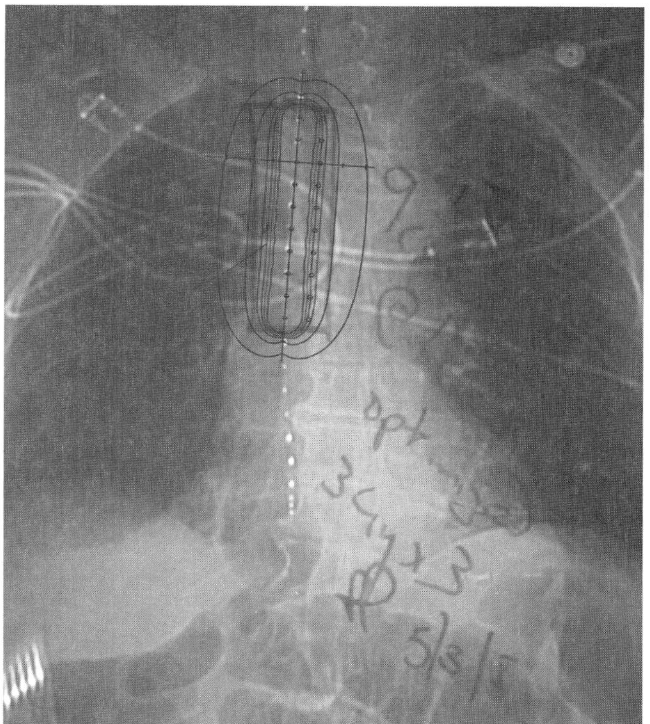

FIGURE 88.2

Anterior radiograph of an intraluminal esophageal applicator with a radio-opaque dummy wire for treatment planning. Treatment isodose lines have been scaled for magnification and overlayed on the radiograph.

high-dose rate brachytherapy can be used (Figure 88.1). In general, for patients with prior EBRT treatment or a short life expectancy, brachytherapy alone as palliation is appropriate. One or 2 fractions of 5 to 7 Gy with HDR or 20 to 25 Gy in a single course of LDR are reasonable (Figure 88.2). For patients with longer life expectancies, additional dose contributions with external beam should be considered.

CONCLUSION

Esophageal cancer continues to be difficult to control and cure, and many patients will require palliation of their symptoms. The most frequent and significant of these is obstruction resulting in dysphagia. External beam radiotherapy and endoluminal brachytherapy can be a safe and effective means of producing durable palliation when offered by a methodical, multidisciplinary team of health care providers.

References

1. DeVita VT, Hellman S, Rosenberg SA, eds. *Principles & Practice of Oncology.* 7th ed. Philadelphia: Lippincott Williams & Wilkens, 2005.
2. Devlin PM, ed. *Brachytherapy: Application and Techniques.* Philadelphia: Lippincott Williams & Wilkens, 2007.
3. Jemal A, Siegel R, Ward E, et al. Cancer Statistics. *CA Cancer J Clin.* 2007;57:43–66.
4. Surveillance Epidemiology and End Results (SEER) Fast Stats. National Cancer Institute. http://seer.cancer.gov/faststats. Accessed October 14, 2008.
5. Al-Sarraf M, Martz K, Herskovic A, et al. Progress report of combined chemoradiotherapy versus radiotherapy alone in patients with esophageal cancer: an intergroup study. *J Clin Oncol.* 1997;15:277–284.
6. Minsky B, Pajak T, Ginsberg R, et al. INT 0123 (Radiation Therapy Oncology Group 94–05) phase III trial of combined-modality therapy for esophageal cancer: high-dose versus standard dose radiation therapy. *J Clin Oncol.* 2002;20:1167–1174.
7. Stahl M, Stuschke M, Lehmann N, et al. Chemoradiation with and without surgery in patients with locally advanced squamous cell carcinoma of the esophagus. *J Clin Oncol.* 2005;23:2310–2317.
8. Petrovich Z, Langholz B, Formenti S, et al. Management of carcinoma of the esophagus: the role of radiotherapy. *Am J Clin Oncol.* 1991;14:80.
9. Caspars RJL, Welvaart K, Verkes RJ, et al. The effect of radiotherapy on dysphagia and survival in patients with esophageal cancer. *Radiother Oncol.* 1988;12:15.
10. Whittington R, Coia LR, Haller DG, et al. Adenocarcinoma of the esophagus and esophago-gastric junction: the effects of single and combined modalities on the survival and patterns of failure following treatment. *Int J Radiat Oncol Biol Phys.* 1990;19:593.
11. Urba SG, Turrisi AT. Split-course accelerated radiation therapy combined with carboplatin and 5-flurouracil for palliation of metastastic or unresectable carcinoma of the esophagus. *Cancer.* 1995;75:435.

12. Coia LR, Soffen EM, Schultheiss TE, et al. Swallowing function in patients with esophageal cancer treated with concurrent radiation and chemotherapy. *Cancer.* 1993;71:281–286.
13. Jager J, Langendijk H, Pannebakker M, et al. A single session of brachytherapy in palliation of oesophageal cancer. *Radiother Oncol.* 1995;37:237–240.
14. Sharma V, Mahanshetty U, Dinshaw K, et al. Palliation of advanced/recurrent esophageal carcinoma with high-dose-rate brachytherapy. *Int J Radiat Oncol Biol Phys.* 2002;52:310–315.
15. Sur RK, Donde B, Levin VC, et al. Fractionated high dose rate intraluminal brachytherapy in palliation of advanced esophageal cancer. *Int J Radiat Oncol Biol Phys.* 1998;40:447–453.
16. Sur RK, Levin CV, Donde B, et al. Prospective randomized trial of HDR brachytherapy as a sole modality in palliation of advanced esophageal carcinoma—an International Atomic Energy Agency Study. *Int J Radiat Oncol Biol Phys.* 2002;53:127–133.
17. Homs MYV, Steyerberg EW, Eijkenboom WMH, et al. Single-dose brachytherapy versus metal stent placement for the palliation of dysphagia from oesophageal cancer: multicentre randomized trial. *Lancet.* 2004;364:1497–504.
18. Bergquist H, Wenger U, Johnsson E, et al. Stent insertion or endoluminal brachytherapy as palliation of patients with advanced cancer of the esophagus and gastroesophageal junction. Results of a randomized, controlled clinical trial. *Dis Esophagus.* 2005;18:131–139.
19. Sargeant IR, Tobias JS, Blackman G, et al. Radiotherapy enhances laser palliation of malignant dysphagia: a randomized study. *Gut.* 1997;40:362–9.
20. Spencer GM, Thorpe SM, Blackman GM, et al. Laser augmented by brachytherapy versus laser alone in the palliation of adenocarcinoma of the oesophagus and cardia: a randomized study. *Gut.* 2002;50:224–227.
21. Gaspar LE, Winter K, Kocha WI, et al. A phase I/II study of external beam radiation, brachytherapy, and concurrent chemotherapy for patients with localized carcinoma of the esophagus (Radiation Therapy Oncology Group Study 9207): final report. *Cancer.* 2000;88:988–995.
22. Gaspar LE, Nag S, Herskovic A, et al. American Brachytherapy Society (ABS) consensus guidelines for brachytherapy of esophageal cancer. *Int J Radiat Oncol Biol Phys.* 1997;38:127–132.

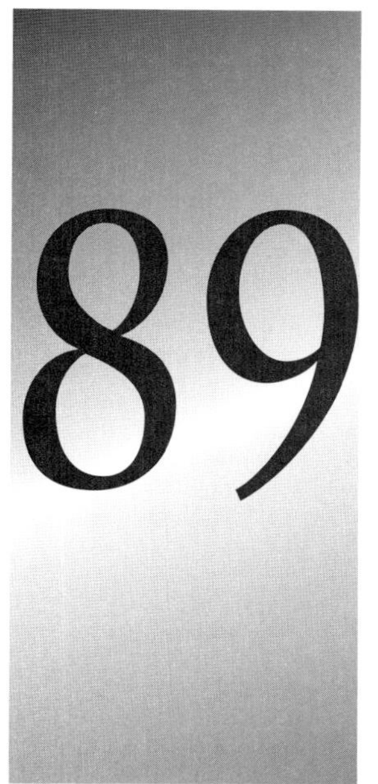

Surgical Palliation: Current Role

Michael Ujiki
Christy M. Dunst

Palliation is an important consideration for those who treat patients with esophageal carcinoma because more than 50% of these patients will present with distant metastases or locally advanced, unresectable disease (1). The goal of palliation in these patients is to improve their quality of life, keeping in mind that only a few will have prolonged progression-free survival. The selection of appropriate palliative methods depends on many factors including expected survival time, the general condition of the patient, and the patient's presenting or associated symptoms.

Consideration for surgical intervention in patients for whom cure cannot be achieved must be made cautiously. Historically, incomplete resections to relieve severe dysphagia or to control a perforation or fistula were acceptable mainly because there were no other options. Esophageal surgeons devised novel operations in an attempt to decrease the extraordinarily high morbidity and in-house mortality observed in these dismal situations. However, with the evolution of advanced endoscopic techniques and improved chemotherapy and radiation protocols, the current role for surgical palliation is limited. For example, successful restoration of the ability to swallow can now be achieved nonsurgically using self-expanding metal stents, photodynamic therapy, or chemoradiation with much lower morbidity and mortality rates (2–4). Palliation for esophageal cancer should not only be safe and effective, it should also be efficient to minimize time spent receiving such treatment.

Surgical intervention may still play a beneficial role in some patients with esophageal carcinoma who present with acute perforation, pulmonary complications from fistulae, or dysphagia unresponsive to endoscopic or other less invasive means, assuming they are acceptable operative candidates with a reasonable predicted survival. Esophageal surgeons should be familiar with potential surgical options for when such situations arise but they should also understand that while palliative esophagectomy and bypass techniques can effectively relieve symptoms, morbidity and mortality rates are high, ranging from 50% to 60% and 0% to 40% respectively (2,5–10). It is imperative that the surgeon have a lengthy, informative discussion with the patient, family, and multidisciplinary team preoperatively so that expectations are realistic.

PALLIATIVE ESOPHAGECTOMY

Currently, palliative resection using a standard esophagectomy approach is not typically considered in patients with distant metastases due to a short life expectancy and the high inherent morbidity and mortality associated with the procedure. Patients with locally advanced unresectable tumors, who do not show evidence of metastatic disease, are also better treated with less invasive means that do not threaten the loss of potentially curative interventions down the road. Resection in these patients is technically challenging and does not improve survival or quality of life. Only in exceptional circumstances should primary resection be performed as a palliative procedure.

PALLIATIVE BYPASS

Although now largely of historic interest, multiple techniques for esophageal bypass have been described. Heimlich and Postlethwait both described using a greater curvature gastric tube as a conduit (11,12). Heimlich preferred a reversed graft, brought in a retrosternal fashion, with an anastomosis in the neck to the cervical esophagus (Figure 89.1). Postlethwait described a similar procedure but postulated that a nonreversed, isoperistaltic tube was more physiologic. Korst and Ginsberg describe using the entire stomach as a gastric tube and excluding the esophagus both proximally and distally (Figure 89.2) (13). In addition, portions of the colon can be used as a conduit to the neck if gastric transposition is not possible. Korst and Ginsberg prefer an isoperistaltic left colon transplant placed in the retrosternal position and based on a left colic arterial pedicle (13).

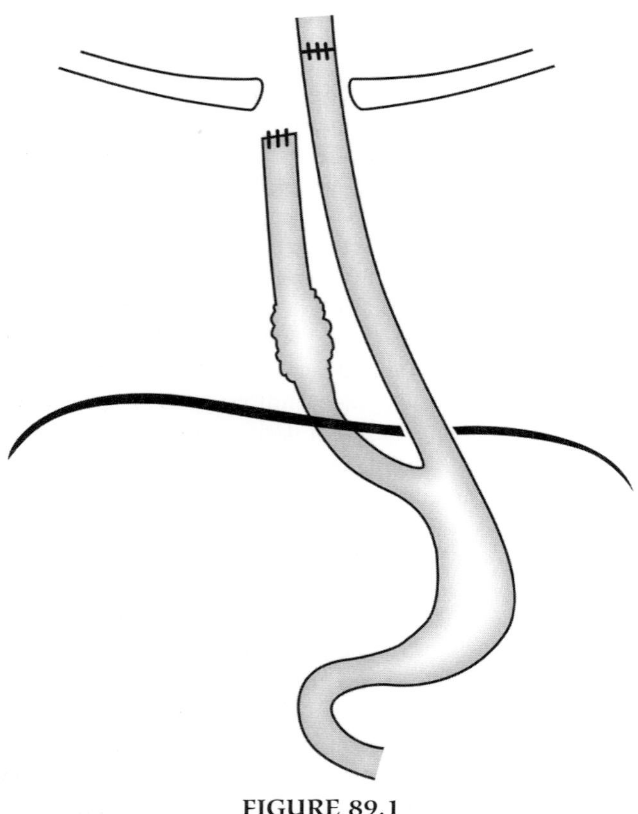

FIGURE 89.1

Retrosternal reversed gastric tube bypass with cervical anastomosis. Illustration by Mark A. Dunst.

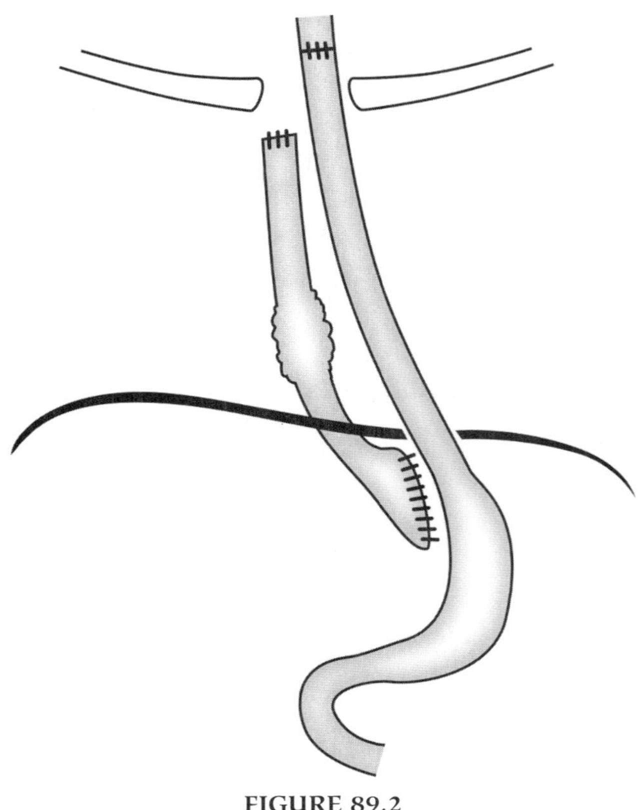

FIGURE 89.2

Retrosternal gastric conduit bypass with total esophageal exclusion. Illustration by Mark A. Dunst.

Techniques that bypass esophageal tumors to the intrathoracic esophagus have also been reported. Kirschner described an intrathoracic gastric bypass with exclusion of the thoracic esophagus proximal to the tumor and distal drainage into a loop of jejunum (Figure 89.3) (14). Ong slightly modified the procedure by using a jejunal conduit and Roux-en-Y configuration, a particularly useful operation for tumors at the gastroesophageal junction (Figure 89.4) (15). This palliative bypass operation has been used in recent reports, and despite improvements in patient selection and postoperative care, morbidity and mortality rates remain excessively high (2,5,6,8). Additional concern for the potential morbidity associated with an anastomotic breakdown in the chest is present when considering these techniques compared to those options that utilize a cervical anastomosis. However, adequate length of the gastric conduit to reach the neck is not always available, and jejunal segments do not work as well with a cervical anastomosis due to its tenuous blood supply.

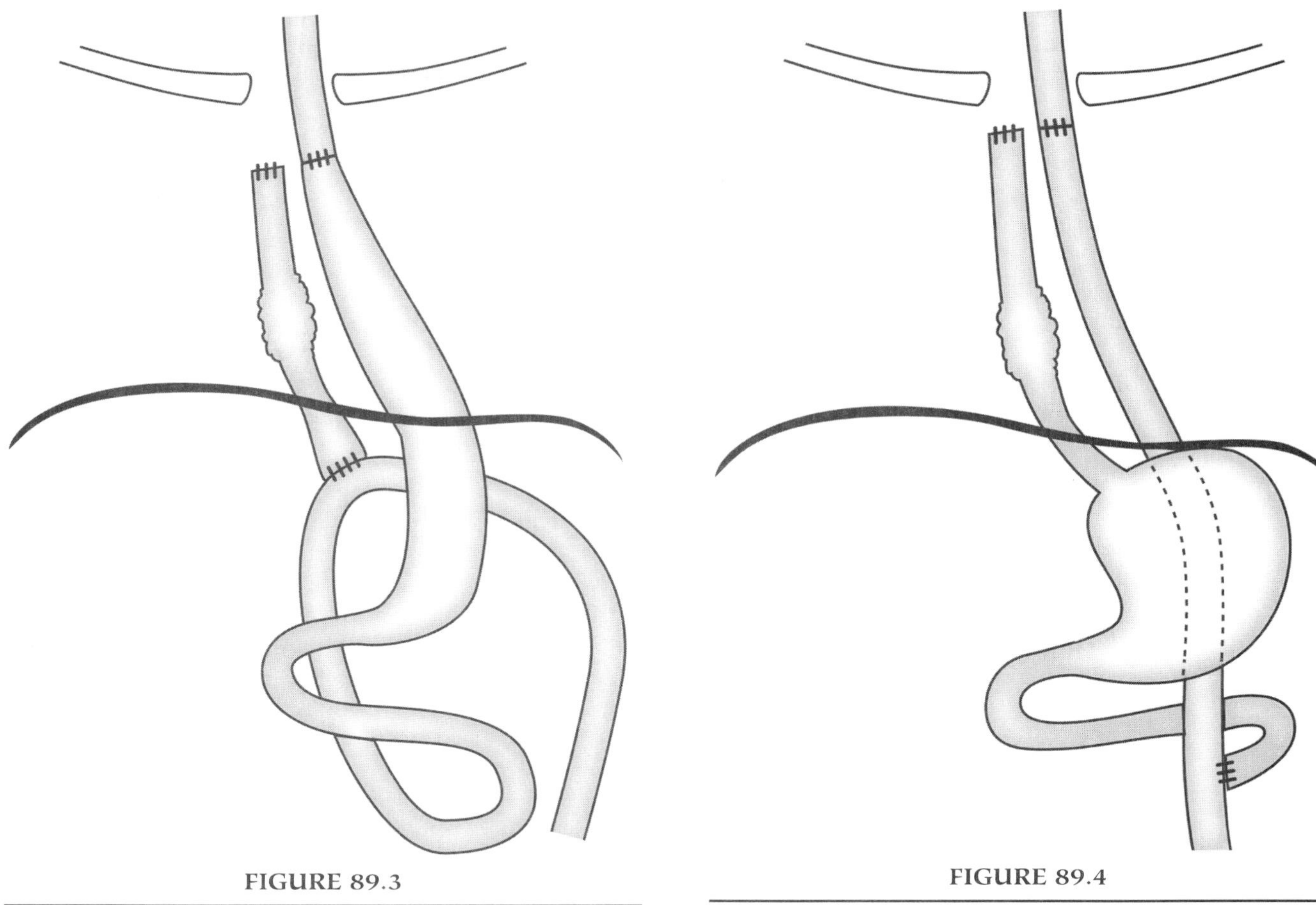

FIGURE 89.3

Intrathoracic gastric bypass with exclusion of the thoracic esophagus proximal to the tumor and distal drainage into a loop of jejunum. Illustration by Mark A. Dunst.

FIGURE 89.4

Intrathoracic jejunal Roux-en-Y bypass. Illustration by Mark A. Dunst.

Another option includes the fundal bypass as described by Popovsky, in which the fundus of the stomach is connected to the distal esophagus (Figure 89.5) (16). This technique can be useful to bypass tumors limited to the gastroesophageal junction and may eliminate the truly intrathoracic suture line and associated complications.

Overall, while these operations are creative and can have excellent palliative results, typical morbidity and mortality rates remain too high to justify their use over current less invasive measures. Even those who regularly performed bypass operations in the past have come to abandon them (17).

FEEDING GASTROSTOMY AND JEJUNOSTOMY

Probably the most applicable operation a surgeon can offer in the palliation of esophageal cancer is that of feeding tube placement. Gastrostomy or jejunostomy tubes placed percutaneously, laparoscopically, or open, can act as a useful adjunct to other palliative procedures. These procedures are rather simple, can be performed with minimal morbidity, and can improve quality of life by improving nutritional status and strength.

CONCLUSION

Whereas surgery was once our only option, advancements in endoscopic techniques and chemoradiation have greatly added to our armamentarium for palliation of esophageal cancer. The role of palliative surgery for this devastating disease has clearly diminished with the introduction of self-expanding metal esophageal stents, photodynamic therapy, and undeniable improvements in the effectiveness of current chemoradiation protocols. Though surgical palliative techniques, such as esophageal bypass, are durable and

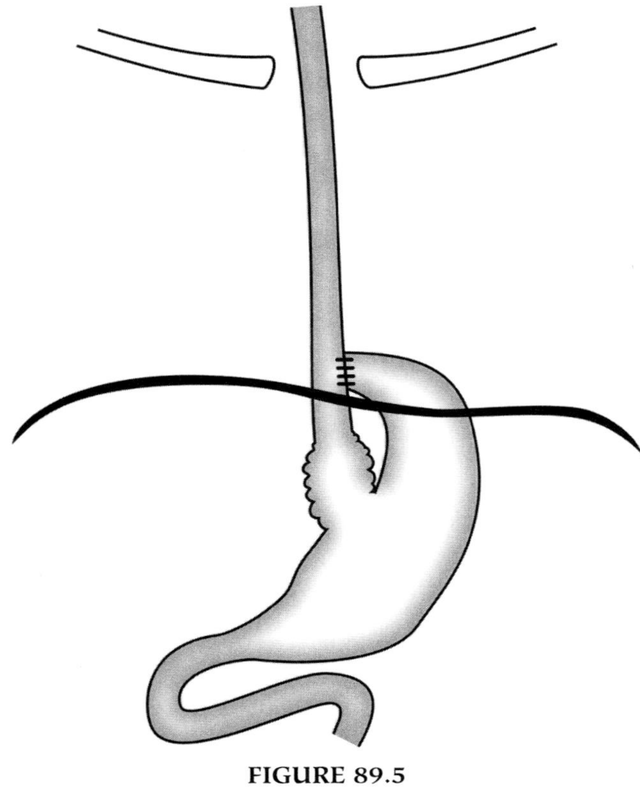

FIGURE 89.5

Distal esophageal fundal bypass. Illustration by Mark A. Dunst.

can improve quality of life, the morbidity and mortality rates are too high to justify their regular use. Only in rare circumstances should the esophageal surgeon consider major noncurative surgery in a patient with a limited life expectancy, and only after a lengthy informative discussion with the patient and multidisciplinary team, in which the appropriate expectations are set.

References

1. Younes M, Henson, DE, Ertan A, et al. Incidence and survival trends of esophageal carcinoma in the United States: racial and gender differences by histological type. *Scand J Gastroenterol.* 2002;37(12):1359–1365.
2. Aoki T, Osaka Y, Takagi Y, et al. Comparative study of self-expandable metallic stent and bypass surgery for inoperable esophageal cancer. *Dis Esophagus.* 2001; 14(3–4):208–211.
3. Ferrante G, De Palma G, Elia S, et al. Endoscopic and surgical palliation of esophageal cancer. *Minerva Gastroenterol Dietol.* 1999;45(4):233–244.
4. Frenken M. Best palliation in esophageal cancer: surgery, stenting, radiation, or what? *Dis Esophagus.* 2001;14(2):120–123.
5. Meunier B, Spiliopoulos Y, Stasik C, et al. Retrosternal bypass operation for unrespectable squamous cell cancer of the esophagus. *Ann Thorac Surg.* 1996; 62(2):373–377.
6. Meunier B, Stasik C, Raoul JL, et al. Gastric bypass for malignant esophagotracheal fistula: a series of 21 cases. *Eur J Cardiothorac Surg.* 1998;13(2):184–188.
7. Seto Y, Yamada K, Fukuda T, et al. Esophageal bypass using a gastric tube and a cardiostomy for malignant esophagorespiratory fistula. *Am J Surg.* 2007;193(6):792–793.
8. Whooley BP, Law S, Murthy SC, et al. The Kirschner operation in unrespectable esophageal cancer: current application. *Arch Surg.* 2002;137(11):1228–1232.
9. Segalin A, Little AG, Ruol A, et al. Surgical and endoscopic palliation of esophageal carcinoma. *Ann Thorac Surg.* 1989;48(2):267–271.
10. Mannell A, Becker PJ, Nissenbaum M. Bypass surgery for unrespectable oesophageal cancer: early and late results in 124 cases. *Br J Surg.* 1988;75(3):283–286.
11. Heimlich HJ. Reversed gastric tube (RGT) esophagoplasty for failure of colon, jejunum, and prosthetic interpositions. *Ann Surg.* 1975;182(2):154–160.
12. Postlethwait RW. Technique for isoperistaltic gastric tube for esophageal bypass. *Ann Surg.* 1979;189(6):673–676.
13. Korst RJ, Ginsberg RJ. Surgical palliation of inoperable carcinoma of the esophagus. In: Shields TW, ed. *General Thoracic Surgery*, 6th ed. Philadelphia: Lippincott, Williams and Wilkins; 2005.
14. Kirschner MB. Ein neues Verfahren der Oesophagoplastik. *Arch Klin Chir.* 1920; 114:606.
15. Ong GB. The Kirschner operation—a forgotten procedure. *Br J Surg.* 1973;60(3):221–227.
16. Popovsky J. Esophagogastrostomy in continuity for carcinoma of the esophagus. Its use for unrespectable tumors of the lower third of the esophagus and cardia. *Arch Surg.* 1980;115(5):637–639.
17. Orringer MB. Substernal gastric bypass of the excluded esophagus-results of an ill-advised operation. *Surgery.* 1984;96(3):467–470.

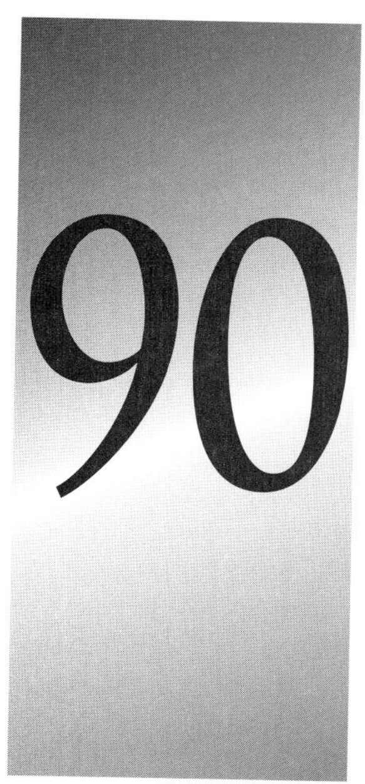

90 Perforated Esophageal Cancer

Lyall A. Gorenstein
Joshua R. Sonett

Perforation of esophageal carcinoma is a life-threatening complication that occurs most frequently during instrumentation of the esophagus. Fortunately, the incidence is low, affecting less than 1% of esophageal cancers. Perforated esophageal cancer is seen in a heterogeneous population of patients that spans a spectrum of prognoses from those with potentially resectable and curable cancers, to those with metastatic disease for whom comfort measures may be the appropriate therapy. Between these 2 extremes are the majority of patients with esophageal cancer. Locally advanced disease may preclude consideration of a curative resection, yet effective non-surgical, treatments can potentially afford prolonged survival. A clinically evident acute esophageal perforation if left untreated is uniformly fatal.

Ideally, a patient with a localized potentially curable cancer and an acute esophageal perforation should undergo urgent esophagectomy and reconstruction. When performed soon after the perforation, the operative mortality is no different than following elective esophagectomy (1–4). However, more often than not, the patients who encounter this complication have locally advanced unresectable tumors, metastatic disease, or severe comorbidities that preclude resection. In this situation, the management of this condition will be determined by several factors including stage of disease, patient comorbidities, the general condition of the patient, time interval to diagnosis, and the technical expertise that is available.

The management of patients with perforated esophageal cancers must therefore be individualized. Treatment options include resection with or without a primary anastomosis, self-expandable covered stents, drainage of the mediastinum or pleural space, or, occasionally, no treatment (23). It may be necessary to combine treatments, i.e., draining the mediastinum or an empyema after placing a self-expanding covered stent across the esophageal perforation (5–7). There are several factors that need to be assessed before instituting definitive therapy, including the site of the perforation, the stage of the cancer, the patient's associated comorbidities and what cancer-related treatment may already have been administered.

ETIOLOGY

Most perforations of esophageal cancers are iatrogenic and occur during attempted dilation, stent insertion, or laser ablation of locally advanced non-resectable tumors (6–8). Tumors arising in the upper or middle thirds of the esophagus that involve the entire thickness of the esophagus or that invade other mediastinal structures are at greater risk of perforation during attempted dilations (6).

Although the risk of esophageal perforation during stent placement for obstructing esophageal cancers is less than 2% (8–12), this accounts for over 40% iatrogenic injuries. Self-expanding stents, which for the most part have replaced the older plastic prostheses, have significantly reduced the incidence of esophageal perforation (8).

Esophageal perforations can also occur during attempted dilation or biopsy during endoscopic evaluation of a patient with an obstructing esophageal cancer. The incidence of perforation during esophageal dilation is approximately 1% to 2% (8–13). Perforations due to esophageal dilation accounts for 20% of esophageal cancer perforations. The liberal use of dilators placed over a guide wire seems to reduce the risk of perforation (9). Spontaneous perforation (Boerhaave's syndrome) of the esophagus in the setting of an underlying cancer, though much less frequent, can also occur (13,14). In patients undergoing active treatment, radiation therapy can lead to rapid tumor necrosis and esophageal perforation resulting in mediastinitis, or fistula formation into other mediastinal structures such as the trachea or aorta (15).

INITIAL MANAGEMENT

It is essential that the diagnosis of esophageal perforation be made expeditiously and resuscitation and treatment be instituted quickly, to afford the best opportunity for a successful outcome. This includes intravenous resuscitation and broad spectrum antibiotic therapy covering oral flora including Candida species. Intravenous H2-blockers or proton pump inhibitors may also be given to reduce acid content and decrease the inflammatory mediastinitis that ensues. Esophageal perforation after instrumentation is often suspected because of technical problems occurring during the procedure. The endoscopist may recognize the perforation before concluding the procedure and, in fact, may be able to manage the perforation with a self-expanding covered stent (7).

More frequently however, a perforation is diagnosed several hours after the injury has occurred. The patient often complains of chest pain, odynophagia, or worsening dysphagia. An upright chest X-ray may show mediastinal emphysema, subcutaneous emphysema, free intraperitoneal air, or a pleural effusion. If the diagnosis of esophageal perforation is suspected only after the endoscopy has been completed, a dilute barium study should be obtained. Gastrograffin may be used as the initial contrast agent but dilute barium more accurately identifies a perforation and defines whether the leak is generalized or contained. Esophagram provides key information regarding the severity and location of the perforation. If there is extension into both pleural spaces, this indicates a more severe injury. Pleural drainage as well as urgent management of the perforation is required.

Often patients with unresectable tumors receive high-dose radiotherapy either alone or combined with systemic therapy. If a radiation stricture develops, dilatations or stenting may be required to palliate dysphagia. Dilatation of a posttreatment stricture may produce a micro perforation, which clinically can mimic a full thickness perforation. The patient usually will complain of pain, and an upright chest X-ray or CAT scan may show mediastinal emphysema. The esophagram provides key information regarding the severity and location of the perforation. The study may be normal, or demonstrate a small fistula or contained leak within the densely scarred mediastinum. If there is no communication with the pleural space, the patient can be managed conservatively, with antibiotics and intravenous fluids. Provided the patient remains clinically well, the esophagram should be repeated after several days, and if unchanged, oral intake can resume.

The esophagram can also provide important information about the site of the perforation. Dilation of gastroesophageal junction (GEJ) tumors can perforate into the peritoneal cavity. Free intraperitoneal air may be present on an upright chest X-ray; however, because this type of perforation occurs more commonly in the lesser sac, only an esophagram will demonstrate the abdominal extension.

Contrast-enhanced computed tomography (CT scan) of the chest and upper abdomen may be necessary to evaluate a patient with a perforated esophageal cancer. If resection is being contemplated, and a CT scan was not done before the perforation, then urgent staging is necessary to exclude metastatic disease to the liver, lungs, or regional lymph nodes that may preclude a curative resection. Although endoscopic ultrasound usually plays a key role on the management in the preoperative staging of patients with esophageal cancer, there is no need to delay definitive management in a patient with an otherwise resectable tumor. Adequate staging can be achieved by simple endoscopic examination of the tumor and a contrast-enhanced CT scan to exclude the presence of metastasis. In patients in whom the injury was not recognized initially and presents with signs of sepsis, a CT scan is crucial in management. This can demonstrate the extent of pleural or mediastinal contamination and can also guide drainage procedures.

SURGICAL MANAGEMENT OF ESOPHAGEAL PERFORATION

Surgical resection of an acutely perforated esophagus can be performed with similar morbidity and mortality as an elective resection (1–3). The decision to resect the perforated esophagus rather than place a self-expanding stent depends on several factors. The tumor must be localized and resectable by CAT criteria, and the patient should be reasonably fit. Advantages to this approach include elimination of a source for ongoing mediastinal and pleural contamination should the stent fail to completely cover the perforation, and providing a potentially curative treatment. In the patient with an early stage cancer, in which the perforation is treated successfully with a stent, delayed resection is technically more complicated because of the mediastinal reaction that results from the injury. Another theoretical disadvantage to delayed resection is dissemination of tumor into the mediastinum; therefore, patients with operable cancers should undergo immediate resection.

There are 2 potential surgical approaches for patients with operable esophageal cancers: a transhiatal esophagectomy or a transthoracic esophagectomy. The decision as to which to use will depend on several factors including location of the tumor, degree of contamination, stability of the patient, and surgical expertise. In a patient with a tumor arising at the GEJ, in whom the diagnosis is made early and there is no hemodynamic instability, the transhiatal route is acceptable (1,2). Often the pleural spaces will be opened during the resection, and chest tubes drainage is required. In a patient with a large, bulky, mid- or distal esophageal cancer in which there is extensive contamination of the pleural space, or mild hemodynamic instability, a transthoracic approach is safest.

Reconstruction can usually be performed with the stomach at the time of resection. In the acute setting, colonic or jejunal interposition is hazardous and should be avoided. If the stomach is not available, than delayed reconstruction with colon several months later should be done. When there is little contamination of the mediastinum and pleura, the stomach can be placed in the esophageal bed. If the diagnosis of a perforation is delayed, and there is extensive contamination of the medistinum, than a substernal route is preferable, thereby eliminating the risk of the gastric staple line breaking down should an abscess develop in the mediastinum. Our preference is to place the esophagogastric anastomosis in the neck, regardless if a transthoracic or transhiatal resection is performed. An intrathoracic anastomosis is inherently at greater risk to leak postoperatively, if the mediastinum has been contaminated. Placing the anastomosis in the neck, out of the mediastinum, reduces the risk of postoperative mediastinitis should the anastomosis fail to heal primarily.

Another option when dealing with a perforated esophageal cancer in a hemodynamically unstable patient is resection without reconstruction, for which there are 2 surgical options. The stomach can be transposed to the neck and a cervical esophagostomy created. Over the next 1 to 2 weeks, scarring between the stomach and surrounding soft tissues closes any potential communication between the neck and the mediastinum. An anastomosis can than be created, without fear that an anastomotic leak may extend down into the mediastinum. Another option in the severely hemodynamically unstable patient is to perform the resection while leaving the stomach in the peritoneal cavity decompressed with a gastrostomy tube and creating a cervical esophagostomy. Delayed reconstruction several months later will require placing the stomach in a substernal location. Though a less ideal location for a gastric conduit compared to the esophageal bed, this is the safest approach in an acutely septic patient. Delayed reconstruction is also appropriate if the viability of the stomach is questionable. The overall mortality in patients undergoing resection and reconstruction is approximately 6% to 10% (1–3,5,17), which is not significantly greater than following elective esophagectomy. Obviously the surgical survival in these small series is skewed by patient selection.

Another option is esophageal exclusion. Rather than resecting the diseased esophagus, a diversion is performed, which theoretically eliminates persistent mediastinal contamination. Different diversion techniques are described whereby diversion is either complete, by dividing the esophagus in the neck and in the abdomen, or partial, when a cervical stoma is created but the esophagus is not divided. These diversion procedures are primarily aimed at managing a benign perforated esophagus, in which primary repair is hazardous because of extensive mediastinal contamination. The need for esophageal diversion occurs most commonly following spontaneous esophageal rupture, in which the diagnosis is delayed. Since most malignant esophageal perforations are iatrogenic, and diagnosed promptly, the need for a diversion procedure is uncommon. However, a situation may arise in that a patient with a potentially resectable perforated esophageal cancer has persistent ongoing mediastinal sepsis, and conservative maneuvers such as stenting and mediastinal drainage have failed to control the leak. Often, in this situation, sepsis has persisted for some time, the mediastinum may be severely inflamed, and resection is no longer a safe option. A diversion procedure performed as a last resort may be life saving. Mortality rates exceed 50% when esophageal diversion is performed for perforated esophageal cancer (17,20–22). However, the high mortality associated with diversion techniques is a reflection of the critical status of these patients, not of the technical approach.

STENTING PERFORATED ESOPHAGEAL CANCERS

With the development of self-expanding covered metal stents (SEMS), the role of stents in managing patients with iatrogenic esophageal perforations has increased, especially in patients with malignancy. To occlude a perforation successfully, a stent must be able to exert sufficient radial force against the wall of the esophagus. Perforations that occur in benign diseases often lack a suitable "shelf" to seat the prosthesis, and migration of the prosthesis is common, whereas in malignant strictures, there is usually an adequate narrowing to achieve a tight seal against the esophageal wall. Because SEMS easily conform to shape of the esophagus, they are more likely to seal the perforation than older rigid plastic stents. When dealing with a perforation, placing a SEMS is less traumatic and more likely effective in occluding the perforation than a rigid plastic stent, which lacks the flexible conforming characteristics of a SEMS (6–8,12–14).

There are several inherent advantages of early stenting. If recognized during the initial procedure, placing a stent reduces mediastinal contamination and may eliminate the need for pleural drainage. An esophageal stent does not preclude further therapy. Neoadjuvant chemotherapy, radiation therapy, or even surgical resection are not contraindicated by the presence of a stent. Once placed, an esophagram should be obtained immediately to confirm successful occlusion of the perforation. Intravenous antibiotics should be administered for several days, and feeding can resume after the esophagram confirms the leak is sealed.

Successful occlusion of an esophageal perforation with a SEMS is dependent on several factors. Mid-esophageal cancers, which more often are squamous cell lesions, provide a better shelf, often have a region of normal esophagus above and below the tumor, and therefore the stent can achieve a better seal. Overlapping stents may be necessary for long tumors. Tumors arising in the GEJ are more difficult to treat, and tumors that have been previously treated with either chemotherapy or radiation may be harder to stent, unless there is sufficient narrowing or a firm posttreatment stricture. If the perforation occurs in the proximal esophagus, remote from the tumor, stenting is unlikely to succeed. Technical experience in placing these stents in the non-emergent situation is certainly advantageous. Reported successful occlusion of malignant perforations with SEMS ranges from 80% to 100%. Despite technical success in placing SEMS across malignant esophageal perforations, the 30-day mortality rate exceeds 25% (6–8,10,12–19). Though this seems high, considering the often-encountered medical comorbidities and extensive locoregional malignant burden in this patient population, survival with SEMS is comparable if not superior to any surgical intervention. It is difficult to compare the results of emergent esophagectomy to SEMS in patients with malignant esophageal perforations, since the patients treated with stents are usually determined to be inoperable because of locally advanced disease. SEMS has replaced emergent esophagectomy or non-operative management in poor risk patients. Older surgical series, prior to SEMS being widely available to treat esophageal perforations, report surgical mortality in unselected patients following emergent esophagectomy in excess of 50% (20–23).

CONCLUSION

Patients with esophageal cancer and an acute esophageal perforation are a complex and heterogeneous group of patients, and treatment must be individualized. Esophageal perforation, left untreated, is a life-threatening complication, which must be acted on quickly if the patient is to survive. Despite aggressive intervention, mortality is high following either insertion of a SEMS or with surgical resection. Many factors need to be evaluated in deciding how best to manage these patients. The following algorithm should be considered:

- Emergent resection should be performed if the patient is a good operative risk, the tumor is localized, and resection is potentially curable.
- In the poor-risk patient, or if the tumor is unresectable, then attempt to place a SEMS across the perforation.
- If the esophageal perforation is recognized during attempted dilatation or stent placement, SEMS should be inserted across the perforation if technically feasible.
- An esophagram is performed following insertion of the SEMS.
- If a persistent leak is seen, a second stent telescoped into the original stent may control the leak. Mediastinal or pleural drainage will be required. Consider emergent resection.
- After placement of a SEMS, any pleural or mediastinal collections should be drained.
- Esophageal diversion is reserved for the very infrequent situation in which a patient with an operable cancer has severe sepsis that precludes resection.

References

1. MacGillivary MC, Etienne HB, Snyder DA, et al. Transhiatal esophagectomy in the management of perforated esophageal cancer. *Military Med*. 1991;156: 634–636.
2. Gupta NM. Emergency transhiatal esophagectomy for instrumental perforation of an obstructed thoracic esophagus. *Br J Surg*. 1996;83(7):1007–1009.
3. Mathews HR, Mitchell IM, McGuigan MA, et al. Emergency subtotal esophagectomy. *Br J Surg*. 1989;76(9):918–920.
4. Adam DJ, Thompson AM, Walker WS, et al. Esophagectomy for iatrogenic perforation of esophageal and cardia carcinoma. *Br. J Surg*. 1996;83(10):1429–1432.
5. Gupta NM, Kaman L. Personal management of 57 consecutive patients with esophageal perforation. *Am J Surg*. 2004;187(1):58–63.
6. Ferguson MK. Esophageal perforation and caustic injury. *Dis Esophagus*. 1997;10:90–94.

7. Johnsson E, Lundell L, Liedman B, et al. Sealing of esophageal perforations or ruptures with expandable metallic stents: a prospective controlled study on treatment efficacy and limitations. *Dis Esophagus*. 2005;18(4);262–266.
8. White RE, Mungatana C, et al. Expandable stents for iatrogenic perforation of esophageal malignancies. *J Gastrointest Surg*. 2003;7:715–720.
9. Boyce HW Jr. Palliation of dysphagia of esophageal cancer by endoscopic lumen restoration techniques. *Cancer Control J*. 1999;6:73–83.
10. Savage AP, Baigrie RJ, et al. Palliation of malignant dysphagia by laser therapy. *Dis Esophagus*. 1997;10:243–246.
11. Bisgaard T, Wajdemann M, Heindorff H, et al. Nonsurgical treatment of esophageal perforations after endoscopic palliation in advanced esophageal cancer. *Endoscopy*. 1197;29(3):155–159.
12. Warren WH. Palliation of dysphagia. *Chest Surg Clin North Am*. 2000;10(3);605–623.
13. Ferri L, Lee JK, Law S, et al. Management of spontaneous perforation of esophageal cancer with covered self-expanding metallic stents. *Dis Esophagus*. 2005;18(1):67–69.
14. Morgan RA, Ellul JP, Denton ER, et al. Malignant esophageal fistulas or perforations: management with plastic covered metallic prostheses. *Radiology*. 1997;204(2):527–532.
15. Mohri N, Akamo Y, Takeyama H, et al. Successful drainage of a mediastinal abscess via an esophago-mediastinal fistula complicating radiotherapy for esophageal cancer: a case report. *Asian J Surg*. 2002;25(1):98–101.
16. Richardson JD. Management of esophageal perforations: the value of aggressive surgical treatment. *Am J Surg*. 2005;190(2):161–165.
17. Watkinson A, Ellul J, Entwisle K, et al. Plastic covered metallic endoprosthesis in the management of esophageal perforation in patients with esophageal carcinoma. *Clin Radiol*. 1995;50(5):304–309.
18. Nicholson AA, Royston CMS, Wedgewood K, et al. Palliation of malignant esophageal perforation and proximal malignant dysphagia with covered metal stents. *Clin Radiol*. 1995;50:11–14.
19. Boyce HW Jr. Palliation of dysphagia of esophageal cancer by endoscopic lumen restoration techniques. *Cancer J*. 1999;6:73–78.
20. Michel L, Grillo HC, Malt RA. Operative and non-operative management of esophageal perforation. *Ann Surg*. 1981;194:57–63.
21. Reeder LB, DeFilippi VJ, Ferguson MK. Current results of therapy for esophageal perforation. *Am J Surg*. 1995;169:615–617.
22. Orringer MB, Sterling MC. Esophagectomy for esophageal disruption. *Ann Thorac Surg*. 1990;49:35–43.
23. Vogel SB, Rout WR, Martin TD, et al. Esophageal perforation in adults. Aggressive, conservative treatment lowers morbidity and mortality. *Ann Surg*. 2005;241: 1016–1023.

91 Radiation

Arta Monir Monjazeb
A. William Blackstock

Outcomes for esophageal cancer patients remain relatively bleak, as most patients present with advanced stages of disease. At presentation only about half of patients are candidates for curative therapy, due to metastatic disease, medical comorbidities, or poor performance status. The vast majority of patients are symptomatic from their disease. Over 90% of patients will have some degree of dysphagia and weight loss stemming from malignant stenosis. Other common symptoms include aspiration, which can result from either dysphagia or tracheoesophageal fistula, and pain. Since many patients are not candidates for curative treatment, palliation of these symptoms becomes an important clinical endpoint and critical to the patients' quality of life. Common palliative interventions include external beam radiotherapy, chemotherapy, enteral nutrition, analgesics, and a number of endoscopic procedures including dilatation, stenting, photodynamic therapy, argon plasma beam, and brachytherapy. These interventions are used both alone and in combination depending on the clinical scenario. The use of palliative esophagectomy is becoming increasingly uncommon given the morbidity and mortality of the procedure and the short life expectancy of these patients. Although a number of case series and prospective nonrandomized trials describing these various techniques have been published, there is a relative paucity of data comparing these techniques and providing guidance as to which intervention may be most appropriate for a given patient. Thus palliative intervention is largely dictated by the physician's discretion, the patient's desires, and institutional practices. A review of available data can, however, provide some general principles to guide our decision making. Many of these interventions are described in great detail in preceding chapters. The focus of this chapter is the administration of external beam radiotherapy (EBRT), either alone or in combination with other therapies, to palliate local symptoms of esophageal cancer. Palliative treatment of distant metastatic disease will not be discussed and should follow the same principles as treating metastatic disease of other origins.

DEFINING PALLIATIVE

Before deciding on a palliative modality, physicians must first decide which patients are appropriate candidates for palliative treatment and which should be treated with curative intent. Many criteria are used to help make this distinction, including operability, age, presence of metastatic disease, medical comorbidities, and performance status. A patient unable to have surgical intervention, either due to locally advanced disease that makes the tumor unresectable or the patient's inability to tolerate surgery, has traditionally been considered incurable. Over the past 2 decades, a number of studies have demonstrated modest but real long-term survival for patients treated with combined modality chemoradiotherapy (CRT) but without esophagectomy (1–3). In the Radiation Therapy Oncology Group (RTOG) 85–01 trial, 5-year overall survival was 26% among the 61 patients randomized to receive combined modality therapy (1). More recent data looking specifically at inoperable patients confirm these findings. In a retrospective review of 90 patients with inoperable esophageal cancer treated with concomitant cisplatin, 5-fluorouracil, and EBRT, Crosby et al. found a 26% 5-year overall survival rate (4). Similarly, a phase III randomized trial from India demonstrates a 5-year overall survival rate of 24.8% for patients with inoperable esophageal cancer treated with CRT (5). Two recent reports also indicate that even very elderly patients with multiple comorbidities who are poor surgical candidates can be treated with curative intent (6,7). In a prospective Japanese trial of Stage I and IIA patients aged 80 or older, Kawashima et al. report a 3-year overall survival of 39% with EBRT (66 Gy) alone (7). A series of 25 patients with a median age of 77 years (range 66–88) from Memorial Sloan-Kettering Cancer Center treated with CRT (5-fluorouracil, mitomycin-C, and EBRT 50.4 Gy) demonstrated a 2-year overall survival of 64% and median survival of 35 months (6). These results demonstrate that many patients may be treated with curative intent despite being inoperable, being of advanced age, or having multiple medical comorbidities. Patients may be appropriately classified as incurable if they have metastatic disease and/or locally advanced disease in conjunction with poor performance status that precludes aggressive intervention. Even in these palliative patients, a wide variety of treatment options have been reported ranging from combined modality therapy similar to that used with curative intent to supportive care alone. In a Swedish multivariate analysis of incurable esophageal cancer patients, both the presence of metastatic disease and the outcome of health-related quality of life surveys are found to strongly correlate with survival. The authors conclude that these factors can aid in the choice of palliative treatment strategy (8).

EXTERNAL BEAM RADIOTHERAPY

The most common symptom requiring palliation in esophageal cancer patients is dysphagia. Often used to palliate malignant dysphagia, EBRT has distinct advantages and disadvantages in comparison to other strategies. In a majority of patients, EBRT alone can provide effective palliation and can achieve durable responses often lasting many months. Palliation of dysphagia is achieved in 55% to 89% of patients treated with EBRT alone (Table 91.1). In contrast to many other palliative approaches, which often provide a short duration of relief and require repeated interventions (reviewed in 9), reports of EBRT with (10–12) or without chemotherapy (13–15) demonstrate median dysphagia-free intervals ranging from 5 to 11.5 months. Most patients (54%–67%) remain dysphagia free until death (10,13). Wara et al. reported on 103 patients who completed 5,000 to 6,000 cGy in 25 to 30 fractions, with 89% having symptomatic improvement and almost all patients reporting an arrest of their previous symptom progression (15). The average duration of palliation was 6.0 months, and 66% of patients maintained relief for at least 2 months. The dysphagia usually improved near the end of therapy.

Palliation can be achieved with EBRT doses ranging from 30 Gy to 64 Gy and various fractionation schemes have been described (Table 91.1). The delivered dose is determined in part by the patient's performance status and ability to tolerate EBRT. Two retrospective series have suggested a dose response for palliation of dysphagia (13,16). Caspers et al. treated 127 patients with unresectable or incurable tumors with EBRT alone (13). They found a 70.5% improvement in dysphagia with 54% of patients able to eat solids until death. The median overall survival and dysphagia-free interval were 7.4 months and 7.5 months respectively. They found that patients treated to doses ≥ 50 Gy had improved overall survival (8.3 vs. 4.8 months) and dysphagia-free interval (8.3 vs. 2.5 months) in comparison to patients treated to less than 50 Gy. This improvement in dysphagia-free interval was not seen for patients with passage scores less than or equal to 1 (unable to tolerate liquids or unable to tolerate any oral intake), and the authors conclude that elevated EBRT doses may not be beneficial to these patients. In another study, the percentage of patients able to tolerate oral intake of solids increased from 36% pretreatment to 68% with EBRT alone (16). Eighty-six percent of patients treated to doses > 45 Gy were able to tolerate solids in comparison to 55% of those receiving 45 Gy or less. The results of both studies should be interpreted with caution given their retrospective, nonrandomized nature. It is likely that healthier patients received more aggressive treatment, making these outcomes biased to some extent.

The treatment delivery technique for palliative EBRT is similar to that used in treatments with curative intent and is described in detail in preceding chapters. Briefly, the target volume is a 5 cm longitudinal and 2 cm radial margin on the primary tumor and a 2 cm radial margin on regional or involved nodes. Target volumes and inclusion of regional or involved nodes should be

TABLE 91.1
Palliation of Dysphagia with Radiotherapy or Chemoradiotherapy

Investigator	# of patients	Radiotherapy	Chemotherapy	Palliation of dysphagia (%)
Langer (32)	44	50–60 Gy	None	55%
Albertsson (16)	67	<45 Gy	None	55% (solids p.o.)
	43	>45 Gy	None	86% (solids p.o.)
Wara (15)	169	50–60 Gy	None	89%
Petrovich (33)	133	55 Gy	None	52%
Kassam (14)	39	40 Gy/20 fx bid	None	69%
Caspers (13)	127	Various	None	70%
Izquierdo (11)	25	50–60 Gy	CDDP/bleo (sequential)	64%
Whittington (34)	165	50–60 Gy	5-FU/MMC	87%
Kavanagh (35)	143	44–60 Gy	CDDP/carbo/VP-16/5-FU	71%
Coia (10)	120	50–60 Gy	5-FU/MMC	88%
Urba (18)	27	40 Gy / 20 fx bid split course	5-FU/carbo	59%
Seitz (12)	122	15 Gy / 5 fx x 3 courses (45 Gy total)	CDDP/5-FU	80%
Kumar (5)	60	66 Gy	None	73%
	65	66 Gy	CDDP	71%
Herskovic/Cooper (1)	62	64 Gy	None	68%
	67	50 Gy	CDDP/5-FU	58%
Roussel (19)	73	56.2 Gy	None	70%
	77	56.2 Gy	MTX	70%

Abbreviations: CDDP = Cisplatinum; 5-FU = 5-fluorouracil; MMC = Mitomycin-C; bleo = Bleomycin; carbo = Carboplatinum; MTX = Methotrexate; VP-16 = Etoposide.

tailored depending on the patient's symptoms, comorbidities, and performance status. Treatment is usually delivery using opposed AP/PA beams, followed by a boost utilizing obliqued fields that exclude the spinal cord after 45 Gy.

Disadvantages of EBRT in comparison to some other palliative strategies include long treatment duration, longer time to onset of symptom palliation, and increased risk of toxicity. Many fractionation schemes have been described attempting to reduce treatment duration for palliative patients. A recent phase I/II trial of 39 patients treated at Princess Margaret Hospital using accelerated fractionation radiotherapy (40 Gy/20 fractions twice a day over 2 weeks) demonstrated a dysphagia response rate of 69% with a median response duration of 5.5 months (14). As opposed to stenting, which can provide immediate symptom relief, EBRT can take 2 to 4 weeks to provide symptomatic response (10,14). With regard to toxicity, palliative EBRT can cause damage to any structure within the treatment field and side effects are similar to those discussed for EBRT with curative intent. Structures at risk may include the esophagus, spinal cord, lungs, heart, stomach, liver, and brachial plexus amongst others. Special care should be taken during treatment planning to minimize as much as possible the toxicity to these structures. Unfortunately, EBRT can cause a worsening of dysphagia symptoms. Transient and self-limited exacerbation of dysphagia due to esophagitis or peritumoral edema usually resolves shortly after treatment completion. Additionally, benign strictures can result from irradiation of esophageal cancers. O'Rourke et al. described a 30% incidence of benign stricture in a series of 80 patients treated with radiation alone, which usually developed 4 to 6 weeks after therapy (17). In 25 patients treated with CRT, Coia et al. observed a 12% incidence of benign strictures that responded to endoscopic dilatation (10).

COMBINED MODALITY TREATMENT: CHEMORADIOTHERAPY

Combined modality CRT is commonly employed in the management of patients. The role of CRT in the palliative setting is less clear. Aggressive radiotherapy and concurrent chemotherapy potentially increase morbidity in patients with incurable disease and a limited life span, but may offer a more effective means of palliation. Palliation of dysphagia is achieved in 59% to 88% of patients treated with CRT (Table 91.1). Coia et al. evaluated the swallowing function in 120 patients receiving mitomycin-C, 5-fluorouracil, and radiotherapy (10). Improvement in dysphagia was reported in 88%, with 67% remaining palliated until the time of death. Urba et al. reported that 59% of patients receiving chemotherapy and split course radiation therapy were able to achieve durable relief of their dysphagia symptoms (18).

RTOG 85–01, a randomized trial of definitive CRT versus EBRT, demonstrates an improvement in 5-year survival for patients treated with CRT (26% vs. 0%) (1). How these findings can be applied to patients treated with palliative intent is a matter of debate. Despite the improvement in survival, CRT does not improve the palliation of dysphagia in this study. Two other randomized studies comparing EBRT and CRT in patients treated with palliative intent report similar findings (5,19). In a recently published trial from India, 125 unresectable patients were randomized to receive EBRT (66 Gy / 33 fractions) alone or with concurrent weekly cisplatin. The authors report an improvement in median and 5-year overall survival (7.1 months vs. 13.4 months and 13.7% vs. 24.8%, respectively) but no significant difference in dysphagia relief (73% vs. 71%) (5). In a randomized trial of 150 palliative patients treated with EBRT (56.25 Gy / 18 fractions) with or without concurrent methotrexate, Roussel et al. (19) detected no difference in median survival (8–9 months) or dysphagia relief (70%). It should be noted that methotrexate is not commonly employed as a first-line agent in the modern-day management of esophageal cancer. A Cochrane Review published in 2008 examining comparing CRT with EBRT alone in the treatment of esophageal cancer only identified 4 randomized studies that reported outcomes on dysphagia relief (20). They found no significant difference in dysphagia relief between the 2 treatment arms. It can thus be concluded that combined modality treatment may improve survival but not dysphagia in comparison to EBRT alone in palliative esophageal cancer patients. Incurable patients can thus be offered CRT on the basis of improved survival if they are able to tolerate aggressive treatment with the understanding that it may exacerbate toxicity and provide no clear improvement of symptoms.

COMBINED MODALITY TREATMENT: RADIOTHERAPY AND OTHER PALLIATIVE INTERVENTIONS

Data comparing EBRT with other palliative modalities are relatively scarce. However, there are some studies examining EBRT in conjunction with or in contrast to other palliative modalities. Wong and colleagues published a case control study of patients with locally advanced or metastatic esophageal squamous cell cancer treated with CRT (36 patients) or endoscopic stenting (36 patients). The groups were well matched in regard to demographics, pretreatment dysphagia score, comorbidities, and tumor characteristics. Not surprisingly, patients receiving CRT had superior median (10.8 vs. 4.0 months) and 5-year survivals (15% vs. 0%). Additionally, only 22% of patients treated with CRT required salvage stenting as compared to 100% of patients treated initially with stenting. The authors suggest that in the palliative setting CRT provides superior survival and prolonged dysphagia palliation in comparison to stenting alone (21). Until a randomized trial addressing this question is performed, the results of this case control study with a small sample size should be interpreted cautiously.

The RTOG conducted a phase I/II study of CRT with an esophageal brachytherapy boost in 49 potentially curable patients (22). Patients received EBRT (50 Gy/25 fractions) with concurrent 5-fluorouracil and cisplatinum, followed by a brachytherapy boost 2 weeks later. The brachytherapy boost was delivered using high-dose rate (15 Gy/3 fractions) or low-dose rate (20 Gy/1 fraction). Patients survived a median of 11 months but there was a significant amount of treatment-related toxicity including 24% grade 4 toxicity, 12% fistula formation, and 10% treatment-related toxicity. A subsequent analysis found that 59% of patients had improved swallowing function (23). Given the toxicity of this strategy, it is not widely used in curative or palliative settings and the use of CRT or brachytherapy alone is much more common.

A retrospective review from Austria examined inoperable patients treated with radiotherapy (brachytherapy and/or EBRT) and/or photodynamic therapy (PDT) (24). Forty-four patients received combined modality therapy and 75 received radiotherapy alone. All patients had an improvement in dysphagia. The median survival for the entire cohort was 7.7 months and the rate of major complications was 9.2%. Survival by treatment groups was 5.6 months for brachytherapy alone, 7.7 months for brachytherapy and EBRT, 6.3 months for PDT and brachytherapy, and 13 months for brachytherapy and EBRT and PDT. Analysis of variance demonstrated a significant improvement for EBRT ($P = 0.0001$) and PDT ($P = 0.0129$).

A randomized prospective trial from India compared EBRT (55–65 Gy) and endoscopic dilatation/intubation versus endoscopic dilatation/intubation alone in 104 patients with stage III or IV disease (25). They found that EBRT improves both median survival (7 vs. 3 months) and quality of life as measured by Eastern Cooperative Oncology Group (ECOG), dysphagia, weight, and several other parameters.

Although no definitive conclusions can be drawn from these studies, they do provide precedence for combining EBRT or CRT with other palliative modalities and provide warning that any added efficacy of combined modality strategies may come at the expense of increased toxicity. Further study is needed to determine the safety and appropriateness of these combined modality treatment strategies.

TRACHEOESOPHAGEAL FISTULA

The development of a malignant fistulous tract between the esophagus and airway (trachea or bronchus) is relatively common because of the anatomic proximity of these 2 structures. Involvement of the trachea with tumor can lead to fistula formation during radiation because of necrosis of the tumor or natural disease progression. Some literature suggests that in cases of malignant fistula between the esophagus and the airway, treatment with radiation should be discontinued. In general, excision, bypass, stenting, or intubation have been recommended in an attempt to prevent further contamination of the airway and provide palliation (26).

Many oncologists accept that irradiation of a fistula worsens the condition because healing may be compromised by radiation. However, for patients who require palliation of a fistula but are otherwise curative candidates, the short survival conferred by supportive measures alone may be inappropriate. Survival following these limited measures can be as brief as 6 to 10 weeks with the procedures themselves resulting in a mortality rate of 10% to 32% (27). Burt et al. found the survival for patients with an untreated fistulous tract to be 4% at 6 months and 1% at 1 year versus 15% and 5% respectively if treated with irradiation (28). Yamada et al. reported on 14 patients with malignant fistulae treated with EBRT. Closure of the fistula occurred in 5 of 8 patients whose fistulae developed before or during radiation (29). A report from Mayo Clinic on 10 patients with fistulae treated with radiation observed a median survival of 4.8 months (30). They did not observe fistula exacerbation with EBRT. There are also some data for the safe use of chemotherapy and/or radiation in managing patients with a tracheoesophageal fistula. Malik et al. observed closure of the fistulae in 2 patients treated with chemoradiation and concluded that the presence of a fistula should not exclude a patient from receiving combined modality therapy (31).

At present, it is difficult to determine whether aggressive combined modality therapy will increase treatment-related morbidity in patients who present with airway/esophageal fistulae or develop them shortly after starting therapy. Palliation of a fistula in a patient treated with curative intent should include EBRT. Once the diagnosis of a fistulous tract into the airway is documented and the process is stabilized, we recommend proceeding with planned curative therapy for selected patients with localized disease. In patients who are incurable, palliation with surgery, expandable stents, or intubation may be more appropriate.

CONCLUSION

Many esophageal cancer patients present with advanced disease and/or poor performance status and are not candidates for curative treatment. The vast majority of patients are symptomatic from their disease and thus palliation is an important endpoint in the treatment of esophageal cancer. EBRT is effective and commonly employed for palliation of esophageal cancers. A number of other effective palliative modalities also exist. Continued advances in radiotherapy and other treatment modalities such as brachytherapy and endoscopic stenting will improve our ability to palliate patients with esophageal cancer. It remains to be determined how targeted therapies such as erlotinib and trastuzumab might be employed in the palliative setting.

There is a relative paucity of prospective randomized data that compare the various palliative strategies. Further studies are needed to help define which patients are most likely to benefit from each of these palliative strategies and when combined modalities should be used for palliation. Although definitive guidelines cannot be established, the available data combined with clinical judgment can provide some general themes to help tailor palliative strategies to each individual patient. For patients who can tolerate aggressive treatment and have a reasonable life expectancy, EBRT appears to provide the longest survival and most durable relief of dysphagia. The addition of chemotherapy may improve survival but it is unclear if it improves palliation of dysphagia. Thus, a relatively healthy patient treated with palliative intent due to a small burden of metastatic disease and mild dysphagia may be a good candidate for EBRT or CRT. If the same patient were to present with complete obstruction, EBRT alone would be inappropriate, as it may take several weeks to relieve dysphagia. In this scenario, enteral nutrition with a percutaneous gastrostomy tube or an endoscopic procedure such as stenting would be more appropriate to provide immediate palliation and then EBRT could be employed afterwards. For patients who have a poor performance status and cannot tolerate aggressive palliative measures, EBRT would be inappropriate and could promote a functional decline. Thus, with a proper assessment of the patient, their goals for treatment, and a thorough knowledge of the various palliative modalities available to achieve those goals, a palliative treatment strategy can be developed for each patient that can improve their quality of life and mitigate their symptoms.

References

1. Cooper JS, Guo MD, Herskovic A, et al. Chemoradiotherapy of locally advanced esophageal cancer: long-term follow-up of a prospective randomized trial (RTOG 85–01). Radiation Therapy Oncology Group. *JAMA.* 1999;281(17):1623–1627.
2. Minsky BD, Pajak TF, Ginsberg RJ, et al. INT 0123 (Radiation Therapy Oncology Group 94–05) phase III trial of combined-modality therapy for esophageal cancer: high-dose versus standard-dose radiation therapy. *J Clin Oncol.* 2002;20(5):1167–1174.
3. Stahl M, Stuschke M, Lehmann N, et al. Chemoradiation with and without surgery in patients with locally advanced squamous cell carcinoma of the esophagus. *J Clin Oncol.* 2005;23(10):2310–2317.
4. Crosby TD, Brewster AE, Borley A, et al. Definitive chemoradiation in patients with inoperable oesophageal carcinoma. *Br J Cancer.* 2004;90(1):70–75.
5. Kumar S, Dimri K, Khurana R, et al. A randomised trial of radiotherapy compared with cisplatin chemo-radiotherapy in patients with unresectable squamous cell cancer of the esophagus. *Radiother Oncol.* 2007;83(2):139–147.
6. Anderson SE, Minsky BD, Bains M, et al. Combined modality chemoradiation in elderly oesophageal cancer patients. *Br J Cancer.* 2007;96(12):1823–1827.
7. Kawashima M, Kagami Y, Toita T, et al. Prospective trial of radiotherapy for patients 80 years of age or older with squamous cell carcinoma of the thoracic esophagus. *Int J Radiat Oncol Biol Phys.* 2006;64(4):1112–1121.
8. Bergquist H, Johnsson A, Hammerlid E, et al. Factors predicting survival in patients with advanced oesophageal cancer: a prospective multicentre evaluation. *Aliment Pharmacol Ther.* 2008;27(5):385–395.
9. Homs MY, Kuipers EJ, Siersema PD. Palliative therapy. *J Surg Oncol.* 2005;92(3):246–256.
10. Coia LR, Soffen EM, Schultheiss TE, et al. Swallowing function in patients with esophageal cancer treated with concurrent radiation and chemotherapy. *Cancer.* 1993;71(2):281–286.
11. Izquierdo MA, Marcuello E, Gomez de SG, et al. Unresectable nonmetastatic squamous cell carcinoma of the esophagus managed by sequential chemotherapy (cisplatin and bleomycin) and radiation therapy. *Cancer.* 1993;71(2):287–292.
12. Seitz JF, Milan C, Giovannini M, et al. Concurrent concentrated radio-chemotherapy of epidermoid cancer of the esophagus. Long-term results of a phase II national multicenter trial in 122 non-operable patients (FFCD 8803) [in]. *Gastroenterol Clin Biol.* 2000;24(2):201–210.
13. Caspers RJ, Welvaart K, Verkes RJ, et al. The effect of radiotherapy on dysphagia and survival in patients with esophageal cancer. *Radiother Oncol.* 1988;12(1):15–23.
14. Kassam Z, Wong RK, Ringash J, et al. A phase I/II study to evaluate the toxicity and efficacy of accelerated fractionation radiotherapy for the palliation of dysphagia from carcinoma of the oesophagus. *Clin Oncol (R Coll Radiol).* 2008;20(1):53–60.
15. Wara WM, Mauch PM, Thomas AN, et al. Palliation for carcinoma of the esophagus. *Radiology.* 1976;121(3 Pt. 1):717–720.
16. Albertsson M, Ewers SB, Widmark H, et al. Evaluation of the palliative effect of radiotherapy for esophageal carcinoma. *Acta Oncol.* 1989;28(2):267–270.
17. O'Rourke IC, Tiver K, Bull C, et al. Swallowing performance after radiation therapy for carcinoma of the esophagus. *Cancer.* 1988;61(10):2022–2026.
18. Urba SG, Turrisi AT III. Split-course accelerated radiation therapy combined with carboplatin and 5-fluorouracil for palliation of metastatic or unresectable carcinoma of the esophagus. *Cancer.* 1995;75(2):435–439.
19. Roussel A, Bleiberg H, Dalesio O, et al. Palliative therapy of inoperable oesophageal carcinoma with radiotherapy and methotrexate: final results of a controlled clinical trial. *Int J Radiat Oncol Biol Phys.* 1989;16(1):67–72.
20. Wong R, Malthaner R. Combined chemotherapy and radiotherapy (without surgery) compared with radiotherapy alone in localized carcinoma of the esophagus. *Cochrane Database Syst Rev.* 2006;(1):CD002092.
21. Wong SK, Chiu PW, Leung SF, et al. Concurrent chemoradiotherapy or endoscopic stenting for advanced squamous cell carcinoma of esophagus: a case-control study. *Ann Surg Oncol.* 2008;15(2):576–582.
22. Gaspar LE, Winter K, Kocha WI, et al. A phase I/II study of external beam radiation, brachytherapy, and concurrent chemotherapy for patients with localized carcinoma of the esophagus (Radiation Therapy Oncology Group Study 9207): final report. *Cancer.* 2000;88(5):988–995.
23. Gaspar LE, Winter K, Kocha WI, et al. Swallowing function and weight change observed in a phase I/II study of external-beam radiation, brachytherapy and concurrent chemotherapy in localized cancer of the esophagus (RTOG 9207). *Cancer J.* 2001;7(5):388–394.
24. Maier A, Tomaselli F, Gebhard F, et al. Palliation of advanced esophageal carcinoma by photodynamic therapy and irradiation. *Ann Thorac Surg.* 2000;69(4):1006–1009.
25. Kharadi MY, Qadir A, Khan FA, et al. Comparative evaluation of therapeutic approaches in stage III and IV squamous cell carcinoma of the thoracic esophagus with conventional radiotherapy and endoscopic treatment in combination and endoscopic treatment alone: a randomized prospective trial. *Int J Radiat Oncol Biol Phys.* 1997;39(2):309–320.
26. Frenken M. Best palliation in esophageal cancer: surgery, stenting, radiation, or what? *Dis Esophagus.* 2001;14(2):120–123.
27. Little AG, Ferguson MK, DeMeester TR, et al. Esophageal carcinoma with respiratory tract fistula. *Cancer.* 1984;53(6):1322–1328.
28. Burt M, Diehl W, Martini N, et al. Malignant esophagorespiratory fistula: management options and survival. *Ann Thorac Surg.* 1991;52(6):1222–1228.
29. Yamada S, Takai Y, Ogawa Y, et al. Radiotherapy for malignant fistula to other tract. *Cancer.* 1989;64(5):1026–1028.
30. Gschossmann JM, Bonner JA, Foote RL, et al. Malignant tracheoesophageal fistula in patients with esophageal cancer. *Cancer.* 1993;72(5):1513–1521.
31. Malik SM, Krasnow SH, Wadleigh RG. Closure of tracheoesophageal fistulas with primary chemotherapy in patients with esophageal cancer. *Cancer.* 1994;73(5):1321–1323.
32. Langer M, Choi NC, Orlow E, et al. Radiation therapy alone or in combination with surgery in the treatment of carcinoma of the esophagus. *Cancer.* 1986;58(6):1208–1213.
33. Petrovich Z, Langholz B, Formenti S, et al. Management of carcinoma of the esophagus: the role of radiotherapy. *Am J Clin Oncol.* 1991;14(1):80–86.
34. Whittington R, Coia LR, Haller DG, et al. Adenocarcinoma of the esophagus and esophago-gastric junction: the effects of single and combined modalities on the survival and patterns of failure following treatment. *Int J Radiat Oncol Biol Phys.* 1990;19(3):593–603.
35. Kavanagh B, Anscher M, Leopold K, et al. Patterns of failure following combined modality therapy for esophageal cancer, 1984–1990. *Int J Radiat Oncol Biol Phys.* 1992;24(4):633–642.

VII

FUTURE DIRECTIONS

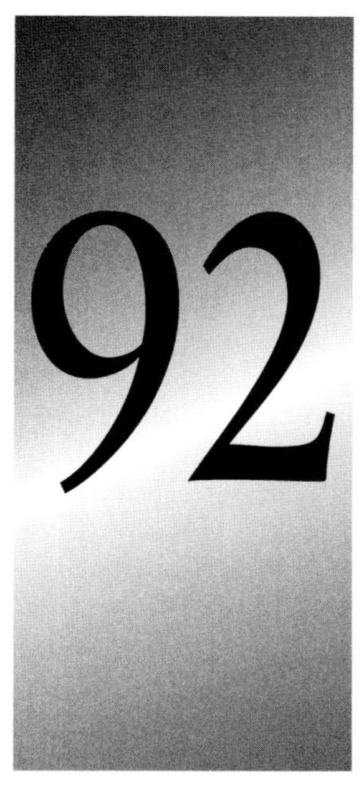

Molecular Outcome Prediction

Harry Yoon
Michael K. Gibson

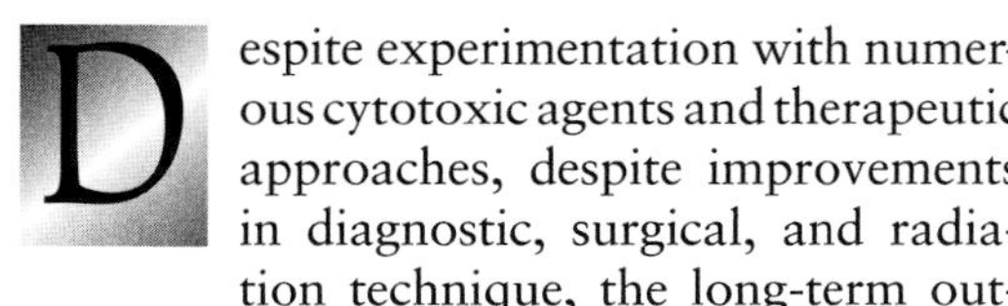

Despite experimentation with numerous cytotoxic agents and therapeutic approaches, despite improvements in diagnostic, surgical, and radiation technique, the long-term outcomes of patients with esophageal cancer remain poor and have improved only modestly in the last few decades. Moreover, the current standard approaches, which commonly involve a combination of surgery, chemotherapy, and radiation, cause considerable toxicity in the vast majority of patients. They are given empirically, with little foreknowledge of outcome. One method to improve outcomes in esophageal cancer is to select patients who are most likely to respond well to a particular therapeutic approach or agent. Such patient stratification holds the potential for maximizing efficacy and minimizing unnecessary toxicity.

Current methods of patient stratification—e.g., tumor grade, lymph node status, and other clinicopathologic traits—provide virtually no help in forecasting the efficacy of a particular therapy. Therefore, the identification of biologic or molecular predictors is a rational next step. The pursuit of identifying such predictive markers in esophageal cancer, though in its infancy, has generated a substantial and growing body of literature. In this chapter, we will try to organize this research vis-à-vis the potential for a marker to be validated in a clinical trial, a necessary step if it is to affect the practical management of patients. With this in mind, we will:

1. Discuss criteria for assessing markers and our approach to classification
2. Assess the literature on marker development in esophageal cancer
3. Discuss some challenges of integrating markers into clinical trials

CRITERIA FOR MARKER ASSESSMENT

The study of outcome markers in esophageal cancer has yielded a considerable body of literature, which is helpful in understanding biologic mechanisms, but somewhat unwieldy when considering how to apply it to the clinic. What confounds accessibility and classification of these data is the great variability across studies in overall design, outcome variables, laboratory methods, patient populations, and therapeutic approaches. This variability in turn complicates any attempt to translate these findings into the design of a prospective, potentially validating clinical trial—which, under current convention, is believed to be necessary before practical patient management is rationally altered.

Outcome markers may be assessed by many axes (e.g., lab method, study population demographics, histopathology, therapeutic approach, and promise as a therapeutic target), but three key axes may be less intuitive (Table 92.1):

1. Whether the marker has *predictive vs. prognostic* value (1). Prognostic and predictive markers differ based on their association with therapy. A marker is *prognostic* if it informs about outcome in the absence of systemic therapy or, if empiric therapy is given, portends an outcome different from that of patients who lack the marker. A simple example of a prognostic marker is cancer stage. On the other hand, a marker is *predictive* if it predicts the differential efficacy of a particular therapy based on marker status. One marker can be predictive, prognostic, both, or neither. A strong predictive marker, whether related to a known therapeutic target (e.g., HER2/neu amplification by fluorescence in situ hybridization [FISH]) or not, carries straightforward clinical implications and is therefore more helpful in patient management. On the other hand, the clinical implication of a prognostic, non-predictive marker—as in most studies in our discussion—is less straightforward. It partly depends on the efficacy/toxicity profiles of current and alternative therapies (see below, "Integration Into Clinical Trials: Challenges").
2. The *timing* of marker ascertainment—that is, before the therapy under question is initiated (most molecular markers fall in this category) versus afterward (e.g., serially, such as fluorodeoxyglucose (FDG)-positron emission tomography [FDG-PET] scan or prostate-specific antigen [PSA]). Disadvantages of marker ascertainment after the initiation of therapy include: (a) patients will have been subjected to toxic, potentially ineffective therapy before the marker is ascertained, (b) initial therapy (prior to marker ascertainment)

TABLE 92.1
Three Axes by Which to Assess Outcome Markers

Axes	Level	Definition	Potential implication in patient management	Example (standard or experimental)
Type	Predictive	Forecasts differently based on which therapy is given	Implies a particular therapeutic option	HER2/neu amplification by FISH in breast cancer implies administration of trastuzumab
	Prognostic	Forecasts differently based on presence vs. absence of marker (irrespective of therapy)	Depends on toxicity and efficacy of alternative therapy	13q deletion in multiple myeloma implies that patient should not undergo bone marrow transplant
Timing of ascertainment	Baseline	Marker obtained at diagnosis (often in pretreatment biopsy specimen)	Directs initial therapy	HER2/neu by FISH
	Serial	Marker obtained in the course of management (e.g., serial biopsies)	Directs management after initial therapy or period, and may serve as an outcome variable itself	• FDG-PET with CT • PSA • CA 125
Outcome variable (esophageal cancer)	pCR	Absence of tumor in the surgical specimen after preoperative therapy	Informs choice of preoperative therapy	NA[a]
	PFS or OS	Long-term outcome after curative neoadjuvant therapy and surgery	Informs choice of pre- or postoperative therapy	NA[a]

[a]In esophageal cancer, no molecular marker has been posited so far as an outcome variable, though the potential conceivably exists, if serially ascertained, for those listed in Tables 92.2 or 92.3. Molecular markers ascertained before preoperative therapy could be assessed against pCR, PFS, or OS, and those ascertained afterward against PFS or OS.
Abbreviations: FISH = fluorescence in situ hybridization; pCR = complete pathologic response; PFS = progression-free survival; OS = overall survival; PSA = prostate-specific antigen.

may theoretically render subsequent therapy less effective (e.g., drug resistance may increase, or a resectable tumor may become inoperable).

3. The particular *outcome variable* by which a marker has been gauged. Ultimately, the incorporation of a particular marker should improve, or promise to improve, a clinically meaningful outcome. All-cause or cancer-related mortality has typically been used as the gold standard outcome variable, because it is meaningful, easily measured, and discrete. However, mortality may be influenced by many factors unrelated to therapy and, as a result, may be too insensitive an outcome measure for assessing the value of a predictive marker. Therefore, complete pathologic response (pCR) rate in the setting of locally advanced esophageal cancer, repeatedly shown to correlate with long-term survival, may better reflect the efficacy of therapy. Some authors have suggested that pCR or overall survival may be used to gauge markers that are used to forecast the efficacy of neoadjuvant or adjuvant therapy, respectively (2).

CLASSIFICATION OF OUTCOME MARKERS

Tables 92.2 and 92.3 describe recent scientific efforts to identify molecular markers that predict outcome in esophageal cancer. The tables differ from one another by the type of *therapy* administered to the study population: chemoradiation followed, in most cases, by surgical resection (Table 92.2) vs. surgery with or without adjuvant therapy (Table 92.3). This division reflects the majority of outcome marker studies in esophageal cancer. We framed the information by treatment approach because, prior to a marker's integration in a large validation trial, it would need to demonstrate promise in a similar therapeutic setting. A marker that is predictive in one therapeutic setting may not generalize to a different one.

In neoadjuvant studies (Table 92.2), the marker is assessed at baseline (e.g., via the diagnostic biopsy specimen or blood) with the ultimate goal of tailoring neoadjuvant chemoradiation to an individual patient. Outcome variables specific to these studies are clinical response (commonly assessed radiographically or endoscopically) after chemoradiation and, if surgery occurred, the pCR rate. By contrast, in studies that use primary surgery followed by adjuvant treatment (Table 92.3), the marker is assessed at surgery (via the resection specimen or blood) and is intended to determine if and what type of chemotherapy should be given postoperatively. Outcome variables used in these studies—i.e., progression-free survival or overall survival—are general and may be used to assess neoadjuvant studies.

The neoadjuvant studies (Table 92.2) apply directly to the chemoradiotherapy followed by surgery, which is the dominant therapeutic approach in the United States. The studies using surgery upfront (Table 92.3) apply most closely to therapeutic settings where surgery is performed first or alone. However, one can argue they also apply to the neoadjuvant paradigm, to influence postoperative therapy, if the effects of neoadjuvant therapy minimally affect the marker.

Second, we emphasized the *lab method* used to assess the marker. The importance of the lab method is illustrated in lung cancer, where substantial variations exist in predictive value, cost, and accessibility when assessing epidermal growth factor receptor (EGFR) status by immunohistochemistry, mutational analysis, or gene copy number (3,4)—all of which affect the marker's ultimate relevance. Therefore, when discussing a marker, we will discuss it by a particular lab method whenever possible. In esophageal cancer, protein expression as evaluated by immunohistochemistry (IHC) was most widely used in earlier studies, despite its shortcomings (e.g., semi-quantitative, limited by antibody sensitivity). More recently, other molecular techniques have been refined or developed, with increasing practical applicability to the clinic, such as gene expression of a particular factor (5–7), genotyping (8), methods to evaluate methylation status (9,10), microarrays (11), and proteomics (12).

Third, we highlighted the *histopathology* of the study population. Squamous cell carcinoma and adenocarcinoma, the 2 dominant histotypes, appear to be distinct clinically, associated with different patterns of risk, recurrence, and perhaps chemosensitivity. As a result, a marker may apply to one histotype, but not the other. The predominance of squamous cell carcinoma in Asian populations is reflected in Asian outcome marker studies, whereas the dramatic rise of adenocarcinoma in the industrialized West is reflected in recent Western studies.

By framing the discussion this way, we hope to clarify the promise, and limitations, of marker development in esophageal cancer in its current state. Our approach has the drawback of de-emphasizing our understanding of biologic pathways (Table 92.4), which are crucial to the development of markers and new therapies, but which are well described elsewhere (2).

REVIEW OF MARKERS AND LIMITS IN INVESTIGATION

In sum, no single marker or panel of markers has emerged as a strong candidate for predicting response or survival. Molecules related to apoptosis (Table 92.4), particularly p53 (which itself also affects DNA repair and cell cycle regulation), comprise one of the most scrutinized groups, in both neoadjuvant- and primary-surgery settings. They have generally been inconsistent

TABLE 92.2

Results of Molecular Outcome Studies in Esophageal Cancer Patients Treated with Chemoradiation with or without Subsequent Surgery

							Association of predictor(s) with: *P Value*[b]			
									Overall survival	
No. of genes	**Lab method**	**Study (year)**	**N**	**AC/SCC (%)**	**Country**	**Predictor(s)**[a]	**Clin. resp.**	**pCR**	**UV**	**MV**
1 to 7	Immuno-histochemistry	Harpole (37) 2001	118	69/31	USA	MT		–	–[c]	–[c]
						GST-π		–	< 0.05[c]	0.07[c]
						P-gp		–	< 0.05[c]	0.08[c]
						TS		–	< 0.05[c]	–[c]
		Izzo (20) 2006	80	93/7	USA	**NF-kB**		0.006	0.009	0.007
		Abdel-Latif (21) 2004	58	100/0	Ireland	**NF-kB**		0.0001	< 0.05	0.07
		Sarbia (14) 1998[d]	38	0/100	Germany	p53	–		–	–
						Bcl-2	–		–	–
						Bcl-X_L	–		–	–
						Bax	–		–	–
		Raouf (13) 2003	48	100/0	Ireland	Bcl-2		–	0.03	
						Bcl-X		–		
						Bax		–		
		Gibson (15) 2003	54	80/20	USA	Bcl-2		–	–	
						Bax		–	–	
		Vallbohmer (16) 2007	59	NA	Germany	survivin		–[f]		
		Gibson (15) 2003	54	80/20	USA	**EGFR**		–	0.009	< 0.05
		Hickey (38) 1994	14	0/100	Ireland	EGFR & PCNA		0.02[f]	0.0003	
		Ribeiro (17) 1998	42	74/26	USA	p53		–	–	
		Muro (18) 1996[e]	20	0/100	Japan	p53	–		< 0.01	
		Shimada (39) 2002[d]	52	0/100	Japan	p53	–		–	–
						TP	0.02		–	–
						VEGF	< 0.001		0.04	0.01
		Sohda (40) 2004[e]	65	0/100	Japan	p53	–		–	
						p21	–		–	
						HIF-1α	0.009		–	

		Hironaka (41) 2002[e]	73	0/100	Japan	**p53**			0.08	0.06
						Ki67			0.07	–
						EGFR			–	
						cyclin D1			–	
						VEGF			–	
						DPD			–	
						GST-π			–	
		Xi (7) 2005	52	39/61	Germany	COX-2		–[f]	–	
		Kulke (42) 2004	46	61/39	USA	COX-2		–	–	
						VEGF		–	–	
	DNA Sequence	Gibson (15) 2003	54	80/20	USA	p53 mutation		–	0.05	–
		Ribeiro (17) 1998	42	74/26	USA	**p53 mutation**		0.01	0.004	0.002
		Ito (43) 2001[e]	40	0/100	Japan	p53 mutation		–	–	
	RT-PCR	Warnecke-Ebertz (19) 2005	51	39/61	Germany	survivin		–[f]	< 0.003	
		Kato (5) 2001[h]	51	0/100	Japan	survivin	0.04		0.03	–
		Warnecke-Ebertz (44) 2004	36	36/64	Germany	ERCC1		< 0.001[f]		
		Miyazono (6) 2004	36	36/64	Germany	HER2/neu		0.02[f]		
					Japan	EGFR		–[f]		
		Xi (7) 2005	52	39/61	Germany	COX-2		–[f]	–	
> 10	Methylation	Hamilton (10) 2006	35	66/33	USA	11 genes[g]		0.03		
	Expression Microarray	Luthra (11) 2006	19	84/16	USA	> 14,500 genes		0.01		
	SNP	Wu (8) 2006	210	83/17	USA	**Genes in CRT pathways**		< 0.05	< 0.05	< 0.05
	Proteomics	Hayashida (12) 2005	42	0/100	Japan	SELDI chip		NAP[f]		

Abbreviations: AC = adenocarcinoma; SCC = squamous cell carcinoma; UV = univariate; MV = multivariate; NA = not available; NAP = not applicable; RT-PCR = real-time polymerase chain reaction; SNP = single nucleotide polymorphism; CRT = chemoradiotherapy; SELDI = surface-enhanced laser desorption and ionization; pCR = complete pathologic response in surgical specimen.

[a]Predictors that contributed independently to survival are shown in bold.

[b]P values < 0.1 are listed. The en dash symbol denotes a P value ≥ 0.1, and a blank space that the statistical test was not performed.

[c]Disease-free survival was used as the endpoint.

[d]Chemoradiotherapy alone was given in a minority of patients.

[e]Chemoradiotherapy alone was given in all or most patients.

[f]As an outcome variable, complete pathologic response was grouped with another outcome category (e.g., minor pathologic response).

[g]Genes involved in tumor biology (Reprimo, CHFR, MGMT, TIMP-3, RUNX-3, p57, p16, p73, COX-2, HPP1, XAF-1).

[h]A minority of patients received preoperative chemotherapy with or without radiation.

TABLE 92.3

Results of Molecular Outcome Studies in Patients with Esophageal Cancer Treated Primarily with Surgery (with or without Subsequent Chemotherapy or Radiation)

						Association of predictor(s) with: *P Value*[b]			
						DFS or PFS		Overall survival	
Lab method	**Study**	**N**	**AC/SCC (%)**	**Country**	**Predictor(s)**[a]	**UV**	**MV**	**UV**	**MV**
Immunohistochemistry	Ikeguchi (45) 2000	191	0/100	Japan	p53			–	–
					pRB			0.001	–
	Makoto (46) 2002	96	0/100	Japan	p53			–	–
					TP			0.04	0.06
	Inada (47) 1999	40	0/100	Japan	p53			–	
					E-cadherin			< 0.01	
					EGFR			< 0.05	
	Ikeguchi (48) 2001	141	0/100	Japan	p53			–[c]	–[c]
					Bax			0.01[c]	–[c]
	Sturm (49) 2001	53	0/100	Germany	p53			–	–
					Bax			0.004	0.02
					p16			0.01	–
	Matsumoto (50) 2001	79	0/100	Japan	p53			–	–
					Rb			–	–
					Bax			0.08	–
					$Bcl\text{-}X_L$			0.05	–
					p21			–	–
	Ikeda (51) 1999	53	0/100	Japan	**p53**			0.002	0.001
					Cyclin D1			–	–
					Ki-67			0.0005	0.02
	Takayama (52) 2001	86	0/100	Japan	Bax			–	–
					Bcl-X			0.001	0.02
					Bcl-2			–	–
	Itami (53) 1999	128	0/100	Japan	**Cyclin D1**			0.02	0.02
					$p27^{Kip1}$			0.09	–
	Shamma (54) 2000	106	0/100	Japan	**$p27^{KIP1}$**			0.001	0.02
					$p16^{INK4}$			–	–
	Inoue (55) 1997	75	0/100	Japan	**VEGF**	0.03		0.02	0.008

	Kitadai (56) 1998	87	NA	Japan	VEGF			–	
	Shih (57) 2000	53	0/100	Japan	**VEGF**			0.04	0.05
	Ogata (58) 2003	92	0/100	Japan	**VEGF**			0.02	0.06
	Fukai (59) 2003	80	0/100	Japan	TGF β1			–[c]	–[c]
					TGF βR1			0.03[c]	–[c]
					TGF βR2			0.02[c]	–[c]
	Han (60) 2005	79	NA	China	**Heparanase**			0.001	< 0.001
					bFGF				0.02
	Kuo (61) 2003	96	0/100	Taiwan	COX-2			–	–
	Mobius (62) 2005	48	100/0	Germany	COX-2			0.01	
	Aloia (63) 2001	61	72/28	USA	**p53**			0.08	0.04
					TGF-α			0.02	0.01
					EGFR			–	–
					Her2/neu			–	–
					P-gp			–	0.004
					MT			–	–
					TS			–	–
					GST-π			0.02	–
	Wang (24) 2007 d	103	100/0	USA	**EGFR**	0.001	0.07	0.004	0.08
	Wilkinson (25) 2004 d	38	100/0	USA	EGFR	0.07		–	
	Krishnadath (64) 1997	65	100/0	Netherlands	**E-cadherin**			0.001	0.04
					α-catenin			0.001	0.09
					β-catenin			0.01	0.03
DNA sequence	Sturm (49) 2001	53	0/100	Germany	p53 mutation			–	–
RT-PCR	Terashita (65) 2004	43	0/100	Japan	ERCC3			0.0003	
Methylation	Brock (9) 2003	41	100/0	USA	**≥ 4 of 7 genes methylated**[e]	0.03	0.03	0.04	0.02
SNP	Izzo (66) 2007	124	100/0	USA	**Cyclin D1**			0.0003	≤ 0.04

Abbreviations: AC = adenocarcinoma; SCC = squamous cell carcinoma; UV = univariate; MV = multivariate; NA = not available; DFS = disease-free survival; PFS = progression-free survival; RT-PCR = real-time polymerase chain reaction; SNP = single nucleotide polymorphism; bFGF = basic fibroblast growth factor; pRB = retinoblastoma protein; TP = thymidine phosphorylase.

[a]Predictors that contributed independently to survival are shown in bold.

[b]P values < 0.1 are listed. The en-dash denotes a P value ≥ 0.1, and a blank space denotes that the statistical test was not performed.

[c]Endpoint was cancer-specific survival.

[d]A minority of cases received pre- or postoperative chemotherapy, radiation, or both.

[e]APC, adenomatous polyposis coli; MGMT, O_6-methylguanine DNA methyltransferase, p16, ER, E-cadherin, TIMP3, DAP-kinase.

TABLE 92.4
Biologic Pathways Implicated in Esophageal Cancer

Pathway	Molecules
Growth regulation	EGFR, TGF-α, Her2/neu, Ki67
Cell cycle control	p16, p21, cyclin D1
Apoptosis	p53, Bcl-2, Bax, Bcl-X, NF-Kb, survivin
Angiogenesis	VEGF, Cox-2, TP
Invasion and metastasis	Cadherins, TIMP, MMP
DNA repair	ERCC1, ERCC3, BRCA
Drug disposition	p-glycoprotein, thymidylate synthase, glutathione S-tranferase, DPD

in predicting therapeutic response or overall outcome (5,13–19), and have rarely been found to be independently predictive in trimodality settings (20,21).

The abundance of null findings may be related to the small sample sizes of most cohorts, which reflect the low overall incidence of this cancer, even with the dramatic rise of adenocarcinoma. Small sample size not only leads to an underpowered study but, just as important, few attempts at replication. To reduce false negatives, we listed *P* values in the tables up to the alpha 0.10 level. Furthermore, efforts at finding markers in the trimodality setting must use (small) pretreatment biopsy specimens, as opposed to in the adjuvant setting, where (large) resection specimens are used. The small size of tumors may make evaluation more difficult and, depending on the analytic method, small tumors may become depleted after only a few markers are evaluated.

Single Gene Approach

NF-kB

Nuclear factor-kB (NF-kB) is a transcription factor that responds to multiple cellular signaling pathways by regulating genes involved in cell survival. It is active in the nucleus and sequestered in the cytoplasm in an inactive state through the binding of inhibitory kB. Physiologically, NF-kB activation is tightly regulated and rapid, initiated by stimuli such as inflammatory cytokines, viruses, carcinogens, and DNA-damaging agents. Aberrant (i.e., constitutive) NF-kB activation has been associated with inflammatory diseases and cancer. Through the activation of survival pathways, it suppresses apoptosis when cancer cells are exposed to radiotherapy or chemotherapy, thus contributing to resistance. Concomitantly, through the enhancement of migratory (e.g., Cox-2, CAM adhesion proteins), invasive (e.g., matrix metalloproteinases), and proangiogenic (e.g., VEGF and Cox-2) properties, NF-kB contributes to metastatic progression. Protein expression of NF-kB[22] (assessed by IHC) is one of the few markers whose independent contribution to prognosis has been replicated at least once (20,21).

One study (20) examined pre- or posttreatment specimens from 80 patients, mostly with adenocarcinoma, treated with various regimens of preoperative chemoradiation (with or without induction chemotherapy). Immunohistochemical staining for activated NF-kB revealed that 7% (2 of 29) of patients with high expression levels had a pCR, compared to 43% (20 of 26) of patients with low expression levels ($P = 0.006$). NF-kB activation remained a substantial risk factor for worse overall survival in multivariate analysis (hazard ration [HR] 0.19, $P = 0.007$).

EGFR

Another promising marker is EGFR protein expression, which, in adenocarcinoma patients, has been independently linked to survival in both neoadjuvant and primary-surgery settings. This transmembrane protein tyrosine kinase growth factor receptor is mutated or overexpressed in many human tumors of epithelial origin, including head and neck, colorectal, pancreatic, lung, and esophageal cancers. In these tumors, overexpression is associated with more aggressive behavior and poor prognosis (23).

In one U.S. study in esophageal cancer of mostly adenocarcinoma patients (15), EGFR expression was assessed immunohistochemically using pretreatment tumors from 54 patients who underwent trimodality therapy with cisplatin and 5-fluorouracil (5-FU). EGFR expression did not correlate with pCR. However, increasing EGFR levels were associated with progressively worse overall survival after adjustment for covariates. Similar findings were obtained in two other studies of adenocarcinoma patients, this time treated typically with surgical resection alone: the larger study (24) included multivariate confirmation, and the smaller, likely underpowered one (25), showed a median survival of 35 months in EGFR-negative patients more than doubled that of EGFR-positive patients ($P = 0.10$). Studies of squamous cell carcinoma patients have also linked EGFR expression with poor prognosis (26,27).

EGFR is an intriguing marker, partly because EGFR-directed drugs are increasingly available. These include the small molecules ZD1839 (Iressa) and OSI-774

(Tarceva) and the monoclonal antibodies C225 (Erbitux) and panitumimab. However, whether such therapy improves outcomes, in a way predicted by EGFR status or not, remains to be seen.

Multigene Approach

Earlier studies often relied on a candidate gene approach (i.e., testing one or a few genes at a time); however, with a growing appreciation of the complexity of interwoven molecular processes, investigators have increasingly examined the effect of cumulative alterations across multiple genes. This has been explored on a genetic, RNA, and epigenetic level.

Single-Nucleotide Polymorphisms

One of the largest studies to date in esophageal cancer patients who received trimodality therapy focused on single-nucleotide polymorphisms (SNPs) as potential predictors (8). SNPs are single-nucleotide variations between individuals that have been associated with cancer susceptibility and chemotherapeutic toxicity. The recent explosion of literature in pharmacogenetics suggests that genetic polymorphisms in genes involved in drug metabolism, drug targets, and DNA repair may contribute significantly to the variability of drug response. Variant alleles have been associated with overall survival in patients with lung (28), colon (29), and head and neck (30) cancer.

For this study, specimens were taken from 210 esophageal cancer patients (1985–2003) treated with cisplatin- and 5-FU–based trimodality therapy. Genotyping was performed for pathways involved in cisplatin, 5-FU, and radiation action, including those related to DNA repair and drug detoxification. In the Cox proportional hazards model, variant alleles in the *MTHFR* gene, involved in folate metabolism, were associated with significantly improved survival (HR 0.56; 95% confidence interval [CI], 0.35 to 0.89) in patients treated with 5-FU. The 3-year survival rates for patients with the variant genotypes and the wild genotypes were 65.26% and 46.43%, respectively. Joint analysis of 5 polymorphisms in three 5-FU pathway genes showed a significant trend for reduced recurrence risk and longer recurrence-free survival as the number of "adverse" alleles decreased ($P = 0.004$). Overall, variant alleles were evidently considered "adverse" or "high risk," unless analysis indicated otherwise. For patients receiving platinum drugs, the *MDR1 C3435T* variant allele was associated with reduced recurrence risk (HR 0.25; 95% CI, 0.10 to 0.64) and improved survival (HR 0.44; 95% CI, 0.23 to 0.85). In nucleotide excision repair genes, there was a significant trend for a decreasing risk of death with fewer high-risk alleles (P for trend = 0.0008). In base excision repair genes, the variant alleles of *XRCC1 Arg399Gln* were associated with the absence of pathologic complete response (odds ratio 2.75; 95% CI, 1.14 to 6.12) and poor survival (HR 1.92; 95% CI, 1.00 to 3.72).

Methylation

A growing body of evidence indicates that abnormal methylation of DNA is an early event in carcinogenesis (31). Methylation of the promoter regions of tumor suppressor genes is commonly found in many human malignancies, including esophageal carcinoma. This methylation leads to the reduced expression of tumor suppressor genes, resulting in unchecked cellular growth, tissue invasion, angiogenesis, and metastases. Multiple studies have shown that promoter methylation of tumor suppressor genes underlies carcinogenesis. In addition, aberrant methylation of multiple genes correlates with prognosis of many cancers. One allure of methylation as a predictive marker is its potential as a target of demethylation therapies to sensitize tumors to chemotherapy and radiation.

In one retrospective study of patients who received trimodality therapy (10), promoter methylation patterns of 11 candidate genes were examined in pretreatment tumor specimens ($n = 35$). The genes were selected according to their known ability to predict responsiveness to chemoradiation and prognosis, or their role in regulating the cell cycle. Somewhat higher than common rates of pCR, 37% of surgical specimens in this cohort demonstrated complete absence of tumor. The number of methylated genes per patient was lower in patients who experienced a pCR than in those that did not (1.4 vs. 2.4 genes per patient; $P = 0.026$). The combined mean level of promoter methylation of *p16, Reprimo, p57, p73, RUNX-3, CHFR, MGMT, TIMP-3,* and *HPP1* was also lower in responders than in nonresponders ($P = 0.003$). The frequency (15% of responders vs. 64% of nonresponders; $P = 0.01$) and level (0.078 in responders vs. 0.313 in nonresponders; $P = 0.037$) of *Reprimo* methylation was significantly lower in responders than in nonresponders. Similarly, a study of esophageal adenocarcinoma patients who received surgical resection alone found that patients whose tumors had 4 or more genes methylated in a 7-gene profile (APC, MGMT, p16, ER, E-cadherin, TIMP3, DAP-kinase) had poorer survival and earlier tumor recurrence compared to patients who did not (9).

Genome-Wide Approach

One disadvantage of looking at a few genes, or a few dozen along several pathways, is that an enormous number of potentially predictive markers may be overlooked. Therefore, some advocate the use of genome-wide strategies to identify new pathways. In the only study to date linking gene expression profiles with treatment and outcome data in esophageal cancer patients receiving trimodality therapy, pretreatment endoscopic cancer biopsies were taken from 19 patients (16 with adenocarcinoma, 2 with squamous cell carcinoma, and 1 with adenosquamous carcinoma) who were enrolled onto a preoperative chemoradiotherapy protocol (11). Patients received 2 cycles of induction chemotherapy (docetaxel [33 mg/m^2], irinotecan [55 mg/m^2], and fluorouracil [2 g/m^2] infusion over 24 hours weekly for 2 weeks, followed by 1 week off, in a 6-week cycle) followed by concurrent radiotherapy (up to 50.4 Gy in 28 fractions) and chemotherapy (docetaxel [20 mg/m^2] IV bolus weekly, irinotecan [30 mg/m^2] IV bolus weekly, and fluorouracil [300mg/m^2/24 hours] as continuous infusion). This was followed by surgical resection.

Pretreatment cancer tissues were subjected to gene expression profiling using an Affymetrix chip of 22,215 non-control probe sets corresponding to > 18,400 distinct transcripts. Unsupervised hierarchic cluster analysis segregated the cancers into 2 molecular subtypes, each consisting of 10 and 9 specimens, respectively. As it turned out, most cancers (5 of 6) that had pathologic complete response (pCR) clustered in molecular subtype I. Moreover, subtype II consisted almost entirely (with one exception) of cancers that had less than pCR (< pCR). Then, the investigators selected and performed RT-PCR on 3 genes (*PERP, S100A2,* and *SPRR3)* whose expression levels were among those which differed by > 2-fold between the 2 subtypes. PERP, a TP53 effector related to peripheral myelin protein 22, is involved in p53-dependent apoptosis. The *S100A2* gene encoding a calcium-binding protein is considered a candidate tumor suppressor gene because of its underexpression in several cancers, including esophageal squamous cell carcinoma, in comparison with healthy epithelia. SPRR3, a proline-rich protein, comprises the cell envelope and is expressed in stratified squamous epithelia during differentiation. This gene has been identified as a marker of esophageal cancer progression. Expression levels of these genes allowed discrimination of pCR from < pCR with high sensitivity and specificity (85%).

The study is limited, given the small sample size, and needs validation. However, it illustrates the potential for identifying markers that are "off our radar," so to speak, but which may help distinguish cancers that are sensitive vs. resistant to therapy.

Serial Ascertainment

Tables 92.2 and 92.3 generally include markers that under current frameworks are ascertained once, before therapy is initiated, but eventually some of them can theoretically be obtained serially (e.g., by repeat biopsy or blood draw) during the course of therapy as well. Serial markers have a dual purpose: (a) forecasting outcomes, and (b) assessing disease status.

A gross example of a serial marker is a CT scan. Tumors that regress on CT are more likely to respond to further therapy than those that have not regressed. In addition, CT scans assess current disease burden. These serial markers, which compare a follow-up image with a baseline image, can also be used to stratify patients for further therapy.

An antiquated version of the CT scan, the barium esophagram, was used to stratify patients in a trial of squamous cell carcinoma patients who had received cisplatin and 5-FU concurrent with radiation (32). This study illustrates the use of delayed ascertainment. Because imaging is less invasive and does not require the standardization of new assays, it may be more easily incorporated into the clinic. Patients who demonstrated <30% response on a restaging esophagram or had unimproved dysphagia were removed from the study. The remaining patients, the responders, were randomized to surgical resection or to further chemoradiation. Overall survival did not differ between the groups, suggesting that surgery does not add benefit to chemoradiation in patients with locally advanced esophageal squamous cell carcinoma who have responded to initial chemoradiotherapy.

INTEGRATION INTO CLINICAL TRIALS: CHALLENGES

Any marker that is rationally integrated into clinical practice should be, if feasible, validated in a prospective trial. By "validation," we do not simply mean *replication* in another retrospective study, which is important; a prospective trial should be designed, at least in part, to establish the role of the marker in patient management. There are numerous options for trial designs; and patient management may or may not be affected by the marker (1). One example in which the marker affects management was performed by the Spanish Lung Cancer Group, using ERCC1 mRNA levels as a means of stratifying non-small cell lung cancer patients (stage IIIB or IV). Patients randomized to the control arm received a cisplatin doublet, whereas patients randomized to the experimental arm received a cisplatin doublet if they had low levels of ERCC1 mRNA and a gemcitabine doublet if they had high levels of ERCC1 mRNA. The study has yielded promising preliminary results (33).

Perhaps the greatest challenge in performing trials intended to validate markers is the large sample size required. Estimated sample sizes depend on several factors, one of which is the anticipated treatment effect of the marker. Samples sizes must be in the range of a few thousand patients for a marker that predicts modest differences in outcome in 1 treatment (perhaps the most likely scenario) or a few hundred patients for a marker that predicts large differences in 2 competing treatments (1). The most simple explanation for the substantial sample size requirement is that these trials, in essence, incorporate planned *subgroup* analyses—with each subgroup representing 1 level of a marker for a specific treatment. Depending on the predictive traits of the marker, this requirement poses substantial challenges in esophageal cancer, which has an annual incidence in the United States of roughly 15,000 (34). Indeed, that the largest trial conducted in the United States enrolled only 440 patients (35) may suggest this requirement is insurmountable unless the marker is strongly predictive.

Our goal, of course, is to develop markers—or a panel of markers—with strong predictive effects across multiple treatments. If we are unable to identify such markers, our options are limited. One, we may need to rely on smaller trials that yield prognostic, not predictive, information, as we have been doing thus far, with one possible exception. While prognostic markers may be important in patient counseling, their impact on therapy is not straightforward; therefore, it would be reasonable for validation studies to focus on identifying predictive markers. The multitude of retrospective studies described above yielded prognostic data at best, because a given marker was not assessed across differing therapies. That is, within each study, patients received largely uniform treatment. As a result, even if a clearly negative prognostic marker emerges through further scientific inquiry, we would theoretically still be in the dark—when confronted with the patient in clinic who possesses the marker—on whether an alternative therapy would fare any better. An exception may be if a marker is able to identify those patients who will do unusually poorly under conventional therapy; NF-kB may be an example. An alternative treatment can be delivered instead, with the grim understanding that it could not do worse.

A second option, suggested elsewhere (36), is to develop pathway-based molecular signatures by using, for example, DNA microarray data to identify activated pathways. These signatures may ultimately permit us to classify cancers irrespective of their site of origin. Ultimately, a drug developed for breast or colon cancer, which targets a specific pathway signature, may be equally effective against a less common cancer having the same signature.

A third option, of course, is continue our empiric approach, emphasizing increased cooperation between investigators for performing clinical trials, in the hope that our growing understanding of tumor biology will lead iteratively to more effective drugs.

SUMMARY

A somewhat nascent approach to improving outcome in esophageal cancer, especially in adenocarcinoma, is to identify molecular markers that stratify patients by their likelihood of success with a particular therapy. As we reviewed markers that have been studied, we focused on their current potential for integration into a validation clinical trial. To date, no single marker or panel of markers has emerged as a strong candidate, but some are promising. Rather than investigating candidate genes, assessing the cumulative effect of many pathways may prove to be more effective in forecasting outcomes. One interest in the field is a genome-wide approach, both to identify unexplored markers and to develop molecular signatures by which to subtype cancers. The main challenge to marker development in esophageal cancer is the requirement for large sample sizes in validation trials. Methods for confronting this barrier in this uncommon disease include pragmatism, increased cooperation, and upturning paradigms.

References

1. Sargent DJ, Conley BA, Allegra C, Collette L. Clinical trial designs for predictive marker validation in cancer treatment trials. *J Clin Oncol.* 2005;23(9):2020–2027.
2. Vallbohmer D, Lenz HJ. Predictive and prognostic molecular markers in outcome of esophageal cancer. *Dis Esophagus.* 2006;19(6):425–432.
3. Raz DJ, Jablons DM. EGFR expression and mutational analysis as a predictive test. *J Clin Oncol.* 2007;25(15):2144; author reply 2145.
4. Dziadziuszko R, Hirsch FR, Varella-Garcia M, Bunn PA Jr. Selecting lung cancer patients for treatment with epidermal growth factor receptor tyrosine kinase inhibitors by immunohistochemistry and fluorescence in situ hybridization—why, when, and how? *Clin Cancer Res.* 2006;12(14 Pt 2):4409s-4415s.
5. Kato J, Kuwabara Y, Mitani M, et al. Expression of survivin in esophageal cancer: correlation with the prognosis and response to chemotherapy. *Int J Cancer.* 2001;95(2):92–95.
6. Miyazono F, Metzger R, Warnecke-Eberz U, et al. Quantitative c-erbB-2 but not c-erbB-1 mRNA expression is a promising marker to predict minor histopathologic response to neoadjuvant radiochemotherapy in oesophageal cancer. *Br J Cancer.* 2004;91(4):666–672.
7. Xi H, Baldus SE, Warnecke-Eberz U, et al. High cyclooxygenase-2 expression following neoadjuvant radiochemotherapy is associated with minor histopathologic response and poor prognosis in esophageal cancer. *Clin Cancer Res.* 2005;11(23):8341–8347.
8. Wu X, Gu J, Wu TT, et al. Genetic variations in radiation and chemotherapy drug action pathways predict clinical outcomes in esophageal cancer. *J Clin Oncol.* 2006;24(23):3789–3798.
9. Brock MV, Gou M, Akiyama Y, et al. Prognostic importance of promoter hypermethylation of multiple genes in esophageal adenocarcinoma. *Clin Cancer Res.* 2003;9(8):2912–2919.
10. Hamilton JP, Sato F, Greenwald BD, et al. Promoter methylation and response to chemotherapy and radiation in esophageal cancer. *Clin Gastroenterol Hepatol.* 2006;4(6):701–708.
11. Luthra R, Wu TT, Luthra MG, et al. Gene expression profiling of localized esophageal carcinomas: association with pathologic response to preoperative chemoradiation. *J Clin Oncol.* 2006;24(2):259–267.
12. Hayashida Y, Honda K, Osaka Y, et al. Possible prediction of chemoradiosensitivity of esophageal cancer by serum protein profiling. *Clin Cancer Res.* 2005;11(22):8042–8047.
13. Raouf AA, Evoy DA, Carton E, Mulligan E, Griffin MM, Reynolds JV. Loss of Bcl-2 expression in Barrett's dysplasia and adenocarcinoma is associated with tumor progression and worse survival but not with response to neoadjuvant chemoradiation. *Dis Esophagus.* 2003;16(1):17–23.

14. Sarbia M, Stahl M, Fink U, Willers R, Seeber S, Gabbert HE. Expression of apoptosis-regulating proteins and outcome of esophageal cancer patients treated by combined therapy modalities. *Clin Cancer Res.* 1998;4(12):2991–2997.
15. Gibson MK, Abraham SC, Wu TT, et al. Epidermal growth factor receptor, p53 mutation, and pathological response predict survival in patients with locally advanced esophageal cancer treated with preoperative chemoradiotherapy. *Clin Cancer Res.* 2003;9(17):6461–6468.
16. Vallboehmer D, Kuhn E, Brabender J, et al. Survivin expression in esophageal cancer: association with histomorphological response to neoadjuvant therapy and prognosis: ASCO Annual Meeting Proceedings Part I. *J Clin Oncol.* 2007;25(18S):4536.
17. Ribeiro U Jr, Finkelstein SD, Safatle-Ribeiro AV, et al. p53 sequence analysis predicts treatment response and outcome of patients with esophageal carcinoma. *Cancer.* 1998;83(1):7–18.
18. Muro K, Ohtsu A, Boku N, et al. Association of p53 protein expression with responses and survival of patients with locally advanced esophageal carcinoma treated with chemoradiotherapy. *Jpn J Clin Oncol.* 1996;26(2):65–69.
19. Warnecke-Eberz U, Hokita S, Xi H, et al. Overexpression of survivin mRNA is associated with a favorable prognosis following neoadjuvant radiochemotherapy in esophageal cancer. *Oncol Rep.* 2005;13(6):1241–1246.
20. Izzo JG, Correa AM, Wu TT, et al. Pretherapy nuclear factor-kappaB status, chemoradiation resistance, and metastatic progression in esophageal carcinoma. *Mol Cancer Ther.* 2006;5(11):2844–2850.
21. Abdel-Latif MM, O'Riordan J, Windle HJ, et al. NF-kappaB activation in esophageal adenocarcinoma: relationship to Barrett's metaplasia, survival, and response to neoadjuvant chemoradiotherapy. *Ann Surg.* 2004;239(4):491–500.
22. Verma A, Mehta K. Transglutaminase-mediated activation of nuclear transcription factor-kappaB in cancer cells: a new therapeutic opportunity. *Curr Cancer Drug Targets.* 2007;7(6):559–565.
23. Nicholson RI, Gee JM, Harper ME. EGFR and cancer prognosis. *Eur J Cancer.* 2001;37(Suppl 4):S9–15.
24. Wang KL, Wu TT, Choi IS, et al. Expression of epidermal growth factor receptor in esophageal and esophagogastric junction adenocarcinomas: association with poor outcome. *Cancer.* 2007;109(4):658–667.
25. Wilkinson NW, Black JD, Roukhadze E, et al. Epidermal growth factor receptor expression correlates with histologic grade in resected esophageal adenocarcinoma. *J Gastrointest Surg.* 2004;8(4):448–453.
26. Kitagawa Y, Ueda M, Ando N, Ozawa S, Shimizu N, Kitajima M. Further evidence for prognostic significance of epidermal growth factor receptor gene amplification in patients with esophageal squamous cell carcinoma. *Clin Cancer Res.* 1996;2(5):909–914.
27. Ozawa S, Ueda M, Ando N, Shimizu N, Abe O. Prognostic significance of epidermal growth factor receptor in esophageal squamous cell carcinomas. *Cancer.* 1989;63(11):2169–2173.
28. Ryu JS, Hong YC, Han HS, et al. Association between polymorphisms of ERCC1 and XPD and survival in non-small-cell lung cancer patients treated with cisplatin combination chemotherapy. *Lung Cancer.* 2004;44(3):311–316.
29. Stoehlmacher J, Park DJ, Zhang W, et al. A multivariate analysis of genomic polymorphisms: prediction of clinical outcome to 5-FU/oxaliplatin combination chemotherapy in refractory colorectal cancer. *Br J Cancer.* 2004;91(2):344–354.
30. Quintela-Fandino M, Hitt R, Medina PP, et al. DNA-repair gene polymorphisms predict favorable clinical outcome among patients with advanced squamous cell carcinoma of the head and neck treated with cisplatin-based induction chemotherapy. *J Clin Oncol.* 2006;24(26):4333–4339.
31. Herman JG, Baylin SB. Gene silencing in cancer in association with promoter hypermethylation. *N Engl J Med.* 2003;349(21):2042–2054.
32. Bedenne L, Michel P, Bouche O, et al. Chemoradiation followed by surgery compared with chemoradiation alone in squamous cancer of the esophagus: FFCD 9102. *J Clin Oncol.* 2007;25(10):1160–1168.
33. Rosell R, Cobo M, Isla D, et al. ERCC1 mRNA-based randomized phase III trial of docetaxel (doc) doublets with cisplatin (cis) or gemcitabine (gem) in stage IV non-small-cell lung cancer (NSCLC) patients (p). ASCO Annual Meeting Proceedings [abstract 7002]. *J Clin Oncol.* 2005;23(16S).
34. Jemal A, Siegel R, Ward E, Murray T, Xu J, Thun MJ. Cancer statistics, 2007. *CA Cancer J Clin.* 2007;57(1):43–66.
35. Kelsen DP, Ginsberg R, Pajak TF, et al. Chemotherapy followed by surgery compared with surgery alone for localized esophageal cancer. *N Engl J Med.* 1998;339(27):1979–1984.
36. Izzo JG, Ajani JA. Thinking in and out of the box when it comes to gastric cancer and cyclooxygenase-2. *J Clin Oncol.* 2007;25(31):4865–4867.
37. Harpole DH, Jr., Moore MB, Herndon JE II, et al. The prognostic value of molecular marker analysis in patients treated with trimodality therapy for esophageal cancer. *Clin Cancer Res.* 2001;7(3):562–569.
38. Hickey K, Grehan D, Reid IM, O'Briain S, Walsh TN, Hennessy TP. Expression of epidermal growth factor receptor and proliferating cell nuclear antigen predicts response of esophageal squamous cell carcinoma to chemoradiotherapy. *Cancer.* 1994;74(6):1693–1698.
39. Shimada H, Hoshino T, Okazumi S, et al. Expression of angiogenic factors predicts response to chemoradiotherapy and prognosis of oesophageal squamous cell carcinoma. *Br J Cancer.* 2002;86(4):552–557.
40. Sohda M, Ishikawa H, Masuda N, et al. Pretreatment evaluation of combined HIF-1alpha, p53 and p21 expression is a useful and sensitive indicator of response to radiation and chemotherapy in esophageal cancer. *Int J Cancer.* 2004;110(6):838–844.
41. Hironaka S, Hasebe T, Kamijo T, et al. Biopsy specimen microvessel density is a useful prognostic marker in patients with T(2–4)M(0) esophageal cancer treated with chemoradiotherapy. *Clin Cancer Res.* 2002;8(1):124–130.
42. Kulke MH, Odze RD, Mueller JD, Wang H, Redston M, Bertagnolli MM. Prognostic significance of vascular endothelial growth factor and cyclooxygenase 2 expression in patients receiving preoperative chemoradiation for esophageal cancer. *J Thorac Cardiovasc Surg.* 2004;127(6):1579–1586.
43. Ito T, Kaneko K, Makino R, et al. Prognostic value of p53 mutations in patients with locally advanced esophageal carcinoma treated with definitive chemoradiotherapy. *J Gastroenterol.* 2001;36(5):303–311.
44. Warnecke-Eberz U, Metzger R, Miyazono F, et al. High specificity of quantitative excision repair cross-complementing 1 messenger RNA expression for prediction of minor histopathological response to neoadjuvant radiochemotherapy in esophageal cancer. *Clin Cancer Res.* 2004;10(11):3794–3799.
45. Ikeguchi M, Oka S, Gomyo Y, Tsujitani S, Maeta M, Kaibara N. Combined analysis of p53 and retinoblastoma protein expressions in esophageal cancer. *Ann Thorac Surg.* 2000;70(3):913–917.
46. Makoto O, Takeda A, Ting-Leig L, et al. Prognostic significance of thymidine phosphorylase and p53 co-expression in esophageal squamous cell carcinoma. *Oncol Rep.* 2002;9(1):23–28.
47. Inada S, Koto T, Futami K, Arima S, Iwashita A. Evaluation of malignancy and the prognosis of esophageal cancer based on an immunohistochemical study (p53, E-cadherin, epidermal growth factor receptor). *Surg Today.* 1999;29(6):493–503.
48. Ikeguchi M, Maeta M, Kaibara N. Bax expression as a prognostic marker of postoperative chemoradiotherapy for patients with esophageal cancer. *Int J Mol Med.* 2001;7(4):413–417.
49. Sturm I, Petrowsky H, Volz R, et al. Analysis of p53/BAX/p16(ink4a/CDKN2) in esophageal squamous cell carcinoma: high BAX and p16(ink4a/CDKN2) identifies patients with good prognosis. *J Clin Oncol.* 2001;19(8):2272–2281.
50. Matsumoto M, Natsugoe S, Nakashima S, et al. Clinical significance and prognostic value of apoptosis related proteins in superficial esophageal squamous cell carcinoma. *Ann Surg Oncol.* 2001;8(7):598–604.
51. Ikeda G, Isaji S, Chandra B, Watanabe M, Kawarada Y. Prognostic significance of biologic factors in squamous cell carcinoma of the esophagus. *Cancer.* 1999;86(8):1396–1405.
52. Takayama T, Nagao M, Sawada H, et al. Bcl-X expression in esophageal squamous cell carcinoma: association with tumor progression and prognosis. *J Surg Oncol.* 2001;78(2):116–123.
53. Itami A, Shimada Y, Watanabe G, Imamura M. Prognostic value of p27(Kip1) and CyclinD1 expression in esophageal cancer. *Oncology.* 1999;57(4):311–317.
54. Shamma A, Doki Y, Tsujinaka T, et al. Loss of p27(KIP1) expression predicts poor prognosis in patients with esophageal squamous cell carcinoma. *Oncology.* 2000;58(2):152–158.
55. Inoue K, Ozeki Y, Suganuma T, Sugiura Y, Tanaka S. Vascular endothelial growth factor expression in primary esophageal squamous cell carcinoma. Association with angiogenesis and tumor progression. *Cancer.* 1997;79(2):206–213.
56. Kitadai Y, Haruma K, Tokutomi T, et al. Significance of vessel count and vascular endothelial growth factor in human esophageal carcinomas. *Clin Cancer Res.* 1998;4(9):2195–2200.
57. Shih CH, Ozawa S, Ando N, Ueda M, Kitajima M. Vascular endothelial growth factor expression predicts outcome and lymph node metastasis in squamous cell carcinoma of the esophagus. *Clin Cancer Res.* 2000;6(3):1161–1168.
58. Ogata Y, Fujita H, Yamana H, Sueyoshi S, Shirouzu K. Expression of vascular endothelial growth factor as a prognostic factor in node-positive squamous cell carcinoma in the thoracic esophagus: long-term follow-up study. *World J Surg.* 2003;27(5):584–589.
59. Fukai Y, Fukuchi M, Masuda N, et al. Reduced expression of transforming growth factor-beta receptors is an unfavorable prognostic factor in human esophageal squamous cell carcinoma. *Int J Cancer.* 2003;104(2):161–166.
60. Han B, Liu J, Ma MJ, Zhao L. Clinicopathological significance of heparanase and basic fibroblast growth factor expression in human esophageal cancer. *World J Gastroenterol.* 2005;11(14):2188–2192.
61. Kuo KT, Chow KC, Wu YC, et al. Clinicopathologic significance of cyclooxygenase-2 overexpression in esophageal squamous cell carcinoma. *Ann Thorac Surg.* 2003; 76(3):909–914.
62. Mobius C, Stein HJ, Spiess C, et al. COX2 expression, angiogenesis, proliferation and survival in Barrett's cancer. *Eur J Surg Oncol.* 2005;31(7):755–759.
63. Aloia TA, Harpole DH Jr, Reed CE, et al. Tumor marker expression is predictive of survival in patients with esophageal cancer. *Ann Thorac Surg.* 2001;72(3):859–866.
64. Krishnadath KK, Tilanus HW, van Blankenstein M, et al. Reduced expression of the cadherin-catenin complex in oesophageal adenocarcinoma correlates with poor prognosis. *J Pathol.* 1997;182(3):331–338.
65. Terashita Y, Ishiguro H, Haruki N, et al. Excision repair cross complementing 3 expression is involved in patient prognosis and tumor progression in esophageal cancer. *Oncol Rep.* 2004;12(4):827–831.
66. Izzo JG, Wu TT, Wu X, et al. Cyclin D1 guanine/adenine 870 polymorphism with altered protein expression is associated with genomic instability and aggressive clinical biology of esophageal adenocarcinoma. *J Clin Oncol.* 2007;25(6):698–707.

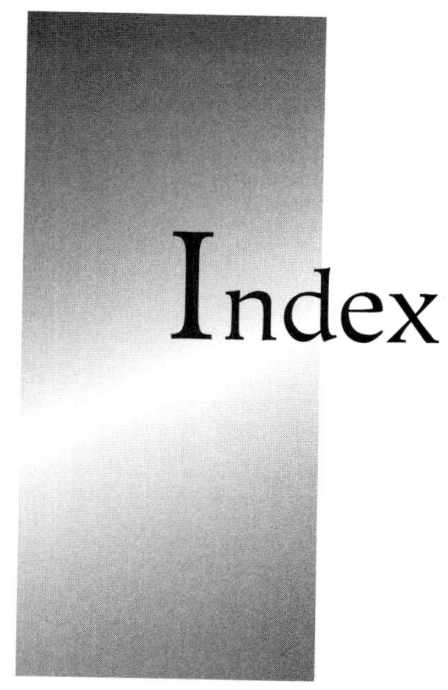

Index